Diagnosis and Management of
Genitourinary Cancer

Donald G. Skinner, M.D.
Professor and Chairman
Department of Surgery, Division of Urology
University of Southern California
Los Angeles, California

Gary Lieskovsky, M.D.
Associate Professor
Department of Surgery, Division of Urology
University of Southern California
Los Angeles, California

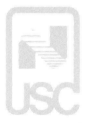

Illustrated by
Theodore Bloodhart

1988
W.B. SAUNDERS COMPANY
Harcourt Brace Jovanovich, Inc.
Philadelphia   London   Toronto   Montreal   Sydney   Tokyo

W. B. SAUNDERS COMPANY
Harcourt Brace Jovanovich, Inc.

West Washington Square
Philadelphia, PA   19105

Library of Congress Cataloging-in-Publication Data

Diagnosis and management of genitourinary cancer.

1. Genito-urinary organs—Cancer.   I. Skinner, Donald G.
   II. Lieskovsky, Gary. [DNLM: 1. Urogenital Neoplasms—
   diagnosis. 2. Urogenital Neoplasms—therapy. WJ 160 D536]

RC280.G4D53 1988   616.99′46   87–4861

ISBN 0–7216–8347–9

Editor: William Lamsback
Designer: W. B. Saunders Company
Production Manager: Carolyn Naylor
Manuscript Editor: Linda Mills
Illustration Coordinator: Walt Verbitski
Indexer: Ellen Murray

Diagnosis and Management of Genitourinary Cancer   ISBN 0–7216–8347–9

Last digit is the print number: 9   8   7   6   5   4   3   2   1

Contributors

THOMAS E. AHLERING, M.D.

Assistant Professor of Surgery/Urology, University of Southern California School of Medicine. Los Angeles, California. Director of Urologic Oncology, City of Hope National Medical Center. Duarte, California.

Diagnosis and Staging of Bladder Cancer; Salvage Options Following Radiotherapy Failures; Management of the Urethra

JEFFREY ASKANAZI, M.D.

Assistant Professor of Anesthesiology, Columbia University, College of Physicians and Surgeons. Director, Pediatric Urology, Columbia-Presbyterian Medical Center, Babies Hospital. Assistant Attending Anesthesiology, Columbia-Presbyterian Medical Center. New York, New York.

Nutritional Support of the Urologic Patient

MALCOLM A. BAGSHAW, M.D.

Catharine and Howard Avery Professor and Chairman, Department of Therapeutic Radiology, Director Division of Radiation Therapy, Stanford University School of Medicine. Chief of Therapeutic Radiology Service, Stanford University Hospital. Stanford, California. Consultant in Radiation Therapy, Palo Alto Veterans Administration Hospital. Palo Alto, California. Associate Medical Staff, Washington Hospital. Fremont, California.

Radiation Therapy for Prostate Cancer

RICHARD BIHRLE, M.D.

Assistant Professor of Urology, Indiana University Medical Center. Staff Surgeon, Indiana University Medical Center, Wishard Memorial Hospital, and Indianapolis Veterans Administration Medical Center. Indianapolis, Indiana.

Transabdominal Retroperitoneal Lymph Node Dissection

DAVID A. BLOOM, M.D.

Associate Professor of Surgery, University of Michigan. Ann Arbor, Michigan. Clinical Associate Professor of Surgery, Uniformed Services University of Health Sciences. Bethesda, Maryland. Chief, Pediatric Urology, Mott Childrens Hospital, University of Michigan. Ann Arbor, Michigan.

Testicular Tumor Management in Children; Turnbull Loop Stoma

WILLIAM D. BOSWELL, JR., M.D.

Associate Professor of Radiology, University of Southern California, School of Medicine. Chief of Diagnostic Radiology, Los Angeles County/University of Southern California Medical Center and Kenneth Norris Jr. Cancer Hospital and Research Institute. Los Angeles, California.

Diagnostic Imaging in Genitourinary Cancer

STUART D. BOYD, M.D.

Assistant Professor of Surgery/Urology, University of Southern California School of Medicine. Attending Urologist, Los Angeles County/University of Southern California Hospital, Good Samaritan Hospital, and Kenneth Norris Jr. Cancer Hospital and Research Institute. Los Angeles, California.

Cutaneous Urinary Diversion; Male Impotency Management; Creation of the Kock Ileal Reservoir

C. EUGENE CARLTON, JR., M.D.

Russell and Mary Hugh Scott Professor and Chairman, Department of Urology, Baylor College of Medicine. Attending, Methodist Hospital, St. Luke's Episcopal Hospital, Texas Childrens Hospital, and Ben Taub General Hospital. Houston, Texas.

Radioactive Isotope Implantation for Prostate Cancer

WILLIAM J. CATALONA, M.D.

Professor of Urologic Surgery, Washington University School of Medicine. Attending Physician, Barnes Hospital, St. Louis Children's Hospital, The Jewish Hospital of St. Louis, John Cochran Veterans Administration Hospital, and St. Louis Regional Medical Center. St. Louis, Missouri.

Management of Superficial Bladder Cancer

ROBERT B. COLVIN, M.D.

Associate Professor of Pathology, Harvard Medical School. Cambridge, Massachusetts. Director, Immunopathology Unit, Massachusetts General Hospital. Boston, Massachusetts.

Renal Tumor Pathology

E. DAVID CRAWFORD, M.D.

Professor and Chairman, Division of Urology, University of Colorado Health Sciences Center. Attending, University Hospital, and Veterans Administration Medical Center. Consultant, Fitzsimmons Army Hospital, and Denver General Hospital. Denver, Colorado.

Cancer of the Penis; Ilioinguinal Lymph Node Dissection

JOHN R. DANIELS, M.D.

Associate Professor of Medicine/Oncology, University of Southern California School of Medicine. Attending, Kenneth Norris Jr. Cancer Hospital and Research Institute, Los Angeles County/University of Southern California Medical Center. Los Angeles, California.

Bladder Carcinoma Chemotherapy

CHARLES J. DAVIS, JR., M.D.

Professor of Pathology, Uniformed Services University of Health Sciences. Bethesda, Maryland. Associate Chairman, Armed Forces Institute of Pathology. Washington, D.C.

Urinary Tract Tumor Pathology

CRAIG A. DAWKINS, M.D.

Attending, Memorial Hospital of Gulfport, Garden Park Community Hospital, and Hancock General Hospital. Jackson, Mississippi.

Cancer of the Penis

G. RICHARD DICKERSIN, M.D.

Associate Professor, Harvard Medical School. Cambridge, Massachusetts. Associate Pathologist, Massachusetts General Hospital. Boston, Massachusetts.

Renal Tumor Pathology

JOHN P. DONOHUE, M.D.

Professor and Chairman, Department of Urology, Indiana University Medical Center. Indianapolis, Indiana.

Diagnosis and Management of Adrenal Tumors; Transabdominal Retroperitoneal Lymph Node Dissection

STEVEN M. DRESNER, M.D.

Chief Resident, Urologic Surgery Training Program, Washington University, and Barnes Hospital. St. Louis, Missouri.

Superficial Bladder Cancer Management

MICHAEL J. DROLLER, M.D.

Professor, Mount Sinai School of Medicine. Director of Urology, Mount Sinai Hospital. Consulting Urologist, Bronx Veterans Administration Hospital, Elmhurst City Hospital, and Beth Israel Medical Center. New York, New York.

Early Urothelial Cancer Pathobiology

LOUIS DUBEAU, M.D., PH.D.

Postdoctoral Fellow, Peter Jones' Laboratory, Urological Research Laboratory, University of Southern California Comprehensive Cancer Center. Los Angeles, California.

Tumor Invasion and Metastasis

LAWRENCE H. EINHORN, M.D.

Professor of Medicine, Indiana University. Indianapolis, Indiana.

Testicular Cancer Chemotherapy

NATHAN B. FRIEDMAN, M.D.

Clinical Professor of Pathology, University of Southern California School of Medicine. Senior Consultant, Cedars-Sinai Medical Center. Consultant, Los Angeles County Medical Center. Los Angeles, California.

Testicular Tumor Pathology

BENAD Z. GOLDWASSER, M.D.

Senior Lecturer, Sackler School of Medicine, Tel-Aviv University. Tel-Aviv, Israel. Acting Chairman, Department of Urology, Chaim Sheba Medical Center. Tel-Hashomer, Israel.

Partial Nephrectomy in Renal Tumor Management

ERIC O. HAAFF, M.D.

Chief Resident, Urologic Surgery Training Program, Washington University, and Barnes Hospital. St. Louis, Missouri.

Superficial Bladder Cancer Management

BRIAN E. HARDY, M.D.

Associate Professor of Surgery/Urology, University of Southern California School of Medicine. Chief, Division of Urology, Childrens Hospital of Los Angeles. Los Angeles, California.

Wilms' Tumor; Pediatric Pelvic Sarcoma Management

BRIAN E. HENDERSON, M.D.

Director, University of Southern California Cancer Center. Professor and Chairman, Department of Preventive Medicine, University of Southern California School of Medicine. Los Angeles, California.

Bladder Cancer Epidemiology; Testis Cancer Epidemiology; Kidney Cancer Epidemiology; Renal Prostate Cancer Epidemiology

TERRY W. HENSLE, M.D.

Associate Professor of Urology, Columbia University, College of Physicians and Surgeons. Director, Pediatric Urology, Columbia-Presbyterian Medical Center, Babies Hospital. Assistant Attending Anesthesiology, Columbia-Presbyterian Medical Center. New York, New York.

Nutritional Support of the Urologic Patient

ROBERT P. HUBEN, M.D.

Chief, Urologic Oncology, Roswell Park Memorial Institute. Buffalo, New York.

Advanced Prostate Cancer Management

PETER A. JONES, PH.D., D.SC.

Professor of Biochemistry, University of Southern California Medical School. Los Angeles, California.

Tumor Invasion and Metastasis

MICHAEL M. LIEBER, M.D.

Professor of Urology, Mayo Medical School. Consultant in Urology, Mayo Clinic. Rochester, Minnesota.

Partial Nephrectomy in Renal Tumor Management

GARY LIESKOVSKY, M.D.

Associate Professor, Department of Surgery, Division of Urology, University of Southern California. Los Angeles, California.

Diagnosis and Staging of Bladder Cancer; Management of Invasive and High-Grade Bladder Cancer; Chemotherapy of Carcinoma of Bladder: Renal Parenchymal Tumor Treatment; Salvage Options Following Radiotherapy Failures; Management of Female Urethra Carcinoma; Management of Early Stage Nonseminomatous Germ Cell Tumors of Testis; Radical Cystectomy Technique; Surgical Treatment of Urethral Cancer in the Male Patient; Cutaneous Urinary Diversion; Turnbull Loop Stoma; Creation of the Continent Kock Ileal Reservoir; Radical Nephrectomy Technique; Management of Renal Cell Carcinoma Involving the Vena Cava; Technique of Radical Retropubic Prostatectomy

MAGED S. MIKHAIL, M.D.

Clinical Assistant Professor of Anesthesiology, University of Southern California School of Medicine. Los Angeles, California.

Intensive Care of the Postoperative Urologic Patient

MALCOLM S. MITCHELL, M.D.

Professor of Medicine and Microbiology, University of Southern California School of Medicine and Comprehensive Cancer Center. Los Angeles, California. Attending Physician, Kenneth Norris Jr. Cancer Hospital and Research Institute, Los Angeles County/University of Southern California Medical Center. Affiliate Attending Staff, Hospital of the Good Samaritan and California Hospital, Los Angeles, and Huntington Memorial Hospital. Pasadena, California.

Immunology and Immunotherapy of Genitourinary Cancers

DAVID L. McCULLOUGH, M.D.

Professor and Chairman, Section of Urology, Bowman Gray School of Medicine, Wake Forest University. Chief of Urology Service, Bowman Gray/North Carolina Baptist Medical Center. Winston-Salem, North Carolina.

Prostatic Cancer Diagnosis and Staging; Endourologic Management of Obstructive Problems in Cancer Patients

F. KASH MOSTOFI, M.D.

Professor of Pathology, Georgetown University. Washington, D.C. Professor of Pathology, University of Maryland. College Park, Maryland. Professor of Pathology, Uniformed Services University of Health Sciences. Bethesda, Maryland. Associate Professor of Pathology, The Johns Hopkins University. Baltimore, Maryland. Chairman, Department of Genitourinary Pathology, Armed Forces Institute of Pathology. Washington, D. C.

Urinary Tract Tumor Pathology

BALFOUR M. MOUNT, M.D., F.R.C.S.(C).

Professor of Surgery, McGill University. Attending, Royal Victoria Hospital. Toronto, Ontario.

Palliative Care of Terminal Cancer Patients

GERALD P. MURPHY, M.D., D.SC.

Professor of Urology, School of Medicine, State University of New York at Buffalo. Buffalo, New York.

Advanced Prostate Cancer Management

PETER NICHOLS, M.D.

Associate Professor of Clinical Pathology, University of Southern California. Laboratory Director, Kenneth Norris Jr. Cancer Hospital. Los Angeles, California.

Penis Tumor Pathology

ANNLIA PAGANINI-HILL, Ph.D.

Associate Professor of Preventive Medicine, University of Southern California School of Medicine. Los Angeles, California.

Bladder Cancer Epidemiology; Renal Cancer Epidemiology; Prostate Cancer Epidemiology

THOMAS E. PALMER, M.D.

Active Staff, Our Lady of the Lake Regional Medical Center, Active Staff, Baton Rouge General Medical Center, Active Staff, Medical Center of Baton Rouge, Active Staff, AMI Riverview Hospital, Active Staff, Women's Hospital of Baton Rouge. Baton Rouge, Louisiana.

Endourologic Management of Obstructive Problems in the Cancer Patient

DAVID F. PAULSON, M.D.

Professor and Chief, Division of Urologic Surgery, Duke University Medical Center. Durham, North Carolina.

Prostate Cancer Surgery; Endocrine Therapy of Prostate Cancer; Radical Perineal Prostatectomy

MALCOLM C. PIKE, Ph.D.

Professor and Director CA Epidemiology Clinical Trials, Imperial CA Research Fund, Oxford University. Oxford, England.

Epidemiology of Testicular Cancer

T. RAND PRITCHETT, M.D.

Fellow in Urological Oncology, University of Southern California School of Medicine. Resident Supervisor, Los Angeles County/University of Southern California Medical Center. Los Angeles, California.

Renal Parenchymal Tumor Treatment; Radical Nephrectomy; Management of Renal Cell Carcinoma Involving the Vena Cava

JEROME P. RICHIE, M.D.

Professor of Surgery (Urology), Harvard Medical School. Cambridge, Massachusetts. Chief, Urologic Oncology, Brigham and Women's Hospital. Boston, Massachusetts.

Renal Pelvis and Ureter Carcinoma; Testicular Tumor Diagnosis and Staging

NICHOLAS A. ROMAS, M.D.

Associate Professor of Clinical Urology, Columbia University College of Physicians and Surgeons. Director, Department of Urology, St. Luke's/Roosevelt Hospital Center. New York, New York.

Early Urothelial Cancer Pathobiology

RONALD K. ROSS, M.D.

Associate Professor of Preventive Medicine, University of Southern California School of Medicine. Los Angeles, California.

Bladder Cancer Epidemiology; Renal Cancer Epidemiology; Prostate Cancer Epidemiology; Testis Cancer Epidemiology

RANDALL G. ROWLAND, M.D.

Associate Professor of Urology, Indiana University School of Medicine. Attending Urologist, Indiana University Hospitals. Consultant Urologist, Wishard Memorial Hospital, Veterans Administration Hospital, and St. Vincent's Hospital. Indianapolis, Indiana.

Transabdominal Retroperitoneal Lymph Node Dissection

PETER T. SCARDINO, M.D.

Professor of Urology, Baylor College of Medicine. Attending Urologist, The Methodist Hospital and St. Luke's Episcopal Hospital. Consulting Urologist, Veterans Administration Hospital, and Ben Taub General Hospital. Houston, Texas.

Thoracoabdominal Retroperitoneal Lymph Node Dissection

JOHN F. SCOTT, M.D.

Assistant Professor of Medicine, University of Toronto and McMaster University. Toronto, Canada.

Palliative Care of the Patient with Terminal Cancer

ISABELL A. SESTERHENN, M.D.

Clinical Assistant Professor of Pathology, Uniformed Services University of Health Sciences. Bethesda, Maryland. Chief, Urogenital Research, Armed Forces Institute of Pathology. Washington, D.C.

Urinary Tract Tumor Pathology

DONALD G. SKINNER, M.D.

Professor and Chairman, Department of Surgery, Division of Urology, University of Southern California. Los Angeles, California.

Diagnosis and Staging of Bladder Cancer; Management of Invasive and High-Grade Bladder Cancer; Chemotherapy of Carcinoma of Bladder; Renal Parenchymal Tumor Treatment; Primary Retroperitoneal Tumors; Salvage Options Following Radiotherapy Failures; Management of Female Urethra Carcinoma; Management of Early Stage Nonseminomatous Germ Cell Tumors of Testis; Radical Cystectomy Technique; Cutaneous Urinary Diversion; Creation of the Continent Kock Ileal Reservoir; Radical Nephrectomy Technique; Management of Renal Cell Carcinoma Involving the Vena Cava

EILA C. SKINNER, M.D.

Resident, Division of Urology, Los Angeles County/University of Southern California Medical Center. Los Angeles, California.

Management of Female Urethra Carcinoma

ROBERT B. SMITH, M.D.

Professor of Surgery/Urology, University of California at Los Angeles. Attending Surgeon, UCLA Medical Center. Chief of Urology, Wadsworth Veterans Administration Hospital. Attending Surgeon, UCLA-Harbor General Hospital, Sepulveda Veterans Administration Hospital, Olive View Medical Center. Los Angeles, California.

Testicular Seminoma

MYRON TANNENBAUM, M.D., PH.D.

Professor of Pathology and Urology, Mount Sinai School of Medicine. Director of Surgical Pathology and Cytology, Bronx Veterans Administration Hospital. Attending Pathologist, Mount Sinai Hospital. New York, New York.

Early Urothelial Cancer Pathobiology

DURAIYAH THANGATHURAI, M.D., F.F.A.R.C.S., F.F.A.R.A.C.S.

Assistant Professor of Clinical Anesthesia, University of Southern California School of Medicine. Director of Intensive Care Unit, Kenneth Norris Jr. Cancer Hospital. Los Angeles, California.

Anesthetic Management in Radical Surgery for Urologic Malignancies; Intensive Care of the Postoperative Urologic Patient

JOHN F. VILJOEN, M.D., F.F.A.R.C.S.

Professor and Chairman, Department of Anesthesiology, University of Southern California School of Medicine. Chief of Anesthesiology, Los Angeles County/University of Southern California Medical Center, Kenneth Norris Jr. Cancer Hospital, and Estelle Doheny Eye Hospital. Los Angeles, California.

Anesthetic Management in Radical Surgery for Urologic Malignancies

JERRY WAISMAN, M.D.

Professor of Pathology, New York University School of Medicine. Director of Laboratories, University Hospital. Consultant, Manhattan Veterans Administration Medical Center. Attending Physician, Bellevue Hospital. New York, New York.

Pathology of Prostate Gland Neoplasms

PATRICK C. WALSH, M.D.

David Hall McConnell Professor and Director, Department of Urology, The Johns Hopkins University School of Medicine. Urologist-in-Chief, The James Buchanan Brady Urological Institute, The Johns Hopkins Hospital. Baltimore, Maryland.

Radical Retropubic Prostatectomy Preserving Sexual Function

NANCY E. WARNER, M.D.

Hastings Professor of Pathology, University of Southern California School of Medicine. Active Staff, Kenneth Norris Jr. Cancer Hospital. Voluntary Attending Staff, Los Angeles County/University of Southern California Medical Center. Affiliate Staff, Hospital of the Good Samaritan. Los Angeles, California.

Adrenal Gland Pathology

PHILLIP G. WISE, M.D.

Resident in Urology, Baylor College of Medicine. Third-year Resident in Urology, The Methodist Hospital, Veterans Administration Hospital, Ben Taub General Hospital, and St. Luke's Episcopal Hospital. Houston, Texas.

Thoracoabdominal Retroperitoneal Lymph Node Dissection

Preface

Diagnosis and Management of Genitourinary Cancer is a comprehensive text designed to give the clinician an in-depth reference to all aspects of genitourinary cancer. Sections on basic science, epidemiology, pathology, diagnosis, and management, as well as descriptive chapters on surgical techniques, present an overview of current concepts for urologists, oncologists, internists, pathologists, and radiologists. At the same time, they provide sufficient detail to serve as a surgical atlas for the physician treating the individual patient. In addition, quality of life issues are addressed, with chapters on alternatives to cutaneous urinary diversion, potency-preserving radical prostatectomy, and on moral and ethical issues relative to management of the patient with incurable disease and intractable pain.

This book addresses all alternatives in management, with selected individuals, with acknowledged leaders in the field of genitourinary cancer offering topics in which they have considerable personal experience. Thus, the reader will benefit from a philosophy of management based on expertise developed from treatment schemes used in the authors' own practice.

Uniformity in illustrations will be evident to the reader, as we were fortunate to engage Mr. Ted Bloodhart to either re-render or provide original illustrations, allowing us to present the highest possible quality and clarity in the depiction of surgical techniques. Ms. Margaret Stevenson served as editor, and her assistance has enhanced the readability of the text without any significant alteration in the style of an individual author.

Portions of several chapters appearing in this book were originally presented at the dedication symposium of the USC Kenneth Norris Jr. Cancer Hospital and Research Institute, and were initially published in *Urological Cancer* by Grune & Stratton (Chapters 2, 3, 4, 5, 13, 14, 17, 30, and 38). It seemed fitting in this current text to utilize these chapters as the foundation on which the authors could add current data. We appreciate the release of this material by Grune & Stratton for publication in *Diagnosis and Management of Genitourinary Cancer*.

We, the editors, would like to acknowledge our own mentors: Drs. Wyland Leadbetter, Willard Goodwin, Hardy Hendren, Joseph Kaufman, William Lakey, and James Metcalfe, whose influence will be passed on through this book to future generations.

Donald G. Skinner, M.D.

Gary Lieskovsky, M.D.

Contents

PART I

Basic Science Concepts of Neoplasia

LOUIS DUBEAU, M.D., Ph.D.
PETER A. JONES, Ph.D., D.Sc.

CHAPTER 1

Tumor Invasion and Ability to Metastasize

The ability of cancer cells to invade surrounding host tissue and to metastasize to distant sites is the hallmark of malignancy. Tumor cells must successfully accomplish several discrete steps before distant metastases can be established (Fig. 1–1). The cells must adapt to growth in a new environment at each step and modify or degrade specific tissue components to allow for invasion. Phenotypic heterogeneity, which appears to be higher in tumors than in normal cells, is probably very important in allowing tumor cells to overcome these biologic obstacles.

It has been suggested that the diversity of phenotypes seen in mature tumors results from the continual evolution of cells that have undergone natural selection for different metabolic, immunologic, and proliferative capacities. The ultimate result is the emergence of tumor cell clones with enhanced autonomy, survival, and growth characteristics.[33, 92] This phenomenon was called tumor progression by Foulds,[33] who concluded that it was characterized by a series of permanent, irreversible cellular changes in each tumor.

One of the central tenets of the concept of tumor progression as advanced by Foulds[33] and Nowell[92] was that genetic alterations are generated by random mutational events. At the time these theories were first promulgated, genetic instability was considered mainly to be the result of base changes in the primary nucleotide sequence of DNA or, alternatively, chromosomal abnormalities and rearrangements. However, recent advances in molecular and cell biology have shown that the genome is far more flexible than previously thought. Thus DNA methylation changes, gene amplification, gene rearrangements, duplications, and deletions are now known to occur, and these may also contribute to the instability of the tumor cell phenotype.

The constant evolution of new phenotypes within tumors might be expected to generate cells with differing invasive or metastatic potentials. In 1973 Fidler[31] published his pioneering study on the selective nature of the metastatic phenotype. He showed that if artificial lung metastases recovered from mice injected with B16 melanoma cells were reinjected into new mice, sublines that showed a much greater capacity to colonize the lungs could be derived. The results were interpreted in favor of the notion that metastases generally arise from minor subpopulations of tumor cells that possess and express the proper set of genes necessary to complete all steps of the metastatic cascade. Thus, metastatic cells were thought to express a spectrum of phenotypic traits that were unexpressed in nonmetastatic cells.[90] This concept of the selective nature of the metastatic phenotype has been challenged by Weiss,[142] and some investigators have arrived at the conclusion that the metastatic phenotype is extremely volatile and can be lost easily. This could be the result of highly unstable genetic alterations leading to a dynamic or rapidly changing phenotype.[49]

The constantly evolving tumor phenotype

3

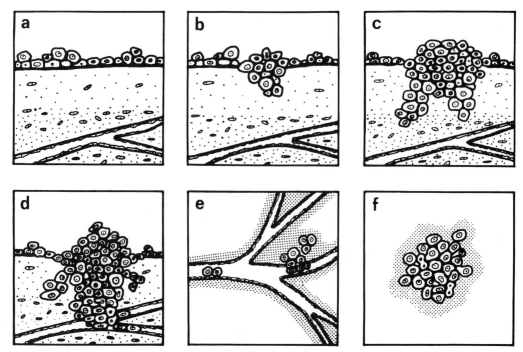

Figure 1–1. Steps of tumor metastasis. In figure 1*a* an epithelial tumor that has not extended beyond the basement membrane (carcinoma in situ) is represented. In Figure 1*b* mesenchymal tissue invasion underneath the basement membrane has occurred (early invasion). The tumor is seen penetrating deeper into the tissue in Figure 1*c* (deep invasion), and Figure 1*d* shows invasion into a blood vessel (vascular invasion). Figure 1*e* represents tumor cells within a blood vessel that are being transported away from the primary tumor and extravasating into a distant organ. In Figure 1*f* tumor cell emboli have left the vascular compartment and are growing as a metastasis.

that results in cells with differing biologic capabilities is therefore likely to constantly generate cells in low numbers that are capable of progressing through the various steps shown in Figure 1–1. The nature of the various biologic obstacles involved at each of these steps of tumor progression will be reviewed in this chapter, and acquired phenotypic properties of cancer cells that are potentially important in overcoming them will be discussed. Comments on potential applications of this knowledge to the management and treatment of cancer patients will also be made.

ROLE OF THE BASEMENT MEMBRANE

Structural and Functional Aspects

With rare exceptions such as hepatocytes, all human epithelial cells rest on a basement membrane. Basement membranes have a unique biochemical composition that differs from other types of extracellular matrices (Table 1–1). Integral components of basement membranes include type IV collagen; the glycoproteins laminin, entactin, and nidogen; and the glycosaminoglycan heparan sulfate.[16, 32, 45, 114, 129, 131] Other macromolecules such as fibronectin and type V collagen are also present,[114] although they are not restricted to this location. The relative ratios of the different macromolecules and the presence or absence of fibronectin varies in basement membranes from different sources.[108, 148, 149] These various components provide anchoring sites for growth and maturation of epithelia and act as a boundary separating the epithelium from underlying stroma.

Laminin is a highly insoluble, multifunctional glycoprotein present in the lamina lucida of most basement membranes; its function appears particularly important.[32] As shown in Figure 1–2, it has three short arms and one long arm arranged in a cross-shape.[29] The end region of each arm is globular; on one or more of the short arms it contains binding sites to type IV collagen and induces cell spreading.[104, 127] The long arm promotes neuritic regeneration[80] and contains a binding site for heparin.[113] The central portion of the molecule, where the four arms meet, is protease resistant[29, 74, 103, 104] and is the recognition site for a specific cell surface receptor.[102, 104, 125, 127] It has been suggested that this cell surface receptor may be altered in number or degree of occupancy in tumor cells.[72, 77] Such alterations may be important in promoting the disorganized type of growth independent of basement membrane that characterizes invasive carcinomas. Evidence for a possible role of this receptor in hematogenous metastases is suggested by the findings that tumor cells selected for their ability to bind to laminin produced 10 times more metastases after intravenous injection[124] and the presence of whole laminin on the tumor cell surface stimulated hematogenous metastases.[137] The presence of laminin receptors on the surface of macrophages may be important in the recognition of metastatic tumor cells by macrophages.[50, 144]

The role of fibronectin has generated much interest, as this protein is also multifunctional, and different biochemical functions can be assigned to different domains on the molecule.[138] It is thought to play a role in cell adhesion, matrix assembly, chemotaxis, and opsonization, as well as in blood coagulation and tissue repair.[111, 136] Recently it has been suggested that fibronectin may also play a role in angiogenesis.[135] The fact that some malignant cells, unlike nonneoplastic cells, fail to deposit fibronectin within the extracellular matrix in vitro has led to much speculation on the importance of this molecule in tumor cell behavior.[111, 136]

A proteolytic fragment of fibronectin, but not the intact molecule, can promote morphologic transformation of virus-transformed fibroblasts in vitro.[23] This same pro-

Table 1–1. ROLE AND DISTRIBUTION OF COLLAGEN ISOTYPE, GLYCOPROTEINS, AND GLYCOSAMINOGLYCANS IN DIFFERENT EXTRACELLULAR MATRICES

	Basement Membranes	Soft Tissue Stroma	Bone	Cartilage	Blood Vessel Wall	Function
Collagen						
Type I		+	+			Provide tensile strength
Type II				+		and bind specifically to
Type III		+			+	other extracellular tissue
Type IV	+					components
Type V	+	+		+	+	
Glycoproteins						
Laminin	+					Adhesion of epithelial or carcinoma cells to collagen, cell spreading, neuritic regeneration
Fibronectin	+	+				Cell adhesion, matrix assembly, chemotaxis, blood coagulation, tissue repair, transformation (?)
Chondronectin					+	Stimulates attachment of chondrocytes to type III collagen
Osteonectin			+			Unknown; may be involved in initiating active mineralization
Microfibrillar proteins		+		(elastic cartilage)	+	Constituents of elastic fibers
Entactin	+					Unknown
Nidogen	+					Unknown
Glycosaminoglycans						
Chondroitin 4- and 6-sulphate		+	+	+	+	Tissue water homeostasis
Keratan sulphate			+	+		
Dermatan sulphate		+	+	+	+	
Heparan sulphate	+	+			+	Heparan sulfate acts as lipoprotein lipase receptor on the surface of vascular endothelial cells
Hyaluronic acid		(ubiquitous)				

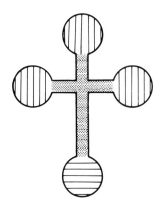

☐☐☐ Type IV collagen binding domain
Cell spreading
Metastatic ability

☐ Heparin binding domain
Neuritic regeneration

▨ Cell binding domain
Decreases metastatic ability

Figure 1–2. The laminin molecule.

teolytic fragment, unlike intact fibronectin, was able to bind effectively to type I collagen at 37°C. Thus, one can hypothesize that tumor cells may induce disorganization of the extracellular matrix by releasing specific proteolytic fragments of the fibronectin molecule. The finding that the transformation-enhancing activity fragment of the fibronectin molecule is present in the serum of most patients with progressive cancer, but only rarely in the serum of normal individuals,[86] has led to the proposal that detection of specific fragments of fibronectin in the serum of patients may provide a useful marker in the diagnosis and follow-up of various types of cancer.[86, 138]

Entactin and nidogen are two recently discovered glycoprotein constituents of basement membranes.[9, 16, 127] Their function is at present unknown.

Type IV collagen is the major structural component of basement membranes and accounts for approximately 20% of the total basement membrane proteins.[61] Unlike collagens I, II, and III, it contains nonhelical segments[128] and has a nonfibrillar ultrastructural appearance.[51] It is thought that the nonhelical segments allow for a greater degree of flexibility, which confers greater elasticity to the basement membrane.[132] Type IV collagen molecules have a unique arrange-

ment that confers both tensile strength and elasticity within the basement membrane.[130, 132, 151]

Heparan sulfate is a glycosaminoglycan found on cell surfaces in various tissues. It is also found within basement membranes, where it provides negative charges that block the passage of other negatively charged macromolecules.[44, 56, 96]

Basement Membrane Dissolution by Cancer Cells

There are no spaces allowing for the free passage of cells from one side of an epithelial basement membrane to the other. Thus, the various components of basement membrane constitute the first major barrier to tumor progression. Invasion of underlying stroma by an early carcinoma necessarily implies that some defects have been introduced in the otherwise continuous basement membrane. In support of this concept, changes in the quality and distribution of basement membrane antigens have been demonstrated during the transition from benign lesions to invasive malignant neoplasms.[7, 14, 116] These studies have shown that although benign breast lesions with a "pseudoinvasive" appearance, such as sclerosing adenosis of the breast, were invariably associated with a continuous basement membrane, the structure was lost in the vicinity of invasive breast carcinomas.

There are two nonmutually exclusive mechanisms whereby such defects in basement membrane could be introduced during the invasive process. There can be alterations in the rate or quality of synthesis of various components of the membrane, or specific components could be actively degraded by the tumor cells. In normal breast tissue the large interlobular ducts are surrounded by a continuous one-cell-thick layer of myoepithelial cells, and it has been suggested that this layer is the source of basement membrane at this location.[41] This hypothesis is supported by the finding that myoepithelial cells can make type IV collagen in vitro,[78] and a parallel has been established between the degree of myoepithelial cell differentiation and the amount of basal lamina deposited in breast tissue.[35, 37–39] In ductal carcinoma in situ of the breast there is loss of the myoepithelial cell layer.[15] Thus, it may be that disruption of the myoepithelial cell layer is at least partly responsible for the decreased amount of basement membrane seen with carcinomas. According to this hypothesis, loss of the myoepithelial cells would result in a discontinuous basement membrane and would allow tumor cells to infiltrate surrounding tissue without having to actively degrade any of the basement membrane components.

The subject of proteolytic enzyme production by tumor cells will be discussed in a later section, and only the data pertinent to the basement membrane will be reviewed here. Metalloproteases that can degrade collagen of types IV and V have been found in human, murine, and amphibian epithelial tumors,[73, 115] and type IV collagenase antigens are present in invasive human breast carcinoma.[8] This enzyme may be important in the process of invasion, since carcinoma in situ and adjacent benign ductal and acinar structures, as well as benign neoplasms such as fibroadenomas, did not contain detectable antigens for the metalloprotease.[8] A possible cooperation between tumor cells and macrophages in the secretion of this enzyme was reported by Henry and colleagues,[48] who found that a type IV collagenase was released in co-cultures of mouse peritoneal macrophages and Lewis lung carcinoma cells but not in cultures of either cell type alone. Many invasive cells also show increased production of plasminogen activator,[145] which could conceivably generate active plasmin in the vicinity of the basement membrane and facilitate glycoprotein and proteoglycan degradation.[55] The exact role of proteolytic enzymes in invasion of the basal lamina by tumor cells and the relative importance of decreased basement membrane synthesis versus active degradation is currently not clear.

LOCAL INVASION

Once malignant epithelial cells have crossed the basement membrane barrier, they must adapt themselves for growth within the subepithelial connective tissue. Table 1–1 lists some of the structural differences between basement membranes and the extracellular stroma of soft tissues. Tumor cells that have penetrated into the subepithelial tissue are subjected to the influence of mesenchymal cells and extracellular matrix components. It is now recognized that various growth factors and oncogene products may play an important role in allowing the cells to grow in this hostile environment. The effect of these growth factors will be discussed in later sections (see Extravasation and Growth into a Distant Organ).

Another important aspect of this phase of tumor progression is that the neoplastic cells not only proliferate within the mesenchymal tissue but also penetrate deeper into it, disrupting its normal architecture and degrading specific extracellular components. This invasiveness characteristic of malignant tumor cells is important in accommodating their expansile growth and in allowing penetration of blood vessels and lymphatic channels. As the cells penetrate deeper into the tissue, the composition of the extracellular matrix may change, resulting in additional selection pressures on the cells. This implies that depth of invasion is not simply a time-related phenomenon but represents different phases of tumor progression. Many types of carcinomas, including transitional cell carcinomas of the urinary bladder, can be separated into those that tend to grow superficially for a long period of time and those that are deeply invasive. A superficial tumor may become large and bulky but will not infiltrate deeper into the tissue unless some cells undergo the necessary phenotypic changes that would allow them to grow into the deeper tissue environment. This has been well documented for superficial spreading malignant melanoma of the skin, where two distinct phases of tumor growth have been identified: an initial phase of radial (superficial) growth followed by a vertical (deeply invasive) growth phase.[19]

This section will deal with mechanisms that are potentially important in allowing tumor cells to penetrate deeper into surrounding tissues. Three such mechanisms are generally invoked: (1) mechanical pressure resulting from rapid proliferation, (2) production of degradative enzymes by the tumor cells, and (3) increased motility and decreased adhesiveness of the tumor cells.

Mechanical Effects

The concept that tumor cell invasiveness could be accounted for entirely by a mechanical process was brought forward by Eaves,[28] from observations on the infiltrative pattern of fluids injected into animal tissues. It already had been shown that the tissue pressure of a malignant tumor was increased compared with that of normal tissue[150] and Eaves argued that because of a higher intracellular pressure, malignant cells were able to force their way into surrounding tissues by following the lines of least resistance. Although such a mechanism could play some role in invasion by certain tumors, it is unlikely to be an important mechanism for most tumors. It fails to explain the frequent finding of infiltrative nests of tumor cells in nonedematous, apparently intact host tissues showing no connection with the main tumor mass.[118] In addition, an invasive tumor does not necessarily follow the lines of least resistance. For example, Mareel[81] pointed out that if this theory were correct, tumor cells arising from epithelia lining body cavities, such as the bladder urothelium, would expand into the lumen rather than infiltrate the underlying tissue. The theory also fails to explain why some of the slower growing tumors such as some breast carcinomas may be highly invasive, in spite of their slow growth.

Role of Degradative Enzymes

Direct observation of invasive tumor cells in patients suggests that actual destruction of the extracellular matrix is a necessary prerequisite for invasion. Many laboratory studies have examined tumor cells for the production of hydrolytic enzymes that might assist in the invasive process. A partial list of these enzymes is given in Table 1–2, and it should be noted that none of them are specific to tumor cells and that all are also produced by normal cells in different physiologic conditions. Thus, the production of these hydrolyses does not itself characterize the malignant state; rather, it is the inappropriate expression or lack of control of the enzymes that might facilitate the invasive process.

Tumor cells are capable of the production of collagenase enzymes that can digest all of the collagens found in the interstitial space and also those collagens specifically confined to basal laminae (see earlier). Studies with explanted tumors have always been complicated by the fact that these tumors contained normal cells, which might in themselves be responsible for the production of the hydrolytic enzymes. However, the use of clonal populations of cells and cell lines (Table 1–2) shows that many tumor cells alone can produce these enzymes.

Table 1–2. HYDROLASES PRODUCED BY TUMOR CELLS

Enzyme	Tumor System	Reference
Interstitial collagenase	Various neoplasms	26
	Osteogenic sarcoma	68
	Malignant melanoma	118
Type IV collagenase	Metastatic fibrosarcoma	74
Type V collagenase	Reticulum cell sarcoma	75
Plasminogen activator	Human tumor cell lines	70
	Human tumors	144
Lysosomal	Human breast carcinoma	98, 105
Proteoglycan degrading activity (glycosidase)	Mouse melanoma	64

Plasminogen activator is another enzyme that is thought to play an important role in tumor cell invasion.[55] The production of small amounts of plasminogen activator by a tumor cell might be expected to result in an amplification of the signal, since this enzyme can generate large amounts of plasmin from the circulating reservoir of protease activity in the form of plasminogen. The production of this nonspecific protease may be important in the degradation of connective tissue glycoproteins and proteoglycan molecules, and indeed this enzyme is often associated in situations in which tissue degradation occurs. Recently Kohga and coworkers[62] used an immunohistochemical approach to study the distribution of urokinase in paraffin-embedded sections of adenomas (polyps) and adenocarcinomas of the colon. Of the two main types of known plasminogen activators, urokinase is the one usually associated with neoplasia. The cells stained intensely with antiurokinase antibody in all adenomas and adenocarcinomas examined, and in sections showing the transition between normal and neoplastic epithelium, cytoplasmic urokinase appeared abruptly in the neoplastic cells. In samples from nonneoplastic colon, the enzyme was seen only in a few goblet cells.[62]

Other nonspecific proteases that may play an important role in matrix destruction, and therefore facilitate the invasive process, include the lysosomal enzymes produced at the invasive edges of human breast carcinoma cells. These enzymes, like plasmin, may be expected to act locally to induce the destruction of matrix glycoproteins and proteoglycans.

Matrix proteoglycans are also thought to play a major role in the physiology of connective tissue and basal laminae (see ref. 133), and enzymes capable of degrading the carbohydrate portions of these molecules recently have been characterized. The data in Table 1–2, which is by no means an exhaustive compilation of work on the production of hydrolyses by tumor cells, clearly show that tumor cells have the potential of degrading all of the subcomponents of the extracellular matrix. However, attempts to correlate the production of specific proteases with the tumorigenic phenotype have shown that simple correlations between these properties are not always evident. The resistance of the normal connective tissues to tumor cell–induced destruction is not a well-understood phenomenon, but it should be realized that there are large numbers of inhibitors of proteases that are present in extracellular fluids and might modulate the metastatic potential in vivo.

Before closing this discussion, it should be pointed out that tumor cells may modify their environment not only by the release of degradative enzymes but also by the secretion of specific stromal components, either directly by the neoplastic cell or via stimulation of normal stromal cells. Merrilees and Finlay[84] recently reported that several human tumor cell lines stimulated synthesis of glycosaminoglycans by human skin fibroblasts in vitro. Phenomena such as tumor-associated desmoplasia could result from modulation of the activity of normal mesenchymal cells by tumors.

Role of Cell Adhesiveness and Motility

The role of decreased adhesiveness and increased motility of cancer cells in promoting invasion of adjacent tissue is highly controversial. It is now several decades since Coman made the observation that cancer cells would detach more easily from host tissue than would normal cells.[20, 21] Although these initial experiments and their interpretations were much criticized,[139, 141] the notion still persists that decreased adhesiveness is a characteristic of cancer cells. Recently, "cell adhesion molecules" were identified and were shown to be reduced in cells transformed by Rous sarcoma virus,

when compared with untransformed cells (see ref. 12 for review). In one such transformed cell line, there was a corresponding increase in cell motility.

Evidence for active movement of cancer cells during the invasive process is also available from a variety of different experimental approaches. As already noted,[118] histologic examination of serial sections of primary tumors has revealed nests of malignant cells completely detached from the parental tumor mass, a phenomenon that must imply cell detachment and migration. Additional evidence came from transmission electron microscopy of mouse mammary carcinoma cells invading liver tissue.[24, 109] Such studies have revealed the presence of cytoplasmic projections of various sizes and shapes on the cancer cells that penetrated through the endothelium of the sinusoids and into the liver parenchyma. These processes were concentrated at the tumor margin, and their orientation was indicative of the future direction of invasion.[24, 109]

Immunohistochemical studies have demonstrated that levels of contractile proteins such as actin and myosin are increased in invasive epithelial tumors, compared with levels in corresponding normal cells, and that this correlated with an increase in the number of microfilaments within the tumor cells.[6, 34, 42, 83, 105, 110] This increase was more prominent in high-grade tumors, and the microfilaments tended to be more concentrated at the growing edges of the tumors and extended into the finger-like cytoplasmic protrusions already described.[6, 83]

More direct evidence for cancer cell movement came from the work of Wood and colleagues,[146, 147] who developed an experimental system in which V2 rabbit carcinoma cells within the mesenchymal tissue of a rabbit ear chamber could be observed directly. After injecting the carcinoma cells into the auricular artery, they were able to observe the movement of the tumor cells through the vessel walls and into the perivascular tissue. Using another approach, Ambrose and Easty[2, 3] did time-lapse filming of the behavior of malignant cells growing on various tissues such as omentum, chick chorioallantoic membrane, and amnion, and they found that although normal fibroblasts and macrophages moved on the surface of those membranes, cells from two types of virus-transformed fibroblasts and from one melanoma cell line anchored on the surface and penetrated into the underlying connective tissue.

From the disorganized pattern of invasion that is observed when malignant tumors are examined histologically, one would expect that cancer cell movement would be multi-directional and relatively uninfluenced by local factors. This conclusion is supported by the various studies mentioned above. However, there is evidence suggesting that cancer cells may respond to chemotactic stimuli. Hayashi and co-workers isolated a tumor product[46] that was chemotactic for tumor cells but not for leukocytes.[94] More recently, various chemoattractants were detected in tissue extracts that stimulated migration of tumor cells in vitro. A particularly powerful chemoattractant in this system was the laminin molecule (see ref. 123).

Thus, the evidence that cancer cells have decreased adhesiveness and increased motility relative to normal cells appears convincing. Although these two properties could theoretically increase the efficiency of invasion, their importance in tumor progression is currently not clear. Since histologic evidence for tumor cell migration away from the main primary tumor mass is more prominent in the most advanced tumors and is usually lacking with microinvasion and superficial tumors, one would expect that such a mechanism of invasion would be more important in the anaplastic tumors and perhaps not significant in the early or less aggressive lesions. In support of this hypothesis, Tullberg and Burger were able to select B16 melanoma cells with increased metastatic potentials by the ability of these cells to penetrate Nucleopore filters.[134] Since certain tumors, such as superficial spreading melanomas of the skin, tend to grow superficially for a prolonged period of time before they become more aggressive,[19] the suggestion that increased cellular motility may play a role in allowing progression to a more invasive lesion in those cases seems appealing.

ESTABLISHMENT OF SECONDARY METASTASES

Invasion of the Vascular Compartments

After local invasion, the next step of tumor metastasis is penetration of the vascular compartments and transportation of the tu-

mor cells to various distant anatomic locations. Although most advanced cancers use both blood vessels and lymphatic channels to achieve this goal, many tumors seem to use one route preferentially for their initial dissemination. It is a well-recognized phenomenon that sarcomas generally tend to have a lower incidence of lymph node metastases and a higher incidence of hematogenous metastasis when compared with carcinomas. In addition, there may be differences between carcinomas of various cell types from the same organ. For example, follicular carcinoma of the thyroid gland spreads preferentially via the blood vessels, whereas thyroid papillary carcinomas metastasize most often to the lymph nodes. Although sarcomas are often closely associated with blood vessels, the factors determining the preferred route of initial spread for any given tumor are not yet clear.

One difference between small lymphatic channels and blood vessels is that only in the latter are endothelial cells lined by a basement membrane. Entry into a blood vessel presumably requires invasion of the vessel wall by a growing tumor mass, whereas free cells that have detached from the primary tumor may have easy access to the lymphatics.[143] Once they have penetrated the vascular space, tumor cells are in an environment that is particularly hostile to their growth. Strong selective pressures are therefore operating, and only those cells that have acquired the ability to cope with these changes will survive.

There is a third mode of spread available for tumors arising from cells lining body cavities. The tumor cells, because of their anatomic location, can shed into such cavities and reimplant on the surface lining of the same or another interconnected cavity at a site distant from that of the primary tumor. This mechanism of spread is seen, for example, with epithelial tumors of the female genital tract and may represent a mechanism for the genesis of multifocal bladder urothelial tumors. An interesting aspect of this particular mode of tumor spread is that prior invasion of the basement membrane is not a prerequisite for tumor dissemination.

Anatomic Distribution of Metastases

After tumor cells have entered the circulation, they are rapidly transported to various organs of the body. Potter and colleagues[101] showed that fluorescein-labeled primary mammary tumor cells injected either intravenously or intra-arterially in mice were present in every organ examined as early as 15 minutes after inoculation. Viable metastases do not, however, become established in every seeded organ, and pathologic examination of a large number of cancer patients suggests that the distribution of metastases is not a random event for most malignant tumors. In other words, a given tumor will tend to metastasize to certain organs more often than to others.

One of the first authors to recognize the nonrandom distribution of metastases was Paget,[96] who in 1889 proposed the "seed and soil" hypothesis to suggest that the environment in which a tumor cell arrested had a substantial influence on its ability to survive. In 1928 Ewing[30] criticized the seed and soil hypothesis and favored the idea that the main determinants of metastatic distribution were mechanical factors related to the anatomy of the circulatory system.

According to Ewing's theory,[30] the organs seeded by the largest number of tumor cells will develop the greater number of metastases. For example, the high frequency of hepatic metastases seen with carcinoma of the colon would be attributed to spread by invasion of the portal vein. Spread of prostatic adenocarcinoma to the vertebral column could also be readily explained by invoking easy access to the vertebral veins. In support of this hypothesis, Gorman and co-workers[36] were recently able to change the pattern of hematogenous dissemination of an anaplastic carcinoma cell line injected into rabbits by constructing a cavoportal shunt prior to tumor inoculation. These authors used VX2 carcinoma cells that normally metastasize exclusively to the lungs. After injection into the hindlimbs of shunted animals, those tumor cells metastasized exclusively to the liver.

However, hemodynamics alone cannot explain many of the observations in both patients and experimental animals. Cases of colon carcinomas metastatic to multiple organs but sparing the liver are known to occur. In addition, certain organs such as the spleen, which are highly perfused by blood, are nevertheless very rarely the site of metastatic growth. The frequently observed spread of gastric carcinoma to the ovary (Krukenberg's tumor) defies any explanation based on that model alone. Observations of patients with malignant ascites treated by peritoneovenous shunts showed that, although this procedure resulted in a large number of tumor cells constantly entering the blood circulation, many patients did not develop hematogenous metastases, and in those who did, the metastatic growths were small and clinically insignificant.[120–122] Additional support for the seed and soil hypothesis came from work with experimental animals, and here the work of Fidler has been determinant. In 1973 this author reported that melanoma cells obtained from pulmonary metastases and injected into the blood stream metastasized to the lung much more readily than cells obtained from the primary tumors.[31] More recently, Hart and Fidler[43] showed that if B16 melanoma cells were injected into syngeneic mice, metastases developed in grafts of pulmonary or ovarian tissue, as well as in the in situ lungs, but failed to develop in grafts of renal tissue.

Thus, the idea put forward nearly a century ago by Paget,[96] that tumor cells metastasize only to the organs that provide the correct microenvironment for their growth, is now recognized as an important determinant of the distribution of metastases, and for many tumors the role of hemodynamic factors is probably a minor one. The putative organophilic factors invoked by this theory are presumably multiple and may represent growth factors, influence of extracellular matrix components, and specific chemotactic substances (see ref. 123), among others. The capillary endothelial cells may also play a role. Alby and Auerback[1] showed that radiolabeled teratocarcinoma cells adhered preferentially to capillaries from mouse ovaries in vitro, whereas glioma cells showed preference for endothelial cells obtained from the mouse brain. Tumor cells may therefore be able to distinguish betwen endothelial cells from different organs.

Extravasation and Growth into a Distant Organ

Once they have arrested within small blood vessels, tumor cells may proliferate until their expansile growth causes disruption of the vessel. However, it seems that the malignant cells more commonly leave the vascular space by invading through the vessel wall (see ref. 89). The sequence of events appears to be attachment of the tumor cells to the surface of endothelial cells, which causes endothelial cell retraction and exposure of the underlying basal lamina.

This is followed by migration of the tumor cells to the basal lamina and migration under adjacent endothelial cells. The cells then destroy the basal lamina and invade the perivascular tissue, with concomitant repair of the capillary endothelium and basal lamina.[89]

What allows the extravasated cancer cells to proliferate within a "foreign" organ is largely unknown and presumably involves many of the factors already discussed under "Local Invasion." One interesting recent development is that the expression of various oncogenes may be related to the metastatic phenotype. Little and colleagues[79] studied amplification of the C-myc oncogene in 18 human lung cancer cell lines. In eight of the lines the gene was amplified. Five of those eight belonged to the variant class of small cell carcinoma, a class associated with more malignant behavior than pure small cell lung carcinoma. Studies with neuroblastoma also showed that the more advanced stages of this disease were associated with amplification of N-myc.[13] More recently, Thorgeirsson and co-workers[126] reported that transfection of human tumor DNA containing different activated ras oncogenes induced the metastatic phenotype in NIH 3T3 cells. Bernstein and Weinberg[10] showed that nonmetastasizing 3T3 mouse fibroblasts transformed by the Ha-ras oncogene became metastatic if they were transfected with DNA obtained from metastatic human tumors. In this last study, the nature of the gene associated with metastatic behavior is not known but could represent an as yet unidentified oncogene or, perhaps, a gene specific for the metastatic phenotype.

The possible role of growth factors also seems interesting. Many growth factors have been identified throughout the body, some with a specific organ distribution (see ref. 52). Cell surface receptors recognized by some growth factors are related to oncogene products (see ref. 68). Cellular responsiveness to growth factors has been shown to correlate with the cell's ability to express the transformed phenotype,[59] and the presence of specific growth factors in certain organs could therefore facilitate tumor growth and invasiveness. In support of this hypothesis, epidermal growth factor has been shown to increase the production of plasminogen activator in A431 epidermoid carcinoma cells,[40] and various growth factors

induced collagenase secretion in human fibroblast cultures.[18] Epidermal growth factor is a mitogen for at least three different bladder carcinoma cell lines in vitro.[85] The epidermal growth factor receptor is related to the v-erb-B oncogene product[25] and is present in increased amounts on the cell surfaces of deeply invasive bladder urothelial tumors, compared with those of superficial tumors.[88]

Other growth factors that can affect tumor behavior are the transforming growth factors (TGFs). TGFs are proteins of low molecular weight that can reversibly induce anchorage, independent growth, and loss of contact inhibition in nonneoplastic cells.[22] Two types have been characterized. TGF-alpha shows amino acid sequence homology with epidermal growth factor.[87] TGF-beta does not act as a mitogen in vitro,[5, 107] but a synergistic effect of both TGF-alpha and -beta are necessary for maximal transforming activity. Another growth factor called platelet-derived growth factor, which does not by itself have transforming activity, was found to modulate the activity of TGF-alpha and -beta.[4]

Although the exact role of TGFs on tumor proliferation is currently not clear, it has been suggested that a cell may maintain its transformed phenotype by autocrine secretion of TGFs.[22, 58, 95] Since it was shown that cellular responsiveness to TGFs correlated with the cell's ability to express the transformed phenotype,[59] tumor cells may respond differently than nonneoplastic cells to those factors in vivo. Interfering with growth-factor activity may therefore be a potentially useful approach for cancer chemotherapy (see later section).

IN VITRO MODELS FOR TUMOR CELL INVASION

The process of tumor cell invasion is ultimately responsible for the lethality of most cancers. Tumor cells must invade through basement membranes, connective tissues, and blood vessel walls or lymphatics in order to establish secondary metastases. The biochemistry of this invasive process is extremely difficult to study either in patients or in animal models because of the difficulty of isolating and characterizing the molecules responsible for this destructive behavior.

Table 1–3. IN VITRO MODELS FOR TUMOR
CELL INVASION

System	Reference
Chicken chorioallantoic membrane	17, 27, 42, 92
Bovine lens capsule basement membrane	116
Chicken embryonic skin	90
Human amnion	112
Hyaline cartilage	97
Dog femoral veins	99
Organ fragments	81
Cultured endothelial cells	62, 63, 66, 69, 139
Artificial blood vessel walls	55
Extracellular matrix substrates	53, 65
Mesenchymal tissue grown on nylon meshes	11

Many experimental systems that allow investigation of the invasive process in isolated culture models have therefore been established so that we can begin to understand both the interactions of tumor cells with basement membranes, stroma, and other tissues and the details of invasive activity.

A partial listing of some of the techniques that have been established is found in Table 1–3. These systems can be divided into two basic groups, those that use connective tissue substrates derived from animal sources and those in which cultured connective tissue cells are used to produce representative connective tissue stroma in vitro.

Examples of the former are studies of the invasive activity of human tumor cells into chicken chorioallantoic membrane, either in ovo or in vitro, using membranes stretched between suitable supports. The interaction of tumor cells with bovine lens capsule basement membranes and chicken embryonic skin have also been examined, but the most common method in use today is the human amniotic membrane system. This method has the advantage that large surface areas of amniotic membrane in an undamaged configuration can be easily obtained and can be kept refrigerated until used in invasion studies. The amnion can be used intact or the epithelial cells can be removed by lysis before tumor cells are added to one side of the membrane. The crossing of the membrane in response to different chemotactic signals has been measured, and cells that have known invasive activities in humans or in animals are capable of traversing the amnion. This suggests the active participation of proteolytic enzymes.

Many investigators have also utilized cultured endothelial cells as substrates for cancer cells with known invasive activities. Tumor cells are capable of attaching to cultured endothelial layers in culture, initiating the retraction of the endothelium, penetrating to the subendothelial area, and subsequently degrading the underlying extracellular material synthesized by the endothelial cells. We have also characterized the details of the degradative activity of tumor cells by the use of subendothelial matrices that have been stripped of their cellular components and have found that collagenase and plasminogen activators play important roles in the dissolution of these complex connective tissue substrates.

It is also possible to construct artificial blood vessel walls in culture by the addition of endothelial cells to pre-existing multilayers of smooth muscle cells.[53] These artificial blood vessel walls can be degraded by tumor cells, although the presence of the endothelial cells markedly inhibits the degradative activity of some cancer cells, suggesting that normal cells may be able to modulate aggressive behavior of tumor cells. Interestingly, the protective effect of endothelial cells can be destroyed by x-irradiation,[47] suggesting that some clinical protocols used to eradicate tumors may in fact increase the possibilities of tumor cell invasion in the irradiated field.

The advantage of culture systems to provide substrates for tumor cell behavior is that the extracellular components can be prelabeled by the inclusion of radioactive precursors in the culture medium at the time that the extracellular matrix is synthesized. This allows much greater freedom in the dissection of the destructive process, since the degradation of a specific component against a background of other components may be easily studied. Recently, a new method to select for highly invasive tumor cells has been developed; it entails the construction of an artificial basement membrane formed by instituting a laminin–type IV collagen barrier compressed onto a matrix[123] of type I collagen. The invasiveness of primary tumor explants grown on multiple layers of mesenchymal cells attached to a nylon mesh has been studied in our laboratory.[11] Figure 1–3 shows that urothelial cells grown from

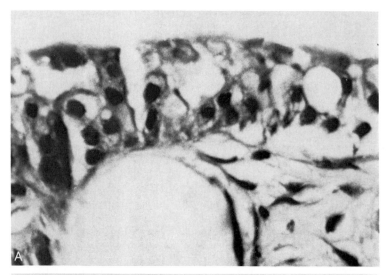

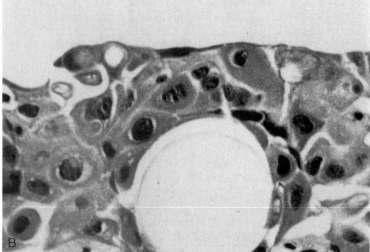

Figure 1–3. In vitro assay for tumor invasiveness. Cells from a line of normal human fibroblast (T–1) were grown on a nylon mesh as described by Bogenmann and Jones.[11] Primary explants from a grossly normal mucosal area of a urinary bladder resected for transitional cell carcinoma (3A) and from a deeply invasive transitional cell carcinoma (3B) were grown on the surface of the mesh and then fixed in buffered formalin, embedded in paraffin, sectioned, and stained with hematoxylin and eosin. The results show penetration of the underlying fibroblast matrix by the invasive tumor but not by the noninvasive urothelium. (× 1430)

the urinary bladder of a patient with invasive transitional cell carcinoma invaded the connective tissue matrix in such a system. Cells grown from the grossly normal area of a urinary bladder with transitional cell carcinoma did not invade the matrix (Fig. 1–3).

These systems should allow us to define the role of tumor cell enzymes in the invasive process. All of them suffer from disadvantages in that they are not exact representations of the kinds of tissues and barriers encountered by invasive tumor cells in the organism, and several of the systems have utilized cultured cell lines for the dissection of the invasive process. These are limita-

tions, and many of the experiments will have to be repeated using cells freshly excised from patients. Nevertheless, the experimental systems have shown that tumor invasion can be recapitulated in vitro and have suggested that tumor-associated enzymes such as specific collagenases, plasminogen activators, and other nonspecific proteases play important roles in the invasive process. If the regulation of these degradative enzymes can be better understood there is, therefore, the possibility of limiting and modulating the invasive process as it occurs in patients. thus diminishing chances of metastatic spread and preventing further invasive activities by secondary tumors.

APPLICATIONS FOR TREATMENT AND MANAGEMENT OF THE CANCER PATIENT

Following this brief review on the mechanisms of tumor metastasis, one may now ask about the potential applications of this knowledge to the clinical management of the cancer patient. It is hoped that understanding the different mechanisms used by tumor cells to infiltrate surrounding tissue and to metastasize to distant organs will suggest new modes of therapy affecting the target cells much more specifically than conventional chemotherapeutic agents. For example, information about the various enzymes and cofactors used by tumor cells during the process of invasion may become the basis for a new class of anticancer drugs interfering specifically with the activity of some of those enzymes. Knowledge of the mode of action of various growth factors and transformation growth factors that affect tumor cells may also give rise to another class of anticancer agents. Tumor cells may differ from nonneoplastic cells in their responsiveness to growth factors and TGFs[59] and could therefore be more directly affected by such chemotherapeutic agents. Some of the in vitro models of tumor invasiveness described in the preceding section may be used as in vitro assays for the sensitivity of tumors to various drugs.

In addition to providing a basis for new chemotherapeutic agents, knowledge of tumor molecular biology could be valuable in cancer diagnosis, in the identification of high-risk individuals, or in having prognostic significance. Amplifications, rearrangements, or other modifications affecting oncogenes may be related to tumor aggressiveness, and detection of such modifications at the level of the cancer cell genome may give reliable prognostic indicators. One candidate for such an approach is the epidermal growth factor receptor gene, which has been found to be expressed in higher titers on the surface of more invasive bladder urothelial tumors.[88] Other specific genomic modifications may be useful in the identification of individuals at risk of developing malignant tumors or of individuals with premalignant disease.[60] The identification of tumor-related products in the circulation (for example, specific proteolytic fragments of macromolecules such as fibronectin) may be useful as screening procedures for diagnosis or as a way to assess response to chemotherapy.

Thus, our understanding of tumor biology has increased rapidly over the last 10 years, and we are much closer to an elucidation of the basic mechanisms involved in tumor progression. It is hoped that new approaches to therapy will be generated by such knowledge.

References

1. Alby L, Auerback R: Differential adhesion of tumor cells to capillary endothelial cells in vitro. Proc Natl Acad Sci USA 81:5739–5743, 1984.
2. Ambrose EJ, Easty DM: Time lapse filming of cellular interactions in organ culture. I. Behavior of non-malignant cells. Differentiation 1:39–50, 1973.
3. Ambrose EJ, Easty DM: Time lapse filming of cellular interactions in organ culture. II. Behavior of malignant cells. Differentiation 1:227–284, 1973.
4. Assoian RK, Grotendorst GR, Miller DM, Sporn MB: Cellular transformation by coordinated action of three peptide growth factors from human platelets. Nature 309:804–806, 1984.
5. Assoian RK, Komoriya A, Meyers CA, et al: Transforming growth factor-beta in human platelets. Identification of a major storage site, purification and characterization. J Biol Chem 258:7155–7160, 1983.
6. Bannasch P, Zerban H, Schmid E, Franke WW: Characterization of cytoskeletal components in epithelial and mesenchymal liver tumors by electron and immunofluorescence microscopy. Virchows Arch [Cell Pathol] 36:139–158, 1981.
7. Barsky SH, Siegal GP, Jannotta F, Liotta LA: Loss of basement membrane components by invasive tumors but not by their benign counterparts. Lab Invest 49:140–147, 1983.
8. Barsky SH, Togo S, Garbisa S, Liotta LA: Type IV collagenase immunoreactivity in invasive breast carcinoma. Lancet 1:296–297, 1983.
9. Bender BL, Jaffe R, Carlin B, Chung AE: Immunolocalization of entactin, a sulfated basement membrane component, in rodent tissues, and comparison with GP-2 (laminin). Am J Pathol 103:419–426, 1981.
10. Bernstein SC, Weinberg RA: Expression of the metastatic phenotype in cells transfected with human metastatic tumor DNA. Proc Natl Acad Sci USA 82:1726–1730, 1985.
11. Bogenmann E, Jones PA: Growth and invasiveness of primary human tumor explants. *In* CC Harris, H Autrup (eds), Human Carcinogenesis. New York, Academic Press, 1983, pp 123–143.
12. Brackenbury R: Molecular mechanisms of cell adhesion in normal and transformed cells. Cancer Metastasis Rev 4:41–58, 1985.
13. Brodeur GM, Seeger RC, Schwab M, et al: Ampli-

fication of N-*myc* in untreated human neuroblastomas correlates with advanced disease stage. Science 224:1121–1124, 1984.

14. Burtin P, Chavanel G, Foidart JM, Martin E: Antigens of the basement membrane and the peritumoral stroma in human colonic adenocarcinomas: an immunofluorescence study. Int J Cancer 30:13–20, 1982.

15. Bussolati G, Botta G, Gugliotta P: Actin-rich (myoepithelial) cells in ductal carcinoma-in-situ of the breast. Virchows Arch [Cell Pathol] 34:251–259, 1980.

16. Carlin B, Jaffe R, Bender B, Chung AE: Entactin: a novel basal-lamina associated sulfated glycoprotein. J Biol Chem 256:5209–5214, 1981.

17. Chambers AF, Ling V: Selection for experimental metastatic ability of heterologous tumor cells in the chick embryo after DNA-mediated transfer. Cancer Res 44:3970–3975, 1984.

18. Chua CC, Geiman DE, Keller GH, Ladda RL: Induction of collagenase secretion in human fibroblast cultures by growth promoting factors. J Biol Chem 260:5213–5216, 1985.

19. Clark WH Jr, Ainsworth AM, Bernardino EA, et al: The developmental biology of primary human malignant melanomas. Semin Oncol 2:83–103, 1975.

20. Coman DR: Decreased mutual adhesiveness: a property of cells from squamous cell carcinomas. Cancer Res 4:625–629, 1944.

21. Coman DR: Mechanisms responsible for the origin and distribution of blood-borne tumor metastases. Cancer Res 13:397–404, 1953.

22. DeLarco JE, Todaro GJ: Growth factors from murine sarcoma virus-transformed cells. Proc Natl Acad Sci USA 75:4001–4005, 1978.

23. De Petro G, Barlati S, Vartio T, Vaheri A: Transformation-enhancing activity of gelatin-binding fragments of fibronectin. Proc Natl Acad Sci USA 78:4965–4969, 1981.

24. Dingemans KP: Invasion of liver tissue by blood-borne mammary carcinoma cells. JNCI 53:1813–1824, 1974.

25. Downward J, Yardon Y, Mayes E, et al: Close similarity of epidermal growth factor receptor and v-erb-B oncogene protein sequences. Nature 307:521–527, 1984.

26. Dresden MH, Heilman SA, Schmidt JD: Collagenolytic enzymes in human neoplasms. Cancer Res 32:993–996, 1972.

27. Easty GC, Easty DM, Tchao R: The growth of heterologous tumor cells in chick embryos. Eur J Cancer 5:287–295, 1969.

28. Eaves G: The invasive growth of malignant tumors as a purely mechanical process. J Pathol 109:233–237, 1973.

29. Engel J, Odermatt E, Engel A, et al: Shapes, domain organizations and flexibility of laminin and fibronectin, two multifunctional proteins of the extracellular matrix. Mol Biol 150:97–120, 1981.

30. Ewing J: Neoplastic Diseases, 3rd ed. Philadelphia, WB Saunders, 1928.

31. Fidler IJ: Selection of successive tumour lines for metastasis. Nature (New Biol) 242:148–149, 1973.

32. Foidart JM, Bere EW Jr, Yaar M, et al: Distribution and immunoelectron microscopic localization of laminin, a noncollagenous basement membrane glycoprotein. Lab Invest 42:336–342, 1980.

33. Foulds L: Neoplastic Development. New York, Academic Press, 1975.

34. Gabbiani G, Csank-Brassert J, Schneeberger JC, et al: Contractile proteins in human cancer cells. Am J Pathol 83:457–474, 1976.

35. Goldenberg VE, Goldenberg NS, Sommers SC: Comparative ultrastructure of atypical ductal hyperplasia, intraductal carcinoma, and infiltrating ductal carcinoma of the breast. Cancer 24:1152–1169, 1969.

36. Gorman JR, Abrahamson J, Mordohovich D, Feldman M: Nonorganophilic, hematogenous dissemination in the presence of positive lymph nodes of a malignant tumor in rabbits. Invest Metastasis 4(Suppl 1):44–59, 1985.

37. Gould VE, Battifora H: Origin and significance of the basal lamina and some interstitial fibrillar components in epithelial neoplasms. Pathol Annu 11:353–386, 1976.

38. Gould VE, Miller J, Jao W: Ultrastructure of medullary, intraductal, tubular and adenocystic breast carcinomas. Comparative patterns of myoepithelial differentiation and basal lamina deposition. Am J Pathol 78:401–416, 1975.

39. Gould VE, Snyder RW: Ultrastructural features of papillomatosis and carcinoma of nipple ducts. The significance of basal lamina and myoepithelial cells in benign, "questionable," and malignant lesions. Pathol Annu 9:441–469, 1974.

40. Gross JL, Krupp MN, Rifkin DB, Lane MD: Downregulation of epidermal growth factor receptor correlates with plasminogen activator activity in human A431 epidermoid carcinoma cells. Proc Natl Acad Sci USA 80:2276–2280, 1983.

41. Hamperl H: The myoepithelia (myoepithelial cells). Normal state; regressive changes; hyperplasia; tumors. Curr Top Pathol 53:161–220, 1970.

42. Hard GC, Toh BH: Immunofluorescent characterization of rat kidney tumors according to the distribution of actin as revealed by specific antiactin antibody. Cancer Res 37:1618–1623, 1977.

43. Hart IR, Fidler IJ: An in vitro quantitative assay for tumor cell invasion. Cancer Res 38:3218–3224, 1978.

44. Hart IR, Fidler IJ: Role of organ selectivity in the determination of metastatic patterns of B16 melanoma. Cancer Res 40:2281–2287, 1980.

45. Hassel JR, Robey PG, Barrach HJ, et al: Isolation of a heparan sulfate-containing proteoglycan from basement membrane. Proc Natl Acad Sci USA 77:4494–4498, 1980.

46. Hayashi H, Yoshida K, Ozaki T, Ushijima K: Chemotactic factor associated with invasion of cancer cells. Nature 226:174–175, 1970.

47. Heisel MA, Laug WE, Stowe SM, Jones PA: Effects of x-irradiation on artificial blood vessel wall degradation by invasive tumor cells. Cancer Res 44:2441–2445, 1984.

48. Henry N, Eeckhout Y, van Lamsweerde AL, Vaes G: Cooperation between metastatic tumor cells and macrophages in the degradation of basement membrane (type IV) collagen. FEBS Lett 161:243–246, 1983.

49. Hill RP, Chambers AF, Ling V, Harris JF: Dynamic heterogeneity: rapid generation of metastatic variants in mouse B16 melanoma cells. Science 224:998–1001, 1984.

50. Huard T, Wood J, Malinoff H, et al: Laminin

promotes macrophage tumor cell binding by specific plasma membrane proteins. Proc Am Assoc Cancer Res 25:196, 1984.

51. Inoue S, Leblond CP, Laurie GW: Ultrastructure of Reichert's membrane, a multilayered basement membrane in the parietal wall of the yolk sac. J Cell Biol: 97:1524–1537, 1983.

52. James R, Bradshaw RA: Polypeptide growth factors. Annu Rev Biochem 53:259–292, 1984.

53. Jones PA: Construction of an artificial blood vessel wall from cultured endothelial and smooth muscle cells. Proc Natl Acad Sci USA 76:1882–1886, 1979.

54. Jones PA, DeClerck YA: Destruction of extracellular matrices containing glycoproteins, elastin and collagen by metastatic human tumor cells. Cancer Res 40:3222–3227, 1980.

55. Jones PA, DeClerck YA: Extracellular matrix destruction by invasive tumor cells. Cancer Metastasis Rev 1:289–317, 1982.

56. Jones PA, Neustein HB, Gonzales F, Bogenmann E: Invasion of an artificial blood vessel wall by human fibrosarcoma cells. Cancer Res 41:4613–4620, 1981.

57. Kanwar YS, Linker A, Farquhar MG: Increased permeability of the glomerular basement membrane to ferritin after removal of glycosaminoglycans (heparan sulfate) by enzyme digestion. J Cell Biol 86:688–693, 1980.

58. Kaplan PL, Anderson M, Ozanne B: Transforming growth factor(s) production enables cells to grow in the absence of serum: an autocrine system. Proc Natl Acad Sci USA 79:485–489, 1982.

59. Kaplan PL, Ozanne B: Cellular responsiveness to growth factors correlates with a cell's ability to express the transformed phenotype. Cell 33:931–938, 1983.

60. Klein G, Klein E: Evolution of tumors and the impact of molecular oncology. Nature 315:190–195, 1985.

61. Kleinman HK, McGarvey ML, Liotta LA, et al: Isolation and characterization of type IV procollagen, laminin, and heparan sulphate proteoglycan from the EHS sarcoma. Biochem 24:6188, 1982.

62. Kohga S, Shashikumar RH, Weaver RM, Markus G: Localization of plasminogen activators in human colon cancer by immunoperoxidase staining. Cancer Res 45:1787–1796, 1985.

63. Kramer RH, Gonzalez R, Nicolson GL: Metastatic tumor cells adhere preferentially to the extracellular matrix underlying vascular endothelial cell. Int J Cancer 26:639–645, 1980.

64. Kramer RH, Nicolson GL: Interactions of tumor cells with vascular endothelial cell monolayers: a model for metastatic invasion. Proc Natl Acad Sci 76:5704–5708, 1979.

65. Kramer RH, Nicolson GL: Invasion of vascular endothelial cell monolayers and underlying matrix by metastatic human cancer cells. In HG Schweiger (ed), Intl Cell Biol. Heidelberg, Springer-Verlag, 1981, pp 794–799.

66. Kramer RH, Vogel KG: Selective degradation of basement membrane macromolecules by metastatic melanoma cells. JNCI 72:889–899, 1984.

67. Kramer RH, Vogel KG, Nicolson GL: Solubilization and degradation of subendothelial matrix glycoproteins and proteoglycans by metastatic tumor cells. J Biol Chem 257:2678–2686, 1982.

68. Kris RM, Libermann TA, Avivi A, Schlessinger J: Growth factors, growth factor receptors and oncogenes. Biotechnology Feb.1985:135–140.

69. Kuettner KE, Soble L, Croxen RL, et al: Tumor cell collagenase and its inhibition by a cartilage-derived protease inhibitor. Science 197:653–654, 1977.

70. Laug WE, DeClerck Y, Jones PA: Degradation of the subendothelial matrix of tumor cells. Cancer Res 43:1827–1834, 1983.

71. Laug WE, Jones PA, Benedict WF: Relationship between fibrinolysis of cultured cells and malignancy. JNCI 54:173–179, 1975.

72. Liotta LA: Tumor invasion and metastases: role of the basement membrane. Am J Pathol 117:339–348, 1984.

73. Liotta LA, Abe S, Robey PG, Martin GR: Preferential digestion of basement collagen by an enzyme derived from a metastatic murine tumor. Proc Natl Acad Sci USA 76:2268–2272, 1979.

74. Liotta LA, Goldfarb RH, Brundage R, et al: Effect of plasminogen activator (urokinase), plasmin, and thrombin on glycoprotein and collagenous components of basement membrane. Cancer Res 41:4629–4635, 1981.

75. Liotta LA, Kleinerman J, Catanzaro P, Rynbrandt D: Degradation of basement membrane by tumor cells. JNCI 58:1427–1431, 1977.

76. Liotta LA, Lanzer WL, Garbisa S: Identification of a type V collagenolytic enzyme. Biochem Biophys Res Commun 98:184–190, 1981.

77. Liotta LA, Rao CN, Barsky SH: Tumor invasion and the extracellular matrix. Lab Invest 49:636–649, 1983.

78. Liotta LA, Wicha MS, Foidart JM, et al: Hormonal requirements for basement membrane collagen deposition by cultured rat mammary epithelium. Lab Invest 41:511–518, 1979.

79. Little CD, Nau MM, Carney DN, et al: Amplification and expression of the c-myc oncogene in human lung cancer cell lines. Nature 306:194–196, 1983.

80. Manthorpe M, Engvall E, Ruoslahti E, et al: Laminin promotes neuritic regeneration from cultured peripheral and central neurons. J Cell Biol 97:1882–1890, 1983.

81. Mareel MM: Recent aspects of tumor invasiveness. Int Rev Exp Pathol 22:65–129, 1980.

82. Mareel M, Kint J, Meyvisch C: Methods of study of the invasion of malignant C3H-mouse fibroblasts into embryonic chick heart in vitro. Virchows Arch [Cell Pathol] 30:95–111, 1979.

83. McNutt NS: Ultrastructural comparison of the interface between epithelium and stroma in basal cell carcinoma and control human skin. Lab Invest 35:132–142, 1976.

84. Merrilees MJ, Finlay GJ: Human tumor cells in culture stimulate glycosaminoglycan synthesis by human skin fibroblasts. Lab Invest 53:30–36, 1985.

85. Messing E: Growth factors in human bladder tumors. J Urol 131:111A, 1984.

86. Mignatti P, Ascari E, Barlati S: Potential diagnostic and prognostic significance of the transforming-enhancing factor(s) in the plasma cryoprecipitate of tumor patients. Int J Cancer 25:727–734, 1980.

87. Murquardt H, Hunkapiller MW, Hood LE, et al: Transforming growth factors produced by retrovirus-transformed rodent fibroblasts and human melanoma cells: amino acid sequence homology

with epidermal growth factor. Proc Natl Acad Sci USA 80:4684–4688, 1983.

88. Neal DE, Bennett MK, Hall RR, et al: Epidermal-growth-factor receptors in human bladder cancer: comparison of invasive and superficial tumors. Lancet 1:366–368, 1985.

89. Nicolson GL: Cancer metastasis. Organ colonization and the cell-surface properties of malignant cells. Biochim Biophys Acta 695:113–176, 1982.

90. Nicolson GL: Generation of phenotypic diversity and progression in metastatic tumor cells. Cancer Metastasis Rev 3:25–42, 1984.

91. Noguchi PD, Johnson JB, O'Donnell R, Petricciani JC: Chick embryonic skin as a rapid organ culture assay for cellular neoplasia. Science 199:980–983, 1978.

92. Nowell PC: The clonal evolution of tumor cell populations. Science 194:23–28, 1976.

93. Ossowski L, Reich E: Changes in malignant phenotype of a human carcinoma conditioned by growth environment. Cell 33:323–333, 1983.

94. Ozaki T, Yoshida K, Ushijima K, Hayashi H: Studies on the mechanisms of invasion in cancer. II. In vivo effects of a factor chemotactic for cancer cells. Int J Cancer 7:93–100, 1971.

95. Ozanne B, Fulton RJ, Kaplan PL: Kirsten murine sarcoma virus transformed cell lines and a spontaneously transformed rat cell line produce transforming factors. J Cell Phys 105:163–180, 1980.

96. Paget S: The distribution of secondary growth in cancer of the breast. Lancet 1:571–573, 1889.

97. Parthasarathy N, Spiro RG: Characterization of the glycosaminoglycan component of the renal glomerular basement membrane and its relationship to the peptide portion. J Biol Chem 256:507–513, 1981.

98. Pauli BU, Memoli VA, Kuettner KE: In vitro determination of tumor invasiveness using extracted hyaline cartilage. Cancer Res 41:2084–2091, 1981.

99. Poole AR, Tiltman KJ, Recklies AD, Stoker TA: Differences in secretion of the proteinase cathepsin B at the edges of human breast carcinomas and fibroadenomas. Nature 273:545–547, 1978.

100. Poste G, Doll J, Hart IR, Fidler IJ: In vitro selection of murine B16 melanoma variants with enhanced tissue-invasive properties. Cancer Res 40:1636–1644, 1980.

101. Potter KM, Juacaba SF, Price JE, Tarin D: Observations on organ distribution of fluorescein-labelled tumor cells released intravascularly. Invasion Metastasis 3:221–233, 1983.

102. Rao CN, Barsky SH, Terranova VP, Liotta LA: Isolation of a tumor cell laminin receptor. Biochem Biophys Res Comm 111:804–808, 1983.

103. Rao CN, Margulies IM, Goldfarb RH, et al: Differential proteolytic susceptibility of laminin alpha and beta subunits. Arch Biochem Biophys 219:65–70, 1982.

104. Rao CN, Margulies IM, Tralka TS, et al: Isolation of a subunit of laminin and its role in molecular structure and tumor cell attachment. J Biol Chem 257:9740–9744, 1982.

105. Raz A, Geiger B: Altered organization of cell-substrate contacts and membrane-associated cytoskeleton in tumor cell variants exhibiting different metastatic capabilities. Cancer Res 42:5183–5190, 1982.

106. Recklies AD, Tittman KJ, Stoker TAM, Poole AR: Secretions of proteinases from malignant and non-malignant human breast tissue. Cancer Res 40:550–556, 1980.

107. Roberts AB, Anzano MA, Meyers CA, et al: Purification and properties of the type beta transforming growth factor from bovine kidney. Biochem 22:5692–5698, 1983.

108. Roll FJ, Madri JA, Albert J, Furthmayr H: Codistribution of collagen types IV and AB2 in basement membranes and mesangium of the kidney: an immunoferritin study of ultra thin frozen sections. J Cell Biol 85:597–616, 1980.

109. Roos E, Dingemans KP, Van de Pavert IV, Van den Bergh-Weerman MA: Mammary carcinoma cells in mouse liver: infiltration of liver tissue and interaction with Kupffer cells. Br J Cancer 38:88–99, 1978.

110. Rungger-Brandle E, Gabbiani G: Human epidermal and mammary carcinoma cells: actin distribution. Eur J Cancer 16:12–13, 1980.

111. Ruoslahti E, Engvall E, Hayman EG: Fibronectin: current concepts of its structure and function. Coll Res 1:95–128, 1981.

112. Russo RG, Thorgeirsson UP, Liotta LA: In vitro quantitative assay of invasion using human amnion. In LA Liotta, IR Hart (eds), Tumor Invasion and Metastases. The Hague, Martinus Nijhoff, 1982, p 173.

113. Sakashita S, Engvall E, Ruoslahti E: Basement membrane glycoprotein laminin binds to heparin. FEBS Lett 114:243–250, 1980.

114. Scott PG: Macromolecular constituents of basement membranes: a review of current knowledge on their structure and function. Can J Biochem Cell Biol 61:942–948, 1983.

115. Shields SE, Ogilvie DJ, McKinnell RG, Tarin D: Degradation of basement membrane collagens by metalloproteases released by human, murine and amphibian tumors. J Pathol 143:193–197, 1984.

116. Siegal GP, Barsky SH, Terranova VP, Liotta LA: Stages of neoplastic transformation of human breast tissue as monitored by dissolution of basement components: an immunoperoxidase study. Invasion Metastasis 1:54–70, 1981.

117. Starkey JR, Hosick HL, Stanford DR, Liggitt HD: Interaction of metastatic tumor cells with bovine lens capsule basement membrane. Cancer Res 44:1585–1594, 1984.

118. Strauli P, Weiss L: Cell locomotion and tumor penetration. Eur J Cancer 131:1–12, 1977.

119. Tane N, Hashimoto K, Kanzaki T, Ohyama H: Collagenolytic activities of cultured human malignant melanoma cells. J Biochem 84:1171–1176, 1978.

120. Tarin D, Price JE, Kettlewell MGW, et al: Clinicopathological observations on metastasis in man studied in patients treated with peritoneovenous shunts. Br Med J 288:749–751, 1984.

121. Tarin D, Price JE, Kettlewell MGW, et al: Mechanisms of human tumor metastasis studied in patients with peritoneovenous shunts. Cancer Res 44:3584–3592, 1984.

122. Tarin D, Vass ACR, Kettlewell MGW, Price JE: Absence of metastatic sequelae during long-term treatment of malignant ascites by peritoneovenous shunting. A clinicopathological report. Invasion Metastasis 4:1–12, 1984.

123. Terranova VP, Hic S, DiFlorio R, Lyall RM: Tumor cell metastasis: the importance of the extracellular matrix. Crit Rev Biochem (in press).

124. Terranova VP, Liotta LA, Russo RG, Martin GR: Role of laminin in the attachment and metastasis of murine tumor cells. Cancer Res 42:2265–2269, 1982.
125. Terranova VP, Rao CN, Kalebic T, et al: Laminin receptor on human breast carcinoma cells. Proc Natl Acad Sci USA 80:444–448, 1983.
126. Thorgeirsson UP, Turpeenniemi-Hujanen T, Williams JE, et al: NIH/3T3 cells transfected with human tumor DNA containing activated *ras* oncogenes express the metastatic phenotype in nude mice. Molec Cell Biol 5:259–262, 1985.
127. Timpl R, Johansson S, Van Delden V, et al: Characterization of protease-resistant fragments of laminin mediating attachment and spreading of rat hepatocytes. J Biol Chem 258:8922–8927, 1983.
128. Timpl R, Martin GR: Components of basement membranes. *In* H Furthmayr (ed), Immunochemistry of the Extracellular Matrix, Vol 2: Applications. Boca Raton, Florida, CRC Press, 1982, pp 125.
129. Timpl R, Martin GR, Bruckner P, et al: Nature of the collagenous protein in a tumor basement membrane. Eur J Biochem 84:43–52, 1978.
130. Timpl R, Oberbaumer I, Furthmayr H, Kuhn K: Macromolecular organization of type IV collagen. *In* K Kuhn (ed), New Trends in Basement Membrane Research. New York, Raven Press, 1982, p 57.
131. Timpl R, Rhode H, Robey PG, et al: Laminin—a glycoprotein from basement membrane. J Biol Chem 254:9933–9937, 1979.
132. Timpl R, Weidmann H, Van Delden V, et al: A network model for the organization of type IV collagen molecules in basement membrane. Eur J Biochem 120:203–211, 1981.
133. Trelstad RL: Glycosaminoglycans: mortar, matrix, mentor. Lab Invest 53:1–4, 1985.
134. Tullberg KF, Burger MM: Selection of B16 melanoma cells with increased metastatic potential and low intercellular cohesion using nucleopore filters. Invasion Metastasis 5:1–15, 1985.
135. Ungari S, Katari RS, Alessandri G, Gullimo PM: Cooperation between fibronectin and heparin in the mobilization of capillary endothelium. Invasion Metastasis 5:193–205, 1985.
136. Vaheri A, Keski-Oja J, Alitalo K, et al: Structure and functions of fibronectin. Devel Biochem 16:161–178, 1980.
137. Varani J, Lovett EJ 3d, McCoy JP, et al: Differential expression of a laminin-like substance by high- and low-metastatic tumor cells. Am J Pathol 111:27–34, 1983.
138. Vartio T, Vaheri A, De Petro G, Barlati S: Fibronectin and its proteolytic fragments. Potential as cancer markers. Invasion Metastasis 3:125–138, 1983.
139. Vassar PS, Seaman GV, Brooks DE: Cell membrane properties in neoplasia. Proc Can Cancer Conf 7:268–291, 1967.
140. Vlodavsky I, Fuks Z, Bar-Ner M, et al: Lymphoma cell-mediated degradation of sulfated proteoglycans in the subendothelial extracellular matrix: relationship to tumor cell metastasis. Cancer Res 43:2704–2711, 1983.
141. Weiss L: The cell periphery and metastasis. Proc Can Cancer Conf 7:292–315, 1967.
142. Weiss L: Random and nonrandom processes in metastasis, and metastatic inefficiency. Invasion Metastasis 3:193–207, 1983.
143. Weiss L, Ward PM: Cell detachment and metastasis. Cancer Metastasis Rev 2:111–127, 1983.
144. Wicha MS, Malinoff HL, Huard TK: Laminin receptors on macrophages: a mechanism for metastatic tumor cell recognition. Proc Am Assoc Cancer Res 24:140, 1983.
145. Wilson EL, Becker MLB, Hoal EG, Dowdle EB: Molecular species of plasminogen activators secreted by normal and neoplastic human cells. Cancer Res 40:933–938, 1980.
146. Wood S Jr: Pathogenesis of metastasis formation observed in vivo in the rabbit ear chamber. Arch Pathol 66:550–568, 1958.
147. Wood S Jr: Mechanism of establishment of tumor metastases. *In* HL Ioachim (ed), Pathobiology Annual, 1971, pp 495–510.
148. Yamada KM: Cell surface interactions with extracellular materials. Annu Rev Biochem 52:761–799, 1983.
149. Yamada KM, Hahn LH, Olden K: Structure and function of the fibronectins. Prog Clin Biol Res 41:797–819, 1980.
150. Young JS, Lumsden CE, Stalker AL: The significance of the "tissue pressure" of normal testicular and of neoplastic (Brown-Pearce carcinoma) tissue in the rabbit. J Pathol Bacteriol 62:313–333, 1950.
151. Yurchenko PD, Furthmayr H: Self-assembly of basement membrane collagen. Biochem 23:1839–1850, 1984.

PART II

Epidemiology of Urologic Tumors

RONALD K. ROSS, M.D.
ANNLIA PAGANINI-HILL, Ph.D.
BRIAN E. HENDERSON, M.D.

CHAPTER 2

Epidemiology of Bladder Cancer*

Epidemiologists have estimated that in the United States, more than 50% of occurrences of bladder cancer in men and more than 35% of cases in women are due either to cigarette smoking or to industrial exposure to carcinogens.[12] In fact, Doll and Peto have estimated that 55% of deaths from bladder cancer are due to cigarette smoking alone.[18] If true, one might expect the incidence of bladder cancer to be increasing due to the growing use of cigarettes and greater industrial pollution since the turn of the century. Time trends in mortality rates in the United States for bladder and lung cancer in white males from 1930 to 1980 are shown in Figure 2–1.[78] During that 50-year period, bladder cancer mortality rates remained relatively stable while lung cancer mortality increased by a factor of more than fifteen. Deaths from lung cancer are almost exclusively attributable to cigarette smoking and industrial exposures.[76] However, apparent trends in cancer mortality can be misleading, since mortality rates are influenced not only by changes in etiologic factors but also by modifications in classification and treatment of diseases. Nonetheless, other demographic characteristics of bladder cancer, especially when compared with those of lung cancer, suggest that environmental factors in addition to

cigarette smoking and industrial exposures make important contributions to the development of bladder cancer.

In this review, we first summarize the descriptive epidemiology of bladder cancer and briefly compare it with that of lung cancer, then review the epidemiologic evi-

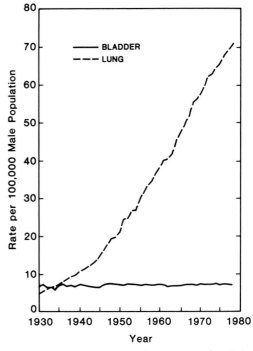

Figure 2–1. Trends in mortality rates in the United States for white males.

*Supported by Grants CA 00652, CA 32197, and CA 17054 from the National Cancer Institute, National Institutes of Health.

dence linking bladder cancer to the major known risk factors, and finally weigh the epidemiologic evidence regarding other etiologic hypotheses.

DESCRIPTIVE EPIDEMIOLOGY OF BLADDER CANCER

By race and sex, the outstanding epidemiologic feature of bladder cancer in the US is the very high incidence rate in white men (Table 2–1). The age-adjusted bladder cancer rate in white men is nearly twice that in blacks, and in men it greatly exceeds that in women for all racial groups, but especially for whites, in whom the sex ratio of affected individuals is 4:1. In the US the age-adjusted rate for lung cancer in white men is lower than in blacks (Table 2–1), who have a high rate of cigarette smoking.[10, 79]

There is a positive social class gradient for bladder cancer incidence in both sexes (Table 2–2). In contrast, lung cancer in men is a disease primarily of the lower social classes; in women, there is a weak positive relationship between social class and incidence.

The distribution of bladder cancer and lung cancer by broad occupational categories closely reflects the social class distribution of the two diseases (Figure 2–2). Bladder cancer rates are highest among those with "white-collar" occupations, such as professionals, managers, and salesmen, and lowest among "blue-collar" workers. Lung cancer displays the opposite pattern, with the highest rates observed among blue-collar workers such as operatives, transportation workers, and laborers. Not only are the high-risk occupations for lung cancer those with the greatest potential for exposure to hazardous chemicals, but also persons employed in

Table 2–1. BLADDER CANCER AND LUNG CANCER AGE-ADJUSTED INCIDENCE RATES* BY RACE AND SEX, LOS ANGELES, 1972–1983

Race	Bladder		Lung	
	Male	Female	Male	Female
Black	19	7	121	32
White	32	8	80	31
Japanese	13	4	48	15

*Per 100,000 population.

Table 2–2. BLADDER CANCER AND LUNG CANCER AGE-ADJUSTED INCIDENCE RATES* BY SOCIAL CLASS AND SEX, WHITES ONLY, LOS ANGELES, 1972–1983

Social Class	Bladder		Lung	
	Male	Female	Male	Female
1 (high)	39	10	72	35
2	37	9	75	32
3	32	9	78	31
4	27	7	80	29
5	24	6	85	28

*Per 100,000 population.

blue-collar occupations are more likely to smoke cigarettes than persons in white-collar occupations.[79]

Incidence data for the US from the Second (1947–1948) and the Third (1969–1971) National Cancer Surveys show an overall increase of 24% in the age-standardized incidence rate of bladder cancer in white men but a 20% decline in white women during the same period.[75] Doll and Peto have suggested that the reported increase of the disease in men may be questionable owing to a

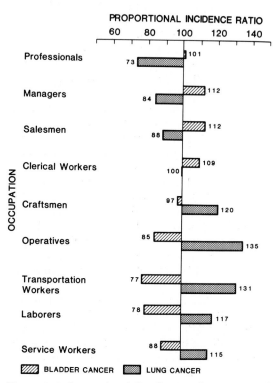

Figure 2–2. Occupational distribution of occurrence of bladder cancer and lung cancer.

progressive tendency to regard as malignant the common papillomas of the bladder, previously classified as benign.[18] This hypothesis could explain the stability in bladder cancer mortality in men in the US at a time when incidence was increasing and survival was improving only slightly (Figure 2–1).[77]

Other than the United States, the only industrialized country in which the bladder cancer mortality rate in males has remained unchanged over the past 30 years is Canada.[16, 54] In other industrialized countries these rates have shown a slow but steady increase, averaging between 25% and 50% since 1950.[44] As in the US, bladder cancer mortality in Canadian women has steadily declined since 1950.[16, 54] In Japanese women, the bladder cancer mortality rate peaked in the mid-1960s, after increasing continually until then; it has since declined.[88] In most other countries, the mortality rate in women, in contrast to that in men, has remained relatively constant. A few such as Scotland, Finland, and Denmark have shown a small but steady increase.[44]

Bladder cancer mortality rates in men and women are only weakly correlated with lung cancer mortality rates. Several populations show particularly high or low mortality from bladder cancer compared with that from lung cancer. In males, US nonwhites and Japanese have very low bladder cancer mortality rates in comparison with deaths in those groups from lung cancer. Conversely, the bladder cancer mortality rate in males in Denmark is far above what would be predicted from the lung cancer rate. Similarly, Danish women have a high bladder cancer mortality rate and Japanese women a low rate relative to lung cancer.

Interestingly, Polynesian men (e.g., native Hawaiians and New Zealand Maoris) have one of the lowest rates of bladder cancer in the world, even though cigarette smoking in that population is quite high. In New Zealand, overall cigarette smoking in Maori men (56%) is measurably greater than among European men (38%).[65] Not surprisingly, the annual age-adjusted lung cancer incidence rate in Maoris (103 per 100,000) is almost twice that of European men (53 per 100,000), but European men have almost three times the incidence of bladder cancer (13 vs. 4 per 100,000).[23]

ETIOLOGIC HYPOTHESES

Cigarette Smoking

The first epidemiologic study of an association between cigarette smoking and bladder cancer was conducted by Lilienfeld and co-workers in 1956.[45] They observed a positive association between cigarette use and bladder cancer risk in men but not in women. The reason for the lack of association in women is unclear; most subsequent studies, beginning with that of Lockwood in 1961,[46] have demonstrated an association between cigarette smoking and increased risk of bladder cancer in both sexes (Table 2–3). Among case-control studies, only that of Anthony and Thomas[1] in England failed to observe a positive association between smoking and bladder cancer in men, and only those of Lilienfeld[45] and Sadeghi[69] did not reveal a positive association in women. Most case-control studies have reported a relative risk of about 2 for cigarette smokers compared with non-smokers, and nearly all have observed steadily higher risks with increasing amounts smoked.[11, 15, 25, 35, 46, 49, 50, 59, 62, 64, 70, 72, 74, 80, 84, 86] Exceptions include the two case-control studies conducted in England,[1, 6] the study by Sadeghi in Iran,[69] and the study by Dunham and colleagues in New Orleans.[21] Since many of these case-control studies have utilized hospital controls as a comparison group, the observed risks might underestimate the true relative risks, since hospitalized patients tend to smoke more than the general population. Nonetheless, the few cohort studies that have considered this association have found comparable risk levels.[19, 26, 27, 38, 82] Cohort analyses to date have been restricted to males (Table 2–4).

Bladder cancer risk appears to be only weakly associated with pipe and cigar smoking and not at all with use of smokeless tobacco.[27] It was recently reported that opium smoking may convey an increased risk of bladder cancer comparable to that of cigarette smoking.[69]

Few studies have addressed the issues of the effects of inhalation patterns and use of filtered cigarettes on risk of bladder cancer. The most detailed information comes from the study of Morrison and co-workers.[62] They found little evidence that the risk of bladder cancer in those who smoke filtered

Table 2–3. CASE-CONTROL STUDIES OF CIGARETTE SMOKING AND BLADDER CANCER

Year	First Author	Location	Relative Risk Male	Relative Risk Female	Type of Controls	Dose Response Male	Dose Response Female
1956	Lilienfeld	New York	1.7	0.7	Hospital	Yes	No
1961	Lockwood	Denmark	2.4	1.5*	Population	Yes	Yes*
1961	Schwartz	France	2.0	—	Hospital	Yes	—
1963	Wynder	New York	3.2	3.8	Hospital	Yes	Yes
1965	Cobb	Seattle	7.3	—	Hospital	Yes	—
1966	Staszewski	Poland	2.7	—	Hospital	Yes	—
1968	Dunham	New Orleans	1.4	1.2	Hospital	No	No
1970	Anthony	England	0.8	—	Hospital	No	—
1971	Cole	Boston	1.9	2.0	Population	Yes	Yes
1974	Morgan	Canada	3.2	1.3	Hospital	Yes	Yes
1974	Makhyoun	Egypt	1.4	—	Hospital	Yes	—
1975	Simon	USA	—	1.6	Hospital	—	Yes
1977	Wynder	USA	2.2	2.2	Hospital	Yes	Yes
1979	Sadeghi	Iran	2.0	0.4†	Hospital	No	—
1980	Howe	Canada	3.9	2.4	Neighborhood	Yes	Yes
1982	Najem	USA	2.0		Hospital	Yes	
1983	Mommsen	Denmark	3.5	3.2	Population	Yes	Yes
1983	Cartwright	England	1.6	1.2	Hospital	No	No
1983	McCredie	Australia	2.7		Population	Yes	
1984	Vineis	Italy	5.1	—	Hospital	Yes	—
1984	Morrison	England	2.2	1.3	Population	Yes	Yes
		USA	1.9	4.2	Population	Yes	Yes
		Japan	1.7	4.3	Population	Yes	No
1985	Gonzalez	Spain	2.3		Hospital	Unknown	
1985	Hartge	USA	2.2	—	Population	Yes	—

*All types of smoking.
†Eleven cases only.

cigarettes differs from the risk in smokers of nonfiltered cigarettes in three study populations: Boston, Massachusetts; Manchester, England; and Nagoya, Japan. However, in a large case-control study in Turin, Italy, Vineis and colleagues found that smokers of filtered cigarettes exclusively had a relative risk of bladder cancer of 0.3 compared with the risk in smokers of nonfiltered cigarettes.[80] Howe and co-workers also found that smokers of nonfiltered cigarettes may be at higher risk.[35] In the study by the Morrison group, deep inhalation increased bladder cancer risk by an additional 30 to 40%, compared with the risk in smokers who inhaled somewhat or not at all,[62] whereas

the Howe group found little effect of inhalation.[35] Both questions require further study.

Another issue related to cigarette smoking and bladder cancer concerns the result of discontinuing smoking. Several studies have found that the risk of bladder cancer in former smokers lies between that of present smokers and those who have never smoked.[28, 35, 61, 80] In the studies headed by Howe[35] and Vineis,[80] risk was inversely related to the number of years since the subject stopped smoking. Again, the most detailed information comes from the study by the Morrison group.[62] There was no clear or consistent relationship between the length

Table 2–4. COHORT STUDIES OF CIGARETTE SMOKING AND BLADDER CANCER

Year	First Author	Population	Relative Risk Smokers: Nonsmokers	Dose Response
1958	Hammond	US white males	2.1	Unknown
1966	Kahn	US veterans	2.2	Yes
1966	Hammond	Volunteers (ACS)		
		<65 years	2.0	Unknown
		≥65 years	3.0	Unknown
1970	Weir	California labor union members	2.0	Yes
1976	Doll	British physicians	2.1	No

of time since stopping smoking and risk in any of their three study areas.

The mechanism by which cigarettes induce bladder cancer is unclear, even though cigarette smoke, especially the particulate matter, is known to contain numerous experimental carcinogens.[85] Aromatic amines, including the human bladder carcinogen β-naphthylamine, are also present in tobacco smoke in small amounts.[66] Mice receiving intraoral tobacco tars have a high likelihood of developing bladder papillomas and carcinomas, and some cyclic N-nitrosamines derived from tobacco alkaloids are bladder-specific carcinogens in animals.[32, 33] If tobacco tars are the etiologic agent for cigarette-induced bladder cancer in man, international variation in the average tar content of cigarettes over time might explain some of the trends in bladder cancer mortality.

Mommsen and co-workers recently proposed that genetic factors might be involved in cigarette-induced bladder cancer.[57] Human liver N-acetyltransferase may be involved in carcinogenic detoxification of aromatic amines.[83] N-acetyltransferase activity in humans is genetically regulated, and those who acetylate slowly are homozygous for an autosomal recessive gene. Several investigators have found that patients with bladder cancer are more likely to be "slow acetylators" than are persons without the disease.[7, 57, 83] Mommsen and colleagues suggest that these "slow acetylators" are unable to detoxify smoking-related aromatic amines, thereby further increasing their risk level.[57] More study is needed to better understand the role of N-acetyltransferase phenotype in bladder cancer susceptibility.

Industrial Exposure

Arylamines compose the class of chemical carcinogens most strongly related to bladder cancer. A comprehensive historic perspective on the association between arylamines and human bladder cancer was recently described by Lower.[47] The first significant exposure to arylamines occurred in the mid-1800s when William Perkin, while attempting to synthesize quinine from aniline, accidentally synthesized aniline purple, an arylamine present in coal tars.[17] This made possible the beginning of the synthetic textile dye industry. In 1895, Rehn reported three cases of bladder cancer among employees in a German chemical dye works.[68] Other case reports of similarly exposed individuals in other European countries followed. In the 1930s, William Hueper, Assistant Director of DuPont Laboratory of Industrial Toxicology, warned the DuPont Corporation that their dye production facility represented a significant health hazard in terms of bladder cancer risk, and 23 cases of bladder cancer were subsequently identified among employees exposed to arylamines. Within a few years, Hueper had demonstrated that oral ingestion by dogs of the industrial arylamine β-naphthylamine could produce bladder carcinomas.[37]

In 1954 in London, Case and coworkers conducted the first epidemiologic cohort study that demonstrated unequivocally that arylamine-exposed chemical workers had a high risk of bladder cancer, about 20 times that of the general population.[9] Simultaneously, they discovered that workers in the rubber tire industry also had a high risk of bladder cancer.[8] Beta-naphthylamine had been used as an antioxidant in the rubber industry, and benzidine, a chemically related compound widely used in the rubber industry, has now been established as a human bladder carcinogen as well. Inordinate deaths from bladder cancer in the rubber industry have been observed among workers involved in tire building, warehousing and shipping, and in compounding, milling, and reclaiming.[51, 58]

In addition to being used in the textile dye and rubber industries, arylamines have been used in hair dyes and paint pigments. Accordingly, some studies have shown hairdressers and painters to be at high risk of bladder cancer.[14, 86]

Other occupations also have been observed to have increased risk of bladder cancer. Several investigators have found an excessive risk in metalworkers and in workers in the leather industry.[14, 46, 71, 81, 86] In the latter group, leather "finishers" who cut, trim, and buff leather skins appear to be at particularly high risk.[14] It was recently suggested by Silverman and colleagues, using data from the National Bladder Cancer Study, that truck drivers may be at high risk.[71] In this study, the risk was related to duration of employment as a truck driver and was especially high in those with a history of operating vehicles with diesel engines.[71] Hoar and Hoover found similar results in a case-control study of truck driving and bladder cancer mortality in rural New England.[31]

OTHER ETIOLOGIC HYPOTHESES

A variety of other potential etiologic factors have been linked to bladder cancer, but supportive epidemiologic evidence is either minimal or absent.

Animal studies have shown that saccharin may cause bladder cancer in rodents.[30] However, if the dose-incidence curve in rodents is extrapolated to humans, calculations show that saccharin users would experience only a 4% increase in bladder cancer occurrence, an effect clearly below the level of detectability by epidemiologic studies.[73] Not surprisingly, therefore, epidemiologic studies of artificial sweeteners and human bladder cancer have, with one exception, been uniformly negative (Table 2–5).[6, 36, 41, 42, 55, 56, 59, 60, 63, 72, 84, 87] Armstrong and Doll found no evidence of unusual occurrence of bladder cancer in diabetics, a group known to consume large amounts of artificial sweetener.[2] The absence of any specific trend in bladder cancer incidence is further assurance that

Table 2–5. CASE-CONTROL STUDIES OF ARTIFICIAL SWEETENERS AND BLADDER CANCER

Year	Authors	Relative Risk Male	Relative Risk Female
Artificial Sweeteners (Combined)			
1974	Morgan and Jain	1.0	0.4
1976	Kessler	0.7	1.7
1977	Wynder and Goldsmith	0.7	0.7
1977	Howe et al	1.6	0.6
1978	Kessler and Clark	1.1	0.8
1978	Miller et al	1.1	0.9
1980	Wynder and Stellman	0.9	0.6
1980	Morrison and Buring		
	Diet beverages	0.8	1.6
	Sugar substitutes	0.8	1.5
1980	Hoover and Strasser	1.0	1.1
Saccharin Only			
1982	Cartwright et al		
	Nonsmokers	2.2	1.6
	Smokers	0.9	1.2
1982	Morrison et al		
	Manchester, England	0.9	0.9
	Nagoya, Japan	0.7	0.5
1982	Najem et al	1.3	
1983	Mommsen et al	—	6.4
Cyclamates Only			
1975	Simon et al	—	1.2

use of artificial sweeteners is having little effect on the occurrence of bladder cancer.

Evidence for an association between coffee drinking and increased bladder cancer risk was initially suggested by a case-control study conducted in Massachusetts in 1971.[13] Cole found that women who drank more than one cup of coffee per day had a relative risk of 2.6, compared with those who drank one cup or less. For men, the relative risk was 1.3. Caffeine is a mutagen in some systems and can increase the transformation rate of cells treated with chemical carcinogens.[20, 43] Other studies of coffee drinking and bladder cancer are summarized in Table 2–6. Although every study finds some increased risk in either men or women, the results are inconsistent and elevations are generally small.[5, 6, 13, 24, 25, 29, 35, 52, 55, 56, 59, 61, 64, 72, 84] However, several case-control studies that have looked simultaneously at coffee drinking and cigarette smoking have found higher relative risks and better evidence of a dose response for coffee drinking than for cigarette smoking.[5, 72, 84]

Heavy use of analgesics, especially those containing phenacetin, has been linked to cancer of the urinary tract, primarily of the renal pelvis.[4] Howe and co-workers found a relative risk of bladder cancer of 1.5 in men who had consumed *aspirin*-containing analgesics "regularly" for at least six months.[35] In women the comparable risk was 1.1. However, no association was observed for *phenacetin*-containing analgesics. McCredie and colleagues in a case-control study of women in New South Wales found a relative risk of 2.6 for consumers of phenacetin-containing analgesics.[50] There was some indication that this risk was dose-related. Unlike the study of the Howe group, this study found no association with use of non-phenacetin-containing analgesics. Similar results were recently reported from a case-control study of 173 women, 20 to 49 years of age, in whom a diagnosis of bladder cancer had been made in New York State over a five-year period. Compared with age-matched random digit-dial controls, these patients were 6.5 times more likely to report regular use of analgesics containing phenacetin.[67] The comparable risk for analgesics containing acetaminophen was 1.5. Fokkens, in a hospital-based case-control study of bladder cancer in the Netherlands, found a fourfold increase in risk of bladder cancer in those who used large amounts of phenacetin.[22]

Table 2–6. CASE-CONTROL STUDIES OF COFFEE DRINKING AND BLADDER CANCER

Year	First Author		Relative Risk Male	Relative Risk Female
1971	Cole		1.2*	2.6*
1971	Fraumeni		2.0*	1.2*
1973	Bross		1.5	1.3
1974	Morgan		0.7	1.3
1975	Simon		—	2.1*
1977	Wynder		1.6	1.1
1978	Miller		1.3	1.6
1979	Mettlin		1.8	1.0
1980	Howe	Regular coffee	1.5	0.8
		Instant coffee	1.5	1.4
1980	Morrison	England	1.0	0.8
		Japan	1.2	0.9
		USA	1.1	1.0
1982	Cartwright		1.1*	0.8*
1982	Najem		1.8	
1983	Hartge		1.6*	1.2*
1983	Mommsen		—	3.7*
1985	Gonzalez		0.6	

*"Adjusted" for cigarette smoking.

Recent evidence suggests that vitamin A and β-carotene may reduce risk of human epithelial cancers, including bladder cancer. In rodents, vitamin A analogues can prevent induction of bladder cancer by chemical carcinogens, including N-nitrosamines.[3] One epidemiologic study has indicated that persons with low intake of vitamin A or β-carotene may have an increased risk of bladder cancer.[56]

As noted above, nitrosamines are chemicals that can produce bladder cancer in mice and rats,[32, 48] and appear in human urine in low concentrations.[39] Nitrosamines can be formed in vivo from tobacco alkaloids or from ingested nitrates and secondary amines by nitrate-reducing bacteria in the human bladder or gut. Consistent with this, several studies have found an association between urinary tract infections and bladder cancer.[34, 40, 86] Kantor and co-workers reported a relative risk of bladder cancer of 2.0 in individuals who reported three or more infections; for squamous cell carcinoma of the bladder, which composed less than 2% of this large case series, the relative risk increased to 4.8.[40] No data was available regarding the time that elapsed from the occurrence of each infection until the diagnosis of bladder cancer. In the study of the Howe group the increase in risk associated with urinary tract infection was limited to the five years prior to diagnosis, suggesting that this association may be due to early signs and symptoms of bladder cancer rather than be part of the causal pathway.[35] Comprehensive dietary studies of foods high in nitrosamine precursors, or in substances (such as vitamin C) that can block in vivo nitrosamine formation, and bladder cancer risk might be useful in elucidating the role of N-nitroso compounds in bladder cancer etiology.

SUMMARY AND CONCLUSIONS

Cigarette smoking and occupational exposure to arylamines are the only well-established risk factors for bladder cancer. Evidence for a weak association between coffee consumption and risk of bladder cancer also exists. Analgesics containing aspirin, caffeine, and phenacetin are potential risk factors that have not been adequately studied. The interaction between cigarette smoking and other known or potential bladder carcinogens also requires further study. More detailed studies are needed on the individual characteristics of cigarettes that influence bladder cancer risk; these factors include tar and nicotine content, brand, and presence or absence of filters.

The effect of cigarette smoking on bladder cancer risk appears to be fundamentally different from the effect of cigarettes on lung cancer risk. Instead of a carcinogen or irritant acting on bladder mucosa directly (as is probable with lung tissue), the effect of cigarettes on the bladder is probably indirect and likely to involve metabolic pathways subject to genetic or environmental influences. Possible examples of these other influences include genetic factors such as N-acetyltransferase phenotypes, dietary factors such as intake of vitamins C or A, and bladder conditions themselves, including presence of bacteria and abnormal urinary pH.

References

1. Anthony HM, Thomas GM: Bladder tumours and smoking. Int J Cancer 5:266–272, 1970.
2. Armstrong B, Doll R: Bladder cancer mortality in diabetics in relation to saccharin consumption and smoking habits. Br J Prev Soc Med 29:73–81, 1975.
3. Becci PJ, Thompson HJ, Grubbs CJ, et al: Inhibitory effect of 13-cis-retinoic acid on urinary bladder carcinogenesis induced in C57BL/6 mice by N-butyl-N-(4-hydroxybutyl)-nitrosamine. Cancer Res 38:4463–4466, 1978.
4. Bengtsson U, Angervall L, Ekman H, Lehman L:

Transitional cell tumors of the renal pelvis in analgesic abusers. Scand J Urol Nephrol 2:145–150, 1968.

5. Bross DJ, Tidings J: Another look at coffee drinking and cancer of the lower urinary bladder. Prev Med 2:445–451, 1973.

6. Cartwright RA, Adib R, Appleyard I, et al: Cigarette smoking and bladder cancer: an epidemiological inquiry in West Yorkshire. J Epidemiol Community Health 37:256–263, 1983.

7. Cartwright RA, Glasham RW, Rogers HJ, et al: Role of N-acetyltransferase phenotypes in bladder carcinogensis: a pharmacogenetic epidemiological approach to bladder cancer. Lancet 2:842–845, 1982.

8. Case RAM, Hosker ME: Tumour of the urinary bladder as an occupational disease in the rubber industry in England and Wales. Br J Prev Soc Med 8:39–50, 1954.

9. Case RAM, Hosker ME, McDonald DM, et al: Tumors of urinary bladder in workmen engaged in manufacture and use of certain dye-stuff intermediates in British chemical industry: role of amiline, benzidine, alpha-naphthylamine, and beta-naphthylamine. Br J Industr Med 11:75–104, 1954.

10. Centers for Disease Control: Morbidity and Mortality Weekly Report 25: August 6, 1976.

11. Cobb BG, Ansell JS: Cigarette smoking and cancer of the bladder. JAMA 193:329–332, 1965.

12. Cole P: A population based study of bladder cancer. In R Doll, I Vodopija (eds), Host Environment Interactions in the Eitiology of Cancer in Man. Lyon, International Agency for Research on Cancer, 1973, pp 83–87.

13. Cole P: Coffee-drinking and cancer of the lower urinary tract. Lancet 1:1335–1337, 1971.

14. Cole P, Hoover R, Friedell GH: Occupation and cancer of the lower urinary tract. Cancer 29:1250–1260, 1972.

15. Cole P, Monson RR, Haning H, Friedell GH: Smoking and cancer of the lower urinary tract. N Engl J Med 284:129–134, 1971.

16. Department of Health and Welfare, Canada. Cancer patterns in Canada, 1931–1974. Vol 15. Ottawa Bureau of Epidemiology, Laboratory Centre for Disease Control, Ottawa, Canada, 1976.

17. Derry TK, Williams TI: A Short History of Technology. Oxford, University Press, 1960, pp 531–556.

18. Doll R, Peto R: The causes of cancer: quantitative estimates of avoidable risks of cancer in the United States today. JNCI 66:1191–1308, 1981.

19. Doll R, Peto R: Mortality in relation to smoking: 20 years' observation on male British doctors. Br Med J 2:1525–1536, 1976.

20. Donovan PJ, DiPaolo JA: Caffeine enhancement of chemical carcinogen-induced transformation of cultured Syrian hamster cells. Cancer Res 34:2720–2727, 1974.

21. Dunham LJ, Rabson AS, Stewart HL, et al: Rates, interview, and pathology study of cancer of the urinary bladder in New Orleans, Louisiana. JNCI 41:683–709, 1968.

22. Fokkens W: Phenacetin abuse related to bladder cancer. Environ Res 20:192–198, 1979.

23. Foster F: New Zealand Cancer Registry Report. In Second Symposium on Epidemiology and Cancer Registries in the Pacific Basin. Natl Cancer Inst Monogr 53. Washington DC, US Govt Printing Office, 1979, pp 79–80.

24. Fraumeni JF Jr, Scotto J, Dunham LJ: Coffee-drinking and bladder cancer. Lancet 2:1204, 1971.

25. Gonzalez CA, Lopez-Abente G, Errezola MP, et al: Occupation, tobacco use, coffee, and bladder cancer in the County of Mataro (Spain). Cancer 55:2031–2034, 1985.

26. Hammond EC, Horn D: Smoking and death rates—report on forty-four months of follow-up of 187,783 men. II. Death rates by cause. JAMA 166:1294–1308, 1958.

27. Hammond EC: Smoking in relation to death rates of 1 million men and women. In Epidemiological Approaches to the Study of Cancer and Other Chronic Diseases. Natl Cancer Inst Monogr 19. Washington DC, US Govt Printing Office, 1966, pp 127–204.

28. Hartge P, Hoover R, Kantor A: Bladder cancer risk and pipes, cigars, and smokeless tobacco. Cancer 55:901–906, 1985.

29. Hartge P, Hoover R, West DW, Lyon JL: Coffee drinking and risk of bladder cancer. JNCI 70:1021–1026, 1983.

30. Hicks RM, Wakefield JS, Chowaniec J: Letters: Cocarcinogenic action of saccharin in the chemical induction of bladder cancer. Nature 243:347–349, 1973.

31. Hoar S, Hoover R: Truck driving and bladder cancer mortality in rural New England. JNCI 74:771–774, 1985.

32. Hoffman D, Schmeltz I, Hecht SS, et al: Tobacco carcinogenesis. In H Gelboin, PO T'so (eds), Polycyclic Hydrocarbons and Cancer, Vol I. New York, Academic Press, 1978, pp 85–117.

33. Holsti LR, Ermala P: Papillary carcinoma of the bladder in mice, obtained after peroral administration of tobacco tar. Cancer 8:679–682, 1955.

34. Hoover RN, Strasser PH: Artificial sweeteners and human bladder cancer. Preliminary results. Lancet 1:837–840, 1980.

35. Howe GR, Burch JD, Miller AB, et al: Tobacco use, occupation, coffee, various nutrients, and bladder cancer. JNCI 64:701–713, 1980.

36. Howe GR, Burch JD, Miller AB, et al: Artificial sweeteners and human bladder cancer. Lancet 2:578–581, 1977.

37. Hueper WC, Wiley FH, Wolfe HD: Experimental production of bladder tumors in dogs by administration of beta-naphthylamine. J Industr Hyg Toxicol 20:46–84, 1938.

38. Kahn HA: The Dorn study of smoking and mortality among United States veterans—report on 8½ years of observation. In Epidemiological Approaches to the Study of Cancer and Other Chronic Diseases. Natl Cancer Inst Monogr 19. Washington DC, US Govt Printing Office, 1966, pp 1–125.

39. Kakizoe T, Wang T-T, Eng VWS, et al: Volatile N-nitrosamines in the urine of normal donors and of bladder cancer patients. Cancer Res 39:829–832, 1979.

40. Kantor AF, Hartge P, Hoover RN, et al: Urinary tract infection and risk of bladder cancer. Am J Epidemiol 119:510–515, 1984.

41. Kessler II: Non-nutritive sweeteners and human bladder cancer: preliminary findings. J Urol 115:143–146, 1976.

42. Kessler II, Clark JP: Saccharin, cyclamate, and human bladder cancer. No evidence of an association. JAMA 20:349–355, 1978.

43. Kuhlmann W, Fromme HG, Heege EM, et al: The

mutagenic action of caffeine in higher organisms. Cancer Res 28:2375–2389, 1968.

44. Kurihara M, Aoki K, Tominaga S (eds): Cancer Mortality Statistics in the World. Nagoya, Japan, University of Nagoya Press, 1984.

45. Lilienfeld AM, Levin ML, Moore GE: The association of smoking with cancer of the urinary bladder in humans. Arch Intern Med 98:129–135, 1956.

46. Lockwood K: On the etiology of bladder tumors in Kobenhavn Frederiksberg. An inquiry of 369 patients and 369 controls. Acta Path Microbiol Scand 51 (Suppl 145):1–166, 1961.

47. Lower GM Jr: Concepts in causality: chemically induced human urinary bladder cancer. Cancer 49:1056–1066, 1982.

48. Magee PN, Barnes JM: Carcinogenic nitroso compounds. Advances Cancer Res 10:163–246, 1967.

49. Makhyoun NA: Smoking and bladder cancer in Egypt. Br J Cancer 30:577–581, 1974.

50. McCredie M, Stewart JH, Ford JM, MacLennan RA: Phenacetin-containing analgesics and cancer of the bladder or renal pelvis in women. Br J Urol 55:220–224, 1983.

51. McMichael AJ, Spirtas R, Gamble JF, et al: Mortality among rubber workers: relationship to specific jobs. J Occup Med 18:178–185, 1976.

52. Mettlin C, Graham S: Dietary risk factors in human bladder cancer. Am J Epidemiol 110:255–263, 1979.

53. Michalek AM, Cummings KM, Pontes JE: Cigarette smoking, tumor recurrence, and survival from bladder cancer. Prev Med 14:92–98, 1985.

54. Miller AB: Recent trends in lung cancer mortality in Canada. Can Med Assoc J 116:28–30, 1977.

55. Miller CT, Neutel CI, Nair RC, et al: Relative importance of risk factors in bladder carcinogenesis. J Chronic Dis 31:51–56, 1978.

56. Mommsen S, Aagaard J: Tobacco as a risk factor in bladder cancer. Carcinogenesis 4:335–338, 1983.

57. Mommsen S, Sell A, Barfod N: Letter: N-acetyltransferase phenotypes of bladder cancer patients in a low risk population. Lancet 2:1228, 1982.

58. Monson RR, Nakano KK: Mortality among rubber workers. I. White male union employees in Akron, Ohio. Am J Epidemiol 103:284–296, 1976.

59. Morgan RW, Jain MG: Bladder cancer: smoking, beverages, and artificial sweeteners. Can Med Assoc J 111:1067–1070, 1974.

60. Morrison AS, Buring JE: Artificial sweeteners and cancer of the lower urinary tract. N Engl J Med 302:537–541, 1980.

61. Morrison AS, Buring J, Verhoek WG, et al: Coffee drinking and cancer of the lower urinary tract. JNCI 68:91–94, 1980.

62. Morrison AS, Buring JE, Verhoek WG, et al: An international study of smoking and bladder cancer. J Urol 131:650–654, 1984.

63. Morrison AS, Verhoek WG, Leck I, et al: Artificial sweeteners and bladder cancer in Manchester, U.K., and Nagoya, Japan. Br J Cancer 45:332–336, 1982.

64. Najem GR, Louria DB, Seebode JJ, et al: Lifetime occupation, smoking, caffeine, saccharine, hair dyes and bladder carcinogenesis. Int J Epidemiol 11:212–217, 1982.

65. New Zealand Census (1976): Age-specific rates per 1,000 population responding to cigarette smoking status question. Wellington, New Zealand, National Health Statistic Centre, 1979.

66. Patrianakos C, Hoffman D: On the analysis of aromatic amines in cigarette smoke. J Anal Toxicol 3:150–154, 1979.

67. Piper JM, Tonascia J, Matanoski GM: Heavy phenacetin use and bladder cancer in women aged 20 to 49 years. N Engl J Med 33:292–295, 1985.

68. Rehn L: Blasengeschwulste bei fuchsin-arbeitern. Arch Clin Chir 50:588–600, 1895.

69. Sadeghi A, Behmard S, Vesselinovitch SD: Opium: a potential urinary bladder carcinogen in man. Cancer 43:2315–2321, 1979.

70. Schwartz D, Flamant R, Lellouch J, Denoix PF: Results of a French survey on the role of tobacco, particularly inhalation, in different cancer sites. JNCI 26:1085–1108, 1961.

71. Silverman DT, Hoover RN, Albert S, Graff KM: Occupation and cancer of the lower urinary tract in Detroit. JNCI 70:237–245, 1983.

72. Simon D, Yen S, Cole P: Coffee drinking and cancer of the lower urinary tract. JNCI 54:587–591, 1975.

73. Smith RJ: Latest saccharin tests kill FDA proposal [News]. Science 208:154–156, 1980.

74. Staszewski J: Smoking and cancer of the urinary bladder in males in Poland. Br J Cancer 20:32–35, 1966.

75. Third National Cancer Survey: Incidence Data. SJ Cutler and JL Young (eds), National Cancer Inst Monogr 41. DHEW Publication No (NIH) 75-787, 1975.

76. UICC Technical Reports Series, Vol 25, Lung Cancer, Chapter 11. Epidemiology, 1976, pp 3–41.

77. U.S. Dept of Health, Education and Welfare, Public Health Service: End Results in Cancer Report No 3. Washington DC, US Govt Printing Office, 1968.

78. U.S. Dept of Health, Education and Welfare, Public Health Service: Vital Statistics of the US, Vol II, Part A. Mortality, 1930–1976.

79. U.S. Dept of Health, Education and Welfare, Public Health Service: National Health Survey—Use habits among adults of cigarettes, coffee, aspirin, and sleeping pills, Series 10, No 131, 1976.

80. Vineis P, Estève T, Terracini B: Bladder cancer and smoking in males: types of cigarettes, age at start, effect of stopping and interaction with occupation. Int J Cancer 34:165–170, 1984.

81. Vineis P, Magnani C: Occupation and bladder cancer in males: a case-control study. Int J Cancer 35:599–606, 1985.

82. Weir JM, Dunn JE Jr: Smoking and mortality: a prospective study. Cancer 25:105–112, 1970.

83. Wolf H, Loer GM Jr, Bryan GT: Role of N-acetyltransferase phenotype in human susceptibility to bladder carcinogenic arylamines. Scand J Urol Nephrol 14:161–165, 1980.

84. Wynder EL, Goldsmith R: The epidemiology of bladder cancer. A second look. Cancer 40:1246–1268, 1977.

85. Wynder EL, Hoffman D: Tobacco. In D Schottenfeld, JF Fraumeni (eds), Cancer Epidemiology and Prevention. Philadelphia, WB Saunders, 1982, pp 277–292.

86. Wynder EL, Onderdonk J, Mantel N: An epidemiological investigation of cancer of the bladder. Cancer 16:1388–1407, 1963.

87. Wynder EL, Stellman SD: Artificial sweetener use and bladder cancer: a case-control study. Science 207:1214–1216, 1980.

88. Yoshiyuki D, Kunio A: Epidemiology of bladder cancer deaths in Japan. Gann 68:715–729, 1977.

ANNLIA PAGANINI-HILL, Ph.D.
RONALD K. ROSS, M.D.
BRIAN E. HENDERSON, M.D.

*Epidemiology of Renal Cancer**

CHAPTER 3

The epidemiology of cancer of the kidney is among the least studied of all major cancers in the United States. In this report, the descriptive epidemiology of renal cancer is summarized and the major etiologic hypotheses is reviewed, using analytical epidemiologic studies and experimental results.

Since tumors in the renal pelvis are anatomically and histologically distinct from the majority of cancers of the kidney, which are of tubular origin, parenchymal "cancer of the kidney" and cancer of the renal pelvis will be considered separately.

EPIDEMIOLOGY

There is about a fivefold difference in the age-adjusted incidence rates between countries at high risk of renal cancer (including renal pelvis), such as Denmark and Sweden, and those at low risk, such as Japan.[51, 58] Countries with intermediate risk levels include the United States and most countries of Western Europe. Despite the high rates of kidney cancer in native Scandinavians, migrants to the western US have incidence rates comparable to other white residents of this area. The renal cancer incidence rate for Japanese immigrants to the United States is intermediate between those for Japanese in Japan and for US whites.[20]

Approximately 20 to 25% of cancers of the kidney in the US occur in the renal pelvis. The most important demographic risk factor for both cancer of the kidney and cancer of the renal pelvis is age. In persons younger than age 35, epithelial cancers of the kidney are rare; after that time there is a steady increase in risk into old age.

The incidence in males predominates both in cancer of the kidney (M:F ratio about 2.1) and cancer of the renal pelvis (M:F ratio about 2.5) in the US, and occurrence of cancer of the renal pelvis (but not cancer of the kidney) is higher in whites than in blacks, especially in men. For kidney cancer the white:black ratio of age-adjusted incidence rates is about 1.0 in men and 0.9 in women. For cancer of the renal pelvis these ratios are 1.9 and 1.3, respectively. Hispanic men and women have kidney cancer rates more than one third higher than those of other whites in the US, but they have similar rates of cancer of the renal pelvis.

Men in higher social classes have a somewhat greater incidence of kidney cancer and cancer of the renal pelvis. This relationship is less clear in women.

Mortality rates of kidney cancer during the past 30 years show a modest increase in consecutive birth cohorts in men but not in women.[55]

*Supported by Grants CA 17054, CA 25669, and CA 00652 from the National Cancer Institute, National Institutes of Health.

ETIOLOGIC HYPOTHESES

Smoking

Since the renal tubules and the renal pelvis are likely to be exposed to many of the same carcinogens as the bladder, one might expect cancers of these organs to have similar risk factors. Cigarette smoking has been well established as a risk factor for bladder cancer[11] and is the only risk factor consistently linked to cancer of the kidney by both epidemiologic case-control and cohort studies (Table 3–1).[4, 5, 16, 21, 22, 28, 29, 59, 62, 64] However, the relative risks observed in some of these studies have been small and a dose-response relationship between smoking and risk has not always been observed.

Five case-control studies have reported on the relationship between cigarette smoking and cancer of the renal pelvis (Table 3–2).[4, 40–42, 49] Although somewhat inconsistent, probably because of the small number of cases, these studies as a group suggest a strong association between cancer of the renal pelvis and cigarette smoking, with the highest risk in the heaviest smokers. We recently completed a population-based case-control study in Los Angeles of cancer of the renal pelvis and ureter. From a preliminary analysis of 188 age- and race-matched case-neighborhood control pairs, we found that persons who had smoked cigarettes regularly had a relative risk of 3.6 for cancer of the renal pelvis and ureter, when compared with persons who had never smoked. For those who had smoked for 25 years or more, this risk increased to 4.8.

The mechanism by which cigarettes might induce kidney cancer is unclear, although cigarette smoke, and the particulate matter especially, is known to contain numerous carcinogens.[61] In addition, the urine of cigarette smokers has been found to contain numerous mutagenic chemicals.[16, 63] A variety of N-nitroso compounds can produce renal adenocarcinomas in rodents.[37, 52] At least one of these, dimethylnitrosamine, is found in tobacco smoke.[37, 52]

The increased risk of kidney cancer in men, compared with that of women, is consistent with the greater use of cigarettes by men during most of this century. The higher mortality from cancer of the kidney in successive birth cohorts of men is also consistent with an etiologic role of cigarettes. However, the rate of increase with age in kidney cancer incidence is not as great as that for other epithelial cancers thought to be caused by cigarette smoking, such as bladder and lung cancer.

Table 3–1. EPIDEMIOLOGIC STUDIES OF CIGARETTE SMOKING AND CANCER OF THE KIDNEY

Cohort Studies

First Author	Year	Population	Relative Risk, Smokers: Nonsmokers	Dose Response
Hammond	1958	US white males	1.6	Unknown
Hammond	1966	US white males aged 45–64	1.4	Unknown
		US white males aged 65–79	1.6	Unknown
Kahn	1966	US veterans	1.5	Yes
Weir	1970	US labor union members	2.5	No
Doll	1976	British physicians	2.7	No
Hirayama	1977	Japanese males	1.2	Unknown

Case-Control Studies

First Author	Year	Location	Type of Controls	Relative Risk, Smokers: Nonsmokers		Dose Response
Bennington	1968	Washington	Hospital	Male	1.6	Yes
				Female	2.0	Unknown
Wynder	1974	US	Hospital	Male	2.0	Yes
				Female	1.5	Yes
Armstrong	1976	England	Outpatient	Male	1.1	No
				Female	1.0	No
Kolonel	1976	New York	Hospital	Male	1.2	Unknown
McLaughlin	1984	Minnesota	Population	Male	1.6	Yes
				Female	1.9	Yes
Yu	1985	California	Population	Male	2.1	Yes
				Female	1.1	Yes

Table 3–2. CASE-CONTROL STUDIES OF CIGARETTE SMOKING AND CANCER OF THE RENAL PELVIS

First Author	Year	Number of Cases	Sex	Relative Risk	
Schmauz	1974	18	Male	Any use	1.8
				≥30/day	2.2
Armstrong	1976	22	Male	Any use	6.2
				≥30/day	20.0
			Female	Any use	0.3
McCredie	1982	11	Male	Any use	1.0*
				Any use	2.8†
		40	Female	Any use	2.2*
				Any use	7.0†
McLaughlin	1983	50	Male	Any use	7.6
				"Heavy"	10.7
		24	Female	Any use	5.8
				"Heavy"	11.1
McCredie	1983	31	Female	Any use	4.7
				$\geq 2 \times 10^5$ Cigarettes	5.2

*Friend controls.
†Screening clinic controls.

Analgesic Use

In 1965 a report from Sweden indicated that six of 106 patients with cancer of the renal pelvis had a history of papillary necrosis associated with heavy usage of phenacetin-containing analgesics.[27] Three years later, Bengtsson described a series of 104 patients with chronic pyelonephritis following extensive use of analgesics.[5] Subsequently, eight of these patients developed transitional cell carcinomas of the renal pelvis, compared with none of 88 patients with chronic pyelonephritis from other causes. A third Swedish study in 1969 found 12 heavy users of phenacetin-containing analgesics in 15 patients with cancer of the renal pelvis.[2] During the early 1970s, similar case reports of cancer of the renal pelvis occurring in heavy analgesic users came from Denmark,[25] Canada,[35] and Australia.[1, 38]

Despite the highly suggestive data from case reports and case series linking analgesic use with cancer of the renal pelvis, the first case-control study was unable to confirm this association (Table 3–3).[4] This study was limited by the small number of cases (n = 33) and the use of hospital controls, who may be unrepresentative of the general population in their frequency of analgesic use.

Subsequent case-control studies of cancer of the renal pelvis have found an association with analgesic use (Table 3–3). In 1982 McCredie and co-workers reported results of a study conducted in New South Wales.[40] Sixty-seven patients were compared with 180 controls drawn from two sources, friends of the patients and participants in a health screening clinic. Regular use of analgesics was strongly associated with risk of cancer of the renal pelvis in both men (RR = 8.3 using friend controls, RR = 4.6 using screening clinic controls) and women (RR = 10.3 using friend controls, RR = 13.5 using screening clinic controls). In women there was a strong dose-response relationship with use of both phenacetin- and non-phenacetin-containing analgesics. The authors estimated that in this population nearly three fourths of all cases of cancer of the renal pelvis in women and one half of the cases in men were attributable to use of analgesics.

In a subsequent case-control study of 31 additional women with cancer of the renal pelvis diagnosed in New South Wales in 1980–1981, McCredie and colleagues reported a relative risk of 4.5 for heavy users of phenacetin-containing analgesics compared with the risk for those who used it in small amounts or not at all.[41] This risk increased to 7.3 for women with a lifetime ingestion of more than 10 kg of phenacetin-containing analgesics. After adjustment for use of phenacetin-containing analgesics, no significant excess risk was observed for use of other analgesics.

In a case-control study of 74 cases of cancer of the renal pelvis and 697 population controls in the Minneapolis–St. Paul area, McLaughlin and co-workers reported a relative risk of 3.9 in males and 3.7 in females for regular long-term (>36 months) users of phenacetin- or acetaminophen-containing drugs, compared with risks to nonusers.[42] Neither result was statistically significant. However, 50% of patients in this study were deceased, and next-of-kin were interviewed.

Based on the preliminary results from our case-control study in Los Angeles, heavy use of over-the-counter analgesics increased the risk of cancer of the renal pelvis and ureter. Any use of aspirin or caffeine-containing analgesics for at least 30 days in any year prior to diagnosis increased risk about twofold. Comparable use of phenacetin- or acet-aminophen-containing analgesics did not increase risk (RR = 1.2). However, more extensive use of these compounds (i.e., at least once daily for 30 or more consecutive days) conveyed some increased risk (RR = 1.7).

The Swedish investigators who first reported the association between analgesic use and renal cancer concluded that phenacetin was the probable cause of the disease even though the analgesics almost always contained several ingredients. The compound 2-hydroxy-4-ethoxyaniline is a urinary metabolite of phenacetin and is a renal and hepatic carcinogen when fed to rats.[9] Nonetheless, other common ingredients of analgesics are also suspect. Aspirin can induce more severe nephrotoxic effects in rats than does phenacetin,[8] and caffeine is a mutagen that has been linked to bladder cancer.[34, 60] The three epidemiologic studies of coffee drinking and cancer of the renal pelvis have been contradictory. One found no association,[4] one a weak association in men but not in women,[42] and the third a strong association.[49] However, the last finding was based on coffee-drinking habits of just 28 persons.

The possible association between heavy use of analgesics and adenocarcinoma of the kidney has been reported by two groups. Armstrong and co-workers reported a relative risk of 10 for cancer of the kidney in persons taking analgesics on a daily basis compared with that for "never users".[4] Although short-term use, possibly related to the presence of prodromes of renal cancer, explained part of this high risk, the residual

risk was still substantial if short-term use was excluded. As with studies of cancer of the renal pelvis, the investigators did not establish with certainty the analgesic ingredient responsible for the increased hazard.

The other study of kidney cancer and analgesic use was a large case-control study of cancer of the kidney in the Minneapolis–St. Paul metropolitan area.[43] Here, McLaughlin and colleagues found a relative risk of 2.2 in males and 2.5 in females for regular long-term (>36 months) users of phenacetin-containing analgesics, compared with non-users. Although neither risk estimate differed significantly from unity, there was a statistically significant trend with increasing duration of use in females. There was evidence that next of kin respondents, making up 50% of the case interviews, greatly overestimated the true prevalence of analgesic use, especially in male respondents.

Although Shennan reported a significant correlation between the per capita consumption of coffee and renal cancer mortality rates,[53] three case-control studies found no association between coffee drinking and cancer of the kidney.[4, 43, 62] However, Yu and co-workers reported a significantly elevated risk for kidney cancer with daily coffee consumption in a population-based study of 160 case-control pairs of women under age 55.[64] After adjustment for other risk factors, the relative risk for daily coffee consumption was 4.2 (p < 0.05), but there was no trend indicating increased risk with expanding consumption.

Table 3–3. CASE-CONTROL STUDIES OF ANALGESIC USE AND CANCERS OF THE RENAL PELVIS AND KIDNEY

First Author	Year	Sex	"Type" of Analgesic	Comparison	Relative Ratio
			Renal Pelvis		
Armstrong	1976	Male and Female	Any	>1/wk vs never	0.7
McCredie	1982	Male	Any	"Regular" vs less often	8.3*
					4.6
		Female	Any	"Regular" vs less often	10.3*
					13.5
McCredie	1983	Female	Phenacetin	"Regular" vs less often	4.5
			Non-Phenacetin	"Regular" vs less often	1.4
McLaughlin	1983	Male	Phenacetin/Acetaminophen	Regular >36 months vs none	3.9
		Female	Phenacetin/Acetaminophen	Regular >36 months vs none	3.7
			Kidney		
Armstrong	1976	Male and Female	Any	Daily vs Never	10.5
McLaughlin	1984	Male	Phenacetin	Regular >36 months vs none	2.2
		Female	Phenacetin	Regular >36 months vs none	2.5

*Top value compares friend controls; bottom value compares screening clinic controls.

Table 3–4. OCCUPATIONS POSSIBLY AT
HIGH RISK OF KIDNEY CANCER

Occupation	Reference	Year	Possible Agent
Coke oven workers	Redmond et al	1972	Aromatic hydro-carbons
Cadmium workers	Kolonel	1974	Cadmium
Asbestos insulation workers	Selikoff et al	1979	Asbestos
Newspaper web-pressmen	Paganini-Hill et al	1980	Lead

Occupational Exposures

Kolonel proposed a role for cadmium exposure in the development of renal cancer (Table 3–4).[29] In a small case-control study he found evidence of an association by using three separate measures of cadmium exposure. The relative risk for persons with a history of employment in industries and occupations with potentially increased exposure to cadmium was 2.5, that for persons with unusually large dietary intakes of cadmium was 1.5, and the risk for persons who smoked cigarettes (which are themselves a source of cadmium) was 1.2. Although cadmium can produce malignant tumors in some organs in rodents, it has never been shown to produce renal tumors in rats.[23] However, the kidney concentrates cadmium more heavily than any other organ and inhibits the action of zinc-containing growth-regulatory enzymes, thereby offering a potential mechanism for carcinogenesis.

In a cohort study of over 4600 coke oven workers, Redmond and colleagues observed eight renal cancer deaths, more than seven times the number expected.[48] Although these authors did not speculate on possible mechanisms, aromatic hydrocarbons can induce renal adenocarcinomas in mice and rats.[19]

In a group of 1361 newspaper web pressmen who were members of the Los Angeles Pressmen's Union,[45] we observed an elevated number of deaths due to kidney cancer (five observed deaths vs 1.6 expected). This excess might be due to exposure to lead pigments in colored printing ink. Although lead is a renal carcinogen in mice and rats,[7, 56] follow-up studies of lead workers have shown no evidence of renal cancer over normal expectation.

Selikoff and co-workers observed 19 deaths due to kidney cancer among 17,800 asbestos insulation workers in the United States and Canada, more than twice the expected number.[50] Asbestos is a proven carcinogen in man,[15] and there is some evidence that asbestos can be absorbed from the gastrointestinal tract and excreted in the urine,[12] suggesting a mechanism for asbestos-induced renal cancer.

Few studies have looked at occupation and cancer of the renal pelvis. Several investigators have found a high risk of cancer of the renal pelvis in dye workers,[36, 47] consistent with the high risk of bladder cancer in such workers.[10] In a small case-control study, Schmauz and Cole found a high risk for leather workers.[49] McLaughlin and colleagues found a significant association between exposure to coal and natural gas (RR = 2.9) and mineral and cutting oils (RR = 2.8) and cancer of the renal pelvis in men.[42]

Obesity

Wynder and co-workers, in a case-control study of 202 patients with adenocarcinoma of the kidney and 394 hospital controls with diseases thought to be unrelated to cigarette smoking, found a strong association between obesity and renal cancer in women.[62] Twenty-nine per cent of 73 female patients had a relative weight (i.e., actual weight relative to ideal weight) greater than 125%, compared with 10% of 138 controls (RR = 3.6). A similar association was found in a case-control study in Minnesota by McLaughlin and colleagues.[43] Women in the highest quartile of body mass index had a more than twofold increased risk of kidney cancer, compared with women in the lowest quartile. Again, no association between obesity and renal cancer was observed in men.

The biologic mechanism for an association between obesity and renal cancer is unclear, although one explanation may be that there is a hormonal basis. Plasma estrogen in the postmenopausal woman is largely derived by peripheral conversion of androstenedione to estrone. The rate of this conversion increases with body weight, since adipose tissue is particularly rich in the necessary enzymes.[54]

A possible role for estrogen in the etiology of renal tumors is supported by experimental data. The first description of an estrogen-induced renal tumor in hamsters was made in 1944.[57] Subsequently, estrogens, especially diethylstilbestrol and estradiol, have been shown to induce renal adenocarcinomas in both intact and castrated male hamsters and in female hamsters under conditions of low progesterone secretion (e.g., following oophorectomy, prior to reproductive maturity, or during late metestrus).[30-32, 39] These tumors are thought to be tubular in origin.[33] However, no epidemiologic studies to date have demonstrated a clear association between exogenous estrogen therapy and renal cancer.

Looking at the descriptive epidemiology of renal cancer in Connecticut from 1935 to 1973, Finger-Kantor and colleagues found that the male:female ratio of renal cell carcinoma was greater during the childbearing years than during the postmenopausal period.[17] The authors suggested that hormone changes in pregnancy might protect women against renal cancer.

In a recent population-based case-control study in Los Angeles, Yu and co-workers found a significant association between obesity and renal cancer in *both* men and women.[64] The relative risk for persons in the upper versus the lowest quartile of Quetelet's Index (weight/height^2) was 2.5 in men and 3.3 in women. They suggested that this association, rather than being specifically related to hormones or to diet, might be explained by use of diuretics and diet pills. In fact, in their study diuretic use was strongly associated with renal cancer in women and partially explained the strong association with obesity.

Other Hypotheses

Armstrong and Doll found a strong correlation between incidence of renal cancer and per capita consumption of animal protein (r = 0.82), and they suggested that this factor might partially explain the geographic distribution of cancer of the kidney.[3] However, a case-control study conducted in England found no evidence that consumption of animal protein conveyed high risk.[4] Wynder and colleagues found a similarly high correlation between renal cancer mortality and per capita animal fat consumption (r = 0.83) and suggested that fat-cholesterol intake contributes to the development of renal cancer.[62] We find little epidemiologic or experimental data to support either hypothesis.[43, 64] Several other factors have been suggested as possible causes of cancer of the renal pelvis. Endemic nephropathy is thought to be responsible for the high incidence of cancer of the renal pelvis in Yugoslavia.[46] The origin of this nephropathy is obscure, but it may be caused by high levels of silicate in the drinking water. Renal pelvis cancers have been reported in patients exposed to the alpha particle emitter Thorotrast, formerly used in retrograde pyelography.[47] In one uncontrolled study of a series of patients with cancer of the renal pelvis, a substantial proportion of cases (23%) reported long-standing urinary obstruction or infection,[38] whereas in another, prostatic hyperplasia was frequent among male patients.[44]

SUMMARY AND CONCLUSIONS

Cigarette smoking is an established risk factor for both cancer of the kidney and cancer of the renal pelvis. However, more epidemiologic studies are needed for better understanding of the strength and nature of this association. Certain occupational exposures also appear to increase risk of cancer of the kidney, but current evidence suggests that only a small proportion of all renal cancers has an occupational origin. Heavy ingestion of analgesics clearly increases risk of cancer of the renal pelvis and possibly cancer of the kidney. The one or more exact components responsible for this increased risk require clarification. In addition, the association between cancer of the kidney and obesity needs confirmation, and alternative mechanisms for this association (e.g., renal damage from obesity-related atherosclerosis or increased use of drugs with renal activity, such as diuretics) need additional study.

References

1. Adam WR, Dawborn JK, Price CG, et al: Anaplastic transitional-cell carcinoma of the renal pelvis in association with analgesic abuse. Med J Austr 1:1108–1109, 1970.
2. Angervall L, Bengtsson U, Zetterlund CG, Zsingmund M: Renal pelvic carcinoma in a Swedish district with abuse of a phenacetin-containing drug. Br J Urol 41:401–405, 1969.

3. Armstrong B, Doll R: Environmental factors and cancer incidence and mortality in different countries with special reference to dietary practices. Int J Cancer 15:617–631, 1975.

4. Armstrong B, Garrod A, Doll R: A retrospective study of renal cancer with special reference to coffee and animal protein consumption. Br J Cancer 33:127–136, 1976.

5. Bengtsson U, Angervall L, Ekman H, et al: Transitional cell tumors of the renal pelvis in analgesic abusers. Scand J Urol Nephrol 2:145–150, 1968.

6. Bennington JL, Laubscher FA: Epidemiologic studies on carcinoma of the kidney. I. Association of renal adenocarcinoma with smoking. Cancer 21:1069–1071, 1968.

7. Boyland E, Dukes CE, Grover PL, Mitchley BC: The induction of renal tumours by feeding lead acetate to rats. Br J Cancer 16:283–288, 1962.

8. Calder IC, Funder CC, Green CR, et al: Comparative nephrotoxicity of aspirin and phenacetin derivatives. Br Med J 4:518–521, 1971.

9. Calder IC, Goss DE, Williams PJ, et al: Neoplasia in the rat inducd by N-hydroxyphenacetin, a metabolite of phenacetin. Pathology 8:1–6, 1976.

10. Case RAM, Hosker ME, McDonald DB, Pearson JT: Tumors of urinary bladder in workmen engaged in manufacture and use of certain dye-stuff intermediates in the British chemical industry: role of aniline, benzidine, alpha-naphthylamine, and beta-naphthylamine. Br J Industr Med 11:75–104, 1954.

11. Cole P, Monson RR, Haning H, Friedell GH: Smoking and cancer of the lower urinary tract. N Engl J Med 284:129–134, 1971.

12. Cook PM, Olson GF: Ingested mineral fibers: elimination in human urine. Science 204:195–198, 1979.

13. Davis DL, Bridbord K, Schneiderman M: Cancer prevention: assessing causes, exposures, and recent trends in mortality for U.S. males, 1968–1978. Teratogenesis Carcinog Mutagen 2:105–135, 1982.

14. Dingwall-Fordyce I, Lane RE: A follow-up study of lead workers. Br J Industr Med 20:313–315, 1963.

15. Doll R: Mortality from lung cancer in asbestos workers. Br J Industr Med 12:162–166, 1973.

16. Doll R, Peto R: Mortality in relation to smoking: 20 years' observations on male British doctors. Br Med J 2:1525–1536, 1976.

17. Finger-Kantor AL, Meigs JW, Heston JF, Flannery JT: Epidemiology of renal cell carcinoma in Connecticut, 1935–1973. JNCI 57:495–500, 1976.

18. Garner RG, Mould AJ, Lindsay-Smith V, et al: Mutagenic urine from bladder cancer patients. JNCI 57:495–500, 1976.

19. Guerin M, Chouroulinkow I, Riviere MR: Experimental kidney tumors. In C Rouiller, RF Muller (eds), The Kidney, Vol 2. New York, Academic Press, 1969, pp 199–268.

20. Haenszel W, Kurihara M: Studies of Japanese migrants. I. Mortality from cancer and other diseases among Japanese in the United States. JNCI 40:43–68, 1969.

21. Hammond EC: Smoking in relation to death rates of 1 million men and women. In Epidemiological Approaches to the Study of Cancer and Other Chronic Diseases. Natl Cancer Inst Monogr No. 19. Washington DC, US Govt Printing Office, 1966, pp 127–204.

22. Hammond EC, Horn D: Smoking and death rates—report on 44 months of follow-up of 187,783

men. II. Death rates by cause. JAMA 166:1294–1308, 1958.

23. Heath JC, Daniel MR: The production of malignant tumours by cadmium in the rat. Br J Cancer 18:124–129, 1964.

24. Hirayama T: Changing patterns in Japan with special reference to the decrease in stomach cancer mortality. In HH Hiatt, JD Watson, JA Winston (eds), Origins of Human Cancer, Book A. Cold Spring Harbor, New York, Cold Spring Harbor Laboratories, 1977.

25. Hoybye G, Nielsen OE: Renal pelvic carcinoma in phenacetin abusers. Scand J Urol Nephrol 5:190–192, 1971.

26. Hubmann R, Hoer PW: Nierenbeckencarcinome nach retrograder Pyelographie mit Thorotrast. Urologe 3:227–237, 1964.

27. Hultengren N, Lagergren C, Ljungqvist A: Carcinoma of the renal pelvis in renal papillary necrosis. Acta Chir Scand 130:314–320, 1965.

28. Kahn HA: The Dorn study of smoking and mortality among United States Veterans—report on 8½ years of observation. In Epidemiological Approaches to the Study of Cancer and Other Chronic Diseases. Natl Cancer Inst Monogr No. 19. Washington DC, US Govt Printing Office, 1966, pp 1–125.

29. Kolonel LN: Association of cadmium with renal cancer. Cancer 37:1782–1787, 1976.

30. Kirkman H, Bacon RL: Renal adenomas and carcinomas in diethylstilbestrol treated male golden hamsters. Anat Rec 103:475–476, 1949.

31. Kirkman H: Estrogen-induced tumors of the kidney. II. Effect of dose, administration, type of estrogen, and age on the induction of renal tumors in intact male golden hamsters. JNCI 13:757–771, 1952.

32. Kirkman H: Estrogen-induced tumors of the kidney. Natl Cancer Inst Monogr 1:1–91, 1959.

33. Kirkman H, Robbins M: Estrogen-induced tumors of the kidney: V. Histology and histogenesis in the Syrian hamster. Natl Cancer Inst Monogr 1:93–139, 1959.

34. Kuhlmann W, Fromme HG, Heege EM, Ostertag W: The mutagenic action of caffeine in higher organisms. Cancer Res 28:2375–2389, 1968.

35. Liu T, Smith GW, Rankin JT: Renal pelvic tumour associated with analgesic abuse. Can Med Assoc J 107:768–771, 1972.

36. Macalpine JB: Papilloma of the renal pelvis in dye workers. Two cases, one of which shows bilateral growth. Br J Surg 35:137–140, 1947.

37. Magee PN, Barnes JM: Induction of kidney tumours in the rat with dimethylnitrosamine (N-nitrosodimethylamine). J Pathol Bacteriol 84:19–31, 1962.

38. Mahony JF, Storey BG, Ibanez RC, Stewart JH: Analgesic abuse, renal parenchymal disease and carcinoma of the kidney or ureter. Aust NZ J Med 7:463–469, 1977.

39. Matthews VS, Kirkman H, Bacon RL: Kidney damage in golden hamster following chronic administration of diethylstilbestrol and sesame oil. Proc Soc Exp Biol Med 66:195–196, 1947.

40. McCredie M, Ford JM, Taylor JS, Stewart JH: Analgesics and cancer of the renal pelvis in New South Wales. Cancer 49:2617–2625, 1982.

41. McCredie M, Stewart JH, Ford JM, MacLennan RA: Phenacetin-containing analgesics and cancer of the bladder or renal pelvis in women. Br J Urol 55:220–224, 1983.

42. McLaughlin JK, Blot WJ, Mandel JS, et al: Etiology

of cancer of the renal pelvis. JNCI 71:287–291, 1983.

43. McLaughlin JK, Mandel JS, Blot WJ, et al: A population-based case-control study of renal cell carcinoma. JNCI 72:275–284, 1984.

44. Ong GB, Leong CH: Carcinoma of the renal pelvis. Br J Urol 44:125–126, 1972.

45. Paganini-Hill A, Glazer E, Henderson BE, Ross RK: Cause-specific mortality among newspaper web pressmen. J Occup Med 22:542–544, 1980.

46. Petković SD: Epidemiology and treatment of renal pelvic and ureteral tumors. J Urol 114:858–865, 1975.

47. Poole-Wilson DS: Occupational tumours of the renal pelvis and ureter arising in the dye-making industry. Proc Soc Med 62:93–94, 1969.

48. Redmond CK, Ciocco A, Lloyd JW, et al: Long-term mortality study of steelworkers. VI. Mortality from malignant neoplasms among coke oven workers. J Occup Med 14:621–629, 1972.

49. Schmauz R, Cole P: Epidemiology of cancer of the renal pelvis and ureter. JNCI 52:1431–1434, 1974.

50. Selikoff IJ, Hammond EC, Seidman H: Mortality experience of insulation workers in the United States and Canada, 1943–1976. Ann NY Acad Sci 330:91–116, 1979.

51. Segi M: Graphic presentation of cancer incidence by site and by area and population. Segi Inst Cancer Epidem, Nagoya, Japan, 1977.

52. Serfontein WJ, Hurter P: Nitrosamines as environmental carcinogens. II. Evidence for the presence of nitrosamines in tobacco smoke condensate. Cancer Res 26:575–579, 1966.

53. Shennan DH: Letter: Renal carcinoma and coffee consumption in 16 countries. Br J Cancer 28:473–474, 1973.

54. Siiteri PK, MacDonald PC: Role of extraglandular estrogen in human endocrinology. In Handbook of Physiology, Sect 7, Vol 2, Part 1. Washington DC, Am Physiol Soc, 1973, pp 615–629.

55. U.S. Dept of Health, Education and Welfare, Public Health Serv: Vital Statistics of the US, Vol II, Part A. Mortality, 1930–1976.

56. Van Esch GJ, Kroes R: The induction of renal tumours by feeding basic lead acetate to mice and hamsters. Br J Cancer 23:765–771, 1979.

57. Vazquez-Lopez E: Reaction of pituitary gland and related hypothalamic centres in hamster to prolonged treatment with oestrogens. J Pathol Bacteriol 56:1–13, 1944.

58. Waterhouse J, Muir C, Shanmugaratnam K, Powell J (eds): Cancer Incidence in Five Continents, Vol IV. IARC Scientific Publications, No. 42, Lyon, International Agency for Research on Cancer, 1982.

59. Weir JM, Dunn JE Jr: Smoking and mortality: a prospective study. Cancer 25:105–112, 1970.

60. Wynder EL, Goldsmith R: The epidemiology of bladder cancer: a second look. Cancer 40:1246–1268, 1977.

61. Wynder EL, Hoffman D: Tobacco. In D Schottenfeld, JF Fraumeni (eds), Cancer: Epidemiology and Prevention. Philadelphia, WB Saunders, 1982, pp 277–292.

62. Wynder EL, Mabuchi K, Whitmore W: Epidemiology of adenocarcinoma of the kidney. JNCI 53:1619–1634, 1974.

63. Yamasaki E, Ames BN: Concentration of mutagens from urine by absorption with the nonpolar resin XAD-2: cigarette smokers have mutagenic urine. Proc Natl Acad Sci USA 74:3555–3559, 1977.

64. Yu MC, Mack TM, Hanisch R, et al: Diuretic use is a risk factor for renal cell carcinoma. JNCI (in press)

RONALD K. ROSS, M.D.
ANNLIA PAGANINI-HILL, Ph.D.
BRIAN E. HENDERSON, M.D.

Epidemiology of Prostatic Cancer*

CHAPTER 4

Cancer of the prostate is the second most common cancer among men in the United States. Despite the relative importance of prostatic cancer, there have been few epidemiologic studies of this disease. In this chapter we provide a brief outline of the demographics of cancer of the prostate and review the epidemiologic and experimental evidence supporting the major etiologic hypotheses.

EPIDEMIOLOGY

Black Americans have the highest incidence of prostatic cancer in the world. It is unlikely that this high rate has an entirely genetic basis, since the disease is much less common in African blacks.[14, 25] White men in the United States have an incidence rate for prostatic cancer that is only one-half that of US blacks, but they have a relatively high rate compared with that for men in other parts of the world (Fig. 4–1).[37] In some parts of the US, blacks have a 30% chance of developing prostatic cancer by age 85.

Among countries with reliable cancer reporting statistics, Japan has the lowest rate of cancer of the prostate. Japanese migrants to the US have a considerably higher prostatic cancer rate than Japanese in Japan, but

this rate is still only about one-half that of US whites (Table 4–1).[11]

Prostatic cancer in the US is rare in men under age 40, but thereafter its incidence continually increases with age. The excess risk in blacks in the US is independent of the lower mean social class of blacks, compared with that of whites, since the ratio of the age-adjusted rates in blacks to whites is similar across all social class strata. In whites, prostatic cancer rates are moderately higher among persons in the upper social class groupings, and there is some indication that a similar relationship exists in blacks (Table 4–2).

ETIOLOGIC HYPOTHESES

Two major hypotheses of the etiology of prostate cancer have been advanced: sexual

Table 4–1. PROSTATIC CANCER: AGE-SPECIFIC AND AGE-ADJUSTED INCIDENCE RATES PER 100,000 BY RACE, LOS ANGELES COUNTY, 1972–1983

	Age				Age-adjusted Rate*
Race	45–55	55–64	65–74	75+	
Black	29	222	866	1825	144
White	11	111	437	901	71
Japanese	5†	50	202	589	39

*Standardized to 1970 US population.
†Fewer than 10 cases.

*Supported by Grants CA 00652, CA 32197, and CA 17054 from the National Cancer Institute, National Institutes of Health.

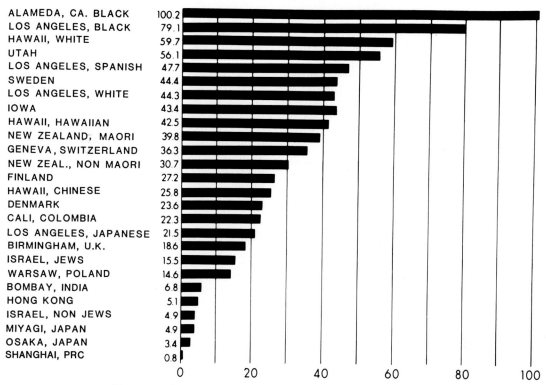

Figure 4–1. Prostate cancer incidence rates in different populations.

transmission by an infectious agent and hormonal stimulation of prostatic tissue by testosterone.

Infectious Agents

Several observers suggest that prostatic cancer might be caused by transmission of an infectious agent through sexual activity. Results from several epidemiologic studies indicate that various measures of sexual activity, including number of sex partners, history of venereal disease, frequency of intercourse, and early age at first intercourse, are associated with high risk of prostatic cancer.[16, 22, 33, 35] In recent case-control studies of prostatic cancer in blacks and whites in Los Angeles, several indices of sexual activity suggest that blacks are more sexually active than whites, but only a history of venereal disease is a strong predictor of risk for cancer of the prostate (RR = 2.8 in whites and 1.7 in blacks).[32] A history of venereal disease was nearly 10 times more common in black controls (37%) than in white controls (4%); frequency of intercourse was 50 to 70% higher in blacks up to age 60; blacks had sexual intercourse, on average, five years

earlier than whites, and spouses of black controls had almost twice as many pregnancies. However, these differences were not adjusted for differences in social class characteristics.

The finding of virus-like particles in human prostatic cancer and the increased incidence of cervical carcinoma in spouses of prostatic cancer patients lend more support to the infectious agent hypothesis.[6, 36] The high rate of cervical cancer in black females in the US suggests a possible common etiology for the two diseases. However, unlike the case for prostatic cancer, the rate of cervical cancer is very high in Spanish-

Table 4–2. PROSTATIC CANCER: AGE-ADJUSTED RATES PER 100,000 BY SOCIAL CLASS AND RACE, LOS ANGELES COUNTY, 1972–1983

Social Class	Whites	Blacks
1 (High)	96	262*
2	82	161
3	70	171
4	60	137
5	60	125

*26 cases.

Table 4–3. ADJUSTED AND UNADJUSTED STANDARD MORTALITY RATIOS (SMR) FOR ALL CAUSES OF DEATH, ALL CANCER DEATHS, AND SELECTED CANCER SITES FOR A COHORT OF LOS ANGELES PRIESTS

Site	Number Expected	Number Observed	SMR	Adjusted SMR
All causes	574.0	459	80	89
All cancers	103.4	82	79	88
Bladder	3.7	1	27	30
Colon	9.8	9	92	102
Esophagus	2.5	2	80	89
Kidney	2.5	1	40	45
Leukemia	4.1	3	73	81
Lung	28.8	13	45*	50*
Pancreas	5.9	5	85	95
Prostate	8.5	13	153	170
Stomach	7.6	9	118	131

*Two-sided $P < 0.01$.

surnamed whites and is strongly associated with low social class. These two facts argue against a hypothesis of common cause for the two diseases and suggest that the factors responsible for the high rate of cervical cancer in black females are not the same as those responsible for the high rate of prostatic cancer in black males.

This sexual-transmission hypothesis was tested by determining the mortality rate of prostatic cancer in a population of celibate males.[30] Nearly 1400 Catholic priests were identified through directories of the Archdiocese of Los Angeles between 1946 and 1955. Such directories list all active priests in the Archdiocese in any given year. Through a variety of sources, we were able to determine the vital status in 1976 in more than 90% of this cohort. Over 500 priests had died by this date. We calculated the expected number of cancer deaths by site, using cause-specific mortality rates for the US white male population from 1946 to 1975. Standard mortality ratios (SMR) were calculated as observed/expected $\times$ 100. Total mortality in the cohort, including only priests with documented deaths, was 85% of that expected, and total cancer mortality was 79% of that expected (Table 4–3). We observed 13 deaths from prostatic cancer in this cohort, compared with only eight expected (SMR = 153). The adjusted SMR in the table includes those 50 priests for whom we had evidence of death but no death certificate. Assuming that the distribution of these deaths by cause was the same for those with death certificates, the adjusted SMR for

prostatic cancer was 170. The absence of a marked deficit of prostatic cancer mortality among celibate men is strong evidence against sexual transmission of the disease.

Endocrine Factors

Normal growth and function of prostatic tissue is largely under hormonal control. The principal trophic hormones regulating this growth are testosterone and its metabolite dihydrotestosterone.[26, 39] We recently proposed that for a variety of tissues whose growth is controlled by hormonal influences, including the prostate, excessive hormonal stimulation can result in neoplasia.[13] One piece of evidence supporting such a hypothesis for cancer of the prostate is the observation by Noble that testosterone alone, given subcutaneously, can produce prostatic adenocarcinomas in rats (Table 4–4).[24, 25] This finding takes on added importance because of the difficulty of inducing adenocarcinoma of the prostate experimentally by any means.[28]

Brown and co-workers were also able to produce adenocarcinoma in intact male rats by joining through parabiosis such rats either to castrated male rats or to oophorectomized female rats, following unilateral nephrectomy in both partners.[4] Very high circulating levels of testosterone were demonstrated in the target male prior to tumor development.

Several studies have compared circulating testosterone levels measured by radioimmunoassay in cases of prostatic cancer with those in controls of similar age (Table 4–5). Ghanadian and colleagues showed that patients with cancer of the prostate had higher levels of serum testosterone than did healthy

Table 4–4. PROSTATIC ADENOCARCINOMA IN Nb RATS AFTER TREATMENT WITH STEROID PELLETS*

Number of Rats	Steroid Treatment†	Incidence of Gross Carcinoma of Prostate (%)
409	None	0.5
13	TPP (1 Pellet)	0.0
30	TPP (2 Pellets)	17.0
55	TPP (3 Pellets)	20.0

*From Noble RL: The development of prostatic adenocarcinoma in Nb rats following prolonged sex hormone administration. Cancer Res 37:1929–1933, 1977.

†TPP pellets contain 90% testosterone proprionate and 10% cholesterol.

Table 4-5. MEAN LEVELS OF SERUM TESTOSTERONE IN CASE-CONTROL STUDIES OF PROSTATIC CANCER

Reference	Cases		Controls		P	Difference (%)
	N	Value (pg/ml)	N	Value (pg/ml)		
Ghanadian et al (1979)	33	6030	42	4820	<0.01	+25
Ahluwalia et al (1981)						
U.S. Blacks	170	4200*	170	3500*	<0.05	+20
African Blacks	55	2000*	55	2200*	<0.05	−9
Drafta et al (1982)	23	6344	63	4011	<0.001	+58
Zumoff et al (1982)†	7	2820	36	4340	<0.001	−35
Wright et al (1985)	26	4440	23	4380	Nonsignificant	+1

*Values not cited in text but interpolated from graphs.
†Subjects are under 65 years of age.

controls.[7] Seven of 33 cases but only one of 42 controls had serum testosterone levels greater than 30 nMol/dl. Ahluwalia and coworkers found levels of serum testosterone significantly higher in patients with prostatic cancer than in age-matched controls in US, but not African, blacks.[1] They also found that both black American patients and controls had substantially higher levels of testosterone than did their black African case and control counterparts. Drafta and colleagues also found significantly higher circulating testosterone levels in 23 patients with prostatic cancer, compared with 63 "normal ambulatory controls."[5]

Although the three aforementioned studies found higher testosterone levels in patients with prostatic cancer than in controls, other groups have not found such differences. Wright and co-workers found no difference in circulating testosterone levels between 23 elderly French urology patients devoid of prostatic disease and 26 elderly men with well-differentiated cancer of the prostate.[40] However, the cancer patients in this study were somewhat older than the control group. Zumoff and colleagues, in a small study of 24-hour serum hormone testosterone levels, actually found prostatic cancer patients under age 65 to have a mean level significantly lower than that of controls without prostatic disease, whereas those over age 65 had a mean level 10% higher.[41] It should be noted that the average age of the controls under age 65 was about 18 years less than that of the patients with prostatic cancer. Hammond and co-workers also found no difference in circulating testosterone levels in their case-control study of only 11 patients with prostatic cancer.[12] Meikle and Stanish found significantly lower testosterone levels in brothers and sons of prostatic cancer patients than in healthy unrelated controls of comparable age.[23]

The hypothesis of a hormonal etiology for prostatic cancer would predict that healthy US black males should have higher testosterone levels than US white males. We recently studied circulating steroid hormone levels in white and black college students in Los Angeles. After adjustment by analysis of covariance for time of sampling, age, weight, alcohol use, cigarette smoking, and use of prescription drugs, the mean testosterone level in blacks was 15% higher than that of whites, and the "free" (i.e., non-protein-bound) testosterone level was 13% higher.[29] Cancer rates tend to increase at approximately the fourth or fifth power of "tissue age."[30] If this "tissue aging" for prostatic cancer begins at puberty, and if a 15% increase in testosterone translates into a 15% increase in "prostatic tissue aging," such an increase could explain nearly all of the twofold increased risk of prostatic cancer in US blacks.[32]

Epidemiologic data relevant to this hypothesis, although not abundant, tend to support it. Increased sexual activity, mentioned earlier in support of the sexual transmission hypothesis, may also be compatible with an increased level of circulating androgens.[38] Autopsy studies have shown that patients with cirrhosis of the liver have lower rates of prostatic cancer than do controls of the same age,[8] and alcohol is known to depress circulating testosterone levels.[9] Castration produces a palliative effect on advanced prostatic cancer,[18] and the disease is seemingly unknown in castrated subjects.[17]

There is a strong correlation between per capita consumption of dietary fat and both prostatic cancer mortality (on an international basis)[2] and prostatic cancer incidence (on a regional basis).[20] Several case-control studies have suggested that patients with prostatic cancer may consume more dietary fat than controls.[10, 19] A cohort study of white male Seventh-Day Adventists produced similar results.[34] In our recent case-control studies of prostatic cancer in whites and blacks in Los Angeles, intake of certain foods, especially fatty foods such as fried meats, pork, and eggs, was a risk factor for prostatic cancer in both populations.[32] The relative risk for cancer of the prostate in controls whose fat intake is above the median, based on all foods, was 1.7 in whites and 1.4 in blacks. The risk in whites was statistically significant ($p < 0.05$). However, there was little difference in mean fat intake between blacks and whites.

It has been hypothesized that dietary fat affects cancer occurrence by altering the hormonal environment.[3] Hill and Wynder studied plasma testosterone levels in four men fed a Western diet (40% calories from fat) for two weeks and then an isocaloric vegetarian low-fat diet (25% calories from fat) for a comparable period.[15] While the men were on the vegetarian diet, their levels of plasma testosterone decreased substantially during each of the six daily sampling periods. An additional 11 men were switched from their usual diets to a vegetarian diet for two weeks; both midmorning and late afternoon testosterone levels decreased about 33% ($p < 0.01$).

SUMMARY

Several areas of evidence suggest that circulating testosterone levels are a major determinant of prostatic cancer risk. These include animal experiments in which exogenous testosterone has produced prostatic adenocarcinoma, findings of higher circulating testosterone levels in patients with prostatic cancer than in healthy controls and also in healthy blacks compared with whites of comparable age, and the important mitotic effect of testosterone and its metabolites on prostatic epithelial cells.

Although greater levels of sexual activity also have been consistently observed in men with prostatic cancer, compared with activity of controls, the absence of a low risk of prostatic cancer in celibate males suggests

that these findings may result from hormonal effects and may not be indicative of a sexually transmitted etiologic agent. The recent observation that dietary fat intake can substantially affect circulating testosterone levels offers a hormonal mechanism for the consistently observed relationship between fat intake and risk of prostatic cancer.

References

1. Ahluwalia B, Jackson MA, Jones GW, et al: Blood hormone profiles in prostate cancer patients in high-risk and low-risk populations. Cancer 48:2267–2273, 1981.
2. Armstrong B, Doll R: Environmental factors and cancer incidence and mortality in different countries, with special reference to dietary practices. Int J Cancer 15:617–631, 1975.
3. Berg JW: Can nutrition explain the pattern of international epidemiology of hormone-dependent cancers? Cancer Res 35:3345–3350, 1975.
4. Brown CE, Warren S, Chute RN, et al: Hormonally induced tumors of the reproductive system of parabiosed male rats. Cancer Res 39:3971–3975, 1979.
5. Drafta D, Proca E, Zamfir V, et al: Plasma steroids in benign prostatic hypertrophy and carcinoma of the prostate. J Steroid Biochem 17:689–693, 1982.
6. Feminella JJ, Lattimer JK: An apparent increase in genital carcinomas among wives of men with prostatic carcinoma: an epidemiologic survey. Pirquet Bull Clin Med 20:3–9, 1974.
7. Ghanadian R, Puah CM, O'Donoghue EPN: Serum testosterone and dihydrotestosterone in carcinoma of the prostate. Br J Cancer 39:696–699, 1979.
8. Glantz GM: Cirrhosis and carcinoma of the prostate gland. J Urol 91:291–293, 1964.
9. Gordon GG, Altman K, Southern AL, et al: Effects of alcohol (ethanol) administration on sex-hormone metabolism in normal men. N Engl J Med 295:793–797, 1976.
10. Graham S, Haughey B, Marshall J, et al: Diet in the epidemiology of carcinoma of the prostate gland. JNCI 70:687–692, 1983.
11. Haenszel W, Kurihara M: Studies of Japanese migrants. I. Mortality from cancer and other diseases among Japanese in the United States. JNCI 40:43–68, 1968.
12. Hammond GL, Kontturi M, Vihko R: Serum steroids in normal males and patients with prostatic diseases. Clin Endocrinol 9:113–121, 1978.
13. Henderson BE, Ross RK, Pike MC, Casagrande JT: Endogenous hormones as a major factor in human cancer. Cancer Res 42:3232–3239, 1982.
14. Higginson J, Oettle AG: Cancer incidence in the Bantu and "Cape Colored" races of South Africa: report of a cancer survey in the Transvaal (1953-1955). JNCI 24:589–671, 1960.
15. Hill PB, Wynder EL: Effect of a vegetarian diet and dexamethasone on plasma prolactin, testosterone, and dehydroepiandrosterone in men and women. Cancer Lett 7:273–282, 1979.
16. Honda GD, Ross RK, Henderson BE: Prostate cancer, vasectomy and cigarette smoking (in review).
17. Hovenanian MS, Deming CL: The heterologous

growth of cancer of the human prostate. Surg Gynecol Obstet 86:29–35, 1948.

18. Huggins C, Hodges CV: Studies on prostatic cancer: effect of castration, of estrogen, and of androgen injection on serum phosphatases in metastatic carcinoma of the prostate. CA 22:232–240, 1972.

19. Kolonel LN, Hankin JH, Lee J: Diet and prostate cancer. (Abstract), Society for Epidemiologic Research, Annual Meeting, Winnipeg, 1983.

20. Kolonel LN, Nomura A, Hinds MV, et al: Role of diet in cancer incidence in Hawaii. Cancer Res 43(Suppl):2397s–2402s, 1983.

21. Kovi H, Heshmat MY: Incidence of cancer in Negroes in Washington D.C. and selected African cities. Am J Epidemiol 96:401–403, 1972.

22. Krain LS: Some epidemiologic variables in prostatic carcinoma in California. Prev Med 3:154–159, 1974.

23. Meikle AW, Stanish WM: Familial prostatic cancer risk and low testosterone. J Clin Endocrinol Metab 54:1104–1108, 1982.

24. Noble RL: The development of prostatic adenocarcinoma in Nb rats following prolonged sex hormone administration. Cancer Res 37:1929–1933, 1977.

25. Noble RL: Production of Nb rat carcinoma of the dorsal prostate and response of estrogen-dependent transplants to sex hormones and tamoxifen. Cancer Res 40:3547–3550, 1980.

26. O'Malley BW: Mechanisms of action of steroid hormones. N Engl J Med 284:370–377, 1971.

27. Pike MC, Krailo MD, Henderson BE, et al: "Hormonal" risk factors, "breast tissue age," and the age-incidence of breast cancer. Nature 303:767–770, 1983.

28. Rivenson A, Silverman J: The prostatic carcinoma in laboratory animals: a bibliographic survey from 1900–1977. Invest Urol 16:468–472, 1979.

29. Ross RK, Bernstein L, Judd H, et al: Serum testosterone levels in healthy young black and white men. JNCI 76:45–48, 1986.

30. Ross RK, Deapen DM, Casagrande JT, et al: A cohort study of mortality from cancer of the prostate in Catholic priests. Br J Cancer 43:233–235, 1981.

31. Ross RK, McCurtis JW, Henderson BE, et al: Descriptive epidemiology of testicular and prostatic cancer in Los Angeles. Br J Cancer 39:284–292, 1979.

32. Ross RK, Shimizu H, Paganini-Hill A, et al: Risk factors for prostate cancer in blacks and whites in Los Angeles. (in press)

33. Schuman LM, Mandel J, Blackard C, et al: Epidemiologic study of prostatic cancer: preliminary report. Cancer Treat Rep 61:181–186, 1977.

34. Snowdon DA, Phillips RL, Choi W: Diet, obesity and risk of fatal prostate cancer. Am J Epidemiol 120:244–250, 1984.

35. Steele R, Lees REM, Kraus AJ, et al: Sexual factors in the epidemiology of cancer of the prostate. J Chronic Dis 24:29–37, 1971.

36. Tannenbaum M, Lattimer JK: Similar virus-like particles found in cancers of the prostate and breast. J Urol 103:471–475, 1970.

37. Waterhouse J, Muir C, Shanmugaratnam K, Power J (eds): Cancer Incidence in Five Continents, Vol. IV. IARC Scientific Publication No. 42. Lyon, International Agency for Research on Cancer, 1982.

38. Williams RH (ed): Textbook of Endocrinology. Philadelphia, WB Saunders, 1974, p 323.

39. Wilson JD: Recent studies on the mechanism of action of testosterone. N Engl J Med 287:1284–1291, 1972.

40. Wright F, Poizat R, Bongini M, et al: Decreased urinary (5 a-androstane-3a, 17B-diol) glucuronide excretion in patients with benign prostatic hyperplasia. J Clin Endocrinol Metab 60:294–298, 1985.

41. Zumoff B, Levin J, Strain GW, et al: Abnormal levels of plasma hormones in men with prostate cancer: evidence toward a "two-disease" theory. Prostate 3:579–588, 1985.

BRIAN E. HENDERSON, M.D.
RONALD K. ROSS, M.D.
MALCOLM C. PIKE, Ph.D.

Epidemiology of Testicular Cancer

Cancer of the testis is relatively uncommon, accounting for less than 1% of all incident cancers and less than 0.5% of all cancer deaths in men. However, several features of the descriptive epidemiology of testicular cancer are particularly striking, including (1) the peak incidence in young men, (2) the rising incidence over the last 50 years in young whites, and (3) the low incidence in young blacks. Recent analytical studies have attempted to "explain" these and other epidemiologic features of testicular cancer in terms of in utero exposure to elevated levels of steroid hormones, particularly estrogens.[9, 15, 16, 31]

DESCRIPTIVE EPIDEMIOLOGY OF TESTICULAR CANCER

The age-specific incidence curve of testicular cancer shows a broad peak between ages 20 and 40, with a subsequent decline in incidence at age 60, followed by a small increase in the older age groups (Fig. 5–1). The majority (95%) of testicular cancers are of germ cell origin and show a continuing decline in incidence after age 40. Embryonal cell cancers account for the largest proportion of testicular cancers to age 35, after which seminomas predominate until age 75. The increase in testicular cancer in old age is due primarily to an increase in lymphomas, which account for more than 50% of

testicular cancers in men after age 75 (Fig. 5–2).

There is a marked variation in the incidence of testicular cancer in different countries (Fig. 5–3). The highest rates have been reported from Scandinavian countries and the lowest from Asian and African countries. In Los Angeles the incidence of testicular

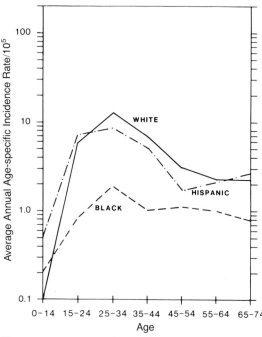

Figure 5–1. Age-specific incidence curves for white, Hispanic, and black males in Los Angeles, 1972–1983.

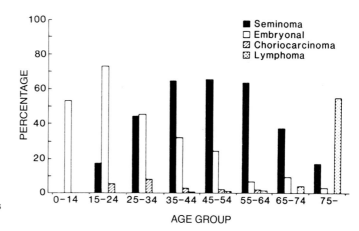

Figure 5-2. Frequency of histologic types of testicular cancer by age.

cancer has remained low in the black population (Fig. 5-4), whereas the incidence rate in Hispanics is now close to the rate in whites. The continued low rate in the black population seems to be unique to that racial group and is unexplained.

Testicular cancer has long been increasing in incidence in young white males in Europe and North America.[4, 25, 31] We are continuing to see that increase in white males in Los Angeles County, primarily because of a continued increase in the incidence rate in young men. Between 1972 and 1983, the age-specific incidence rate tripled in men 25 to 34 years of age, whereas the overall age-adjusted rate doubled (Fig. 5-4).

The incidence of testis cancer is highest in men of the highest socioeconomic classes (Table 5-1), and rates in the highest social class approximately double those in the lowest. Within individual socioeconomic classes, the age-adjusted incidence rate in Hispanics is essentially identical to that of whites. Among black males, there appears

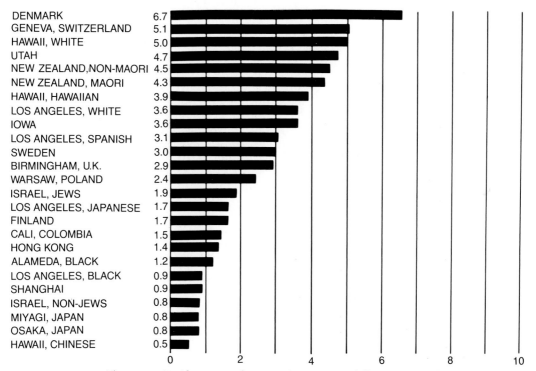

Figure 5-3. Incidence rates for testicular cancer in different areas and races.

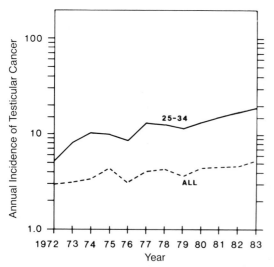

Figure 5–4. Age-specific and age-adjusted incidence rates for testicular cancer in white males in Los Angeles, 1972–1983.

to be a similar gradient from highest to lowest class, although within any particular class, the rate in blacks is still less than one-third the rate in whites.

RISK FACTORS FOR TESTICULAR CANCER

Cryptorchidism

A cryptorchid testis is at increased risk for testicular cancer. Recent epidemiologic studies have reported relative risks of testicular cancer from 3 to 14 for persons with a cryptorchid testis.[5, 9, 15, 21, 22, 26, 31] A similar association with a relative risk of 14 has been found in dogs.[13]

A persistently undescended testis is accompanied by considerable structural abnormalities. The testis is smaller and, histologically, tubule development and spermatogenesis are retarded. Sertoli cell development is delayed, and there are abnormalities of the Leydig cells.[19]

It is clearly not just the abdominal location of the undescended testis that increases the risk of cancer in this gonad. Surgically descended testes, particularly those moved after childhood, retain a high risk of cancer.[11, 26] More importantly, the contralateral descended testis in patients with cryptorchidism has been reported to have a twofold increased risk of cancer,[15, 18, 21] although Pottern and co-workers[26] found substantially different results in a recent study. In their

study of 271 patients and 259 controls, no increased risk of testicular cancer was found in the normally descended testis among those with unilateral cryptorchidism. However, because of the small numbers, the 95% confidence intervals around this risk were very broad (0.1 to 7.0) and are certainly compatible with the small elevated risk observed by us and others.[15, 18, 21] Consistent with elevated risk, endocrine dysfunction and histologic abnormalities in spermatogenesis in men without testicular cancer persist in both testicles for 15 to 30 years after unilateral orchiopexy.[19]

Normal descent of the testis is under hormonal control.[12] Animal experiments have shown that nonsteroidal estrogen treatment of pregnant mice can lead to undescended and hypogenetic testes.[24] Similar abnormalities have been reported in male offspring of women exposed to diethylstilbestrol (DES)[6, 10] and to oral contraceptives[30] during pregnancy. In the study by Depue,[10] gestational exposure to exogenous estrogens increased the risk of cryptorchidism (RR = 3.3, p = 0.04).

As rates for testicular cancer have increased, so apparently have rates of cryptorchidism. An increase in cryptorchidism in army recruits during the past 50 years has been reported,[2] and there was an increase in the incidence of cryptorchidism in white infant males in Atlanta, Georgia, during the period from 1968 to 1977.[3] A recent report from England documents a doubling of the frequency of undescended testis between 1962 and 1981.[7] An increasing trend in rates of other congenital malformations of the male external genitalia (e.g., hypospadias) has also been reported.[8] There is also a threefold excess risk in whites of undescended testis, compared with the risk in blacks,[14] analogous to the excess risk of testis cancer observed in whites.

Table 5–1. AGE-ADJUSTED INCIDENCE RATES FOR TESTICULAR CANCER BY SOCIOECONOMIC CLASS, LOS ANGELES COUNTY, 1972–1983

Socioeconomic Class	Other Whites	Hispanics	Blacks
1 (high)	5.0	5.4	*
2	4.5	3.8	*
3	4.0	3.9	1.6
4	3.6	3.8	0.7
5 (low)	3.0	2.7	0.5

*Fewer than five cases.

Exogenous Estrogens

As stated above, experimental studies in animals and observational studies in humans have suggested a possible role for sex steroids in cryptorchidism. The use of estrogens for threatened abortion and other complications of pregnancy was a common practice between 1940 and 1960 in the United States. Women also have taken estrogens (and progestins) as a test for pregnancy, as a method of birth control, and as a "supplementary" therapy during their reproductive years. The reported experience of the daughters of women who had received DES during pregnancy offers an intriguing parallel to the epidemiology of testicular cancer. The incidence of adenocarcinoma of the lower genital tract in these girls rises sharply after age 14, peaks at 19, and begins to decline in the early 20s. Essentially all the reported excess risk of vaginal adenocarcinoma occurs in offspring exposed during the first trimester of gestation.[17]

The relationship between exogenous sex steroids in pregnancy and the risk of testicular cancer in offspring has been examined in three case-control studies (Table 5–2). All three studies found an increased risk in the male offspring of women exposed to DES, estrogen, or the estrogen-progestin combinations used in pregnancy tests. The relative risks ranged from 2.8 to 5.3. In the most recent study,[9] all hormone use began in the first two months of the pregnancy. Of the nine exposed women, five had only a single exposure as a result of a pregnancy test.

Other Risk Factors

Many other possible risk factors for testicular cancer have been investigated. An elevated risk (RR = 2.0) has been found for inguinal hernia, presumably another reflection of the interference with normal testicular descent that seems to be characteristic

Table 5–3. OTHER RISK FACTORS ASSOCIATED WITH TESTICULAR CANCER

Risk Factor	Reference Number	Matched Relative Risk	One-sided P Value
Excessive nausea	15	4.00	0.06
Treated nausea	9	5.00	0.02
Mother's Quetelet index value before index pregnancy:	9		
Less than 19		1.0	0.02
19 to 21		1.9	
Greater than 21		2.86	

of patients with cancer of the testis. Testicular cancer patients do not appear to be infertile. Depue and colleagues[9] calculated an index of fertility by dividing the number of children by the number of years married and found values of 0.24 for men with testicular cancer and 0.23 for controls. No evidence has been found for an increased risk associated with childhood infectious diseases such as mumps or chickenpox nor with medical x-ray exposure during the pregnancy.

We have found in two studies that excessive nausea during pregnancy is associated with an increased risk of testicular cancer in sons born to these women (Table 5–3).[9, 15] The risk was highest for children whose mother's nausea required medical treatment and was most noticeable for those who were the product of the first full-term pregnancy.

The cause of nausea in pregnancy is not definitely known, but it almost invariably starts in the first two months of gestation. This is a period of rapidly rising estrogen levels in the mother, which has been suggested as the inciting event, since exogenous estrogens commonly produce nausea. The mechanism to explain maternal nausea as a risk factor for testicular cancer in offspring may thus be related to that for the risk factors of hormone administration and cryptorchidism. If estrogens are the cause of the nausea, it may be the circulating level of "unbound" estrogen, rather than simply the total level of estrogen, that determines risk. It is generally accepted that hormones bound to sex-hormone-binding globulin (SHBG) are unavailable to tissues.[36] Therefore, decreased estrogen binding by SHBG will increase the hormone's biologic activity. The role of albumin, the other major binding protein, on tissue availability of estrogens remains unclear. The production of SHBG,

Table 5–2. RELATIVE RISKS FOR HORMONE USE DURING PREGNANCY OF MOTHERS OF PATIENTS WITH TESTICULAR CANCER AND CONTROLS FROM THREE CASE-CONTROL STUDIES

Reference	No. Used/Total Case	Control	Unmatched Relative Risk
Schottenfeld et al[31]	11/190	3/141	2.8
Henderson et al[15]	5/78	1/78	5.3
Depue et al[9]	9/107	2/108	4.9

an estrogen-inducible protein synthesized by the liver, may lag behind the rapidly increasing estrogen synthesis during the first trimester of pregnancy, the critical period for urogenital differentiation. Such an effect would likely be greatest and most frequent during the first pregnancy, which is often a woman's first experience with high levels of circulating estrogen. In this regard, in both of our studies of testicular cancer, we have found some evidence of an increased risk in the first-born, and Swerdlow[33] reported an elevated risk for cryptorchidism in primigravidae.

The increasing risk observed with increasing values of Quetelet's index in the mothers of sons who develop testicular cancer[9] as well as mothers of sons who have cryptorchidism[10] prior to the index pregnancy (Table 5–3) likewise may be a reflection of an excess of "free" estrogen. It is known that SHBG levels are decreased and "free" estrogen levels increased in obese women.[32] A low birth weight and premature delivery have been reported to be risk factors for both cryptorchidism[10] and testicular cancer.[9, 15]

There have been many reports of familial testicular cancer, and Tollerud and co-workers[34] recently have summarized the literature on this subject. The age at onset and histologic type of testicular cancer are more similar in cases from the same generation than in father-son pairs. Approximately 2% of the relatives of testicular cancer patients also have higher rates of urogenital anomalies (cryptorchidism, inguinal hernia, and hydrocele).

ETIOLOGIC HYPOTHESIS

We propose a unifying hypothesis for the pathogenesis of germ cell neoplasms of the testis. The initial event occurs in utero, if elevated levels of "free" estrogens, and perhaps other sex steroids, are present when the primordial germ cells of the gonad are beginning differentiation (Fig. 5–5). The excess estrogen somehow permanently alters the germ cell, which then remains dormant until stimulated to multiply by the rising levels of leutinizing hormone (LH) and follicle-stimulating hormone (FSH) that accompany puberty. The "abnormal" primitive germ cells must either produce a growing neoplasm within the first germ cell divi-

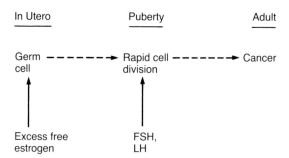

Figure 5–5. Pathogenesis of testicular cancer.

sions, die, or revert to normal, since the age-specific incidence curve rises rapidly after puberty, peaks, and then falls. Such an effect would be analogous to that of in utero exposure to DES, which also appears to be most carcinogenic during the first trimester and results in an abrupt rise in the incidence of urogenital adenocarcinoma after puberty and a subsequent fall by the end of the third decade.[17]

Excess "free" estrogen in the first trimester of pregnancy may be the result of exogenous administration, as in the case of DES or a hormonal test of pregnancy. It is intriguing that a single pregnancy test can confer risk of testicular cancer that is not manifested until 20 to 40 years later. We have observed that the hormone-associated cases in our two studies[9, 15] encompass the full range of germ cell neoplasms (embryonal cell carcinoma, teratocarcinoma, choriocarcinoma, and seminoma). This observation is consistent with the view that all these cell types have a common cellular origin and that the rate of cell division, and perhaps other age-related host factors, are the important determinants of histologic pattern.

Excess free estrogen may also result from a temporary increase in free endogenous estrogen that accompanies the early part of pregnancy, particularly in the first pregnancy. The rapid rise in hormone secretion rates temporarily exceeds the binding capacity of circulating sex-hormone-binding globulins producing an excess of free hormone. Excess weight, as measured by increased value for Quetelet's index, will produce a similar net increase in free estrogen, as discussed earlier.

The decline after age 40 in the age-specific incidence of testicular cancer of germ cell origin mitigates against any substantial neoplastic risk for the many generations of germ cells formed during the adult life of the male.

We have argued[16] that random chromosome copying errors can lead to neoplastic transformation of normally proliferating cells such as those of the prostate and breast, and, as such, would expect these generations of germ cells to produce neoplasms. It has been shown that there is a mechanism for selective destruction of presumably abnormal germ cells during spermatogenesis in many animal species, including humans.[1, 28] We think that this mechanism may actively eliminate those germ cells with neoplastic chromosomal changes as it does those with teratogenic potential.

References

1. Barr AB, Moore DJ, Paulsen CA: Germinal cell loss during human spermatogenesis. J Reprod Fert 25:75–80, 1971.
2. Campbell HE: The incidence of malignant growth of the undescended testicle: a reply and re-evaluation. J Urol 81:663–668, 1959.
3. Center for Disease Control: Congenital malformation surveillance report, January–December 1978. Atlanta GA, September 1979 DHEW publ no. [CDC] 80-8262.
4. Clemmesen J: A doubling of morbidity from testis carcinoma in Copenhagen, 1943–1962. Acta Path Microbiol Scand 72:348–349, 1968.
5. Coldman AJ, Elwood JM, Gallagher RP: Sports activities and risk of testicular cancer. Br J Cancer 46:749–756, 1982.
6. Cosgrove MD, Benton B, Henderson BE: Male genitourinary abnormalities and maternal diethylstilbestrol. J Urol 117:220–222, 1977.
7. Chilvers C, Forman D, Pike MC, et al: Apparent doubling of frequency of undescended testis in England and Wales in 1962–81. Lancet 2:330–332, 1984.
8. Czeizel A: Increasing trends in congenital malformations of male external genitalia. Lancet 1:462–463, 1985.
9. Depue RH, Pike MC, Henderson BE: Estrogen exposure during gestation and risk of testicular cancer. JNCI 71:1151–1155, 1983.
10. Depue RH: Maternal and gestational factors affecting the risk of cryptorchidism and inguinal hernia. Int J Epidemiol 13:311–318, 1984.
11. Dow JA, Mostofi FK: Testicular tumors following orchiopexy. S Med J 60:193–195, 1967.
12. Goodman LS, Gilman A (eds): The Pharmacological Basis of Therapeutics. London, Macmillan, 1970, p 1528.
13. Hayes HM Jr, Pendergrass TW: Canine testicular tumors: epidemiologic features of 410 dogs. Int J Cancer 18:482–487, 1976.
14. Heinonen OP, Slone D, Shapiro S: Malformation of the genitourinary system. In DW Kaufman (ed), Birth Defects and Drugs in Pregnancy. Littleton, MA, Publishing Sciences Group, 1977, pp 176–199.
15. Henderson BE, Benton B, Jing J, et al: Risk factors for cancer of the testis in young men. Int J Cancer 23:598–602, 1979.
16. Henderson BE, Ross RK, Pike MC, Casagrande JT: Endogenous hormones as a major factor in human cancer. Cancer Res 42:3232–3239, 1982.
17. Herbst AL, Cole P, Norusis MJ, et al: Epidemiologic aspects and factors related to survival in 384 registry cases of clear cell adenocarcinoma of the vagina and cervix. Am J Obstet Gynecol 135:876–886, 1979.
18. Johnson DE, Woodhead DM, Pohl DR, Robison J: Cryptorchidism and testicular tumorigenesis. Surgery 63:919–922, 1968.
19. Lipshultz LI, Caminos-Torres R, Greenspan CS, et al. Testicular function after orchiopexy for unilaterally undescended testis. N Engl J Med 295:15–18, 1976.
20. Mack TM, Henderson BE: Cancer registries for general and special uses. In US-USSR Monograph, NIH publ no. 80-2044, 1980, pp 57–61.
21. Morrison AS: Cryptorchidism, hernia and cancer of the testis. JNCI 56:731–733, 1976.
22. Mostofi FK: Testicular tumors. Epidemiological, etiologic, and pathologic features. Cancer 32:1186–1201, 1973.
23. Nethersell ABW, Drake LK, Sikora K. The increasing incidence of testicular cancer in East Anglia. Br J Cancer 50:377–380, 1984
24. Nomura T, Kanzaki T: Induction of urogenital anomalies and some tumors in the progeny of mice receiving diethylstilbestrol during pregnancy. Cancer Res 37:1099–1104, 1977.
25. Petersen GR, Lee JA: Secular trends of malignant tumors of the testis in white men. JNCI 49:339–354, 1972.
26. Pottern LM, Brown LM, Hoover RN, et al: Testicular cancer risk among young men: role of cryptorchidism and inguinal hernia. JNCI 74:377–381, 1985.
27. Pugh RCB: Testicular tumors—introduction. In RCB Pugh (ed), Pathology of the Testis. Oxford, Blackwell Scientific Publications, 1976, p 140.
28. Roosen-Runge EC: Germinal-cell loss in normal metazoan spermatogenesis. J Reprod Fert 35:339–348, 1973.
29. Ross RK, McCurtis JW, Henderson BE, et al: Descriptive epidemiology of testicular and prostatic cancer in Los Angeles. Br J Cancer 39:284–292, 1979.
30. Rothman KJ, Louik C: Oral contraceptives and birth defects. N Engl J Med 299:522–524, 1978.
31. Schottenfeld D, Warshauer ME, Sherlock S, et al: The epidemiology of testicular cancer in young adults. Am J Epidemiol 112:232–246, 1980.
32. Siiteri PK, MacDonald PC: Role of extraglandular estrogen in human endocrinology. In Handbook of Physiology, Sec 7, Vol 2, Part 1. Washington DC, American Physiological Society, 1973, pp 615–629.
33. Swerdlow AJ, Wood KH, Smith PG: Case-control study of the aetiology of cryptorchidism. J Epid Comm Health 37:238–244, 1983.
34. Tollerud DJ, Blattner WA, Fraser MC, et al: Familial testicular cancer and urogenital development anomalies. Cancer 55:1849–1854, 1985.
35. Waterhouse J, Muir C, Shanmugaratnam K, Power J (eds). Cancer Incidence in Five Continents, Vol IV. IARC Scientific Publications No. 42. Lyon, International Agency for Research on Cancer, 1982.
36. Vermeulen A: Transport and distribution of androgens at different ages. L Martini, M Motta (eds), Androgens and Antiandrogens. New York, Raven Press, 1977.

PART III Pathology of Genitourinary Tumors

MYRON TANNENBAUM, M.D., Ph.D.
NICHOLAS A. ROMAS, M.D.
MICHAEL J. DROLLER, M.D.

CHAPTER 6

The Pathobiology of Early Urothelial Cancer

The classification and histopathologic characteristics of urinary bladder carcinomas have been extensively described by numerous authors.[13, 27] In addition, Mostofi has clarified histologically the multitudinous patterns that urothelial cancers demonstrate on conventional light histologic methods.[22] Traditionally, the classifications of bladder biopsy material have been based on the cytologic details and histologic architecture of the urothelium. In recent years, however, *cytology* and *flow cytometry* have provided additional prognostic information on the so-called urothelial state of affairs. Less frequently employed, but equally useful diagnostic tools such as transmission electron microscopy (TEM) and scanning electron microscopy (SEM), also have assisted in delineating the status of urothelial disease.

Despite all of these diagnostic tools, there is much about neoplasms of the urothelial tract that remains enigmatic. In this chapter, we will discuss why confusion persists about the pathologic features of the urothelium and why evaluation of the data by various investigators continues to generate controversy.

DYSPLASIA, OR UROTHELIAL ATYPIA

Although it might be assumed that the pathogenesis of urothelial malignancy in groups of patients at high risk for the development of bladder cancer is quite similar to that of the general population, this may not always be the case. For example, in one high-risk group, patients with spinal cord injuries, three of seven,[7] seven of 11,[21] and six of six[11] developed bladder cancers with squamous cell involvement. Indeed, of the 24 tumors, 16 were purely of squamous cells, whereas the remainder were of mixed squamous and transitional cell composition. This poses the question as to whether such differences reflect a pathogenesis of disease that is different from that in the general population or whether this is a form of disease actually quite common in bladder cancer but simply accentuated in these types of populations. We used bladder-mapping techniques in our own group of patients with spinal cord injuries because of our interest in determining whether such differences might provide a clue in the pathogenesis of transitional cell carcinoma. In view of previous observations on the squamous nature of tumors in this population, we were surprised to find an adenocarcinoma with some areas of high-grade transitional cell carcinoma and well-differentiated squamous cell carcinoma in one of three cystectomy specimens. We also observed these findings in random biopsies from three additional patients without endoscopically visible cancer. In eight additional patients, biopsies demonstrated areas of severe adenomatous hyperplasia (nephrogenic adenoma type) and numerous focal areas of severe *urothelial atypia (urothelial dysplasia)* and *carcinoma in situ.* The presence of the nephrogenic adenomas clearly demonstrates the great metaplastic ability of the urothelium to respond to various stimuli that may be present within the urinary system.

Urothelial atypia and *urothelial dysplasia* are relatively recent terms that will need further clinical definition with increased recognition of this pathologic lesion. There is now considerable evidence to suggest that *urothelial atypia* and *dysplasia* as a pathologic diagnosis may precede clinically overt urothelial cancer. In fact, they may describe a spectrum of histologic abnormalities that are interposed between normal urothelium and frank carcinoma in situ.[24] Some have suggested that such lesions are, in effect, *preneoplastic.* In a retrospective study of resected flat urothelium adjacent to exophytic urothelial cancer, Althausen and associates found that nine of 25 patients (36%) with urothelial atypia (dysplasia) developed invasive cancers within a five-year follow-up period.[1] Similarly, Murphy and co-workers studied prospectively selected urothelial biopsies from patients followed for urothelial cancer.[23] Eleven of 29 patients (38%) with epithelial dysplasia had superficial recurrences after the appearance of these apparently *premalignant lesions,* compared with only five of 32 (16%) individuals with "normal urothelium" at the selected biopsy sites. It must be remembered that different tumor courses were reported in these studies, possibly indicating that different types of urothelial atypia or dysplasia were examined in the first report. In the second report, simple recurrence and not necessarily tumor progression was documented. Attempts to document characteristics within so-called urothelial atypia or dysplasia that may distinguish potentially different tumor courses might therefore be important. Moreover, these lesions can usually be subdivided into three degrees of morphologic severity—mild, moderate, and severe. Lesions of the lowest grade may not be readily distinguishable from reactive, regenerating, or reparative urothelium. Correspondingly, the highest grade of dysplasia may be difficult to distinguish from unequivocal carcinoma in situ.

Like carcinoma in situ, urothelial atypia or urothelial dysplasia may be multifocal

and may frequently be encountered in those patients who have had a previous diagnosis of bladder cancer or are at high risk for development of the disease. It is found quite frequently in cystectomy specimens removed for tumors and in urothelial biopsies from bladders with gross tumors but with urothelium otherwise seemingly free of clinical disease.[5, 13, 23] Such lesions may not be visualized cystoscopically.

These lesions, like carcinoma in situ, commonly exfoliate cells into the urine. Therefore, it is not surprising that patients with urothelial atypia may also complain of frequent urination and dysuria. Unfortunately, such cells in the urine cannot be readily differentiated by means of ordinary light-microscopic examination from the atypical cells commonly found in urine when there is regenerating urothelium associated with catheter-induced trauma, the presence of stones, or infection. It is hoped that newer histochemical immunoperoxidase techniques and flow cytometry may more clearly define those cells that are truly preneoplastic.

CARCINOMA IN SITU, NONPAPILLARY CARCINOMA IN SITU, AND ATYPICAL HYPERPLASIAS

It has now been over three decades since the term carcinoma in situ was first applied to urothelium that showed cytologic evidence of neoplasia and was interposed between surrounding exophytic papillary tumors that had led to the removal of the bladder.[19, 20] The clinical significance of these neoplastic lesions was realized when urinary cytologic examination was used to identify a group of patients, selected out of an even larger group that had cancers of the urinary bladder, whose only evidence of persistent neoplasia was the presence of neoplastic cells in the urine.[17] When these patients were examined cystoscopically, they were found to be free of visible tumors. It was only after they were followed by urinary cytologic testing for a period of three months to seven years that any visible cytoscopic lesions became apparent. Preneoplastic lesions were undoubtedly present during these intervals. Today, it is a common practice to obtain random cold-cup biopsies from the lateral and posterior walls of the bladder above the trigone in order to detect early preneoplastic lesions.

At the Mount Sinai Hospital and the Bronx VA Medical Center, a similar disease pattern has also been seen. It has become routine in many urologic centers to obtain biopsies of the bladder mucosa in a random fashion. In those patients who have positive results of urinary cytologic tests, it is not unusual to detect not only carcinoma in situ but also microscopically invasive lesions in their biopsies. In addition, the carcinoma in situ, in some instances, contains intraepithelial blood vessels, suggesting an angiogenic reaction that may represent the earliest phase in the development of fibrovascular stalks.

In biopsy specimens, cells of carcinoma in situ usually can be shown to be pleomorphic when compared cytologically with normal cells present within the same microscopic field. In such specimens, abnormal cells can be readily demonstrated to be juxtaposed, not only beneath the normal surface urothelial cells but also above the basement membrane. They also are present in Brunn's nests, regions of cystitis cystica, and, in many instances, in periurethral prostatic ducts. The nuclei of these cells are usually two to three times the nuclear size of the adjacent normal urothelial cells.

A low-power magnification photomicrograph demonstrates that the urothelial lesion usually is in close proximity to a highly vascularized area (Fig. 6–1). This is seen on the left side of the photomicrograph. On the right side of the figure, the upper third of the urothelium is normal. The middle third contains both carcinoma in situ and an early papillary lesion in which there are already the histologic beginnings of an exophytic tumor. However, it is doubtful that this would be visible cystoscopically. In addition, the lower third of the urothelium on the right side is markedly atypical where the basal cells and some of the intermediary cells already appear to be neoplastic (Fig. 6–2).

Urothelial cancers are generally believed to begin in the basal cell layer and then to extend outward toward the lumen, replacing the intermediary cell layer as well as the surface cell layer (Figs. 6–2 and 6–3). Each of the three cell layers that compose the normal urothelium has certain ultrastructural characteristics that readily identify it as originating from that particular layer (Fig. 6–4). However, transmission electron microscopy, when used in conjunction with scanning electron microscopy, reveals cellular characteristics that can label these cells as malignant even before conventional light histologic and cytologic observations. Thus, the surface of the normal bladder cell (Fig. 6–5) has microridges (Fig. 6–6A and B) that disappear when the cell has become committed to develop in the direction of cancer (Figs. 6–6C and D and 6–7). The intermediate and basal cells also have these changes but as yet they have not been studied extensively.

Koss performed bladder mappings from 20 surgically removed radical cystectomy specimens that were studied by light-microscopic sections.[16] He has demonstrated nonpapillary carcinoma in situ and related lesions (i.e., atypical hyperplasias or dysplasias) in areas adjacent to or distant from visible tumors. He also has found numerous areas of occult invasive carcinoma that seemingly have been derived from such abnormal epithelium. The areas of the bladder most frequently involved by these precancerous lesions are the left and right lateral walls and the posterior wall. The trigone and the dome areas were less frequently involved.

In a retrospective histologic study of 140 patients with various grades of carcinoma in situ of the urinary bladder who had no previous history of urothelial or bladder cancer and who were followed for a period of 14 to 21 years, 40% were observed to progress from Stage A to B_1 in a period of four to six years.[31] In this time 10% went from Stage B_2 to C. After 10 years, 60% of the patients advanced from Stage A to B_1, 20% progressed from Stage B_2 to C, and the remaining patients expired either of their disease or other causes. At 15 to 21 years after initial documentation of carcinoma in situ, 40% had died from their disease, whereas the remaining 60% had bladder cancer ranging from Stages B_1 to D. These results would suggest that urothelial carcinoma in situ is a biologically aggressive and nonretrogressive disease. Although the carcinoma in situ was not graded in any of these patients, most (72%) appeared to be of low grade. It is only through cytologic studies and random biopsies of the cystoscopically normal urothelium under the most fastidious of cystoscopic conditions and proper pathologic fixation (see methods below) that these early urothelial cancers could be documented.

Text continued on page 65

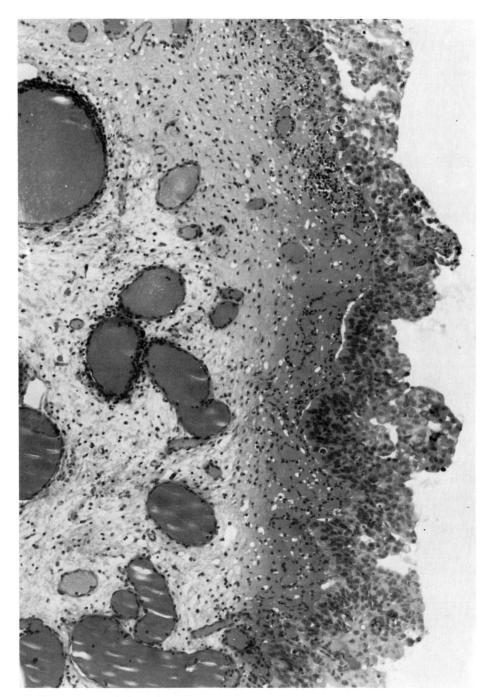

Figure 6–1. Photomicrograph of early bladder cancer. Numerous blood vessels are on the left, and the upper third of the urothelium on the right is normal. The middle third is carcinoma in situ and the beginning of early papillary transitional cell carcinoma because of new blood vessels. The lower third of the urothelium is markedly atypical in the basal layer of cells. (× 160)

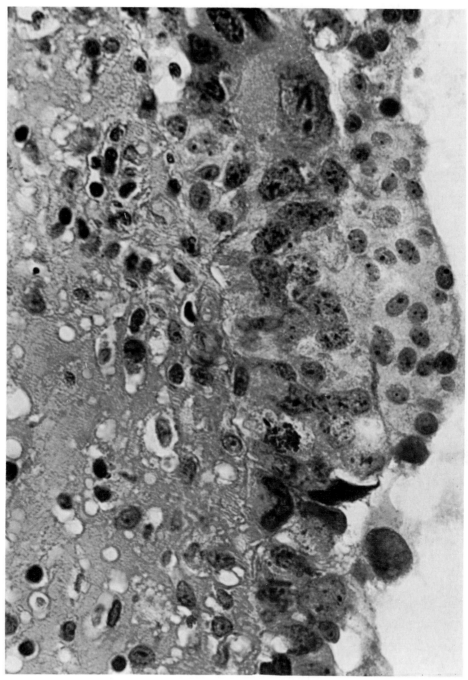

Figure 6–2. Photomicrograph of early carcinoma in situ in which the basal layer of cells is already neoplastic and is covered in part by normal urothelial cells. Note in the upper half of the photomicrograph on the right that the neoplastic nuclei are from three to ten times the size of the normal nuclei. (× 857)

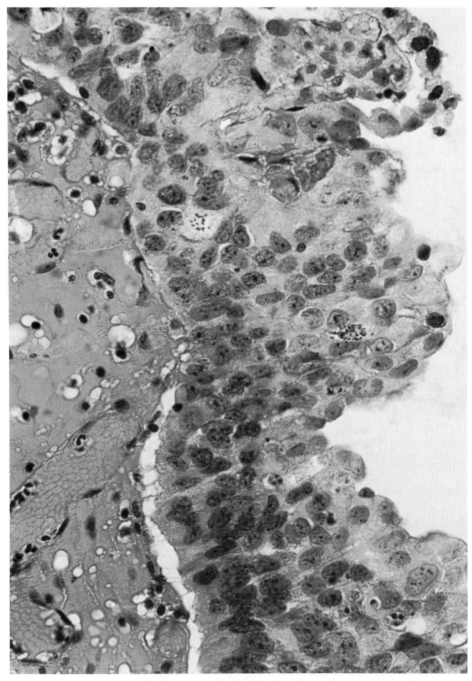

Figure 6–3. Photomicrograph of early papillary tumor in upper half of picture; the lower half of the urothelium is represented by mild urothelial atypia due to abnormality in the basal cells. Notice that the urothelium is beginning to separate from the basement membrane and lamina propria by a hollow space. This specimen was taken with a cystoscopy fluid of distilled water and is a cold punch biopsy. (× 558)

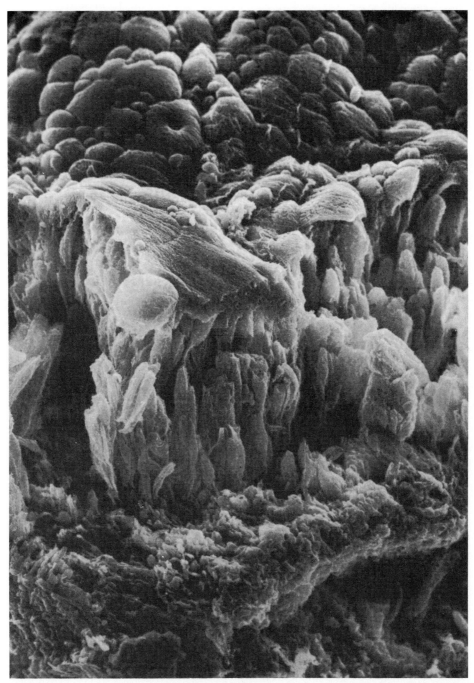

Figure 6–4. Scanning electron micrograph of normal bladder mucosa in which the upper third of the photomicrograph is represented by normal surface cells. The middle third is constituted by intermediary cells, and the lower third by basal cells that are attached to the basement membrane. (× 612)

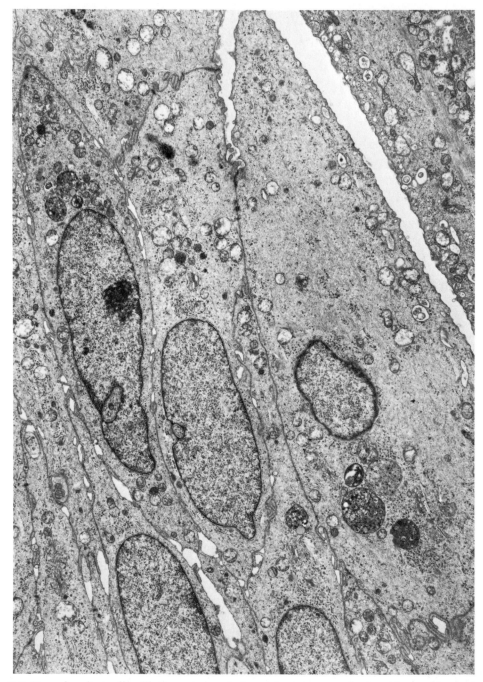

Figure 6–5. Normal surface cells with transmission electron microscopy reveal microridges, subluminal vesicles, fibrillar cytoplasm, and mitochondria. (× 13,000)

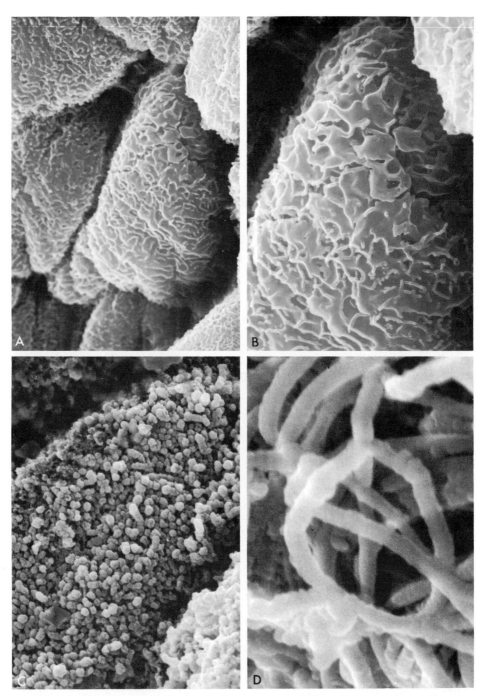

Figure 6–6. Scanning electron micrograph of normal urinary and neoplastic urinary cells. A, Normal urothelial cells with numerous microridges. (× 3200) B, Photomicrograph of a higher power view of one of the cells seen in A. Note the platelike microridges covering the surface of these normal urothelial cells. (× 6600) C, Scanning electron microscopy surface of a malignant urothelial cell. Note that the surface is covered by an almost uniform sea of microvilli. (× 10,000) D, Extreme high power magnification of microvilli in C. (× 50,000) Scanning electron micrograph of neoplastic urothelial cells.

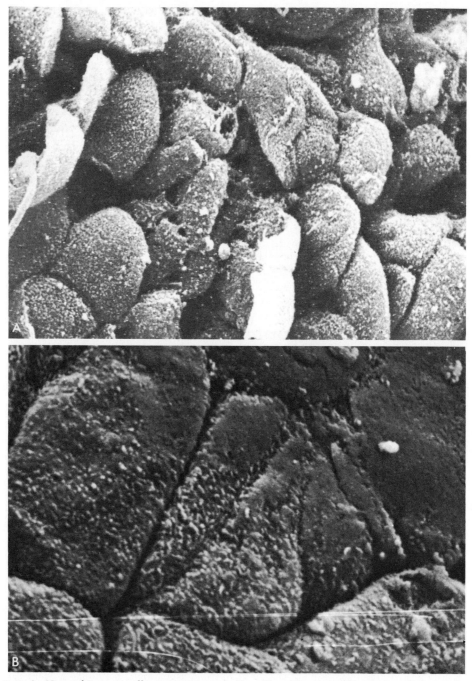

Figure 6–7. A, Note white cap cells covering neoplastic cells with microvilli. Many cellular junctions have disappeared between these cells. (× 1800) B, The surface of these neoplastic cells is partially covered by microvilli, whereas other parts are devoid of them. (× 3400)

Similar morphologic and clinical observations were made in lesions that were detected by positive urinary cytologic results in patients without previous urothelial neoplasms.[5] The evolution of these tumors was similarly found to be considerably longer than had been previously documented.[33]

The greatest incidence of carcinoma in situ appears to be at the lateral and posterior walls above the trigone of the urinary bladder. As a result, random biopsies of the bladder mucosa are now obtained routinely from these sites. If multiple tissue levels are then taken of the areas of carcinoma in situ, a microinvasive urothelial cancer will be found in approximately 30% of the cases. These areas may represent those instances in which the carcinoma in situ is the precursor lesion for those cancers that become deeply invasive without first declaring themselves in an exophytic form.

The natural history of this lesion has yet to be resolved. On the basis of serial biopsies and mapping studies of cystectomy specimens, it is readily recognized that there may be a progression of normal urothelium to flat carcinoma in situ (recognizable cystoscopically as a flat erythematous area) through possible stages of *hyperplasia* and *atypia*.[3, 14–17] Hyperplasia is characterized by an increase in the number of cells in each of the three cellular layers of the urothelium. The intermediary and the basal cell compartments will be more than one cell layer in thickness and will demonstrate an increase in mitotic figures with a normal configuration.

Atypia may also be characterized by an increase in cellular numbers but, in addition, will have varying degrees of pleomorphism of the nuclei. In urothelial atypia or dysplasia, there are also varying degrees of loss of polarity of differentiation of the basal, intermediary, and surface cells of the urothelium. The basal cells do not mature in a normal way into the intermediary cell layer, nor does the latter mature into the surface cells; instead, there are varying degrees of atypical urothelial hyperplasia or dysplasia.

Generally the various histologic features that constitute carcinoma in situ also exemplify those features found in higher grade papillary transitional cell tumors (i.e., Grades 2 or 3). This is seen in the loss of the superficial umbrella cells as well as greater pleomorphism of the nuclei in the remaining layers of the urothelium. Although there appear to be no specific histologic features diagnostic for the early phases of low-grade carcinoma in situ (nonexophytic), several characteristics might be considered for further examination. For example, the vascular pattern in the underlying lamina propria may be a feature providing valuable early histologic identification of a potentially dangerous hyperplastic or atypical urothelium that might progress to carcinoma in situ.[14, 15] The inexorable nature of this sequence has not been well documented. It is anticipated that a combined effort by the urologist and the pathologist will define, with the aid of immunologic and ultrastructural probes, the various pathologic and clinical early stages of urothelial cancer.

Cytology

Although exfoliative urinary cytologic examination is a relatively simple diagnostic tool for following the pathobiologic features of urothelial cancers,[14] for many reasons it has failed to attain wide acceptance as a routine diagnostic laboratory procedure. The principal reason is that most tissue pathologists do not devote sufficient time to urinary cytologic studies; ten years ago it was thought to be unreliable and unnecessary. The now well recognized need to assess the urothelium, and the concomitant importance of the role of urinary cytology in the diagnosis of bladder cancer, has changed this thinking. With many more training programs in urinary cytology, more pathologists provide consistently accurate cytologic diagnoses. A second reason is that some collection procedures may cause spurious results. Although the traditional method for processing voided or catheterized specimens has been to fix each urine specimen with an equal volume of 50% ethyl alcohol, we have found that if alcohol is used, the slides reveal (1) fewer cells adhering to the glass slides; (2) the presence of hemolyzed blood, which obscures the structural elements of the cells; and (3) fewer nuclear and cytoplasmic details. We therefore encourage the collection of a total voided specimen rather than a fractionated one, obtained late in the morning or early afternoon and sent immediately to the cytology laboratory for definitive processing. If this is impossible, we and others refrigerate the specimen overnight and have the cytology laboratory process it early the next morning rather than fix the urine specimens in alcohol.[14] This latter procedure should be used only as a last resort.

If these suggestions are followed, it is common to see, in the practice of urinary cytology, adequate numbers of malignant cells from the urinary tract one to seven years before there is any cystoscopic or radiologic documentation of tumor. Generally it is preferable to send a freshly voided urine specimen for cytologic study before any instrumentation procedures are done, because artifacts can be introduced by various cystoscopy fluids and can be caused by the instruments themselves. Distilled water and even isotonic saline can cause cytologic abnormalities. It should also be noted that one should wait two to three months after any instrumentation procedure before sending another urine specimen to the cytology laboratory. Instrumentation may cause papillary clusters to be dislodged from the prostatic urethra, thereby causing a false-positive cytologic interpretation of urothelial cancer. Instrumentation, like stones, can cause abnormalities in cytologic features because of anaplasia associated with urothelial repair. Other factors that could conceivably influence cytologic interpretation, such as a history of stones, bladder biopsy, chemotherapy, or pelvic radiation, should be reported on the specimen transmittal slip.

In addition to conventional light-microscopic cytologic techniques, other morphologic and immunologic tools have been applied to the study of cells in the urine. Several investigators have used the scanning electron microscope (SEM). This instrument allows examination of the surface of cells that are either shed or brushed off into the urine. It has been noted that the luminal membranes of surface cells in the urinary bladder have a definite microridge pattern, whereas tumor cells do not. Consequently, SEM may reveal *conformational membrane changes* in bladder cells from cytologic washings and brushings and in the urinary exfoliated cells from bladders that contain cancer.[4, 12] The applicability of SEM to the study of cytology in the clinical situation was also investigated by Jacobs, who examined bladder washings from 50 patients.[10] Twenty of these patients had transitional cell carcinoma, and 15 of these had Grade 1 or 2 noninvasive carcinomas that were subsequently treated by transurethral resection (TUR). Of these 15 patients, 12 had cells

with *pleomorphic microvilli* in their SEM cytological preparations. Light-microscopic evaluation of samples from these 15 patients showed only six to be positive for malignant cells, three to be suspect, and six to be negative. This included one case that was positive by light microscopy and negative by SEM, although the biopsy specimens examined by SEM showed that there were pleomorphic microvilli present on the luminal cells. The cells that were positive by light-microscopic cytologic examination were not the same cells that were examined in the SEM. All of these methods have a sampling error. The urine specimen containing cells that permitted the cytologists to call the urine positive for malignancy probably could not provide the additional malignant cells with pleomorphic microvilli for SEM. The other five patients with bladder carcinoma had high-grade lesions, and all of them had cells with pleomorphic microvilli in their cytologic specimens. We also have recently observed pleomorphic microvilli on cells collected by *brushings from bladders of paraplegics* and on many exfoliated urothelial cells, provided they are properly oriented on the slide for SEM (unpublished observation).

In Jacobs's study, sequential cytologic specimens from 12 of the 15 patients with low-grade, low-stage bladder carcinoma contained cells with pleomorphic microvilli.[10] When any patients developed a recurrence, pleomorphic microvilli were present even when the results of light-microscopic cytologic testing were negative or only suggestive of disease. In addition, five patients had cells with pleomorphic microvilli at follow-up examination after TUR, even though cystoscopy did not reveal any evidence of recurrence and light microscopic cytologic results were negative. Although these findings at first were considered to be "false-positive," two of five patients were found to have recurrent disease within one to six months after pleomorphic microvilli were observed by SEM. These conformational membrane changes may be an indication of neoplastic change in the urothelium that can be visualized by SEM even before conventional light-microscopic cytologic methods can reveal them. Twelve other patients in this study with other urinary tract diseases included 10 with bacterial cystitis and two with cyclophosphamide-induced hemorrhagic cystitis. Urine specimens from 18 persons without urinary tract disease were also examined. None of these 30 samples contained cells with pleomorphic microvilli.

These studies are associated with conditions that can cause difficult diagnostic problems in evaluating the urinary cytologic specimen. Squamous cells in the urine also can cause diagnostic difficulties in interpretation. They can be present in such conditions as stones in the urinary system, chronic cervicitis or squamous cell carcinoma of the cervix, trigonitis of the urinary bladder, and associated urinary tract infections; they can also occur as a result of chemotherapy. Suzuki and associates observed squamous cells with pleomorphic microvilli in seven of 40 patients with neoplastic as well as nonneoplastic urinary bladder conditions.[28] In the urinary tract, squamous cells generally originate in the stratified squamous epithelium of the urethra and the trigone region of the bladder, especially in females.[8] Since the specimens in Suzuki's study were from urine obtained by catheterization or bladder washings, the squamous cells presumably originated in the trigone.[28] By cystoscopic examination, four of the six female patients did not have bladder lesions or a history of bladder cancer. However, the other two female patients had evidence in their urine specimens of recurrent papillary transitional cell carcinomas of the bladder as well as transitional cells with pleomorphic microvilli in addition to squamous cells with pleomorphic microvilli. The squamous cells observed by conventional light-microscopic cytologic methods appeared benign. There was slight atypia of some of the transitional cells, but none were considered to be neoplastic by light microscopy. There were no squamous cells with pleomorphic microvilli found in 33 of 40 patients.

It therefore appears that benign squamous cells with pleomorphic microvilli on their surface are occasionally seen in exfoliative cytologic specimens from the urinary bladder.[6, 12] Transitional cells with pleomorphic microvilli, however, seem to be more significant diagnostically or prognostically than squamous cells with pleomorphic microvilli. Therefore, care must be taken to identify the cell types presenting pleomorphic microvilli on their surfaces, so that SEM may have greater clinical usefulness in detecting low-grade flat and papillary transitional cell carcinomas of the lower urinary tract. This is especially important because low-grade lesions cannot be diagnosed effectively by exfoliative cytologic methods using conventional light microscopy. Consequently, additional morphologic or immunologic techniques are required to detect these earlier lesions.

Flow Cytometry and Detection of Bladder Cancer

By means of flow cytometry and specific fluorescent dyes, the various nuclear and cytoplasmic constituents in individual urothelial cells can be analyzed. This method has great clinical potential. Most importantly, a large number of urothelial cells can be assessed in a much shorter time than is needed for routine urinary cytologic techniques. The number of cells to be analyzed from the various cytologic preparations can vary from a few thousand to several hundred thousand, with an average of about 35,000. In addition, the cells that are studied can be from bladder washing, freshly voided urine specimens, or from needle aspirates of various urologic organs.[32]

These methods permit not only assessment of DNA levels of a particular cell population but also examination of the proportion of cells in various phases of the cell cycle. It is also possible to document the percentage of cells that are in the S-phase or chromosomal reduplication phase of the cycle, which is then a reflection of the proliferative potential of the urothelial cell population.

There is considerable evidence that chromosomal studies as well as single cell DNA photometry provide diagnostic value, along with conventional morphologic and clinical assessment of genitourinary tract tumors. The following work, by Tribukait,[32] confirms this impression.*

1. *The DNA histogram can provide clinically useful cytologic information.* In general, experience from various laboratories indicates that it is impossible to distinguish normal urothelial cells from tumor cells that have a small deviation from the normal number of chromosomes. Continuously dividing

---

*The material in this section has been taken from Tribukait B: Flow cytometry in surgical pathology and cytology of tumors of the genitourinary tract. In LG Koss, DV Coleman (eds), Advances in Clinical Cytology, Vol 2. Paris, Masson, 1984, pp 163–189, with permission.

tumor cells follow a cell cycle from one mitosis to the next. That portion of the cell cycle that exists between mitosis (M phase) and chromosomal reduplication phase (S phase) is called G_1 phase. That portion of the cell cycle between the S phase and the M phase is the G_2 phase. An arrest of cells in the G_2 phase results in the appearance of polyploid cells. Consequently, if the urothelial cells in the G_1 peak of the cell cycle deviate less than 10% from the internal standard lymphocyte values, they are considered to be a diploid population. An aneuploid urothelial cell population is discernible if there is, in addition to the G_1 peak, another distinct peak that deviates more than 10% from the internal standard lymphocyte values. Many of the urinary samples have lymphocytes in them, which then serve as an internal control in the flow cytometry measurements. However, more commonly, an aneuploid urothelial cell population occurs with a tetraploid amount of DNA if there is a discernible peak that exceeds by three standard deviations the G_2 + M peak found in normal urothelial cells. The percentage of cells in the various phases of the cell cycle can be calculated by using the simplified method described by Baisch and associates.[2] Cytologic preparations from normal bladder mucosa provided a G_2 + M peak of 3.9% ± 1.3. This amount can be subtracted from the tetraploid G_1 peak when the proportion of cells in the various phases of the cell cycle is calculated.[32]

The S *phase* indicates the number of cells that are in the process of reduplicating their chromosomes in preparation for the mitotic phase, which can be readily recognized by means of light microscopy. The value for the S *phase* of the cell cycle in which there is chromosomal reduplication is only approximate. However, these S-phase values are indicative of the proliferative potential of the neoplastic or normal urothelium.

A DNA histogram of a diploid type is illustrated in Figure 6–8. It is not possible to distinguish a diploid type of urothelial cancer from that of normal urothelium. The large peak at 2c (diploid number of chromosomes) represents G_1 cells with the same DNA content as that in normal lymphocytes. The smaller peak at 4c (tetraploid) represents G_2 + M cells. Between these two peaks is an area where approximately 6% of all the cells present are in the S phase of the cell

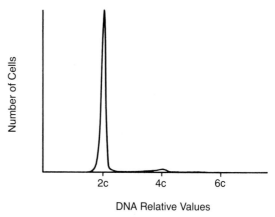

Figure 6–8. DNA histogram from a patient with no urothelial tumor or dysplasia.

cycle. In contrast, Figure 6–9 is an example of the G_1 peak found about 5c of an aneuploid urothelial cell population from a bladder tumor.[32] An aneuploid urothelial cell population contains chromosomal numbers that are more or less than the normal diploid number of chromosomes.

2. *DNA histograms can provide information on newly detected urothelial cancers.* There is a definite relationship between the degree of ploidy, the tumor stage (T categories or Jewett stage), and the tumor grade. The majority of diploid tumors are found to be Stages 0 and A (Ta to T1). Of the aneuploid tumors in Stages 0 to A (Ta to T1), a third were observed to be tetraploid. Tetraploid tumors in Stages B_1, B_2, and C (T2 to T4) were infrequently found; however, multiple aneuploid urothelial cell lines were found in 15% of tumors in Stages 0 to A (Ta to T1) and in 40% of tumors in other stages.

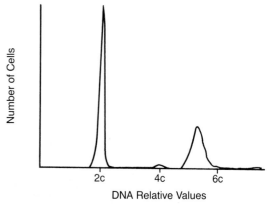

Figure 6–9. DNA histogram from a patient with a Grade 2 aneuploid urothelial tumor.

Thus, there may be several malignant cell lines with various degrees of chromosomal abnormalities present within the same individual tumor. When examined by flow cytometry, tumor (carcinoma) in situ (TIS) was exclusively aneuploid, of nontetraploid type, and often with multiple cell lines. It is possible that diploid and tetraploid types of TIS may also exist. Thus tumors evaluated by flow cytometry can be arranged in the order of increasing grade of malignancy: (1) diploid tumors, (2) tetraploid tumors, (3) nontetraploid aneuploid tumors, and (4) tumors with several aneuploid cell lines within each stage of bladder tumor (Fig. 6–10).[32]

The pattern of ploidy can also be correlated with the grade of the urothelial carcinomas. Most Grade 1 tumors have been found to be diploid. In the large group of Grade 2 tumors, half were diploid and the remainder were aneuploid, either of the tetraploid or the nontetraploid type. Most importantly, 15% of the aneuploid Grade 2 tumors had multiple aneuploid cell lines. The Grade 3 tumors were predominantly aneuploid of the nontetraploid type, with approximately 50% having several aneuploid cell lines.

The degree of ploidy expressed by number of chromosomes of the G_1 peak (the so-called c-value) can be definitely related to the stage of the tumor (Table 6–1). Stage 0 (Ta) tumors were almost entirely diploid. There were a few aneuploid tumors, and they were similar to the Stage A (T1) tumors. These few tumors were either diploid or aneuploid, with the largest number of cases in the tetraploid region. When the aneuploid Stage A (T1) tumors were compared with those of Stage B_2 or C (T3), there was a definitive shift of the Stage B_2 or C to the aneuploid region. Of

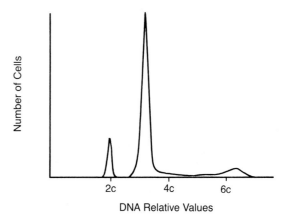

Figure 6–10. DNA histogram from a patient with a Grade 2 urothelial tumor but with several aneuploid cell lines.

the stage B_2 or C (T3) tumors, only one of the 72 aneuploid cell lines was tetraploid, whereas 26 of 85 Stage A (T1) tumors were tetraploid. It thus appears that the DNA pattern or chromosomal composition is highly indicative of a tumor's being superficial or invasive. The Stage B_1 (T2) tumors as a group had characteristics of both the Stage 0 (or TIS) and Stage B_2–C (T3) tumors. The TIS cases that were not associated with exophytic tumors had, by flow cytometry, very similar DNA patterns to Stage C (T3), with values between 3c and 4c. It has been suggested that, because of the similarities between TIS and Stage B–C (T3) tumors, Stage C (T3) tumors might be derived from TIS.[32]

A relationship also appears to exist between the percentage of cells in S phase and the tumor stage and grade. As the stage (T category) increases, the percentage of cells in S phase also increases. Aneuploid tumors in Stage A (T1) are, however, significantly different from aneuploid tumors in Stages C

Table 6–1. FREQUENCY OF DIPLOID AND ANEUPLOID CELL LINES IN UNTREATED BLADDER CARCINOMAS RELATED TO TUMOR STAGE*

Tumor Stage	Diploid	Tetraploid	Aneuploid Nontetraploid	Multiple	Total
Ta, T1	82 (51%)	25 (16%)	40 (25%)	13 (8%)	160 (58%)
T2	2 (8%)	3 (13%)	11 (46%)	8 (33%)	24 (9%)
T3	5 (9%)	1 (2%)	29 (51%)	22 (38%)	57 (20%)
T4		2 (16%)	5 (42%)	5 (42%)	12 (4%)
TIS			11 (46%)	13 (54%)	24 (9%)
Total	89 (32%)	31 (11%)	96 (35%)	61 (22%)	277

*From Tribukait B: Flow cytometry in surgical pathology and cytology of tumors of the genitourinary tract. In LG Koss, DV Coleman (eds), Advances in Clinical Cytology, Vol 2. Paris, Masson, 1984, pp 163–189.

and D (T3–T4). The S phase in half of the aneuploid tumors in Stage A make up less than 10% of all the cells, whereas in the majority of tumors in Stages C and D (T3 and T4), their proportion exceeds 10%. The percentage of cells in S phase in the TIS is slightly lower than that in tumors in Stages C and D (T3 and T4). Diploid tumors have almost the same percentage of cells in S phase as do normal mucosa. In general, superficial tumors have lower S phase value than invasive tumors. Tetraploid tumors have a lower S phase value than do the nontetraploid aneuploid tumors. The lowest percentage of S phase cells has been found in diploid tumors and is slightly higher than in normal mucosa (6.9% ± 0.27 and 4.7% ± 0.22). A linear increase can be seen in the S phase cells with a change in ploidy from tetraploid to triploidy, and also from tetraploidy to higher ploidy levels.[32] The proportion of S phase cells increases to a maximum for tumors that are in 3c. Based on this, it therefore appears that flow cytometry can be applied quite reliably to diagnostic and prognostic evaluation of urothelial cells.[32]

Biopsies of Early Lesions

It is imperative that all biopsy specimens be taken as cold biopsies when there is positive cytologic evidence of cancer or a strong clinical suspicion of bladder cancer that may or may not be visible cystoscopically. This will prevent the possibility of introducing cautery artifact. The cystoscopic fluid should have sufficient osmolarity (osmotic pressure) to permit a proper cytologic and histopathologic evaluation of the cystoscopically normal bladder.[30]

The proper nature of the cystoscopic fluids, however, remains partially unsettled. When a biopsy of the bladder mucosa is obtained with either distilled water or with various buffered glycine solutions, cytologic and architectural distortion can easily be demonstrated (Figs. 6–11 and 6–12). For example, Figure 6–11A shows a carcinoma in situ over an inflamed and vascular stroma. There is an exuberant urothelial proliferation that contains intraepithelial blood vessels. The cytologic characteristics of these cells are further demonstrated to be pleomorphic and anaplastic when compared with cytologically normal cells found in a urothelial inclusion cyst of cystitis cystica

(Fig. 6–11C and D). In these pictures, the nuclei in the carcinoma in situ are two to three times the size of those in normal urothelium. There is intense vacuolization and fine chromatin dispersion in both the neoplastic and normal urothelial cells. This finding is due to the fact that when these biopsy specimens were taken, the osmotic pressure was less than normal (greater than distilled water but less than urine).

Transmission electron microscopy of a similar type of urothelial neoplasm obtained in this manner is seen in Figure 6–12. There is intense vacuolization within the cytoplasm of the cells. The vacuoles are lined by a distinct limiting membrane. The mitochondria have dense bodies in them, which is the sign of irreversible cell damage to the cytoplasmic machinery that generates the energy for repair of various parts of the cell. These features are indicative of the effect of distilled water on the urothelial bladder cells during cystoscopy. When cystoscopy fluids that do not contain distilled water are used, these architectural disturbances do not appear. Another distinctive feature is the disappearance of the normal basement membrane as well as the partial appearance of electron-dense deposits beneath the cells of the carcinoma in situ (Fig. 6–13). Although these electron-dense deposits are reminiscent ultrastructurally of those found in the basement membranes of glomeruli in kidneys with various immune glomerulonephropathies, their significance in the present context is unclear.

When biopsy specimens are not taken as cold cup specimens, cells that are of an inflammatory cell origin can easily be misdiagnosed as tumor. Frequently the tumor cells are so distorted that it is impossible to differentiate a tumor cell from a tissue macrophage or histiocyte. This is especially important when the depth of invasion has to be evaluated. Many squamous cell and urothelial tumors of the urinary bladder exfoliate into the urine not only tumor cells but also histiocytes with nuclei that appear malignant on cytologic screening. In addition, we have noted a crush or cautery artifact which, in many instances, has led to a false diagnostic biopsy. Not only can the urothelial cells that are invading be destroyed beyond recognition but also the multinucleated cells that are present can be distorted so that they are misdiagnosed as tumor cells. These cells are ubiquitous and

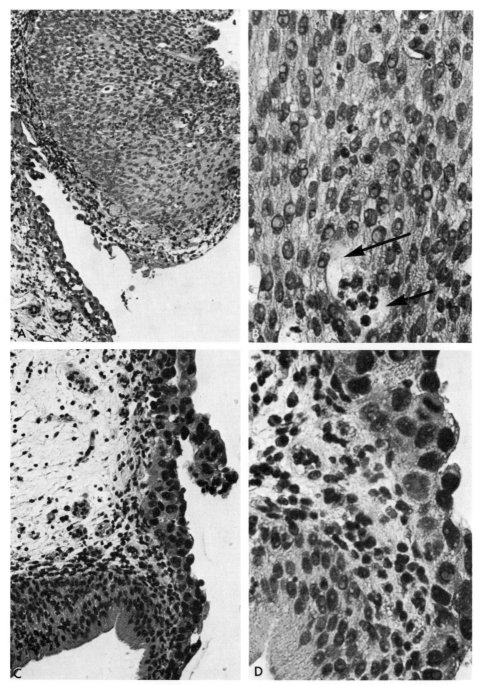

Figure 6–11. A, Light histology photomicrograph of bladder mucosa removed in cystoscopy fluid of glycine. Note epithelial proliferation with small blood vessels in it in upper portion of photomicrograph. Lower portion contains urothelium that is consistent with carcinoma in situ. (× 100) B, Higher power photograph of upper portion of urothelium seen in A. Note small capillaries filled with blood cells scattered throughout urothelium. Nuclei are also vacuolated. (× 428) C, Carcinoma in situ urothelium covering inflamed and edematous lamina propria. Urothelium which is normal lines cystitis cystica in lower portions. (× 175) D, Higher power photomicrograph of C demonstrating increased nuclear size of carcinoma in situ when compared with normal urothelial nuclei in lower portion of picture. Both neoplastic and normal nuclei are partially vacuolated. (× 428)

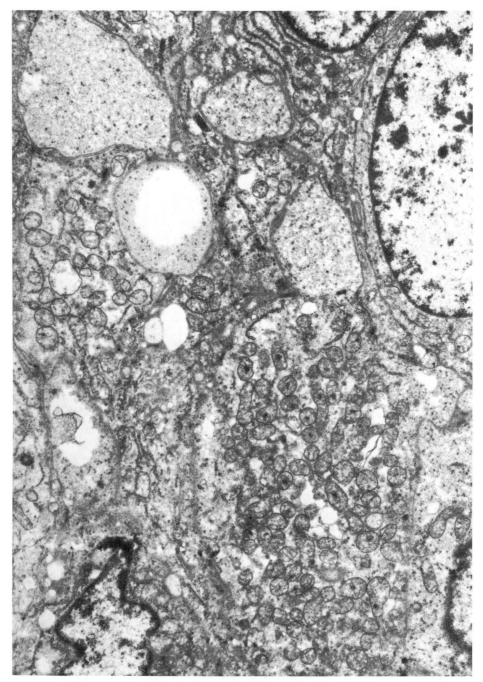

Figure 6–12. Transmission electron micrograph of intermediary cells subjected to a cystoscopy fluid of glycine with an osmotic pressure of 150 mOsm. Note the electron-dense bodies in the mitochondria and the areas of cytoplasmic swelling surrounded by double layered membranes. There is also swelling of the nuclei with some vacuolization of it and the surrounding cytoplasm. ($\times$ 9000)

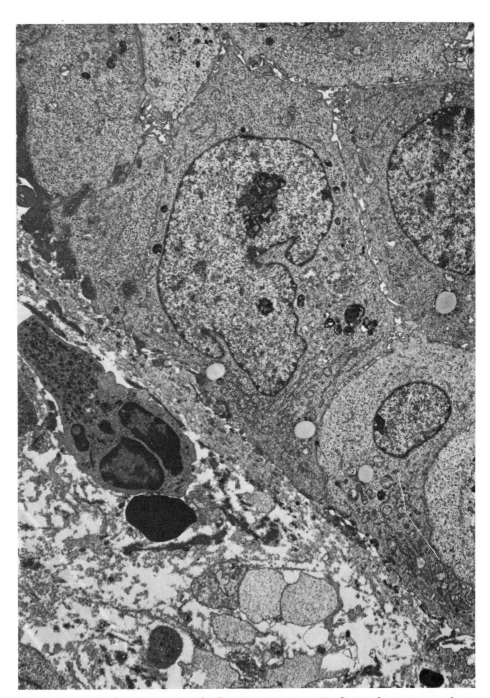

Figure 6–13. Transmission electron micrograph of carcinoma in situ. No distinct basement membrane is noted beneath neoplastic cells that are sending pseudopods into surrounding lamina propria. Note electron-dense material in lamina propria next to these cells on the left side of the picture. There is a polymorphonuclear leukocyte in stroma. Tumor cells have numerous cell connections between them. (× 4500)

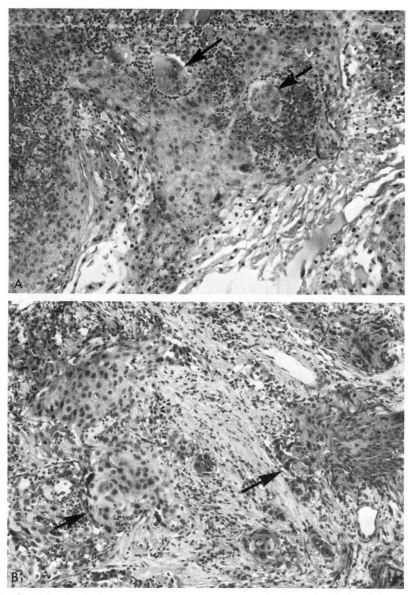

Figure 6–14. A, Photomicrograph showing squamous cells desquamating into lumen of bladder. There are numerous histiocytes (arrows), inflammatory cells, and invading tumor. (× 156) B, Undifferentiated and invading part of exophytic squamous cell tumor. Surrounding individual clusters of tumor are numerous dark cells (arrows). (× 154)

seem to increase in numbers when there have been (1) previous biopsies of the urinary bladder, (2) prior radiotherapy to the bladder, (3) instillation of chemotherapeutic agents into the bladder, and (4) invading tumor.

An example of this can be seen in Figure 6–14A. Extensive squamous cell changes are evident in the urothelium abutting on the lumen of the bladder. In the lamina propria beneath this squamous urothelium are numerous inflammatory cells as well as invading tumor cells and multinucleated giant cells. If the last cells are distorted, they can

easily be misinterpreted as tumor cells, especially when they appear in large numbers, as may occur in many inflammatory processes. On the other hand, the appearance of these cells under the transmission electron microscope is very distinctive and differs from the appearance of invading bladder tumor cells. The syncytium of histiocytes or macrophages has several nuclei and a markedly vacuolated cytoplasm or numerous vesicles that are lined by either a single or a double layer of membranes. The cytoplasm may contain mitochondria, dense bodies, and phagolysosomes, but the Golgi appara-

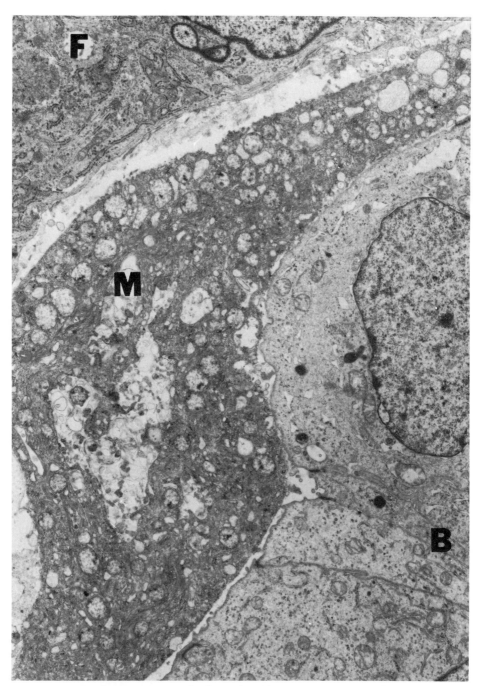

Figure 6–15. Transmission electron micrograph of invading bladder tumor. Dark cell (M) adjacent to bladder tumor cells (B) and fibroblast (F). (× 7500)

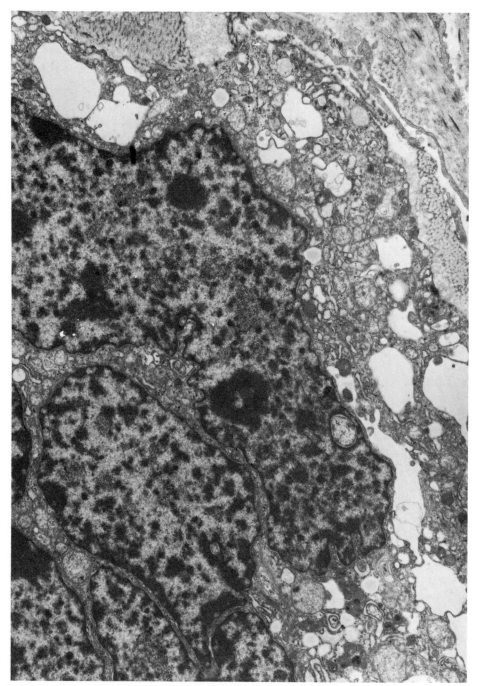

Figure 6–16. Electron micrograph of multinucleated giant cell. This syncytium of histiocytes or macrophages contains at least four nuclei. It is adjacent to collagen at top of picture. (× 7500)

tus in these cells is hard to find (Figs. 6–15, and 6–16). The giant cells are almost always adjacent to collagen and tumor cells, but they do not appear to fuse to them. The nuclei have prominent chromocenters that are sometimes multiple, with margination of some of the chromatin at the nuclear membrane (Fig. 6–16). There are also fine, granular, dense bodies in their nuclei. Sometimes it is almost impossible to distinguish these types of cells from invading tumor cells. If the biopsy material is examined in the best of circumstances, usually it is possible to distinguish these cells from invading tumor cell clusters, especially if the former have cytoplasmic inclusions that are of a foreign body nature. Therefore, it is most important that these biopsies be obtained cold and the bladder cystoscopy fluids be isotonic.

Another variant of these cells appears to be clearly juxtaposed on the epithelial tumor cells and, on light microscopy, can be easily ignored or misdiagnosed as a part of the tumor cell cluster (Fig. 6–14B). Transmission electron microscopy of these clusters reveals that these cells have cytoplasm similar to that of the multinucleated giant cells or histiocytes seen in Figure 6–16. These cells, or macrophages (M), are not attached to the epithelial tumor cells (B) (Fig. 6–15). In contrast, the tumor cells have numerous cell attachments of various sorts, including desmosomes. The macrophages seen in these figures are also found in normal urothelium, but in extremely small numbers.[29] These histiocytes or macrophages are morphologically identical to those found in lymph nodes when there is prominent sinus histiocytosis.

In the evaluation of the first bladder biopsy, grading of the tumor is of paramount importance. However, grading of the same urothelial tumor on different occasions by the same pathologist and by different pathologists has not been consistently reproducible. In one study, 57 transurethrally resected bladder tumors were analyzed to determine whether different pathologists graded the same bladder tumor differently (interindividual consistency) and whether the same pathologist graded a bladder tumor differently at different times (intraindividual consistency).[25] Disturbingly, high interindividual and intraindividual inconsistencies in the grading of bladder tumors were found.

In clinical decision-making, such inconsistencies might invalidate the usefulness of bladder tumor grading. When morphometric grading of bladder tumors was compared with subjective histologic grading of the same tumor by different pathologists, the nuclear sizes of the tumor cells obtained from superficial and deep cell layers of each carcinoma and from giant tumor cells were found to be increased as higher grades of tumor were seen.[26] However, tumors of Grades 1 and 2 showed significant differences only in the size of the large cells. Morphometry may therefore be a valuable tool in the objective grading of bladder tumors. Carcinoma in situ, however, may remain an exception. The measurement of these areas is difficult because there is great variation in the size of the cells as well as their nuclei. It varies greatly from one microscopic field to another that may be just 100 μm away. It also is important that the biopsy material for grading should be as free as possible from crush, cautery, and distilled water artifacts. Fixation in nonbuffered formalin should also be avoided, since this causes marked nuclear distortion. The best fixative is Bouin's solution for reproducible grading of malignant urothelial lesions.

PATHOBIOLOGY OF UNTREATED INVASIVE UROTHELIAL TUMORS

Once the tumor is detected, a variegated pattern of tumor spread is observed. Melicow has worked out a schematic life cycle of untreated tumors of the urinary bladder (Fig. 6–17).[18]

Many of these tumors extend beyond the basement membrane into the lymphatics. Frequently, these solid nonpapillary cancers tend to spread laterally. At the same time, they perforate the submucosa and spread as finger-like projections into the muscularis propria of the bladder. At first, the papillary tumors are exophytic into the urinary bladder lumen and can readily be seen cystoscopically. Both the in situ and exophytic forms of cancer shed cells and thus provide evidence of tumor by means of urinary cytologic tests. The papillary form of tumor also breaks through the basement membrane and invades the lamina propria (Fig. 6–18). However, it is often very difficult to dem-

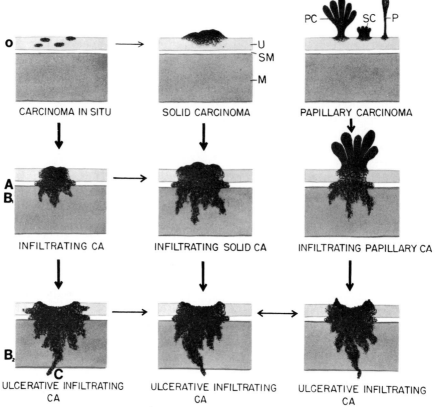

Figure 6–17. *Schematic representation of the natural history of bladder tumors. From Melicow MM: Tumors of the bladder: a multifaceted problem. J Urol 112:467, 1974.*

onstrate direct histologic evidence of invasion from the overlying neoplastic urothelium into the muscularis propria. Melicow noted that almost all types of urothelial tumors eventually become both ulcerated and infected.[18] When the bladder becomes filled with multiple tumors it can be difficult at times to determine whether the tumors were originally solid or papillary. Melicow also noted that with the judicious use of cytologic studies, many of these tumors could be detected before they reached the stages shown in the lower third of the diagram (Fig. 6–17), that is, to Stages B_2 and C. Consequently, they can be detected cytologically in urine at an early stage, as represented in the upper third of the diagram. At all times it is extremely difficult for any pathologist to critically separate the advanced Stage B_1 lesions from the early B_2 lesions. This difficulty is compounded when the specimens are cauterized, making it very difficult to orient the biopsy specimen for proper histologic sectioning.

The topographic distribution and cell types of bladder tumors are seen in Figure 6–19.[18] The majority of bladder tumors (70%) are located on the posterior and lateral walls of the bladder near the ureteral orifices. Most tumors (80%) in this category are papillary with fibrovascular stalks. The remaining 20% are of the solid invasive form with no stalk formation. A varying amount of carcinoma in situ is also found to be associated with these bladder neoplasms. The incidence of carcinoma in situ associated with solid or papillary exophytic lesions may be considerably greater than 3%, but this may depend upon many factors, such as the fixative, the methods of handling the specimen, and whether the pathologist obtains sufficient numbers of histologic sections and spends the time looking for these lesions.

A small proportion (10%) of the tumors are distributed in the dome, and a certain significant percentage of these tumors are seen in the bladder trigone (20%). According

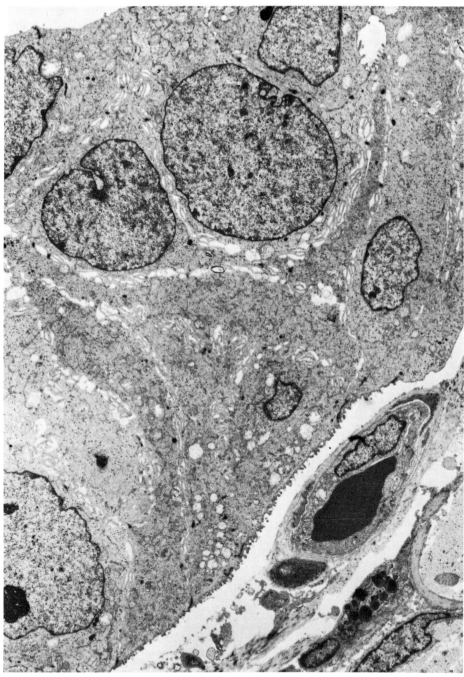

Figure 6–18. Electron micrograph of invading bladder tumor. The lower right hand corner reveals stroma abutting at the advancing edge of the tumor with capillaries and fibroblasts. No basement membrane is noted. The advancing edge of the tumor contains numerous microvilli and tripartite junctional complexes. The luminal surface in the upper left corner does not contain any microvilli. This configuration is a demonstration of reversal of polarity of differentiation. (× 2800)

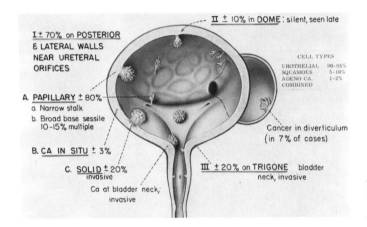

Figure 6–19. Usual sites and shapes of bladder neoplasms. From Melicow MM: Tumors of the bladder: a multifaceted problem. J Urol 112:467, 1974.

to Melicow, the majority of the cell types are urothelial (90 to 95%), with 5 to 10% being squamous cell and the rest adenocarcinoma.[18] However, it is not uncommon to find varying percentages of each of these cell types mixed with the other. The more sections that are taken of these tumors, the greater will be the percentages of different cell type combinations. However, it is rare that all three cell types are found together.

Melicow studied 840 primary vesical tumors over a period of 10 years and showed varying distributions of grades, incidence, age group, and sex (Fig. 6–20). It was noted that 97% of the tumors developed after the patient was over 40 years old and that the greatest incidence occurred between the ages of 50 and 79. The male to female ratio was approximately 3:1. The extremely well differentiated tumors of Grades 1 and 2 reached

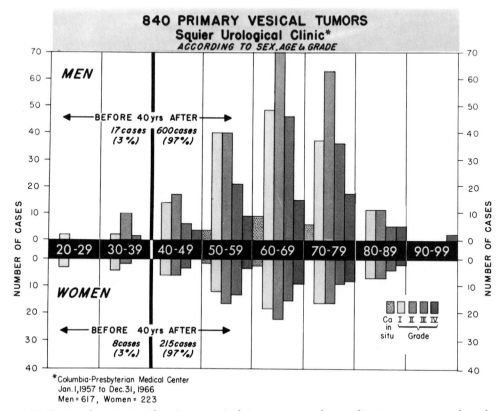

Figure 6–20. Series of patients with primary vesical tumors grouped according to sex, age, and grade. From Melicow MM: Tumors of the bladder: a multifaceted problem. J Urol 112:467, 1974.

a peak incidence within the sixth to seventh decades of life, and then there was a relative decrease within the next decade. Tumors in Grades 3 and 4 were fewer in number but continued to be relatively prominent from the seventh decade on. Melicow also included papillomas with the Grade 1 tumors. Evidence for carcinoma in situ was probably greater than indicated by the dotted columns in Figure 6–20.

SUMMARY

The early detection and clinical characterization of human urothelial tumors can be readily determined by the use of urinary cytologic studies and examination of numerous total freshly voided specimens. The procedure can then be followed by cold punch biopsies examined by light histologic or other techniques, such as immunohistochemical or transmission electron microscopy, to ascertain whether the urothelial cancer cells have already broken through the basement membrane into the lamina propria. Therefore, it is possible to detect these tumors early enough to permit the patient to be rendered cytologically free of tumor by surgical intervention or by chemotherapy. Cytologic examination and flow cytometric determinations can then detect the harbingers of any new accruing tumor.

References

1. Althausen AF, Prout GR Jr, Dal JJ: Non-invasive papillary carcinoma of the bladder associated with carcinoma in situ. J Urol 116:575–580, 1976.
2. Baisch H, Göhde W, Linden WA: Analysis of PCP data to determine the fraction of cells in the various phases of cell cycle. Rad Environ Biophys 12:31–39, 1975.
3. Cooper PH, Waisman J, Johnston WH, Skinner DG: Severe atypia of transitional epithelium and carcinoma of the urinary bladder. Cancer 31:1055–1060, 1973.
4. Domagala W, Kahan AV, Koss LG: The ultrastructure of surfaces of positively identified cells in the human urinary sediment. A correlative light and scanning electron microscopic study. Acta Cytol 23:147–155, 1979.
5. Farrow GM, Utz DC, Rife CC: Morphological and clinical observations of patients with early bladder cancer treated with total cystectomy. Cancer Res 36:2495–2501, 1976.
6. Gilchrist KW, Benson RC Jr, Albrecht RM, et al: Scanning electron microscopy after cytologic examination of urinary cells: lack of diagnostic advantage using combined microscopy. Acta Cytol 26:92–95, 1982.
7. Hoffman CA Jr, Bunts RC: Present urologic status of the World War II paraplegic: fifteen year followup; comparison with status of five year Korean War paraplegic. J Urol 86:60–68, 1961.
8. Holmquist ND: Diagnostic cytology of the urinary tract. In GL Wied (ed), Monographs in Clinical Cytology, Vol 6. New York, S Karger, 1977, p 3.
9. Ionescu G, Romas NA, Ionescu L, et al: Carcinoembryonic antigen and bladder cancer. J Urol 115:46, 1976.
10. Jacobs JB: The potential of scanning electron microscopic (SEM) exfoliative cytology in the clinical management of human cancer. In W Bonney, G Prout (eds), Bladder Cancer, AUA Monograph, Vol 1. Baltimore, Williams & Wilkins, 1982, p 95.
11. Kaufman JM, Fam B, Jacobs SC, et al: Bladder cancer and squamous metaplasia in spinal cord injury patients. J Urol 118:967–971, 1977.
12. Kenermans P, Davina JHM, deHaan RW, et al: Cell surface morphology in epithelial malignancy and its precursor lesion. In O Johari et al (eds), Scanning Electron Microscopy, 1981, Pt III. Chicago, Scanning Electron Microscopy, 1981, p 23.
13. Koss LG: Tumors of the urinary bladder. In Atlas of Tumor Pathology. Second Series, Part II. Washington, DC, Armed Forces Institute of Pathology, 1974.
14. Koss LG: Cytology in the diagnosis of bladder cancer. In EH Cooper, RE Williams (eds), The Biology and Clinical Management of Bladder Cancer. Oxford, Blackwell Scientific, 1975, p 111.
15. Koss LG: Mapping of the urinary bladder: its impact on the concepts of bladder cancer. Hum Pathol 10:533–548, 1979.
16. Koss LG, Nakanishi I, Freed SZ: Nonpapillary carcinoma in situ and atypical hyperplasia in cancerous bladders: further studies of surgically removed bladders by mapping. Urology 9:442–455, 1977.
17. Melamed MR, Voutsa NG, Grabstald H: Natural history and clinical behavior of in situ carcinoma of the human urinary bladder. Cancer 17:1533–1545, 1964.
18. Melicow MM: Tumors of the bladder: a multifaceted problem. J Urol 112:467–478, 1974.
19. Melicow MM: Histological study of vesical urothelium intervening between gross neoplasms in total cystectomy. J Urol 68:261–279, 1952.
20. Melicow MM, Hollowell JW: Intra–urothelial cancer: carcinoma in situ, Bowen's disease of urinary system: discussion of 30 cases. J Urol 68:763–772, 1952.
21. Melzak J: The incidence of bladder cancer in paraplegia. Paraplegia 4:85–96, 1966.
22. Mostofi FK: Pathobiology of malignant tumours of urinary bladder. In EH Cooper, RE Williams (eds), The Biology and Clinical Management of Bladder Cancer. Oxford, Blackwell Scientific, 1975, p 87.
23. Murphy WM, Nagy GK, Rao MK, et al: "Normal" urothelium in patients with bladder cancer: a preliminary report from The National Bladder Cancer Collaborative Group A. Cancer 44:1050–1058, 1979.
24. Murphy WM, Soloway MS: Developing carcinoma (dysplasia) of the urinary bladder. In SC Sommers, PP Rosen (eds), Pathology Annual, Vol 17. New York, Appleton-Century-Crofts, 1982, p 1.
25. Ooms EC, Anderson WA, Alons CL, et al: Analysis of the performance of pathologists in the grading of bladder tumors. Hum Pathol 14:140–143, 1983.
26. Ooms EC, Kurver PH, Veldhuizen RW, et al: Mor-

phometric grading of bladder tumors in comparison with histologic grading by pathologists. Hum Pathol 14:144–150, 1983.

27. Pugh RCB: The pathology of bladder tumors. *In* DM Wallace (ed), Tumours of the Bladder, Vol 2. Edinburgh, Livingstone, 1959, p 116.

28. Suzuki T, St. John M, Cohen SM, Friedell GH: Benign squamous cells with pleomorphic microvilli in urine or bladder washings. Acta Cytol 27:497–499, 1983.

29. Tannenbaum M: Differential diagnosis: invading urothelial tumor cells versus tissue macrophage or histiocyte. Urology 8:273, 1976.

30. Tannenbaum M: Light and electron microscopy of urothelial cancer: carcinoma in situ. Urology 8:498–501, 1976.

31. Tannenbaum M, Romas NA: The pathobiology of early urothelial cancers. *In* DG Skinner, JB de-Kernion (eds), Genitourinary Cancer. Philadelphia, WB Saunders, 1978, p 232.

32. Tribukait B: Flow cytometry in surgical pathology and cytology of tumors of the genitourinary tract. *In* LG Koss, DV Coleman (eds), Advances in Clinical Cytology, Vol 2. Paris, Masson, 1984, pp 163–189.

33. Utz DC, Hanash KA, Farrow GM: The plight of the patient with carcinoma in situ of the bladder. J Urol 103:160–164, 1970.

F. KASH MOSTOFI, M.D.
CHARLES J. DAVIS, JR., M.D. COL., M.C., U.S.A.
ISABELL A. SESTERHENN, M.D.

CHAPTER 7

Pathology of Tumors of the Urinary Tract

TUMORS OF THE BLADDER

Since epithelial tumors of the urinary bladder are the most frequent neoplasms of the urinary tract, since they have by far much greater socioeconomic impact than other neoplasms of the urinary tract, and since these tumors have been more extensively studied, we plan to discuss carcinomas of bladder in great detail and to follow this by a discussion of tumors of urethra, ureters, and renal pelvis.

The urinary bladder is lined by transitional epithelium sometimes referred to as urothelium. The thickness of the epithelial layer depends on whether the viscus-bladder, ureters, and renal pelvis are collapsed or distended. In its collapsed state the epithelium is five to seven layers thick; in the distended state it is two to three cell layers.

The luminal surface is lined by large "umbrella" cells. The configuration of these cells varies from flat to cuboidal, depending on distention or contraction of the bladder. They cover the intermediate and basal layers of transitional epithelial cells. Tannenbaum and colleagues (Chapter 6) have presented the ultrastructure of the epithelial layer. The epithelial layer rests on a thin, delicate basement membrane, the existence of which has been questioned but is demonstrable by electron microscopy. The basement membrane is the first line of defense, and it is the interaction of the epithelium and the base-

ment membrane that determines whether the tumor will have a good or bad prognosis. As long as the basement membrane is intact, the carcinoma is noninvasive and cannot gain access to capillaries and lymphatics.

The lamina propria (sometimes called submucosa) consists of loose fibrovascular tissue which, more or less, blends into the muscularis. The muscularis is arbitrarily divided into superficial and deep layers. Although the distinction between the two is often difficult, many urologists consider it of clinical importance. The muscularis is surrounded by a layer of fibroadipose tissue, and all but the anterior surface is covered by peritoneum. Once there is invasion of perivesical tissue, the prognosis is very grave.

These comments apply equally to renal pelvis, ureters, and urethra.

Criteria for Diagnosis of Carcinoma

Pathologic criteria for diagnosis of carcinoma of bladder have long been controversial. As part of its program of standardization of criteria and nomenclature for tumors, the World Health Organization (WHO) convened a panel of experts* to develop an

*Drs. E. Dahme, M. Gazayerli, A. C. Jain, A. Ljunguist, V. McGovern, F. K. Mostofi, A. M. Pamukcu, R. C. B. Pugh, and H. Usizima.

83

international histologic classification of these tumors.[72] Certain epithelial abnormalities were adopted as evidence of anaplasia: increased cellularity, nuclear crowding, disturbances of cellular polarity, failure of differentiation from the base to the surface, polymorphism, irregularity in the size of cells, variation of shape and chromatin pattern of nuclei, and displaced or abnormal mitotic figures and giant cells. Any cytologic anaplasia as defined was considered as evidence of malignancy. Although the panel recognized that certain inflammatory, reactive, or regenerative conditions may result in the presence of some of these changes, it proposed that diagnosis of carcinoma could and should be made on the basis of such anaplastic changes, even though there was no invasion.

Pathology of Epithelial Tumors

In addition to rendering a diagnosis of carcinoma, the pathologist must provide information on the following important factors:

Growth Pattern. On gross and microscopic examination the tumors can be separated into papillary, infiltrating, papillary and infiltrating, or nonpapillary and noninfiltrating (i.e., carcinoma in situ, CIS) categories. At initial examination, about 70% of tumors are papillary, about 25% are invasive, and 3 to 5% are nonpapillary and noninvasive (CIS). The distinction is valuable because papillary tumors have a better prognosis.

Cell Type. Disagreement exists in the pathologic designation of the cell type. Although it is generally accepted that most of the tumors consist of transitional cells, a number of laboratories label the tumors as epidermoid carcinoma, others as urothelial, and still others as transitional cell carcinoma—a term that we prefer. In practice, carcinoma indicates transitional or urothelial tumor. In the Western Hemisphere, over 90% of tumors are of transitional cell type. About 7% are squamous (in endemic bilharzial areas, nearly 80% are squamous), about 2% are glandular, and about 1% are undifferentiated. A number (20 to 30%) of transitional cell carcinomas show areas of squamous or glandular differentiation, or both. Some pathologists ignore such areas; others refer to them as metaplastic tumors. We prefer to list the components that are present.

We also recognize whether the cells are small or large.

That a number of tumors consist of spindle cell carcinoma or sarcoma of some type has been a source of much pontification. The availability of keratin and epithelial membrane stains resolves the problem. However, it should be remembered that positive keratin stain does not necessarily indicate a carcinoma.

Grade. It has been customary to grade carcinomas of the bladder but, again, no agreement exists as to criteria for grading or the number of grades. Some base grading on differentiation; others, on anaplasia. We prefer to base grading on nuclear anaplasia. Some pathologists use four grades—1, 2, 3, and 4. Some use only three grades, some use seven, and some use four designated 1, 2A, 2B, and 3. Grading on the same slides has been said to vary from 1 to 4.[68] We prefer three grades and code all the grades that are present but consider grading based on current hematoxylin and eosin stains as entirely unsatisfactory since it implies homogeneity of neoplastic cells, which does not exist in fact. Cutler and co-workers[17] have reported that at initial examination 35% of tumors were Grade 1, 35% were Grade 2, and 30% were Grade 3.

The role of grade in recurrence, speed of recurrence, and progression to invasion and metastasis has long been recognized.

Heterogeneity of Cell Population. Prout has called attention to the "extreme heterogeneity" of bladder cancer, considering the grade, stage, multicentricity, recurrence, and various types of therapy.[78] Heterogeneity of cell population in each grade and stage has received scant attention. For example, in grading tumors, some grade according to the most prominent element and some grade according to the most malignant element. Application of modern techniques, especially blood group isoantigens and tumor ploidy, has demonstrated that most tumors have a heterogeneous cell population.

To date, the level at which the presence of the other element, the anaplastic component, affects the behavior is unknown.

Pathologic Staging. Although the two are sometimes confused, pathologic staging is different from clinical staging. Clinical staging is an estimation of depth of infiltration. Pathologic staging is a precise observation of the depth of infiltration as determined by the examination of the tissue.[10, 43, 56, 77, 92]

Cutler and co-workers[17] have recorded that 48% of newly diagnosed tumors were limited to mucosa, 31% had invasion of lamina propria, 2% had invasion of muscularis, and 12% were already outside the bladder.

Pathologic staging and grading are two different measurements, and although there is an 80% correlation between the two, we have seen Grade 1 tumors that were deeply invasive. Secondly, the predictive value of histologic grade within the same tumor stage is weak.[29]

Mode and Location of Spread. The manner in which the carcinoma spreads in the wall of the bladder is often entirely ignored by pathologists. The significance of recognizing and recording these observations is that tentacular types are more aggressive neoplasms, more apt to be incompletely removed, and more apt to invade blood vessels and lymphatics. We recognize four methods of spread. (1) In tentacular types of invasion, the tumor infiltrates in strands, nests, and as individual cells insinuating themselves in between normal structures. This is most often seen in invasive tumors. (2) In cases of *en bloc invasion*, the tumor advances along a broad front. This is seen more frequently in papillary neoplasms. (3) *Lymphatic or vascular invasion*, especially in tissue removed by cautery, is often difficult to recognize, since shrinkage of carcinoma cells following cautery may create a false space around the cell nests. It should be emphasized that although tumors with muscle invasion show a 40% frequency of lymphatic and vascular invasion, 7 to 10% of superficial tumors also show such invasion.[44] (4) *Intraepithelial spread* also occurs and will be discussed later.

Tumor Recurrence. Bladder tumors have a remarkable propensity for recurrence,[84, 88] which is most often seen in the bladder in the original tumor site or elsewhere; however, it may occur in some other area in the urinary tract. Recurrence in the original site would indicate incomplete removal of the initial tumor. Factors that may contribute to this are the presence of tentacular invasion, resulting in incomplete removal of the tumor, and failure to histologically recognize premalignant lesions and CIS in cystoscopically normal mucosal margins of the excised specimen, especially in transurethral resection (TUR) tissue. Tumor recurrence, sometimes referred to as occurrence, elsewhere in the bladder is more frequent in the dome but it may be seen in the lateral, anterior, or posterior walls. Recurrence is less frequent in patients who had no prior tumor. Forty-nine per cent of patients with no prior tumor showed recurrence, compared with 66.7% of those with prior tumors.[88] The median time to first recurrence was 31 months from successful treatment of the first recurrence to the diagnosis of the second. From the second to third recurrence the interval was 12 months.[17]

Recurrence elsewhere in the urinary tract will be discussed later.

Two mechanisms have been proposed to explain the frequency of recurrence. Since the entire urinary tract is covered by transitional epithelium, circulating carcinogenic agents may affect one or more sites synchronously or consequently. The bladder is constantly exposed to urine, which may contain carcinogenic agents and affect different parts of the vesical mucosa at different times. In this situation, recurrence is a manifestation of the field effect of carcinogenic agents. The second hypothesis is that recurrence is the result of seeding of viable tumor cells. Implantation of syngeneic tumor cells in traumatized or inflamed mouse bladder[95] lends experimental support to this hypothesis. It is also conceivable that when the bladder is emptied after surgery, the contracted epithelial layer entraps some of the floating viable tumor cells and they may grow. We believe that probably both factors—field effect and seeding—may be present in recurrence.

The role of chromosomes in detection of potentiality of recurrence is discussed later.

Inflammatory Cell Infiltrate in the Tumor. Lymphoplasmocytic infiltration of lamina propria adjacent to a tumor is not an uncommon finding. Rarely, a bladder tumor is associated with monocytic and lymphoplasmocytic cells that surround and infiltrate the tumor to such an extent as to mask the neoplastic cells. Such inflammatory cell infiltrate seems to result in good prognosis.

Status of the Adjacent Mucosa. Urologists generally remove "adequate margin," but many pathologists tend to ignore the adjacent mucosa. The tissue at the margins and the random biopsies that are now being taken show proliferative and papillary cystitis, atypia, "dysplasia," hyperplasia, and carcinoma in situ. Althausen and co-workers reported that the presence of atypical cells at the margins of superficial tumors was associated with eventual progression to cancer in 36% of cases and, when CIS was reported, the frequency rose to 83%, compared with 7% when the epithelium was normal.[2] Atypical cells in random biopsies from endoscopically normal mucosa have been associated with a higher rate of recurrence.[94, 111] On the other hand, the Cutler group found no consistent predictive pattern for cancer development in atypia of random biopsies.[17] We believe all such changes are indicative of sick, agitated mucosa and should be reported.

Transmission (TEM) and Scanning (SEM) Electron Microscopy. These techniques, discussed elsewhere in this book (Chapter 6), are helpful primarily in recognition of malignant cells but also in prognosis.[1, 39, 75] By TEM the luminal side of the umbrella cells consist of an asymmetrical unit membrane. In carcinomas the density of desmosomes is significantly reduced in the plasma membrane. However, the amount of cell surface occupied by desmosomes is greater in carcinomas than in controls. Desmosomes are abundant in invading nests of tumor cells.[1, 75] On SEM examination, the umbrella cells show a pavement-like arrangement with microridges covering the surface. Small bleb-like microvilli are present along all cell junctions. In carcinoma the asymmetrical membrane unit is lost. The pavement-like arrangement is replaced by a cobblestone appearance of round cells of varying sizes. The microridges are replaced by irregular microvilli of varying sizes (villous transformation).

The number of cell junctions has been correlated with the behavior of tumor cells. Pleomorphic microvilli were present in tumor cells in all cases regardless of grade or stage of the tumor, but the degree of pleomorphism of the microvilli and the cells tend to increase with the grade of the tumor.[42]

TEM is not very practical because it requires special fixation, but SEM can easily be done in formalin-fixed, paraffin-embedded tissues.

Transitional Cell Tumors

There are many systems of pathologic classification of bladder tumors. The classification in use in the Bladder Tumor Registry is presented in Table 7–1.

Table 7–1. EPITHELIAL TUMORS OF THE BLADDER

Transitional Cell Tumors
Superficial Tumors
Inverted papilloma
Papilloma
Papillary noninfiltrating tumors
Papillary carcinomas with invasion of lamina propria
Carcinoma in situ of any grade (noninfiltrating)

Infiltrating Tumors
Papillary and infiltrating carcinomas
Sessile nodular infiltrating carcinomas

Nontransitional Cell Carcinomas
(May be superficial, papillary, in situ, and/or infiltrating carcinomas)

Squamous Carcinomas

Adenocarcinomas
Primary vesical
Urachal
Exstrophy
Mesonephric
Metastatic

Undifferentiated Carcinomas

Carcinomas With More Than One Histologic Type
(Specify cell types and growth pattern)

Superficial Epithelial Tumors

This category includes inverted papilloma, papilloma, papillary noninfiltrating tumors (pTa), papillary tumors with invasion of lamina propria but not beyond (A, PT1), and nonpapillary, noninfiltrating tumors (CIS, TIS, PIS).

Inverted Papilloma
(Fig. 7–1)
Grossly, the tumor may be pedunculated or sessile with a smooth, nonpapillary surface. Microscopically, the characteristic feature of inverted papilloma is that the surface is covered by a continuous layer of normal, thin or thick benign transitional epithelium. The tumor consists of anastomosing cords and sheets of transitional epithelium. Some areas may show glandular and squamous differentiation and even mucin production. Mitotic figures and giant cells are rare. The adjoining mucosa shows varying numbers of Brunn's nests.

Inverted papilloma is benign. However, at times it may be associated with a carcinoma.

Papillary Noninfiltrating Tumors
Incidence. Papillary tumors constitute about 75% of primary epithelial tumors of the bladder.

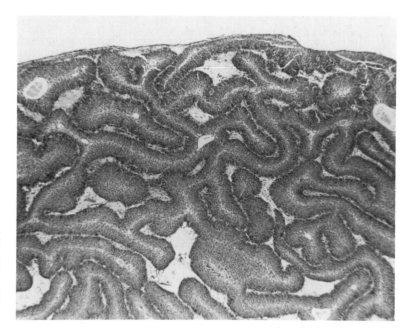

Figure 7–1. Inverted papilloma. The surface is covered by a continuous layer of thin transitional epithelium. The tumor is made up of anastomosing cords and sheets of transitional epithelium, Brunn's nests, and cystitis cystica. (AFIP Neg. 86-46, H & E, × 40)

Pathology. The cystoscopic and gross appearances of these tumors are characteristic. They are red, sea anemone–like structures attached to a fibrovascular stalk. There may be secondary and tertiary stalks.

Papillary tumors may be single or multiple, confined to one area or distributed over several areas, or, rarely, diffusely involving the entire mucosa (diffuse papillomatosis); they may be large in height or width, and they may have a broad or narrow base. Tumors larger than 2.5 cm in diameter have generally been considered to have a less favorable prognosis. Larger tumors appear to be more frequently accompanied by changes in the adjoining mucosa than do the smaller ones.

The most common sites are the lateral walls and the trigone. The most frequent age groups manifesting papillary tumors are those in the sixth and seventh decades of life.

Categories. Papillary tumors may be classified as papilloma or papillary carcinoma. The distinction between the two, especially when the latter is of a low grade of malignancy (Grade 1) has been controversial. Some centers have diagnosed all papillary tumors as carcinoma; others have tended to call them papillary tumors; still others have designated all papillary noninfiltrating tumors as papilloma. We distinguish between papilloma and papillary carcinoma.

Papilloma
(Fig. 7–2)

Definition. The WHO Scientific Advisory Panel on Bladder Tumors recommended that the diagnosis of papilloma be reserved for papillary tumors covered by epithelium that is indistinguishable from normal vesical mucosa, is not more than six layers in thickness, and has normal maturation of the cells from the base to the surface. They also recommended that papilloma should not be characterized as benign since a significant number of these tumors are followed by carcinoma.[72] Defined as such, papilloma makes up 3% of all bladder tumors.

Clinical Course. Patients in whom the diagnosis of papilloma is made have a good prognosis. Miller and associates found no recurrence in 26 patients followed for five years.[65] In 138 patients with papilloma, Marshall reported 50% recurrence after five years, histologic carcinoma in 17, and five-year survival in 79%.[57] In 35 patients, Nichols and Marshall reported 60% recurrence in five years and 85% five-year survival.[73] Marshall and McCarron[58] reported that between 1960 and 1971 they saw 203 patients with papillomas and there was a five-year survival of 64%—considerably lower than that reported by Beall and Marshall[57] from the same institution. The incidence of carcinoma was about the same in both groups, 14% and 17%. The reasons for increased

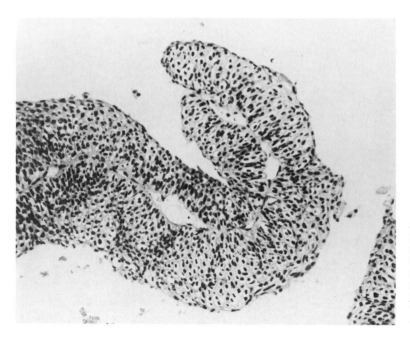

Figure 7–2. *Transitional cell papilloma. The papillary tumor is covered by a layer of transitional epithelium that is five to seven layers thick and resembles normal bladder mucosa. The fronds consist of delicate fibrovascular stroma. (AFIP Neg. 86-47, H & E, × 160)*

mortality were not apparent. In 321 patients with papillomas, Pyrah and colleagues reported 69% recurrence in three years and progression into carcinoma in about 10%.[80] The survival rate was 85%. In 125 patients, Lerman and co-workers showed that single tumors had a 31% five-year recurrence, whereas multiple lesions had a 66% recurrence, giving an overall recurrence rate of 47%.[53] In 74 patients whom they followed, 9.6% developed carcinoma and 88% survived. Olsson and White have reported a recurrence rate of 47% and development of carcinoma in 10%.[74] It must be noted that, as mentioned above, in these reports the designation of papilloma has been used for a variety of lesions.

In summary, about half of all papillomas recur and some may progress to carcinoma, but papillomas are not fatal. In fact, many are discovered incidentally in patients having other neoplasias, and recurrences are treated by simple cautery.

Papillary Carcinomas
(Figs. 7–3 to 7–7)

Definition. Papillary carcinoma is a papillary tumor covered by a layer of transitional epithelium demonstrating varying degrees of anaplasia as defined by WHO.[57] The number of cell layers is usually, but not invariably, more than seven, and the stroma is delicately fibrovascular.

Pathology. The tumor is recognizable as transitional cell carcinoma. The papillae are covered by eight to 10 layers of epithelium. Three grades are recognized, based on nuclear anaplasia. Those with slight anaplasia, constituting 70 to 75% of tumors, are Grade 1. Those with moderate anaplasia, constituting about 20% of tumors, are classified as Grade 2. They are also still readily recognizable as transitional cell carcinoma. Koss has identified five variants: (1) the small cell variant, composed of densely packed, small hyperchromatic cells; (2) a variant with columnar and spindle cells; (3) a variant with a rosette-like arrangement of cells; (4) a clear cell variant; and (5) a spindle cell variant.[48] The rare Grade 3 papillary carcinomas show marked anaplasia. Friedell has reported 10 cases in 348 patients with transitional cell carcinoma.[30]

Categories. In all papillary carcinomas we try to determine whether the basement membrane has been broken through or not and, if it has, the depth of invasion. Jewett and Eversole have emphasized the significance of the distinction that there are no lymphatics in the epithelial layer—lymphatics are in the lamina propria and muscularis.[43] Vascular and lymphatic invasion can occur only after invasion of lamina propria. With few exceptions, Grade 1 papillary carcinomas are initially noninvasive or invade only the lamina propria. About half of Grade 2 carcinomas are initially invasive of lamina propria

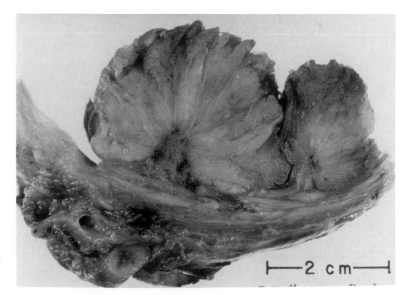

Figure 7–3. Papillary carcinoma (transitional cell). Section of the bladder shows two large arborescent tumors. (AFIP Neg. 86-53)

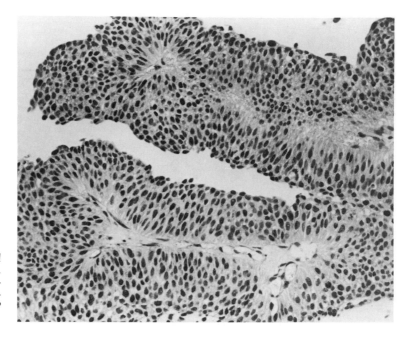

Figure 7–4. Transitional cell carcinoma, Grade 1, papillary. The epithelium shows slight anaplasia and failure of maturation from base to surface. (AFIP Neg. 86-48, H & E, × 160)

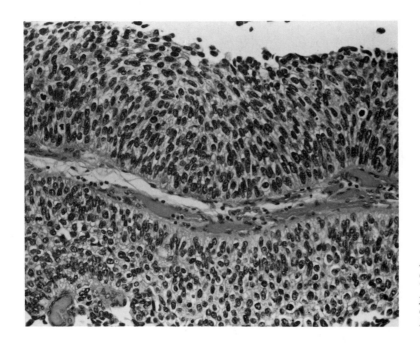

Figure 7–5. Transitional cell carcinoma, Grade 2, papillary. There is moderate anaplasia and failure of differentiation. Note condensation of nuclei. (AFIP Neg. 86-49, H & E, × 160)

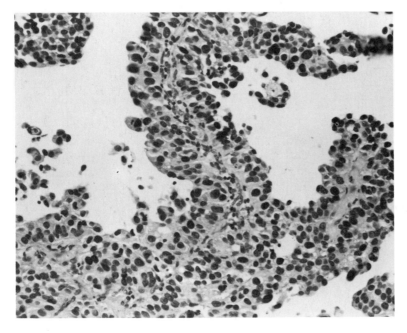

Figure 7–6. Transitional cell carcinoma, Grade 3, papillary. There is marked anaplasia of the cells and loss of cohesiveness. (AFIP Neg. 86-50, H & E, × 160)

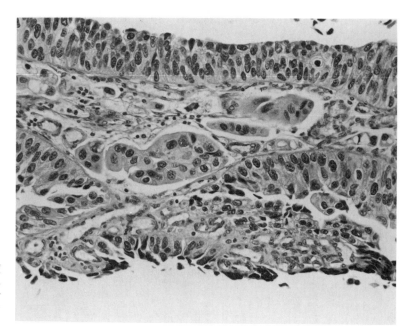

Figure 7–7. *Transitional cell carcinoma, Grade 2, papillary, with invasion of stalk of a papillary frond and vascular spaces. (AFIP Neg. 86-51, H & E, × 160)*

and, later, of superficial muscle. The invasive tumors usually originate as invasive neoplasms but may develop in a papillary carcinoma. It must be emphasized that lymphatic and vascular invasion occurs in 7 to 10% of these papillary (P_1 and P_2) tumors.

Clinical Course. The course of papillary carcinomas is that many of them recur, with the rate of recurrence higher in Grade 2 tumors. Multiple or large tumors have a higher risk of recurrence than do single or small tumors. They may also become more anaplastic. Melicow has reported a 75% recurrence, with the majority tending toward anaplasia.[63] Mostofi reported 46% recurrence in five years, 65% in 10, and 81% in 15 years.[66]

Although the tumors recur, they tend to remain essentially localized; only 20% progress to infiltrating tumors, but it is possible that even some of these started as papillary and infiltrating tumors. About 10% invade lymphatics and 17% metastasize; these occur only in tumors that have invaded the lamina propria.

The course of these tumors, as of all bladder tumors, is complicated by multicentricity, aggressive potential of the cell, existence of preneoplastic changes and CIS elsewhere in the bladder, and iatrogenic seeding that may occur when the tumor is resected transurethrally. These have been or will be discussed elsewhere.

Nonpapillary, Noninfiltrating Tumors (Carcinoma in Situ, CIS)

(Figs. 7–8 to 7–12)

Definition. CIS may be defined as anaplasia of surface epithelium and Brunn's nests of varying grades but nonpapillary and noninfiltrating. This definition is at variance with that of Friedell[30] and Cohen and associates[12] in several points. These authors have restricted CIS to flat lesions with marked anaplasia involving the entire thickness of the mucosa and have categorized all other alterations as dysplasia. Secondly, Friedell has used CIS to define papillary, noninfiltrating tumors of any grade.[31]

Since the existence of Grade 1 and Grade 2 papillary and infiltrating vesical carcinomas is universally recognized, limiting the diagnosis of CIS only to Grade 3 lesions seems inconsistent, especially since at least 30% of atypias and dysplasias progress to carcinoma. We believe the same criteria that are applied to papillary and infiltrating tumors should be applied to flat lesions. These include variations in size, shape, and staining of nuclei; the presence of nucleoli; failure of maturation from the base to the surface; crowding of nuclei; and presence of mitotic figures in other than the basal layer. These changes may be slight, moderate, or marked. In accordance with these criteria, we grade our in situ carcinomas by a procedure that has been used by the Mayo

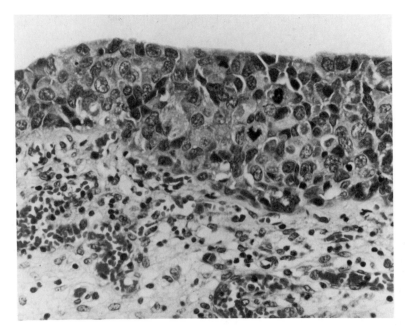

Figure 7–8. Transitional cell carcinoma, Grade 3, in situ. There is marked anaplasia involving the full thickness of epithelial layers. Note misplaced mitotic figures. (AFIP Neg. 86-52, H & E, × 160)

Clinic for many years (Farrow, personal communication). In practice we tend to limit the diagnosis of CIS Grade 1 to flat lesions accompanying papillary or infiltrating carcinoma, or both, if the histologic features of the flat mucosal changes are identical to that of the tumor. For Grades 2 and 3 CIS we apply the same criteria that we do for frank carcinomas. Many pathologists, however, do not grade CIS; some use the term "high grade."

A second and more serious risk in the use of the term "dysplasia" is that the patient is misled to believe that he has nothing to worry about. We have seen several such patients who have returned four to five years later with invasive and metastatic tumors.

Categories. There are two categories of CIS: (1) those seen in association with clinical carcinoma of bladder that may be found simultaneously with initial diagnosis of carcinoma or sequentially during follow-up of

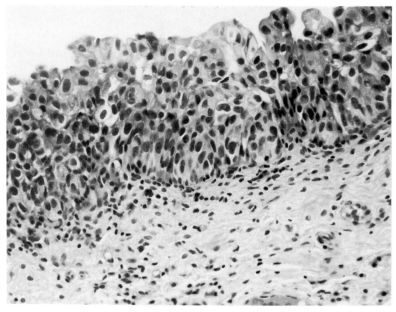

Figure 7–9. Transitional cell carcinoma, Grade 2, in situ. There is moderate anaplasia of the epithelium. (AFIP Neg. 86-53, H & E, × 250)

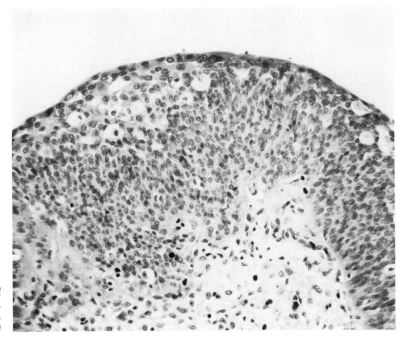

Figure 7–10. Transitional cell carcinoma, Grade 1, in situ. There is slight anaplasia of cells. (AFIP Neg. 86-54, H & E, × 250)

the patients treated for carcinoma of the bladder, and (2) those that occur initially and de novo. Melicow was the first to call attention to the neoplastic changes in the mucosa adjoining frank carcinoma.[63] Eisenberg and co-workers found "proliferative lesions" in 60% of patients with infiltrating carcinoma and in 20% of those with papillary tumors.[23] Schade and Swinney found

"atypia" in 86% of 100 patients with carcinoma of bladder severe enough in 40% to justify the diagnosis of CIS.[87] Groups headed by Cooper[15] and Skinner[92] have reported incidences ranging from 33 to 100%, depending on the degree of anaplasia of the associated carcinoma. Friedell,[30] Koss and associates,[50] and Farrow,[27] by study of total bladders of patients with frank carcinoma,

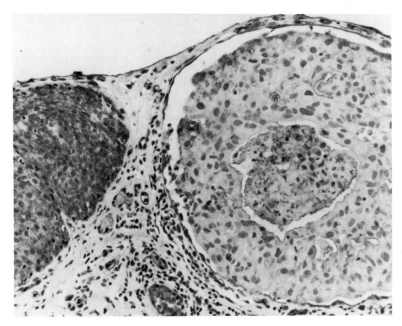

Figure 7–11. Transitional cell carcinoma, Grade 2, in situ, involving Brunn's nests. (AFIP Neg. 86-56, H & E, × 250)

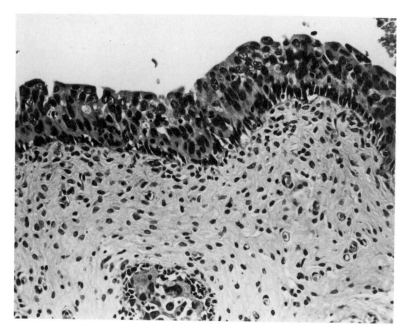

Figure 7–12. Transitional cell carcinoma, Grade 2, in situ, with invasion of lymphatics. The surface epithelium, viewed by itself, would be categorized by some pathologists as dysplasia. (AFIP Neg. 86-69, H & E, × 250)

have reported abnormality of varying degrees in almost every patient. Many pathologists tend to ignore such mucosal changes. Recognition and reporting of these mucosal changes at the margins of frank carcinomas will alert the urologists to the probability of incomplete removal of the neoplastic and preneoplastic lesions and lead to the proper management of the patient. Such patients are at high risk, and, if left alone, may manifest carcinoma of bladder many years later.

Carcinoma in situ may also be encountered in the follow-up biopsy of patients who have been treated for carcinoma of the bladder. In such patients it is essential to compare the biopsy results to the previous cancer and, if the histologic findings are identical, to diagnose the lesion as carcinoma and not dismiss it as atypia and dysplasia. In fact, any abnormality of the epithelium should be reported, as there definitely is a high incidence of carcinoma in such patients.

In the second group, noted above, the initial CIS is discovered usually by cytologic or biopsy examination of a patient with irritative bladder symptoms or in an asymptomatic patient in whom hematuria is either observed or found incidentally. This category may also be seen in individuals who are at risk because of prolonged exposure to carcinogenic agents. In the course of screen-

ing 35,000 patients with urine cytologic examinations, Farrow and colleagues found 106 patients who had no cystoscopically visible bladder tumor.[27, 28] Sixty-nine were proved by biopsy to have CIS—all were transitional and anaplastic. In 503 men who had been exposed to vesical carcinogenic substances, Koss and co-workers found 13 cases of CIS.[49]

Cystoscopy may show nothing, some thickening, or an erythematous and swollen mucosa but no frank carcinoma. Ultraviolet fluorescence is not helpful.[61]

Although CIS is more often seen in the trigone and the ureteral orifices and the lesion may be focal, more often it is a diffuse process involving 50 to 85% of the bladder, indicating a field effect.

In most instances positive cytologic findings lead to the diagnosis of CIS. Such findings are seen more frequently in Grade 3 CIS than in Grade 2. Patients whose CIS has been downgraded because of chemotherapy are at risk because negative cytologic results may mislead to a false sense of security.

Pathology. We recognize several growth patterns in CIS. In the *first* the entire thickness of the mucosa is involved, and the growth may be generalized or localized. In the *second* form the neoplastic change may be confined to the basal layers of the epithelium, pushing up the normal mucosa and eventually sloughing off of the benign surface epithelium, leaving two layers of neoplastic cells. The *third* form is a pagetoid appearance with clusters of distinct malignant epithelial cells scattered amidst apparently benign epithelium. A *fourth* form is neoplasia involving the surface layers with the subjacent epithelium appearing benign. Whether these represent variable manifestations of the response of the epithelium to carcinogenesis or indicate intraepithelial spread of CIS has not been resolved.

Carcinoma in situ may involve not only the surface layer but also Brunn's nests and cells of cystitis cystica. These changes may be seen in tissues with denuded or intact surface epithelium, and recognition of abnormalities is important in denuded areas.

Most CIS consists of transitional epithelium. A few examples may be squamous, and since many of these are well differentiated, the diagnosis of CIS may be difficult; however, slight to moderate anaplasia should be looked for. The diagnosis of in situ adenocarcinoma is often difficult for these are usually well differentiated neoplasms.

An important feature of CIS Grade 3 and sometimes of Grade 2 is the tendency of the epithelial layer to have lost its cohesiveness, resulting in positive cytologic findings. Biopsy in such cases may show a denuded surface, a thin layer of anaplastic basal cells regarded as undiagnosable by some pathologists. Severe congestion and edema of the lamina propria and lymphoplasmocytic infiltration are almost invariably present and lead to the erroneous diagnosis of cystitis. Occasionally, although often overlooked, a Brunn's nest that may or may not show cellular anaplasia may be seen.

In summary, we limit the diagnosis of CIS to flat lesions, and we diagnose as CIS lesions that show varying degrees of anaplasia that may or may not involve the entire thickness of the epithelial layer.

Clinical Course. Information relative to the course of CIS is quite confusing. The two categories of CIS as defined above have not been separated from each other. Another difficulty stems from the fact that since the initial reports of CIS were in follow-up of patients with frank carcinoma, and the course of the disease was unfavorable, it had been customary to do an immediate total cystectomy on every patient on whom CIS was diagnosed, irrespective of whether it was an initial CIS or one that followed a frank carcinoma. Third, since CIS of low grade of anaplasia has not been recognized, the available information is based mostly on the experience with Grade 3 or high-grade in situ carcinomas. Fourth, the distinction between symptomatic and asymptomatic CIS, focal and diffuse CIS, and those that involve the bladder neck has not been observed.

Melamed and associates reported 25 patients with flat CIS, 24 of whom had prior tumors.[60] In 12 of these treated with resection and radiation but not cystectomy, nine progressed to invasive carcinoma.

In 503 patients exposed to a carcinogen, Koss and co-workers[49] and Melamed and associates[59] found 13 with CIS. These patients had a period of negative cytologic results that lasted from several months to eight years. After the diagnosis of CIS was made, seven of the 13 who had developed positive cytologic test results progressed into invasive carcinoma.

Tannenbaum and co-workers reported 140 cases of CIS with follow-up periods of 14 to 21 years.[98] None of these patients had prior carcinoma. The details are given elsewhere; suffice it to say that examination at intervals of 14 to 21 years after their initial documentation of CIS revealed that 40% of these patients had died from their disease and the remaining majority were classified as having tumors in Stages B_2 to D.

Utz and colleagues recorded that from January 1, 1950, through December 31, 1963, about 2300 new patients with carcinoma of bladder were admitted to Mayo Clinic.[102] On initial biopsy, 62 had CIS. In 12 of these there had been an earlier diagnosis of carcinoma of bladder. Recurrence after treatment in 82% was accompanied by deterioration in grade in 52% and by infiltration in 73%.

Yates-Bell[112] reported that three of five patients progressed to invasive carcinoma, and Barlebo and associates noted three patients, one who developed invasive carcinoma, one who persisted with CIS, and one who was disease-free.[4] Anderson reported 15 patients with CIS, 12 of whom developed invasive carcinoma in three years.[3]

Riddle found that nine of 12 patients with symptomatic and extensive CIS had invasion of lamina propria.[82] Of 11 patients treated with radiation alone, only one survived 18 months. Daly observed that 11 of 18 patients who had positive cytologic test results and no cystoscopic evidence of tumor subsequently developed overt invasive carcinoma after an average interval of 19 months.[18] Cytologic findings in six others were later classified as doubtful or negative.

Farrow and co-workers found that 17 of the 21 patients in whom cytologic diagnosis of carcinoma was made without cystoscopic evidence had CIS of moderate to high degree of anaplasia.[27] In four, microinvasion was already present, and step sectioning demonstrated widespread mucosal involvement. Extension to the prostatic duct was found in seven of 19 patients, and extension into the mucosa of one or both distal ureters occurred in 12 patients. Premalignant atypia of the mucosa was widespread, particularly along prostatic ducts and ureters. There were no deaths from tumors; 17 patients were living and well one month to 66 months after radical cystectomy.

In the course of screening 35,000 urological outpatients with urine cytologic tests between March 1970 and September 1976, Farrow and associates found 106 with positive results; 69 of these had biopsy-proven CIS.[28] Follow-up data were available in 58 patients treated by various means. These all had tumors of Grades 3 and 4, according to Broder's scale. Invasive carcinoma developed in 37 within five years and, in most of these, in three years. In both reports, the Farrow groups were impressed by the remarkably long duration of symptoms and the prolonged course of the lesion.[27, 28]

We have endeavored to focus attention on CIS of lower grades of malignancy. We have demonstrated that CIS Grade 2 (generally dismissed as dysplasia) has definite invasive potential as manifested by vascular and lymphatic invasion. Comparing Grade 2 and Grade 3 CIS, we found that of 28 patients with Grade 2 CIS, four went to infiltrating and three to papillary and infiltrating carcinomas; in 49 with CIS of Grade 3, 16 progressed to infiltrating and two to papillary and infiltrating carcinomas. In 30 to 80% of patients, diffuse CIS is associated with symptoms and progression to infiltrating carcinomas.[110]

In both grades, especially in Grade 2, the evolution of the lesion is considerably longer than previously claimed. The situation has been reviewed by Farrow and co-workers,[27] Weinstein and associates[107, 108] and by Droller.[22] Suffice it to say that there may be two forms of CIS: one that has invasive and metastatic potential and one that does not (a comment that is true for all cancers). The extent and location also affect the behavior. We must distinguish between those lesions that involve one area and those that involve extensive areas of the mucosa. The latter group may involve the bladder and urethral and ureteral orifices, and the other does not.

The risk involved in CIS (as in all superficial carcinomas) is invasion of the lamina propria, the lymphatics and blood vessels, the prostate ducts, the ureters, and the urethra. Much research is now going on to detect the invasive potential of CIS—blood group isoantigens (ABO, Kell, and T), tumor ploidy, morphometry, and chromosomal analysis. These will be disussed later.

In summary, the evidence shows that although all carcinomas begin as CIS, only 30 to 35% progress to invasive carcinoma, even among those of high-grade malignancy and involving the entire thickness of the mucosa. A smaller number of lesions diagnosed as dysplasia, severe atypia, or CIS Grade 2 have a similar course, although in many the course is prolonged.

Infiltrating and Metastatic Tumors

Definition. Invasive tumors are defined as those that have invaded muscularis (B_1, B_2, or T_2, T_{3a}); perivesical fibroadipose tissue (C or T_{3b}); the prostate, uterus, cervix, or vagina (T_{4a}); or pelvic or abdominal wall (T_{4b}). Metastatic tumors are defined as those that have metastasized to regional (D_1, any T + N_1) or distant nodes (any T + N_2) or distant sites.

Some urologists separate superficial from deep muscle invasion, but Richie and associates,[81] Skinner,[92] and Chisholm and colleagues[10] maintain that the distinction is meaningless.

In the United States urologists generally categorize T_4 with the metastatic group (D_1 and D_2), as most T_4 tumors show metastasis. There is a strong tendency to place all Grade 3 tumors in invasive (even deeply invasive) categories, irrespective of stage. The two are different.

Incidence. At the time of the initial examination, 24% of bladder tumors showed muscle invasion; 12% had further extension.[17]

Pathology. Two categories may be recognized: those that start as papillary carcinoma and progress to infiltrating carcinoma, and those that are infiltrating at the outset. The

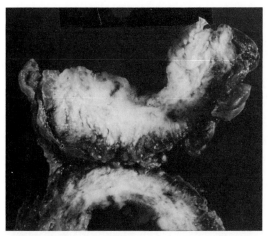

Figure 7–13. Sessile nodular infiltrating tumor. Cut section of a bladder tumor showing deep infiltration. (AFIP Neg. 86-59)

former constitute about 10%, and the latter make up 20% of bladder tumors. This group must start as CIS, but this cannot be demonstrated in the majority of cases.

Grossly, the tumors are sessile, nodular, and bulky (Fig. 7–13). The tumor may fill the bladder, but it is obviously infiltrating the bladder wall; the depth of infiltration is easily recognizable by its grayish white appearance, the firmness of the tissue, and the loss of muscular architecture.

Histologically, although most of the tumors are transitional, there is usually con-siderable variation in size, shape, and staining of the cells, so that it may be difficult to identify the transitional nature of the cells. The cells may be large or small. In contrast to papillary tumors and tumors that are papillary and infiltrating (which are usually pure transitional cell character with some tubular or acinar structures), invasive carcinomas have foci of squamous and glandular structures or spindle cells. About one fourth are undifferentiated. The tumors are mostly Grade 3 (Fig. 7–14) but may be Grade 2 or even, rarely, Grade 1.

In papillary and infiltrating tumors the depth of penetration of muscularis is more superficial than in sessile nodular tumors.[77, 95] Also, the mode of infiltration is usually different. In the former the infiltration is usually along a broad front—maintaining the papillary architecture—whereas in invasive tumors the infiltration is more often tentacular. Both subjacent and lateral invasion may be seen in this group. Vascular and lymphatic invasion is found in more superficially invasive tumors half as often as in more deeply invasive tumors.[7, 93]

Neoplastic, preoplastic, and reactive changes are more frequent at the margins of invasive tumors than at those of superficial tumors.

Clinical Course. Whether papillary and invasive tumors are invasive from the start or begin as papillary tumors and progress to

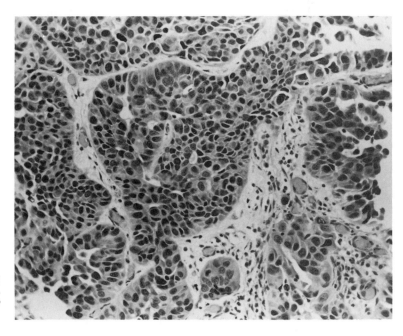

Figure 7–14. Transitional cell carcinoma, Grade 3, deeply infiltrating bladder wall. (AFIP Neg. 86-58, H & E, × 160)

invasion has not been resolved, but such tumors may have clones of cells with invasive potential not recognized in routine hematoxyline and eosin stains. On the other hand, the available evidence strongly suggests that invasive carcinomas usually begin as sessile, nodular tumors or as CIS, and that most of the deaths from carcinoma of bladder occur in this group. The course of invasive tumors includes a high rate of recurrence, extravesical extension, metastasis, and death from renal failure, extensive local neoplastic involvement, or widespread metastases. Multicentricity, aggressive potential of the cell, and the existence of CIS elsewhere in the bladder will be discussed later.

The histologic characteristics of the tumor have considerable bearing on the course of the disease. Jewett and associates reported that in their series of Stage C tumors, metastases developed in two of five low-grade transitional cell carcinomas, three of nine low-grade squamous carcinomas, nine of 22 high-grade transitional cell carcinomas, 45 of 67 squamous cell carcinomas, 22 of 31 undifferentiated carcinomas, and in both patients with adenocarcinoma.[43, 44]

Wallace observed that solid anaplastic tumors had an infiltration rate of 90%, compared with solid differentiated tumors, and an 82% rate of infiltration, compared with papillary anaplastic (62%) and papillary differentiated (19%) tumors.[105]

From data available, Slack and Prout reported that lymphatic invasion was present in 74% of all patients who had solid tumors, compared with 25% of those with papillary and invasive neoplasms.[93]

Cooling noted that 55% of patients with infiltration of muscle showed vascular or lymphatic invasion, or both, and 27% had metastasis.[13] In tumors that had extended beyond the bladder, the figures were 85% and 60%. Cooling also reported that vascular and lymphatic invasion alone was seen in 65% of patients at autopsy, but lymphatic invasion only was seen in 23% and vascular invasion alone in 12%. Metastases were found in lymph nodes (88%), liver (51%), lung (39%), bones (22%), and peritoneum (13%). It must be emphasized that no organ is spared.

Factors That Affect Recurrence and Progression of Bladder Tumors

History of Prior Bladder Tumors. Schulman and colleagues reported that in 39 pa-

tients without a prior history of tumors, 16 (41%) developed recurrence, whereas 20 (66%) of 30 patients who had previous tumor had recurrence.[88]

Single Tumors Confined to Mucosa. These were associated with 67% likelihood of recurrence, compared with 90% in those with multiple tumors. In patients with multiple tumors, the interval between initial and recurrent tumors was shorter than in those with single tumors. Comparable findings have been reported for tumors not confined to mucosa.[6, 17, 35, 103]

Size. Patients with tumors less than 3 cm in diameter were more likely to remain disease-free for at least 24 months than were patients with larger tumors. Of patients with large tumors (5 cm or larger), 79% were disease-free, compared with 98% of those with small tumors (less than 1 cm).[17]

Presence or Absence of Invasion at Initial Examination Affects Progression. Of 120 patients with initial carcinomas confined to the mucosa, 65% remained disease-free at 12 months, 52% at 24 months, and 46% at 36 months. Three per cent had recurrent tumors with muscle invasion. On the other hand, of 78 patients with tumors that initially showed invasion of lamina propria, 24% progressed to muscle invasion, two thirds during the first year.[17, 38] Cutler and associates have made other observations as follows:[17]

Depth of invasion: Disease-free state was reported in 98% of mucosal tumors, 90% of those with invasion of lamina propria, and 72% of those with muscle invasion. These authors reported 24-month disease-free indices as follows:

No invasion	$0.98 \times 0.55 = 0.54$
Lamina propria	$0.90 \times 0.48 = 0.43$
Muscle	$0.72 \times 0.51 = 0.37$

Growth Pattern. Ninety-four per cent of patients with papillary tumors achieved disease-free status, compared with 71% of those with invasive tumors; the number of the latter was too small for reliable assessment.[17]

Grade. One of 90 patients with Grade 1 tumors failed to achieve a disease-free state, compared with 16% of patients with Grade 2 and 14% of patients with Grade 3 tumors.[17]

"Worse Nontumor Abnormality." Of 100 patients with no mucosal abnormality, 58% were disease-free, compared with 52% of 55 patients with hyperplasia or mild dysplasia,

or both, and 40% of 31 patients with moderate or severe dysplasia.[17]

Tumor Progression. Prout and associates reported that total cystectomy usually leaves the pelvis free from disease unless the lymph nodes are positive or there is extensive lymphatic involvement. Three quarters of the time, metastases were found in bone, lungs, and liver, and metastases appeared in one year in 65 to 75% of patients. Most patients for whom carcinoma of bladder is fatal will be dead within two years, and the rest will die in the next six months.[79]

Invasive and Malignant Potential of the Tumor. Weinstein had discussed this in detail.[107] Four theories have been proposed; they involve mechanical aspects of neoplasms, membrane alterations, increased motility of the tumor cells, and compromise of natural host barriers. Whatever the mechanism (and more than one mechanism may be at play), the aggressive potential of the cell is manifested clinically by change in stage and pathologically by possible change in grade but, more specifically, by change in pathologic stage and development of vascular and lymphatic invasion. Whether the aggressive cell was present but undetected in a heterogeneous cell population or resulted from a change in cell phenotype from a cell with limited growth and invasive capability to one of unlimited growth and invasive potential (extending locally, invading lymphatics and blood channels, metastasizing, and growing in the metastasis) remains to be resolved. Irrespective of how it occurs, the tumor progresses to a higher stage. Without such expression of the malignant potential of the cell, superficial tumors rarely kill the patient.

Most of the deaths from carcinoma of bladder occur in patients who have high-grade, high-stage tumors, and there is considerable evidence that this potentiality is present at the time of initial appearance of clinical symptoms; in only a few does this develop subsequently. The challenge is to prevent the appearance of invasive tumors and to detect malignant potential in noninvasive tumors before invasion has become clinically apparent.

Attempts to predict more accurately the malignant potential of vesical carcinomas have led to application of a host of modern techniques undreamed of 10 to 20 years ago: cell surface markers, tumor-associated antigens, tumor ploidy, chromosomal analysis, and morphometry.

The discovery that malignant transformation is associated with alterations of cell membrane has led to extensive research of this phenomenon. A detailed discussion of structure and composition of cell membrane is beyond the scope of this presentation, and the reader is referred to several excellent reviews (Singer and Nicholson,[91] Weinstein,[107] and Weinstein[108]).

Blood group antigens are glycolipids or proteins not only expressed in erythrocytes but also in cell membranes of a wide variety of tissues. Davidsohn and associates were among the first to investigate the expression of blood group (BG) antigens in tumors.[19] They observed that in contrast to normal epithelium, the antigens were either not demonstrable or weakly present in some carcinomas.

Hakomori has described the chemical properties of blood group (BG) isoantigens A, B, and O (H-structure).[36, 37] The H-structure is the precursor for types A and B. The addition of N-acetylgalactosamine to the H-structure by a specific glycosyltransferase results in BG-A; when galactose is added, the product is BG-B. Since glycolysation is incomplete, most persons with antigens A or B, or both, also express some H antigen. The expression of ABH antigens on epithelial cells is dependent on the secretor status of an individual.

The A, B, and H antigens occur in tissue in two forms: the alcohol-soluble form is present in erythrocytes, endothelial cells, and epithelial cells; the water-soluble form is found in epithelial mucin. In nonsecretors and tumor cells the alcohol-soluble form of ABH antigen appears to be more sensitive to lipid solvents used in the fixation and embedding process.[52, 54] Most studies of the status of BG antigens in carcinoma of the bladder are based on specific red blood cell adherence (SRCA) tests. More recently, preference has been given to the more sensitive and simple immunoperoxidase technique, utilizing either homologous or heterologous antibodies, especially monoclonal antibodies against BG-A and BG-B. The H-substance is demonstrated by a plant lectin, *Ulex europaeus.*

The discovery by Decenzo and associates that the expression of BG antigens in the initial bladder tumor could be correlated with subsequent behavior led to a number of clinical studies.[21] Most carcinomas show a heterogeneous cell population in respect to BG isoantigens. It has been customary to designate carcinomas as BG antigen–positive if at least 30 to 35% of the cells retain their respective blood groups.

About 66% of carcinomas that are BG isoantigen–negative are said to infiltrate the muscle within five years, in contrast to 5% of BG isoantigen–positive tumors. Ninety per cent of negative tumors have recurrences, in contrast to 50% of positive tumors. It is not clear, however, if the latter consist of carcinomas with a mixed cell population. We prefer to record the estimated percentages of positive and negative cell populations so that the data relative to the behavior of these lesions can be better analyzed. Most carcinomas in situ have a predominantly negative cell population.

The limited prognostic acumen of the system has led to application of another surface antigen, referred to as Thomsen-Friedenreich (T) antigen. The T antigen is a precursor of the MN blood group system and is present in erythrocytes, endothelial cells, and epithelial cells. Normally, T antigen is masked by sialic acid residues and can only be demonstrated after pretreatment of the sections with neuraminidase. Therefore, the masked T antigen is referred to as cryptic T antigen. The T antigen can be demonstrated by the use of peanut lectin (Arachis hypogaea).[14, 55, 89, 109] Carcinomas showing alterations from normal (i.e., either spontaneous appearance of the T antigen or loss of cryptic T antigen) are associated with aggressive behavior. Coon and associates found that only 10% of cryptic T antigen-positive tumors developed invasion, in contrast to 39% of either cryptic T antigen–negative or T antigen–positive tumors.[14]

As with BG antigens A, B, and O, the predictive value is best in low-stage tumors, and most tumors show a heterogeneous cell population with respect to T antigen expression. If a carcinoma that is BG isoantigen–negative also shows alterations in the T antigen expression, the prognostic accuracy is greater than with either of the BG systems alone. The status of BG isoantigens is not necessarily related to the grade or the stage of the tumor, as a number of invasive carcinomas have retained the appropriate blood group isoantigens.

The development of monoclonal antibodies enables investigation of a host of other tumor-associated antigens, some of which appear to occur predominantly in aggressive tumors.[16]

Lamb reported the first comprehensive study of chromosomes in bladder cancer.[51] Twenty-nine transitional cell carcinomas were studied, and well-differentiated carcinomas had chromosome counts in the diploid or near-diploid range. All noninvasive tumors and only two of the invasive tumors had a diploid chromosome count. Loss of differentiation was associated with an increase in the number of chromosome numbers to a nearly tetraploid range. However, banding techniques have shown that tumors that have diploid values with respect to modal numbers of chromosomes actually have abnormal karyotypes or marker chromosomes.

Studies by Falor of a number of noninvasive carcinomas revealed that these tumors had more than 50% of cells with modal numbers near diploid counts, in contrast to invasive carcinomas, in which 80% of cells showed hypodiploid or hypertetraploid counts with abnormal karyotypes and marker chromosomes.[25] Sandberg found that the presence of marker chromosomes in noninvasive papillary carcinomas was followed by recurrence in over 90% of cases; there was only 5% recurrence rates in tumors lacking marker chromosomes.[84, 85] The five-year survival rate in patients with noninvasive papillary or papillary and superficially infiltrating carcinomas without marker chromosomes was about 95%, in comparison to a five-year survival of 40% when marker chromosomes were present. The potential value of finding a marker chromosome in a noninvasive bladder cancer is obvious. As Falor and Ward have indicated, the triad of tetraploidy, markers, and submucous invasiveness in moderately well differentiated carcinomas appears to carry such poor prognosis as to indicate early radical resection.[26] Falor and Ward[26] and Sandberg[85] have demonstrated that "benign" papillary tumors were found to be preponderantly diploid. In two of these that recurred, there were a few karyotypically abnormal cells at the initial examination. The modal chromosome number in papillary carcinomas was usually in the diploid range from 44 to 49, varying in individual tumors. The invasive tumors were accompanied by a large number of marker chromosomes with many complicated karyotypes.

The most frequently found marker chromosomes are an isochromosome of the short arm of 5, monosomy of chromosome 9, involvement of chromosome 8 as an isochromosome of the long arm or loss of short arm, and interstitial deletion of chromosome 13. The reader is referred to the excellent summary of the situation by Sandberg.[84]

Flow cytometry has the great advantage that it allows investigation of thousands of tumor cells for their DNA and RNA contents in a matter of minutes. Barlogie,[5] Klein,[47] Tribukait,[100] Melamed,[62] and their co-workers have demonstrated a correlation between aneuploid cell lines and grade and stage of bladder carcinomas. Tribukait and associates found that the presence of several aneuploid cell lines was associated with a more aggressive tumor behavior than that found in tumors with only one aneuploid cell line.[100] The reader is referred to several excellent reviews.[5, 101]

Flow cytometry has the disadvantage that it cannot be correlated with the specific cell type. On the other hand, cytophotometry on paraffin-embedded and Feulgen-stained sections has the advantage that tumor cells can be evaluated in situ to enable the morphologist to identify the specific cell type. In preliminary studies of 106 patients with carcinoma of bladder, we found that cytophotometry correlates well with grade based on hematoxylin and eosin section but, understandably, not with growth pattern, as the latter may manifest any grade. The prognostic value appears to be limited, especially in comparing the behavior of CIS lesions of the same grade.

Nontransitional Cell Carcinomas

(Figs. 7–15 to 7–19)

Transitional cell carcinomas constitute 90% of all carcinomas of bladder. About 10% of tumors consist of squamous carcinomas, adenocarcinomas, and undifferentiated carcinomas. These cell types may be seen in pure form as the sole manifestation of neoplasia. More frequently, squamous, glandular, and tubular areas are seen in transitional cell carcinomas. This group will be discussed later.

Squamous Cell Carcinomas

Two categories are recognized—the nonbilharzial and the bilharzial. The nonbilharzial form seen in the Western Hemisphere constitutes about 5% of bladder tumors.

Most often it is associated with long-standing chronic infection, vesical calculi, vesical diverticuli, chronic use of Foley catheters, and cyclophosphamide treatment. Grossly, the tumors are bulky, often with ulceration and necrosis. We limit the diagnosis of squamous cell carcinoma to tumors that are purely squamous. The tumor may vary from well differentiated with large polyhedral prickle cells and squamous pearls to poorly differentiated tumors. The well-differentiated lesions that are confined to the mucosa are sometimes difficult to distinguish from severe squamous metaplasia. The distinction can be made if there is invasion of lamina propria. Two unusual features of squamous cell carcinoma are that the cell nests have pointed or angular outlines and there is considerable stromal reaction.

The squamous cell carcinoma associated with bilharzial infection is the most common cell type seen in Egypt, parts of Africa, and the Middle East, where *Schistosoma haematobium* is prevalent. It constitutes about 60% of bladder tumors. Grossly, these tumors may be fungating, infiltrative, or ulcerative. Most, if not all, of these tumors are well differentiated, but by the time they are seen by a urologic surgeon they show invasion of muscle and, in over two thirds, have extended beyond the bladder.[41] Although deeply infiltrating, these tumors tend to remain well differentiated and confined to the bladder.

Poorly differentiated squamous carcinomas have poor prognosis.

Adenocarcinoma

In pure form, adenocarcinoma constitutes about 2% of bladder tumors.[70] Categories recognized are primary vesical, primary urachal, mesonephric, and metastatic tumor.

Primary vesical adenocarcinoma may occur anywhere in the bladder, but most often it is in the trigone or the posterior wall. These tumors are usually preceded by a long history of cystitis, mucin in the urine, glandular cystitis, and mucous metaplasia. In the early stages primary vesical adenocarcinomas are often difficult to diagnose. The biopsy may consist only of benign-appearing, columnar, mucous-producing epithelium or lakes of mucin. Invariably, there is associated glandular cystitis. Unless invasion can be demonstrated, it is impossible to determine malignancy. Sooner or later

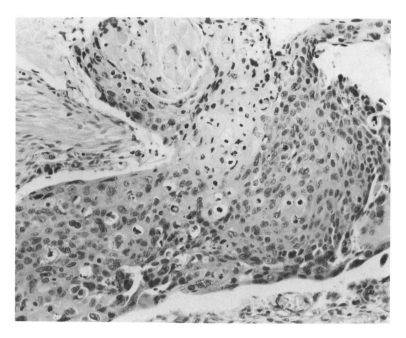

Figure 7–15. Squamous cell carcinoma, well differentiated, Grade 2. (AFIP Neg. 86-61, H & E, × 250)

there is anaplasia of the cells or invasion of muscularis, or both, but even before this occurs the presence of lakes of mucin in the muscle layer should lead to suspicion of malignancy. Histologically, the tumor may resemble colonic carcinoma with tall, columnar, mucus-producing epithelium or signet-ring cells. The behavior of primary vesical adenocarcinoma is roughly that of

infiltrating transitional cell carcinoma, but the tumors are not radiosensitive.

Urachal adenocarcinomas are confined to the dome or the anterior wall. They are primarily and principally intramural, with secondary involvement of the mucosa. There is usually little or no change of adjoining mucosa. Although most urachal tumors are adenocarcinomas, we have seen a number

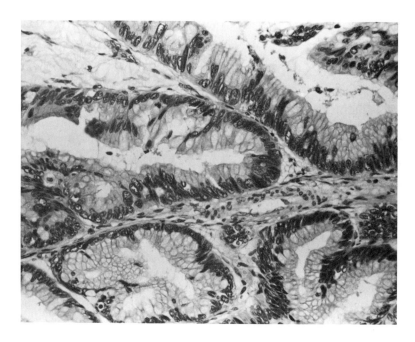

Figure 7–16. Mucinous adenocarcinoma, Grade 2. This histologic picture may be seen in primary vesical adenocarcinoma, in urachal adenocarcinoma, and in exstrophy. (AFIP Neg. 86-60, H & E, × 250)

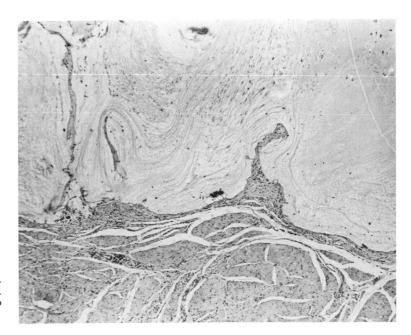

Figure 7–17. Mucinous adeno-carcinoma. Lakes of mucin infil-trate the bladder wall. (AFIP Neg. 86-62, H & E, × 40)

that had areas of transitional cell carcinoma or consisted entirely of transitional cell carcinoma. The proper management of these tumors must take into account the ramifications of the urachal tract, not only in the wall of bladder but in the space of Retzius and the anterior abdominal wall.[69]

Carcinomas in *exstrophy* are usually mucinous adenocarcinomas. Carcinoembryonic antigen is readily demonstrable in these tumors.

An unusual and very rare form of primary adenocarcinoma is the *mesonephric* type. The tumor consists of tubular structures lined by cuboidal or flattened epithelium. The tumor may involve the entire thickness of the bladder and may be the malignant counterpart of nephrogenic adenoma.

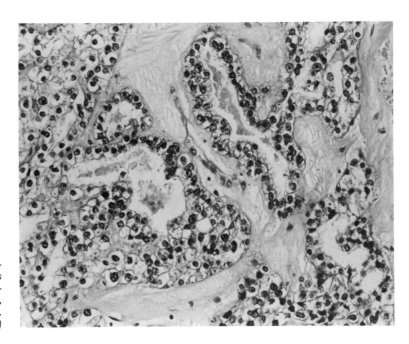

Figure 7–18. Mesonephric ade-nocarcinoma. The tumor is made up of tubules lined by vac-uolated cuboidal epithelium, suggesting renal cell carcinoma. (AFIP Neg. 86-63, H & E, × 250)

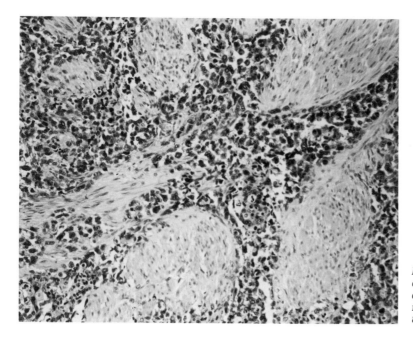

Figure 7–19. Undifferentiated carcinoma, Grade 3. The cells are neither transitional, squamous, nor glandular. (AFIP Neg. 86-64, H & E, × 250)

The bladder is frequently involved in adenocarcinomas that are primary in the cervix, uterus, prostate, and colon, but it is rare to have such metastatic tumors initially manifest bladder symptoms.

Undifferentiated Carcinoma of the Bladder

This form of tumor is very rare. Instead of transitional, squamous, or glandular elements, the cells are primitive and undifferentiated. Histologically, the cells may be small or large. The spindle cell variety simulates sarcoma. In these cases, keratin and epithelial membrane antigen stains are positive. The tumor may be radiosensitive, but experience with this lesion is limited. Such carcinomas often show areas of squamous differentiation.

Rarely, an undifferentiated tumor may show marked anaplasia with multi- and mononuclear giant cells. Some of these may produce heterotopic human chorionic gonadotropin (HCG). The presence of giant cells and demonstration of HCG in the cells simulate choriocarcinoma. Histologically, the distinction from choriocarcinoma can readily be made by the fact that the giant cells do not resemble syncytiotrophoblasts in any stage of their development and HCG is present not only in the giant cells but in small cells as well.

Carcinomas of More Than One Cell Type
(Figs. 7–20 to 7–22)

In many bladder tumors, especially infiltrating and recurrent carcinomas, more than one cell type may be seen. Most commonly it is transitional cell carcinoma with squamous, glandular, or tubular areas. This category has been subject to some confusion. Some pathologists ignore such areas, others diagnose the tumors as squamous carcinomas or adenocarcinomas, others refer to them as metaplastic tumors, and still others refer to them as transitional cell carcinomas with squamous or glandular differentiation. We prefer to designate them as areas of squamous, glandular, tubular, or undifferentiated carcinomas. The tumor may show one or more of such areas. Not infrequently, especially in older patients, a tumor that consisted of transitional cell carcinoma with or without squamous or glandular areas may present with spindle cell areas. In most cases these are spindle cell carcinomas, and this can be confirmed by keratin and epithelial membrane antigen stains.

The pleomorphic cell population is simply indicative of the potentiality of vesical epithelium, which will be discussed later.

Histogenesis of Bladder Tumors

Although many, if not all, bladder cancers are environmentally and occupationally induced (by smoking and exposure to carcinogenic chemicals, respectively) and although the lesion can readily be produced in experimental animals, we have very little factual information on the origin and progression of these tumors in humans.

In bladders that have been exposed to chronic inflammation or irritation, certain mucosal abnormalities are observed. These may be grouped under the broad headings of proliferative, metaplastic, and neoplastic changes. These changes may be seen individually or collectively, simultaneously or consecutively.

Proliferative Changes

Proliferation may be manifested by epithelial hyperplasia. Hyperplasia is defined as an increase in the number of cell layers without a loss of polarity but with differentiation and maturation from the base to the surface. It is conceivable that such hyperplasia may progress to neoplasia, but this has not been proved.

Another form of epithelial hyperplasia is

manifested by outpocketing of epithelium into lamina propria to form Brunn's nests. These may become cystic, to form cystitis cystica. Whether Brunn's nests are premalignant or not has been controversial. Weiner and associates found that Brunn's nests in normal bladders appear to increase with age.[106] This observation plus the fact that Brunn's nests have not been demonstrated to progress invariably and inevitably into neoplasia would seem to indicate that the nests are reactive and not preneoplastic. On the other hand, since these nests are present at the margins of frank carcinoma, since they are seen in patients exposed to carcinogenic agents before carcinoma has developed, and since they are present in experimental tumors, it is possible that at least in some cases they are preneoplastic. Irrespective of this, the presence of Brunn's nests would seem to indicate a sick, agitated mucosa. Progression of Brunn's nests to inverted papilloma seems noncontroversial, but to date no information is available on long-term follow-up of patients with Brunn's nests.

It has been customary to include papillary cystitis under proliferative lesions. In this entity the mucosa forms papillary projections. The appearance is due to edema, swelling, and proliferation of the lamina propria, but the epithelium is entirely normal. Conceptually, papillary cystitis may progress to papilloma and papillary carci-

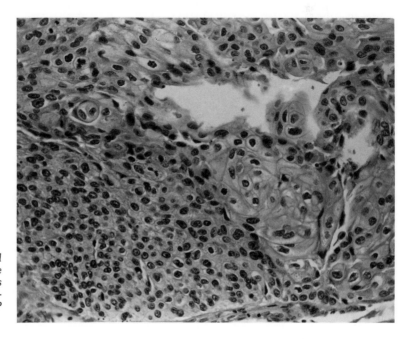

Figure 7–20. Transitional and squamous cell carcinoma, Grade 2. An island of squamous cells is seen in the midst of transitional cell carcinoma. (AFIP Neg. 86-85, H & E, × 250)

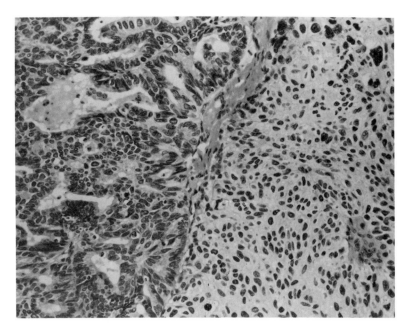

Figure 7–21. Transitional cell carcinoma and adenocarcinoma. *(AFIP Neg. 86-85, H & E, × 250)*

noma, but such progression has not been proved in humans.

Metaplastic Changes
(Fig. 7–23)

The transitional epithelium may transform into squamous epithelium with or without keratinization, to glandular epithelium with or without mucin formation, or to tubular (cuboidal) epithelium. Such changes are generally referred to as metaplasia, which may be a misnomer. Squamous "metaplasia" of the trigone is most frequently observed in young women during the height of estrogen production. The epithelial layer is thickened, the superficial cells are vacuolated, and the basal cells are squamous. There is no keratinization. This is a physiologic change, and although it may give some

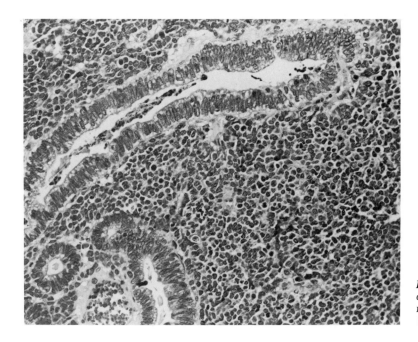

Figure 7–22. Undifferentiated carcinoma and adenocarcinoma. *(AFIP Neg. 86-67, H & E, × 250)*

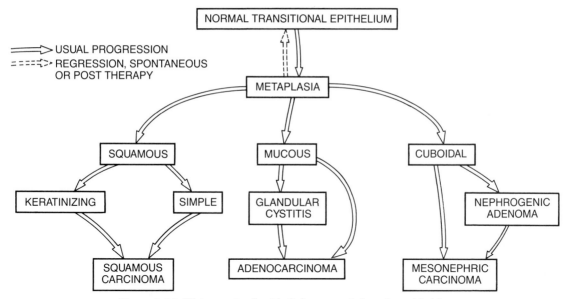

Figure 7–23. *Histogenesis of epithelial tumors of the urinary bladder.*

symptoms, it is a reversible change without significance.

A papilloma resembling condyloma may be seen, usually in young men and almost invariably associated with urethral condyloma, generally attributed to viral infection. Squamous "metaplasia" with keratinization is a more serious occurrence. It is seen in association with chronic infection, vesical calculi, diverticuli, chronic use of Foley catheters, and so forth, and is generally regarded as preneoplastic.

Glandular metaplasia and cystitis glandularis are usually mucinous. Most commonly observed in vesical infection of long standing, these conditions are quite frequently seen in exstrophy, urachal cysts, and remnants.

Tubular "metaplasia," commonly referred to as nephrogenic adenoma, denotes the presence of tubules lined by cuboidal or hobnail epithelium and sometimes surrounded by hyalinized basement membrane. The surface epithelium may also show similar changes and, frequently, papillation.

It is not infrequent to see all three phenomena in the bladder (and renal pelvis and ureters), even in the same section. We believe that these metaplastic changes are simply an expression of the potentialities of transitional epithelium.[67]

These metaplastic changes are benign, but they may progress to neoplasia, usually a process that takes many years. From the pathologic point of view, although the two extremes (benign and malignant) are readily distinguishable, the exact transition from benign to malignant tissue is often difficult to determine. The key to distinguishing between the two is recognition of anaplasia and detection of invasion.

Neoplastic Changes
(Fig. 7–24)

Neoplastic change may develop in proliferative, metaplastic, or normal epithelium. It will be recalled that proliferation may take the form of a thickened epithelial layer or formation of Brunn's nests, and neoplastic change may be superimposed on hyperplastic epithelium perhaps as a result of a promoting factor. In many carcinomas of the bladder, the surface epithelium may show not only more than seven layers of epithelium but anaplasia of the cells as well. Similarly, anaplasia may appear in Brunn's nests. Conceptually, papilloma may progress to papillary carcinoma, as evidenced by the fact that at times both entities may be seen in the same section.

Metaplastic changes per se are benign, but anaplasia may supervene and lead to the appearance of squamous, glandular, or tubular (mesonephric) carcinoma. Simultaneously, the carcinogenic initiator-promotor may act on the adjacent transitional epithelium to show transitional cell carcinoma as well.

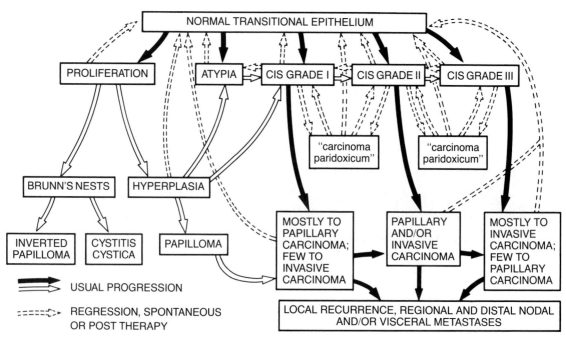

Figure 7–24. Histogenesis of epithelial tumors of the urinary bladder.

Anaplasia may occur de novo in the normal surface epithelium. Conceptually, the surface can be entirely normal but in a period of time assume the appearance of Grade 3 carcinoma involving the full thickness of the epithelial layer. Thus it is quite conceivable that the initial reaction may be marked anaplasia of the entire epithelial layer.

We believe that such Grade 3 anaplastic change may involve the entire thickness of the epithelial layer, or more likely, be initially manifested in the basal layer, superficial layer, or scattered individual cells. The recognition, identification, and recording of alterations that do not involve the full thickness of the epithelial layer have been controversial. Irrespective of the degree of cellular anaplasia, some pathologists persist in labeling such changes as dysplasia, even though cytologically, biochemically, and biophysically such cells are malignant.

It is also quite possible, if not probable, that the epithelial layer goes through a series of morphologic (biochemical and biophysical) alterations that are steps in the development of carcinoma. It is the recognition and designation of these steps that also have been controversial.

We believe that the earliest change may be atypia or low-grade carcinoma. By atypia we mean alteration of the epithelium in which there is epithelial thickening with preservation of cell polarity but some nuclear crowding and nuclear atypia (Fig. 7–25). Since alterations in the nucleus have a limited reaction to any injury, morphologically similar changes may be seen in reactive, inflammatory, or regenerative epithelium. Therefore, if such changes are encountered at the margins of an ulcer or where there is an intraepithelial inflammatory reaction, they are dismissed as reactive. On the other hand, if there is no apparent cause for the alterations, we designate the changes as atypia, indicating that they do not fulfill the criteria for diagnosis of carcinoma.

Progression of these changes could conceptually lead to low- or high-grade carcinoma. In low-grade carcinomas the epithelium may be thickened. There is cellular crowding, loss of polarity, nuclear hyperchromasia and crowding, occasional giant cells, and misplaced mitotic figures. The umbrella cells may be present or absent. These changes may be slight or moderate (Fig. 7–26). If the slight changes are identical to those of Grade 1 papillary or infiltrating carcinoma, we recognize them as such. If the changes are moderate, resembling Grade 2 papillary or infiltrating carcinoma, we label them as such. Some pathologists, how-

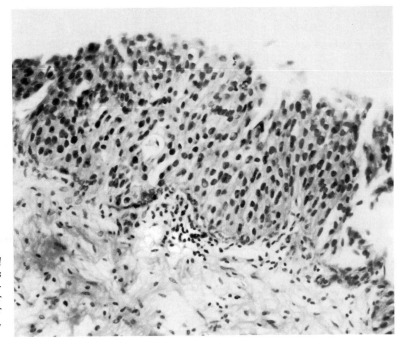

Figure 7–25. *Atypia of vesical epithelium. The mucosa is thickened. Cell polarity is preserved. There is some nuclear crowding and minimal nuclear atypia. (AFIP Neg. 86-68, H & E, × 250)*

ever, designate such lesions as dysplasia. Obviously, dysplasia has been applied to the entire spectrum of epithelial abnormalities. These range from those in which the cellular alterations viewed alone would be diagnosed as Grade 3 carcinoma, but they are dismissed because the entire thickness is not involved, to the other extreme in which the changes are minimal or moderate. Therefore, we have refrained from using the term dysplasia in reference to the bladder—a position adopted by WHO Panel of Experts on Bladder Tumors.[72]

We believe that if progression occurs, low-grade in situ carcinomas progress into papillary carcinomas but rarely into infiltrating

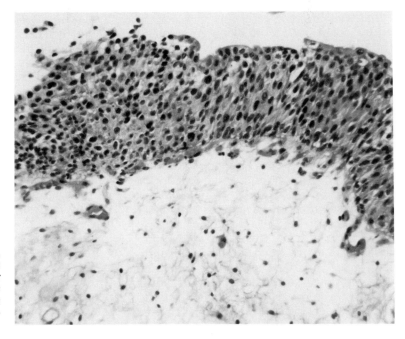

Figure 7–26. *Carcinoma in situ, Grades 1 and 2. The mucosa is thickened. There is cellular crowding and misplaced mitotic activity. Note that umbrella cells are still present. (AFIP Neg. 86-70, H & E, × 250)*

carcinomas. On the other hand, high-grade in situ carcinomas usually tend to advance into infiltrating carcinomas but rarely into papillary tumors. When this occurs the tendency is for early invasion. Invasive carcinomas may show squamous, glandular, tubular, or undifferentiated areas, recapitulating the potentialities of agitated normal transitional epithelium to metaplasia, as mentioned earlier.

At any point these processes may revert to the normal state spontaneously or as a result of treatment. Our concepts are illustrated in Figure 7–24.

Sarcoma of the Bladder

Sarcomas of the bladder constitute about 2% of its malignant tumors. They are most often in the trigone but may occur anywhere. Originating intramurally, they may grow intravesically to form a polypoid mass or extravesically to invade adjacent organs or structures or to fill the pelvis. The overlying mucosa is usually intact, smooth, and pinkish gray. As the tumor enlarges it may ulcerate and bleed easily. At times the surface may be covered by a necrotic, calcified membrane.

About half of the vesical sarcomas consist of rhabdomyosarcomas and leiomyosarcomas. Rhabdomyosarcoma is the most common neoplasm, and although it may be seen in later life, it is most frequently confined to the childhood period.

Rhabdomyosarcomas of the bladder constitute about 4% of rhabdomyosarcomas. They are usually manifested by obstructive symptoms rather than hematuria, which occurs only with ulceration. They present as polypoid grape-like growths, occasionally with gelatinous consistency. Histologically, over 90% are embryonal rhabdomyosarcomas, and only 5% are of the alveolar type. The histologic appearance of the tumor has been described in detail elsewhere.[71] Suffice it to say that the epithelial layer may be normal or hyperplastic or even squamous. The lamina propria is edematous and myxomatous. Biopsies at this stage are difficult to interpret. A Masson trichrome and immunochemical stains (myoglobin and desmin) may reveal the true identity of the spindle cells. In others and in later stages there is generally a zone of cellularity of three to four cell layers. These cellular areas consist of small, round, lymphocyte-like cells, oval or spindle cells with darkly staining nuclei, and indistinct cytoplasm. The nuclei vary in size and shape, may have one or two nucleoli, and show frequent mitoses. More differentiated forms contain varying numbers of round or oval rhabdomyoblasts with distinct eosinophilic cytoplasm and more deeply staining, fibrillary, or stringy material arranged concentrically around the nucleus. Cross striations are rare. Others, especially in later stages, may consist of spindle-shaped cells with varying degrees of anaplasia.

Unipolar, racket-shaped cells with single nuclei located in the broader end taper to a single spindle. Other cells are elongated at both ends with double spindles. Still other cells are larger and show cross striations, but these may be difficult to demonstrate. Giant cells of various types are common, and they may be multi- or mononucleated. At times the tumor may consist entirely of rhabdomyoblasts.

The alveolar type consists of poorly differentiated round or oval cells, forming irregular "alveolar" spaces, with necrotic cells in the center and viable cells at the periphery occurring in a single layer and suggesting an adenocarcinoma. The cell masses are supported by hyalinized fibrous septae.

Leiomyosarcomas are seen in older patients and constitute about 30% of sarcomas. They are solid, fibrillar, and grayish pink. They may protrude into the lumen, sometimes filling the cavity. Histologically, the tumors consist of interlacing bands of spindle-shaped cells containing varying numbers of nonstriated myofibrils. The nuclei are cigar-shaped, often with a "bird's eye" nucleolus. Many leiomyosarcomas are well differentiated with slight or no anaplasia, but they are invasive.

Myosarcomas are somewhat more primitive tumors.

Granular cell myoblastomas are distinguished by a polymorphous cell population with large hyperchromatic nuclei. The cells usually form a mosaic but may be spindle. The tumors are mostly benign but may be malignant.

Fibrosarcomas constitute 14% of vesical sarcomas and occur in older patients. Grossly, they present a grayish-white whorled appearance, and microscopically they consist of interlacing spindle-shaped fibroblasts. The cells show varying degrees of atypia, mitotic activity, intercellular connective tissue fibers, and collagen deposition. The more cellular areas may have a herringbone pattern. Trichrome stains distinguish fibrosarcoma from leiomyosarcoma.

In differential diagnoses of any spindle cell lesion of the bladder, consideration should be given to a reactive process, consisting of plump spindle cells associated with inflammatory cell infiltrate of varying degrees and areas of granulation tissue. This process is seen most often at the site of prior surgery or trauma. The lesion is referred to as postsurgical spindle cell nodule.

"Myxosarcomas" are mostly rhabdomyosarcomas. About 6% of sarcomas are osteo- or chondrosarcomas, which occur usually in patients over the age of 60, and should be distinguished from sarcomas or carcinomas, which may have metaplastic cartilage or bone. The cartilage and bone must be obviously malignant.

Many of these are, in fact, carcinosarcomas that begin as carcinomas, often with areas of transitional, glandular, or squamous carcinomas later becoming replaced by malignant cartilage or bone. Carcinosarcomas constitute less than 1% of vesical malignancies and should be distinguished from carcinoma with spindle areas. To diagnose carcinosarcoma, we insist that the sarcomatous element should be differentiated and identifiable as rhabdo-, osteo-, or chondrosarcoma. Keratin and epithelial membrane antigen stains are mandatory to rule out a spindle cell carcinoma.

Mixed mesenchymal tumors show areas of myosarcoma, fibrosarcoma, liposarcoma, and so forth. Hemangiopericytomas and fibrous histiocytomas are rarely encountered.

Malignant lymphomas and Hodgkin's disease rarely involve the bladder and constitute about 1% of sarcomas. Differentiation between malignant lymphoma and severe follicular cystitis may be difficult. In the former the follicular pattern and secondary follicles are usually absent and the infiltrate invades the muscle fibers. Differentiation between malignant lymphoma and small cell carcinoma may be difficult if the tissue is cooked or poorly preserved. Hodgkin's disease may be difficult to distinguish from certain forms of cystitis, but the latter lack characteristic Reed-Sternberg cells.

Pheochromocytomas, carcinoids, and malignant melanomas are rarely seen in the bladder. Pheochromocytomas are benign but rarely they may recur and metastasize.

CARCINOMA OF THE URETHRA

Male Urethra

The incidence of the various types of urethral carcinoma cited by Sullivan and Grabstald[97] is representative of that which may be found in the literature: 78% squamous, 15% transitional, 6% adenocarcinoma, and 1% undifferentiated. The incidence by location is 55% for bulbomembranous urethra, 36% for penile urethra, and 9% for prostatic urethra.

The type of carcinoma that may be expected to arise in a given location is largely dependent upon the type of epithelium normally present. It is commonly stated that the prostatic urethra is lined by transitional epithelium. This is partly true. Like the prostatic ducts, this area, including the surface of the verumontanum, is usually lined in part by prostatic secretory epithelial cells, and small prostatic acini open directly into the urethra. Thus, two types of carcinoma occur in the prostatic urethra: transitional cell carcinoma and prostatic carcinoma. The figure of 9% for the relative frequency of tumors in the prostatic urethra does not take into consideration the large number of patients who, in the course of being treated and followed for bladder carcinoma, eventually develop urethral carcinoma as a part of the multifocal process previously discussed. Koss believes that urethral involvement is no less common than ureteral carcinoma in such patients, a view with which we fully agree.[50] However, as an initial presentation, these tumors are rare.

The second type of prostatic urethral carcinoma is prostatic carcinoma. For the past 15 years or so, certain tumors in this area were designated as "endometrioid" carcinomas. This was based on the view that they originated in the utricle, and since this structure embryologically derives from the müllerian duct, and since the tumors bore some resemblance to endometrial carcinoma, they were thus diagnosed and estrogen therapy withheld. In reality, both the precursor cell and the tumor cell morphologically and functionally resemble the prostatic secretory cell. That such tumors are papillary rather than microacinar is due to the fact that their growth is largely luminal. The tumors are invariably positive for both prostatic acid phosphatase and prostate-specific antigen. The findings of Epstein and Woodruff are similar to our experience—that the so-called endometrioid carcinoma is associated with the more common microacinar growth patterns of prostatic carcinoma more often than not, and that a marked clinical response to estrogen may be achieved.[24]

The bulbomembranous urethra is the most common location for de novo urethral carcinoma. That the great majority of these are squamous cell carcinomas is doubtless due to squamous metaplasia of the transitional epithelium of this area, which is the expected result following urethritis and strictures with scarring that so often precede tumors in this location. These squamous carcinomas tend to be higher grade and aggressive. A few adenocarcinomas arise in this area, either from periurethral glands or glandular metaplasia of the mucosa.

Tumors of the penile urethra, like those in the bulbomembranous urethra, are largely of the squamous type. In both sites, transitional cell carcinoma is occasionally seen. The chief difference between the two sites is that penile urethral lesions are detected earlier, at a lower stage, and have a much better prognosis. Most tumors in the meatal and parameatal area are benign papillomas and condylomata acuminata. The latter may be multiple and recurrent, but only rarely have they been associated with, or followed by, the development of carcinoma.

Female Urethra

The anterior two thirds of the female urethra is lined by squamous epithelium, and the posterior third is a continuation of the transitional epithelium from the bladder. The most frequent type of carcinoma is squamous cell (70%), followed by adenocarcinoma (18%), transitional cell (10%), and undifferentiated carcinoma (2%).[97] Not uncommonly, tumors have a mixed transitional-squamous appearance. As in the male urethra, chronic irritation is believed to be an etiologic factor in many cases. Tumors originating in the meatal and adjacent anterior urethral region are generally squamous,

transitional, or mixed, and present as papillary excrescences or nodules. They may protrude through the meatus and mimic a caruncle.

Tumors of the middle third of the urethra are histologically similar. These, too, may protrude through the meatus; they often are ulcerated and produce fistulas into the vagina.

Tumors of the posterior third, as in the prostatic urethra, often are first discovered in the course of examining cystectomy specimens from patients with bladder cancer, but many of the de novo tumors in this region are adenocarcinomas. Most of the latter have a tubular pattern of growth, with the cells having clear, sometimes eosinophilic cytoplasm. These lesions are aggressive and often spread to bone. We agree with Young and Scully that it is important to distinguish these from the benign nephrogenic adenoma.[113] Unlike the nephrogenic adenoma, the carcinomas lack basement membranes around the tubules, have mitotic figures and anaplastic cells, often show stratification of cells, and penetrate the tissues beyond the zone of inflammation.

Most female urethral carcinomas are diagnosed in advanced stage. Eighty-four per cent have invaded the periurethral muscularis (Stage B or higher) at the time of discovery.[97]

CARCINOMA OF THE URETER AND RENAL PELVIS

As in the urinary bladder, the vast majority of neoplasms of the upper urinary tract, excluding the renal parenchyma, are malignant tumors that originate from the transitional epithelium of the lining. The general morphologic features and etiology are similar to those of bladder tumors, so this section will focus largely on certain unique aspects of transitional cell carcinoma and its variant forms, as seen in the upper tracts.

Multicentric and Bilateral Lesions

That the patient who develops carcinoma of the urinary tract is at risk for the development of another lesion is well known. Synchronous or metachronous occurrence of carcinoma in one or both ureters or renal pelvises in such a patient is not at all uncommon. Indeed, one occasionally will find malignancy involving essentially the entire tract from the pelvis to the urethra and prostatic ducts.

The incidence of multifocal lesions in the patient with carcinoma of the ureter or pelvis is said to be nearly 50%.[8] The findings of Hvidt and Feldt-Rasmussen are of particular interest in this regard.[40] Thirty per cent of their cases of pelvic carcinoma had synchronous tumor elsewhere, with 26% in the ureter and 4% in the bladder. In their series of ureteral carcinomas, 40% exhibited synchronous lesions, with 32% in the pelvis, 6% in other parts of the ureter, and 2% in the bladder. Groups headed by Grabstald[33] and Wagle[104] found that 3.5% and 4%, respectively, of patients with pelvic carcinomas had similar lesions in the contralateral pelvis.

The incidence of bilateral ureteral carcinoma was reported as 15% by Schade and associates[86] and 23% by Sharma and colleagues.[90] Both of these studies are of further significance since they address the common problem of evaluating the status of the ureters in patients treated by cystectomy for bladder cancer. Sharma and associates found ureteral carcinoma in 17 of 205 such patients (8.5%).[90] The highest incidence was in those patients with multifocal, high-grade, and high-stage bladder tumors. In their series of 30 cystectomy specimens, Schade and associates found ureteral carcinoma in 10—either in situ, papillary, or invasive.[86] These lesions were most commonly found in that part of the ureter nearest the bladder, and many others of these 60 ureteral stumps showed epithelial abnormalities that many would regard as premalignant or low-grade in situ carcinoma. Koss and co-workers found carcinoma in situ in one or both distal ureters in six of 10 cases of bladder carcinomas examined by total histologic study.[50]

Kimball and Ferris provide information on the sequential development of carcinoma.[46] Of 74 patients with renal pelvic tumors and similar lesions in the bladder or ureter, the lesions were present synchronously in 24 and developed later in 50. Clayman and associates found that only 1% of patients have synchronous lesions, whereas 2.1% eventually develop contralateral ureteral or pelvic carcinomas.[11] Over 80% of such "recurrences" develop within

the first three years after surgery but, occasionally, they may take up to 20 years. These observers also noted that a patient with ureteral or pelvic carcinoma has a 1% chance of developing contralateral carcinoma, if predisposing factors are absent.

Predisposing Factors

In general, the environmental and carcinogenic factors that are applicable to bladder carcinoma apply also to carcinomas of the ureter and renal pelvis. There are three diseases, however, that are associated with a significant increase in the incidence of upper tract carcinoma: Balkan nephropathy, analgesic abuse nephropathy, and sickle cell trait nephropathy.

Since 1953, a dramatic increase in the development of renal pelvic and ureteral carcinoma has occurred in part of Yugoslavia and adjacent Balkan countries. This coincided with the discovery of an idiopathic form of interstitial nephritis characterized by progressive renal failure. The tumors tend to be low grade, and most deaths are apparently related to the nephritis, but 10% of the tumors are bilateral, and the sexes are equally affected. The magnitude of the problem is such that upper tract tumors now exceed those of the renal parenchyma in frequency. Petkovic cited the discovery of 205 renal tumors, compared with 214 of the pelvis and 105 of the ureter.[76] In some villages, there was one pelvic tumor per 200 inhabitants. By comparison, the incidence in the United States is more nearly one in 100,000.

Analgesic nephropathy, resulting from the long-term ingestion of large amounts of phenacetin, occurs more commonly in Australia, South Africa, Switzerland, and Sweden. In the last country, it is said to affect one of every 156,000 people, of whom about 4 to 8% will develop renal pelvic carcinoma.

For some years, we have noted a possible relationship between renal pelvic carcinoma and sickle cell trait. Although such tumors are very uncommon in persons under the age of 30 years, of the relatively small number that occur, an interesting proportion has proved to be in patients who also have sickle cell trait. The apparent association is in need of further study, but based on the limited data now available, it is clear that these are very aggressive tumors that seemingly are not associated with multifocal tumors in the lower urinary tract.

Pathology

Carcinoma of the renal pelvis and ureter are classified, as are those of the bladder, as papillary, invasive, in situ, and as any combination of these.[69] Grossly, one invariably finds hydroureter and hydronephrosis associated with papillary ureteral carcinoma, since the lumen is quickly filled with tumor. Papillary tumors of the pelvis may produce hydronephrosis if the ureteropelvic junction becomes obstructed or, if situated in a calyx, segmental hydronephrosis may result. It should be noted also that complete obstruction of the upper tract may lead to a cessation of hematuria and a false sense of security. Infiltrating carcinomas are characterized by thickening and induration of the wall of the ureter or pelvis with closure of the lumen in a constricting fashion. Where the tumor infiltrates renal parenchyma, there is invariably a pyelointerstitial nephritis and often some degree of tumor-associated fibrosis. The resulting admixture of inflammation, fibrosis, and neoplasm may make difficult the task of defining the extent of the tumor. In situ carcinoma will not usually be grossly apparent but, when dealing with an overt carcinoma (papillary or infiltrating, or both), mucosal areas that appear to be hyperemic, hemorrhagic, or thickened should be sectioned for histologic study. Carcinomas of the upper urinary tract exhibit the same histologic spectrum that has already been described for the urinary bladder. The four basic cell types—transitional, squamous, glandular and undifferentiated—may be found in pure form or combinations. The great majority are transitional cell carcinomas. Less than 10% of pelvic tumors are pure squamous carcinoma. Since these have such a poor prognosis, they should be distinguished from transitional cell carcinoma showing areas of squamous change. About half of them have been associated with calculi and squamous metaplasia. Squamous carcinoma should also be distinguished from the so-called cholesteatoma of kidney. This is essentially a keratinizing squamous metaplasia of pelvic and calyceal mucosa in a hydronephrotic kidney. The deeper recesses of the cornified calyceal pockets will mimic a low-grade squamous carcinoma in the substance of the kidney. Unlike the case in the bladder, pure mucinous carcinoma of the pelvis is rare. Because of this, a primary lesion elsewhere, such as in the colon, should always be considered. Most of these tumors have been in females and have been associated with calculi and chronic infection.

Grading and Pathologic Staging

Grading of upper urinary tract tumors is the same as that used for bladder tumors. Grade 1 tumors are those in which the tumor cells show but little variation from normal (benign) cells. Grade 3 tumors show marked variation (or anaplasia), and Grade 2 lesions show intermediate changes.

A widely accepted system for the pathologic staging of renal pelvic and ureteral tumors has not been devised, although Bennington and Beckwith have proposed the following:[8]

Stage I. Papillary or in situ carcinoma without evidence of stromal invasion.

Stage II. As above, but with stromal invasion, which is limited to lamina propria.

Stage III. Papillary or in situ carcinoma in which invasion is into muscularis. This includes those calyceal tumors that invade into but not beyond the kidney.

Stage IV. Those tumors that extend to the adventitial surface, adjacent structures, or exhibit metastases.

Metastases

Unlike renal parenchymal tumors, which spread chiefly by the hematogenous route, pelvic and ureteral tumors involve the local lymphatics and, initially, regional lymph nodes. Later, frequent sites of spread are lung, liver, and bones.[99]

Prognosis

In general, renal pelvic tumors have a relatively poor prognosis, with five-year survival rates of 30 to 45%. To some extent, this is due to the squamous carcinomas, which have an extremely poor prognosis.

The opinions or assertions contained herein are the private views of the authors and are not to be construed as official or as reflecting the views of the Department of the Army or the Department of Defense.

Johansson and Wahlquist achieved a five-year survival of 84% by adopting an aggressive approach: transabdominal perifascial nephroureterectomy with a cuff of bladder and homolateral adrenalectomy.[45] As a group, ureteral carcinomas present as lower grade tumors, and at a lower stage. In spite of this, however, the overall five-year survival is no better than 50%.[8]

References

1. Alroy J, Pauli BU, Weinstein RS: Correlation between numbers of desmosomes and the aggressiveness of transitional cell carcinoma in human urinary bladder. Cancer 47:104–112, 1981.
2. Althausen AF, Prout GR Jr, Daly JJ: Non-invasive papillary carcinoma of the bladder associated with carcinoma in situ. J Urol 116:575–580, 1976.
3. Anderson CK: Current topics on the pathology of bladder cancer. Proc R Soc Med 66:283–286, 1973.
4. Barlebo H, Sorensen BL: Flat epithelial changes in urinary bladder in patients with prostatic hypertrophy. Scand J Urol Nephrol Supplement 15:121–128, 1972.
5. Barlogie B, Johnston DA, Smallwood L, et al: Prognostic implication of ploidy and proliferative activity of human solid tumors. Cancer Genet Cytogenet 6:17–28, 1982.
6. Barnes RW, Bergman RT, Hadley HL, et al: Control of bladder tumors by endoscopic surgery. J Urol 97:864–868, 1967.
7. Bell JT, Burney SW, Friedell GH: Blood vessel invasion in human bladder cancer. J Urol 105:675–678, 1971.
8. Bennington JL, Beckwith JD: Tumors of the Kidney, Renal Pelvis, and Ureter. Atlas of Tumor Pathology, Second Series, Fascicle 12. Washington, DC, Armed Forces Institute of Pathology, 1975.
9. Bolduan JP, Farah RN: Primary urethral neoplasms: review of 30 cases. J Urol 125:198–200, 1981.
10. Chisholm GD, Hindmarsh JR, Howatson AG, et al: TNM (1978) in bladder cancer. Use and abuse. Br J Urol 52:500–505, 1980.
11. Clayman RV, Lange PH, Fraley EE: Cancer of the upper urinary tract. In N Javadpour (ed), Principles and Management of Urologic Cancer, 2nd ed. Baltimore, Williams & Wilkins, 1983, pp 544–559.
12. Cohen SM, Greenfield RE, Jacobs RB, Friedell GH: Precancerous and noninvasive lesions of the urinary bladder. In RL Carter (ed), Precancerous States. New York, Oxford Press, 1984, pp 278–303.
13. Cooling CJ: Review of 150 postmortems of carcinoma of the urinary bladder. In DM Wallace (ed), Tumors of Bladder. London, Livingstone, 1959, pp 171–186.
14. Coon JS, Weinstein RS, Summers JL: Bladder group precursor T-antigen expression in human urinary bladder carcinoma. Am J Clin Pathol 77:692–699, 1982.
15. Cooper PH, Waisman J, Johnston WH, Skinner DG: Severe atypia of transitional epithelium and carcinoma of the urinary bladder. Cancer 31:1055–1060, 1973.
16. Cordon-Cardo C: Monoclonal antibodies in the diagnosis of solid tumors: studies of renal cell carcinomas, transitional cell carcinomas and melanoma. In J Russo (ed), Immunohistochemistry in Tumor Diagnoses. Boston, Martinus Nijhoff, 1984, pp 281–292.
17. Cutler SJ, Heney NM, Friedell GH: Longitudinal study of patients with bladder cancer: factors associated with disease recurrence and progression. In AUA Monographs, Vol 1. WW Bonney, GR Prout, Jr. (eds), Bladder Cancer. Baltimore, Williams & Wilkins, 1982, pp 35–46.
18. Daly JJ: Carcinoma-in-situ of the urothelium. Urol Clin North Am 3:87–105, 1976.
19. Davidsohn I, Kovarik S, Lee CL: A, B, and O substances in gastrointestinal carcinoma. Arch Pathol 81:381–390, 1966.
20. Davidsohn I, Stejskal R, Lill P: The loss of iso-antigens A, B, and H in carcinoma of urinary bladder (Abstr). Lab Invest 28:382, 1973.
21. Decenzo JM, Howard P, Irish CE: Antigenic deletion and prognosis of patients with stage A transitional cell bladder carcinoma. J Urol 114:874–878, 1975.
22. Droller MJ: Transitional cell cancer: upper tract and bladder. In P Walsh, B Gittes, A Perlmutter, T Stamey (eds), Campbell's Urology. Baltimore, Williams & Wilkins, 1986, pp 1343–1440.
23. Eisenberg RB, Roth RB, Weinberg MH: Bladder tumors and associated proliferative mucosal lesions. J Urol 84:544–550, 1960.
24. Epstein JI, Woodruff JM: Adenocarcinoma of the prostate with endometrioid features. A light microscopic and immunohistochemical study of ten cases. Cancer 57:111–119, 1986.
25. Falor WH: Chromosomes in noninvasive papillary carcinoma of the bladder. JAMA 216:791–794, 1971.
26. Falor WH, Ward RM: Prognosis in early carcinoma of the bladder based on chromosomal analysis. J Urol 119:44–48, 1978.
27. Farrow GM, Utz DC, Rife CC: Morphological and clinical observations of patients with early bladder cancer treated with total cystectomy. Cancer Res 36:2495–2501, 1976.
28. Farrow GM, Utz DC, Rife CC, Green L: Clinical observations on sixty-nine cases of in situ carcinoma of the urinary bladder. Cancer Res 37:2794–2798, 1977.
29. Fossa SD, Reitan JB, Ous S, et al: Prediction of tumor progression in superficial bladder carcinoma. Eur Urol 11:1–5, 1985.
30. Friedell GH: Carcinoma, carcinoma in situ, and "early lesions" of the uterine cervix and the urinary bladder. Introduction and definitions. Cancer Res 36:2482–2484, 1976.
31. Friedell GH: Current concepts of the aetiology, pathogenesis, and pathology of bladder cancer. Urol Res 6:179–182, 1978.
32. Gibas Z, Prout GR Jr, Connolly JG, et al: Nonrandom chromosomal changes in transitional cell carcinoma of the bladder. Cancer Res 44:1257–1264, 1984.
33. Grabstald H, Whitmore WF Jr, Melamed MR: Renal pelvis tumors. JAMA 218:845–854, 1971.
34. Grabstald H: Tumors of the urethra in men and women. Cancer 32:1236–1255, 1973.
35. Greene LF, Hanash KA, Farrow GM: Benign pap-

illoma or papillary carcinoma of the bladder? J Urol 110:205–207, 1973.

36. Hakomori EI: Glycolipids of tumor cell membrane. Adv Cancer Res 18:265–351, 1973.

37. Hakomori EI: (Philip Levine Award Lecture). Blood group glycolipid antigens and their modifications as human cancer antigens. Am J Clin Pathol 82:635–648, 1984.

38. Heney NM, Nocks BN, Daly JJ, et al: Ta and T1 bladder cancer: location, recurrence, and progression. Br J Urol 54:152–157, 1982.

39. Hicks RM, Newman J: Scanning electron microscopy of urinary sediment. In LG Koss, VV Coleman (eds), Advances in Clinical Cytology, Vol 2. New York, Masson, 1984, pp 235–261.

40. Hvidt V, Feldt-Rasmussen K: Primary tumours in the renal pelvis and ureter with particular attention to the diagnostic problems. Acta Clin Scand 433(Suppl):91–101, 1973.

41. Ishak KG, LeGolvan PC, El Sebai I: Malignant bladder tumors associated with schistosomiasis. A gross and microscopic study. In FK Mostofi (ed), Bilharziasis. Springer Verlag, 1967, pp 58–92.

42. Jacobs JB: The potential of scanning electron microscopic explorative cytology on the clinical management of human bladder cancer. In AUA Monographs, Vol 1. WW Bonney, GB Prout, Jr. (eds), Bladder Cancer. Baltimore, Williams & Wilkins, 1982, pp 95–109.

43. Jewett HJ, Eversole SL Jr: Carcinoma of the bladder. Characteristic modes of local invasion. J Urol 83:383–389, 1960.

44. Jewett HJ, King LR, Shelley WM: A study of 365 cases of infiltrating bladder cancer: relation of certain pathological characteristics to prognosis after extirpation. J Urol 92:668–678, 1964.

45. Johansson S, Wahlqvist L: A prognostic study of urothelial renal pelvic tumors: comparison between the prognosis of patients treated with intrafascial nephrectomy and perifascial nephroureterectomy. Cancer 43:2525–2531, 1979.

46. Kimball FN, Ferris HW: Papillomatous tumor of the renal pelvis associated with similar tumors of ureter and bladder: review of literature and report of 2 cases. J Urol 31:257–304, 1934.

47. Klein FA, Herr HW, Sogani PC, et al: Detection and follow-up of carcinoma of the urinary bladder by flow cytometry. Cancer 50:389–395, 1982.

48. Koss LG: Tumors of the urinary bladder. Atlas of Tumor Pathology, Fascicle II, 2nd Series. Washington, DC, Armed Forces Institute of Pathology, 1975.

49. Koss LG, Melamed MR, Kelly E: Further cytologic and histologic studies of bladder lesions in workers exposed to para-aminodiphenyl: progress report. JNCI 43:233–243, 1969.

50. Koss LG, Tiamson EM, Robbins MA: Mapping cancerous and precancerous bladder changes. A study of the urothelium in ten surgically removed bladders. JAMA 227:281–286, 1974.

51. Lamb D: Correlation of chromosome counts with histological appearances and prognosis in transitional-cell carcinoma of bladder. Br Med J 1:273–277, 1967.

52. Lange PH, Limas C: Molecular markers in the diagnosis and prognosis of bladder cancer. Urology 23(Suppl 4):46–54, 1984.

53. Lerman RI, Hutter RVP, Whitmore WF Jr: Papilloma of the urinary bladder. Cancer 25:333–342, 1970.

54. Limas C, Lange P, Fraley EE, Vessella RL: A, B, H antigens in transitional cell tumors of the urinary bladder: correlation with the clinical course. Cancer 44:2099–2107, 1979.

55. Lotan R, Skutelsky E, Danon D, Sharon N: The purification, composition, and specificity of the anti-T lectin from peanut (Arachis hypogaea). J Biol Chem 250:8518–8523, 1975.

56. Marshall VF: The relation of preoperative estimate in the pathologic demonstration of the extent of vesical neoplasms. J Urol 68:714–717, 1952.

57. Marshall VF: Symposium on bladder tumors: current clinical problems regarding bladder tumors. Cancer 9:543–550, 1956.

58. Marshall VF, McCarron JP Jr: The curability of vesical cancer: greater now or then? Cancer Res 37:2753–2755, 1977.

59. Melamed MR, Koss LG, Rocci A, Whitemore RW Jr: Cystohistological observations on developing carcinoma of the urinary bladder in man. Cancer 13:67–74, 1960.

60. Melamed MR, Voutsa NG, Grabstald H: Natural history and clinical behavior of in situ carcinoma of the human urinary bladder. Cancer 17:1533–1545, 1964.

61. Melamed MR, Grabstald H, Whitmore WF Jr: Carcinoma in-situ of bladder. Clinico-pathological study of case with a suggested approach for detection. J Urol 96:466–471, 1966.

62. Melamed MR, Klein FA: Flow cytometry of urinary bladder irrigation specimens. Hum Pathol 15:302–305, 1984.

63. Melicow MM: Histological study of vesical urothelium intervening between gross neoplasms in total cystectomy. J Urol 68:261–279, 1952.

64. Melicow MM: Tumors of the urinary bladder: clinicopathological analyses of over 2500 specimens and biopsies. J Urol 74:498–521, 1955.

65. Miller A, Mitchell JP, Brown NJ: The Bristol Bladder Tumour Registry. Br J Urol 41(Suppl):1–64, 1969.

66. Mostofi FK: A study of 2678 patients with initial carcinoma of the bladder: I. survival rates. J Urol 75:480–491, 1956.

67. Mostofi FK: Potentialities of bladder epithelium. J Urol 71:705–714, 1954.

68. Mostofi FK: Standardization of nomenclature and criteria for diagnosis of epithelial tumors of urinary bladder. Acta Union Int Cancer 16:310–314, 1968.

69. Mostofi FK, Davis CJ: Tumors and tumor-like lesions of kidney. In R Hickey (ed), Current Problems in Cancer. Chicago, Year Book Medical Publisher, 1986.

70. Mostofi FK, Thomson RV, Dean AL Jr: Mucous adenocarcinoma of the urinary bladder. Cancer 8:741–758, 1955.

71. Mostofi FK, Morse WH: Polypoid rhabdomyosarcoma (sarcoma botryoides) of bladder in children. J Urol 67:681–687, 1952.

72. Mostofi FK, Sobin LH, Torloni H: Histological typing of urinary bladder tumors. Geneva, WHO, 1973.

73. Nichols JA, Marshall VF: The treatment of bladder carcinoma by local excision and fulguration. Cancer 9:559–565, 1956.

74. Olsson CA, White RWD: Cancer of bladder. In N Javadpour (ed), Principles and Management of Urologic Cancer. Baltimore, Williams & Wilkins, 1979, pp 337–375.

75. Pauli BU, Cohen SM, Alroy J, Weinstein RS:

Desmosome ultrastructure and the biological behavior of chemical carcinogen-induced urinary bladder carcinomas. Cancer Res 38:3276–3280, 1978.

76. Petkovic SD: Conservation of the kidney in operations for tumours of the renal pelvis and calyces: a report of 26 cases. Br J Urol 44:1–8, 1972.

77. Prout GR Jr: Classification and staging of bladder carcinoma. In AUA Monographs, Vol 1. WW Bonney, GR Prout Jr (eds), Bladder Cancer. Baltimore, Williams & Wilkins, 1982, pp 133–146.

78. Prout GR Jr: Heterogeneity of superficial bladder cancer. In AUA Monographs Vol 1. WW Bonney, GR Prout Jr (eds), Bladder Cancer. Baltimore, Williams & Wilkins, 1982, pp 149–155.

79. Prout GR Jr, Griffin PP, Shipley WU: Bladder carcinoma as a systemic disease. Cancer 43:2532–2539, 1979.

80. Pyrah LH, Raper FP, Thomas GM: Report of a follow-up of papillary tumours of the bladder. Br J Urol 36:14–25, 1964.

81. Richie JP, Skinner DG, Kaufman JJ: Radical cystectomy for carcinoma of bladder: 16 years of experience. J Urol 113:186–189, 1975.

82. Riddle PR, Chisholm DG, Trott PA: Flat carcinoma in situ of bladder. Br J Urol 47:829–833, 1975.

83. Roberts TW, Melicow MM: Pathology and natural history of urethral tumors in females: review of 65 cases. Urology 10:583–589, 1977.

84. Sandberg AA: Chromosome markers and progression in bladder cancer. Cancer Res 37:2950–2956, 1977.

85. Sandberg AA: Chromosomes in bladder cancer. In AUA Monographs, Vol 1, WW Bonney, GR Prout Jr (eds), Bladder Cancer. Baltimore, Williams & Wilkins, 1982, pp 81–93.

86. Schade ROK, Serck-Hanssen A, Swinney J: Morphological changes in the ureter in cases of bladder carcinoma. Cancer 27:1267–1272, 1971.

87. Schade ROK, Swinney J: Pre-cancerous changes in bladder epithelium. Lancet 2:943–946, 1968.

88. Schulman C, Sylvester R, Robinson M, et al: Adjuvant therapy of T1 bladder carcinoma: preliminary results of an EORTC randomized study. Urol Res (as quoted in Slack & Prout, ref. 93).

89. Sesterhenn I, Mostofi FK, Davis CJ Jr: Immunopathology of prostate and bladder tumors. In J Russo (ed), Immunocystochemistry in Tumor Diagnosis. Boston, Martinus Nijhoff, 1984, pp 337–361.

90. Sharma TC, Melamed MR, Whitmore WF Jr: Carcinoma in-situ of the ureter in patients with bladder carcinoma treated by cystectomy. Cancer 26:583–587, 1970.

91. Singer SJ, Nicholson GL: The fluid mosaic model of the structure of cell membranes. Science 175:720–731, 1972.

92. Skinner DG: Current state of classification and staging of bladder cancer. Cancer Res 37:2838–2842, 1977.

93. Slack NH, Prout GR Jr: Heterogeneity of invasive bladder carcinoma and different responses to treatment. In AUA Monographs, Vol 1. WW Bonney, GR Prout, Jr (eds), Bladder Cancer. Baltimore, Williams & Wilkins, 1982, pp 213–232.

94. Smith G, Elton RA, Beynon LL, et al: Prognostic significance of biopsy results of normal-looking mucosa in cases of superficial bladder cancer. Br J Urol 55:665–669, 1983.

95. Soloway MS: The management of superficial bladder cancer. Cancer 45:1856–1863, 1980.

96. Stellner K, Hakomori S, Warner GS: Enzymic conversion of "H1-glycolipid" to A or B glycolipid and deficiency of these enzyme activities in adenocarcinoma. Biochem Biophys Res Commun 55:439–445, 1973.

97. Sullivan J, Grabstald H: Management of carcinoma of the urethra. In DG Skinner, JB deKernion (eds), Genitourinary Cancer. Philadelphia, WB Saunders, 1978, pp 419–429.

98. Tannenbaum M, Romas NA: The pathobiology of early urothelial cancer. In DG Skinner, G Lieskovsky (eds), Diagnosis and Management of Genitourinary Cancer, Chapter 6. Philadelphia, WB Saunders, 1987.

99. Thackray AC: Malignant tumors of the urothelium—tumors of the renal pelvis. In ED Riches (ed), Tumors of Kidney and Ureter. London, Livingstone, 1965, pp 87–89.

100. Tribukait B, Gustafson H, Esposti PL: The significance of ploidy and proliferation in the clinical and biological evaluation of bladder tumours: a study of 100 untreated cases. Br J Urol 54:130–135, 1982.

101. Tribukait B: Flow cytometry in surgical pathology and cytology of tumors of the genitourinary tract. In LG Koss, DV Coleman (eds), Advances in Clinical Cytology, Vol 2. New York, Masson, 1984, pp 163–189.

102. Utz DC, Hanash KA, Farrow GM: The plight of the patient with carcinoma in situ of the bladder. J Urol 103:160–164, 1970.

103. Varkarakis MJ, Gaeta JF, Moore RH, et al: Superficial bladder tumors: aspect of clinical progression. Urology 4:414–420, 1974.

104. Wagle DG, Moore RH, Murphy GP: Primary carcinoma of the renal pelvis. Cancer 33:1642–1648, 1974.

105. Wallace DM: Clinicopathological behavior of bladder tumors. In D Wallace (ed), Tumors of Bladder. London, Livingstone, 1959, pp 157–170.

106. Weiner DP, Koss LG, Sablay B, Freed SW: The prevalence and significance of Brunn's nests, cystitis cystica, and squamous metaplasia in normal bladder. J Urol 122:317–321, 1979.

107. Weinstein RS: Origin and dissemination of human urinary bladder carcinoma. Semin Oncol 6:149–156, 1979.

108. Weinstein RS: Intravesical dissemination and invasion of urinary bladder carcinoma. In AUA Monographs, Vol 1. WW Bonney, GR Prout, Jr (eds), Bladder Cancer. Baltimore, Williams & Wilkins, 1982, pp 27–33.

109. Weinstein RS, Miller AW, Coon JS: Tissue blood group ABH and Thomsen-Friedenreich antigens in human urinary bladder carcinoma. Prog Clin Biol Res 153:249–260, 1984.

110. Whitmore WF Jr: Management of bladder cancer. Curr Probl Cancer 4:1–48, 1979.

111. Wolf H, Hojgaard KE: Urothelial dysplasia concomitant with bladder tumours as a determinant factor for future new occurrences. Lancet 2:134–136, 1983.

112. Yates-Bell AJ: Carcinoma-in-situ of the bladder. Br J Surg 58:359–364, 1971.

113. Young RH, Scully RE: Clear cell adenocarcinoma of the bladder and urethra. Am J Surg Pathol 9:816–826, 1985.

G. RICHARD DICKERSIN, M.D.
ROBERT B. COLVIN, M.D.

Pathology of Renal Tumors CHAPTER 8

Renal cell carcinoma
Adenoma
  Oncocytoma
Nephroblastoma (Wilms' tumor)
Nephroblastomatosis (persistent renal
  blastema, nodular renal blastema)
Congenital mesoblastic nephroma
Fetal rhabdomyomatous nephroblastoma
Cystic, partially differentiated nephroblas-
  toma
Clear cell sarcoma of the kidney
Malignant rhabdoid tumor of the kidney
Miscellaneous sarcomas
Angiomyolipoma
Juxtaglomerular tumor (reninoma)

Malignant tumors of the renal parenchyma rank thirteenth in frequency among all cancers and account for about 3% of human malignant tumors overall.[13] Pathologic analysis has permitted more accurate classification of benign and malignant variants and is an essential basis for proper choice of therapy. Furthermore, even among the more common types of parenchymal tumors (renal cell carcinoma and nephroblastoma), certain pathologic features have a significant influence on prognosis. Here we will emphasize those pathologic features that are of diagnostic or prognostic value, particularly in renal cell carcinoma and nephroblastoma. Less common renal tumors of importance in differential diagnosis or therapy will be described briefly. Other chapters in this volume discuss renal pelvic tumors and the clinical and therapeutic aspects of renal tumors. In general, landmark articles and pertinent recent work are cited; further refer-

ences can be found in comprehensive reviews.[6, 13, 95, 106]

RENAL CELL CARCINOMA

Renal cell carcinoma, variously called hypernephroma, renal adenocarcinoma, clear cell carcinoma, and other less common terms,[13] is the most common renal tumor in adults, representing 85% of all primary renal malignancies[6] and accounting for 1000 female and 2300 male deaths per one hundred million persons under the age of 65 in the United States in 1978.[35] We estimate over 7000 new cases per year in the United States. Since the tumor cells generally share ultrastructural (described later) and antigenic[65, 69, 142] features with normal proximal tubular cells, we prefer the term renal cell (or, more precisely, renal tubular cell) carcinoma.

Gross Features

The tumors are roughly spherical masses that are usually based in the cortex but expand into the perinephric tissue (Fig. 8–1). They have no true capsule but may have a condensation of fibrous tissue and inflammatory cells around the periphery. Gerota's fascia often seems to form a barrier to penetration into the perinephric fat. There is no apparent predilection for either left or right sides or different segments of the kidney. Bilateral tumors are extremely rare and are found in about 1% of cases.[6, 93] The presence of multiple tumors in one or both

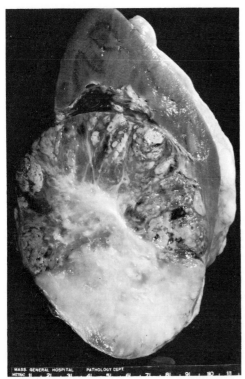

Figure 8–1. This typical renal cell carcinoma has destroyed one pole of the kidney but is still covered with Gerota's fascia (the perinephric fat was removed for photography). The nodules in the upper portion of the tumor were bright yellow; the whiter portion below consisted chiefly of fibrous tissue.

kidneys should suggest the possibility of von Hippel–Lindau disease.[59, 79] Growth into renal veins is found in about 40% of the surgical specimens in patients who have no evidence of metastasis.[125] The tumors are quite variegated and show hemorrhage, necrosis, cystic areas, calcification, and fibrosis. Lipid in the cells usually imparts a yellow-orange color to the tumor. Tumors rich in granular cells are brown, probably due to the cytochrome enzymes in the abundant mitochondria (see section on electron microscopy). Tumors consisting of less differentiated "sarcomatous" cells are often less pigmented and appear gray or tan. At times viable tumor may be present as a small yellow-brown plaque or nodule in the wall of an otherwise typical benign cyst.[143] This finding is common in our experience in von Hippel–Lindau disease. The tumors rarely invade the pelvis and ureters,[112] and malignant cells can be identified in the urine in less than 7% of the patients.[136]

Histologic Features

By light microscopy, several patterns of growth can be found, often in the same tumor. Typical patterns are trabecular (cords) (Figs. 8–2 and 8–3), alveolar, papillary, and solid sheets. The tubular pattern (Figs. 8–4 and 8–5), which resembles normal tubules, occurs infrequently. Although cells may border a lumen that may contain mucopolysaccharides, intracellular mucus is not seen and, if present, suggests another origin for the tumor, either the renal pelvis or a metastasis. There are three common cell types: clear cells, granular cells, and spindle cells; rarer variants have also been described.[94] Clear cells (Figs. 8–2 and 8–3) are rounded or polygonal cells with abundant cytoplasm that stains poorly in routine sections. This is the cell type in about 25 to 51% of renal cell carcinoma.[6, 125] The cytoplasm stains with the periodic acid–Schiff technique. This staining is inhibited by prior digestion with diastase, which indicates the presence of glycogen, as opposed to glycoprotein or glycosaminoglycans. The cytoplasm in frozen sections also stains well with oil red O and Sudan black,[13] which demonstrates the presence of neutral lipids and phospholipids. Cholesterol has been found by extraction, and spaces that suggest cholesterol crystals can be found by electron microscopy (see later). Granular cells contain much less glycogen and neutral lipid, and their cytoplasm is eosinophilic, coarsely granular (Figs. 8–4 and 8–5), and rich in mitochondria. About 9 to 12% of renal cell carcinomas consist principally of granular cells,[6, 125] but as many as half contain both granular and clear cells. The spindle cell tumors that account for about 3 to 14% of renal cell tumors grow in solid sheets and often resemble pleomorphic mesenchymal cells (Fig. 8–6). The cells usually can be distinguished from fibrosarcoma cells by the presence of neutral lipid and glycogen.

Hemorrhage is common in renal cell carcinomas and may relate to vascular fragility. Other features include necrosis, fibrosis, hemosiderin deposits, lipid-filled macrophages, and psammoma bodies.[13] A sparse mononuclear cell infiltrate sometimes is present, usually at the periphery, but these tumors rarely incite a prominent inflammatory response except in areas of necrosis. The nuclei vary from those resembling normal tubular cell nuclei to enlarged bizarre

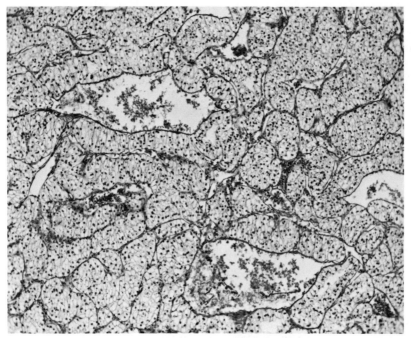

Figure 8–2. The thin-walled, dilated capillaries separate the cords of clear cells in this renal cell carcinoma. This and other light micrographs are stained with hematoxylin and eosin. (× 120)

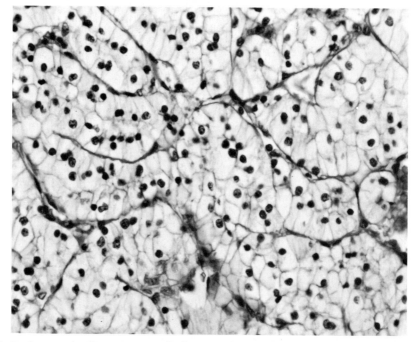

Figure 8–3. A Grade 2 renal cell carcinoma with clear cytoplasm and a trabecular pattern of growth. The nuclei are not enlarged but do demonstrate hyperchromatism. (× 390)

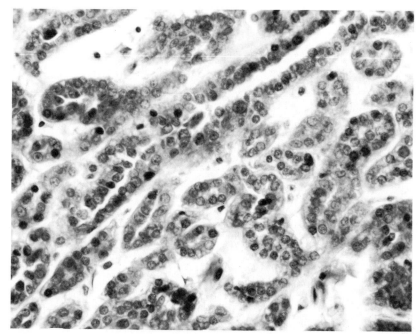

Figure 8–4. A Grade 1 renal cell carcinoma with granular cytoplasm and a tubular pattern of growth. The nuclei are indistinguishable from normal tubular cell nuclei. (× 390)

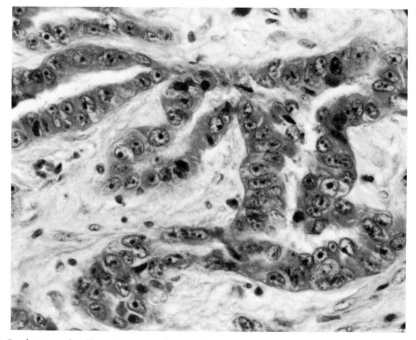

Figure 8–5. A Grade 3 renal cell carcinoma with granular cytoplasm and a tubular pattern of growth. The nuclei are enlarged (compare with Fig. 8–4), moderately irregular, and have prominent nucleoli. (× 390)

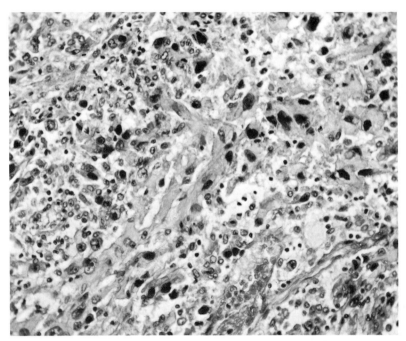

Figure 8–6. A Grade 4 renal cell carcinoma with a spindle pattern of growth. The nuclei are enlarged, hyperchromatic, and bizarre. (× 390)

nuclei. The grade of the tumors based on nuclear appearance correlates with survival and is discussed further below. Mitoses, except in Grade 4 tumors, are infrequent. Mixtures of cell types commonly occur, and multiple sections may be necessary to appreciate the full spectrum present. The biologic basis for the heterogeneity in cell type and growth pattern is unknown. It is tempting to speculate that differences in the cell of origin as well as the etiologic agents may be partly responsible. It has been shown that the majority of renal cell carcinomas contain brush border and other antigens characteristic of proximal tubular cells and lack distal tubule antigens (Tamm-Horsfall protein).[41, 69, 142] Most of these tumors also have been demonstrated to contain cytokeratins of the epidermal and parenchymal types and vimentin.[65, 69] The immunofluorescent and immunocytochemical approaches used by these workers have value, therefore, in the diagnosis as well as classification of suspected renal cell tumors.

These tumors are highly vascular, and the cords of cells are separated by a lattice of thin-walled blood vessels (Fig. 8–2) that often have fenestrations similar to the normal peritubular capillaries (see Electron Microscopy, later). Tumor may grow into these vessels and gain access to the venous drainage. When this occurs, a tumor thrombus may form that can extend into the renal vein and even cephalad through the vena cava to the heart.[126] We believe that this usually is due not to true vascular "invasion" of the walls of the larger veins but more likely to a process of herniation into the small and fragile thin-walled tumor vessels. Growth into arteries is not common in our experience, but it does occur.[13]

Electron Microscopy

The ultrastructural features of the cells in renal cell carcinoma first made it apparent that they resembled the epithelium of renal tubules and not that of adrenal cortex.[97] Since then, a number of other ultrastructural investigations on humans and lower animals have confirmed the impression that the convoluted tubule, and more specifically the proximal tubule, is the probable origin of this neoplasm.[13, 42, 117, 120, 130, 131] The normal proximal tubular epithelium has a more complex cytoplasm and plasmalemma than the epithelium in the more distal parts of the nephron. Characteristically, the free or apical surface of the cell has long and numerous microvilli. The crypts of the villi are coated with a glycocalyx, and the apical cytoplasm contains numerous pinocytotic vesicles and vacuoles. Features common to both proximal and distal tubules include parallel infoldings of the basal cell membrane and numerous mitochondria,[120] as well as a basal lamina surrounding the tubule, lateral cell junctions and interdigitations, and varying proportions of cytoplasmic glycogen, lipid, microbodies, and lysosomes.

In renal cell carcinoma, all these features of normal tubular cells may be present to some degree, but even the most highly differentiated tumor will have certain differences from normal cells (Figs. 8–7 to 8–9). The brush borders usually are not fully and orderly developed and are present only in a proportion of the tumor cells (Fig. 8–7). Moreover, ectopic brush borders may occur on the nonapical surface of the cell, and microacinar formation may be present between the lateral borders of adjacent cells or apparently within the cytoplasm of individual cells (Fig. 8–9). Cellular junctions and basal border infoldings are usually decreased, and basal lamina material may be found around individual cells and groups of cells.

The ultrastructure of clear cells is distinctly different from that of granular cells. Clear cells have abundant glycogen and lipid and a paucity of cytoplasmic organelles (Figs. 8–7 and 8–8). The glycogen is not completely preserved by some processing methods for electron microscopy and is identifiable as empty, escalloped, cytoplasmic spaces (Fig. 8–7). However, when specimens are processed to preserve the glycogen, cells manifest numerous electron-dense particles larger than ribosomes and about 200 to 400 Å in diameter (Fig. 8–8). Similar material is found in the extracellular space (Fig. 8–8). The lipid occurs as unbound droplets of light or medium osmiophilia, and clefts suggesting cholesterol crystals also can be found (Fig. 8–8). The granular cells have very little glycogen and fat, and the cytoplasm is almost completely occupied by mitochondria (Fig. 8–9). The mitochondria may be pleomorphic and have elongated, parallel layering of their cristae. The Golgi apparatus usually is well developed, and free ribosomes and lysosomes may be numerous.

The ultrastructural characteristics of the spindle cell type of renal carcinoma are incompletely elucidated. However, there is sufficient ultrastructural evidence that it is of epithelial and not mesenchymal origin because of the presence of cell junctions, basal lamina, occasional brush borders, and intracytoplasmic lumens.[32, 131] Resemblance of the spindle cells to granular cells with altered mitochondria also has been reported.[6] The epithelial features in spindle cell tumors help to distinguish this renal cell variant from the soft tissue type of sarcomas, such as fibrosarcoma and malignant fibrous histiocytoma, which may arise in the kidney on rare occasions.

We have found that the blood vessels in these tumors typically have fenestrated endothelium (Figs. 8–8 and 8–9), just as the normal peritubular capillaries. This highly differentiated feature also has been described by others, in a metastasis to the brain.[67] These observations may have potential diagnostic usefulness and, furthermore, they show clearly that the neoplasm exerts profound control, not just on the growth[43] but also on the differentiation of the tumor vessels.

Features with Prognostic Significance

Numerous studies have shown that prognosis correlates with the stage of the tumor.[68, 111, 121, 125] In particular, when tumor is confined to the kidney (Stage I), patients have a significantly better survival (Table 8–1), and reported results vary from 60 to 80% at five years. As expected, those patients with distant metastases (Stage IV) survive for shorter times on the average (10% at five years), but three of our 42 patients survived after excision of metastatic lesions; another had spontaneous regression of a pulmonary infiltrate, thought to represent tumor but never proved histologically.

The significance of renal vein invasion is controversial. It is commonly held, with data to support the conclusion,[3, 12, 96, 104] that renal vein "invasion" worsens prognosis. However, when large numbers of cases are analyzed in more detail, it appears that the excessive mortality is not related to renal vein invasion but rather to the inclusion of tumors that extend into perinephric fat or lymph nodes. In our own series of 272 patients, those patients in whom the tumor involved renal veins but did not extend beyond the capsule had the same five-year

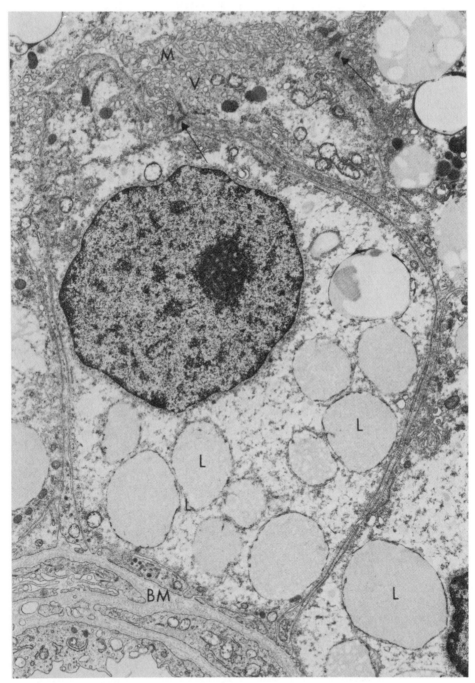

Figure 8–7. Electron micrograph of a clear cell in a renal cell carcinoma. The microvilli (M), apical vesicles (V), cell junctions (arrows), and basement membrane (BM) resemble normal proximal tubular cells. Numerous lipid droplets (L) are in the cytoplasm. The lucent areas represent the spaces filled with glycogen that was not preserved in this tissue. (× 8410)

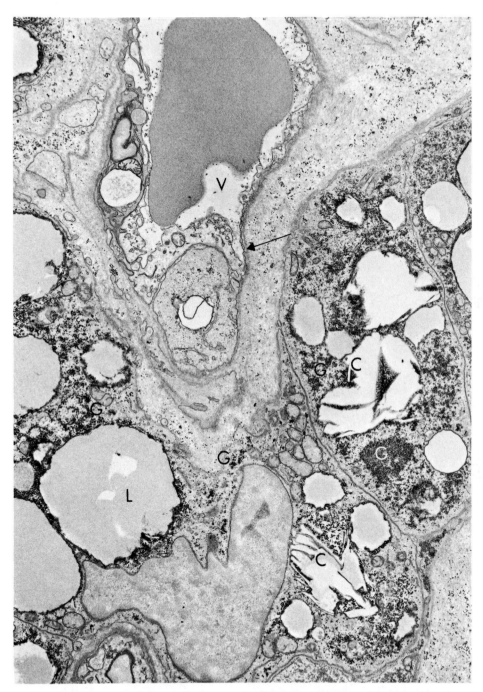

Figure 8–8. Electron micrograph of clear cells in a renal cell carcinoma processed in potassium ferrocyanide to preserve the glycogen granules that appear as dense particles (G) in cells, particularly around the lipid droplets (L). The irregular clefts (C) in the cytoplasm suggest cholesterol crystals. The endothelium of the small tumor vessel (V) is fenestrated (arrow), a feature of normal peritubular capillaries. This suggests that the tumor controls the differentiation of these vessels. (× 6840)

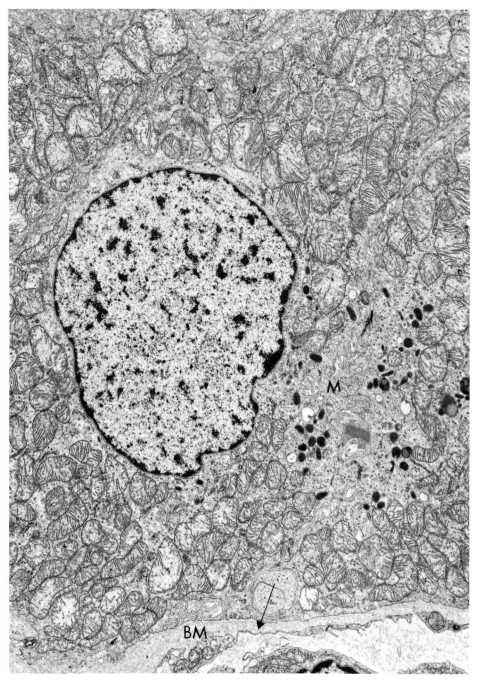

Figure 8–9. Electron micrograph of a granular cell in a renal cell carcinoma. The cytoplasm is filled with mitochondria. Microvilli are present between cells (M) and ectopically against the basement membrane (BM). The nearby tumor vessel has fenestrated endothelium (arrow) as in Fig. 8–8. (× 6840)

Table 8–1. SURVIVAL OF PATIENTS WITH RENAL CELL CARCINOMA
BY STAGE OF TUMOR AT NEPHRECTOMY*

Stage	Number of Patients	Five-year Survival (%)	Ten-year Survival (%)
Confined to kidney			
Without renal vein involvement	91	65	56
With renal vein involvement	81	66	49
Extension into perinephric fat	57	44	26
Metastases to regional lymph nodes	19	16	8
Distant metastasis	62	10	9
Contiguous viscera involved	15	0	0

*From Skinner DG, et al: Diagnosis and management of renal cell carcinoma. A clinical and pathologic study of 309 cases. Cancer 28:1165, 1971.

survival rate (66%) as those without renal vein involvement (65%) (Table 8–1). Other, more recent, studies have yielded similar results.[121, 124] Although surprising at first, consideration of the close association of tumor with dilated thin-walled vessels (Fig. 8–2) suggests that this tumor has ready access to the circulation. Furthermore, as noted above, infrequent actual "invasion" through the walls of veins and arteries suggests that growth into vessels may represent merely a "prolapse" of the tumor and does not have the same significance as it does in other tumors.

Certain microscopic features correlate with survival, and others, such as necrosis, calcification, hemorrhage, or the pattern of growth (such as sheets, cords, and alveoli), generally do not.[94, 125] However, the papillary pattern, which typically is poorly vascular by angiography, had a better prognosis in one series.[86] The cell type has some influence on prognosis.[94, 121, 125] In our series, patients with pure clear cell tumors had a five-year survival rate of 58%, whereas the presence of granular cells lowered the survival rate slightly, to 46%. Others also have found clear cell tumors to carry a better prognosis than neoplasms of the other cell types.[133] Spindle cell tumors, the most anaplastic form, have the worst prognosis (23% survival at five years) in our study.

We found that nuclear appearance was correlated with survival, even among patients with tumors of the same stage (Table 8–2).[121] Grade 1 nuclei (Fig. 8–4) resemble those of normal tubular cells and the usual cells in tubular adenomas (described later) and thus indicate a tumor of low malignant potential. However, Grade 1 tumors can invade perinephric fat (Table 8–2) and, to this extent, manifest malignant behavior. Patients with tumors with bizarre, enlarged nuclei (Grade 4, found usually in spindle cell tumors, Fig. 8–6) have the worst prognosis. Even as one goes from hyperchromatic but normal-sized nuclei (Grade 2, Fig. 8–3) to moderately enlarged nuclei with prominent nucleoli (Grade 3, Fig. 8–5) in Stage I and Stage III tumors, respectively, the prognosis worsens from 81% to 58%, and 70% to 40% ($p < 0.05$). Other studies[3, 18, 47, 52, 66, 116, 121] also have found correlation between microscopic features, especially nuclear grade and cell type, and survival. We believe that careful grading and notation of cell type should prove valuable in prospective studies by allowing the physician both to estimate the prognosis more precisely than by stage alone and to choose the therapy more judiciously. Obviously, recognition of Grade 1 tumors that have low malignant potential is of significant clinical relevance. It should be

Table 8–2. FIVE-YEAR SURVIVAL (%) OF PATIENTS WITH RENAL CELL CARCINOMA BY GRADE AND STAGE*

Nuclear Grade‡	Stage†			
	I	II	III	IV
1	(75)	(100)	—	—
2	81	38	70	22
3	58	62	40	3
4	67	(33)	27	(5)

*From Skinner DG, et al: Diagnosis and management of renal cell carcinoma. A clinical and pathologic study of 309 cases. Cancer 28:1165, 1971.

†Stage I, confined to kidney; Stage II, local extension; Stage III, regional nodes or vein involved; Stage IV, involvement of contiguous or distant organs. Parentheses indicate fewer than five patients at risk. One patient with a Grade 1 lesion died from a pulmonary embolism.

‡See text.

pointed out that while the evidence for the importance of nuclear grading is rather convincing, clinical staging of renal cell carcinoma is more important than histologic grading in regard to predicting the biological behavior of the tumors (Table 8–2).[132]

Metastases from renal cell carcinoma spread most commonly by the blood stream and are found in the lung or other sites in 23 to 33% of patients at the time of presentation.[58, 125] Moreover, almost 5% of the patients may present first with signs related to the metastasis,[109] which may involve skin, brain, bone, or other organs.[13, 28, 108] Even metastases to sites as remote as the uvula have been the first sign or symptom of renal cell carcinoma.[77] Careful study of the urinary tract is obviously warranted in patients with unknown primary tumors[26] or unexplained systemic symptoms.[22]

The rare occurrence of spontaneous regression of metastases has been reported more frequently from renal cell carcinomas than from any other tumor.[38] It should be emphasized that long survival has been reported after surgical excision of a primary renal cell carcinoma and its metastases, which are usually solitary pulmonary nodules[126] but may also involve the brain.[78]

The differential diagnosis of renal cell carcinoma can be difficult, particularly in metastatic lesions when clear cells are not prominent. The presence of lipid and glycogen and the absence of mucus (mucicarmine-positive) are helpful in distinguishing these tumors from adenocarcinomas, other clear cell tumors (ovary, uterus, lung), and sarcomas. As noted above, antibody to brush border, which detects proximal tubular antigens,[65, 69, 142] may be of diagnostic value in identifying a neoplasm as renal in origin. In difficult cases, electron microscopy is desirable, since the characteristic features of brush borders, cell junctions, basal lamina, glycogen, lipid, and fenestrated endothelium would be highly suggestive of renal cell carcinoma.

Adenomas frequently arise in scarred kidneys, but no similar correlation has been proved for renal cell carcinoma.[21, 23] However, in our experience, we have become impressed with the high incidence of asymptomatic renal cell carcinomas in severely scarred (end-stage) kidneys removed from transplant recipients (Fig. 8–10). We have had five examples in the nephrectomies from 115 transplant recipients, about 10 times the expected frequency based on five per 1000 autopsies (unpublished data). Others have described renal cell carcinoma in end-stage kidneys from over 60 dialysis patients.[36, 70, 98] In the 24 found incidentally in transplant recipients collected by Penn,[102] none had caused death, but one had spread into the perinephric fat. In Dunnill's series of 30 dialysis patients, five had renal cell tumors (not necessarily malignant), one of which had metastasized. All of the five patients with tumors had acquired cystic disease.[36] None of our patients has developed evidence

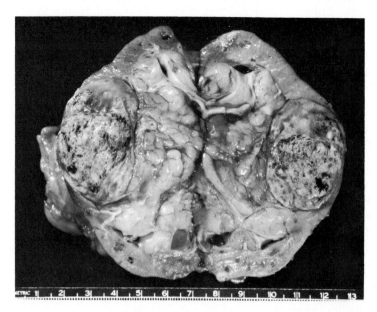

Figure 8–10. A renal cell carcinoma in an end-stage pyelonephritic kidney removed from a 43-year-old transplant recipient.

of recurrence after 11 years of follow-up. Hypothetically, the reactive changes in tubules, or the uremic state when present for a long period of time, favor the development of carcinoma. Further studies are needed to determine whether and when bilateral nephrectomy of end-stage kidneys may be beneficial as preventive surgery in dialysis and transplant patients.

ADENOMA

Adenomas present a special problem. Since the work of Bell,[12] size has become a criterion of malignancy. Indeed, in Bell's autopsy series there was a clear correlation between size and metastasis. However, Bell himself noted that three of 62 tumors under 3 cm in diameter had metastasized. Although size is of prognostic value, it obviously has little diagnostic value, since malignant tumors do not arise fully formed from the renal cortex, as Athena from Zeus's head, measuring 3.1 cm. Arguments for the extreme opposite view, that all tubular cell adenomas are malignant, have been presented by Bennington and Beckwith[13] and by Tannenbaum.[132] This dilemma has been more a reflection of ignorance than knowledge of the criteria of malignancy for these tumors. Our own belief is that nuclear grading separates more satisfactorily those tumors with low malignant potential from those more likely to metastasize.

Oncocytoma

In recent years, much attention has been directed to the oncocytic adenoma, or "oncocytoma." Approximately 200 of these tumors have been reported in the medical literature, and 90% of them have appeared since Klein and Valensi's landmark report of the first sizable series, in 1976.[137, 147] Oncocytomas characteristically are composed of sheets or nests of cells arranged in a solid or tubular pattern. The cells are of a uniform size and of a round or polygonal shape. They have abundant eosinophilic and granular cytoplasm as well as small nuclei without prominent nucleoli and without mitoses. Ultrastructurally, the cytoplasm is filled with mitochondria and contains a paucity of other organelles and inclusions (lipid and glycogen). These tumors are further defined as being grossly tan, devoid of hemorrhage and

necrosis, and small and noninvasive. In addition, many of them have a central area of fibrosis. They may be multicentric and bilateral.

Unfortunately, the foregoing classical definition has proved to be too restrictive, for there are occasional examples of oncocytomas that are large, invasive of perirenal fat, and even metastatic to distant sites.[137] A reasonable explanation for occasional exceptional behavior in this otherwise benign group of neoplasms is that oncocytomas and other adenomas probably represent the benign side of a spectrum of renal cell tumors, with renal cell carcinoma being at the other extreme. Although some authors[37, 92] believe that electron microscopy enables a difference to be recognized between oncocytomas and granular cell carcinomas, we feel there is too much overlap in the ultrastructural features of these two lesions for a reliable distinction to be made. The main difference cited is that the cytoplasm in oncocytomas is filled with mitochondria at the expense of other organelles and inclusions, whereas in granular cell carcinomas there are many mitochondria but also a prominent Golgi apparatus and a moderate number of other structures.[37, 92] If the "spectrum" concept for adenomas and carcinomas is correct, then it could be expected that there would also be an overlap in some of the light microscopic characteristics of these benign and malignant tumors. Indeed, this has been the experience of a number of investigators who have identified Grade 2 nuclei in small foci of some of the oncocytomas they studied.[7, 37, 81, 92, 147] In addition, oncocytoma and renal cell carcinoma have been seen contralaterally in the same patient,[147] and adenomas are known to occur more frequently in kidneys containing renal cell carcinomas.[13]

Finally, an actual category of renal tumors believed to lie clinically and pathologically between oncocytomas and renal cell carcinomas has been defined by Barnes and Beckman.[7] In their review of 257 primary renal cortical tumors, 241 were accepted as carcinomas and 10 as oncocytomas. Six others that had previously been called carcinomas were difficult to reclassify as malignant because of areas that resembled oncocytomas. These tumors were termed "congeners of renal oncocytoma." Atypical for classical oncocytomas, they exhibited various combinations of large size (5 to 24 cm), lighter than mahogany color, focal hemorrhage and necrosis, microscopic sheets of cells with no nesting pattern, foci of clear cells, foci of cells with Grade 2 or 3 nuclei, rare mitoses, and metastasis (one case).

NEPHROBLASTOMA (WILMS' TUMOR)

Over forty terms have been applied to this unusually pleomorphic tumor,[13] although nephroblastoma and Wilms' tumor are now the most widely used. In the first National Wilms' Tumor Study, the peak incidence of nephroblastoma was between the ages of one and two years, and less than 2% of patients were over the age of 12.[13] A genetic influence has been suggested in the incidence of Wilms' tumor, and a number of families having multiple tumors has been described.[73, 101] Knudson and Strong have presented a mathematical model consistent with the available data, that the combination of two genetic (or mutation) factors is required for tumor development.[73] Among the genetic associations with Wilms' tumor are trisomy 18,[50] XX/XY mosaicism,[129] a depletion in chromosome 8,[75] and a deletion near the oncogene c-Ha-rasl on chromosome 11.[138] Among the phenotypic associations are sporadic aniridia;[73] hemihypertrophy;[91] Beckwith-Wiedemann syndrome, which consists of macroglossia, gigantism, umbilical hernia, and hyperplasia of kidneys and pancreas;[9] Klippel-Trenaunay syndrome, which includes multiple nevi, hemangiomas, mental retardation, and seizures;[101] genitourinary malformations, including the external genitalia and the collecting system;[101] and an unclassified glomerular disease with nephrotic syndrome.[129]

Gross Features

On gross examination nephroblastomas are typically multilobulated, bulging, gray-tan tumors with focal areas of necrosis and hemorrhage. The resemblance to brain tissue led to the old term "encephaloid" for these tumors. Calcification is unusual and is of diagnostic value in distinguishing them from neuroblastomas. Cystic areas may be related to hemorrhage or necrosis. Extension into perinephric fat and contiguous organs may occur. Venous invasion is less common in this lesion than in renal cell carcinoma. In many instances there are multiple nodules,

and 5.8% of the tumors are bilateral.[13] This finding is more frequent in patients with a genetic predisposition and with multiple primary lesions. These patients also tend to present at a younger age.[25, 73]

Histologic Features

By light microscopy, nephroblastomas most typically have three components: epithelium, blastema, stroma. The epithelium usually forms tubules that have an embryonic appearance (Fig. 8–11) and, less commonly, glomeruloid structures lacking in endothelial and mesangial cells (Fig. 8–12). The blastema consists of oval, densely packed cells with dark nuclei and scant cytoplasm (Figs. 8–11 and 8–13), which resemble the normal metanephric blastema of the embryo and fetus. The stroma is composed of stellate and spindle cells loosely arranged in a pale matrix (Fig. 8–11).

Not all Wilms' tumors show the three types of tissue described; some are composed just of blastema and stroma and others are made up of blastema alone (Fig. 8–13). There are also examples of nephroblastomas that contain heterologous elements including various types of differentiated epithelium, striated muscle, smooth muscle, cartilage, bone, and nerve. The heterologous elements exist as cellular constituents (e.g., squamous epithelium) rather than as organoid structures (e.g., skin, complete with epidermis, dermis, and appendages) and therefore differ from teratomas.[10]

Occasionally, especially in adolescents and young adults, the tubular differentiation in a nephroblastoma may be focally or diffusely similar to or indistinguishable from renal cell carcinoma, only one of more than a dozen types of renal neoplasms that may be related to Wilms' tumor, as Beckwith has emphasized.[11] Persistent renal blastema (nephroblastomatosis), congenital mesoblastic nephroma, cystic partially differentiated Wilms' tumor, sarcomatous nephroblastoma, true renal sarcoma, angiomyolipoma, and juxtaglomerular cell tumor are examples of this group of neoplasms, and will be described following this passage on the more usual form of Wilms' tumor.

Electron Microscopy

Prior to our first edition of this chapter,[27] there were relatively few electron micro-

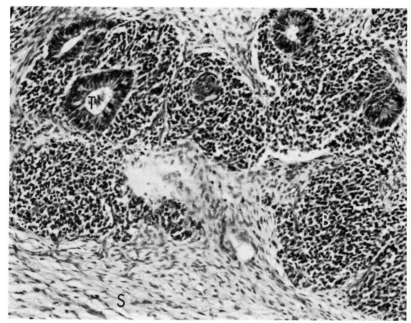

Figure 8–11. A moderately well-differentiated Wilms' tumor shows the three classic components: epithelial tubules (T), blastema (B), and stroma (S). (× 170)

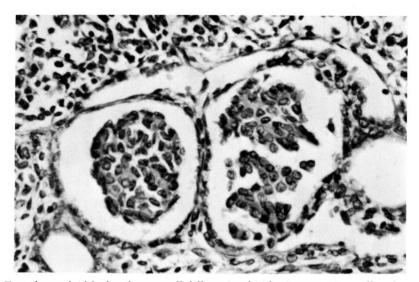

Figure 8–12. Two glomeruloid bodies from a well-differentiated Wilms' tumor. No capillary loops are seen, but both parietal and visceral epithelium are present. (× 390)

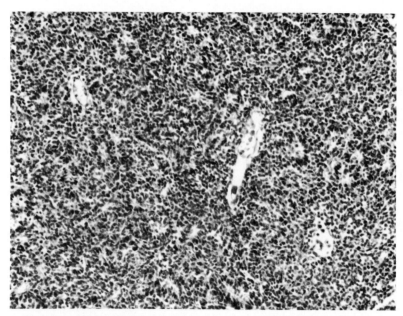

Figure 8–13. A poorly differentiated Wilms' tumor with a barely discernible rosette pattern, the only suggestion of epithelial differentiation in this case. (× 170)

scopic reports of nephroblastoma.[4, 5, 105, 114, 131, 134, 146] Since then, we have had the opportunity to perform detailed ultrastructural studies on a relatively large group of these tumors, gathered from several institutions.[118] These reports, plus experimental studies on avian virus-induced nephroblastomas,[34, 64] support the prevalent opinion that nephroblastomas derive from the totipotential primitive mesenchymal cells of the metanephric blastema. The blastema of the neoplasm (Fig. 8–14) in turn differentiates into both the epithelial and stromal elements, which have the same basic ultrastructural features as their counterparts in the normal kidney but with several exceptions: the cells are simultaneously in different stages of maturation, there are varying degrees of development of organoid structures, and the final stage of differentiation is never perfect or "mature." For example, solid clusters of epithelial cells are sometimes not separated from adjacent blastema by basal lamina, but the cells do have junctions. Tubules with lumens may have cell junctions and apical vesicles but lack microvilli, lateral border interdigitations, and basal border infoldings. Glomeruloid structures may have almost normal parietal and visceral epithelial cells (podocytes), the latter with foot processes,[5] but mesangial cells, endothelial cells, and cap-

illary lumens are not apparent. Unusual paired cisternae of rough endoplasmic reticulum in association with chromatin particles have been noted during and after mitosis, but their significance is uncertain.[131]

Interesting recent information to support the dual line of differentiation that blastema follows has resulted from the immunohistochemical analysis of intermediate filaments. Altmannsberger and associates examined 10 nephroblastomas using antibodies to cytokeratin and vimentin, and they observed that in seven tumors blastema was positive for both antibodies.[1] Furthermore, nephroblastomatous tubules were positive only for cytokeratin, and stromal cells were positive only for vimentin. Two neoplasms were composed completely of blastema, and these were negative for cytokeratin and positive for vimentin. The final neoplasm among the 10 was a clear cell sarcoma and this was vimentin-positive.

The stromal component of some Wilms' tumors consists focally or diffusely of cells that differ from the stellate, or spindle, fibroblastic type cell seen in most examples of this neoplasm. These heterologous secondary mesenchymal elements, as has been noted already, may be skeletal muscle, smooth muscle, cartilage, bone, and adipose tissue. Examples of some, but not all, of

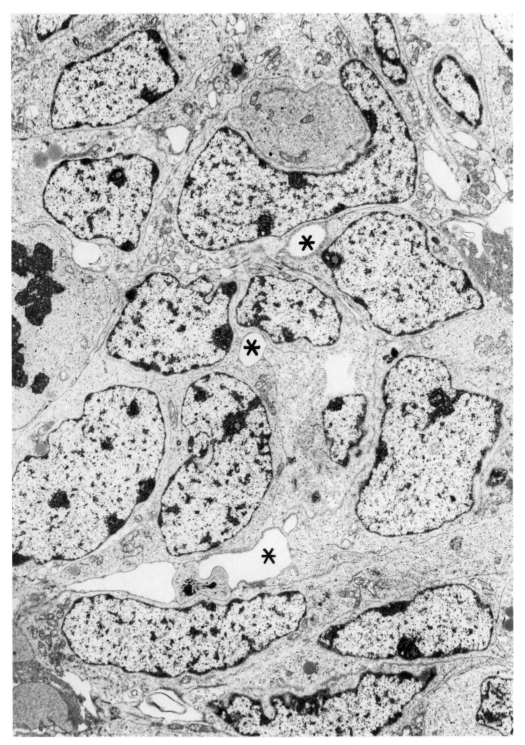

Figure 8–14. A blastematous area of a Wilms' tumor contains small intercellular spaces (*) lined by a fuzzy basal lamina–like material. This probably represents one of the earliest signs of differentiation of blastema into tubules. (× 4000)

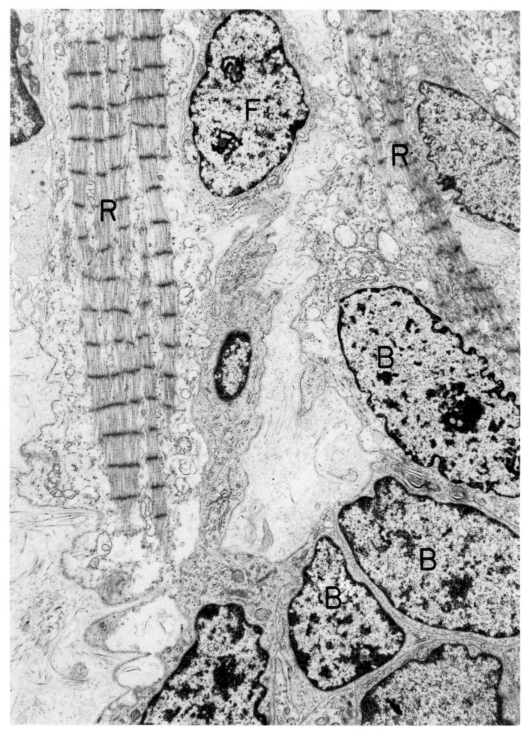

Figure 8–15. This field illustrates one type of heterologous mesenchymal element that may make up the stroma of Wilms' tumors; namely, rhabdomyoblasts (R). The more usual component, fibroblasts (F) are also present. The stroma is separated from the blastema or early-stage epithelial cells (B) by basal lamina. (× 7100)

these mesenchymal components have been confirmed in the electron microscopic studies of Wilms' tumors. Tremblay first verified the coexistence of fibroblasts and skeletal muscle cells in varying stages of differentiation in one case,[134] and we subsequently identified fibroblasts, rhabdomyoblasts, and chondroblasts among the Wilms' tumors in our study (Fig. 8–15).

Features with Prognostic Significance

As a result of the National Wilms' Tumor Studies,[8, 29, 30] there has been a refinement in the criteria for predicting prognosis in patients with this neoplasm. Extension of the tumor beyond Gerota's fascia and invasion of veins had been considered previously to be poor prognostic signs,[103] but now it is evident that appropriate surgery and chemotherapy can negate the importance of these findings. Additional features that no longer are considered important prognostic signs, provided surgery and chemotherapy are complete, include the age of the patient, the size of the tumor, and operative spillage of tumor.

Findings that portend an unfavorable outcome, even with optimal therapy, are a high histologic grade, the presence of metastatic tumor, and the metachronous involvement of both kidneys.[122] Histologic grade, which consists primarily of nuclear anaplasia, is especially important, whether focal or diffuse, regardless of the cell type.[11] The anaplasia is defined as nuclear enlargement, hyperchromatism, and multipolar mitotic figures. However, nuclear anaplasia in the skeletal muscle component does not change the favorable prognosis in an otherwise low-grade tumor.[11] High-grade tumors are uncommon in children under two years of age, and they represent only about 6% of all nephroblastomas.[10]

Studies similar to the National Wilms' Tumor Studies have been taking place in England (Medical Research Council), and the tentative conclusions are generally similar. However, one difference is in the importance attributed to the degree of tubular differentiation. Tumors having many tubules (3+) were correlated with 100% survival, and those with no tubules, a 68% survival.[89] No mention is made in that report of how the degree of anaplasia varied with the extent of tubular differentiation, albeit anapla-

sia was assessed independently to be a poor prognostic factor.

NEPHROBLASTOMATOSIS (PERSISTENT RENAL BLASTEMA, NODULAR RENAL BLASTEMA)

This lesion consists of retained metanephric blastema after nephrogenesis is complete, at about 36 weeks of gestation. It tends to be multifocal and bilateral and is found in association wih trisomy 18 with Wilms' tumors.[13, 19, 113] Futhermore, this retained tissue is probably the source from which Wilms' tumors arise, since it is found in almost half of the kidneys containing these neoplasms and in all the kidneys of patients having bilateral Wilms' tumors.[84] As originally described, nephroblastomatosis occurred in the superficial, or subcapsular, region of the kidney,[19, 107] and consisted mostly of blastema and partly of epithelial nests, tubules, and glomeruloid structures, without much or any stroma (Fig. 8–16). This histologic picture, except for being better differentiated, has a definite resemblance to Wilms' tumor itself. More recently, retained blastema has been identified in the deep cortical, or intralobar, location of the kidney,[63, 84, 85] where it is associated with a different range of congenital defects and has a different histologic composition from that of the superficial form. It is composed of blastema, tubules lined by benign-appearing epithelium, and stroma separating the blastema and tubules. This histologic picture may be mistaken for Wilms' tumor because of a tendency for a high degree of mitotic activity in the blastema and for the stromal component to form heterologous elements. In addition, the area of retained blastema is not well demarcated from the surrounding renal parenchyma. Deep nephroblastomatosis also appears to be associated with two particular histologic subtypes of Wilms' tumor, "fetal rhabdomyomatous nephroblastoma," and "cystic, partially differentiated nephroblastoma,"[84] both of which are stromal-predominant neoplasms (see below).

Nephroblastomatosis, in addition to being a multifocal condition, has been recognized to have a rare, diffuse form that may involve large zones of renal parenchyma or even entire kidneys.[31, 83] Although more information on this entity is necessary, it also ap-

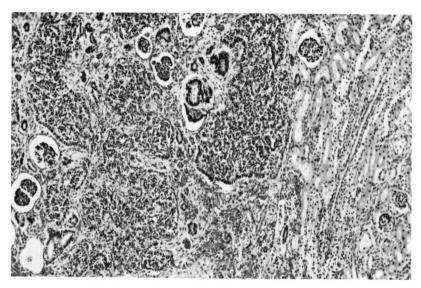

Figure 8–16. *Nodular renal blastema. This microscopic focus was present in otherwise normal kidneys in this newborn. (× 120) Courtesy of David L. Gang, MD.*

pears to be related to genetic malformations and to the development of Wilms' tumors.[83]

CONGENITAL MESOBLASTIC NEPHROMA

This tumor was the first of several to be separated from nephroblastoma by its distinctive morphologic features and its low-grade malignancy.[16] It arises typically in the first year of life, and many are detected at birth. This tumor probably accounts for the early observation that congenital Wilms' tumors had a better prognosis than those occurring later in infancy and childhood.[16]

On gross examination, the tumor is solid, round, gray-tan, and whorled, resembling a uterine leiomyoma (Fig. 8–17). Careful inspection reveals an indistinct border with the cortex and diffuse extension of the tumor into the surrounding normal cortical tissue. The infiltration is by insinuation rather than destruction, much as a neurofibroma behaves, and invasion into peripelvic fat is uncommon. Microscopically, the cells are spindle shaped and form interlacing bundles resembling fibroblasts or smooth muscle cells (Fig. 8–18). Nuclei may be pleomorphic and mitoses numerous. Fibrous tissue may be present.

Of the more than 100 cases of congenital mesoblastic nephroma reported in the literature,[14] at least 10 (including the case illustrated in Figs. 8–17 to 8–19) have been studied by electron microscopy.[33, 40, 46, 49, 80, 123, 128, 144] In all instances the neoplastic cells were of mesenchymal, not epithelial, type. The differentiation in the majority of cases was in the direction of fibroblasts (Fig. 8–19), although in one neoplasm the cells were quite primitive and resembled mesenchyme. Three cases had some neoplastic cells with cytoplasmic filaments and dense aggregates of filaments suggestive of smooth muscle, but fibroblastic elements predominated.[40, 46, 123] The cells containing smooth muscle–like features may actually have been myofibroblasts, as was observed by Snyder and associates in one case,[128] and by us in two others. Other findings, in two cases, were intercellular junctions; zona adherens and broad attachment sites, respectively; and cilia in one case. These observations were interpreted as a residual potential of mesenchyme to differentiate into epithelium.[46, 144] Paired cisternae of rough endoplasmic reticulum, similar to that described in classic Wilms' tumor, were an additional interesting observation in the latter case, and they occurred both in mitotic and nonmitotic cells.

The differential diagnosis of congenital mesoblastic nephroma is chiefly with Wilms' tumor. Morphologically, the best evidence for a Wilms' tumor is the presence of

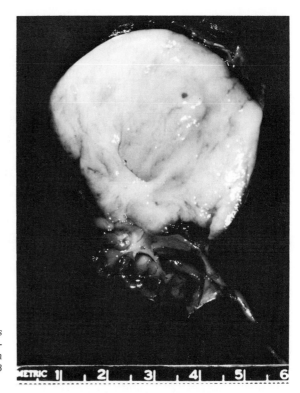

Figure 8–17. Congenital mesoblastic nephroma. This mass was removed from an infant. The tumor was gray-yellow and had an indistinct border with the much smaller but normal-sized kidneys. This and Figs. 8–18 and 8–19 are from the same case.

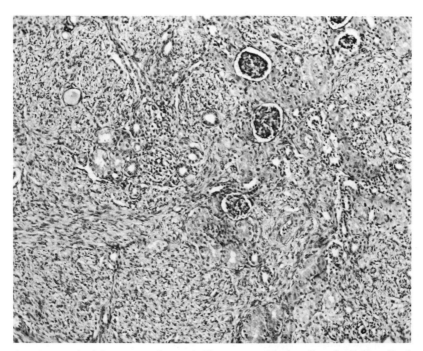

Figure 8–18. Light micrograph of the same patient as in Figure 8–17. The bundles of spindle cells characteristically dissect between and entrap normal glomeruli and tubules in the border between the tumor and the cortex. ($\times$ 120)

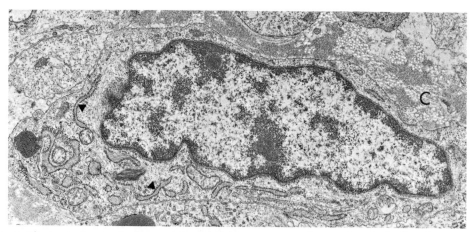

Figure 8–19. Electron micrograph of same patient as in Figures 8–17 and 8–18. A typical cell with extensive rough endoplasmic reticulum (arrowheads) and no evidence of epithelial or smooth muscle differentiation is illustrated. Dense amorphous material and collagen bundles (C) surround the cell. (× 9450)

tubules formed of tumor cells (not just trapped normal tubules), and multiple sections may be necessary to find these elements. An interdigitating border around the tumor is quite characteristic of congenital mesoblastic nephroma. The presence of cross striations in the cells would favor the rhabdomyoblastic form of Wilms' tumor.

The prognosis in congenital mesoblastic nephroma is much better than in Wilms' tumor. Patients treated by nephrectomy have generally done well, although inadequate excision may lead to local persistence and, rarely, death.[46, 141] Marsden and Lawler[88] described three "atypical mesoblastic nephromas" that displayed dense cellularity, nuclear atypia, increased mitotic activity, and focal polygonal cells. However, these behaved as other mesoblastic nephromas (patients were alive after 11 to 21 years), as did two other examples of atypical congenital mesoblastic nephroma.[128] On the other hand,

there is one recent case reported in which a congenital mesoblastic nephroma–like lesion did metastasize.[53, 54] The authors termed this, and a similar neoplasm that did not metastasize, as "malignant mesenchymal nephroma," since they were grossly necrotic and microscopically anaplastic.

Potent chemotherapy and radiotherapy seem unnecessary for this usually benign-behaving tumor, and for that reason it is important for the pathologist to recognize the entity.

FETAL RHABDOMYOMATOUS NEPHROBLASTOMA

In 1976, Wigger described a variant of Wilms' tumor that was composed of a fetal type of nonmalignant-appearing skeletal muscle.[145] He had seen five examples of this

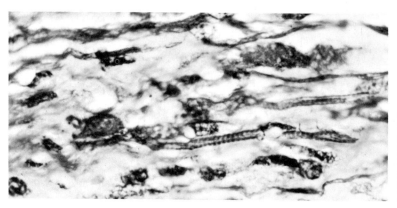

Figure 8–20. A rhabdomyomatous variant of Wilms' tumor. Striations are seen in this phosphotungstic acid–stained section, and the striated muscle origin was confirmed by electron microscopy. (× 630) Courtesy of David L. Gang, MD.

type of neoplasm and had collected 15 from the literature. Six similar cases were found among 32 renal neoplasms occurring in children under one year of age, in a study by Ugarte and co-workers.[135] In these cases of fetal rhabdomyomatous nephroblastoma, 30 to 80% of the tissue volume was composed of long, eosinophilic muscle cells and interspersed fibroblasts and collagen (Fig. 8–20). This microscopic picture recapitulated the pattern of skeletal muscle development in the 8- to 10-week-old fetus. The remaining nonmuscular portion of each tumor was composed of varying amounts of blastema and tubular epithelium. Three of the tumors were bilateral, all of the patients were older than three months, and there was a high rate of coexistence with hypertension and congenital anomalies. One tumor metastasized (to the lung), and the metastatic lesion contained the same type of anaplastic skeletal muscle that had been present in the primary tumor. Of 20 patients known to date to have fetal rhabdomyomatous nephroblastoma, 20% have died of the disease,[84] indicating that the original opinion of a good prognosis for these neoplasms is in need of reassessment.

In summary, this special category of nephroblastoma having a high component of skeletal muscle is currently classified separately from classical Wilms' tumor, but it should not be confused with the rarely occurring rhabdomyosarcoma of the kidney, which contains no blastema or epithelium.

CYSTIC, PARTIALLY DIFFERENTIATED NEPHROBLASTOMA

This rare renal neoplasm of infants and young children occurs deep within the kidney and consists of varying proportions of epithelium-lined cysts and intervening septae, with the septae being composed of the tissues found in Wilms' tumor (Fig. 8–21). These tissues include blastema, tubular and glomeruloid epithelial components, and fibrous stroma with skeletal muscle.[17, 71] The lesion has been viewed as falling on a spectrum halfway between benign multilocular renal cyst and potentially malignant polycystic Wilms' tumor.[2] Gonzalez-Crussi and associates[55] feel strongly that "cystic nephroma," as they term this entity, is more closely related to Wilms' tumor than to any form of non-neoplastic, cystic malformation, such as polycystic disease and renal dysplasia. Furthermore, they have defined certain criteria, in addition to the presence of Wilms' tissue in the septae, for its diagnosis: (1) the lesion must be solitary and cystic (usually unilateral); (2) one main cyst contains multiple locules; (3) individual locules do not interconnect with each other or with

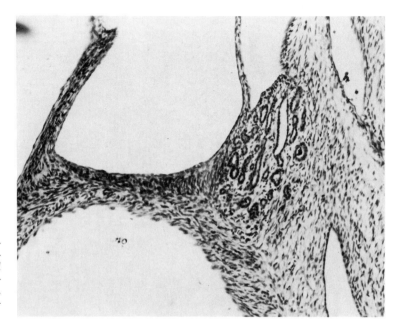

Figure 8–21. Cystic partially differentiated nephroblastoma. Epithelium-lined cysts are separated by tissue composed of the elements found in Wilms' tumor, here depicted as blastema, tubules, and stroma. (× 200)

the pelvocalyceal system; (4) no normal renal parenchyma is found in the septae; (5) some normal, uninvolved kidney must be present.

Among the neoplasms classified as cystic, partially differentiated nephroblastoma, there may be differences in the degree of differentiation of the Wilms' components, although the prognosis is usually considered to be good. The tumor is often associated with deep nephroblastomatosis and with rhabdomyomatous nephroblastoma.[84]

CLEAR CELL SARCOMA OF THE KIDNEY

Clear cell sarcoma of the kidney is one of two neoplasms (rhabdoid tumor being the other—see below) that, until recently, have been considered as sarcomatous variants of Wilms' tumor.[11] It has now been separated from the true Wilms' group of tumors, since it is composed of a single type of cell of unknown origin that is not obviously from blastema, epithelium, or stroma. The neoplastic cell is polygonal or stellate, has pale or clear cytoplasm, and has poorly discernible cell borders. Nuclei are oval, nucleoli are not prominent, and mitoses are infrequent (Fig. 8–22). The tumor typically forms nests of uniform cells in a network of regularly interspersed blood vessels. Variant patterns are less frequent and include trabecular and pseudotubular, cystic, angiectatic, neu-

rilemmoma-like, and hyalinized stroma.[11] To date, ultrastructural examination of the neoplastic "clear" cells has not revealed any distinguishing features of a particular cell line. Haas and co-workers[61] performed electron microscopy on 12 of the 75 examples of clear cell sarcomas in the National Wilms' Tumor Studies file. They found mitochondria and rough endoplasmic reticulum to be the most prominent cytoplasmic organelles. Some cells had dense collections of intermediate filaments, and some had cytoplasmic processes enwrapping pale matrix; both features were interpreted by the authors to account for the clear spaces seen by light microscopy. The cells were also noted to differ in various ultrastructural ways from those in certain other clear cell neoplasms with which they might be confused by light microscopy, including clear cell sarcoma of tendons and aponeuroses, clear cell carcinoma of the ovary and uterus, and clear cell carcinoma of the kidney. Other possible cells of origin for the clear cell sarcoma of kidney that the authors thought they could rule out were blastemal, mesangial, and neurilemmal. Gonzalez-Crussi and Baum[57] also performed electron microscopic studies on clear cell sarcoma of the kidney and found the cytoplasm of some cells to be electron-lucent and sparsely populated by organelles. Filaments were present to a significant degree in only one tumor, that of a patient who had undergone chemotherapy. These authors emphasized the extracellular, amorphous

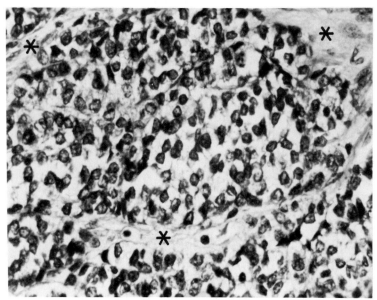

Figure 8–22. Clear cell sarcoma of kidney. Nests of uniform cells with clear cytoplasm and oval nuclei are separated by a network of blood vessels in a scant, fibrous stroma (*). (× 500) Courtesy of Gordon F. Vawter, MD.

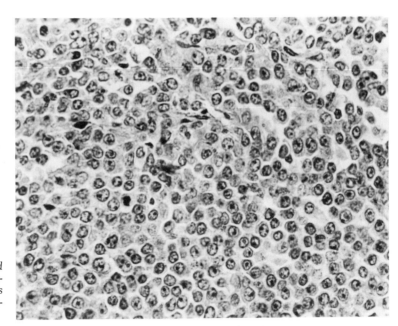

Figure 8–23. Malignant rhabdoid tumor of kidney. Diffusely arranged, oval, and elongate cells have abundant cytoplasm and nuclei with large nucleoli. (× 500)

material abutting plasmalemmas, similar to that seen in classical Wilms' tumor.

In England, clear cell sarcoma has also been called bone-metastasizing renal tumor of childhood[87] because of its propensity to spread to bone. It is a highly malignant neoplasm; bone metastases have occurred in 13 of 31 cases, and tumor-related death has ensued in about 15 of 31 cases in the first and second National Wilms' Tumor Studies.[10] Since then, the incidence of bone metastasis has averaged downward to 17% of cases.[61] There seems to be no better prognosis for clear cell sarcoma in children under the age of two years, and about half of these tumors are discovered prior to that age. They usually do not occur prior to the age of one year. Males outnumber females by at least 3:1 in harboring this neoplasm, and the total incidence among all childhood renal tumors is about 4%.

MALIGNANT RHABDOID TUMOR OF THE KIDNEY

Malignant rhabdoid tumor of kidney occurs in young infants and is highly malignant; it was lethal in 19 of 21 patients in the first and second National Wilms' Tumor Studies.[11] This neoplasm was originally classified in the first National Wilms' Tumor Study as a rhabdomyosarcomatoid form of Wilms' tumor because of the myoblastic ap-

pearance of the cells by light microscopy.[8] Characteristically, the cells have a diffuse arrangement, are ovoid and elongate, contain abundant eosinophilic cytoplasm, and have large nucleoli (Fig. 8–23). A hallmark in some cells is a round, eosinophilic, perinuclear globule that stains with PAS reagents (Fig. 8–24).

More recently, these primitive neoplasms have been reclassified as "rhabdoid," since cytoplasmic cross striations cannot be demonstrated by light microscopy, thick filaments and Z-band material are not discerned on ultrastructural examination, and myoglobin is not evident by immunochemical marking.[11, 57, 60, 115, 119]

Cells showing the typical cytoplasmic globules, in our experience and that of some others,[88] may be very scant, and in random samples for electron microscopy they may be completely absent (Fig. 8–25). When present, these perinuclear globules are striking and consist of large whorls of filaments (Fig. 8–26) that have been reported to be of the thin type (6 nm) by some observers,[57, 82, 119] and of the intermediate size (12 nm) by others.[60, 140]

Other ultrastructural features of rhabdoid cells are not particularly helpful in determining the cell of origin and consist of varying combinations of small groups of filaments not in whorls, a moderate number of mitochondria, a few cisternae of rough endoplasmic reticulum, large Golgi appara-

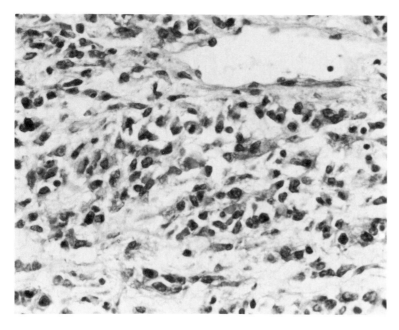

Figure 8–24. Malignant rhabdoid tumor of kidney. A characteristic of some of the cells in this neoplasm, depicted in this field, is a dense, perinuclear globule (eosinophilic with H & E staining and positive with PAS reagents). (× 500)

tuses, a few lysosomes, and occasional lipid droplets. Small intercellular junctions may be visible.

In regard to the histogenetic lineage of rhabdoid tumors, a recent cytochemical study employing immunoperoxidase staining of intermediate filament proteins has provided new information.[140] Rhabdoid tumor cells were positive for vimentin and for a 54-kilodalton cytokeratin, the former being a marker for mesenchymal cells and the latter for nonsquamous epithelial cells. Furthermore, the vimentin staining appeared to be in the perinuclear whorls of filaments, whereas the cytokeratin marking was elsewhere in the cytoplasm. These investigators also were able to culture the neoplastic cells in vitro and to produce rhabdoid tumors in athymic (nude) mice by injecting the cultured cells. The resulting neoplastic cells contained identical filamentous inclusions as in the original rhabdoid tumor but stained slightly differently. The globular inclusions stained for vimentin and the remainder of the cytoplasm for cytokeratin, similar to the native tumor, but the globular inclusions of the cultured cells also stained for cytokeratin. Antibodies to neurofilaments and desmin did not react with the native or cultured rhabdoid cells, evidence against neuroectodermal and muscular origins. Thus, rhabdoid tumor of the kidney appears to possess the immunologic markers both for mesenchymal and epithelial differentiation. Vogel

and associates[140] point out that this dual lineage has been noted also in renal cell carcinomas. Since renal cell carcinoma and Wilms' tumor appear to have an interrelationship (see earlier section on Nephroblastoma), the question arises as to whether the rhabdoid tumor is actually a special form of one or the other of those two entities. Against this concept is that primary rhabdoid tumors have occurred in sites other than the kidney, including subcutaneous tissue, paravertebral soft tissue, thymus, central nervous system, and pelvic soft tissue.[11, 45, 56, 82] Obviously, further studies will be necessary to identify the complete histogenetic nature of rhabdoid tumor cells.

MISCELLANEOUS SARCOMAS

In addition to clear cell sarcoma and rhabdoid tumor, sarcomas of various types may occur rarely in the kidney. These include rhabdomyosarcoma (embryonal and spindle-cell forms), leiomyosarcoma, and fibrosarcoma.[57, 100] In addition, incompletely classified sarcomas, including a type with a diffuse, hyalinized stroma ("sarcoma with sclerosing features") have been described.[57] A single case of malignant mesenchymoma also has been reported.[90]

These various sarcomas have no special histologic or ultrastructural features that are related to their location in the kidney, and

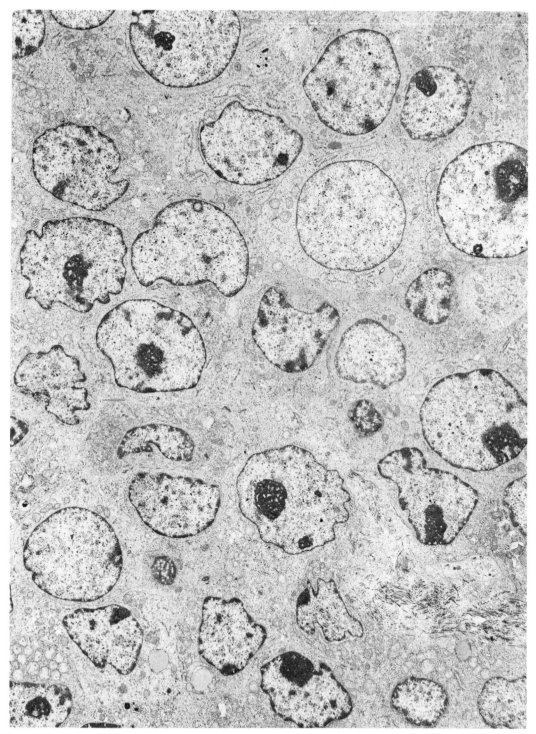

Figure 8–25. Malignant rhabdoid tumor of kidney. A solid arrangement of oval cells having large nucleoli is quite characteristic of this neoplasm, and whorls of cytoplasmic filaments are not present in this randomly chosen field. (× 4350)

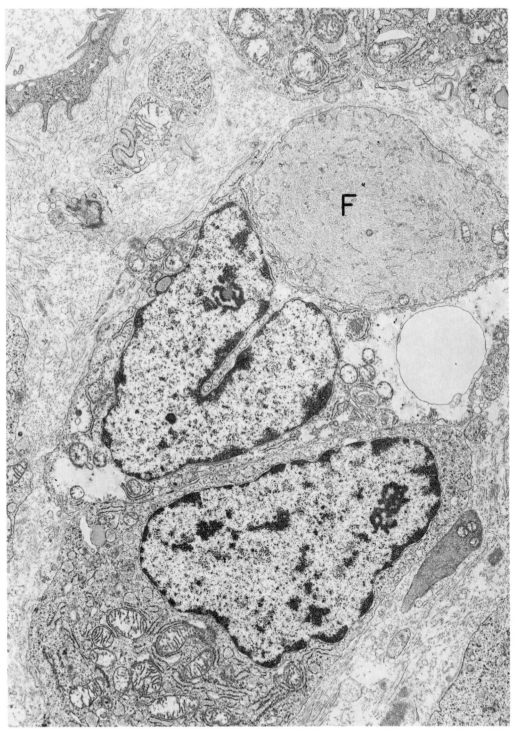

Figure 8–26. *Malignant rhabdoid tumor of kidney. Corresponding to the perinuclear eosinophilic globules, seen at light microscopy in this neoplasm, are the whorls of densely arranged filaments (F), discernible at the electron-microscopic level of magnification. (× 7700)*

when differentiated into a recognizable cell line (skeletal muscle, smooth muscle, or fibrous tissue), they have the same appearance as they do elsewhere in the body. The main point in classifying them is to rule out the presence of blastema and epithelial components, thereby separating them from the Wilms' group of neoplasms.

ANGIOMYOLIPOMA

These benign tumors are commonly found in patients with tuberous sclerosis (80%), but in about 40% of the cases there is no other evidence of this syndrome.[62] Grossly, the tumors may be as large as 20 cm, and they are often multiple and bilateral. They are yellow and gray and are sometimes hemorrhagic. On microscopic examination the tumors are found to consist of benign-appearing adipocytes and malformed muscular blood vessels (Fig. 8–27). Sheets of smooth muscle cells, fibroblasts, and lymphatic vessels may be found. Mitoses are rare, but the pleomorphism of the nuclei may cause concern.[39] Complete excision seems to be curative;[39, 62] however, in three cases the tumor could not be removed because of local ex-

tension.[74] Ten cases have been described with angiomyolipoma in regional nodes.[15] None of the five with follow-up (one to 11 years) has shown evidence of recurrence. Whether this represents "benign metastasis" or a multicentric benign tumor is unknown.

JUXTAGLOMERULAR TUMOR (RENINOMA)

Fifteen cases have been described since the report of Robertson and associates[110] of a renin-secreting tumor believed to be derived from the juxtaglomerular cells.[76] The patients have all presented with hypertension, typically have been young (average age 23 years), and had hyperaldosteronism and hyperreninemia. Of importance, some cases had a normal result on intravenous pyelogram and arteriogram.[99] The great inequality of the renal vein renin concentration led to the diagnosis in most cases (renal vein renin ratios of $\geq 1.5:1$). Some Wilms' tumors also have secreted renin,[48] which indicates that these totipotential tumors can also differentiate toward juxtaglomerular cells.

The cortical tumors found are solitary, small (8 to 40 mm), and usually gray-yellow

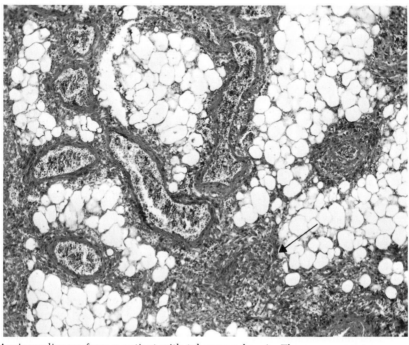

Figure 8–27. Angiomyolipoma from a patient with tuberous sclerosis. Three components are present: adult fat cells, tortuous abnormal vessels, and sheets of smooth muscle proliferation (arrow). Similar multiple tumors were present bilaterally. (× 120)

with areas of vascularity or hemorrhage. Microscopically, the tumor resembles hemangiopericytomas found elsewhere in the body. However, the distinctive, sometimes laminated granules of the juxtaglomerular cells that contain renin by immunofluorescence[76] can be seen by electron microscopy or be stained by the Bowie technique. The tumor extracts in several cases contained high concentrations of renin, sometimes over 30 times that of the normal cortex. None of these lesions underwent malignant change, and resolution of the hypertension occurred in all the patients. Since the tumors are solitary and benign, local excision, when the lesions can be located at surgery, is the most appropriate therapy.

References

1. Altmannsberger M, Osborn M, Schäfer H, et al: Distinction of nephroblastomas from other childhood tumors using antibodies to intermediate filaments. Virchows Arch [Cell Pathol] 45:113–124, 1984.
2. Andrews MJ Jr, Askin FB, Fried FA, et al: Cystic partially differentiated nephroblastoma and polycystic Wilms' tumor: a spectrum of related clinical and pathologic entities. J Urol 129:577–580, 1983.
3. Arner O, Blanck C, von Schreeb T: Renal adenocarcinoma; morphology-grading and malignancy-prognosis. A study of 197 cases. Acta Chir Scand [Suppl] 346:1–51, 1965.
4. Badini A, Buffa D, Micheletti V, Tanzi A: Morphologic studies using the optical and electron microscope and short histogenetic considerations in 8 cases of Wilms' tumor. Pathologica 68:137, 1976.
5. Balsaver AM, Gibley CW Jr, Tessmer CF: Ultrastructural studies in Wilms' tumor. Cancer 22:417–427, 1968.
6. Bannayan GA, Lamm DL: Renal cell tumors. Pathol Annu 15:271–308, 1980.
7. Barnes CA, Beckman EN: Renal oncocytoma and its congeners. Am J Clin Pathol 79:312–318, 1983.
8. Beckwith JB, Palmer NF: Histopathology and prognosis of Wilms' tumor: results from the first National Wilms' Tumor Study. Cancer 41:1937–1948, 1978.
9. Beckwith JB: Macroglossia, omphalocele, adrenal cytomegaly, gigantism, and hyperplastic visceromegaly. Birth Defects: Original Article Series 5:188, 1969.
10. Beckwith JB: Histopathological aspects of renal tumors in children. In Renal Tumors: Proceedings of the First International Symposium on Kidney Tumors, Progress in Clinical and Biological Research. New York, Alan R. Liss, 1982.
11. Beckwith JB: Wilms' tumor and other renal tumors of childhood: a selective review from the National Wilms' Tumor Study Pathology Center. Hum Pathol 14:481–492, 1983.
12. Bell ET: Renal Disease, 2nd ed. Philadelphia, Lea & Febiger, 1959, p 435.
13. Bennington JL, Beckwith JB: Tumors of the kidney, renal pelvis, and ureter. Atlas of Tumor Pathology. Washington DC, Armed Forces Institute of Pathology, 1975, Fasc. 12.
14. Biggers RD: Congenital mesonephric blastoma. Urology 21:302–304, 1983.
15. Bloom DA, Scardino PT, Ehrlich RM, Waisman J: The significance of lymph nodal involvement in renal angiomyolipoma. J Urol 128:1292–1295, 1982.
16. Bolande RP: Congenital mesoblastic nephroma of infancy. Perspect Pediatr Pathol 1:227–250, 1973.
17. Bolande RP: Commentary: Multicystic nephroma, what it is and its relationship to Wilms' tumor. Pediatr Radiol 12:46, 1982.
18. Böttiger LE: Prognosis in renal carcinoma. Cancer 26:780–787, 1970.
19. Bove KE, Koffler H, McAdams AJ: Nodular renal blastema: definition and possible significance. Cancer 24:323–332, 1969.
20. Bove KE, McAdams AJ: The nephroblastomatosis complex and its relationship to Wilms' tumor: a clinicopathologic treatise. Perspect Pediatr Pathol 3:185–223, 1976.
21. Buddin RD, McDonnell PJ: Renal cell neoplasms: their relationship to arterionephrosclerosis. Arch Pathol Lab Med 108:138, 1984.
22. Casirola G, Ippoliti G, Marini G, Ascari E, Recalde HR: Para-neoplastic syndromes due to a urologically silent Grawitz tumor. Recenti Prog Med 58:198–214, 1975.
23. Choi H, Almagro UA, McManus JT, et al: Renal oncocytoma. A clinicopathological study. Cancer 51:1887–1896, 1983.
24. Chung-Park M, Ricanati E, Lankerani M, Kedia K: Acquired renal cysts and multiple renal cell and urothelial tumors. Am J Clin Pathol 79:238–242, 1983.
25. Cochran W, Froggatt P: Bilateral nephroblastoma in two sisters. J Urol 97:216–220, 1967.
26. Coffman CS, Schreiber MH: Unusual manifestations of metastatic renal cell carcinoma. Tex Med 71:60–68, 1975.
27. Colvin RB, Dickersin GR: Pathology of renal tumors. In DG Skinner, JB deKernion (eds), Genitourinary Cancer. Philadelphia, WB Saunders, 1978.
28. Conner DH, Taylor HB, Helwig EB: Cutaneous metastasis of renal cell carcinoma. Arch Pathol 76:339, 1963.
29. D'Angio GJ, Evans AE, Breslow N, et al: The treatment of Wilms' tumor: results of the National Wilms' Tumor Study. Cancer 38:633, 1976.
30. D'Angio GJ, Evans AE, Breslow N, et al: The treatment of Wilms' tumor: results of the second National Wilms' Tumor Study. Cancer 47:2302–2311, 1981.
31. de Chadarévian JP, Fletcher BD, Chatten J, Rabinovitch HH: Massive infantile nephroblastomatosis: a clinical, radiological and pathological analysis of four cases. Cancer 39:2294–2305, 1977.
32. Deitchman B, Sidhu GS: Ultrastructural study of a sarcomatoid variant of renal cell carcinoma. Cancer 46:1152–1157, 1980.
33. Dickersin GR: Ultrastructural studies of congenital mesoblastic nephroma. (Unpublished data).
34. Dmochowski L, Grey CE, Burmester BR, Walter WG: Submicroscopic morphology of avian neoplasms. V. Studies on a nephroblastoma. Tex Rep Biol Med 19:545–579, 1961.

35. Doll R, Peto R: The Causes of Cancer: Quantitative Estimates of Avoidable Risks of Cancer in the United States Today. Oxford, England, Oxford University Press, 1981, p 1284.

36. Dunnill MS, Millard RP, Oliver D: Acquired cystic disease of the kidneys: a hazard of long-term intermittent maintenance haemodialysis. J Clin Pathol 30:868–877, 1977.

37. Eble JU, Hull MT: Morphologic features of renal oncocytoma: a light and electron microscopic study. Hum Pathol 15:1054, 1984.

38. Everson TC: Spontaneous regression of cancer. Ann NY Acad Sci 114:721–735, 1964.

39. Farrow GM, Harrison EG Jr, Utz DC, Jones DR: Renal angiomyolipoma. A clinicopathologic study of 32 cases. Cancer 22:564, 1968.

40. Favara BE, Johnson W, Ito J: Renal tumors in the neonatal period. Cancer 22:845–855, 1968.

41. Finstad CL, Cordon-Cardo C, Bander NH, et al: Specificity analysis of mouse monoclonal antibodies defining cell surface antigens of human renal cancer. Proc Natl Acad Sci USA 82:2955, 1985.

42. Fisher ER, Horvat B: Comparative ultrastructural study of so-called renal adenoma and carcinoma. J Urol 108:382–386, 1972.

43. Folkman J: Tumor angiogenesis. Adv Cancer Res 43:175, 1985.

44. Folkman J, Merler E, Abernathy C, Williams G: Isolation of a tumor factor responsible for angiogenesis. J Exp Med 132:275–288, 1971.

45. Frierson HF Jr, Mills SE, Innes DG Jr: Malignant rhabdoid tumor of the pelvis. Cancer 55:1963–1967, 1985.

46. Fu Y, Kay S: Congenital mesoblastic nephroma and its recurrence. Arch Pathol 96:66–70, 1973.

47. Furham SA, Lasky LC, Limas C: Prognostic significance of morphological parameters in renal cell carcinoma. Am J Surg Pathol 6:655, 1982.

48. Ganguly A, Gribble J, Tune B, et al: Renin-secreting Wilms' tumor with severe hypertension: report of a case and brief review of renin-secreting tumors. Ann Int Med 79:835–837, 1973.

49. Garcia-Bunuel R, Brandes D: Fetal hamartoma of the kidney: case report, with ultrastructural cytochemical observations. Hopkins Med J 127:213–221, 1970.

50. Geiser CF, Schindler AM: Long survival in a male with 18-trisomy syndrome and Wilms' tumor. Pediatrics 44:111–116, 1969.

51. Giangiacomo J, Penchansky L, Monteleone PL, Thompson J: Bilateral neonatal Wilms' tumor with B-C chromosomal translocation. J Pediatr 86:98–102, 1975.

52. Gilchrist KW, Hogan TF, Harberg J, Sonneland PRL: Prognostic significance of nuclear sizing in renal cell carcinoma. Urology 24:122–124, 1984.

53. Gonzalez-Crussi F, Sotelo-Avila C, Kidd JM: Malignant mesenchymal nephroma of infancy: report of a case with pulmonary metastasis. Am J Surg Pathol 4:185–190, 1980.

54. Gonzalez-Crussi F, Sotelo-Avila C, Kidd JM: Mesenchymal renal tumors in infancy: a reappraisal. Hum Pathol 12:78–85, 1981.

55. Gonzalez-Crussi F, Kidd JM, Hernandez RJ: Cystic nephroma: morphologic spectrum and implications. Urology 20:88–93, 1982.

56. Gonzalez-Crussi F, Goldschmidt RA, Hsueh W, Trujillo YP: Infantile sarcoma with intracytoplasmic filamentous inclusions: distinctive tumor of possible histiocytic origin. Cancer 49:2365–2375, 1982.

57. Gonzalez-Crussi F, Baum ES: Renal sarcomas of childhood. A clinicopathological and ultrastructural study. Cancer 51:898–912, 1983.

58. Graham AP: Malignancy of kidney: survey of 195 cases. J Urol 58:10–21, 1947.

59. Greene LF, Rosenthal MH: Multiple hypernephromas of the kidney in association with Lindau's disease. N Engl J Med 244:633–634, 1951.

60. Haas JE, Palmer NF, Weinberg AG, Beckwith JB: Ultrastructure of malignant rhabdoid tumor of the kidney. A distinctive renal tumor of children. Hum Pathol 12:646–657, 1981.

61. Haas JE, Bonadio JF, Beckwith JB: Clear cell sarcoma of the kidney with emphasis on ultrastructural studies. Cancer 54:2978–2987, 1984.

62. Hajdu SI, Foote FW Jr: Angiomyolipoma of the kidney: report of 27 cases and review of the literature. J Urol 102:396–401, 1969.

63. Harms D, Zeidler H: Histopathology of nephroblastomas. Klin Padiatr 193:206–212, 1981.

64. Heine U, DeThe G, Ishiguro H, et al: Multiplicity of cell response to the BAI strain A (myeloblastosis) avian tumor virus. II. Nephroblastoma (Wilms' tumor): ultrastructure. JNCI 29:41–105, 1962.

65. Herman CJ, Moesker O, Kant A, et al: Is renal cell (Grawitz) tumor a carcinosarcoma? Evidence from analysis of intermediate filament types. Virchows Arch [Cell Pathol] 44:73–83, 1983.

66. Hermanek P, Sigel A, Chlepas S: Histological grading of renal cell carcinoma. Eur Urol 2:189–191, 1976.

67. Hirano A, Zimmerman HM: Fenestrated blood vessels in metastatic renal carcinoma in the brain. Lab Invest 26:465–468, 1972.

68. Holland JM: Cancer of the kidney—natural history and staging. Cancer 32:1030–1042, 1973.

69. Holthofer H, Miettman A, Paasivuo R, et al: Cellular origin and differentiation of renal carcinomas. A fluorescence microscopic study with kidney-specific antibodies, anti-intermediate filament antibodies, and lectins. Lab Invest 49:317–326, 1983.

70. Hughson MD, Hennigar GR, McManus JFA: Atypical cysts, acquired renal cystic disease, and renal cell tumors in end stage dialysis kidneys. Lab Invest 42:475–480, 1980.

71. Joshi VV: Cystic partially differentiated nephroblastoma: an entity in the spectrum of infantile renal neoplasia. Perspect Pediatr Pathol 5:217–235, 1979.

72. Klein MJ, Valensi QJ: Proximal tubular adenomas of kidney with so-called oncocytic features. Cancer 38:906–914, 1976.

73. Knudson AG Jr, Strong LC: Mutation and cancer: a model for Wilms' tumor of the kidney. JNCI 48:313–324, 1972.

74. Kragel PJ, Toker C: Infiltrating recurrent renal angiomyolipoma with fatal outcome. J Urol 133:90–91, 1985.

75. Ladda R, Atkins L, Littlefield J, et al: Computer-assisted analysis of chromosomal abnormalities: detection of a deletion in aniridia–Wilms' tumor syndrome. Science 185:784–787, 1974.

76. Lam ASC, Bedard YC, Buckspan MB, et al: Surgically curable hypertension associated with reninoma. J Urol 128:572–575, 1982.

77. Lansigna NC Jr, Benisch BM, Sidoti JS: Renal carcinoma presenting as metastasis to uvula. Urology 2:449–451, 1973.

78. Lapin AL, Hermann HB, Pinto Z: Hypernephroma with solitary cerebral metastasis: six-year survival following nephrectomy. NY J Med 65:1037–1040, 1965.

79. Lauritsen JG: Lindau's disease. A study of one family through six generations. Acta Chir Scand 139:482–486, 1973.

80. Levin NP, Damjanov I, Depillis VJ: Mesoblastic nephroma in an adult patient. Recurrence 21 years after removal of primary lesion. Cancer 49:573–577, 1982.

81. Lieber MM, Tomera KM, Farrow GM: Renal oncocytoma. J Urol 125:481–485, 1981.

82. Lynch HT, Shurin SB, Dahms BB, et al: Paravertebral malignant rhabdoid tumor in infancy: in vitro studies of a familial tumor. Cancer 52:290–296, 1983.

83. Machin GA: Persistent renal blastema (nephroblastomatosis) as a frequent precursor of Wilms' tumor; a pathological and clinical review. Part 2. Significance of nephroblastomatosis in the genesis of Wilms' tumor. Am J Pediatr Hematol Oncol 2:253–261, 1980.

84. Machin GA, McCaughey WT: A new precursor lesion of Wilms' tumour (nephroblastoma): intralobar multifocal nephroblastomatosis. Histopathology 8:35–53, 1984.

85. Mahoney JP, Saffos RO: Fetal rhabdomyomatous nephroblastoma with a renal pelvic mass simulating sarcoma botryoides. Am J Surg Pathol 5:297–306, 1981.

86. Mancilla-Jimenez R, Stanley RJ, Blath RA: Papillary renal cell carcinoma: a clinical, radiologic, and pathologic study of 34 cases. Cancer 38:2469–2480, 1976.

87. Marsden HB, Lawler W, Kumar S: Bone metastasizing renal tumor of childhood: morphological and clinical features and differences from Wilms' tumor. Cancer 42:1922–1928, 1978.

88. Marsden HB, Lawler W: Primary renal tumours in the first year of life. A population based review. Virchows Arch [A] 399:1–9, 1983.

89. Marsden HB, Lawler W, Carr T, Kumar S: A scoring system for Wilms' tumour: pathological study of the Second Medical Research Council (MRC) Trial. Int J Cancer 33:365–368, 1984.

90. Mead JH, Herrera G, Kaufman MF, Herz JH: Case report of a primary cystic sarcoma of the kidney, demonstrating fibrohistiocytic, osteoid, and cartilaginous components (malignant mesenchymoma). Cancer 50:2211–2214, 1982.

91. Meadows AT, Lichtenfield JL, Koop CE: Wilms' tumor in three children of a woman with congenital hemihypertrophy. N Engl J Med 291:23–24, 1974.

92. Merino MJ, Livolsi VA: Oncocytomas of the kidney. Cancer 50:1852–1856, 1982.

93. Moertel CG, Dockerty MB, Baggenstoss AH: Multiple primary malignant neoplasms. III. Tumors of multicentric origin. Cancer 14:238–248, 1961.

94. Mostofi FK: Pathology and spread of renal cell carcinoma. In JS King Jr (ed), Renal Neoplasia. Boston, Little, Brown, 1967, p 41.

95. Mostofi FK: Tumors of the renal parenchyma. Monogr Pathol 20:356–412, 1979.

96. Myers GM, Fehrenbaker LG, Kelalis PP: Prognostic significance of renal vein invasion by hypernephroma. J Urol 100:420–423, 1968.

97. Oberling C, Riviere M, Haguenau F: Ultrastructure of the clear cells in renal carcinomas and its importance for the demonstration of their renal origin. Nature 186:402, 1960.

98. Olsson PJ, Fierer JA, Kelly CE, et al: Renal carcinoma and dialysis in end-stage renal disease. South Med J 78:507, 1985.

99. Orjavik OS, Fauchald P, Hovig T, et al: Renin-secreting renal tumour with severe hypertension. Case report with tumour renin analysis, histopathological and ultrastructure studies. Acta Med Scand 197:329–335, 1975.

100. Penchansky L, Gallo G: Rhabdomyosarcoma of the kidney in children. Cancer 44:285–291, 1979.

101. Pendergrass TW: Congenital anomalies in children with Wilms' tumor. Cancer 37:403–409, 1976.

102. Penn I: Transplantation in patients with primary renal malignancies. Transplantation 24:424–434, 1977.

103. Perez CA, Kaiman HA, Keith J, et al: Treatment of Wilms' tumor and factors affecting prognosis. Cancer 32:609–617, 1973.

104. Petkovic S: Significance of venous invasion in renal parenchymal tumor for prognosis. Urol Nephrol 69:707–712, 1976.

105. Pinchuk VG, Chudakov VG, Goldschmid B, Monastyrshaia B: Morphology and ultrastructure of Wilms' tumor in children. Arkh Patol 36:42–48, 1974.

106. Pochedly C, Miller D (eds): Wilms' Tumor. New York, John Wiley & Sons, 1976.

107. Potter EL: Pathology of the Fetus and Infant, 2nd ed. Chicago, Year Book Medical Publishers, 1961.

108. Reidy JF: Osteoblastic metastases from a hypernephroma. Br J Radiol 48:225–227, 1975.

109. Riches E: On carcinoma of the kidney. Ann R Coll Surg Engl 32:201–208, 1963.

110. Robertson PW, Klidjian A, Harding LK, et al: Hypertension due to a renin-secreting renal tumour. Am J Med 43:963–976, 1967.

111. Robson CJ, Churchill BM, Anderson W: The results of radical nephrectomy for renal cell carcinoma. J Urol 101:297–301, 1969.

112. Roller MF, Stuppler SA, Kandzari SJ, Milam DF: Hypernephroma and associated ureteral involvement. Urology 8:575–578, 1976.

113. Rous SN, Bailie MD, Kaufman DB, et al: Nodular renal blastema, nephroblastomatosis, and Wilms' tumor. Different points on the same disease spectrum. Urology 8:599–604, 1976.

114. Rousseau MF, Nabarra B: Embryonic kidney tumors; ultrastructure of nephroblastoma. Virchows Arch [A] 363:149, 1974.

115. Rutledge J, Beckwith JB, Benjamin D, Hass JE: Absence of immunoperoxidase staining for myoglobin in the malignant rhabdoid tumor of the kidney. Pediatr Pathol 1:93, 1983.

116. Sarjanen K, Hjelt L: Grading of human renal adenocarcinoma. Scand J Urol Nephrol 12:49, 1978.

117. Sarjanen K, Hjelt L: Ultrastructural characteristics of human renal cell carcinoma in relation to the light microscopic grading. Scand J Urol Nephrol 12:57, 1978.

118. Schmidt D, Dickersin GR, Vawter GF, et al: Wilms' tumor: review of ultrastructure and histogenesis. Pathobiol Annu 12:281–300, 1982.

119. Schmidt D, Harms D, Zieger G: Malignant rhab-

doid tumor of the kidney. Histopathology, ultrastructure and comments on differential diagnosis. Virchows Arch [A] 398:101–108, 1982.

120. Seljelid R, Ericsson JL: Electron microscopic observations on specialization of the cell surface in renal clear cell carcinoma. Lab Invest 14:435–447, 1965.

121. Selli C, Hinshaw WM, Woodard BH, Paulson DF: Stratification of risk factors in renal cell carcinoma. Cancer 52:899–903, 1983.

122. Shaw A, Konrad PN: Pediatric surgical oncology: update on Wilms' tumor, neuroblastoma and rhabdomyosarcoma. Curr Probl Cancer 8:1–44, 1984.

123. Shen SC, Yunis EJ: A study of the cellularity and ultrastructure of congenital mesoblastic nephroma. Cancer 45:306–314, 1980.

124. Siminovitch JM, Montie JE, Straffon RA: Prognostic indicators in renal adenocarcinoma. J Urol 130:20–23, 1983.

125. Skinner DG, Colvin RB, Vermillion CD, et al: Diagnosis and management of renal cell carcinoma. A clinical and pathologic study of 309 cases. Cancer 28:1165, 1971.

126. Skinner DG, Pfister RC, Colvin RB: Extension of renal cell carcinoma into the vena cava: the rationale for aggressive surgical management. J Urol 107:711–716, 1972.

127. Skinner DG, Vermillion CD, Colvin RB: The surgical management of renal cell carcinoma. J Urol 107:705–710, 1972.

128. Snyder HM, Lack EE, Chetty-Baktavizian A, et al: Congenital mesoblastic nephroma: relationship to other renal tumors of infancy. J Urol 126:513–516, 1981.

129. Spear GS, Hyde TP, Gruppo RA, Slusser R: Pseudohermaphroditism, glomerulonephritis with the nephrotic syndrome, and Wilms' tumor in infancy. J Pediatr 79:677–681, 1971.

130. Sun CN, Bissada NK, White HJ, Redman JF: Spectrum of ultrastructural patterns of renal cell adenocarcinoma. Urology 9:195–200, 1977.

131. Tannenbaum M: Ultrastructural pathology of human renal cell tumors. Pathol Annu 6:249–277, 1971.

132. Tannenbaum M: Surgical and histopathology of renal tumors. Semin Oncol 10:385–389, 1983.

133. Tomera KM, Farrow GM, Lieber MM: Well differentiated (grade 1) clear cell renal carcinoma. J Urol 129:933–937, 1983.

134. Tremblay M: Ultrastructure of a Wilms' tumour and myogenesis. J Pathol 105:269–277, 1971.

135. Ugarte N, Gonzalez-Crussi F, Hsueh W: Wilms' tumor: its morphology in patients under one year of age. Cancer 48:346–353, 1981.

136. Umliker W: Accuracy of cytologic diagnosis of cancer of the urinary tract. Acta Cytol 8:186, 1964.

137. van der Walt JD, Reid HA, Risdon RA, Shaw JH: Renal oncocytoma. A review of the literature and report of an unusual multicentric case. Virchows Arch [A] 398:291–304, 1983.

138. van Kessel AG, Nusse R, Slater R, et al: Localization of the oncogene c-Ha-rasl outside the aniridia–Wilms' tumor–associated deletion of chromosome 11 (del 11p13) using somatic cell hybrids. Cancer Genet Cytogenet 15:79, 1985.

139. Vaziri ND, Darwish R, Martin DC, Hostetler J: Acquired renal cystic disease in renal transplant recipients. Nephron 37:203–205, 1984.

140. Vogel AM, Gown AM, Caughlan J, et al: Rhabdoid tumors of the kidney contain mesenchymal specific and epithelial specific intermediate filament proteins. Lab Invest 50:232–238, 1984.

141. Walker D, Richard GA: Fetal hamartoma of the kidney: recurrence and death of patient. J Urol 110:352–353, 1973.

142. Wallace AC, Nairn RC: Renal tubular antigens in kidney tumors. Cancer 29:977–981, 1972.

143. Weitzner S: Clear cell carcinoma of the free wall of a simple renal cyst. J Urol 106:515–517, 1971.

144. Wigger H: Fetal mesenchymal hamartoma of kidney. A tumor of secondary mesenchyme. Cancer 36:1002–1008, 1975.

145. Wigger HJ: Fetal rhabdomyomatous nephroblastoma—a variant of Wilms' tumor. Hum Pathol 7:613–623, 1976.

146. Williams AO, Ajayi OO: Ultrastructure of Wilms' tumor (nephroblastoma). Exp Mol Pathol 24:35–47, 1976.

147. Zhang G, Monda L, Wasserman NF, Fraley EE: Bilateral renal oncocytoma: report of 2 cases and literature review. J Urol 133:84–86, 1985.

JERRY WAISMAN, M.D.

Pathology of Neoplasms of the Prostate Gland

This review of the pathology of neoplasms of the prostate gland includes a description of the microscopic features of the gland in normal, hyperplastic, and neoplastic states. Representing its rate of occurrence, a discussion of adenocarcinoma occupies much of the text. Photomicrographs supplement the narrative description, and references to electron microscopy are provided when available and relevant. Several rare neoplasms are illustrated, and unusual or new features of adenocarcinoma, including the effects of treatment, the results of new diagnostic techniques, and the importance of grading are described. Both classic and recent references are noted for unusual or controversial topics.

NORMAL STRUCTURE

Gross Features

The normal prostate gland (Fig. 9–1) is a small, firm organ shaped like an inverted and flattened pyramid, with a central urethra running from the superior (cranial) base to the inferior (caudal) apex. In the young adult, the gland weighs 15 to 20 gm and measures roughly 4 cm across.[239] The superior surface abuts the neck of the urinary bladder, the apex rests on the urogenital diaphragm, the lateral surfaces are narrowly separated from the levator ani muscles by a venous plexus, the anterior face lies against the fat and blood vessels of the retropubic space, and the posterior surface is separated from the rectum by Denonvilliers' fascia. A dense, fibrous fascia surrounds the gland, distinct from the false "surgical capsule" of compressed glandular tissue frequently found in nodular hyperplasia. The prostate gland is penetrated posteriorly and superiorly by the ejaculatory ducts, which end next to the blind pouch of the utricle on the posterior urethral swelling known as the verumontanum. A shallow midline depression called the median furrow, as well as the superiorly placed seminal vesicles, usually are palpable landmarks on rectal examination.

Internally, the prostate gland in the adult has no obvious true lobar divisions.[5, 80, 171] Despite this, some authors[173, 239, 246] have described five artificial partitions (anterior, medial, posterior, and two lateral lobes) based on Lowsley's fetal studies.[210] Recent studies on adult glands have led to conflicting suggestions of three paired lobes in an onion-skin arrangement around the urethra[331] and two disc-like parts with a separate "peri-urethral organ."[225, 226] In view of the unresolved differences concerning the internal structure of the gland, the simplest approach is to regard the prostate gland as having a central area (submucosal and periurethral zone, "female" area, area of hyperplasia) and a horseshoe-shaped peripheral area (prostate proper, "male" area, area of carcinoma). This concept correlates with the distribution of disease and responsiveness to hormones, though not necessarily to anatomic divisions.[80, 112, 159, 203] The arterial supply to the prostate gland is provided by branches of

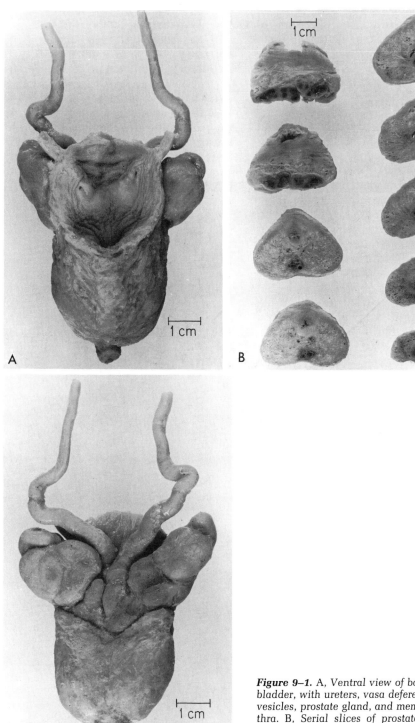

Figure 9–1. A, Ventral view of base of urinary bladder, with ureters, vasa deferentia, seminal vesicles, prostate gland, and membranous urethra. B, Serial slices of prostate gland from base to apex. C, Dorsal view of prostate gland and related structures.

the internal pudendal, inferior vesical, and middle rectal arteries. Abundant venous plexuses empty chiefly into the internal iliac veins but also enter tributaries of vertebral veins, which may be important to the spread of cancer.[18] Lymphatic drainage is to internal iliac and presacral nodes, with secondary connections to the external iliac chains.[19, 315]

Microscopic Features

The prostate gland itself contains several subtypes of glands. Small central or peri-urethral glands, which account for the prostate enlargement of aged men, empty separately into the anterior region of the prostate urethra.[30, 160] The embryonic origin of these small periurethral glands is distinct from that of the remaining prostate glands. Other central glands are larger and drain to lateral ducts, which open into each urethral sinus to the side of the verumontanum. The glands of the verumontanum surround a dilated cavity or utricle and may represent an accessory sexual organ. The large peripheral or proper prostate glands have a major secretory function. These glands converge into large ducts, which also drain into the urethral sinuses (Fig. 9–2).

The prostate gland is composed of many lobules connected by interlobular ducts and defined by bands of connective tissue. Acini and intralobular ducts comprise the lobules and are generally lined by tall columnar cells with small, round, basal nuclei and clear, apical cytoplasm (Fig. 9–3). These cells are rich in acid phosphatase.[132] Indifferent basal or reserve cells are present irregularly between the columnar cells and a delicate basement membrane. Argentaffin and argyrophilic cells also have been identified in the basal position,[185] and some contain somatostatin,[74] ACTH,[45] or serotonin.[104] In acini, the columnar epithelium is thrown into folds or delicate papillae. In dilated or atrophic acini, the columnar epithelium is replaced by cuboid or squamous cells, and the large ducts, particularly near the urethra, may be lined by transitional epithelium. Acini and ducts may contain exfoliated cells and secretions. Enlarging masses of condensed secretions become laminated and form the corpora amylacea. The corpora amylacea share certain features with amyloid, including the characteristic staining properties.[142]

The prostate stroma contains smooth muscle cells, collagenous fibers, and a few elastic

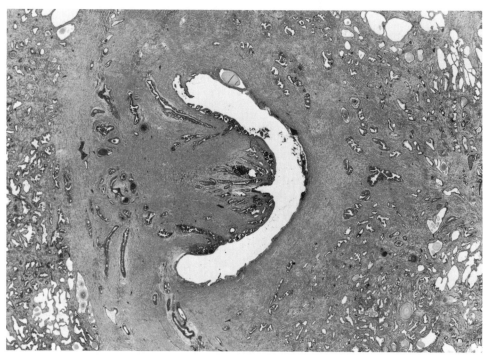

Figure 9–2. Prostatic urethra with verumontanum, major ducts, and hyperplastic periurethral glands. (Hematoxylin and eosin stain, × 9)

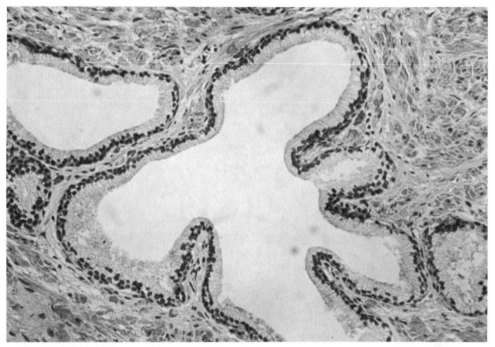

Figure 9–3. *Prostate gland, from a young adult man, that shows acinus lined by columnar cells and surrounded by smooth muscle cells. (H & E, × 250)*

fibers. The muscle is prominent about the urethra, whereas condensed fibrous tissue forms a capsule at the periphery. Blood vessels and nerves are prominent at the periphery, and striated muscle fibers may also be found in this region. The presence of lymphatic vessels within the prostate gland has been debated; however, they have been found by electron microscopy in human prostate glands between the muscle fibers and in the fibrous stroma but not beneath the epithelium.[117] There are no perineural lymphatic vessels.[151]

Descriptions of transmission and scanning electron microscopy of the prostate gland are available.[75, 105, 119, 347, 348]

COMMON DIAGNOSTIC PROCEDURES

Sampling Techniques

Aspiration

Transrectal aspiration of the prostate gland with a fine needle is a simple procedure that can be performed rapidly on an outpatient basis without anesthesia and usu-ally without risk of infection. The aspirates are spread on standard glass slides similar to the procedure used for the preparation of smears of blood and bone marrow, and they are stained by any of the common methods, including the Papanicolaou stain and hematologic stains such as the May-Grünwald-Giemsa (MGG) stain. I use a commercial stain (Diff-quik). In addition to standard diagnostic microscopy, special studies such as the immunoperoxidase technique,[181] electron microscopy,[202] and flow cytometry[334] can easily be performed upon the aspirated cells.

Smears of benign lesions (e.g., nodules in nodular hyperplasia) contain sheets of uniform cells with sharp borders and small regular nuclei (Fig. 9–4). Smears of prostate adenocarcinoma contain sheets of atypical cells or many free atypical cells (Fig. 9–5). The sheets of neoplastic cells may have small acini with a central cytoplasmic mass and a rim of nuclei (microacinar pattern). Often the nuclei overlap and are molded. Nuclear pleomorphism and fragility and the presence, number, and size of nucleoli are other variable features catalogued in a scheme for classification of prostate adenocarcinoma according to grade of differentia-

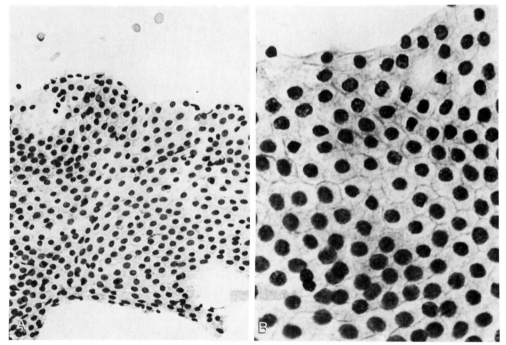

Figure 9–4. A, Smear of prostatic aspirate, showing monolayer of regular epithelial cells, characteristic of nodular hyperplasia. (Papanicolaou stain, × 250) B, Classic honeycomb appearance of nodular hyperplasia. (Papanicolaou stain, × 675)

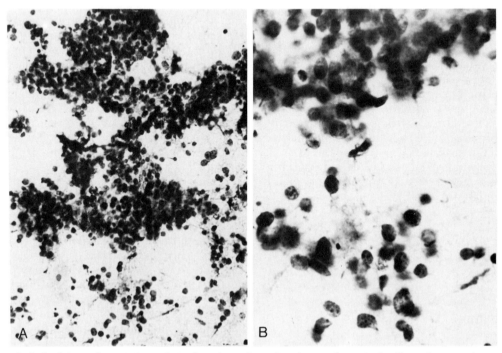

Figure 9–5. A, Smear of prostatic aspirate that shows irregular cluster of atypical cells and many pleomorphic bare nuclei, characteristic of poorly differentiated acinar adenocarcinoma. (Papanicolaou, × 250) B, Same area of same smear. (× 675)

tion. Although the reliability of grading has been questioned,[92] grading of aspirates from prostate adenocarcinoma has been formalized,[196, 341] and cytologic grading of prostate adenocarcinoma has clinical relevance.[352]

The technique of prostate aspiration was developed in the United States,[102] but the procedure did not gain local acceptance until recent years. In fact, references to the technique in the American literature were limited although laudatory[110, 209] until the present decade.[182, 193, 194, 230] The role of transrectal aspiration in the diagnosis of prostate adenocarcinoma was established in Sweden[95] and has found widespread acceptance outside the United States.[153, 316] Aspiration is considered reliable when compared with transrectal needle biopsy,[211] and the two procedures give a combined accuracy rate of 96% in the diagnosis of adenocarcinoma.[92] Other cytologic procedures have not proved so valuable in the diagnosis of prostate adenocarcinoma,[183, 304] with the exception of one enthusiastic report about the examination of prostate fluid aspirated through the urethra.[161]

Needle Biopsy

The needle biopsy is a common means of obtaining tissue from suspicious areas of the prostate gland. The approach can be either transperineal or transrectal, and several cylinders of tissue should be obtained at one sitting. They should be handled delicately because crush artifact can easily ruin the specimen. There is obviously a problem in taking small samples from a large gland, but a positive biopsy result is always meaningful. Conversely, a negative result is an indication for a repeat biopsy when there is a suspicious nodule. The diagnostic accuracy of this technique exceeds 70 to 80% and improves with the experience of the surgeon.[15, 183, 184, 242]

Transurethral Biopsy

Transurethral biopsy or resection of prostate tissue yields multiple, curled fragments of tissue, 2 to 4 cm in size. Most pathologists examine only a sample of these "chips" of prostate tissue, although some claim that the yield of cancer diagnoses increases with the amount of tissue examined.[69, 204] One recent study reported a 99% probability of identifying a cancer when four blocks were submitted,[280] and another group found that all clinically significant adenocarcinomas were found when 10 gm of tissue were submitted for microscopic examination.[67] Others have recommended embedding all of the tissue.[237] Another report indicates that the incidence of metastasis has been tied to the fraction of chips containing adenocarcinoma.[99] Prostatic cancer occurs predominantly in the "outer zone" and might be missed by a central biopsy; however, Denton showed that the transurethral method yields more accurate information than the perineal needle biopsy if the resection is deep.[70] A transurethral resection gives the pathologist more tissue with less compression than a needle biopsy, but the electrocautery may produce a disturbing thermal artifact (Fig. 9–6).

Open Biopsy

Open perineal biopsy is considered the most accurate biopsy technique,[64, 158, 165] and provides the best specimen for microscopic examination; however, it may carry a greater risk of complication for the patient.

Non-neoplastic Alterations

Non-neoplastic diseases of the prostate gland often enter the differential diagnosis of prostate cancer, particularly when they cause induration or hard nodules that are noticed on rectal examination.[166] These lesions include inflammatory processes, nodular hyperplasia, infarction with metaplasia, melanosis, and calculi.

Acute and Chronic Prostatitis

Most aging prostate glands contain small foci of acute inflammatory cells and collections of lymphocytes and plasma cells, particularly in association with nodular hyperplasia.[255] True acute prostatitis is generally bacterial and is characterized by collections of neutrophils within acini and stroma, often with foci of necrosis leading to abscesses (Fig. 9–7). Chronic prostatitis is a doubtful entity clinically, bacteriologically, and microscopically. Aerobic and anaerobic cultures usually reveal no pathogens,[250, 256, 260] and microscopic examination shows nonspecific changes including lymphoid infiltrates, dilated ducts and acini, desquamation of acinar cells, and an increase in fibrous

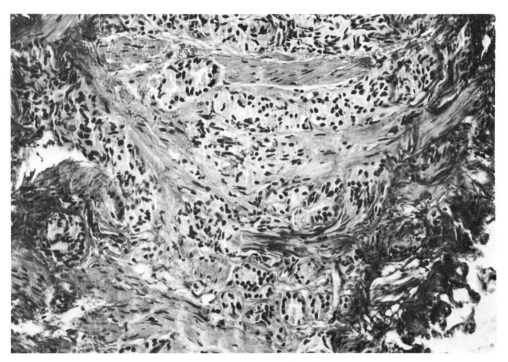

Figure 9–6. Adenocarcinoma of prostate gland, obtained by a transurethral resection, showing peripheral thermal artifact. (H & E, × 250)

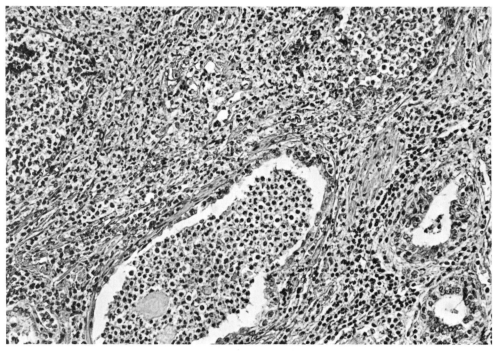

Figure 9–7. Acute prostatitis, showing exudate in acini and through stroma. Microabscesses are seen in upper left corner. (H & E, × 250)

tissue. Similar microscopic changes are common in nonsymptomatic patients.

Granulomatous prostatitis is an uncommon disease[329] that may resemble adenocarcinoma on rectal examination.[186] The blockage of ducts with subsequent rupture and leakage of prostate secretions is thought to cause poorly defined, noncaseous granulomas. Numerous vacuolated histiocytes, lymphocytes, plasma cells, and foreign-body giant cells are present,[186, 323] and the histiocytic component can be mistaken for poorly differentiated adenocarcinoma in biopsy specimens.[109] A distinctive subgroup is that in which small stellate foci of fibrinoid necrosis, sometimes with acute vasculitis and peripheral concentrations of eosinophils, are present (Fig. 9–8). This subtype of granulomatous prostatitis has been considered an allergic or autoimmune phenomenon, and some of the patients indeed may have asthma or systemic vasculitis.[187, 333] One patient with simple eosinophilic granulomatous prostatitis was also recently described.[272] However, most examples of eosinophilic, necrotizing granulomatous prostatitis occur following transurethral resection of the prostate gland.[89, 97, 101, 195, 232, 263, 293]

Tuberculosis, fungal infections, protozoal infestations, and malacoplakia occasionally affect the prostate gland (Fig. 9–9), producing granulomatous inflammation.

Nodular Hyperplasia and Involution

Age-related changes in the prostate gland include both hyperplasia and atrophy, and these two processes frequently coexist in different parts of the same gland. Benign prostate hypertrophy is the popular name for this extremely common nodular enlargement of aged glands; however, nodular hyperplasia is a more appropriate term.[240] The process begins in the fourth decade and affects almost 80% of the male population by the ninth decade.[112, 240] Clinical symptoms are considerably less frequent, since very large glands may produce no obstruction. The origin of nodular hyperplasia remains obscure, although most observers favor some endocrine disturbance; Mostofi has reviewed this topic.[244]

The hyperplastic prostate gland often weighs in excess of 100 gm and exhibits an irregular nodularity centered on the periurethral area, generally adjacent or cephalad to the verumontanum (Fig. 9–10).[240] Randall has divided the gross patterns of enlargement into eight types, but the common feature is an enlargement of the inner zone, which compresses the nonhyperplastic peripheral tissue into a "false" surgical capsule.[270] Microcysts and calculi are common.

Microscopically, the very earliest nodules may consist of mixed glandular and stromal tissues or either component separately;[112, 179, 244] however, a few authors maintain that the initial lesion is always stromal hyperplasia into which acini subsequently penetrate.[203, 240, 275] Franks has listed five major types of hyperplastic nodules: fibrous or fibrovascular, fibromuscular, muscular, fibroadenomatous, and fibromyoadenomatous.[112] The fibroadenomatous pattern was recently reviewed;[172] a sixth purely adenomatous form is rarely seen. Thus, nodular hyperplasia consists of all combinations of stromal and epithelial elements, including "pure" fibrous and smooth muscle lesions, which would be considered benign neoplasms in other locations.

The fully developed larger nodules can be surprisingly difficult to distinguish from surrounding prostate tissue. These large nodules usually contain mixed epithelial and stromal elements that maintain a lobular pattern (Fig. 9–11). The hyperplastic stroma lacks elastic fibers but retains other components.[240] Tall, double-layered "active" epithelium as well as cuboid "inactive" epithelium may line the acini, which frequently have papillary intraluminal projections (Fig. 9–12) or appear dilated. Inflammatory foci and infarcts are common. Electron microscopy reflects this light-microscopic picture and shows no significant ultrastructural difference between the hyperplastic and normal cells.[35, 105]

Atrophy or senile involution usually develops in the peripheral portion of the gland concurrent with the nodular hyperplasia of the inner gland. This peripheral involution is manifested by an increase in collagen (particularly in trabeculae between acini), a relative decrease in smooth muscle, enlarged acini, and an "inactive" epithelium (Fig. 9–13). The so-called secondary senile hyperplasia presents the same pattern, but the epithelium has been secondarily stimulated and is composed of tall, active-appearing cells.

Basal Cell Hyperplasia. Recognized as one pattern of nodular hyperplasia, this form is

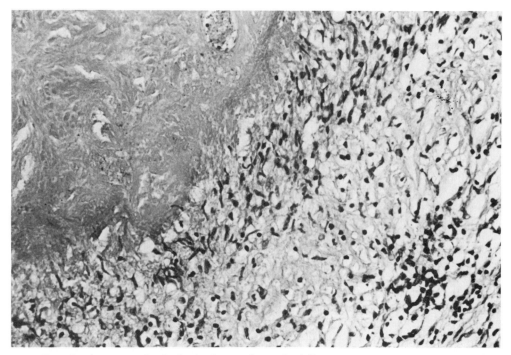

Figure 9–8. Sample of prostate gland, obtained several months following transurethral resection of the gland, showing a granuloma with central necrosis and characteristic palisade of epithelioid cells. (H & E, × 250)

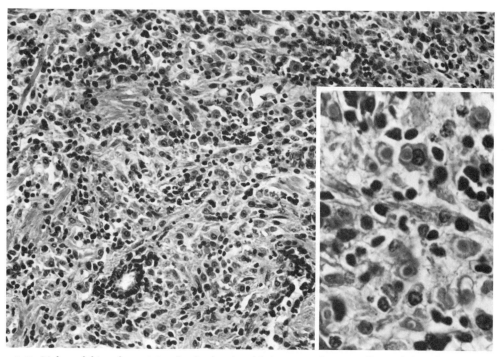

Figure 9–9. Malacoplakia of prostate gland, showing histiocytes, plasma cells, and lymphocytes. Insert is enlargement of central area, which has several Michaelis-Gutmann bodies. (H & E, × 250; insert, × 675)

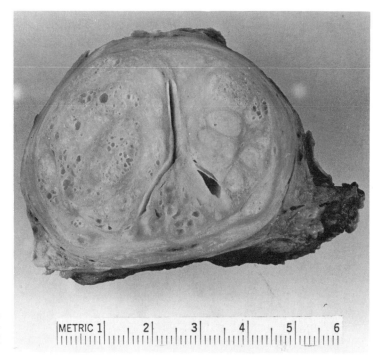

Figure 9–10. Cross section of hyperplastic prostate gland. Note distortion of urethra, cystic glands, and nodules. (× 1.5)

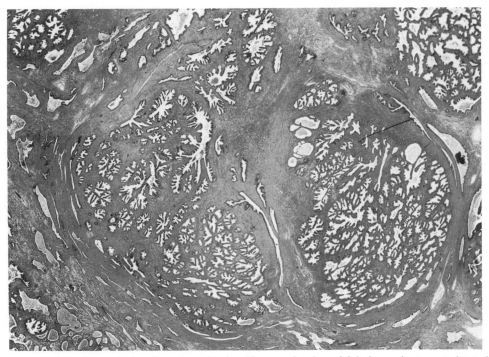

Figure 9–11. Nodular hyperplasia of prostate gland, with several enlarged lobules and attenuated interlobular ducts. (H & E, × 9)

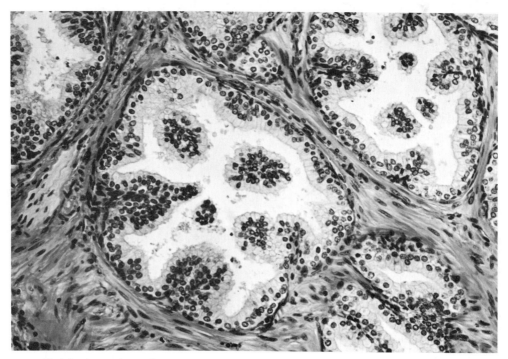

Figure 9–12. Nodular hyperplasia of prostate gland, with characteristic epithelial papillae and "active" columnar epithelium. (H & E, × 250)

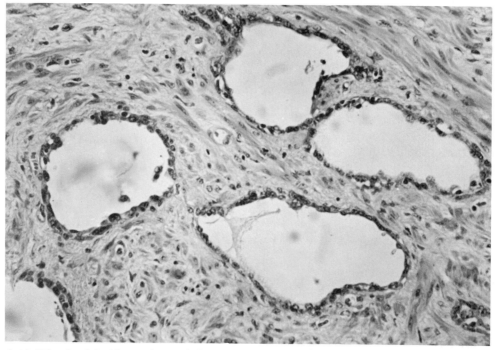

Figure 9–13. Dilated acini with atrophic epithelium, from a prostate gland showing nodular hyperplasia. (H & E, × 250)

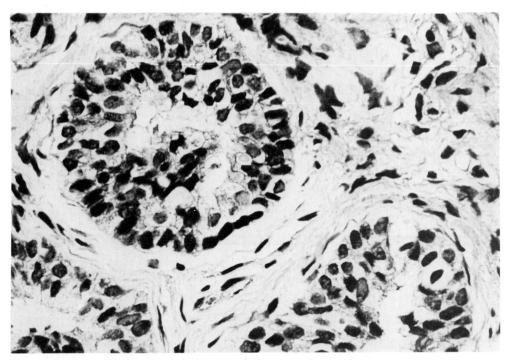

Figure 9–14. Prostate gland showing hyperplasia of basal or reserve cells, which nearly fill the small, regular acini. (H & E, × 675)

thought by some to be a true proliferation of undifferentiated basal or reserve cells.[71] It can occur as a separate nodule or as part of a lobule with otherwise classic acinar cell hyperplasia.[54] The small acini of basal cell hyperplasia are filled or nearly filled by small cells with round or oval nuclei and scant, pale blue-gray cytoplasm (Fig. 9–14). The cells do not appear atypical, and the acinar-lobular pattern is intact. The stroma may be loose and cellular or inconspicuous. This process has also been called a basal cell adenoma and has been mistaken for adenocarcinoma. One variant, apparently distinguished by loose stroma, has been termed embryonal hyperplasia.[26] Basal cell hyperplasia has been described as a precursor of an adenoid basal cell tumor, otherwise known as adenoid cystic carcinoma of the prostate gland.[273]

Atypical Hyperplasia. Focal atypical epithelial hyperplasia also occurs in this setting, and both Franks[112] and McNeal[224] have suggested that this atypical "active" epithelium is premalignant. Recently, this position was restated and supported in a study of 180 adenocarcinomas, wherein almost 60%

had associated atypical hyperplasia.[175] Atypical hyperplasia has also been designated dysplasia, carcinoma in situ, and adenosis.[37] Several microscopic patterns are seen with the designation of atypical hyperplasia, but the common finding is that of nuclear atypia, usually of a mild or moderate degree, in the hyperplastic epithelium. Often the epithelium is papillary, has a saw-toothed appearance, and at low magnification looks bluer than hyperplastic epithelium without atypia (Fig. 9–15). It is blue because nuclei are enlarged and crowded. Small nucleoli are present in some cells (Fig. 9–16). Atypical hyperplasia may have a cribriform pattern; however, I believe that not all acini with this pattern are atypical, having seen the cribriform pattern in the absence of nuclear atypia. Sometimes, atypical nuclei are seen in small, crowded acini in the absence of invasion or even distortion of the lobules, and I have also designated this as atypical hyperplasia. So far, I have found atypical hyperplasia only in prostate glands with an invasive adenocarcinoma, although on several occasions it has been necessary to look painstakingly for a small adenocarcinoma.

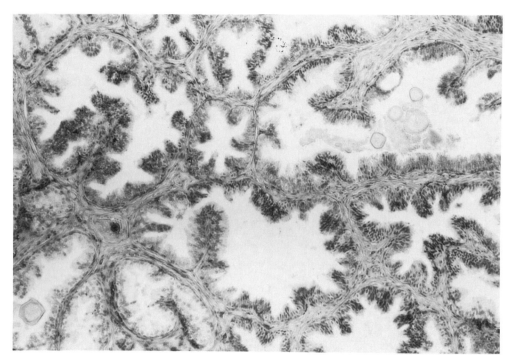

Figure 9–15. Hyperplastic prostatic acini showing atypia. (H & E, × 100)

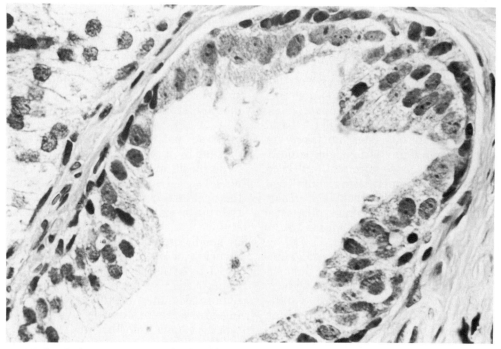

Figure 9–16. Atypical prostatic acini (right) lined by epithelium showing crowded, large, pleomorphic nuclei with small nucleoli. Compare these with the small, uniform nuclei on the far left of the field. (H & E, × 675)

Infarction and Squamous Metaplasia

Prostatic infarction occurs almost exclusively in nodules of benign hyperplasia, and up to 25% of hyperplastic glands contain recent or healed infarcts.[240] Patients commonly present with transient, acute urinary retention secondary to swelling of damaged tissue or with hematuria, should the urethra be involved.[157] Prior urethral instrumentation sometimes seems to be a contributing factor.[245]

On gross examination, the infarct appears as a spherical, hemorrhagic or mottled gray, bulging area, and multiple lesions are present in 10% of the cases.[245] The microscopic picture was first described by Abeshouse,[1] who emphasized the zonal pattern of healing infarcts with central coagulative necrosis, a narrow halo of neutrophils and lymphocytes, and an outer rim composed of distorted acini and solid cords of metaplastic ductal epithelium. This metaplasia is characteristically squamous and occasionally shows intercellular bridges and even keratin pearls (Fig. 9–17). Less frequently the metaplasia occurs in transitional epithelium or in low cuboidal cells resembling Brunn's nests.[245] The healed infarct is a collagenous scar containing irregular clumps of metaplastic epithelium. Unfortunately, the bizarre appearance of the peripheral zone of metaplasia has led many pathologists to make an erroneous diagnosis of cancer.[1, 245, 282] The differential diagnostic points include the lack of cellular atypia, the lack of invasion, and the adjacent infarct itself. Squamous and transitional metaplasia are also noted in the periurethral and major ducts as a spontaneous phenomenon or secondary to infection, chronic irritation, or estrogen therapy.[13]

Melanosis

Melanosis of the prostate gland may be generalized or local, and when local may simulate a neoplasm.[121] Melanosis is applied to the occurrence of melanin-bearing stromal and epithelial cells, whereas the term blue nevus describes melanin limited to dendritic stromal cells.[201] In one case, melanin was confined to the prostate epithelium,[131] and it also has been observed in the cells of adenocarcinoma.[3] Electron microscopy has been employed in the diagnosis of an example of blue nevus of the prostate gland.[163] Melanin-like pigment also has been described in prostatic epithelium.[302]

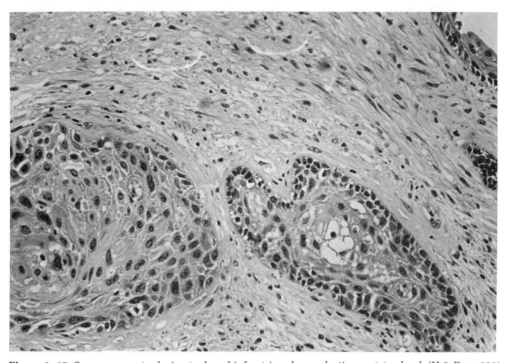

Figure 9–17. Squamous metaplasia at edge of infarct in a hyperplastic prostate gland. (H & E, × 250)

Calculi and Other Non-neoplastic Alterations

Calculi are extremely common, although most are too small to be detected clinically. They may occasionally be large enough to occupy the entire prostate area.[63, 84, 152] Chronic inflammation, obstructed ducts, and "pressure" atrophy may be seen in the adjacent tissue. Other non-neoplastic space-occupying lesions include acquired or developmental (usually müllerian) cysts and amyloid deposits.

BENIGN NEOPLASMS

Lesions identified as benign neoplasms at other sites are generally considered part of the spectrum of nodular hyperplasia in the prostate gland. Thus, erstwhile fibromas and leiomyomas represent a one-sided local growth as part of the general proliferation of prostate stroma in nodular hyperplasia. Two remote reports illustrate the prior misconception about benign neoplasms of the prostate gland;[218, 220] similar cases are not found in the current literature, although other benign stromal tumors such as hemangiopericytoma have been reported.[356]

An outgrowth of prostate tissue, possibly from a duct, presents rarely as a polyp in the prostate urethra and is a cause of hematuria in young men.[149] This prostatic tissue is generally considered ectopic and not neoplastic,[16, 62, 241] although the diagnostic term papillary adenoma properly describes the features. Prosoplasia of urethral epithelium also has been suggested,[343] and this better explains the occurrence of similar lesions in the urinary bladder.[276] The surface of this lesion is often papillary (Fig. 9–18), but in other respects the microscopic appearance is identical to hyperplastic prostate glands, including the presence of corpora amylacea. One cystic, benign papillary neoplasm that was designated a cystic adenoma was observed within the prostate gland,[191] and there is a recent report of an intraprostatic, intraductal papilloma.[362] One malignant variant has been reported; however, the diagnosis of malignancy in this case is questionable.[128]

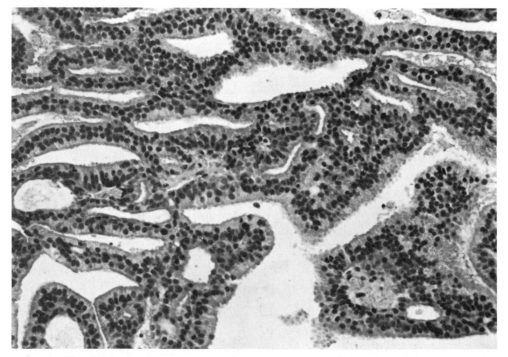

Figure 9–18. Papillary adenoma of major prostatic duct and urethra of a young man with hematuria. (H & E, × 250)

MALIGNANT NEOPLASMS

Malignant neoplasms of the prostate gland are extremely common, particularly in the older age groups. The majority of these tumors are adenocarcinomas of the common or acinar type. Accordingly, prostatic acinar adenocarcinoma will be covered in some detail, with discussion of gross and microscopic features, special diagnostic techniques, the effects of treatment, microscopic grading, and metastatic spread. A brief survey of the rarer cancers will follow.

Acinar Adenocarcinoma

Gross Features

On gross appearance alone, it is frequently impossible to differentiate adenocarcinoma from other common lesions in the prostate gland, such as nodular hyperplasia, recent or healed infarcts, tuberculosis, or other chronic inflammatory processes. Pathologists continue to use the time-honored features including yellow coloration, firmness, loss of the lobular pattern, and hemorrhagic foci in an attempt to identify cancers macroscopically; yet when Kahler applied similar criteria to 631 prostate glands containing 195 cancers, he was able to detect only 102 of the adenocarcinomas by gross examination. He missed 93 adenocarcinomas and wrongly identified 62 hyperplastic glands as malignant. A yellow color was noted in only 21% of the cancers.[173]

The preferred site for adenocarcinoma within the gland has long been a point of contention. The "posterior lobe" contained the majority of the tumors in three series;[238, 278, 360] however, Kahler found more cancer in the "lateral lobes" than in the "posterior lobes."[173] Others detected no predilection for the "posterior lobe."[31, 223] The argument is probably futile, since no distinct "posterior lobe" exists in the adult gland. To complicate the matter, prostatic adenocarcinoma is often multifocal;[40, 222, 238] in one large series 85% of the glands had more than one lesion.[43] These contradictions and complications aside, there is a consensus that adenocarcinoma occurs with greatest frequency in subcapsular peripheral regions of the gland.[31, 35, 43, 114, 238] The division of the prostate gland into "inner" and "outer" zones therefore correlates with a predilection for adenocarcinoma to occur in the "outer" zone, whereas hyperplasia occurs in the "inner" zone.

Microscopic Features

The microscopic appearance of prostate adenocarcinoma is one of the topics on which there is general agreement.[173, 246, 300] The diagnosis is based on evaluation of three criteria: cellular atypia, architectural disturbances, and invasion. The latter two traditionally have been paramount.

The cellular atypia in many prostatic adenocarcinomas often is of a minimal degree, and this criterion is accordingly difficult to apply. Bizarre cells with great variation in size and shape are seen chiefly in the poorly differentiated tumors, where there is little doubt as to the diagnosis on any basis. The majority of tumors are composed of regular, single layers of cuboid or low columnar cells with clear or dense cytoplasm and distinct cell borders. Nuclei are rounded and surprisingly bland, except for occasional prominent nucleoli (Fig. 9–19). Mitotic figures are rare. Irregular clumping of nuclear chromatin and thickening of the nuclear membrane may be present, but these features are better appreciated on cytologic, as opposed to histologic, preparations.

The most important architectural disturbance is loss of the regular lobular pattern with interposed whorls of smooth muscle and connective tissue. In adenocarcinoma, this pattern is replaced by a haphazard arrangement of closely packed, irregularly shaped, and variably sized acini that assume no lobular pattern and are not bound by the regular sweep of stroma (Fig. 9–20). This random acinar growth has been referred to as "stromal invasion"[243, 246] and is a hallmark of prostatic adenocarcinoma. Other alterations in the pattern include microacini, macroacini, intraductal growth, cribriform or other complex glands, and loss or accentuation of papillae (Fig. 9–21). A clear-cell variant resembling renal tubular adenocarcinoma also has been noted, usually as a focal change.[129] In poorly differentiated lesions, there may be a total loss of acinar structure with a diffuse spread of individual cells or formation of solid cords or sheets of cells (Fig. 9–22). Mucinous and xanthomatous variants are seen occasionally. Some degree of microscopic variability within the indi-

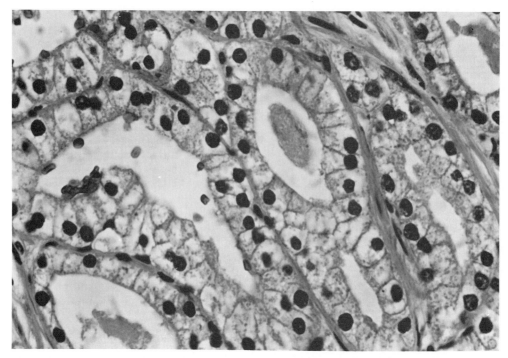

Figure 9–19. Crowded glands of well-differentiated (acinar) adenocarcinoma of the prostate gland. Cells are cuboid or columnar with slightly irregular hyperchromatic nuclei and a few nucleoli. Stroma is inconspicuous. (H & E, × 675)

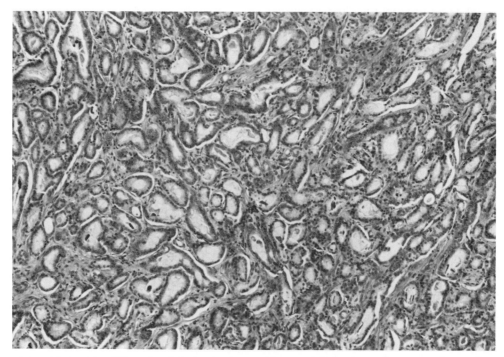

Figure 9–20. Moderately differentiated (acinar) adenocarcinoma with haphazardly arranged irregular glands "invading" stroma. (H & E × 100)

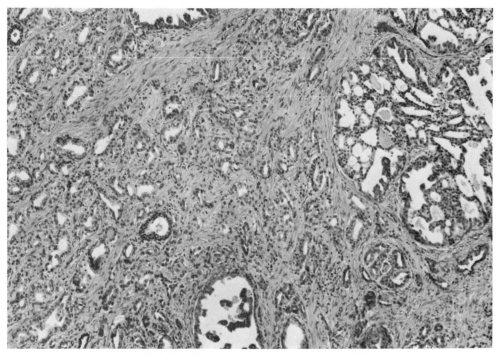

Figure 9–21. Moderately differentiated (acinar) adenocarcinoma of prostate gland, demonstrating morphologic variation with large cribriform glands on right and small, irregular glands on left. (H & E, × 100)

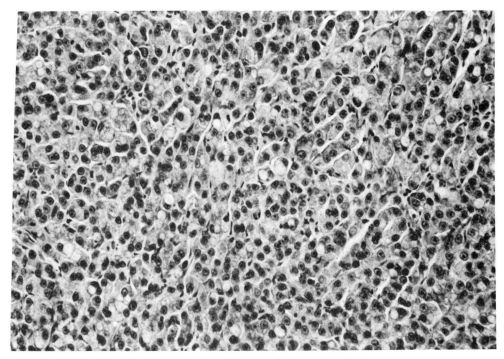

Figure 9–22. Poorly differentiated (acinar) adenocarcinoma of prostate gland, showing sheets of small, round cells. Nucleoli are prominent. (H & E, × 250)

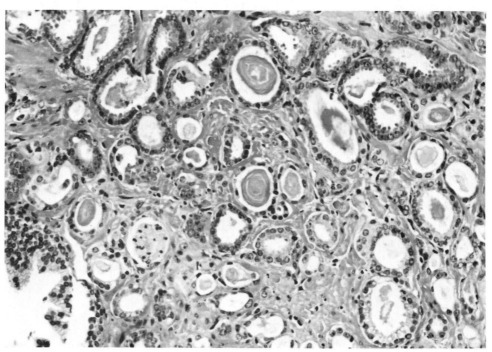

Figure 9–23. *Corpora amylacea within small acini of moderately differentiated (acinar) adenocarcinoma. (H & E, × 250)*

vidual tumor is the general rule, and, in occasional large growths, all patterns may coexist.[43, 339]

An interesting minor finding is the presence of well-formed corpora amylacea within obviously malignant acini (Fig. 9–23). Moore, writing on early adenocarcinoma, stated that "a formed corpus amylaceum has never been observed in these small acini."[238] Unfortunately, this erroneous view has enjoyed a long life. My observations agree with Kahler's;[173] corpora amylacea, albeit occasionally poorly formed, are common in neoplastic acini.

Some corpora amylacea contain central eosinophilic crystals, and similar crystals are observed in the acini of prostatic adenocarcinoma (Fig. 9–24). These crystals are characteristic of well-differentiated adenocarcinoma or, at least, a well-defined acinar component of adenocarcinoma. In a series of 57 patients with Stage B adenocarcinoma of the prostate gland, 23 of the adenocarcinomas contained crystals, and none with crystals progressed.[125] Crystals have been seen in hyperplastic acini adjacent to adenocarcinomas,[164] and they also have been found in 10% of a series of cases of atypical hyperplasia.[25] These crystals resemble crystalline Bence-Jones protein and may represent one form of immunoglobulin, whereas corpora amylacea are the usual deposits of prostatic immunoglobulin.[155]

Invasion is a useful diagnostic criterion in all cancers, but tumors of the prostate exhibit a uniquely helpful example. This is perineural invasion, in which malignant epithelial cells or acini are found adjacent to nerves with no intervening collagenous fibers (Fig. 9–25). Roughly 90% of prostatic adenocarcinomas show perineural invasion[31, 43] and a search for perineural invasion in an otherwise "borderline" lesion stands a good chance of success. "Benign perineural invasion" recently has been reported in the prostate gland,[47] and such a finding has been descibed at other sites.[135] The presence of hyperplastic prostatic acini adjacent to intraprostatic nerves is rare, in my experience (Fig. 9–26). In any case, perineural growth does not represent vascular invasion.[151]

Invasion of true lymphatic vessels, blood vessels, capsule, and seminal vesicles may also be seen and is diagnostic of malignancy. Caution must be used in interpreting lymphatic invasion, since acini commonly pull away from surrounding stroma during tissue

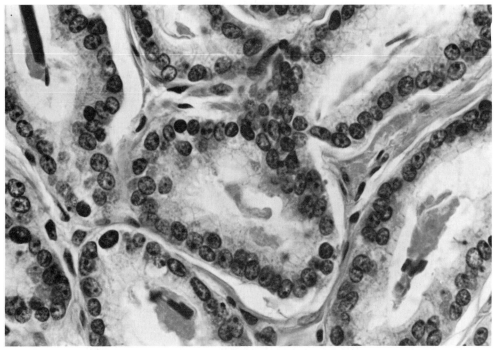

Figure 9–24. Well-differentiated (acinar) adenocarcinoma of prostate gland, showing hyaline, eosinophilic luminal crystals. (H & E, × 675)

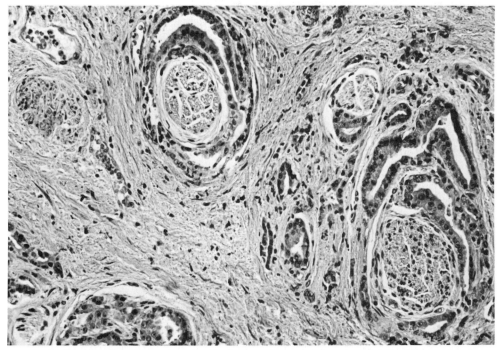

Figure 9–25. Moderately differentiated (acinar) adenocarcinoma of prostate gland, with extensive perineural involvement. (H & E, × 250)

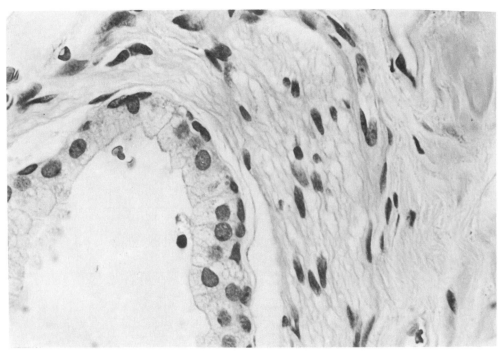

Figure 9–26. Nerve at periphery of prostate gland with perineural hyperplastic acinar epithelium, an example of "benign perineural invasion." (H & E, × 675)

fixation, leaving an artifactual "lymphatic space" into which the "tumor" appears to project. The presence of free epithelial cells within blood vessels, without attachment to the wall, should also be viewed skeptically, as cutting the specimen may displace various components through the tissue. Lastly, the presence of acini between striated muscle bundles is not conclusive evidence of invasion, since striated muscle is normally present in certain areas of the prostate gland.[197, 212]

Prognostically, invasion of the vasculature,[246] penetration through the capsule,[23, 43, 166, 222, 339] and invasion of the seminal vesicle are all associated with decreased survival. There is no prognostic significance to perineural invasion.[43, 222, 339]

Special Diagnostic Techniques

The diagnosis of prostatic adenocarcinoma is based chiefly on the routine microscopic examination of tissue. There are other diagnostic methods that play a supporting role, but in the past they were rarely definitive. These include histochemistry,[36, 116, 190, 206, 268] immunology,[235, 236, 309] and electron microscopy.[35, 105, 214, 258] The cited references should be consulted for a discussion of the individual methods. These techniques were least effective in those instances in which they should be most helpful (for example, in well-differentiated "borderline" lesions), but they may establish the prostatic origin of metastases from an occult primary tumor. Two historical methods deserve mention. The acid phosphatase reaction in serum or on frozen sections of tissue can help to distinguish paraprostatic or extraprostatic tumors (acid phosphatase–negative) from primary intraprostatic cancers (acid prosphatase–positive).[229] The second method is the immunodiffusion test for metastatic cancer of the prostate.[235] Specific antiserum raised against prostatic acid phosphatase will form an arc of precipitate with homogenates of lymph nodes or bone marrow containing prostatic cancer, but no arcs are formed against tissue without cancer or with nonprostatic neoplasms.

Immunohistochemistry has become a major diagnostic technique that can be performed upon fresh-frozen tissue or routinely fixed and embedded tissue. The latter is more useful in a clinical setting, wherein routine samples of tissue can be examined retrospectively without special preservation or preparation. This involves the use of the immunoperoxidase technique and a variety of antibodies, including those to prostate-specific acid phosphatase (PAP) and prostate-specific antigen (PSA).[253, 254] The technique has been especially recommended to distinguish metastatic adenocarcinoma of the prostate from other metastatic cancers,[29] and it can be performed upon smears of aspirates as well as routine samples of tissue.[188] Some have related positive staining for PAP to the grade of the adenocarcinoma,[17, 306, 319] but others have found no suggested relation (or none at all) between the presence of PAP and the differentiation of the adenocarcinoma.[29, 88, 124] Using the same immunoperoxidase technique, prolactin-binding sites have been located in the human prostate gland,[354] and androgen-binding sites that may predict response to hormonal therapy have been descibed in prostatic adenocarcinoma.[262] By using the red blood cell adherence test, investigators have been able to identify blood group antigens on the surface of normal but not neoplastic prostatic epithelial cells, and these antigens presumably can be identified by the immunoperoxidase technique.[344] Chorioembryonic antigen (CEA) has been reported in prostatic adenocarcinoma,[297] and I recently have seen one case that was weakly positive for CEA.

In all instances in which the immunoperoxidase technique is used, positive results appear the same. Colored granular deposits mark the site of the antigen, and usually the positive marker is a coarse, brown granule (Fig. 9–27). Results should be interpreted with caution and common sense and compared with positive and negative controls. Spurious false-positive staining is often obtained on the surfaces of pieces of tissue, and some commercial antibodies have proven capricious. Clinical application of prostate marker studies in general also have been questioned.[266]

Histochemistry is often overlooked in the diagnosis of prostatic adenocarcinoma, but it is occasionally useful. Acidic mucoproteins have been described in the lumens of the neoplastic acini of adenocarcinomas but not in normal or hyperplastic acini.[114, 325] This feature may be useful in separating hyperplastic acini from neoplastic acini in borderline cases of well-differentiated adenocarcinoma. I have not examined a large series of cases of prostatic acinar adenocarcinomas, but almost every case examined focally contained mucin as demonstrated by mucicarmine, PAS, and alcian blue stains.

The prostate gland contains neuroendocrine cells, both in ducts and acini,[185] and these cells may be argyrophilic or argentaf-

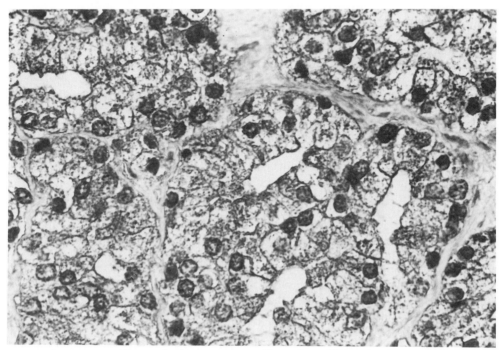

Figure 9–27. Immunoperoxidase stain for prostate-specific antigen (PSA), showing many coarse "positive" cytoplasmic granules in a moderately differentiated prostatic (acinar) adenocarcinoma. (× 675)

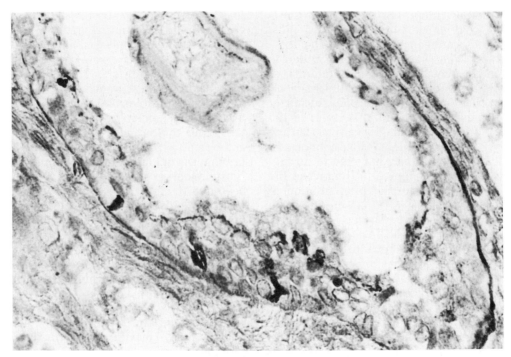

Figure 9–28. Hyperplastic prostatic acinus showing several "neuroendocrine" cells with coarse, dense granules; one cell is dendritic. (Argyrophil stain, × 675)

fin-positive, although argyrophilic cells are more common.[45] The cells appear dendritic (Fig. 9–28) and contain membrane-bound neurosecretory granules when examined by electron microscopy.[75] Somatostatin or similar substances[74] and serotonin[104] have been demonstrated in these cells by immunohistochemical methods. Argentaffin-positive and argyrophilic cells were present in about one half of a series of 50 prostatic adenocarcinomas[185] and in one third of another series.[45] The techniques of histochemistry and immunohistochemistry and their application to the diagnosis of prostatic cancer have been recently reviewed.[233]

Cytometry has been applied to the study of prostatic adenocarcinoma. This method can be used on tissue or aspirated cells and involves flow methods or in situ measurements. For example, measurement of nuclear DNA by flow cytometry revealed adenocarcinomas that were diploid, tetraploid, or aneuploid other than tetraploid; and there is hope that these measurements will provide reliable indicators of the behavior of the tumors.[303, 334] The methods and applications seem sound and are under intense study as related to mammary and thyroid cancer as well as to prostatic adenocarcinomas, al-

though I have no direct experience with these techniques.

Prognosis and Grading

Prognostic microscopic features of adenocarcinoma of the prostate are the subject of an extensive and, at times, confusing literature. Many of the published studies suffer from small numbers of patients, lack of critical analysis, short follow-up, variations in therapy, and other problems common in clinical studies. However, it appears that sufficient evidence has been collected to demonstrate a positive and useful correlation between the microscopic appearance or grade of prostatic adenocarcinoma and the survival of patients. The extent or stage of the neoplasm at the time of treatment likewise indicates the outcome. There are several timely and thoughtful overviews of the topics of grading (and staging) of prostatic adenocarcinoma.[120, 138, 175, 251]

The grading of primary prostatic adenocarcinoma for predictive purposes has been controversial, and a few authors deny its applicability.[43, 106, 115, 283, 294, 326] Most studies have shown a positive correlation between the microscopic grade and survival of patients.[15, 20, 23, 60, 65, 85, 94, 98, 130, 234, 248, 267, 295, 305, 327, 339, 351] A correlation also has been demonstrated between grade and the incidence of metastases[173, 271, 295, 339] and grade and the extent of tumor.[14, 20, 23, 38, 65, 166, 271, 337, 339] As an impressive illustration, Pool and Thompson followed 1469 patients, unclassified as to age or stage, after transurethral resection; and patients with Grade 1 through Grade 4 lesions had five-year survival rates of 59.5%, 34.1%, 16.2%, and 5.6%, respectively. No Grade 4 patient lived for 10 years.[267] Additional prognostic significance is obtained by combining the grade and certain clinical features;[130, 339] Gleason's results are particularly noteworthy.[130]

Grading of latent (incidental or Stage A) cancers may assist physicians in the treatment of these controversial lesions. Conservative therapy has been recommended for all latent tumors on the basis of a presumed benign biologic potential,[44, 68, 148] yet many clinical Stage A cancers have actually spread beyond the prostate gland.[43, 72, 221] A discriminate approach to Stage A carcinoma has been suggested in which the grade or number of neoplastic foci or both factors would determine the need for radical treatment in these tumors.[20, 59, 189] Using the Gleason system of grading biopsies in localized adenocarcinoma, investigators found that the biopsy findings predicted the final grade at prostatectomy in almost 75% of more than 100 patients.[122] Gleason's system also has been used to predict the behavior of localized prostatic adenocarcinoma.[108] Brawn has, however, shown a loss of differentiation in prostatic adenocarcinoma over several years when followed by transurethral resection,[38] and similar results were found in another study.[33]

At present one of the major problems is the question of which system of grading to use. Published series have utilized multiple approaches, varying from Broders' four grades of cellular differentiation to the poorly defined "well-differentiated" versus "poorly differentiated" classifications, to Gleason's five major patterns of growth. Each author champions his own method. For example, the group at Roswell Park has devised a system of evaluating the "glands" and nuclei, each on a scale of 1 through and including 4.[118] The worst grade in each category is assigned if it is significant in amount. A similar but more complex system of evaluating patterns and nuclei predicted

survival and proved 91% reproducible among four pathologists.[33] The question of ease of use and reproducibility for any such system is important but is not often assessed. Reproducibility of Gleason's system, for example, has been tested several times and is not always so satisfactory.[12, 321] A further evaluation of Gleason's system indicates that the highest (worst) grade has the greatest prognostic importance, contrary to the initial description of the system.[219] The Mostofi system of combining an evaluation of patterns (architecture) and nuclear aberrations has been critically analyzed, and both components (i.e., pattern and nuclear atypia) apparently are necessary to assign a meaningful grade.[296] The system at MD Anderson is based on an estimate at low magnification of the extent of "glands," and three grades of glandular differentiation proved relevant in regard to survival.[39]

Several studies have emphasized nuclear features in grading. For example, prognosis of localized prostate adenocarcinoma is related to nuclear roundness as analyzed by a computer[49, 87] and in a limited study the presence of nucleoli was associated with progression to distant metastases.[252]

I prefer classifying adenocarcinoma in three grades, whether expressed numerically (I through III) or as well differentiated, moderately differentiated, and poorly differentiated.[247] The well-differentiated acinar adenocarcinomas are composed of small uniform acini that are closely but haphazardly packed (Fig. 9–29). The cells have round nuclei that are larger than normal but are uniform in size and shape and have small inconspicuous nucleoli. The moderately differentiated adenocarcinomas show irregular acinar patterns, including complex or papillary arrangements (Fig. 9–30). The nuclei are variable in shape and size as well as enlarged, and nucleoli are conspicuous. In poorly differentiated adenocarcinoma the acinar pattern is lost, and cells may be large or medium-sized with very atypical, hyperchromatic nuclei (Fig. 9–31). Mitotic figures are present, and nucleoli are often large and multiple.

Effects of Treatment

The treatment of adenocarcinoma may alter the structure. It is important to be aware of these changes in order to avoid misdiagnosis and to evaluate the efficacy of ther-

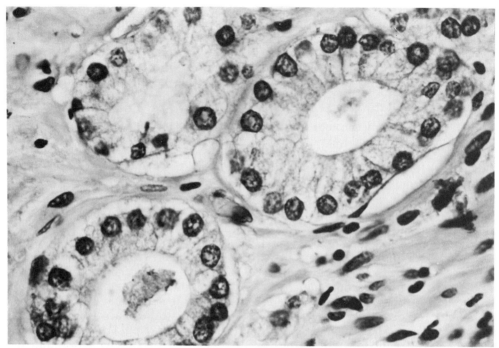

Figure 9–29. Several neoplastic acini of a well-differentiated prostatic (acinar) adenocarcinoma that are lined with a single layer of regular cells with minimally atypical nuclei. (H & E, × 675)

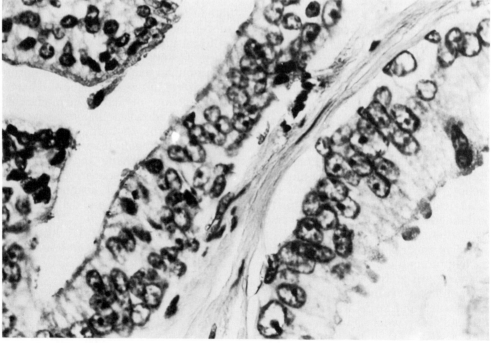

Figure 9–30. Irregular neoplastic acini with multilayered, obviously atypical cells and conspicuous nucleoli, in a moderately differentiated (acinar) adenocarcinoma. (H & E, × 675)

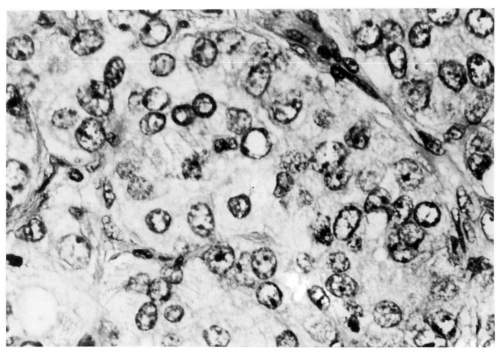

Figure 9–31. Sheets of atypical cells with pleomorphic atypical nuclei, characteristic of poorly differentiated (acinar) adenocarcinoma. (H & E, × 675)

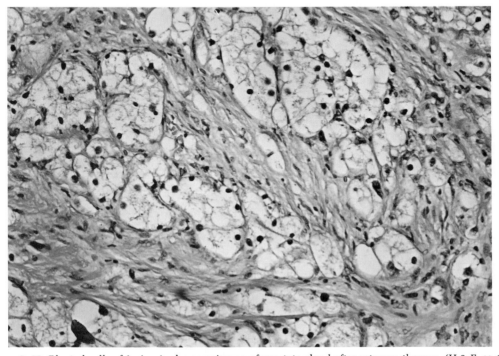

Figure 9–32. Bloated cells of (acinar) adenocarcinoma of prostate gland after estrogen therapy. (H & E, × 250)

apy. Operative therapy will alter the gross structure of the gland and complicate the already difficult task of macroscopically localizing the tumor. Microscopically, the fibrosis and distortion of an operation may make determination of capsular invasion impossible in subsequent biopsies. Estrogen has a marked effect on the neoplastic cells themselves, at least the responsive population. Sensitive cells develop basal vacuoles with apical displacement of the nucleus (Fig. 9–32). The basal vacuoles expand and eventually coalesce, whereas the nucleus shrinks to a small dark mass and may disintegrate. Cell membranes break, and the malignant acinus ends as a clear space containing a few pyknotic nuclei.[113, 291] Poor fixation may occasionally produce a similar picture. The non-neoplastic epithelium and some neoplastic cells may show focal squamous metaplasia in response to estrogen.[103] This alteration should not be mistaken for epidermoid carcinoma.

When radiation therapy is added to estrogen treatment, additional changes are produced. These include nuclear gigantism and nuclear degeneration within epithelial cells and a marked stromal fibrosis with thickening of walls of blood vessels.[177, 317] Marked changes are evident after interstitial radia-

tion, and the atypia of ductal or acinal epithelium is easily mistaken for that of adenocarcinoma (Fig. 9–33).[154, 279] Bostwick and associates summarized the effects of radiation upon normal and neoplastic prostate glands by stating that architectural features rather than cellular changes are most important in distinguishing residual adenocarcinoma from radiation-induced atypia of prostate epithelium, an opinion with which I concur.[34] Residual adenocarcinoma following radiation is usually obvious clinically and microscopically, and a few scattered atypical acinar or ductal cells in the absence of clinically obvious cancer have little, if any, meaning. The microscopic effects of radiation plus chemotherapy (other than hormone therapy) are similar to those induced by radiation and hormones.[336]

Metastases

Adenocarcinoma of the prostate gland spreads through lymphatic channels and blood vessels to distant sites. Metastases to lymph nodes appear in most patients with terminal cancer.[83] A third of the patients with early cancer (that is, clinically limited to the prostate gland) have evidence of metastases to the pelvic lymph nodes.[7] These

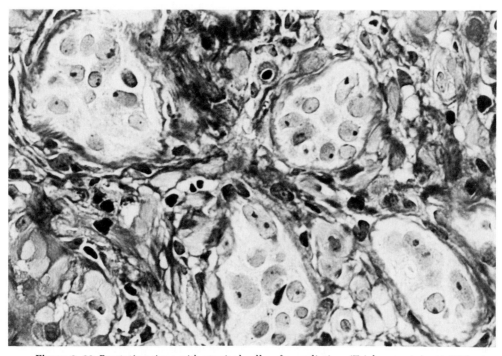

Figure 9–33. Prostatic acinus with atypical cells, after radiation. (Trichrome stain, × 675)

deposits may be microscopic (less than 2 mm) and may escape detection even after rapid evaluation of selected lymph nodes by frozen sections.[221] In two recent studies, up to 20% of pelvic nodes judged negative for cancer at frozen section contained microscopic deposits of secondary prostatic adenocarcinoma,[50, 199] raising the question of whether frozen sections are appropriate in these circumstances. There is also some question as to the importance of the volume of metastatic adenocarcinoma, both in regard to the number of lymph nodes involved or the extent of replacement of any given lymph node.[314] Many recent encouraging reports about the value of transabdominal fine-needle aspiration in identifying metastatic cancer, including prostatic adenocarcinoma in pelvic lymph nodes, obviate the need for staging operations (and frozen sections) in many patients.[58, 81, 134, 265, 340, 342] Regional lymphatic metastases are said to be more common in patients with poorly differentiated adenocarcinomas, and the microscopic appearance of the secondary site often resembles that of the primary neoplasm,[217] although Gleason's categories of prostate adenocarcinoma did not serve to predict metastases in one recent study.[284] Nuclear atypia and microscopic evidence of capsular invasion also correlate with metastases to regional lymph nodes, whereas perineural invasion is not a prognostic feature.[221]

The lymphatic drainage of the prostate gland in humans was studied by the intraprostate injection of a soluble dye,[315] and the conclusion was that the prostate gland of the adult does not contain lymphatic vessels. Male rats possess a rich periprostatic lymphatic plexus but no intraprostatic vessels.[216] Recent electron microscopic studies have, however, indicated intraprostatic lymphatic vessels in humans.[117] There is no evidence of human perineural lymphatic channels,[151] although perineural invasion by adenocarcinoma is common.[281, 353] Perhaps the prostate gland is an "immunologically privileged site."[127]

The lymph from the pelvis flows through the thoracic duct to the confluence of the left subclavian and internal jugular veins, and lymph nodes in the supraclavicular area lie adjacent to the veins in direct communication with the thoracic duct. Thus, patients with widespread (inoperable) adenocarcinoma of the prostate gland often have metastatic cancer in the supraclavicular or scalene lymph nodes.[8] In rare patients the initial sign of prostatic adenocarcinoma is a large left supraclavicular lymph node.[41] On microscopic examination, the supraclavicular deposits are usually poorly differentiated adenocarcinoma with acinar, solid, or combined patterns. These adenocarcinomas contain atypical cells with mitotic figures and a small amount of mucin.[107] Immunohistochemistry may be helpful in identifying the prostatic origin of metastatic adenocarcinoma in supraclavicular lymph nodes,[357] although mammary adenocarcinoma in women occasionally stains weakly positive for PAP.[207]

Spread of prostatic adenocarcinoma to the rectum is infrequently seen, even in postmortem studies. Thus, the rare patient with prostatic adenocarcinoma presenting as a rectal mass is a diagnostic dilemma.[66, 274] With disregard to the arguments about the mechanism of spread and reasons why it is so uncommon, the presence of a submucosal rectal mass with the classic microscopic appearance of prostatic acinar adenocarcinoma or of a poorly differentiated type should be clues to the correct diagnosis. Obviously, it is important to differentiate between adenocarcinoma arising in the rectum and in the prostate gland because of differences in treatment and behavior, and this is one problem for which immunohistochemistry offers a ready solution.

The hematogenous spread of prostatic adenocarcinoma is a feature of the terminal phase of the disease and typically involves the lungs, liver, and kidneys as well as miscellaneous sites throughout the body. For example, up to half of the fatal cases exhibit pulmonary metastases at postmortem examination. Unsuspected spread of prostatic adenocarcinoma to the testis is rarely found at orchiectomy. This may be part of a general spread of the cancer;[167] however, survival is not necessarily related to the incidental finding of metastatic prostatic adenocarcinoma in the testis.[349] On the other hand, patients with cutaneous or subcutaneous deposits do poorly,[180, 338] and intracranial spread is a poor sign.[21, 48] Epididymal metastasis occurs rarely.[2] An overview of metastasis from almost 2000 cases studied by postmortem examination provides some insight into the patterns of spread of prostatic adenocarcinoma.[286]

Recently, there has been concern about the iatrogenic spread of prostatic adenocar-

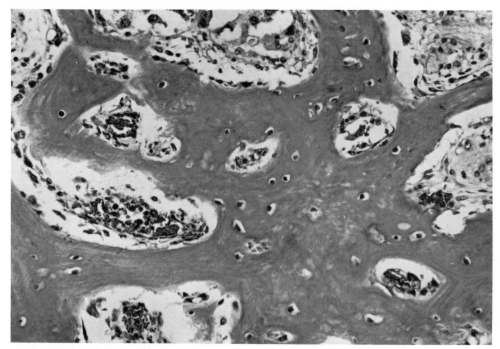

Figure 9–34. New bone formation in osteoblastic metastasis to ilium from prostatic adenocarcinoma. Carcinoma cells are difficult to recognize. (H & E, × 250)

cinoma by biopsy, but one study of over 500 patients showed no relation between the number of transrectal needle biopsies and the risk of metastatic spread.[162] Transurethral resection in one series also did not significantly increase the risk of metastasis to bone.[200]

Metastases to bone are observed in two thirds of the patients with advanced disease, and involvement of bone is commonly observed at postmortem examination.[337] Multiple neoplastic deposits occur in the vertebrae, pelvis, skull, and long bones. Osteosclerosis usually accompanies the deposits in such frequency that adenocarcinoma of the prostate gland is the most common cause of osteoblastic metastatic cancer. Often the bone is so dense that microscopic evidence of the adenocarcinoma is inconspicuous (Fig. 9–34). The mechanism by which the adenocarcinoma reaches bone is uncertain, although spread by blood, by lymphatic channels, along nerves, and by direct extension occurs in individual cases.[346]

Age and Adenocarcinoma

An unresolved controversy concerns the common opinion that young patients (50 years and under) with prostatic cancer have a worse prognosis than old men.[23, 55, 115, 148, 170, 332] Recent studies have concluded that young men may fare as well as, if not better than, older patients.[42, 150, 156, 267, 311, 312] From the viewpoint of the surgical pathologist, there is no significant gross or microscopic difference between adenocarcinomas in the two age groups that might reflect difference in behavior. Adenocarcinoma of the prostate gland has also been reported in children and very young men.[307, 350]

Ductal Adenocarcinoma

Adenocarcinomas of the prostate gland rarely arise from the major ducts.[46, 289, 299, 322] When ductal adenocarcinomas occur, they usually are not isolated neoplasms but more often are associated with acinar adenocarcinoma. The ductal tumors project into the prostate urethra and may cause urethral obstruction with hematuria. Microscopically, ductal adenocarcinomas are usually papillary and are composed of tall columnar cells with basal nuclei and eosinophilic cytoplasm (Fig. 9–35). In one case a papillary ductal adenocarcinoma had a hyaline stroma

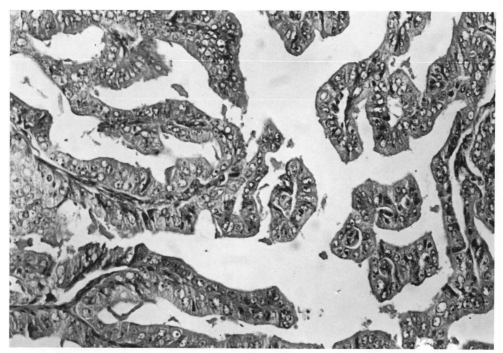

Figure 9–35. Papillary (ductal) adenocarcinoma of prostate gland, resembling endometrial adenocarcinoma. (H & E, × 250)

and was associated with papillomatosis of the primary ducts.[24] Dube and his associates divided the ductal adenocarcinomas into those of primary and those of secondary ducts, depending upon location and microscopic appearance.[78] The cancers of primary ducts were papillary, cribriform, or both. Zaloudek and his associates added a third type of ductal adenocarcinoma, those that microscopically resemble endometrial adenocarcinoma.[361] This type of lesion was originally thought to arise from the prostate utricle, a müllerian remnant.[228] Contrary to expectation, one such tumor regressed after a bilateral orchiectomy.[359] Two tumors had ultrastructural features consistent with origin in prostatic ducts, and one contained acid phosphatase.[93, 361] One recent small series of ductal adenocarcinomas confirmed the presence of prostate-specific acid phosphatase in the neoplastic cells,[91] and this and another study showed prostate-specific antigen in the neoplastic cells.[264] Clearly, the majority of prostate ductal adenocarcinomas are not derived from müllerian remnants and are not endometrioid in spite of their superficial microscopic resemblance to endometrial adenocarcinoma. Although the number of cases is small, ductal adenocarcinomas of the prostate gland are probably similar in behavior to acinar adenocarcinomas.[139]

Mucinous Adenocarcinoma

Criteria proposed for the diagnosis of primary prostatic mucinous adenocarcinoma are (1) the neoplastic cells secrete abundant mucin that is acidic or neutral, (2) the adenocarcinoma does not arise in major ducts or the urethra, (3) the adenocarcinoma has a colloid pattern, and (4) no other site of origin of the mucinous adenocarcinoma can be found.[82] Others say that at least 25% of a prostatic adenocarcinoma should have lakes of extracellular mucin in order to be called mucinous.[90] These rare prostatic mucinous adenocarcinomas may be derived from seromucinous acini, which have been observed in the prostate gland,[73] or from mucin-producing cells scattered in the gland.[206] On microscopic examination, mucinous adenocarcinoma of the prostate gland (Fig. 9–36) resembles mucinous adenocarcinoma from other sites, including the rectum; at times the distinction between mucinous adenocarcinoma of the prostate gland and of the rectum may be difficult or impossible.[208, 259] In these difficult cases, the neoplastic cells are suspended in pools of mucin, whereas a merging of the mucinous adenocarcinoma with typical acinar adenocarcinoma reveals the prostatic origin in others.[310]

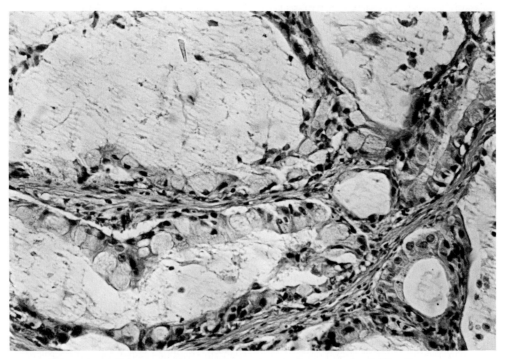

Figure 9–36. Primary mucinous adenocarcinoma of prostate gland. (H & E, × 250)

All six mucinous prostatic adenocarcinomas studied in a recent series were positive for PAP and PSA, and several also had argyrophilic cells.[90] The behavior of mucinous prostatic adenocarcinoma is uncertain, but most of the reported patients had advanced disease and did not respond to treatment.[90]

A recent report of nonmucinous, signet-ring–celled adenocarcinoma of the prostate gland is noted.[126]

Several examples of adenoid cystic carcinoma displayed the characteristic cylindromatous and cribriform patterns.[111, 198, 308] One of these cases proved negative for PSA.[308] A case of malignant mixed tumor of prostatic origin has also been reported.[213] Reed has written that these so-called salivary gland patterns of carcinoma are really adenoid basal cell tumors that arise from areas of basal cell hyperplasia in the prostate gland.[273]

Epidermoid Carcinoma

Epidermoid (squamous) carcinoma rarely involves the prostate gland, and in these few cases the carcinoma is usually secondary to a primary neoplasm in the urethra or urinary bladder. Epidermoid carcinoma of the prostate gland representing metaplasia of adenocarcinoma has been recorded[176] and, in one instance, followed radiation and estrogen therapy.[27] Adenosquamous carcinoma of the prostate gland has also been reported following radiation for adenocarcinoma.[285] There remain several reports of primary epidermoid carcinoma of the prostate gland.[57, 137] At UCLA Medical Center, I found two examples of primary epidermoid carcinoma of the prostate gland. The microscopic appearance of epidermoid carcinoma of the prostate gland resembles the carcinoma at other sites. Thus, well-differentiated, keratinized neoplasms and neoplasms composed of undifferentiated basal cells have been observed (Fig. 9–37).[328] Squamous metaplasia following infarction of a hyperplastic gland or after estrogen therapy must be distinguished from epidermoid carcinoma.

Transitional Carcinoma

Transitional carcinoma occurs within the ducts and, to a lesser extent, the acini of the prostate gland. In some patients, the transitional prostatic carcinoma is an isolated finding. In other patients, the prostatic car-

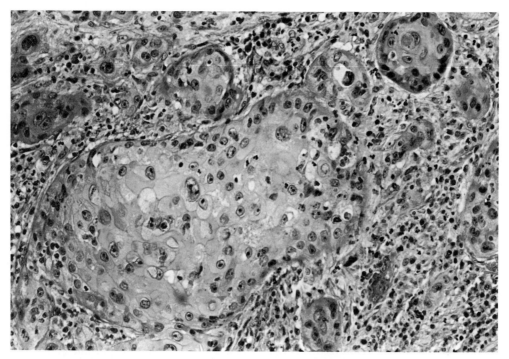

Figure 9–37. Primary epidermoid carcinoma of prostate gland. (H & E, × 250)

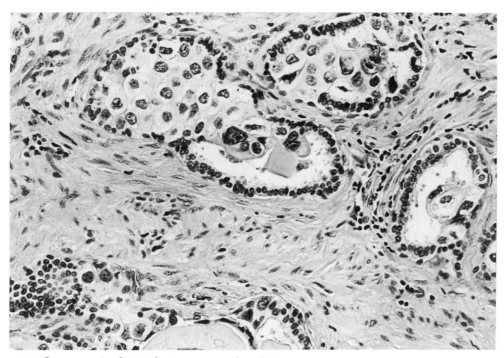

Figure 9–38. Severe atypia of metaplastic transitional epithelium in prostate gland from patient with transitional carcinoma of urinary bladder. (H & E, × 250)

cinoma occurs with or follows a similar cancer in the urinary bladder.[100, 301] Concurrent transitional carcinomas of the urinary bladder and prostate gland are often in situ lesions in which the normal epithelium is replaced by a thick or thin layer of atypical transitional cells that have large angular nuclei, prominent nucleoli, and mitotic figures (Fig. 9–38). The atypical epithelium is disorderly and often ragged. Occasionally, the atypical cells are sprinkled through an otherwise unremarkable transitional epithelium in the fashion of Paget's disease of the breast.[100] The prostatic involvement may be extensive and, rarely, invasive.[301] In a group of nine patients, a spectrum of changes from hyperplasia to severe atypia representing carcinoma in situ was observed in transitional epithelium lining the primary prostatic ducts.[335] The atypia of the transitional epithelium probably represents a field of change through the urinary tract and portends a poor prognosis.[56, 136, 290]

Transitional carcinoma isolated in the prostate gland—that is, not associated with transitional carcinoma of the urinary bladder—grows through the prostatic ducts and focally invades the stroma, lymphatic channels, and blood vessels.[140] The intraductal growth features central necrosis with dystrophic calcification resembling comedocarcinoma of the female breast. The majority of the neoplasms are poorly differentiated,[169] and only a rare tumor is well differentiated and papillary.[174] Hyperplastic and atypical transitional epithelium may or may not be found in nearby prostatic ducts.[169, 277] Some tumors are mixed transitional carcinoma and adenocarcinoma.[86, 140, 277] Separate acinar adenocarcinomas are also found in patients with transitional prostatic carcinoma.[169]

Many of the patients with primary transitional carcinoma of the prostate gland have severe prostatitis, urinary obstruction, and hematuria. The prostate gland is large, and transurethral biopsies offer the best means of diagnosis. The prognosis is poor,[140, 141, 324, 355] especially with invasion.[52]

Neuroendocrine Tumors

Small-celled carcinomas or tumors resembling carcinoid tumors have recently been described in the prostate gland. Some of them appeared pure, but some cells contained PAP and PSA in addition to argyrophilic granules.[4, 11] Others were clearly mixed with or evolved from acinar adenocarcinomas.[45, 123, 297] Cushing's syndrome was observed in several of these patients. The microscopic appearance is that of the usual carcinoid tumor with sheets of small, uniform cells or small cells in a trabecular or ribbon-like pattern (Fig. 9–39). Cytoplasm is described as acidophilic and granular and nuclei as small, uniform, and round. Most of the reported cases were highly malignant fatal neoplasms, but there are too few cases to generalize about the behavior of neuroendocrine tumors arising in the prostate gland.

Sarcomas

Sarcomas of the prostate gland, exclusive of malignant lymphoma (lymphosarcoma), account for less than 1% of all prostatic neoplasms. The majority of the sarcomas are myosarcomas,[313] and they fall into two groups related to the age of the patients and the microscopic differentiation of the neoplasms.[292] In boys and young men, almost all of the myosarcomas are embryonal rhabdomyosarcomas.[330] These are large, fleshy tumors of diffuse growth that alter urination and cause hematuria. The tumors often fill the pelvis, and most patients are dead within months,[133] although one patient recently survived seven years after local removal of the tumor.[79] The neoplasms contain both small, round, undifferentiated cells with scanty eosinophilic cytoplasm and large cells with abundant eosinophilic cytoplasm, rarely showing striations (Fig. 9–40). The neoplastic cells may be sparse in a loose stroma or concentrated without obvious orientation. The ultrastructural features of both types of cells have been recorded.[288]

Many of the prostatic sarcomas of middle-aged or old men are leiomyosarcomas, although rhabdomyosarcomas also occur in this group.[176, 178] The leiomyosarcomas are firm and often circumscribed, in contrast to rhabdomyosarcomas. They cause urinary obstruction.[51] The characteristic microscopic appearance of leiomyosarcoma is that of a neoplasm of fusiform cells arranged in alternate bundles (Fig. 9–41); however, pleomorphic, bizarre, and giant cells are observed.[320] Electron microscopy has been obtained and reported in at least one case.[257]

Several examples of malignant schwannoma (neurogenic sarcoma) have been re-

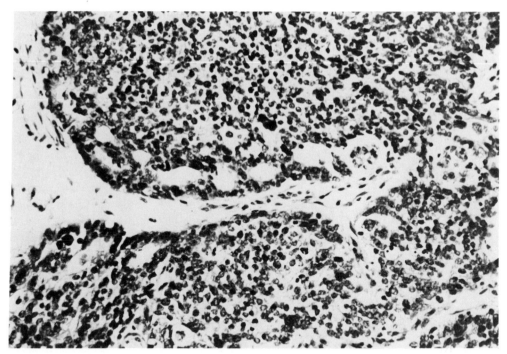

Figure 9–39. Carcinoma of prostate gland with pattern of a neuroendocrine carcinoma (scattered cells are silver positive). (H & E, × 250)

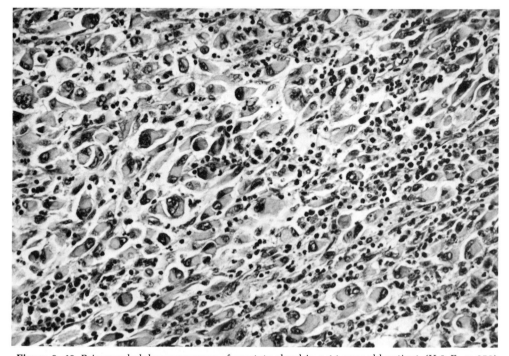

Figure 9–40. Primary rhabdomyosarcoma of prostate gland in a 14-year-old patient. (H & E, × 250)

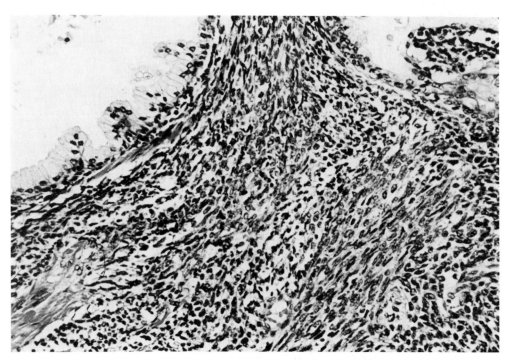

Figure 9–41. Sample of prostate gland from a 48-year-old man with a leiomyosarcoma, composed of bundles of atypical fusiform cells infiltrating prostatic acini and smooth muscle. (H & E, × 250)

ported in patients with von Recklinghausen's disease or as an isolated finding.[298] A primary osteosarcoma of the prostate gland has been reported, including the results of aspiration, but the diagnosis is not well supported by illustration.[249] These authors also report a rare hemangiopericytoma of the prostate gland.[356] There is a report of an atypical but benign fibromyoid tumor of the prostate gland that has features of a botryoid tumor and lacks markers for muscle or Schwann cells.[145]

Carcinosarcoma and Cystosarcoma Phyllodes

For years pathologists have debated the propriety of the diagnostic term carcinosarcoma. These proceedings reached a peak with Saphir's review of the subject, which led to general skepticism about the existence of a single neoplasm with malignant glandular and stromal elements.[287] Although many neoplasms seemingly with both components may be explained otherwise, there remain a few convincing examples of carcinosarcoma of the prostate gland. Mostofi and Price limit the term to malignant neoplasms

with glandular components and "neoplastic" bone or cartilage.[246] Perhaps striated muscle should be added to the list of stromal components, qualifying other cases as true carcinosarcomas.[144, 147, 215, 269] A report of leiomyosarcoma and adenocarcinoma in ·the same prostate gland is controversial but is deserving of consideration in the context of a discussion of carcinosarcoma.[261]

Three reports of cystosarcoma phyllodes (phylloides)[9, 143, 358] and two other reports of unusual, benign combined tumors[61, 77] of the prostate gland provide an interesting footnote to the discussion of carcinosarcoma. In two of the examples of cystosarcoma phyllodes, the prostate urethra was obstructed by a bulky prostate neoplasm and the other tumor was diffuse. Microscopically, the prostate neoplasm consisted of hyperplastic glands in an expanded stroma containing spindle-shaped or polygonal cells, including giant and bizarre forms (Fig. 9–42). A recurrent and possibly malignant expression of one of these neoplasms consisted of the stromal component, analogous to cystosarcoma phyllodes of the breast.[205] An editorial comment appended to one of these reports describes the similarity between micro-

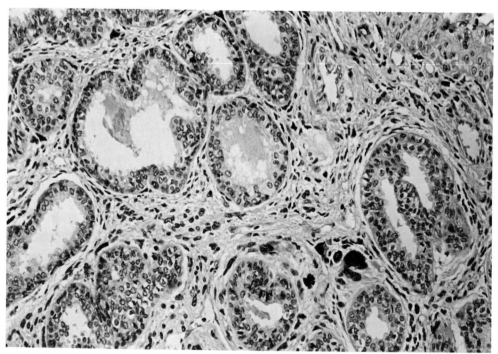

Figure 9–42. Cystosarcoma phylloides of prostate gland with hyperplastic epithelium and bizarre stromal cells with giant hyperchromatic nuclei. (H & E, × 250)

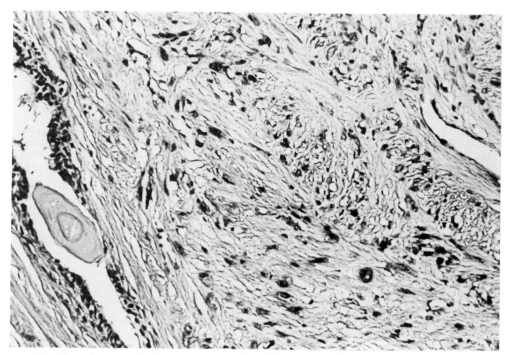

Figure 9–43. Edge of an atypical prostatic stromal nodule composed of pleomorphic fusiform cells, with compression of an adjacent acinus and stroma on the left. (H & E, × 250)

scopic patterns of certain lesions in the female breast and in the prostate gland.[9] A report of atypical stromal hyperplasia in the prostate gland also calls attention to the similar stromal lesions of the breast, especially in fibroadenomas.[10] These lesions contain stromal cells with large and irregular nuclei (Fig. 9–43) but lack mitotic figures and do not recur or metastasize. I, too, am struck by certain common gross and microscopic features of mammary dysplasia and nodular prostatic hyperplasia and by the comparable structural features of other lesions at both sites.

Secondary Neoplasms

Secondary cancer of the prostate gland rarely presents a clinical problem and is of only minor concern to the pathologist. Advanced cancer of the urinary bladder grows into the prostate gland, and adenocarcinoma of the rectum or sigmoid colon spreads to the prostate gland during the terminal phase of the disease. The latter may represent direct infiltration or metastasis through lymphatic channels.[328] In a recent series of almost 1500 patients with cancer of the prostate gland, 18 tumors were secondary to a distant primary neoplasm. Only three of these caused urinary obstruction, and six consisted of microscopic foci as part of disseminated disease.[168] Malignant melanoma of the skin and bronchial carcinoma account for many of the metastatic deposits in the prostate gland; however, most of the metastatic neoplasms are leukemia or malignant lymphoma.[231, 318] Relatively few patients with leukemia have prostatic involvement, either in operative specimens or at postmortem examination, and these patients usually have chronic lymphocytic leukemia.[227] Involvement of the prostate gland during acute leukemia has been reported in a young man.[22] The older literature contains isolated reports of prostatic involvement in malignant lymphoma,[192, 345] and several recent reports, including a series of nine cases, are available.[76, 313] Two examples of a plasma cell tumor (multiple myeloma) in the prostate gland were found,[96] and one case of renal tubular adenocarcinoma presenting as a secondary deposit in the prostate gland has been noted.[53]

References

1. Abeshouse BS: Infarct of the prostate. J Urol 30:97–112, 1933.
2. Addonizio JC, Thelmo W: Epididymal metastasis from prostatic carcinoma. Urology 18:490–491, 1981.
3. Aguilar M, Gaffney EF, Finnerty DP: Prostatic melanosis with involvement of benign and malignant epithelium. J Urol 128:825–827, 1982.
4. Almagro UA: Argyrophilic prostatic carcinoma: case report with literature review on prostatic carcinoid and "carcinoid-like" prostatic carcinoma. Cancer 55:608–614, 1985.
5. Andrews GS: Histology of human foetal and prepubertal prostates. J Anat 85:44–54, 1951.
6. Anson BJ: Morris' Human Anatomy, 12th ed. New York, McGraw-Hill, 1966, p 898.
7. Arduino LJ, Glucksman MA: Lymph node metastases in early carcinoma of the prostate. J Urol 88:91–93, 1962.
8. Arduino LJ: Scalene node excision-biopsy in stages 3 and 4 carcinoma of prostate: background notes and preliminary report. J Urol 103:458–461, 1970.
9. Attah EB, Nkposong EO: Phyllodes type of atypical prostatic hyperplasia. J Urol 115:762–764, 1976.
10. Attah EB, Powell ME: Atypical stromal hyperplasia of the prostate gland. Am J Clin Pathol 67:324–327, 1977.
11. Azumi N, Shibuya H, Ishikura M: Primary prostatic carcinoid tumor with intracytoplasmic prostatic acid phosphatase and prostate-specific antigen. Am J Surg Pathol 8:545–550, 1984.
12. Bain GO, Koch M, Hanson J: Feasibility of grading prostatic carcinomas. Arch Pathol Lab Med 106:265–267, 1982.
13. Bainborough AR: Squamous metaplasia of prostate following estrogen therapy. J Urol 68:329–336, 1952.
14. Barnes RW, Hirst A, Rosenquist R: Early carcinoma of the prostate: comparison of stage A and B. J Urol 115:404–405, 1976.
15. Barnes RW, Ninan CA: Carcinoma of the prostate: biopsy and conservative therapy. J Urol 108:897–900, 1972.
16. Baroudy AC, O'Connell JP: Papillary adenoma of the prostatic urethra. J Urol 132:120–122, 1984.
17. Bates RJ, Lin CW, Chapman CM, Prout GR Jr: Immunohistochemical identification of prostatic acid phosphatase: correlation of tumor grade with acid phosphatase distribution. J Urol 127:574–580, 1982.
18. Batson OV: The function of the vertebral veins and their role in the spread of metastases. Ann Surg 112:138–149, 1940.
19. Battezzati M, Donini I: The Lymphatic System. New York, John Wiley & Son, 1972, p 387.
20. Bauer WC, McGavran MH, Carlin MR: Unsuspected carcinoma of the prostate in suprapubic prostatectomy specimens. Cancer 13:370–378, 1960.
21. Baumann MA, Holoye PY, Choi H: Adenocarcinoma of prostate presenting as brain metastasis. Cancer 54:1723–1725, 1984.

22. Belis JA, Lizza EF, Kim JC, Raich PC: Acute leukemic infiltration of the prostate. Successful treatment with radiation. Cancer 51:2164–2167, 1983.

23. Belt E, Schroeder FH: Total perineal prostatectomy for carcinoma of the prostate. J Urol 107:91–96, 1972.

24. Belter LF, Dodson AI Jr: Papillomatosis and papillary adenocarcinoma of prostate ducts: a case report. J Urol 104:880–883, 1970.

25. Bennett B, Gardner WA Jr: Crystalloids in prostatic hyperplasia. Prostate 1:31–35, 1980.

26. Bennett BD, Gardner WA Jr: Embryonal hyperplasia of the prostate. Am J Clin Pathol 82:368, 1984.

27. Bennett RS, Edgerton EO: Mixed prostatic carcinoma. J Urol 110:561–563, 1973.

28. Bentz MS, Cohen C, Demers LM, Budgeon LR: Immunohistochemical demonstration of prostatic origin of metastases. Urology 19:584–586, 1982.

29. Bentz MS, Cohen C, Demers LM, Budgeon LR: Immunohistochemical acid phosphatase level and tumor grade in prostatic carcinoma. Arch Pathol Lab Med 106:476–480, 1982.

30. Blacklock NJ: Surgical anatomy of the prostate. Sci Foundations Urol 2:113–125, 1976.

31. Blennerhassett JB, Vickery AL Jr: Carcinoma of the prostate gland—an anatomical study of tumor location. Cancer 19:980–984, 1966.

32. Bloom W, Fawcett DW: A Textbook of Histology, 10th ed. Philadelphia, WB Saunders, 1975, pp 848–850.

33. Böcking A, Kiehn J, Heinzel-Wach M: Combined histologic grading of prostatic carcinoma. Cancer 50:288–294, 1982.

34. Bostwick DG, Egbert BM, Fajardo LF: Radiation injury of the normal and neoplastic prostate. Am J Surg Pathol 6:541–551, 1982.

35. Brandes D, Kirchheim D, Scott WW: Ultrastructure of the human prostate: normal and neoplastic. Lab Invest 13:1541–1560, 1964.

36. Braunstein H: Staining lipid in carcinoma of the prostate gland. Am J Clin Pathol 41:44–48, 1964.

37. Brawn PN: Adenosis of the prostate: a dysplastic lesion that can be confused with prostate adenocarcinoma. Cancer 49:826–833, 1982.

38. Brawn PN: The dedifferentiation of prostate carcinoma. Cancer 52:246–251, 1983.

39. Brawn PN, Ayala AG, von Eschenbach AC, et al: Histologic grading study of prostate adenocarcinoma: the development of a new system and comparison with other methods. A preliminary study. Cancer 49:525–532, 1982.

40. Butler J, Braunstein H, Freiman DG, Gall EA: Incidence, distribution, and enzymatic activity of carcinoma of the prostate gland. Arch Pathol 68:243–251, 1959.

41. Butler JJ, Howe CD, Johnson DE: Enlargement of the supraclavicular lymph nodes as the initial sign of prostatic carcinoma. Cancer 27:1055–1063, 1971.

42. Byar DP, Mostofi FK: Cancer of the prostate in men less than 50 years old: an analysis of 51 cases. J Urol 102:726–733, 1969.

43. Byar DP, Mostofi FK: Carcinoma of the prostate—prognostic evaluation of certain pathologic features in 208 radical prostatectomies. Cancer 30:5–13, 1972.

44. Byar DP: Survival of patients with incidentally found microscopic cancer of the prostate. J Urol 108:908–913, 1972.

45. Capella C, Usellini L, Buffa R, et al: The endocrine component of prostatic carcinomas, mixed adenocarcinoma, carcinoid tumours and non-tumour prostate. Histochemical and ultrastructural identification of the endocrine cells. Histopathology 5:175–192, 1981.

46. Carney JA, Kelalis PP: Endometrial carcinoma of the prostatic utricle. Am J Clin Pathol 60:565–569, 1973.

47. Carstens PH: Perineural glands in normal and hyperplastic prostates. J Urol 123:686–688, 1980.

48. Castaldo JE, Bernat JL, Meier FA, Schned AR: Intracranial metastases due to prostatic carcinoma. Cancer 52:1739–1747, 1983.

49. Catalona WJ: Grading and staging of prostate cancer. J Urol 128:747–748, 1982.

50. Catalona WJ, Stein AJ: Accuracy of frozen section detection of lymph node metastases in prostatic carcinoma. J Urol 127:460–461, 1982.

51. Chatterjee AC: Leiomyosarcoma of the prostate. Br J Urol 47:577, 1975.

52. Chibber PJ, McIntyre MA, Hindmarsh JR, et al: Transitional cell carcinoma involving the prostate. Br J Urol 53:605–609, 1981.

53. Cihak RW, Haas R Jr, Koenen CT, Chinchinian H: Metastatic renal carcinoma to the prostate gland: presentation as prostatic hypertrophy. J Urol 123:791–792, 1980.

54. Cleary KR, Choi HY, Ayala AG: Basal cell hyperplasia of the prostate. Am J Clin Pathol 80:850–854, 1983.

55. Cook GB, Watson FR: A comparison by age of death rates due to prostate cancer alone. J Urol 100:669–671, 1968.

56. Cooper PH, Waisman J, Johnston WH, Skinner DG: Severe atypia of transitional epithelium and carcinoma of the urinary bladder. Cancer 31:1055–1060, 1973.

57. Corder MP, Cicmil GA: Effective treatment of metastatic squamous cell carcinoma of the prostate with adriamycin. J Urol 115:222, 1976.

58. Correa RJ Jr: Lymphangiography with fine-needle aspiration biopsy of pelvic and abdominal lymph nodes in cancer staging. Urol Clinics North Am 9:153–155, 1982.

59. Correa RJ Jr, Anderson RG, Gibbons RP, Mason JT: Latent carcinoma of the prostate—why the controversy? J Urol 111:644–646, 1974.

60. Corriere JN Jr, Cornog JL, Murphy JJ: Prognosis in patients with carcinoma of the prostate. Cancer 25:911–918, 1970.

61. Cox R, Dawson IMP: A curious prostatic tumor: probably a true mixed tumour (cysto-adeno-leiomyofibroma). Br J Urol 32:306–311, 1960.

62. Craig JR, Hart WR: Benign polyps with prostatic-type epithelium of the urethra. Am J Clin Pathol 63:343–347, 1975.

63. Cristol DS, Emmett JL: The incidence of coincident prostatic calculi, prostatic hyperplasia, and carcinoma of the prostate gland. JAMA 124:646, 1944.

64. Culp OS: Significance and treatment of prostatic nodules. J Mich State Med Soc 58:585–594, 1959.

65. Culp OS, Meyer JJ: Radical prostatectomy in the

treatment of prostatic cancer. Cancer 32:1113–1118, 1973.

66. Davis JM: Carcinoma of the prostate presenting as disease of the rectum. Br J Urol 32:197–203, 1960.

67. Dean PJ, Murphy WM, Brasfield JA: Evaluation of transurethrally resected prostatic tissue for detection of clinically significant adenocarcinoma of the prostate. Lab Invest 42:18A, 1985.

68. del Regato JA: Topics in radiology: cancer of the prostate. JAMA 235:1727–1730, 1976.

69. Denton SE, Choy SH, Valk WL: Occult prostatic carcinoma diagnosed by the step-section technique of the surgical specimen. J Urol 93:296–298, 1965.

70. Denton SE, Valk WL, Jacobson JM, Kettunen RC: Comparison of the perineal needle biopsy and the transurethral prostatectomy in the diagnosis of prostatic carcinoma: an analysis of 300 cases. J Urol 97:127–129, 1967.

71. Dermer GB: Basal cell proliferation in benign prostatic hyperplasia. Cancer 41:1857–1862, 1978.

72. Dhom G, Hautumm B: Die Morphologie der klinischen Stadiums O des Prostatacarcinoms. Urologe [Ausg A] 14:105–111, 1975.

73. Dikman SH, Toker C: Seromucinous gland ectopia within the prostatic stroma. J Urol 109:852–854, 1973.

74. di Sant'Agnese PA, de Mesy Jensen KL: Somatostatin and/or somatostatinlike immunoreactive endocrine-paracrine cells in the human prostate gland. Arch Pathol Lab Med 108:693–696, 1984.

75. di Sant'Agnese PA, de Mesy Jensen KL: Endocrine-paracrine cells of the prostate and prostatic urethra: an ultrastructural study. Hum Pathol 15:1034–1041, 1984.

76. Doll DC, Weiss RB, Shah S: Lymphoma of the prostate presenting as benign prostatic hypertrophy. S Med J 71:1170–1171, 1978.

77. Douillet M, Cabanne F, Couderc P, Coste M: Cystadenome papillaire de la prostate. J Urol Nephrol 69:339–343, 1963.

78. Dube VE, Farrow GM, Greene LF: Prostatic adenocarcinoma of ductal origin. Cancer 32:402–409, 1973.

79. Dupree WB, Fisher C: Rhabdomyosarcoma of prostate in adult: long-term survival and problems of histologic diagnosis. Urology 19:80–82, 1982.

80. Edwards CN, Steinthorsson E, Nicholson D: An autopsy study of latent prostatic cancer. Cancer 6:531–554, 1953.

81. Efremidis SC, Dan SJ, Nieburgs H, Mitty HA: Carcinoma of the prostate: lymph node aspiration for staging cancer. AJR 136:489–492, 1981.

82. Elbadawi A, Craig W, Linke CA, Cooper RA Jr: Prostatic mucinous carcinoma. Urology 13:658–666, 1979.

83. Elkin M, Mueller HP: Metastases from cancer of the prostate. Autopsy and roentgenological findings. Cancer 7:1246–1248, 1954.

84. Emmett JL: Transurethral removal of large prostatic calculi. Mayo Clin Proc 16:289–293, 1941.

85. Emmett JL, Green LF, Papantoniou A: Endocrine therapy in carcinoma of the prostate gland—10-year survival studies. J Urol 83:471–484, 1960.

86. Ende N, Woods LP, Shelley HS: Carcinoma originating in ducts surrounding the prostatic urethra. Am J Clin Pathol 40:183–189, 1963.

87. Epstein JI, Berry SJ, Eggleston JC: Nuclear roundness factor. A predictor of progression in untreated stage A$_2$ prostate cancer. Cancer 54:1666–1671, 1984.

88. Epstein JI, Eggleston JC: Immunohistochemical localization of prostate-specific acid phosphatase and prostate-specific antigen in stage A$_2$ adenocarcinoma of the prostate. Hum Pathol 15:853–859, 1984.

89. Epstein JI, Hutchins GM: Granulomatous prostatitis: distinction among allergic, nonspecific, and posttransurethral resection lesions. Hum Pathol 15:818–825, 1984.

90. Epstein JI, Lieberman PH: Mucinous adenocarcinoma of the prostate gland. Am J Surg Pathol 9:299–308, 1985.

91. Epstein JI, Woodruff JM: Adenocarcinoma of the prostate with endometrioid features: a light microscopic and immunohistochemical study of 10 cases. Lab Invest 52:20A, 1985.

92. Epstein NA: Prostatic carcinoma, correlation of histologic features of prognostic value with cytomorphology. Cancer 38:2071–2077, 1976.

93. Epstein NA: Primary papillary carcinoma of the prostate: report of a histopathologic, cytologic, and electron microscopic study on one case. Acta Cytol 21:543–546, 1977.

94. Epstein NA, Fatti LP: Prostatic carcinoma—some morphological features affecting prognosis. Cancer 37:2455–2465, 1976.

95. Esposti PL: Cytologic malignancy grading of prostatic carcinoma by transrectal aspiration biopsy. Scand J Urol Nephrol 5:199–209, 1971.

96. Estrada PC, Scardino PL: Myeloma of the prostate: a case report. J Urol 106:586–587, 1971.

97. Evans CS, Goldman RL, Klein HZ: More on prostatic granulomas. Am J Surg Pathol 8:798, 1984.

98. Evans N, Barnes RW, Brown AF: Carcinoma of the prostate—correlation between the histologic observations and the clinical course. Arch Pathol 34:473–483, 1942.

99. Fan K, Peng C-F: Predicting the probability of bony metastasis through histologic grading of prostate carcinoma: a retrospective correlative analysis of 81 autopsy cases with antemortem transurethral resection specimen. J Urol 130:708–711, 1983.

100. Farrow GM, Utz DC, Rife CC: Morphological and clinical observations of patients with early bladder cancer treated with total cystectomy. Cancer Res 36:2495–2501, 1976.

101. Feiner HD, Avitabile AM: Reparative granulomas of the prostate. Am J Surg Pathol 8:797–798, 1984.

102. Ferguson RS: Prostatic neoplasms. Their diagnosis by needle puncture and aspiration. Am J Surg 9:507–511, 1930.

103. Fergusson JD, Franks LM: The response of prostatic carcinoma to estrogen treatment. Br J Surg 40:422–428, 1952.

104. Fetissof F, Dubois MP, Arbeille-Brassart B, et al: Endocrine cells in the prostate gland, urothelium, and Brenner tumors. Immunohistological and ultrastructural studies. Virchows Arch [Cell Pathol] 42:53–64, 1983.

105. Fisher ER, Sieracki JC: Ultrastructure of human normal and neoplastic prostate. Pathol Annu 5:1–26, 1970.

106. Foot NC, Humphreys GA, Coats EC: Carcinoma of the prostate—a review of 162 cases with a pathologic classification. NY State J Med 50:84–88, 1950.

107. Foster EA, Levine AJ: Mucin production in metastatic carcinomas. Cancer 16:506–509, 1963.

108. Fowler JE Jr, Mills SE: Operable prostatic carcinoma: correlations among clinical stage, pathological stage, Gleason histological score and early disease-free survival. J Urol 133:49–52, 1985.

109. Fox H: Nodular histiocytic prostatitis. J Urol 96:372–374, 1966.

110. Frable WJ: Newer techniques in clinical cytology: aspiration biopsy and brushing cytology. MCV Quar 9:310–316, 1973.

111. Frankel K, Craig JR: Adenoid cystic carcinoma of the prostate. Report of a case. Am J Clin Pathol 62:639–645, 1974.

112. Franks LM: Benign nodular hyperplasia of the prostate: a review. Ann R Coll Surg Engl 14:92–106, 1954.

113. Franks LM: Estrogen-treated prostatic cancer—the variation in responsiveness of tumor cells. Cancer 13:490–501, 1960.

114. Franks LM: Etiology, epidemiology, and pathology of prostatic cancer. Cancer 32:1092–1095, 1973.

115. Franks LM, Fergusson JD, Murnaghan GF: An assessment of factors influencing survival in prostatic cancer—the absence of reliable prognostic features. Br J Cancer 12:321–326, 1958.

116. Franks LM, O'Shea JD, Thomson AER: Mucin in the prostate: a histochemical study in normal glands, latent, clinical and colloid cancers. Cancer 17:983–991, 1964.

117. Furusato M, Mostofi FK: Intraprostatic lymphatics in man: light and ultrastructural observations. Prostate 1:15–30, 1980.

118. Gaeta JF, Asirwatham JE, Miller G, Murphy GP: Histologic grading of primary prostatic cancer: a new approach to an old problem. J Urol 123:689–693, 1980.

119. Gaeta JF, Berger JE, Gamarra MC: Scanning electron microscopic study of prostatic cancer. Cancer Treat Rep 61:227–253, 1977.

120. Gardner WA Jr: Histologic grading of prostate cancer: a retrospective and prospective overview. Prostate 3:555–561, 1982.

121. Gardner WA Jr, Spitz WU: Melanosis of the prostate gland. Am J Clin Pathol 56:762–764, 1971.

122. Garnett JE, Oyasu R, Grayhack JT: The accuracy of diagnostic biopsy specimens in predicting tumor grades by Gleason's classification of radical prostatectomy specimens. J Urol 131:690–693, 1984.

123. Ghali VS, Garcia RL: Prostatic adenocarcinoma with carcinoidal features producing adrenocorticotropic syndrome. Immunohistochemical study and review of the literature. Cancer 54:1043–1048, 1984.

124. Ghazizadeh M, Kagawa S, Maebayashi K, et al: Prostatic origin of metastases: immunoperoxidase localization of prostate-specific antigen. Urol Int 39:9–12, 1984.

125. Gibbons RP, Elder JS, Wheelis RF, et al: Carcinoma of the prostate: clinical and pathological staging and prognosis. Prostate 4:441–446, 1983.

126. Giltman LI: Signet ring adenocarcinoma of the prostate. J Urol 126:134–135, 1981.

127. Gittes RF, McCullough DL: Occult carcinoma of the prostate: an oversight of immune surveillance—a working hypothesis. J Urol 112:241–244, 1974.

128. Glancy RJ, Gaman AJ, Rippey JJ: Polyps and papillary lesions of the prostatic urethra. Pathology 15:153–157, 1983.

129. Gleason DF: Classification of prostatic carcinomas. Cancer Chem Rep 50:125–128, 1966.

130. Gleason DF, Mellinger GT: Prediction of prognosis for prostatic adenocarcinoma by combined histologic grading and clinical staging. J Urol 111:58–64, 1974.

131. Goldman RL: Melanogenic epithelium in the prostate gland. Am J Clin Pathol 49:75–78, 1968.

132. Gomori G: Distribution of acid phosphatase in the tissues under normal and under pathologic conditions. Arch Pathol 32:189–199, 1941.

133. Goodwin WE, Mims MM, Young HJ: Rhabdomyosarcoma of the prostate in a child: first 5-year survival (combined treatment by preoperative, local irradiation; actinomycin D; intra-arterial nitrogen mustard and hypothermia; radical surgery and ureterosigmoidostomy). Trans Am Assoc Genito-Urin Surg 59:186–190, 1967.

134. Göthlin JH, Höiem L: Percutaneous fine-needle biopsy of radiographically normal lymph nodes in the staging of prostatic carcinoma. Radiology 141:351–354, 1981.

135. Gould VE, Rogers DR, Sommers SC: Epithelial-nerve intermingling in benign breast lesions. Arch Pathol 99:596–598, 1975.

136. Grabstald H: Prostatic biopsy in selected patients with carcinoma in situ of the bladder: preliminary report. J Urol 132:1117–1118, 1984.

137. Gray GF Jr, Marshall VF: Squamous carcinoma of the prostate. J Urol 113:736–738, 1975.

138. Grayhack JT, Assimos DG: Prognostic significance of tumor grade and stage in the patient with carcinoma of the prostate. Prostate 4:13–31, 1983.

139. Greene LF, Farrow GM, Ravitz JM, Tomera FM: Prostatic adenocarcinoma of ductal origin. J Urol 121:303–305, 1979.

140. Greene LF, Mulcahy JJ, Warren MM, Dockerty MB: Primary transitional cell carcinoma of the prostate. J Urol 110:235–237, 1973.

141. Greene LF, O'Dea MJ, Dockerty MB: Primary transitional cell carcinoma of the prostate. J Urol 116:761–763, 1976.

142. Gueft B: The x-ray diffraction pattern of prostatic corpora amylacea. Acta Pathol Microbiol Immunol Scand [A-80] 233(Suppl):132–134, 1972.

143. Gueft B, Walsh MA: Malignant prostatic cystosarcoma phyllodes. NY State J Med 75:2226–2278, 1975.

144. Haddad JR, Reyes EC: Carcinosarcoma of the prostate with metastasis of both elements. J Urol 103:80–83, 1970.

145. Hafiz MA, Toker C, Sutula M: An atypical fibromyxoid tumor of the prostate. Cancer 54:2500–2504, 1984.

146. Ham AW: Histology, 7th ed. Philadelphia, JB Lippincott, 1974, pp 926–929.

147. Hamlin WB, Lund PK: Carcinosarcoma of the prostate: a case report. J Urol 97:518–522, 1967.

148. Hanash KA, Utz DC, Cook EN, et al: Carcinoma of the prostate: a 15-year followup. J Urol 107:450–453, 1972.

149. Hara S, Horie A: Prostatic caruncle: a urethral papillary tumor derived from prolapse of the prostatic duct. J Urol 117:303–305, 1977.

150. Harrison GS: The prognosis of prostatic cancer in the younger man. Br J Urol 55:315–320, 1983.

151. Hassan MO, Maksem J: The prostatic perineural

space and its relation to tumor spread. Am J Surg Pathol 4:143–148, 1980.

152. Hassler O: Calcifications in the prostate gland and adjacent tissues: a combined biophysical and histological study. Pathol Microbiol 31:97–107, 1968.

153. Hendry WF, Williams JP: Transrectal prostatic biopsy. Br Med J 4:595–597, 1971.

154. Herr HW, Whitmore WF Jr: Significance of prostatic biopsies after radiation therapy for carcinoma of the prostate. Prostate 3:339–350, 1982.

155. Holmes EJ: Crystalloids of prostatic carcinoma: relationship to Bence-Jones crystals. Cancer 39:2073–2080, 1977.

156. Huben R, Natarajan N, Pontes E, et al: Carcinoma of prostate in men less than fifty years old. Urology 20:585–588, 1982.

157. Hubly JW, Thompson GJ: Infarction of the prostate and volumetric changes produced by the lesion. J Urol 43:459–467, 1940.

158. Hudson PB, Finkle AL, Trifilio A, Wolan CT: Value of transurethral biopsy in search of early prostatic cancer. Surgery 35:897–900, 1954.

159. Huggins C, Webster WO: Duality of human prostate in response to estrogen. J Urol 59:258–266, 1948.

160. Hutch JA, Rambo ON Jr: A study of the anatomy of the prostate, prostatic urethra and the urinary sphincter systems. J Urol 104:443–457, 1970.

161. Ichijo S, Katagose K, Koguchi M, et al: Exfoliative cytology of prostatic carcinoma using a prostatic fluid collecting catheter. J Urol 133:416–420, 1985.

162. Jacobi GH, Lonne C, Riedmiller H, Hohenfellner R: Iatrogenically induced metastases in prostate cancer? Analysis of 509 transrectal biopsies. Aktuel Urol 13:317–323, 1982.

163. Jao W, Fretzin DF, Christ ML, Prinz LM: Blue nevus of the prostate gland. Arch Pathol 91:187–191, 1971.

164. Jensen PE, Gardner WA Jr, Piserchia PV: Prostatic crystalloids: association with adenocarcinoma. Prostate 1:25–30, 1980.

165. Jewett HJ: Radical perineal prostatectomy for early cancer. Bull NY Acad Med 34:26–33, 1958.

166. Jewett JH, Bridge RW, Gray GF Jr, Shelley WM: The palpable nodule of prostatic cancer. JAMA 203:403–406, 1968.

167. Johansson JE, Lannes P: Metastases to the spermatic cord, epididymis, and testicles from carcinoma of the prostate—five cases. Scand J Urol Nephrol 17:249–251, 1983.

168. Johnson DE, Chalbaud R, Ayala AG: Secondary tumors of the prostate. J Urol 112:507–508, 1974.

169. Johnson DE, Hogan JM, Ayala AG: Transitional cell carcinoma of the prostate. A clinical morphological study. Cancer 29:287–293, 1972.

170. Johnson DE, Lanieri JP Jr, Ayala AG: Prostatic carcinoma occurring in men under 50 years of age. J Surg Oncol 4:207–216, 1972.

171. Johnson FP: The later development of the urethra in the male. J Urol 4:447–501, 1920.

172. Kafandaris PM, Polyzonis MB: Fibroadenoma-like foci in human prostatic nodular hyperplasia. Prostate 4:33–36, 1983.

173. Kahler JE: Carcinoma of the prostate gland: a pathologic study. J Urol 41:557–574, 1939.

174. Karpas CM, Moumgis B: Primary transitional cell carcinoma of prostate gland: possible pathogenesis and relationship to reserve cell hyperplasia of prostatic periurethral ducts. J Urol 101:201–205, 1969.

175. Kastendieck H: Prostatic carcinoma: aspects of pathology, prognosis, and therapy. J Cancer Res Clin Oncol 96:131–156, 1980.

176. Kastendieck H, Altenahr E: Das Plattenepithelcarcinom der Prostata als Beispiel einer Tumor Metaplasie. Z Krebsforsch 82:335–340, 1974.

177. Kastendieck H, Altenahr E, Burchardt P: Zur Ultrastruktur des behandelten Prostatacarcinoms. Virchows Arch [A] 366:287–304, 1975.

178. Kastendieck H, Altenahr E, Geister H: Das Myosarkom der Prostata. Dtsch Med Wschr 99:392–394, 1974.

179. Kato T: Histological study on hyperplasia of the prostate with special reference to histogenesis of nodule. Nippon Hinyokika Gakkai Zasshi 58:469–483, 1967.

180. Katske FA, Waisman J, Lupu AN: Cutaneous and subcutaneous metastases from carcinoma of prostate. Urology 19:373–376, 1982.

181. Katz RL, Raual P, Brooks TE, Ordonez NG: Role of immunocytochemistry in diagnosis of prostatic neoplasia by fine-needle aspiration biopsy. Diagn Cytopathol 1:28–32, 1985.

182. Kaufman JJ, Ljung BM, Walther P, Waisman J: Aspiration biopsy of prostate. Urology 19:587–591, 1982.

183. Kaufman JJ, Rosenthal M, Goodwin WE: Methods of diagnosis of carcinoma of the prostate: a comparison of clinical impressions, prostatic smear, needle biopsy, open perineal biopsy, and transurethral biopsy. J Urol 72:450–465, 1954.

184. Kaufman JJ, Schultz JI: Needle biopsy of the prostate: a reevaluation. J Urol 87:164–168, 1962.

185. Kazzaz BA: Argentaffin and argyrophil cells in the prostate. J Pathol 112:179–193, 1974.

186. Kelalis PP, Greene LF, Harrison EG Jr: Granulomatous prostatitis: a mimic of carcinoma of the prostate. JAMA 191:287–289, 1965.

187. Kelalis PP, Harrison EG Jr, Greene LF: Allergic granulomas of the prostate in asthmatics. JAMA 188:963–967, 1964.

188. Keshgegian AA, Kline TS: Immunoperoxidase demonstration of prostatic acid phosphatase in aspiration biopsy cytology (ABC). Am J Clin Pathol 82:586–589, 1984.

189. Khalifa NM, Jarman WD: A study of 48 cases of incidental carcinoma of the prostate followed 10 years or longer. J Urol 116:329–331, 1976.

190. Kirchheim D, Niles NR, Frankus E, Hodges CV: Correlative histochemical and histological studies on thirty radical prostatectomy specimens. Cancer 19:1683–1696, 1966.

191. Kirkland KL, Bale PM: A cystic adenoma of the prostate. J Urol 97:324–327, 1967.

192. Kirshbaum JD, Larkin HS, Culver H: Retothel sarcoma of prostate gland: report of case. J Urol 50:597–607, 1943.

193. Kline TS, Kannan V: Prostatic aspirates. A cytomorphologic analysis with emphasis on well-differentiated carcinoma. Diagn Cytopathol 1:13–18, 1985.

194. Kline TS, Kohler FP, Kelsey DM: Aspiration biopsy cytology (ABC). Its use in diagnosis of lesions of the prostate gland. Arch Pathol Lab Med 106:136–139, 1982.

195. Kopolovic J, Rivkind A, Sherman Y: Granulomatous prostatitis with vasculitis. A sequel to transurethral prostatic resection. Arch Pathol Lab Med 108:732–733, 1984.

196. Koss LG, Woyke S, Schreiber K, Kohlberg W,

Freed SZ: Thin-needle aspiration biopsy of the prostate. Urol Clin North Am 11:237–251, 1984.

197. Kost LV, Evans GW: Occurrence and significance of striated muscle within the prostate. J Urol 92:703–704, 1964.

198. Kramer SA, Bredael JJ, Krueger RP: Adenoid cystic carcinoma of the prostate: report of a case. J Urol 120:383–384, 1978.

199. Kramolowsky EV, Narayana AS, Platz CE, Loening SA: The frozen section in lymphadenectomy for carcinoma of the prostate. J Urol 131:889–890, 1984.

200. Kuban DA, El-Mahdi AM, Schellhammer PF, Babb TJ: The effect of transurethral prostatic resection on the incidence of osseous prostatic metastasis. Cancer 56:961–964, 1985.

201. Langley JW, Weitzner S: Blue nevus and melanosis of prostate. J Urol 112:359–361, 1974.

202. Lazzaro AL: Technical note: Improved preparation of fine-needle aspiration biopsies for transmission electron microscopy. Pathology 15:399–402, 1983.

203. LeDuc IE: The anatomy of the prostate and the pathology of early benign hypertrophy. J Urol 42:1217–1241, 1939.

204. Lefer DG, Rosier RP: Increased prevalence of prostatic carcinoma due to more thorough microscopical examination (Letter). N Engl J Med 296:109, 1977.

205. Lester J, Stout AP: Cystosarcoma phyllodes. Cancer 7:335–353, 1954.

206. Levine AJ, Foster EA: The relation of mucicarmine-staining properties of carcinoma of the prostate to differentiation, metastasis, and prognosis. Cancer 17:21–25, 1964.

207. Li C-Y, Lam WK, Yam LT: Immunohistochemical diagnosis of prostatic cancer with metastasis. Cancer 46:706–712, 1980.

208. Lightbourn GA, Abrams M, Seymour L: Primary mucoid adenocarcinoma of the prostate gland with bladder invasion. J Urol 101:78–80, 1969.

209. Linsk JA, Axilrod HD, Solyn R, Delaverdac C: Transrectal cytologic aspiration in the diagnosis of prostatic carcinoma. J Urol 108:455–459, 1972.

210. Lowsley OS: The development of the human prostate gland with reference to the development of other structures at the neck of the urinary bladder. Am J Anat 13:299–349, 1912.

211. Maier W, Czerwenka K, Neuhold N: The accuracy of transrectal aspiration biopsy of the prostate: an analysis of 452 cases. Prostate 5:147–151, 1984.

212. Manley CB Jr: The striated muscle of the prostate. J Urol 95:234–240, 1966.

213. Manrique JJ, Albores-Saavedra J, Orantes A, Brandt H: Malignant mixed tumor of the salivary gland type, primary in the prostate. Am J Clin Pathol 70:932–937, 1978.

214. Mao P, Nakao K, Angrist A: Human prostatic carcinoma: an electron microscope study. Cancer Res 26:955–973, 1966.

215. Martin SA, Fowler M, Catalona WJ, Boyarsky S: Carcinosarcoma of the prostate: report of a case with ultrastructural observations. J Urol 122:709–711, 1979.

216. McCullough DL: Experimental lymphangiography. Experience with direct medium injection into the parenchyma of the rat testis and prostate. Invest Urol 13:211–219, 1975.

217. McCullough DL, Prout GR Jr, Daly JJ: Carcinoma of the prostate and lymphatic metastases. J Urol 111:65–71, 1974.

218. McGavran HG: Giant prostate without symptoms: neurofibroma. J Urol 60:254–259, 1948.

219. McGowan DG, Bain GO, Hanson J: Evaluation of histological grading (Gleason) in carcinoma of the prostate: adverse influence of the highest grade. Prostate 4:111–118, 1983.

220. McIntyre DW: Massive leiomyoma of prostate: case report. J Urol 59:1198–1202, 1948.

221. McLaughlin AP, Saltzstein SL, McCullough DL, Gittes RF: Prostatic carcinoma: incidence and location of unsuspected lymphatic metastases. J Urol 115:89–94, 1976.

222. McNeal JE: Regional morphology and pathology of the prostate. Am J Clin Pathol 49:347–357, 1968.

223. McNeal JE: Origin and development of carcinoma in the prostate. Cancer 23:24–34, 1969.

224. McNeal JE: Age related changes in prostatic epithelium associated with carcinoma. In K Griffiths, CG Pierrepoint (eds): Third Tenovus Workshop. Cardiff, Wales, Alpha Omega Alpha Publishers, 1970, pp 23–32.

225. McNeal JE: Structure and pathology of the prostate. In M Goland (ed): Normal and Abnormal Growth of the Prostate. Springfield, Illinois, Charles C Thomas, 1975, pp 55–68.

226. McNeal JE: Anatomy of the prostate: an historical survey of divergent views. Prostate 1:3–13, 1980.

227. Melchior J, Valk WL, Foret JD, Mebust WK: The prostate in leukemia: evaluation and review of literature. J Urol 111:647–651, 1974.

228. Melicow MM, Tannenbaum M: Endometrial carcinoma of uterus masculinus (prostatic utricle). Report of 6 cases. J Urol 106:892–902, 1971.

229. Melicow MM, Uson AC: A spectrum of malignant epithelial tumors of the prostate gland. J Urol 115:696–700, 1976.

230. Melograna F, Oertel YC, Kwart AM: Prospective controlled assessment of fine-needle prostatic aspiration. Urology 19:47–51, 1982.

231. Merimsky E, Baratz M, Kahn Y: Leukaemic infiltration of the prostate. Br J Urol 53:150–151, 1981.

232. Mies C, Balogh K, Stadecker M: Palisading prostate granulomas following surgery. Am J Surg Pathol 8:217–221, 1984.

233. Miller GJ: The use of histochemistry and immunohistochemistry in evaluating prostatic neoplasia. Prog Surg Pathol 5:115–129, 1983.

234. Mobley TL, Frank IN: Influence of tumor grade on survival and on serum acid phosphatase levels in metastatic carcinoma of the prostate. J Urol 99:321–323, 1968.

235. Moncure CW, Johnston CL Jr, Smith MJ, Koontz WW Jr: Immunological and histochemical evaluation of marrow aspirates in patients with prostatic carcinoma. J Urol 108:609–611, 1972.

236. Moncure CW, Prout GR Jr, Blaylock K: The immunological detection of prostatic acid phosphatase in dog and man (Abstr). Fed Proc 26:574, 1967.

237. Moore GH, Lawshe B, Murphy J: Sampling of transurethral prostatectomy specimens in the diagnosis of adenocarcinoma. Lab Invest 52:45A, 1985.

238. Moore RA: The morphology of small prostatic carcinoma. J Urol 33:224–234, 1935.

239. Moore RA: The evolution and involution of the prostate gland. Am J Pathol 12:599–624, 1936.

240. Moore RA: Benign hypertrophy of the prostate, a morphologic study. J Urol 50:680–710, 1943.

241. Mori K, Spiro LH, Hecht H, Orkin LA: Recurrent intraurethral proliferation of ectopic prostatic tissue associated with hematuria. J Urol 114:316–318, 1975.

242. Mosca P, Roy JB: Outpatient needle-biopsy of the prostate: a retrospective study. Okla State Med Assoc J 73:3–6, 1980.

243. Mostofi FK: Criteria for pathologic diagnosis of carcinoma of the prostate. Proceedings of the Second National Cancer Conference, Philadelphia, American Cancer Society, 1952, pp 332–344.

244. Mostofi FK: Benign hyperplasia of the prostate gland. In MF Campbell, JH Harrison (eds): Urology, 3rd ed, Vol 2. Philadelphia, WB Saunders, 1970, pp 1065–1129.

245. Mostofi FK, Morse WH: Epithelial metaplasia in "prostatic infarction." Arch Pathol 51:340–345, 1951.

246. Mostofi FK, Price EB Jr: Tumors of the Male Genital System. Washington, DC, Armed Forces Institute of Pathology, 2nd Series, 1973.

247. Mott LJ, Waisman J, Boxer RJ, Skinner DG: Significant microscopic features of prostatic adenocarcinoma with a comparison of current methods of grading. Lab Invest 40:274, 1979.

248. Muir EG, Lond MS: Carcinoma of the prostate. Lancet 1:667–672, 1934.

249. Müller H-A, Wünsch PH: Features of prostatic sarcomas in combined aspiration and punch biopsies. Acta Cytol 25:480–484, 1981.

250. Murnaghan GF, Tynan AP, Farnsworth RH, Harvey K: Chronic prostatitis—an Australian view. Br J Urol 46:55–59, 1974.

251. Murphy GP, Whitmore WF Jr: A report of the workshops on the current status of the histologic grading of prostate cancer. Cancer 44:1490–1494, 1979.

252. Myers RP, Nevis RJ, Farcow GM, Utz DC: Nucleolar grading of prostatic adenocarcinoma: light microscopic correlation with disease progression. Prostate 3:423–432, 1982.

253. Nadji M, Tabei SZ, Castro A, et al: Prostatic origin of tumors: an immunohistochemical study. Am J Clin Pathol 73:735–739, 1980.

254. Nadji M, Tabei SZ, Castro A, et al: Prostatic-specific antigen: an immunohistologic marker for prostatic neoplasms. Cancer 48:1229–1232, 1981.

255. Nielsen ML, Christensen P: Inflammatory changes of the hyperplastic prostate. Scand J Urol Nephrol 6:6–10, 1972.

256. Nielsen ML, Justesen T: Studies on the pathology of prostatitis. Scand J Urol Nephrol 8:1–6, 1974.

257. Ohmori T, Arita N, Tabei R: Prostatic leiomyosarcoma revealing cytoplasmic virus-like particles and intranuclear paracrystalline structures. Acta Pathol Jpn 34:631–638, 1984.

258. Ohtsuki Y, Seman G, Maruyama K, et al: Ultrastructural studies of human prostatic neoplasia. Cancer 37:2295–2305, 1976.

259. Olsen BS, Carlisle RW: Adenocarcinoma of the prostate simulating primary rectal malignancy. Cancer 25:219–222, 1970.

260. O'Shaughnessy EJ, Parrino PS, White JD: Chronic prostatitis: fact or fiction? JAMA 160:540–542, 1956.

261. Palma PCR, Netto NR Jr, Ikari O, et al: Leiomyosarcoma in association with incidental adenocarcinoma of the prostate. J Urol 129:156–157, 1983.

262. Pertschuk LP, Rosenthal HE, Macchia RJ, et al: Correlation of histochemical and biochemical analyses of androgen binding in prostatic cancer: relation to therapeutic response. Cancer 49:984–993, 1982.

263. Pieterse AS, Aarons I, Jose JS: Focal prostatic granulomas rheumatoid-like—probably iatrogenic in origin. Pathology 16:174–177, 1984.

264. Pillarisetti SG, Espinoza CG, Richman AV: Prostatic adenocarcinoma with focal "endometrioid" features: histopathologic and immunocytochemical findings. Lab Invest 48:68A, 1983.

265. Piscioli F, Leonardi E, Reich A, Luciani L: Percutaneous lymph node aspiration biopsy and tumor grade in staging of prostatic carcinoma. Prostate 5:459–468, 1984.

266. Pontes JE: Biological markers in prostate cancer. J Urol 130:1037–1047, 1983.

267. Pool TL, Thompson GJ: Conservative treatment of carcinoma of the prostate. JAMA 160:833–837, 1956.

268. Prout GR Jr: Chemical tests in the diagnosis of prostatic carcinoma. JAMA 209:1699–1700, 1969.

269. Quay SC, Proppe KH: Carcinosarcoma of the prostate: case report and review of the literature. J Urol 125:436–438, 1981.

270. Randall A: Surgical Pathology of Prostatic Obstruction. Baltimore, Williams & Wilkins, 1931.

271. Ray GR, Pistenma DA, Castellino RA, et al: Operative staging of apparently localized adenocarcinoma of the prostate: results in fifty unselected patients. Cancer 38:73–83, 1976.

272. Redman JF, Downs RA: Simple eosinophilic granulomatous prostatitis. J Urol 132:358, 1984.

273. Reed RJ: Consultation case. Am J Surg Pathol 8:699–704, 1984.

274. Reeves LJ, Wheatley IC: Carcinoma of the prostate with rectal symptoms. Med J Aust 2:500–501, 1978.

275. Reischauer F: Die Entstehung der sogenannten Prostatahypertrophie. Virchows Arch [A] 256:357–389, 1925.

276. Remick DG Jr, Kumar NB: Benign polyps with prostatic-type epithelium of the urethra and the urinary bladder. Am J Surg Pathol 8:833–839, 1984.

277. Rhamy RK, Buchanan RD, Spalding MJ: Intraductal carcinoma of the prostate gland. J Urol 109:457–460, 1973.

278. Rich AR: On the frequency of occurrence of occult carcinoma of the prostate. J Urol 33:215–223, 1935.

279. Riley RS, Gnepp DR, Kandzari S, Belis JA: Prostatic adenocarcinoma: histological effects of treatment with ^{125}I-seed implantations. Am J Clin Pathol 78:269–270, 1982.

280. Rismyhr B, Eide TJ, Stalsberg H: The diagnosis of carcinoma in transurethral resectates of the prostate. A study of the probability of overlooking malignant tissue when only part of the material is embedded for histological examination. Acta Pathol Microbiol Scand [A] 88:211–215, 1980.

281. Rodin AE, Larson DL, Roberts DK: Nature of the perineural space invaded by prostatic carcinoma. Cancer 20:1772–1779, 1967.

282. Roth RB: Prostatic infarction. J Urol 62:474–479, 1949.

283. Rous SN, Mallouh C: Prostatic carcinoma: the

relationshp between histologic grade and incidence of early metastases. J Urol 108:905–907, 1972.

284. Sagalowsky AI, Milam H, Reveley LR, Silva FG: Prediction of lymphatic metastases by Gleason histologic grading in prostatic cancer. J Urol 128:951–952, 1982.

285. Saito R, Davis BK, Ollapally EP: Adenosquamous carcinoma of the prostate. Hum Pathol 15:87–89, 1984.

286. Saitoh H, Hida M, Shimbo T, et al: Metastatic patterns of prostatic cancer: correlation between sites and number of organs involved. Cancer 54:3078–3084, 1984.

287. Saphir O, Vass A: Carcinosarcoma. Am J Cancer 33:331–361, 1938.

288. Sarkar K, Tolnai G, McKay DE: Embryonal rhabdomyosarcoma of the prostate. An ultrastructural study. Cancer 31:442–448, 1973.

289. Satter EJ, Blumenfeld CM: Endometrial carcinoma of the prostatic utricle. J Urol 112:505–506, 1974.

290. Sawczuk I, Tannenbaum M, Olsson CA, White R deV: Primary transitional cell carcinoma of prostatic periurethral ducts. Urology 25:339–343, 1985.

291. Schenken JR, Burns EL, Kahle PJ: The effect of diethylstilbestrol and diethylstilbestrol diproprionate on carcinoma of the prostate gland. J Urol 48:99–112, 1942.

292. Schmidt JD, Welch MJ Jr: Sarcoma of the prostate. Cancer 37:1908–1912, 1976.

293. Schned AR: Prostatic granulomas. Am J Surg Pathol 8:797, 1984.

294. Schoonees R, Palma LD, Gaeta JF, et al: Prostatic carcinoma treated at categorical center. NY State J Med 72:1021–1027, 1972.

295. Schroeder FH, Belt E: Carcinoma of the prostate: a study of 213 patients with stage C tumor treated by total perineal prostatectomy. J Urol 114:257–260, 1975.

296. Schroeder FH, Blum JHM, Hop WCJ, Mostofi JK: Grading of prostatic cancer: (1) an analysis of the prognostic significance of single characteristics. Prostate 6:81–100, 1985.

297. Schron DS, Gipson T, Mendelsohn G: The histogenesis of small cell carcinoma of the prostate. An immunohistochemical study. Cancer 53:2478–2480, 1984.

298. Schuppler J: Malignant neurilemmoma of prostate gland. J Urol 106:903–905, 1971.

299. Scott MB, Goldstein AM, Onofrio RC, Cosgrove MD: Papillary adenocarcinoma of prostate. Urology 8:277–230, 1976.

300. Scott WW, Schirmer HKA: Carcinoma of the prostate. In MF Campbell, JH Harrison (eds), Urology, Vol 2. Philadelphia, WB Saunders, 1970, pp 1143–1189.

301. Seemayer TA, Knaack J, Thelmo WL, et al: Further observations on carcinoma in situ of the urinary bladder: silent but extensive intraprostatic involvement. Cancer 36:514–520, 1975.

302. Semen G, Gallager HS, Johnson DE: Melanin-like pigment in the human prostate. Prostate 3:59–72, 1982.

303. Seppelt U, Sprenger E: Nuclear DNA cytophotometry in prostate carcinoma. Cytometry 5:528–262, 1984.

304. Sharifi R, Shaw M, Ray V, et al: Evaluation of cytologic techniques for diagnosis of prostate cancer. Urology 21:417–420, 1983.

305. Shelley HS, Auerbach SH, Classen KL, et al: Carcinoma of the prostate—a new system of classification. Arch Surg 77:751–758, 1958.

306. Shevchuk MM, Romas NA, Ng PY, et al: Acid phosphatase localization in prostatic carcinoma. A comparison of monoclonal antibody to heteroantisera. Cancer 52:1642–1646, 1983.

307. Shimada H, Misugi K, Sasaki Y, et al: Carcinoma of the prostate in childhood and adolescence: report of a case and review of the literature. Cancer 46:2534–2542, 1980.

308. Shong-San C, Walters MNI: Adenoid cystic carcinoma of prostate: report of a case. Pathology 16:337–338, 1984.

309. Shulman S, Mamrod L, Lang RW, et al: Measurement of prostatic acid phosphatase by gel diffusion methods. J Reprod Fertil 10:55–60, 1965.

310. Sika JV, Buckley JJ: Mucus-forming adenocarcinoma of prostate. Cancer 17:949–952, 1964.

311. Silber I, McGavran MH: Adenocarcinoma of the prostate in men less than 56 years old: a study of 56 cases. J Urol 105:283–285, 1971.

312. Smedley HM, Sinnot M, Freedman LS, et al: Age and survival in prostatic carcinoma. Br J Urol 55:529–533, 1983.

313. Smith BH, Dehner LP: Sarcoma of the prostate gland. Am J Clin Pathol 58:43–50, 1972.

314. Smith JA Jr, Middleton RG: Implications of volume of nodal metastasis in patients with adenocarcinoma of the prostate. J Urol 133:617–619, 1985.

315. Smith MJV: The lymphatics of the prostate. Invest Urol 3:439–444, 1966.

316. Sonnenschein R: The effectiveness of transrectal aspiration cytology in the diagnosis of prostatic carcinoma. Eur Urol 1:189–192, 1975.

317. Spieler P, Gloor F, Egle N, Bandhauer K: Cytological findings in transrectal aspiration biopsy on hormone- and radio-treated carcinoma of the prostate. Virchows Arch [A] 372:149–159, 1976.

318. Sridhar KN, Woodhouse CR: Prostate infiltration in leukaemia and lymphoma. Eur Urol 9:153–156, 1983.

319. Stein BS, Vangore S, Petersen RO, Kandall AR: Immunoperoxidase localization of prostate-specific antigen. Am J Surg Pathol 6:553–557, 1982.

320. Stenram W, Holby LA: Case of circumscribed myosarcoma of the prostate. Cancer 24:803–806, 1969.

321. Svanhohm H, Mygind H: Prostatic cancer. Reproducibility of histologic grading. Acta Pathol Microbiol Immunol Scand [A] 93:67–71, 1985.

322. Tannenbaum M: Endometrial tumors and/or associated carcinomas of prostate. Urol 6:372–375, 1975.

323. Tanner FH, McDonald JR: Granulomatous prostatitis. Arch Pathol 36:358–370, 1943.

324. Taylor HG, Blom J: Transitional cell carcinoma of the prostate. Response to treatment with adriamycin and cis-platinum. Cancer 51:1800–1802, 1983.

325. Taylor NS: Histochemistry in the diagnosis of early prostatic carcinoma. Hum Pathol 10:513–520, 1979.

326. Terry R: Some questions raised by histologic study of RTOG protocols 75–06 and 77–06 as illustrated by selected samples. Prostate 3:543–554, 1982.

327. Thompson GJ: Transurethral resection of malignant lesions of prostate gland. JAMA 120:1105–1109, 1942.

328. Thompson GJ, Albers DD, Broders AC: Unusual carcinomas involving prostate gland. J Urol 69:416–425, 1953.

329. Thybo E, Zdravkovic D, Zdravkovic M: Granulomatous prostatitis. Scand J Urol Nephrol 7:111–114, 1973.

330. Timmons JW Jr, Burgert EO Jr, Soule EH, et al: Embryonal rhabdomyosarcoma of the bladder and prostate in childhood. J Urol 113:694–697, 1975.

331. Tisell LE, Salander H: The lobes of the human prostate. Scand J Urol Nephrol 9:185–191, 1975.

332. Tjaden HB, Culp DA, Flocks RH: Clinical adenocarcinoma of the prostate in patients under 50 years of age. J Urol 93:618–621, 1965.

333. Towfighi J, Sadeghee S, Wheeler JE, Enterline HT: Granulomatous prostatitis with emphasis on the eosinophilic variety. Am J Clin Pathol 58:630–641, 1972.

334. Tribukait B, Rönström L, Esposti PL: Quantitative and qualitative aspects of flow DNA measurements related to the cytologic grade in prostatic carcinoma. Anal Quant Cytol 5:107–111, 1983.

335. Ullman AS, Ross OA: Hyperplasia, atypism, and carcinoma in situ in prostatic periurethral glands. Am J Clin Pathol 47:497–504, 1967.

336. Uyama T, Moriwaki S: Histological evaluation of radiochemotherapy for prostatic cancer: early results of a pilot study. Prostate Suppl 1:59–64, 1981.

337. Varkarakis MJ, Murphy GP, Nelson CM, et al: Lymph node involvement in prostatic carcinoma. Urol Clin North Am 2:197–212, 1975.

338. Venable DD, Hastings D, Misra RP: Unusual metastatic patterns of prostate adenocarcinoma. J Urol 130:980–985, 1983.

339. Vickery AL Jr, Kerr WS Jr: Carcinoma of the prostate treated by radical prostatectomy. Cancer 16:1598–1608, 1963.

340. von Eschenbach AC, Zornoza J: Fine-needle percutaneous biopsy. A useful evaluation of lymph node metastasis from prostate cancer. Urology 20:589–590, 1982.

341. Waisman J, Löwhagen T: Fine-needle aspiration of the prostate gland. Tutorials Cytol (Chicago) 36:1–33, 1984.

342. Wajsman Z, Gamarra M, Park JJ, et al: Fine-needle aspiration of metastatic lesions and regional lymph nodes in genitourinary cancer. Urology 19:356–360, 1982.

343. Walker AN, Mills SE, Fechner RE, Perry JM: Epithelial polyps of the prostatic urethra. A light-microscopic and immunohistochemical study. Am J Surg Pathol 7:351–356, 1983.

344. Walker PD, Karnik S, deKernion JB, Pramberg JC: Cell surface blood group antigens in prostatic carcinoma. Am J Clin Pathol 81:503–506, 1984.

345. Waller JI, Shullenberger WA: Lymphosarcoma of the prostate. J Urol 62:480–487, 1949.

346. Warren S, Harris PN, Graves R: Osseous metastasis of carcinoma of the prostate. Arch Pathol 22:139–160, 1936.

347. Webber MM: Ultrastructural changes in human prostatic epithelium grown in vitro. J Ultrastruct Res 50:89–102, 1975.

348. Webber MM, Bouldin TR: Ultrastructure of human prostatic epithelium. Secretion granules or virus particles? Invest Urology 14:482–487, 1977.

349. Weitzner S: Survival of patients with secondary carcinoma of prostate in testis. Cancer 32:447–449, 1973.

350. Weitzner S, Sarikaya H, Furness TD: Adenocarcinoma of prostate in a twenty-seven-year-old man. Urology 16:286–288, 1980.

351. Wiederanders RE, Stuber RV, Mota C, et al: Prognostic value of grading prostatic carcinoma. J Urol 89:881–888, 1963.

352. Willems JS, Löwhagen T: Transrectal fine-needle aspiration biopsy for cytologic diagnosis and grading of prostatic carcinoma. Prostate 2:381–395, 1981.

353. Willis RA: The Spread of Tumours in the Human Body, 3rd ed. London, Butterworths, 1973, pp 121–122.

354. Witorsch RJ: The application of immunoperoxidase methodology for the visualization of prolactin binding sites in human prostate tissue. Hum Pathol 10:521–532, 1979.

355. Wolfe JH, Lloyd-Davies RW: The management of transitional cell carcinoma in the prostate. Br J Urol 53:253–257, 1981.

356. Wünsch PH, Müller HA: Hemangiopericytoma of the prostate. A light-microscopic study of an unusual tumor. Pathol Res Pract 173:334–338, 1982.

357. Yam LT, Winkler CF, Janckila AJ, et al: Prostatic cancer presenting as metastatic adenocarcinoma of undetermined origin. Immunodiagnosis by prostatic acid phosphatase. Cancer 51:283–287, 1983.

358. Yokota T, Yamashita Y, Okuzomo Y, et al: Malignant cytosarcoma phylloides of prostate. Acta Pathol Jpn 34:663–668, 1984.

359. Young BW, Lagios MD: Endometrial (papillary) carcinoma of the prostatic utricle—response to orchiectomy. A case report. Cancer 32:1293–1300, 1973.

360. Young HH: Cancer of the prostate: a clinical, pathological, and postoperative analysis of 111 cases. Ann Surg 50:1144–1233, 1909.

361. Zaloudek C, Williams JW, Kempson RL: "Endometrial" adenocarcinoma of the prostate. A distinctive tumor of probably prostatic duct origin. Cancer 37:2255–2262, 1976.

362. Zimmerman A, Zeltner T: Papillom der Prostata. Urologe [Ausg A] 18:109–111, 1979.

NANCY E. WARNER, M.D.

CHAPTER 10

Pathology of the Adrenal Gland

EMBRYOLOGY, ANATOMY, HISTOLOGY, FUNCTION

The adrenal gland originates from two quite separate primordia. The cortex arises from mesoderm of the genitourinary ridge on the posterior body wall in close proximity to the developing gonads and kidneys. As a consequence of this juxtaposition, adrenal cortical rests may become incorporated in the gonadal adnexae (hilus of the testis, or the broad ligament, where they are known as Marchand bodies), retroperitoneum, or the renal cortex.[42, 64] The medulla is a derivative of the neural crest, arising from neuroblasts that migrate ventrolaterally from the primitive autonomic ganglia to colonize the adrenal medulla. This specialized subpopulation of ganglion cells differentiates successively into sympathicoblasts, pheochromoblasts, and, finally, pheochromocytes. Some of the migrating neuroblasts destined to become pheochromocytes fail to make the journey to the adrenal gland but lodge instead in other paravertebral locations, forming the system of extra-adrenal chromaffin bodies that accounts for the occurrence of extra-adrenal pheochromocytomas. The neuroblastoma series of adrenal medullary neoplasms apparently arises from the same population of specialized neuroblasts that have failed to differentiate as pheochromocytes. The word *pheochromocyte* is derived from Greek roots: *phaios*, meaning dusky, and *chroma*, color. The term refers to the fact that the cells turn dark upon exposure to oxidizing agents, a transformation known as the chromaffin reaction. The reaction is based on the oxidation and polymerization of intracellular adrenalin and noradrenalin (catecholamines), with formation of dark brown pigments (adrenochromes).

The normal adrenal in the adult weighs 4 to 5 gm at operation and 6 gm at autopsy.[54] Careful assessment of the weight is important in the diagnosis of hyperplasia.

The adrenal gland has three equal parts, designated the head, body, and tail.[56] The central longitudinal ridge on the dorsal aspect of the gland is termed the crest, and the lateral extensions are known as the alae. In the fresh state, the cortex is greater than 0.1 cm but less than 0.2 cm in thickness. The outer two thirds is bright yellow, corresponding to the zona glomerulosa and the zona fasciculata. The innermost portion is brown, corresponding to the zona reticularis. The medulla is pale gray. Normally, the medulla is confined to the head and body (crest and one ala) of the gland, and does not extend into the tail (Fig. 10–1).[18]

With light microscopy, three zones are apparent in the adrenal cortex. The zona glomerulosa is the discontinuous narrow outer zone that lies just beneath the capsule. It consists of small clusters ("glomerules") of cells with foamy cytoplasm; these cells elaborate aldosterone. Their function is regulated by the renin-angiotensin system. The zona fasciculata is the widest of the three zones. Its cells are slightly larger, and they are arranged in parallel columns. This zone produces glucocorticoids, chiefly cortisol.

195

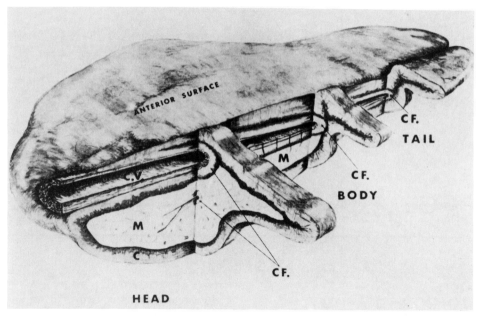

Figure 10–1. Diagram of adrenal showing distribution of normal medulla (confined to head and body of the gland). Key: M, medulla; C, cortex; C.V., central vein; C.F., perivenous adrenal cortex. From Neville AM, and O'Hare MJ in VHT James (ed), The Adrenal Gland. New York, Raven Press, 1979, with permission.

The zona reticularis is the innermost zone. Its cells have compact granular acidophilic cytoplasm, and they produce sex steroids. The functions of the zona fasciculata and zona reticularis are regulated by ACTH secreted by the adenohypophysis. Electron microscopy reveals features consistent with steroid hormone synthesis but has not been of much help in defining nuances of hormone secretion.

The medulla is composed of pheochromocytes, polygonal or elongated cells arranged in clusters and groups, separated by delicate fibrous septa, and supplied with a rich network of small vascular spaces. Scattered sympathetic ganglion cells, singly or in clusters, also are present. The pheochromocytes produce adrenalin and noradrenalin. These catecholamines are readily oxidized to produce insoluble, colored compounds known as adrenochromes. This histochemical transformation is the basis for the familiar screening test known as the chromaffin reaction, and it is the reason why pheochromocytes also are known as chromaffin cells. In hematoxylin-eosin–stained sections, the cytoplasm of pheochromocytes is faintly basophilic following formalin fixation or yellowish-brown after dichromate fixation.

Cytoplasmic hyaline globules of unknown significance may be present. Electron microscopy reveals characteristic membrane-bound secretory granules, designated type I (noradrenaline) and type II (adrenaline).

HYPERPLASIA OF ADRENAL CORTEX

In this condition, both glands are enlarged due to overgrowth of the cortex. Hyperplasia of the adrenal cortex is associated with (1) hypercortisolism, or Cushing's syndrome; (2) hypersecretion of androgens, with virilization (occurring almost exclusively in childhood); and (3) hyperaldosteronism, or Conn's syndrome. Feminization associated with hyperplasia of the cortex has not been reported.

Hyperplasia with hypercortisolism is the most common of the three types. The underlying problem usually is an ACTH-secreting basophil microadenoma of the adenohypophysis.[59] Ectopic production of ACTH by a variety of extra-adrenal neoplasms accounts for a significant number of cases. Nowadays, the diagnosis of idiopathic hyperplasia as the cause of hypercortisolism is rare.

It has been well documented that hypercortisolism with Cushing's syndrome may occur in patients with adrenal glands of normal weight and gross and microscopic appearances. It follows that examination of frozen sections is of no value in the intraoperative assessment of non-neoplastic hyperfunctioning adrenals in Cushing's syndrome.

Adrenal hyperfunction with virilism is known as the adrenogenital syndrome. Adrenal cortical hyperplasia is the most common cause of virilization in childhood.[2] The underlying cause of the hyperplasia is an enzyme defect in the adrenal cortex, and the treatment is medical.

Primary hyperaldosteronism due to hyperplasia is uncommon, and only a few cases have been reported.[43] Unilateral adrenocortical hyperplasia is a rare but well-documented cause of this disorder.[53]

Gross Features. Hyperplastic glands may each weigh up to 15 gm or more and have blunt contours and a cortex 3 or 4 mm in thickness. Hyperplasia may be diffuse or nodular, interspersed with nonencapsulated nodules up to several millimeters across in the thickened cortex. Thickening of the crest is a significant surgical landmark in the intraoperative recognition of this disorder. In congenital adrenal hyperplasia, the thickened cortex is brown. In all forms, the medulla is unaffected and shows no change. As described (see earlier), the glands in some patients with hypercortisolism may be entirely normal in appearance and weight.

Microscopic Features. In Cushing's syndrome, the width of the zona reticularis usually is disproportionately increased, and compact cells make up the inner half of the cortex; the outer cortex is composed of clear cells of fascicular type. In adrenogenital syndrome due to hyperplasia, the cortex is composed entirely of acidophilic compact cells. In hyperaldosteronism due to hyperplasia, the zona glomerulosa is focally or diffusely thickened, forming a continuous layer.

ADENOMA

Functioning adenomas correspond to the three major cell types of the normal cortex and thus may be associated with hyperaldosteronism, hypercortisolism, or excess of adrenal sex steroids (almost always androgens). Feminizing adenomas have been reported but are very rare.[29]

Cortisol Adenoma

These tumors are the most common of the adrenal adenomas. They produce excess cortisol and are responsible for Cushing's syndrome, with its distinctive clinical features that include moon facies, truncal obesity, hirsutism, cutaneous striae, hypertension, hyperglycemia, and osteoporosis.

Gross Features. Adenomas producing cortisol are discrete, circumscribed, solid tumors. They generally range from 10 to 70 gm, though cortisol adenomas up to 3.0 kg have been described. Cut surfaces are yellow and slightly bulging; brown mottling may be present. Hemorrhage, necrosis, and calcification are distinctly uncommon. Rarely, the cut surfaces are black—the so-called black adenoma.[38, 61] The residual cortex adjacent to the tumor and the cortex of the contralateral gland invariably are atrophic as a consequence of the "reverse feedback" effect of excess cortisol on the corticotroph cells of the adenohypophysis.

Microscopic Features. The tumors are composed of nests and cords of lipid-laden clear cells separated by fine fibrovascular trabeculae. The nuclei are orderly, mitoses are rare, and cytoplasm is abundant. Brown areas observed grossly correspond to regions with cells having granular pink cytoplasm (Fig. 10–2). In the rare variant known as black adenoma, the cytoplasm is stuffed with lipofuscin granules.[4]

Aldosterone Adenoma

The tumors produce excess aldosterone, and as a consequence the patient suffers from hypokalemia, sustained hypertension, weakness, paresthesias, polyuria, alkalosis, and low levels of plasma renin.

Gross Features. The typical aldosterone adenoma is a small, soft, well-circumscribed, bright yellow tumor. As a rule, these tumors are only a few centimeters in diameter and weigh less than 5 gm. Aldosterone adenomas are almost always solitary and unilateral.[43]

Microscopic Features. In hematoxylin-eosin–stained sections, the cells form cords and solid nests separated by thin fibrovascular septa, with an appearance that may closely resemble the clusters of cells in the normal zona glomerulosa. The nuclei are regular and orderly, and the cytoplasm is abundant and foamy. Cells of the type seen in fasciculata or reticularis may be inter-

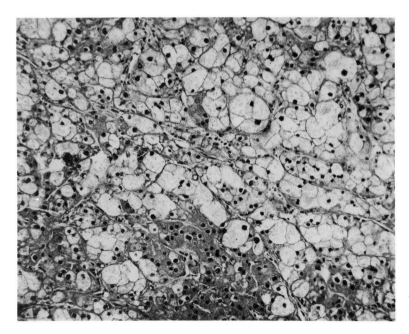

Figure 10–2. Cortisol adenoma, showing admixture of clear cells and compact cells. (× 125)

spersed. "Hybrid" cells having features of both glomerulosa and fasciculata may be numerous.[45] Usually, the zona glomerulosa of the uninvolved cortex in the attached gland and also in the contralateral adrenal show hyperplasia of microscopic proportions, forming a focally or diffusely thickened zone at the periphery of the cortex.[45]

Virilizing Adenoma

Virilizing tumors are rare; fewer than 500 cases have been reported. Although they affect both sexes and may occur at any age, the tumors are more common in females.[56] These neoplasms produce androgens and cause masculinization in women; in men, symptoms of androgen excess usually are lacking.

Gross Features. Virilizing adenomas vary widely in size, ranging from 30 gm to 1.5 kg.[56] The tumors are encapsulated, with soft, brown, bulging cut surfaces. Large lesions usually have foci of necrosis and hemorrhage, and areas of calcification may be present. Unlike the cortisol adenoma, virilizing tumors are not accompanied by atrophy of the contralateral and uninvolved ipsilateral adrenal cortex.

Microscopic Features. The tumors are composed of compact cells with granular cytoplasm resembling those in the zona re-

ticularis. The nuclei tend to be small and uniform, though in the larger tumors nuclear enlargement and pleomorphism are a feature. The cells are arranged in nests and cords. According to Symington, nuclear pleomorphism and the presence of giant or bizarre nuclei portend the onset of malignancy, and prognosis must be guarded.[56]

Feminizing Adenoma

Feminizing adenoma is the rarest of the adrenal adenomas. Fewer than a dozen cases have been reported, almost all in boys.[8, 24, 29, 41] Long follow-up is necessary to substantiate the diagnosis, since metastases can be delayed up to eight years.[3] Findings include elevated levels of estrogens, advanced bone age, gynecomastia in boys, and isosexual precocity in girls.

Gross Features. Feminizing adenomas vary widely in size, and weights of 10 gm to 2 kg have been reported.[52, 56] The tumors are encapsulated and have soft, bulging, brown cut surfaces. In larger tumors, calcification and foci of hemorrhage and necrosis may be present. Atrophy of the uninvolved cortex is not observed.

Microscopic Features. The tumors are composed of nests, cords, or sheets of cells with variable-sized nuclei and abundant acidophilic cytoplasm. Neville and Mackay noted that larger tumors tend to have enlarged nuclei and cellular pleomorphism, and the distinction between benign and malignant tumors can be extremely difficult.[43] More recently, Neville and O'Hare have recommended that all feminizing tumors be treated as carcinoma, irrespective of histologic features.[44]

CARCINOMA

The majority of adrenal cortical carcinomas are functional, most often causing Cushing's syndrome or virilization; rarely, feminization or hyperaldosteronism are produced. Nonfunctioning tumors present with pain, abdominal mass, or weight loss. Some of these nonfunctioning tumors are known to produce inactive steroidal precursors. The carcinomas invade locally to involve retroperitoneum, diaphragm, kidney, renal vein or inferior vena cava, and pancreas.[11, 26, 31, 39, 55] Metastatic spread commonly involves regional lymph nodes, liver, lungs, and bone.

Gross Features. The usual carcinoma of adrenal cortex is a bulky, soft, spherical or ovoid lobulated tumor. The mean weight of reported cases is approximately 800 gm.[57] However, weights of 57 to 4,500 gm have been recorded.[33, 35] The presence of a capsule is an inconstant feature. The cut surfaces are variegated; yellow regions predominate, with foci of hemorrhage, necrosis, and calcification.

Microscopic Features. The cells are arranged in sheets, nests, or cords, and they tend to be pleomorphic with hyperchromatic nuclei and prominent nucleoli (Fig. 10–3). Mitoses are present and usually are numerous. Fields with more orderly neoplastic cells may be encountered, but the cells are more crowded than those of an adrenal adenoma. Microscopic foci of necrosis are characteristic (Fig. 10–3). Areas with enlarged bizarre cells having pleomorphic, giant nuclei may be interspersed. Invasion of blood vessels, vascular spaces, and the capsule (if present) is characteristic.

Differential diagnosis of benign and malignant adrenal cortical tumors can be difficult, and the subject has been much debated. Although the diagnosis of carcinoma may be obvious in the case of a large adrenal tumor with evidence of capsular or vascular invasion, increased mitotic activity, and cellular pleomorphism, the borderline tumor with respect to size or cellular abnormality can present a problem. Symington recommends that patients with tumors weighing 100 gm or more should have close follow-up and a guarded prognosis.[56] Feminizing tumors are a particularly difficult problem and, as pre-

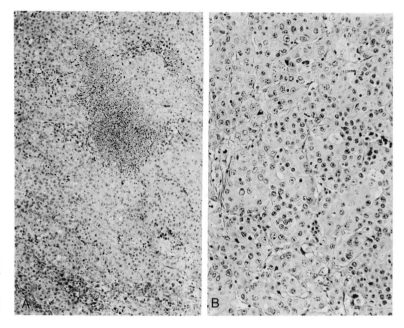

Figure 10–3. Carcinoma of adrenal cortex. A, Microscopic foci of necrosis. B, Sheets of closely packed, somewhat pleomorphic neoplastic cells. Compare with Figure 10–2. (A, × 75; B, × 125)

viously noted, Neville and O'Hare advise that all of them should be treated as carcinomas, irrespective of histologic features.[44]

Hough, Hollifield, and associates identified 12 clinical and pathologic criteria that were statistically significant in predicting metastasis; they include weight loss, tumor weight, presence of fibrous bands, diffuse pattern (growth of cells in sheets), vascular invasion, and cell necrosis.[28] No single criterion, including weight, reliably separated benign from malignant tumors.

Weiss did a comparative histologic study of 43 adrenocortical tumors and identified criteria useful in differentiating adenoma and carcinoma (nuclear grade, mitotic rate, atypical mitoses, clear cells, diffuse architecture, microscopic necrosis, and vascular or capsular invasion).[62] No tumor meeting fewer than three of these criteria metastasized, whereas 18 of 19 tumors meeting four or more criteria recurred or metastasized.

Slooten and co-workers analyzed seven microscopic criteria in 60 adrenocortical tumors and found that mitotic activity (greater than two per 10 high-power fields) and moderate or extensive regressive changes (necrosis, hemorrhage, fibrosis, calcification) were the best histologic predictors of malignancy.[50]

METASTATIC CARCINOMA

Although the incidence of metastatic cancer in the adrenal at autopsy is sizable, it is uncommon for a metastasis from an undiagnosed primary tumor in another organ to masquerade as primary carcinoma of the adrenal. Rarely, renal cell carcinoma may metastasize to the contralateral adrenal and simulate a nonfunctioning primary neoplasm of adrenal cortex. Adrenal carcinoma and renal cell carcinoma have many microscopic features in common, and differentiation on histologic grounds can be quite difficult. Metastatic renal cell carcinoma often has clear cells with abundant glycogen, but this feature may be lacking. According to Foucar and Dehner, the presence of papillations, tubules, or well-formed glands containing erythrocytes and debris suggests the diagnosis of metastatic renal cell carcinoma.[23] Intraoperative frozen sections are not likely to be helpful in differentiating the two neoplasms.

HYPERPLASIA OF ADRENAL MEDULLA

Hyperplasia may be defined as enlargement of the medulla with expansion into both alae and the tail of the gland (where medulla is not found normally) and decreased corticomedullary ratio. Hyperplasia has been firmly established as a clinicopathologic entity only in the last decade.[14, 17, 60] The condition is associated with multiple endocrine neoplasia (MEN) type II syndrome (see later). Medullary hyperplasia is responsible for excess secretion of catecholamines and their metabolites and may cause paroxysmal hypertension.

Gross Features. Medullary hyperplasia can be unilateral or bilateral. The gland may appear normal or enlarged; weights from 3.8 to 9.5 gm have been recorded.[14, 60] The medulla is pale gray with the usual consistency. Enlargement may be diffuse or nodular.[13] Size of the nodules is important; those greater than 1 cm should be diagnosed as pheochromocytoma.[13] Distribution of the medulla must be noted carefully; extension into the tail and both alae of the body is considered diagnostic.[60] To carry out planimetric analysis, the adrenal must be carefully transected by multiple parallel slices made at right angles to the long axis, at intervals of 3 to 4 mm, yielding 10 to 12 slices. Orientation of the slices must be maintained meticulously during processing. A random or indiscriminate cut at any juncture will preclude planimetry and can jeopardize the diagnosis.

Microscopic Features. Morphometric analysis of the medulla by light microscopy is crucial: demonstration of reduced corticomedullary ratio by planimetry and extension of the medulla into the tail of the gland and both alae of the crest are diagnostic.[17, 44, 60] Enlarged medullary cells with increased mitotic activity, nuclear pleomorphism, and cytoplasmic vacuoles or PAS-positive hyaline droplets also have been described, but none of these findings is considered specific since the changes also may be present in the normal medulla.[9, 17, 60]

PHEOCHROMOCYTOMA

Pheochromocytoma is a tumor of pheochromocytes, the specialized cells of the adrenal medulla that produce adrenalin and noradrenalin. The tumor has distinctive clinical manifestations that include paroxysmal or sustained hypertension, with attacks of headache, palpitation, and sweating. Pheochromocytoma is unquestionably a rare tumor. Nonetheless, it is a curable cause of hypertension, a fact that continues to stimulate screening of hypertensive patients.

Pheochromocytoma occurs as an isolated, sporadic tumor[32] or as part of a familial syndrome known as multiple endocrine neoplasia type II (MEN II), in association with medullary carcinoma of thyroid, first described by Sipple.[49] Subsequently, it has become clear that pheochromocytoma in MEN II arises in the setting of nodular or diffuse medullary hyperplasia of the adrenals and is likely to be bilateral.[13, 20, 36] MEN II is inherited as an autosomal dominant, and screening of relatives is mandatory.

Pheochromocytoma is known as the "10% tumor" because 10% are bilateral and 10% are extra-adrenal. Bilateral tumors may be synchronous or asynchronous. Ten per cent of pheochromocytomas also are said to be malignant. However, Neville and O'Hare[44] cite the incidence of malignancy as approximately 1% of all cases, a figure that coincides more closely with this author's experience. The extra-adrenal pheochromocytomas also are known as chromaffin paragangliomas; most of them arise in the para-vertebral regions in association with the system of chromaffin paraganglia. Common locations include the organ of Zuckerkandl, the retroperitoneum in the vicinity of the adrenal glands, the mediastinum, and the cervical region.

Some prefer the term *chromaffinoma* for the tumors of pheochromocytes that arise outside the adrenal medulla, but Sloper and Fox make the point that dual terminology for tumors of the same lineage has no particular merit and has the disadvantage of obscuring the identity of the extra-adrenal neoplasms.[51]

Pheochromocytoma also can arise in the urinary bladder;[16] in this site, it may cause attacks related to micturition, with compression of the tumor and release of catecholamines.

Gross Features. Pheochromocytomas vary widely in size, ranging from 1.4 gm to 3.6 kg.[44] The average weight is said to be 100 gm.[30] The tumors generally are encapsulated and well circumscribed; an attenuated remnant of cortex often can be identified at the periphery. Cut surfaces are bulging, soft, and pale gray, gray-pink, or reddish brown. Cysts, calcific areas, and foci of old hemorrhage may be encountered, and a central fibrous scar may be present. Upon exposure to dichromate solution between pH 5 and 6, pheochromocytoma promptly turns dark brown owing to formation of adreno-

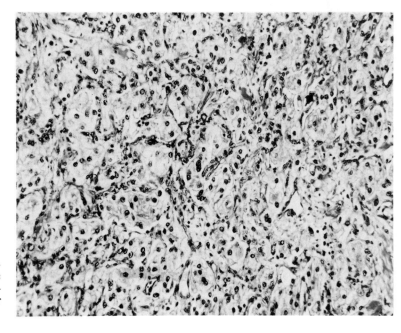

Figure 10–4. Pheochromocytoma of adrenal. Nests and cords of pheochromocytes are separated by thin fibrovascular septa. (× 250)

chromes, colored compounds formed by oxidation of the catecholamines contained within the tumor. If extraction and assay of catecholamines is to be performed, tissue should be frozen and stored at −20°C.

Microscopic Features. The tumors are composed of pleomorphic polyhedral or spindle cells that more or less resemble normal pheochromocytes and are arranged in cords and nests separated by thin fibrous septa with abundant vascular channels and sinusoidal spaces lined by tumor cells (Fig. 10–4). Alveolar patterns also may occur. Pleomorphism may be striking, with giant nuclei and bizarre cells, and mitotic figures, capsular invasion, and vascular invasion may be present. However, the only conclusive proof of malignancy is the presence of tumor in locations where pheochromocytes and chromaffin paraganglion cells are not normally found (see later).

With electron microscopy, the cells contain distinctive membrane-bound secretory granules in the cytoplasm, resembling those seen in the normal medulla.

Malignant Pheochromocytoma

Benign and malignant pheochromocytoma are indistinguishable in their gross and microscopic appearances. This fact has led to the dictum that the only absolute criterion for diagnosis of malignant pheochromocytoma is the presence of metastases in locations where chromaffin tissue is not found normally.[44] This view now is widely accepted. The usual sites of metastasis are liver, lymph nodes, lungs and bone. Successful removal of a malignant pheochromocytoma and its osseous metastasis has been reported.[48]

NONCHROMAFFIN TUMORS OF ADRENAL MEDULLA

The nonchromaffin tumors of the adrenal medulla are neuroblastoma, ganglioneuroblastoma, and ganglioneuroma. These neoplasms arise from elements of the sympathetic nervous system in the adrenal medulla. In normal development, neuroblasts migrate from the neural crest and colonize the adrenal medulla to give rise to the chromaffin and nonchromaffin cells (pheochromocytes and ganglion cells). The

neuroblasts differentiate successively into sympathicoblasts, sympathogonia, and, ultimately, the ganglion cells. Their neoplastic counterparts are neuroblastoma (a tumor of cells resembling neuroblasts), ganglioneuroblastoma (a mixture of neuroblasts and immature ganglion cells), and ganglioneuroma (a tumor of mature ganglion cells and their processes).

The histogenesis of nonchromaffin tumors parallels their embryogenesis. The concept that neuroblastoma, ganglioneuroblastoma, and ganglioneuroma represent stages of maturation in a spectrum of neural crest tumors is supported by morphologic evidence, experimental observations, and survival data. Signs of differentiation (including nuclear enlargement, increased cytoplasm, presence of cytoplasmic processes, formation of rosettes, and presence of mature ganglion cells) correlate well with survival.[40]

Neuroblastoma

The peak incidence of neuroblastoma is in the first few years of life. The most common site is the adrenal gland, but the neoplasm also occurs in association with sympathetic trunks and has been found in pelvis, abdomen, thorax, and neck. The tumor may secrete catecholamines, and vanillylmandelic acid (VMA) is found in the urine in a high percentage of cases.

In general, neuroblastoma is a highly malignant neoplasm, but, in a small group of patients, mortality is dramatically reduced by spontaneous regression of the tumor. In this subgroup (designated Stage IV-S), metastases are confined to liver, skin, or marrow.

Gross Features. Neuroblastoma is a discrete, soft, friable tumor that is usually encapsulated. Cut surfaces are bulging and pale gray and may exhibit scattered fresh hemorrhages. Foci of calcification are common, and areas of necrosis are observed in larger tumors.

Microscopic Features. Neuroblastoma is composed of small cells with hyperchromatic nuclei, scanty cytoplasm, and variable mitotic activity that are arranged in clusters or sheets in a loose fibrillar stroma. The cells resemble primitive neuroblasts but may show signs of differentiation with formation of cytoplasmic processes or nuclear enlargement and variation in size. The hallmark of

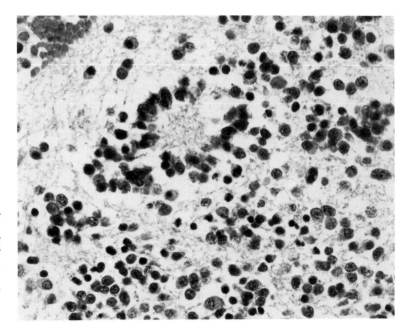

Figure 10–5. Neuroblastoma of adrenal. The Homer Wright rosette shows a peripheral rim of nuclei and a central mass of tangled neurofibrils. (× 500) From Warner NE: Basic Endocrine Pathology. Chicago, Year Book Medical Publishers, 1971, p 93, with permission.

the neuroblastoma is the Homer Wright rosette,[66] a spherical aggregate of neoplastic cells enclosing a central tangle of neurofibrils (Fig. 10–5). Though not consistently present, it is a valuable diagnostic feature.

Electron microscopy demonstrates diagnostic features in undifferentiated neuroblastoma, including dense-core neurosecretory granules of norepinephrine type and cytoplasmic filaments, neurotubules, and processes.

Ganglioneuroblastoma

Ganglioneuroblastoma is a rare malignant tumor of older children and adults. It contains elements of both neuroblastoma and ganglioneuroma, with gradations of malignant to benign histologic types. The presence of ganglion cells is associated with improved prognosis.

Gross Features. The appearance reflects the mixture of components that are present, and cut surfaces may range from soft, pale gray, and focally hemorrhagic to firm and pearly gray or white tissue. Calcific foci are characteristic.

Microscopic Features. The tumor has mixed patterns, with numerous rosettes, nerve fibers, and groups of elements resembling immature ganglion cells. The appear-

ance suggests a neuroblastoma that has undergone some degree of differentiation.

Ganglioneuroma

Ganglioneuroma is a benign tumor occurring mainly in older children and adults.

Gross Features. The tumor is encapsulated, firm, and pale gray or white, with firm cut surfaces that may have a watered-silk appearance.

Microscopic Features. Ganglioneuroma is composed of haphazardly arranged bundles of nerve fibers with interspersed ganglion cells scattered singly or in clusters. Mitoses are absent. The ganglion cells may be quite sparse. A careful search should be made for neuroblastic foci; their presence changes the diagnosis to neuroblastoma, which carries a much graver prognosis.

MYELOLIPOMA

Myelolipoma is a rare, benign adrenal tumor of uncertain histogenesis and composed of a mixture of fat and hematopoietic tissue. The tumor is almost always nonfunctioning and asymptomatic, presenting as an incidental finding at autopsy, surgery, or diagnostic imaging. The first removal of a symptomatic myelolipoma was recorded in 1957, when a 1100-gm tumor with recent hemorrhage was removed from a patient with a short history of acute abdominal pain.[19] More than a dozen examples have been reported since, associated with pain or dyspnea,[10, 21, 46, 47] hematuria,[6, 58, 63] nephrotic syndrome,[15] or Cushing's disease.[7] For the silent adrenal tumor discovered by CAT scan ("incidentaloma"), observation may be the treatment of choice.[25]

Gross Features. Myelolipomas range from minute nodules to large tumors weighing 2 kg or more.[21] They are well circumscribed, and the larger tumors are well demarcated from surrounding tissues. Cut surfaces are firm and variegated, with yellow zones intermixed with darker red areas.

Microscopic Features. The tumors are composed of a mixture of mature fat (yellow areas) and hematopoietic tissue (red areas) resembling normal marrow, with all three lines represented. Adipose tissue generally predominates. Foci of calcification or ossification may be encountered, and nodules of adrenocortical tissue have been described.[7]

CYST

Cysts of the adrenal are uncommon; most are encountered as an incidental finding at autopsy. With the advent of newer imaging techniques, asymptomatic cysts are being recognized more frequently during life,[12, 25, 65] and at least one cyst has been drained successfully by directed needle aspiration.[12] Four types are described: endothelial (basically lymphangioma or hemangioma), pseudocyst (secondary to adrenal hemorrhage in a previously normal gland or within an adrenal tumor), parasitic (most commonly echinococcal), and epithelial (due to malformation or to cystic change in an adenoma).[1, 5] These categories overlap, and a better classification may be the simple division into true cyst and pseudocyst.[27] Lymphangiomatous cyst and pseudocyst are the most common types.

Gross Features. Adrenal cysts are unilocular or multilocular; frequently, the wall has focal calcification.[34] Most are 10 cm or less, but cysts may achieve large sizes, and a diameter of 33 cm has been recorded.[22] Lymphangiomatous cysts are thin walled with a smooth lining and contain thin milky or clear fluid. Pseudocysts have a thick fibrous wall and a pigmented shaggy lining and contain pasty semisolid material.

Microscopic Features. Large cysts have a wall consisting of dense fibrous tissue; adrenal cortical tissue may be present focally. In the case of cyst arising in pheochromocytoma or adrenal adenoma, careful search may reveal islands of residual tumor in the wall. In the case of hemorrhagic pseudocyst, material consistent with organizing hematoma may be present.

References

1. Abeshouse GA, Goldstein RB, Abeshouse BS: Adrenal cysts: review of the literature and report of three cases. J Urol 81:711–719, 1959.
2. Ackerman LV, Rosai J: Surgical Pathology, 6th ed. St Louis, CV Mosby, 1981, p 703.
3. Bacon GE, Lowrey GH: Feminizing adrenal tumor in a six-year-old boy. J Clin Endocr Metab 25:1403–1406, 1965.
4. Bahu RM, Battifora H, Shambaugh G 3rd: Functional black adenoma of the adrenal gland. Light and electron microscopical study. Arch Pathol 98:139–142, 1974.
5. Barron SH, Emanuel B: Adrenal cyst. A case report and a review of the pediatric literature. J Pediatr 59:592–599, 1961.
6. Behan M, Martin EC, Muecke EC, Kazam E: Myelolipoma of the adrenal: two cases with ultrasound and CT findings. AJR 129:993–996, 1977.
7. Bennett BD, McKenna TJ, Hough AJ, et al: Adrenal myelolipoma associated with Cushing's disease. Am J Clin Pathol 73:443–447, 1980.
8. Bhettay E, Bonnici F: Pure oestrogen-secreting feminizing adrenocortical carcinoma. Arch Dis Child 52:241–243, 1977.
9. Bialestock D: Hyperplasia of the adrenal medulla in hypertension of children. Arch Dis Child 36:465–473, 1961.
10. Boudreaux D, Waisman J, Skinner DG, Low R: Giant adrenal myelolipoma and testicular interstitial cell tumor in a man with congenital 21-hydroxylase deficiency. Am J Surg Pathol 3:109–123, 1979.
11. Bradley EL 3rd: Primary and adjunctive therapy in carcinoma of the adrenal cortex. Surg Gynecol Obstet 141:507–516, 1975.
12. Buchino JJ, Dougherty HK, Shearer LT: Adrenal cyst. Arch Pathol Lab Med 109:377–379, 1985.
13. Carney JA, Sizemore GW, Sheps SG: Adrenal medullary disease in multiple endocrine neoplasia, type 2: pheochromocytoma and its precursors. Am J Clin Pathol 66:279–290, 1976.
14. Carney JA, Sizemore GW, Tyce GM: Bilateral adrenal medullary hyperplasia in multiple endocrine neoplasia, type 2: the precursor of bilateral pheochromocytoma. Mayo Clin Proc 50:3–10, 1975.
15. Damjanov I, Katz SM, Catalano E, et al: Myelolipoma in a heterotopic adrenal gland. Light and electron microscopic findings. Cancer 44:1350–1356, 1979.
16. Das S, Bulusu NV, Lowe P: Primary vesical pheochromocytoma. Urology 21:20–25, 1983.

17. DeLellis RA, Wolfe HJ, Gagel RF, et al: Adrenal medullary hyperplasia. A morphometric analysis in patients with familial medullary thyroid carcinoma. Am J Pathol 83:177–196, 1976.
18. Dobbie JW, Symington T: The human adrenal gland with special reference to the vasculature. J Endocrinol 34:479–489, 1966.
19. Dyckman J, Freedman D: Myelolipoma of the adrenal gland with clinical features and surgical excision. J Mount Sinai Hosp 24:793, 1957.
20. Farndon JR, Fagraeus L, Wells SA Jr: Recent developments in the management of phaeochromocytoma. In IDA Johnston, NW Thompson (eds), International Medical Reviews. Endocrine Surgery. London, Butterworths, 1983, pp 189–202.
21. Filobbos SA, Seddon JA: Myelolipoma of the adrenal. Br J Surg 67:147–148, 1980.
22. Foster DG: Adrenal cysts. Review of the literature and report of case. Arch Surg 92:131–143, 1966.
23. Foucar E, Dehner LP: Renal cell carcinoma occurring with contralateral adrenal metastasis: a clinical and pathological trap. Arch Surg 114:959–963, 1979.
24. Gabrilove JL, Sharma DC, Wotiz HH, Dorfman RI: Feminizing adrenocortical tumors in the male. A review of 52 cases including a case report. Medicine 44:37–79, 1965.
25. Geelhoed GW, Druy EM: Management of the adrenal "incidentaloma." Surgery 92:866–874, 1982.
26. Harrison JH, Mahoney EM, Bennett AH: Tumors of the adrenal cortex. Cancer 32:1227–1235, 1973.
27. Hodges FV, Ellis FR: Cystic lesions of the adrenal glands. Arch Pathol 66:53, 1958.
28. Hough AJ, Hollifield JW, Page DL, Hartmann WH: Prognostic factors in adrenal cortical tumors. A mathematical analysis of clinical and morphological data. Am J Clin Pathol 72:390–399, 1979.
29. Howard CP, Takahashi H, Hayles AB: Feminizing adrenal adenoma in a boy. Mayo Clin Proc 52:354–357, 1977.
30. Hume DM: Pheochromocytoma in the adult and in the child. Am J Surg 99:458–496, 1960.
31. Huvos AG, Hajdu SI, Brasfield RD, Foote FW Jr: Adrenal cortical carcinoma. Clinicopathologic study of 34 cases. Cancer 25:354–361, 1970.
32. Kalff V, Shapiro B, Lloyd R, et al: Bilateral pheochromocytomas. J Endocrinol Invest 7:387–392, 1984.
33. Kay S: Hyperplasia and neoplasia of the adrenal gland. Pathol Annu 11:103–139, 1976.
34. Kearney GP, Mahoney EM, Maher E, Harrison JH: Functioning and nonfunctioning cysts of the adrenal cortex and medulla. Am J Surg 134:363–368, 1977.
35. Lewinsky BS, Grigor KM, Symington T, Neville AM: The clinical and pathologic features of "non-hormonal" adrenocortical tumors. Report of twenty new cases and review of the literature. Cancer 33:778–790, 1974.
36. Lips CJ, Minder WH, Leo JR, et al: Evidence of multicentric origin of the multiple endocrine neoplasia syndrome type 2a (Sipple's syndrome) in a large family in the Netherlands. Diagnostic and therapeutic implications. Am J Med 64:569–578, 1978.
37. Lipsett MB, Hertz R, Ross GT: Clinical and pathophysiologic aspects of adrenocortical carcinoma. Am J Med 35:374–383, 1963.
38. Macadam RF: Black adenoma of the human adrenal cortex. Cancer 27:116–119, 1971.
39. Macfarlane DA: Cancer of the adrenal cortex. Ann R Coll Surg Engl 23:155, 1958.
40. Mäkinen J: Microscopic patterns as a guide to prognosis of neuroblastoma in childhood. Cancer 29:1637–1646, 1972.
41. Mitschke H, Saeger W, Breustedt HJ: Feminizing adrenocortical tumor. Histological and ultrastructural study. Virchows Arch [A] 377:301–309, 1977.
42. Nelson AA: Accessory adrenal cortical tissue. Arch Pathol 27:955–965, 1939.
43. Neville AM, Mackay AM: The structure of the human adrenal cortex in health and disease. Clin Endocrinol Metab 1:361, 1972.
44. Neville AM, O'Hare MJ: Aspects of structure, function, and pathology. In VHT James (ed), The Adrenal Gland. New York, Raven Press, 1979, pp 32, 52–55.
45. Neville AM, Symington T: Pathology of primary aldosteronism. Cancer 19:1854–1868, 1966.
46. Newman PH, Silen W: Myelolipoma of the adrenal gland. Report of the third case of a symptomatic tumor and review of the literature. Arch Surg 97:637–639, 1968.
47. Parsons L Jr, Thompson JE: Symptomatic myelolipoma of the adrenal gland. Report of a case and review of the literature. N Engl J Med 260:12–15, 1959.
48. ReMine WH, Estes JE Jr, Dockerty MB, Priestley JT: Hemiplegia resulting from pheochromocytoma; report of case. JAMA 152:808–811, 1953.
49. Sipple JH: The association of pheochromocytoma with carcinoma of the thyroid gland. Am J Med 31:163–166, 1961.
50. Slooten HV, Schaberg A, Smeenk D, Moolenaar AJ: Morphologic characteristics of benign and malignant adrenocortical tumors. Cancer 55:766–773, 1985.
51. Sloper JC, Fox B: The adrenal glands and the extra-adrenal chromaffin tissue. In W St C Symmers (ed), Systemic Pathology, Vol 4. London, Churchill Livingstone, 1978, p 1965.
52. Snaith AH: A case of feminizing adrenal tumor in a girl. J Clin Endocrinol Metab 18:318, 1958.
53. Sommers SC: Adrenal glands. In JM Kissane (ed), Anderson's Pathology, Vol 2. St Louis, CV Mosby, 1985, p 1441.
54. Studzinski GP, Hay DC, Symington T: Observations on the weight of the human adrenal gland and the effect of preparations of corticotropin of different purity on the weight and morphology of the human adrenal gland. J Clin Endocrinol Metab 23:248–254, 1963.
55. Sullivan M, Boileau M, Hodges CV: Adrenal cortical carcinoma. J Urol 120:660–665, 1978.
56. Symington T: Functional Pathology of the Human Adrenal Gland. Edinburgh, Livingstone, 1969, pp 13, 90, 97, 101, 158–159.
57. Tang CK, Gray GF: Adrenocortical neoplasms. Prognosis and morphology. Urology 5:691–695, 1975.
58. Tulcinsky DB, Deutsch V, Bubis JJ: Myelolipoma of the adrenal gland. Br J Surg 57:465–467, 1970.
59. Tyrrell JB, Brooks RM, Fitzgerald PA, et al: Cushing's disease. Selective trans-sphenoidal resection of pituitary microadenomas. N Engl J Med 298:753–758, 1978.
60. Visser JW, Axt R: Bilateral adrenal medullary hy-

perplasia: a clinicopathological entity. J Clin Pathol 28:298–304, 1975.

61. Visser JW, Boeijinga JK, Meer CV: A functioning black adenoma of the adrenal cortex: a clinocopathological entity. J Clin Pathol 27:955–959, 1974.

62. Weiss LM: Comparative histologic study of 43 metastasizing and nonmetastasizing adrenocortical tumors. Am J Surg Pathol 8:163–169, 1984.

63. Whittaker LD: Myelolipoma of the adrenal gland. Surgical removal. Arch Surg 97:628–631, 1968.

64. Willis RA: The Borderland of Embryology and Pathology. London, Butterworth, 1958, pp 326–329.

65. Wilson JM, Woodhead DM, Smith RB: Adrenal cysts. Diagnosis and management. Urology 4:248–253, 1974.

66. Wright JH: Neurocytoma or neuroblastoma, a kind of tumor not generally recognized. J Exp Med 12:556, 1910.

PETER NICHOLS, M.D.

CHAPTER 11   *Pathology of Cancer of Penis*

EMBRYOLOGY, ANATOMY, AND HISTOLOGY

The penis is composed of three parallel cylindrical erectile bodies, the right and left corpus cavernosum and the corpus cavernosum urethrae (or corpus spongiosum). The three corpora and the glans are all covered by a tunica albuginea, except for the more proximal portion of the corpus spongiosum in the area of the bulbous urethra. Proximally, the tunica albuginea of the corpora cavernosa are fused to the inferior rami of the ischium and pubis. The corpus cavernosum urethrae begins as the bulbous urethra and lies beneath the corpora cavernosa in a groove created by the fusion of the two. The three corpora unite anteriorly and inferiorly to the pubic symphysis to form the mobile portion of the penis. They terminate in the glans penis, which covers all three distally. On the mobile part of the penis the integument separates a thin, delicate, hairless skin from the tunica albuginea. Interestingly, this integument is almost devoid of fat.[56]

Development of the external male genitalia, including the penis, is complete at about 12 weeks of gestation (crown-rump embryonal length of 50 mm). The genital tubercle, which arises ventral to the cloacal membrane early in the fourth week, is the first recognizable sign of the penis. The urethra develops from the endodermal cloacal membrane via a structure known as the endodermal urethral plate, which migrates along the ventral surface of the developing phallus. All of the urethra is derived from

endoderm except for the most distal portion, which is ectodermal in origin and is created by growth of superficial epithelium into the glans, where it meets the urethral plate. The bulbourethral glands and the glands of Littre also are believed to be endodermal in origin. The corpus cavernosum urethrae is of mesodermal origin and develops as a result of proliferation of mesenchyme around the penile urethra. The corpora cavernosa also are of mesodermal derivation.[24]

The blood supply to the penis is derived almost entirely from the internal pudendal artery, a branch of the internal iliac artery. The former gives rise to variably named branches, one of which is referred to by some as the penile artery. This in turn gives rise to four branches: the artery of the penile bulb, the spongiosal artery, the cavernosal artery, and the dorsal artery of the penis.[20, 56]

The venous outflow occurs via the deep veins of the penis, which drain from the proximal portions of the corpora cavernosa; the deep dorsal vein, which drains the glans, the corpus spongiosum, and the peripheral portion of the corpus cavernosum; and the superficial dorsal vein, which drains the skin and subcutaneous structures.[20, 56]

Because most tumors of the penis spread by means of lymphatics, the lymphatic drainage is most important in predicting sites of metastasis and therefore planning therapy. The areas drained include skin and subcutaneous tissue, corpora, and the glans. Lymphatics draining each of these sites anastomose with lymphatics draining the others. Lymphatic vessels within the glans form a plexus that drains ventrally and then

207

passes on the sides of the penis to join lymphatics along the deep dorsal vein. These lymphatics drain to a plexus at the root of the penis and then to the external iliac lymph nodes, superficial inguinal lymph nodes, and deep inguinal lymph nodes in the femoral canal. Lymphatics draining the skin lie along the superficial dorsal vein, decussate freely at the base of the penis, and drain to the superficial inguinal lymph nodes on either side. These lymphatics also anastomose with those along the deep dorsal vein. Lymphatics of the distal portions of the corpora are distributed in a pathway similar to those of the glans. The lymphatics of the proximal corpora and urethra, including the membranous and the prostatic portions, drain to the internal iliac lymph nodes.[20, 56]

PRENEOPLASTIC LESIONS OF EPITHELIUM

Squamous cell carcinoma in situ is the most significant preneoplastic lesion found on the penis. When this disease occurs on the mucosal surface (including the prepuce, sulcus, corona, frenulum, urethral meatus, or glans) it is called erythroplasia of Queyrat.[22] When it occurs on the cutaneous surface, the condition is referred to as Bowen's disease.[6, 7]

Bowen's disease (Fig. 11–1) was first described in 1912 with a report of two cases, one on the buttock and another on the right calf.[6, 7] Since that time numerous cases have been described, and some of these have occurred on the penis. The disease affects all races and usually presents in middle or old age. The lesions appear grossly as crusting or ulcerating plaques 1 to 2 cm in diameter. About a third of the patients have multiple lesions.[5, 21]

Microscopically, Bowen's disease has all the features of squamous carcinoma in situ. The epidermis is acanthotic with broadening and lengthening of the rete ridges to the point where dermal papillae are effaced. Parakeratosis is marked and irregular, and there is disarray of the normal maturing epithelial cells. The neoplastic cells are highly varied in their appearance, and mitoses are prominent throughout all layers. Dyskeratotic cells, or cells with abundant eosinophilic cytoplasm and hyperchromatic nuclei, are also present throughout all cell layers. The lesion can extend into adnexal structures but is usually well demarcated from the underlying dermis by a distinct basement membrane. All agree that the tendency for invasion is low; Graham and Hel-

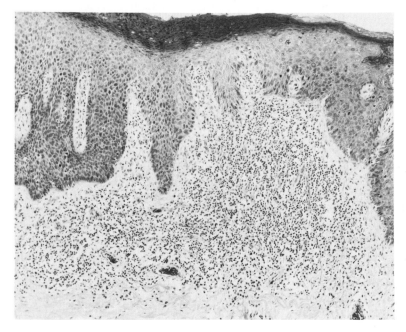

Figure 11–1. Bowen's disease. The epidermis is thickened, with prominent parakeratosis; the cells are disorganized and pleomorphic, with mitoses in the most superficial layer.

wig report microinvasion in 5.2% of patients in their series.[21] Invasion appears to occur only after a long history of a lesion, and metastases are likely only if the lesion has become deeply invasive.[21] Once invasion is identified, the prognosis becomes that of squamous cell carcinoma.

Erythroplasia of Queyrat is a lesion histologically identical to Bowen's disease, and it is found on mucosal surfaces of uncircumcised men. Because of its virtually identical morphologic appearance, some choose to classify this lesion as Bowen's disease. The primary argument for keeping these lesions separate comes from Graham and Helwig, who identified a strong relationship with systemic cancer in Bowen's disease but found no such association with erythroplasia of Queyrat.[21, 22] Subsequent studies have not resolved the question. Peterka suggested an association with visceral cancer only when the Bowen's lesions were on skin normally protected from the sun.[45] A study by Andersen and associates indicated that there was no association between Bowen's disease and visceral cancer,[3] whereas the findings of Callen and Headington[9] supported the contention of Graham and Helwig.

Evidence at this time seems to favor the observation by Graham and Helwig, and it appears most reasonable to continue to distinguish between Bowen's disease and erythroplasia of Queyrat. Because of identical morphologic appearance it is important to clinically document the site of the lesion. The pathologist can make a clear distinction only if there are skin appendages in the biopsy, affirming its skin origin.

Clinically, erythroplasia of Queyrat occurs in middle-aged or older noncircumcised men; 65% of patients in the series of Graham and Helwig were between the ages of 40 and 69. The range was 20 to 80 years, with a median of 51 years. In almost half the patients, the lesions were multiple, with an average size of 1.0 to 1.9 cm (ranging from 0.2 to 3.5 cm). The lesion is usually described as a bright red, shiny, velvety plaque. Despite this distinctive clinical appearance, only 15 of 100 patients reported by Graham and Helwig had the correct diagnosis made prior to biopsy. Like Bowen's disease, the tendency to invade is low (10% from the Graham and Helwig series), but once the

invasion was present, the tumor could metastasize.[22]

One of the most common lesions clinically confused with erythroplasia of Queyrat is balanitis circumscripta plasmacellularis.[64] Morphologically, balanitis is characterized by a thin epidermis, diamond-shaped keratinocytes, and erythrocytes in the epidermis. In addition, there is a dense band-like chronic inflammatory infiltrate in the upper dermis.

Recently Wade, Kopf, and associates described a lesion they named bowenoid papulosis of the penis. Histologically, it showed squamous cell carcinoma in situ, but it was clinically distinct from Bowen's disease or erythroplasia of Queyrat.[30, 59, 60] The 28 men they first described ranged in age from 21 to 38, and all but one had been circumcised as infants. The patients presented with multiple erythematous papules (from 2 to 10 mm in diameter) on the glans or shaft of the penis or in both areas. Only one patient had symptoms of pruritus, and in no case was a diagnosis of carcinoma in situ clinically considered. All patients had resolution of these lesions following surgical excision or topical therapy.

Since the first report, accounts of additional cases have been published, and in only one instance has progression to Bowen's disease been noted.[15] This patient was atypical because he was 42 at the time that bowenoid papulosis was first diagnosed. Kao and Graham suggest that the lesions can be distinguished from carcinoma in situ histologically.[28] They claim that atypical keratinocytes are not found throughout the epidermis in bowenoid papulosis. The clinical history is important, and a diagnosis of bowenoid papulosis should not be made without it.

The histogenesis of the lesion is still uncertain. About one third of patients reported have had genital herpes, and another third have had condylomata acuminata. The lesions occur in clusters or in a linear distribution, suggesting an infectious origin. A recent review by Kimura argues for a viral etiology and suggests that the most probable cause is a human papilloma virus.[29] Viral particles have been demonstrated with electron microscopy.

The therapeutic approach for patients with this disorder is clearly a conservative one. Studies should better define the malignant potential of this lesion in the near future.

NEOPLASMS OF EPITHELIUM

Carcinoma of the penis is a relatively rare tumor in the United States and represents less than 1% of cancers.[41, 54] Worldwide, the tumor is common in many Latin,[52] African,[16] and southeast Asian countries. The tumor is rare in young men, and in most series the peak occurrence is around the age of 60.

A definite association has been shown between the occurrence of this tumor and circumcision, and uncircumcised men have the highest incidence of disease. The age at circumcision appears to play a role. In the Muslim faith, circumcision is performed just prior to puberty, and in those patients (circumcised around 10 years of age) the tumor does occur but at a lower frequency than in uncircumcised men. The tumor is virtually nonexistent in men circumcised at birth, and reports of penile cancers rarely occur in this group.[40]

A less clear but perhaps significant association is that of carcinoma of the uterine cervix and carcinoma of the penis. Several studies have suggested a definite relationship.[23, 32–34] An increased risk of cervical cancer in wives of men with penile cancer has been reported.[23] Because of the low incidence of penile carcinoma in this country, the converse would be difficult to demonstrate, but in China, where both cancers are common, a link is suggested.[33, 34] It would be useful to study the association in uncircumcised men in this country.

Patients usually present with a large, exophytic fungating mass, a nonhealing ulcer, or a verrucous lesion. Carcinoma is almost always found on the mucosal surfaces of the penis and is rare on the skin. In many patients it is difficult to determine the exact site of origin because of the size of the tumor. It is common for the lesion to be infected, leading to local induration and regional lymphadenopathy. Such lymphadenopathy results in inaccurate clinical staging of the lymph nodes, making pathologic evaluation of regional lymph nodes critical to proper staging of these carcinomas. In contrast, patients also have been observed with clinically unsuspected metastatic carcinoma in lymph nodes.[14]

The majority of penile carcinomas are of squamous cell type, usually well or moderately well differentiated. The tumors occur in two basic patterns: infiltrating cords of tumor with an adjacent stromal reaction and rounded solid masses with a pushing border.[18] Both basal cell carcinoma and melanoma may occur on the penis, but these conditions are rare.[19, 58]

Accurate pathologic and clinical staging is important in evaluating patients with penile carcinoma because it offers prognostic information. Jackson has proposed a staging system, the value of which has been demonstrated by deKernion et al.[14, 27] In that system, Stage I tumors are confined to the glans or prepuce and Stage II tumors extend onto the shaft of the penis. Stage III tumors have operable involvement of lymph nodes of the groin, and Stage IV tumors have distant metastasis, inoperable groin lymph nodes, or extension beyond the penile shaft. Using this system, deKernion showed the following three-year disease-free survival: Stage I, 95%; Stage II, 67%; Stage III, 29%; and Stage IV, 0%.

Verrucous carcinoma is a rare variant of squamous cell carcinoma (Fig. 11–2). Patients with this neoplasm typically present with a large, bulky tumor that has a mushroom appearance. Histologically, it is characterized by papillary fronds surfaced by densely keratinized, well-differentiated squamous epithelium. The deep margin is sharply outlined and composed of well-oriented but expanded rete ridges. The squamous epithelium must be well differentiated throughout to be considered a verrucous carcinoma.[2, 31]

Giant condyloma acuminatum of Buschke and Löwenstein is strikingly similar in appearance to verrucous carcinoma.[12, 36] Ackerman[2] believes that in fact they are the same tumor.[12, 31, 53] Mostofi, on the other hand, suggests that the two tumors are distinct and can usually be differentiated by using subtle histologic criteria.[43] Despite the controversy concerning their separation, the two lesions behave in a similar manner. That is, they recur locally, have the potential to invade deeply, and rarely metastasize.[8, 31] In addition, both lesions are ineffectively treated by podophyllin; in fact, podophyllin induces a cytologic change, making the distinction from a more conventional squamous carcinoma difficult.[37]

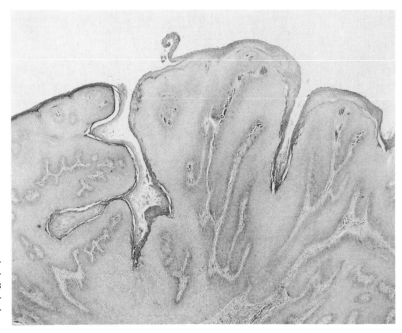

Figure 11–2. Verrucous carcinoma. The lesion is characterized by broad papillary fronds surfaced by thickened, well-differentiated hyperkeratotic epithelium.

SOFT TISSUE TUMORS

Soft tissue neoplasms of the penis are uncommon. In a literature review published in 1984, only 23 leiomyosarcomas were found.[26] Almost all soft tissue tumors have been observed in the penis; however, it is interesting that no lipomas or liposarcomas have been reported. A single report of an angiomyolipoma was published by Chaitin and associates in 1984.[10]

As one might expect, based on the vascularity of the penis, vascular neoplasms are the most common mesenchymal tumors.[13, 49] In the largest report of soft tissue tumors of the penis, Dehner and Smith identified 19 out of a total of 46 as angiomatous tumors.[13] Of these, most were benign, occurred on the glans of young patients, and were hemangiomas. Seven were malignant: four Kaposi's sarcomas and three malignant hemangioendotheliomas.

Kaposi's sarcoma involving the penis usually appears first on the glans as a purplish to red-brown, irregular, flat cutaneous lesion measuring from several millimeters to several centimeters.[11, 35] It then progresses through a plaque stage and eventually forms a nodular lesion. Histogenetically, the cells appear to originate from endothelium or perhaps from the vascular wall. The presence of factor VIII antigen in the cytoplasm and the ultrastructural features of the cells support this concept.[39] Histologically, the tumors are composed of groups or cords of cells with a predilection for adnexal structures. The cells are spindle-shaped and are separated by slit-like spaces that often contain erythrocytes. With progression, the groups and cords of cells take on the configuration of nodules of disorganized spindle cells (Fig. 11–3). Hemosiderin, usually lying free or in macrophages, is a characteristic feature. Cells that contain small eosinophilic globules are almost always present.

Recently, Kaposi's sarcoma has taken on increased significance because of its relationship to the acquired immunodeficiency syndrome (AIDS). The incidence of the neoplasm has dramatically increased and can be expected to continue to rise. Presentation on the penis has not increased disproportionately to presentation at other sites. The biologic behavior of this tumor in AIDS patients appears to be similar to the most aggressive form of Kaposi's sarcoma that occurs in young patients without AIDS. In the AIDS patient, Kaposi's sarcoma does not appear to be a morphologically distinct tumor.

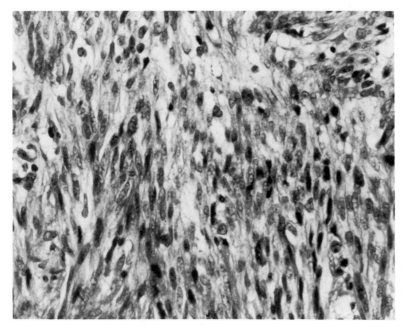

Figure 11–3. Kaposi's sarcoma. Atypical spindle cells are characteristic of Kaposi's sarcoma and are separated by slit-like vascular spaces.

A second vascular tumor reported in Dehner's review of sarcomas, malignant hemangioendothelioma, appears in the last several years to have been partially clarified in the literature. None of Dehner's three patients died of the tumor, although a malignant course has been reported with these lesions.[63] Weiss and Enzinger reported three penile tumors that they designated as epithelioid hemangioendotheliomas.[61] These tumors are associated with a vessel (the dorsal vein when it occurs in the penis) and are frequently mistaken for metastatic carcinoma. The cell of origin appears to be an endothelial cell, and a "salient" feature is the "epithelial quality of the endothelial cells." Weiss and Enzinger were able to predict a malignant course from the microscopic appearance in many, but not all, of the tumors they reported. Therefore, they placed the tumor in a borderline category with regard to its malignant potential. They suggest a possible relationship between this lesion and a rare tumor on the penis diagnosed as epithelioid hemangioma or Kimura's disease.[51, 57]

In Dehner's series, neural tumors were the second most common soft tissue neoplasms. These tumors occurred in patients up to 36 years of age and were usually on the penile shaft. The only malignant neural tumors they reported were schwannomas in patients with probable von Recklinghausen's disease.

Tumors of muscle origin include leiomyoma, leiomyosarcoma, and rhabdomyosarcoma, which are extremely rare.[4, 50] None had unusual or distinctive histologic features that separated them from other tumors of muscular origin occurring in different locations. A recent report by Isa and associates reviewed all cases of leiomyosarcoma in the literature[26] and found that they could be divided into superficial and deep tumors. Those that were superficial tended to be smaller, grow more slowly, recur locally, and have a good prognosis. The deep tumors had an aggressive behavior in spite of radical surgery. Deep tumors disseminated widely, and most patients were dead of disease within one to two years. These observations confirm the findings reported by Pratt and Ross.[48]

Fibrous tumors and lymphomas are rare, but both have presented as penile tumors. An unusual tumor known as epithelioid sarcoma, described in the early 1970s by Enzinger,[17] has rarely been reported on the penis. In one instance this tumor mimicked Peyronie's disease in its clinical presentation. This interesting case report emphasizes the importance of distinguishing sarcomas from Peyronie's disease,[42] a benign disorder that appears to begin in the loose areolar tissue between the corpora and the tunica albuginea.[55] Microscopically, the changes are a progressive fibrosis associated with perivascular inflammation, sometimes with areas of ossification and bone formation.

In summary, soft tissue tumors are unusual in the penis. The only fatty tumor is an angiomyolipoma.[9] In older patients, sarcomas are more likely to occur on the penile shaft, where they most often present as a rapidly growing tender mass. Interestingly, most sarcomas are unlikely to metastasize, but they do recur locally. On the other hand, benign tumors tend to occur on the prepuce or glans, are not tender, and usually are found in younger patients.[13]

METASTATIC LESIONS

Metastatic tumor to the penis is unusual.[47] Pond and Wade speculate that the vascularity in the spleen (another organ in which tumor metastases are uncommon) and in the penis may be similar and that this vascularity somehow protects against metastases.[46] Most often, patients present with priapism or edema, which may obscure a tumor mass. Bladder and prostatic cancers account for about 60% of the reported cases of metastatic carcinoma, with the gastrointestinal tract, kidney, testis, and respiratory tract accounting for almost all of the remaining cases. The greatest significance of a penile metastasis is its prognostic implication: with few exceptions, patients die within six months of the discovery of the metastasis.

Although all regions of the penis have been described as sites of metastasis, the corpora cavernosa seem to be the most commonly reported sites. Review of the literature revealed no case with involvement of the corpus spongiosum without involvement elsewhere.[62] This observation is used by some for evidence to suggest that instrumentation does not play a role as a cause of metastasis.[44] Several authors have extensively reviewed possible mechanisms of metastasis.[1, 44]

It is unusual for metastasis to occur without a history of the patient having carcinoma elsewhere. However, it has been pointed out by several authors that it is not unusual to mistake a metastasis for "Peyronie's disease, edema, thrombosis of the corpora cavernosa or deep dorsal vein, primary carcinoma, and inflammatory lesions."[25, 38]

References

1. Abeshouse BS, Abeshouse GA: Metastatic tumors of the penis: a review of the literature and a report of two cases. J Urol 86:99–112, 1961.
2. Ackerman LV: Verrucous carcinoma of oral cavity. Surgery 23:670–678, 1948.
3. Andersen SL, Nielsen A, Reymann F: Relationship between Bowen disease and internal malignant tumors. Arch Dermatol 108:367–370, 1973.
4. Ashley DJB, Edwards EC: Sarcoma of the penis. Leiomyosarcoma of the penis: report of a case with a review of the literature on sarcoma of the penis. Br J Surg 45:170–179, 1957.
5. Berger BW, Hori Y: Multicentric Bowen's disease of the genitalia: spontaneous regression of lesions. Arch Dermatol 114:1698–1699, 1978.
6. Bowen JT: Precancerous dermatoses: a study of two cases of chronic atypical epithelial proliferation. J Cutan Dis 30:214–255, 1912.
7. Bowen JT: Precancerous dermatoses: a sixth case of a type recently described. J Cutan Dis 33:787–802, 1915.
8. Boxer RJ, Skinner DG: Condylomata acuminata and squamous cell carcinoma. Urology 9:72–78, 1977.
9. Callen JP, Headington J: Bowen's and non-Bowen's squamous intraepidermal neoplasia of the skin. Relationship to internal malignancy. Arch Dermatol 116:422–426, 1980.
10. Chaitin BA, Goldman RL, Linker DG: Angiomyolipoma of penis. Urology 23:305–306, 1984.
11. Cox FH, Helwig EB: Kaposi's sarcoma. Cancer 12:289–298, 1959.
12. Dawson DF, Duckworth JK, Bernhardt H, Young JM: Giant condyloma and verrucous carcinoma of the genital area. Arch Pathol 79:225–231, 1965.
13. Dehner LP, Smith BH: Soft tissue tumors of the penis. A clinicopathologic study of 46 cases. Cancer 25:1431–1447, 1970.
14. deKernion JB, Tynberg P, Persky L, Fegen JP: Carcinoma of the penis. Cancer 32:1256–1262, 1973.
15. De Villez RL, Stevens CS: Bowenoid papules of the genitalia. A case progressing to Bowen's disease. J Am Acad Dermatol 3:149–152, 1980.
16. Dodge OG, Linsell CA: Carcinoma of the penis in Uganda and Kenya Africans. Cancer 16:1255–1263, 1963.
17. Enzinger FM: Epithelioid sarcoma. A sarcoma simulating a granuloma or a carcinoma. Cancer 26:1029–1041, 1970.
18. Frew ID, Jefferies JD, Swinney J: Carcinoma of the penis. Br J Urol 39:398–404, 1967.
19. Fronstin MH, Hutcheson JB: Malignant melanoma of the penis: a report of two cases. Br J Urol 41:324–326, 1969.
20. Goldstein I, Krane RJ: Blood vessels and lymphatics of the penis. In DI Abramson, PB Dorbin (eds). Blood Vessels and Lymphatics in Organ Systems. Orlando, FL, Academic Press, 1984, pp 552–560.
21. Graham JH, Helwig EB: Bowen's disease and its relationship to systemic cancer. Arch Dermatol 83:738–758, 1961.
22. Graham JH, Helwig EB: Erythroplasia of Queyrat. A clinicopathologic and histochemical study. Cancer 32:1396–1414, 1973.
23. Graham S, Priore R, Graham M, et al: Genital cancer in wives of penile cancer patients. Cancer 44:1870–1874, 1979.
24. Hamilton WJ, Boyd JD, Mossman HW: Human Embryology: Prenatal Development of Form and Func-

tion, 4th ed. Cambridge, W Heffer & Sons; Baltimore, Williams & Wilkins, 1982, pp 354–355, 413–419.

25. Hayes WT, Young JM: Metastatic carcinoma of the penis. J Chronic Dis 20:891–895, 1967.

26. Isa SS, Almaraz R, Magovern J: Leiomyosarcoma of the penis. Case report and review of the literature. Cancer 54:939–942, 1984.

27. Jackson SM: The treatment of carcinoma of the penis. Br J Surg 53:33–45, 1966.

28. Kao GF, Graham JH: Bowenoid papulosis. Int J Dermatol 21:445–446, 1982.

29. Kimura S: Bowenoid papulosis of the genitalia. Int J Dermatol 21:432–436, 1982.

30. Kopf AW, Bart RS: Tumor Conference No. 11: Multiple Bowenoid papules of the penis: a new entity? J Dermatol Surg Oncol 3:265–269, 1977.

31. Kraus FT, Perez-Mesa C: Verrucous carcinoma. Clinical and pathologic study of 105 cases involving oral cavity, larynx and genitalia. Cancer 19:26–38, 1966.

32. Levine RU, Crum CP, Herman E, et al: Cervical papillomavirus infection and intraepithelial neoplasia: a study of male sexual partners. Obstet Gynecol 64:16–20, 1984.

33. Li JY, Li FP, Blot WJ, et al: Correlation between cancers of the uterine cervix and penis in China. JNCI 69:1063–1065, 1982.

34. Li JY, Li FP, Blot WF, et al: Correlation between cancers of the uterine cervix and penis. JNCI 71:427–428, 1983.

35. Linker D, Lieberman P, Grabstald H: Kaposi's sarcoma of genitourinary tract. Urology 5:684–687, 1975.

36. Loewenstein LW: Carcinoma-like condylomata acuminata of penis. Med Clin North Am 23:789–795, 1939.

37. Machacek GF, Weakley DR: Giant condylomata acuminata of Buschke and Lowenstein. Arch Dermatol 82:41–47, 1960.

38. McCrea LE, Tobias GL: Metastatic disease of the penis. J Urol 80:489–500, 1958.

39. McNutt NS, Fletcher V, Conant MA: Early lesions of Kaposi's sarcoma in homosexual men. An ultrastructural comparison with other vascular proliferations in skin. Am J Pathol 111:62–77, 1983.

40. Melmed EP, Pyne JR: Carcinoma of the penis in a Jew circumcised in infancy. Br J Surg 54:729–731, 1967.

41. Merrin CE: Cancer of the penis. Cancer 45:1973–1979, 1980.

42. Moore SW, Wheeler JE, Hefter LG: Epithelioid sarcoma masquerading as Peyronie's disease. Cancer 35:1706–1710, 1975.

43. Mostofi FK, Price EB Jr: Tumors and tumor-like lesions of the penis. In Tumors of the Male Genital System. Washington, DC, Armed Forces Institute of Pathology. 2nd series. Fasc. 11, 1973, pp 277–283.

44. Paquin AJ Jr, Roland SI: Secondary carcinoma of the penis: a review of the literature and a report of nine new cases. Cancer 9:626–632, 1956.

45. Peterka ES, Lynch FW, Goltz RW: An association between Bowen's disease and internal cancer. Arch Dermatol 84:623–629, 1961.

46. Pond HS, Wade JC: Urinary obstruction secondary to metastatic carcinoma of the penis: a case report and review of the literature. J Urol 102:333–335, 1969.

47. Powell BL, Craig JB, Muss HB: Secondary malignancies of the penis and epididymis: a case report and review of the literature. J Clin Oncol 3:110–116, 1985.

48. Pratt RM, Ross RTA: Leiomyosarcoma of the penis. A report of a case. Br J Surg 56:870–872, 1969.

49. Rabson SM: Angioma of corpus cavernosum penis. J Urol 45:111–117, 1941.

50. Ramos JZ, Pack GT: Primary embryonal rhabdomyosarcoma of the penis in a 2-year-old child. J Urol 96:928–932, 1966.

51. Rao RN, Spurlock BO, Witherington R: Angiolymphoid hyperplasia with eosinophilia: report of a case with penile lesions. Cancer 47:944–949, 1981.

52. Riveros M, Lebrón RF: Geographical pathology of cancer of the penis. Cancer 16:798–811, 1963.

53. Rosai J: Ackerman's Surgical Pathology, Vol 1. St Louis, CV Mosby, 1981, pp 911–912.

54. Skinner DG, Leadbetter WF, Kelley SB: The surgical management of squamous cell carcinoma of the penis. J Urol 107:273–277, 1972.

55. Smith BH: Peyronie's disease. Am J Clin Pathol 45:670–678, 1966.

56. Spalteholz W (translated by LF Barker): Hand Atlas of Human Anatomy, Vol 3. Philadelphia, JB Lippincott, 1921, pp 610–615.

57. Srigley JR, Ayala AG, Ordóñez NG, van Nostrand AW: Epithelioid hemangioma of the penis. A rare and distinctive vascular lesion. Arch Pathol Lab Med 109:51–54, 1985.

58. Staubitz WJ, Lent MH, Oberkircher OJ: Carcinoma of the penis. Cancer 8:371–378, 1955.

59. Wade TR, Kopf AW, Ackerman AB: Bowenoid papulosis of the penis. Cancer 42:1890–1903, 1978.

60. Wade TR, Kopf AW, Ackerman AB: Bowenoid papulosis of the genitalia. Arch Dermatol 115:306–308, 1979.

61. Weiss SW, Enzinger FM: Epithelioid hemangioendothelioma: a vascular tumor often mistaken for a carcinoma. Cancer 50:970–981, 1982.

62. Weitzner S: Secondary carcinoma in the penis. Report of three cases and literature review. Am J Surg 37:563–567, 1971.

63. Williams JJ, Mouradian JA, Hagopian M, Gray GF: Hemangioendothelial sarcoma of penis. Cancer 44:1146–1149, 1979.

64. Zoon JJ: Balanoposthite chronique circonscrite bénigne à plasmocytes (contra érythroplasie de Queyrat). Dermatologica 105:1–7, 1952.

NATHAN B. FRIEDMAN, M.D.

CHAPTER 12

Pathology of Testicular Tumors

Nowhere in pathology is an appreciation of embryology more important than in the understanding of tumors in general and of testicular neoplasms in particular. A survey of the structures of the adult testis for homologues of the new growths of this organ, as has been the conventional approach to most tumors, could lead only to insight into the nature of Leydig cell and tubular Sertoli cell growths, but these represent only a small fraction of testicular tumors. The germ cell teratoid neoplasms that form the majority of the group are not explicable in terms of the tissues of the adult testis. They can be understood only in terms of the potentialities of embryonal testicular elements. Cohnheim recognized as far back as 1889 that there is "a close agreement between entire categories of tumors and embryonic forms of tissue."[17] Such an approach leads to a simplification of oncologic concepts and yields classifications that are meaningful histogenetically and useful both therapeutically and prognostically.

It is to be noted that the testis is formed from a somatic blastema to which the primordial germ cells migrate. Its tumors can therefore express the potentialities of primordial germ cells in the form of germinomas (seminomas, dysgerminomas), which can transform into neoplasms of somatic and extraembryonic tissues, as in the embryonal carcinomas, teratocarcinomas, teratomas, yolk sac tumors, and choriocarcinomas. They also manifest the somatic capacities of the gonadal blastema in Leydig cell growths,

tubular neoplasms, and theca-granulosa tumors. Both the somatic apparatus and the germinal elements of the gonad are expressed in the gonadoblastomas.

Finally, there exists that unique growth, the spermatocytic seminoma, which is germinal but in its differentiation moves towards the gamete. Its cells apparently do not become totipotent elements unless they are involved, in some manner not understood, in the parthenogenetic activation that precedes the evolution of other tumors from the germinomas. Spermatocytoma does not occur in the prepubertal testis or in the ovary or in the germinal teratoid tumors of the thymus and pineal gland, which otherwise reproduce all the other types seen in the testis and ovary.

Possible roles of genetic predisposition and steroid exposure have been implicated.[22, 40, 41, 125] Newbold and associates[85] have produced rete carcinoma in mice with diethylstilbestrol. The association with cryptorchism, even after orchiopexy, is well known.[2, 21, 30, 59, 66, 71]

When tumors are bilateral, as in cryptorchism, germinomas dominate.[48, 114] Berthelsen and colleagues found a high incidence in situ in contralateral testes.[5]

As the use of markers for clinical purposes has developed, so has the employment of immunoperoxidase techniques to identify cell types. Although some have suggested[91] that classifications and concepts must be changed to accommodate immunoperoxidase findings, in actuality they support the

Table 12–1. SIMPLIFIED CLASSIFICATION OF
TESTICULAR TUMORS

Germ Cell Tumors
Germinoma in situ
Germinoma
  Spermatocytoma
Embryonal carcinoma
  Yolk sac carcinoma
  Choriocarcinoma
Teratocarcinoma
Teratoma
  Secondary teratocarcinoma
  Secondary teratosarcoma
Somatic Tumors
  Interstitial cell tumor
  Sertoli cell tumor
  Androblastoma
  Gynoblastoma
  Gynandroblastoma
Gonadoblastoma

histogenetic concepts of American workers from 1946 to date.[46, 61, 81] Although there is a long list,[63] the most useful for germ cell tumors are alpha-fetoprotein and chorionic gonadotropin and, for somatic tumors, the steroids.[62] There are also markers for the in situ intratubular cells.

Histologic evaluation of vascular invasion may be aided by immunoperoxidase procedures.[38] Fine-needle aspiration techniques have more usefulness in the diagnosis of metastatic lesions than in evaluation of primary testicular tumors.[29]

Table 12–1 lists a simple classification of testicular tumors.

GERMINOMA

The germinoma (seminoma) is one of the most easily recognized of all growths. Its cellular elements are generally rounded or polyhedral, loosely grouped in clumps, strands, or pseudotubules, but almost never in frankly epithelial complexes. The monotonous uniformity is striking and accounts for its gross appearance with the encephaloid coalescent grayish nodules reminiscent of lymphoma. The nuclear and cytoplasmic membranes are distinct, the cytoplasm clear to granular and containing both glycogen and alkaline phosphatase (Fig. 12–1). Frequent central nucleoli give the cell and nucleus a bull's eye–target appearance. Areas of necrosis are common, with ghost cells sometimes still recognizable. The stroma is as unique as the tumor. The characteristic lymphocytic infiltrate that led to the old designation, "embryonal carcinoma with lymphoid stroma," progresses to epithelioid granulomas with giant cells (Fig. 12–2). The last phase of stromal development results in fibrosis. The stromal granulomas may efface the tumor tissues almost completely in exceptional cases and can result in a misdi-

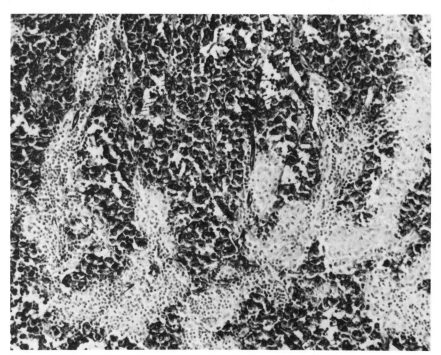

Figure 12–1. Testicular germinoma. Histochemical preparation demonstrating alkaline phosphatase. (× 175)

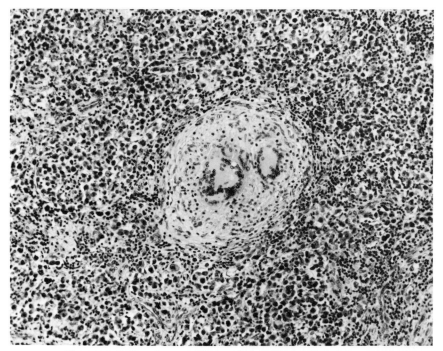

Figure 12–2. Germinoma with pseudosarcoid granuloma. (× 175)

agnosis of granulomatous orchitis. Whether the granulomas are nonspecific, reactant to mycolic acid,[130] or representative of an immune response[70] is not known.

An anaplastic variant of germinoma with bizarre nuclei, increased mitotic activity, and cytologic atypia has been described,[82] although this might represent an early stage of embryonal carcinomatous transformation. Confirmation of "anaplastic" seminoma as a transition between germinoma and embryonal carcinoma has come from several workers.[54, 78, 101, 102] Mitoses have had too great a significance ascribed to them.[128] Tumors that are partly germinomatous and partly carcinomatous are not rare (Fig. 12–3). Infre-

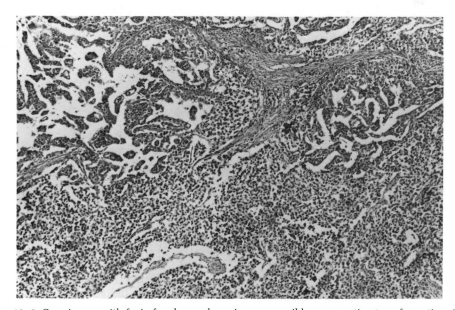

Figure 12–3. Germinoma with foci of embryonal carcinoma, possibly representing transformation. (× 68)

quently one may even encounter unquestioned syncytial trophoblastic giant cells amidst an otherwise uniform germinoma.

The spermatocytic variant has special interest and significance; it is the only true seminoma. Despite a superficial resemblance to germinoma, it is characterized by three cell types of varying size, paralleling the spermatocytic series in normal seminiferous epithelium. The characteristic filamentous chromatin of meiotic prophase and the synaptonemal complex can be seen by electron microscopy.[105] The tumor's tendency to occur in tubular clusters can lead to confusion with intratubular germinoma.

Spermatocytoma occurs in relatively older patients and can metastasize, but rarely.[108, 118, 129] It is not as radiosensitive as germinoma. Origin from primordial germ cells is as likely as from spermatogonia. The spermatocytic appearance can be the result of differentiation rather than an indication of origin. There is no association with teratoid germ cell neoplasms.

The presence of germinomatous elements within testicular tubules[112] at the edge of any of the germinal teratoid tumors, taken in the past as evidence of the seminiferous epithelial nature of the germinoma, is now believed to represent the earliest phase in the development of the germ cell neoplasms (Fig. 12–4). Such cells were occasionally seen retrospectively in biopsies after tumors had developed.[88]

Skakkebaek,[112] who was the first to recognize the significance of the in situ intratubular process, prefers the term carcinoma in situ, whereas Coffin and co-workers[16] use the designation intratubular neoplasia. Müller and colleagues[83] also traced in situ elements found in a patient at age 10 to a frank germinoma over 10 years later. This in situ change can be present in testicular feminization.[113] The progression from the intratubular phase to extratubular invasion and growth has achieved recognition.[35, 109] Since the cells in the tubules are identical to those of classical germinoma, I prefer the term germinoma in situ. These cells are the precursors of all the germinal teratoid tumors and the spermatocytomas, although Skakkebaek considers the latter of spermatocytic origin. It is of interest that the Stevens mouse tumor also begins within tubules.

EMBRYONAL CARCINOMA

Embryonal carcinoma is both a histologic diagnosis and a conceptual entity. It has been confused in the past with germinoma. It is composed of primitive epithelium with all the appearances of carcinomas. Grossly, too, embryonal carcinoma looks like a carcinoma in that it is gray-yellow or chalky white with granular or friable solid tissue manifesting much more variegation than the uniform germinoma. It may be in the form

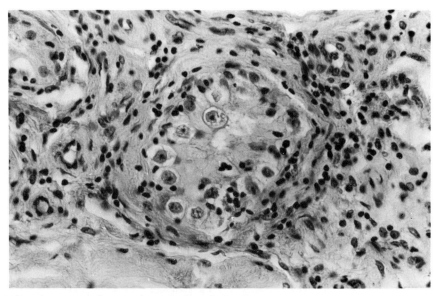

Figure 12–4. Germinomatous elements in testicular tubules that are easily confused with spermatogonia. These represent the earliest stage of germ cell tumors. ($\times$ 420)

of sheets, cords, glands, papillations, or other morphologic patterns. Large bizarre and hyperchromatic nuclei and mitotic figures with abnormal forms are characteristic. The cells cohere as they do in other epithelial tumors rather than present the loose appearance of germinomas. A characteristic pattern occurs when growth within testicular tubules undergoes necrosis and resembles a mammary comedocarcinoma. This may calcify and can remain as a marker in the scars of regressed tumors.[100]

The embryonic epithelium may resemble primitive neuroepithelium, entoderm, or trophoblastic or vitellicular epithelium. At times an entire early embryo may be manifest, sometimes reduplicated many times over, in the so-called embryoid bodies.[92] Mostofi[79, 82] has segregated this as a special subtype, polyembryoma. Marin-Padilla[69] has divided the embryonal carcinomas into those manifesting embryonic ectoderm, mesoderm, or endoderm and those consisting of extraembryonic mesoderm, endoderm, or trophoblast and combinations of these. The most generally recognizable carcinomas are the embryoid, the trophoblastic, and the yolk sac patterns. There are probably other as yet unrecognized types. If teratoid differentiation takes place, the embryonal carcinoma becomes first a teratocarcinoma and then, if differentiation continues, a teratoma. This change can occur in the primary growth, in the metastases, or in both.

CHORIOCARCINOMA

Trophoblastic differentiation is first manifest by the appearance in an embryonal carcinoma of cells resembling cytotrophoblast. Then a second set of elements appears, marginal to clusters of cytotrophoblastic elements, and fuses to form the syncytia that mark choriocarcinoma. Syncytiotrophoblastic elements are more easily recognized than cytotrophoblastic elements since they are large, multinucleated, and have a strikingly heavily stained amphophilic cytoplasm. They are the supposed source of chorionic gonadotropin,[9] at least in normal trophoblast, but one can encounter what appears to be a pure embryonal carcinoma that is nevertheless associated with hormone production. The occasional occurrence of syncytial elements focally in tumors largely of other cytologic types does not alter the ca-

tegorization of the growth by the dominant pattern and does not appear to enhance the aggressiveness of the tumor.

The designation of choriocarcinoma is generally reserved for the fully formed tumor that is composed of both cytotrophoblast and syncytiotrophoblast, arranged with the latter ensheathing the former. Some resemblance to chorionic villi does exist, but the pathologic pseudovilli of choriocarcinoma, whether in the testis or ovary, or even in the gestational uterine and extrauterine lesion, lack the stromal core of the physiologic chorionic villus. Grossly, the choriocarcinoma is characterized by conspicuous hemorrhage and necrosis. This is due to its florid angioinvasiveness. Some attribute the occasional regression of this tumor to this process of self-infarction, although senescence of trophoblast is a still unexcluded possibility.[32]

YOLK SAC CARCINOMA

Another extraembryonic pattern of differentiation in certain embryonal carcinomas is the reproduction of structures seen in the yolk sac or its homologues.[121] In Teilum's endodermal sinus tumor, alpha-fetoprotein has been identified in the hyaline bodies seen in the meshes of the tumor.[123] In addition to a loose reticular network with eosinophilic bodies and the polyvesicular vitelline form[106] is a pattern with small buds into spaces originally misinterpreted as mesonephric. This neoplasm is characteristic of the infantile testis.[11, 94]

TERATOCARCINOMA

The most primitive teratocarcinoma, the polyembryoma with its embryoid bodies, is generally classed with the embryonal carcinomas. The presence of any other histologic evidence of differentiation places the tumor into the category of teratocarcinoma. There is little difficulty in recognizing the fully fledged example, with its mixtures of differentiated tissues, as seen in adult teratomas, intermingled with embryonal carcinomatous complexes of varying types. Early teratoid differentiation can be seen in stroma, epithelium, or both. The stroma around carcinomatous epithelial structures becomes dense and specialized, culminating most commonly as recognizable muscle or cartilage. At times there is no relationship to epithelium and a mesenchymal lobule appears alone as a chiefly myxoid but partly adipose structure, mimicking immature lobulated fat. The embryonic epithelium changes in whole or in part to recognizable enteric, respiratory, transitional, or other membranes, with or without specialized stromal supporting tissues. A common type is fetal epiderm with its clear cells; ectoderm and neuroectoderm often form a continuous layer.

Some pathologists call teratocarcinoma embryoma, whereas the British school refers to it as malignant teratoma. Actually, since the carcinoma precedes the teratoma, the term *carcinoteratoma* would be more appropriate. *Teratocarcinoma* is also useful to designate other mixtures of teratoid and monocellular growths.

TERATOMA

The terms *adult, mature,* and *differentiated teratoma* are preferable to *benign,* since such a growth can be associated with metastatic disease. It is not the mature tissue that metastasizes but the embryonal carcinomatous epithelium from which it has developed and that disseminated while in that phase of its evolution and subsequently matured.

Teratomas of the testis differ from those in the ovary in that they do not tend to be so overtly cystic. Grossly, they are variegated and generally multinodular, with microcysts and often cartilage. The tissues do not usually attain the degree of differentiation of the ovarian homologue but remain at what might be called a histoid rather than organoid level. It is of great interest that adult ovarian teratomas are the commonest of germ cell tumors in women during their reproductive period but are only fourth in frequency in testes, in which malignant germ cell tumors are most frequently encountered.

These differences in male and female germ cell tumors have fascinated many workers. One suggestion had been that trophoblastic tissue in choriocarcinoma stemmed from the male gamete.[47] The tendency of neoplastic germ cells to form adult teratomas in the ovary and embryonal carcinomas in the testis might be rooted in a genetic basis or due to differing environmental influences in the

male scrotum and female pelvis.[32] More recent studies have been stimulated by work such as that of Linder and colleagues,[64] who demonstrated that ovarian teratomas arise from single germ cells after the first meiotic division. Hypotheses involving recessive mutation[103, 104] appear in conflict with the concept that the malignant potential of teratomas has to do with gene control rather than mutational events; even the possibility that the male gamete and a Y chromosome are involved has been resurrected.[27]

An apparently pure epidermoid cyst also exists. Although some would regard it in the same light as a more complex teratoma, many have placed it in a category of its own as a "benign" cyst without any teratoid overtones.[96, 111]

Malignant tumors arising from the secondary carcinomatous growth of one of the somatic components of a teratoma are rare. Neuroepithelial growths and myosarcomas have been seen, although differentiation between embryonal neural tissues and neoplastic neuroblastic structures may be almost impossible. These might be called secondary teratocarcinoma or teratosarcoma.

Ulbright and associates[126, 127] have collected a variety of carcinomas and sarcomas arising from germ cell tumors following therapy. The possibility that this is due to destruction of the more responsive tissues must be given consideration, but it may be more plausible that treatment encourages somatic maturation, as is discussed later.

Carcinoids and neuroepithelial growths are being reported more frequently,[4] with "first report" of the latter both by Nocks and Dann[87] and by Aguirre and Scully.[1] These are comparable to the neural proliferations in "immature" ovarian teratomas, which should not be so designated since they are secondary growths arising in teratomas and are not precursor tissues. Both neurocrine and hepatic elements have been found.[7, 10, 52]

Any combination of the main histologic patterns (germinoma, embryonal carcinoma, choriocarcinoma, and teratoma) can occur. These combined growths may be intermingled, adjacent, or separate. Although for purposes of diagnosis small foci of other tumor types can be ignored in favor of the dominant tissue expression, such mixtures are crucial in an understanding of the interrelationships in this closely knit group of tumors. Combinations that comprise equal or nearly equal components of differing types present greater difficulties in nomenclature. What should one call a tumor combining germinoma and embryonal carcinoma? The mixture of teratoma and embryonal carcinoma is well served by "teratocarcinoma"; can mixed germinoma and teratoma be "teratogerminoma?" When it comes to tumors with three or four patterns and in addition includes the subtypes, a brief and precise designation becomes next to impossible.

METASTASES

Metastases of germinoma occur via lymphatics or direct extension, as along the spermatic cord and peritoneal surfaces. Most of these may be of the so-called anaplastic variety. The lack of cellular cohesiveness is manifested by the numerous artifactual "strays" seen in microscopic sections of germinomas and attached structures. Metastases need not remain germinomatous but can evolve to other types. Metastases of choriocarcinoma are largely hematogenous, especially to the lungs. Choriocarcinoma also has the capacity to provide bizarre metastases, such as to the spleen and other sites not common to the usual run of carcinomatous metastases. Teratocarcinoma, teratoma, and embryonal carcinoma are intermediate between germinoma and choriocarcinoma in their degree of aggressiveness. The evolution of both primary and metastatic tumors to more complex and differentiated types is one of the strongest pieces of evidence from which modern concepts of pathogenesis were derived[36] and now have been so soundly worked out by animal experimentation.

Germinomas metastasize as germinomas two thirds of the time, while in the remaining third other patterns emerge, with embryonal carcinoma predominating. Embryonal carcinoma generally remains embryonal carcinoma when it metastasizes, but in about 10% of all instances choriocarcinomatous or teratomatous patterns are seen. Teratomas and teratocarcinomas give rise to metastases that are roughly evenly divided between embryonal carcinoma and teratocarcinoma, with some choriocarcinomatous admixtures.[23] The incidence of choriocarcinoma in metastases is higher than that found in primary tumors. Furthermore, these metastases may be purely trophoblastic even though the primary tumor contained only

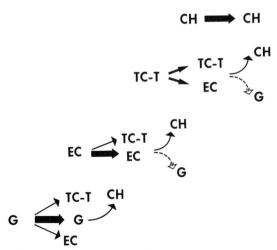

Figure 12–5. Evolution of different patterns in metastases from precursor primary growths. G = germinoma; EC = embryonal carcinoma; TC = teratocarcinoma; T = teratoma; CH = choriocarcinoma. Thickness of arrows indicates frequency of change. Note tendency for choriocarcinoma to appear in metastases and rarity of germinomatous metastases except from germinoma. From Friedman NB: Pathogenesis and histogenetic classification of testicular germ cell tumors. In DG Skinner (ed), Urological Cancer. New York, Grune & Stratton, 1983.

small foci or no identifiable choriocarcinomatous elements (Fig. 12–5).

Although it is true that small foci exist that differ from the predominant pattern, it is equally true that multiple block surveys of entire tumors have shown that many tumors are purely of one type. It seems more reasonable to accept the transformation and evolution of tumor types than to assume that experienced and sophisticated pathologists have overlooked part of the tumor every time a change occurs in the neoplastic tissues.

PATHOGENESIS

The germ cell origin[19] of the testicular teratoid growths[80] is a prime example of the stem cell origin of tumors.[95] The primordial germ cell is ancestor to the gamete and, through fertilization, to the next generation of germ cells and the somatic and extraembryonic structures of the conceptus.[37] The suggested relationship in that study between the primordial germ cells and the hematopoietic stem cells makes the report by the Jacobsens[51] of hemoglobin F in germ cell tumors of great interest. In tumors the primordial germ cell can reproduce itself (germinoma) and can differentiate as a gamete (spermatocytoma), but the latter occurs only in the testis. Usually conversion to teratocarcinoma, teratoma, choriocarcinoma, yolk sac carcinoma, or combinations takes place through an intermediate embryonal carcinoma phase, with or without embryoid bodies. Occasionally, however, intermediate stages may be telescoped, as in germinoma with syncytial trophoblast.[45] If one understands these continua and spectra of differentiation there is no necessity to categorize individually the legions of subtypes.[12]

What has been called the American classification is based on the work of Teilum,[120, 122] Friedman and Moore,[36] Dixon and Moore,[23] Melicow,[74, 75] Mostofi,[79] and Marin-Padilla.[69] The basic concept maintains that the teratoid tumors of the testis derive from primordial germ cells, which, through processes not unlike parthenogenesis and embryogenesis, differentiate into tumor types that parallel the somatic tissues of the embryo and the associated extraembryonic structures (Figs. 12–6 and 12–7).

The British school has been in opposition in that it has not granted diplomatic recognition to the primordial germ cells, insists on separating seminomas from teratomas, and considers the origin of teratomas to be unknown. They do not consider it "realistic to trace the histogenesis of adult neoplasms to so primitive a past."[18] The British characterizations of the various histologic types leave nothing to be desired, as they provide excellent morphologic descriptions of the same neoplastic patterns described in this

chapter; only the names differ. Table 12–2, which compares the British classification with the one most commonly used in the United States, demonstrates the main differences and explains why a comparison of survival figures between the two classifications can be confusing. For instance, malignant teratoma, intermediate group B (MTIB) combines embryonal tumors demonstrating epithelial differentiation with those also containing primitive tridermal components such as primitive cartilage, loose groups of muscle cells, or fatty tissues. The latter group of tumors would be classified as teratocarcinoma in the United States,[36] even though they do not contain mature tissue or demonstrate organoid differentiation. Therefore, Pugh's recent proposal to include the MTIB and MTA (malignant teratoma, anaplastic) groups under the term malignant teratoma, undifferentiated (MTU), does not resolve the problem, although a review of the percentages of tumors falling under the various categories suggests that there is probably only a minor discrepancy.[98] Happily, there are signs of reconciliation. Pugh's new treatise[98] includes the familiar Teilum diagram; a recent paper by Brown[11] features the Teilum diagram, and a drawing of the Keimbahn appears on the cover of the Journal of Clinical Pathology.

The British classification[33] has been hampered from the start by Willis's[132] view of the germ cell origin of teratoid tumors as a disguised version of the fetus-in-fetu concept, and he considered the "theory of the

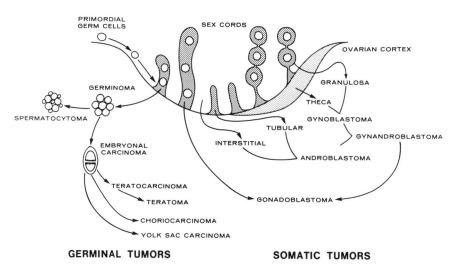

GERMINAL TUMORS   **SOMATIC TUMORS**

Figure 12–6. Pathways of differentiation and transformation in testicular tumors. Oncogenesis recapitulates ontogenesis.

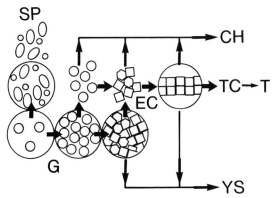

Figure 12–7. Pathogenesis of germ cell tumors. Intratubular germinomatous in situ change progresses to solid tubular growth. Transformation to embryonal carcinoma occurs either before or after invasion of interstitium. Final teratogenesis (TC–T), trophogenesis (CH), and vitelliculogenesis (YS) occur via embryonal body or bypassing it. Spermatocytoma side branch is seen at upper left. From Friedman NB: Pathogenesis and histogenetic classification of testicular germ cell tumors. In DG Skinner (ed), Urological Cancer. New York, Grune & Stratton, 1983.

primordial germ cells a fallacy." Collins and Pugh[18] rejected histogenetic concepts completely. In 1976, Pugh and Cameron actually equated fetal-form teratoma and tumors of germ cell origin but were reluctantly forced to accept the conceptual correctness of the germ cell theory in the experimental animal.[98] However, to them, the histogenesis of these tumors in humans was still uncertain and speculative. By 1983, Pugh finally acknowledged that seminomas and non-seminomas may arise from a common stem cell.[98a]

The evidence for authenticity of the American view of the germ cell tumors consists of data from the accumulated knowledge of the primordial germ cells, the behavior of metastases, comparison with ovarian and extragonadal tumors, experimental and spontaneous animal tumors, and ultrastructural and genetic studies.

The early separation of the primordial germ cells from those cells destined to produce somatic and extraembryonic structures makes it possible to maintain the continuity of the germ plasm. An examination of the embryonic material in which these cells are seen in the process of migration shows a striking resemblance between the primordial elements (Fig. 12–8) and the cells of the germinoma. They are both rich in glycogen and alkaline phosphatase. Their migrations throughout the body account for the occurrence of the germinal teratoid growths in such places as the pineal[107] and thymus.[31] The designation *germinoma* has achieved acceptance in the case of the extragonadal tumors, although the term *seminoma* hangs on stubbornly in the testis. In view of Robert Meyer's early recognition of the nature of the "seminoma" cells,[76] it seems appropriate to use the term *dysgerminoma*, but without the prefix, in preference to Masson's "gonioma"[72] or the "gonocytoma" of Teilum.[120]

The patterns and types of testicular tumors in animals vary from species to species. Rodents in general manifest interstitial cell tumors, whereas teratomas are not infrequent in horses. In the dog, however, teratomas are uncommon, since the monocellular tumor that does occur is more comparable to the human spermatocytoma than to germinoma or embryonal carcinoma; it would consequently not be expected to be a precursor of teratoma. In studies of experimental teratoma of the testis produced by injections of caustic metallic compounds, teratomas are preceded by intratubular monocellular growths.[13]

By culturing cells from teratomas (ovarian), Linder and co-workers[64] have deter-

Table 12–2. CLASSIFICATIONS OF NON-SEMINOMATOUS GERMINAL CELL TUMORS OF THE TESTIS

Friedman and Moore, 1946	Teratoma	Teratocarcinoma		Embryonal carcinoma	Choriocarcinoma
Collins and Pugh, 1964	TD	MTIA (malignant teratoma, intermediate group A)	MTIB (malignant teratoma, intermediate group B)	MTA (malignant teratoma, anaplastic)	MTT (malignant teratoma, trophoblastic)
Pugh, 1976	TD	MTI (malignant teratoma, intermediate)	MTU (malignant teratoma, undifferentiated)		MTT (malignant teratoma, trophoblastic)

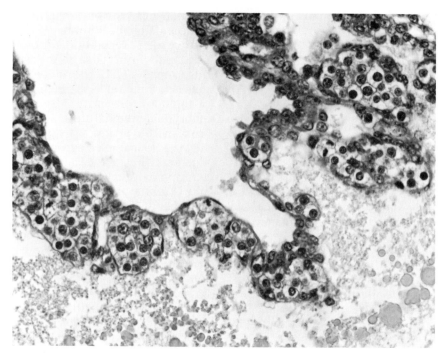

Figure 12–8. Primordial germ cells in early embryonic human yolk sac. Note resemblance to cells of germinomas. (× 300)

mined, through a study of chromosomal and enzymatic patterns, that the cell of origin must be a germ cell after the first meiotic division. The homologous tumors of the testis are believed to arise by a different mechanism,[103] and Erickson and Gondos[27] have attempted to explain the benign nature of ovarian teratomas and the malignancy of testicular tumors by genetic mechanisms.

The work of Pierce and Abell[93] with the Stevens mouse tumor[115] confirmed the predictions based on the observations of human testicular tumors.[36] The growth from even single cells of embryonal carcinomas and their differentiation into either somatic teratomas or tumors of extraembryonic tissues is indisputable evidence of germ cell origin. The remarkable demonstration by Mintz and Illmensee[77] of the possibilities inherent in the differentiation of malignant teratocarcinoma into normal tissues of genetically mosaic mice opens broad vistas. Human tumors include a number of examples of spontaneous differentiation, and the germinal teratoid tumors provide the most striking instances. It may be only a matter of time before physiologic means will replace destructive agents in the treatment of forms of human cancer.

Spontaneous maturation of germ cell tumors has been known for a long time and

accounts for the discrepancies occasionally encountered between a primary growth and its metastases. The phenomenon has attracted renewed interest since the recent success of chemotherapy.[14, 35, 49, 67, 68, 90] Some have attributed maturation to therapy, whereas others have felt that the preferential chemical destruction of the undifferentiated component was responsible. However, adult teratoma cannot metastasize but undifferentiated cells can, and when malignant transformation of adult teratoma takes place it is not in the form of embryonal carcinoma.

Regression of tumors is a phenomenon as well known as maturation and has been brought into sharper focus by recent therapeutic advances. Both spontaneous and presumably therapeutic regressions in metastases are now added to long-documented regression of primary tumors. Calcification is seen not only in scars but in tumors; some calcific bodies are seen in dysgenetic gonads and cryptorchid testes.

The calcifying "comedonecrosis" of regressing intratubular tumors is discussed in an overview of calcification by Wurster and Menges.[133] They also portray psammomatous concretions, which resemble the bodies of cryptorchid hypoplastic tubules and in calcifying Sertoli cell tubular growths.

The extreme extent of differentiation seen

in ovarian teratoids (struma ovarii) but not seen in testicular tumors has been attributed to differences in male and female gametes.[47, 50]

OTHER TUMORS

Angiomas and neuromas can arise in the testis, but they are rare. Lymphomas can be part of systemic disease or a special presentation.[44] In addition to lymphomas,[116] leukemic involvement of the testis as a sanctuary site has necessitated biopsies in the follow-up of childhood leukemia.[3] The association between testicular lymphoma and head and neck involvement[25] was also observed by Hamlin and co-workers.[44] Metastatic adenocarcinoma, particularly from the prostate, not only can involve the testis but can simulate tubular androblastomas. Signet-cell mucinous adenocarcinomatous metastasis, homologous to the ovarian Krukenberg tumor, can also occur (Fig. 12–9).[65]

Ectopic accessory spleens are generally adnexal, but accessory adrenocortical tissue can give rise to either hyperplastic or neoplastic proliferation not only in the accessory structures but within the testis itself.

The tunica vaginalis can be the site of pseudofibromas and mesotheliomas; the latter may be malignant as well. Brenner tumors have been described (Fig. 12–10).[43] The papillary adenocarcinomas of the rete testis appear to me to be mesotheliomas. The only rete tumors I have seen were instances of small hilar germinomas in which the epithelium of the rete was studded with germinomatous elements (Fig. 12–11).

The difficulty in differentiation between mesothelioma and rete carcinoma has been pointed out by others,[86] and sometimes ignored,[42] despite asbestosis. The first reported case[28] when seen by me at the Armed Forces Institute of Pathology during the war was clearly mesothelioma, although I am incorrectly cited to the contrary. There may be such a tumor and it is claimed to have been produced in animals,[84] but I have never encountered one. Mesotheliomas, however, are established entities.[15, 53]

Tiltman's review[124] of tumors metastatic to the testis includes pleural mesothelioma. I reported such a case but with the primary growth in the tunica and the secondary growth in the pleura.[34] Recently, I have seen a tumor similar to the one interpreted as an intratesticular müllerian growth,[26] but I have reservations on both.

The gonadal stromal tumors form the largest group outside of the germ cell tumors and will be considered somatic tumors.

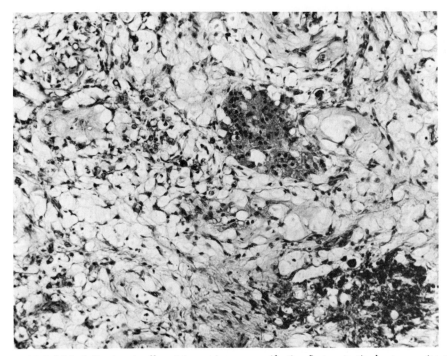

Figure 12–9. Metastatic signet cell gastric carcinoma manifesting first as testicular tumor. ($\times$ 175)

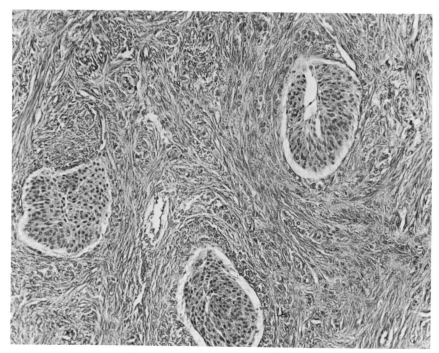

Figure 12–10. Brenner tumor. (× 175)

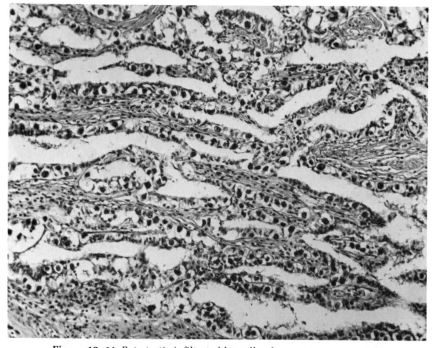

Figure 12–11. Rete testis infiltrated by cells of a germinoma. (× 175)

SOMATIC TUMORS

Although the tumors of somatic tissues of the testis have been designated as gonadal stromal tumors or sex cord mesenchymal tumors, use of the term *somatic* seems more appropriate to separate them histogenetically from the germ cell tumors. They may be composed of tubular complexes, called tubular or Sertoli cell adenomas and adenocarcinomas, or they can consist of interstitial (Leydig) cells. If both Leydig cells and tubules are present, the growth can be termed *androblastoma* to indicate that the structures are male.

On the other hand, if the structures formed are female, consisting of thecal stroma or granulosal complexes, the growth can be designated *gynoblastoma*.[131] If both male and female tissues are represented, the term *gynandroblastoma* is appropriate. *Gonadoblastoma* designates a combined somatic and germ cell tumor.

It should be emphasized that a "male" tumor can produce estrogen and a "female" neoplasm can produce androgen, and either is capable of producing a wide range of steroids. Naming a tumor according to the hormone it produces and ignoring its structure can be confusing. Such confused tumors could be called masculinizing gynoblastoma or feminizing androblastoma or corticoid-producing interstitial cell tumor so that the clinician is not confused by the pathologist.[39]

INTERSTITIAL CELL TUMOR

The Leydig cell tumor is composed of elements similar to normal interstitial cells. They are generally polygonal, darkly eosinophilic units with relatively small nuclei but are not infrequently vacuolated and fatty. In addition, the presence of crystalloids in the cytoplasm helps to separate interstitial cells from adrenocortical elements, with which they are easily confused. The characteristic mitochondria associated with steroid production are present, as well as membranous whorls.[57] The separation of interstitial cell adenomas from instances of marked interstitial cell hyperplasia is simpler at times in theory than in practice. In fact, the differentiation of hyperplasia from the mere contraction of interstitial cell mass that accompanies tubular atrophy is also difficult.

Interstitial cell carcinomas are rare.[20, 89] Here, as in many endocrine tissues, an apparently well-differentiated tumor may be angioinvasive and malignant (Figs. 12–12 and 12–13). Occasionally, a frank carcinoma, with typically malignant appearance,

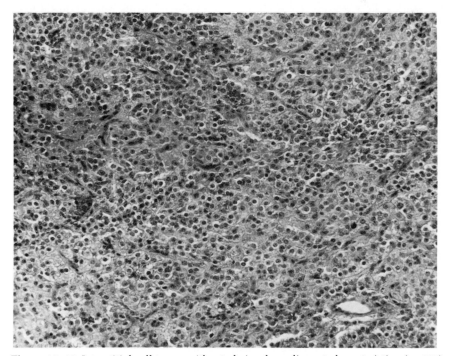

Figure 12–12. Interstitial cell tumor without obviously malignant characteristics. (× 215)

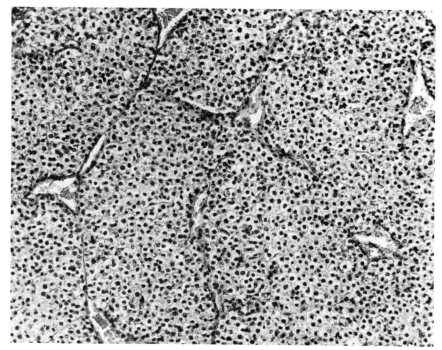

Figure 12–13. Inguinal metastasis 25 years later from tumor illustrated in Figure 12–11. (× 175)

may occur. Since accessory interstitial cells or adrenocortical tissue may be present all along the spermatic cord and in the testicular adnexa, one must avoid misinterpreting these as metastases.

In a testis bearing a Leydig cell tumor, local humoral effects were manifested by maturation of Sertoli cells.[60] This is reminiscent of local interstitial cell differentiation adjacent to HCG-producing embryonal carcinoma.[32] Warner (personal communication) studied an angioma of the testis with local proliferation of Leydig cells, possibly due to a thermal effect.

In dogs, interstitial cell tumors frequently accompany estrogen-producing Sertoli cell tubular tumors existing in the same testis. Concomitantly, certain strains of mice regularly develop interstitial cell tumors when treated with estrogen and adrenocortical tumors if they were previously castrated.

Finally, an interesting "adrenogenital" syndrome exists in which adrenocortical hyperplasia is accompanied by bilateral testicular hilar masses of hyperplastic elements (Fig. 12–14) that resemble the adrenal elements more than they do interstitial cells.[56] This entity has been updated by Kirkland and associates,[58] who showed that these cells were responsive to ACTH. Association with

pituitary tumor[55] and adrenal myelolipoma[8] has also been reported.

SERTOLI CELL TUMOR

Tubular or Sertoli cell adenomas are made up of glandular tubular or fused solid epithelial complexes lined by immature Sertoli cells (Fig. 12–15). In their more differentiated forms they are practically identical to prepubertal testicular tubules, such as are found in solitary or multiple foci in the undescended testis (Fig. 12–16). Here, too, the lines between hamartium, hamartoma, hyperplasia, and neoplasia are not clearly drawn. Intratubular bodies have had special significance ascribed to them in the past but have now been identified as infolded thickened basement membranes cut tangentially. The large tumors that arise from the testes in the phenotypically female instances of testicular feminization are tubular or Sertoli cell neoplasms. If the gonad is small, the diagnosis of neoplasia may be hazardous. All degrees of differentiation exist, from these well-differentiated examples to those in which some tubular complexes still can be made out to those in which they become lost in specialized thecoid stroma. Mixed

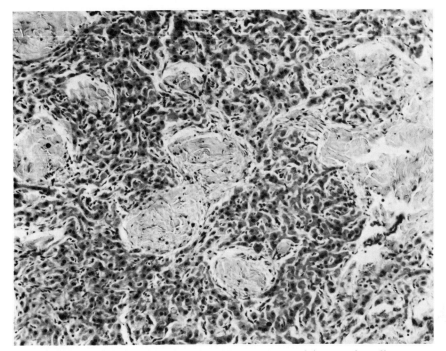

Figure 12–14. Hilar hyperplasia of adrenocortical elements simulating Leydig cell tumor. (× 175)

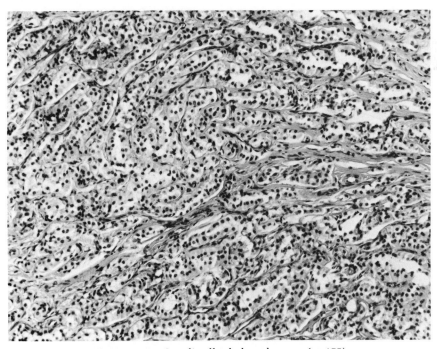

Figure 12–15. Sertoli cell tubular adenoma. (× 175)

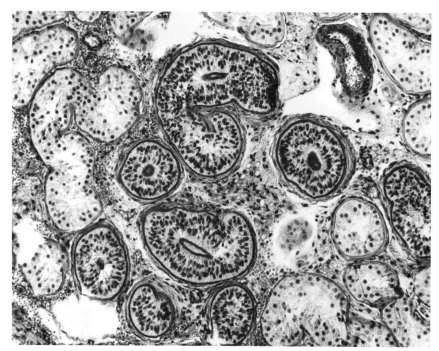

Figure 12–16. Hypoplastic tubules in cryptorchid testis. Other tubules are atrophic. (× 175)

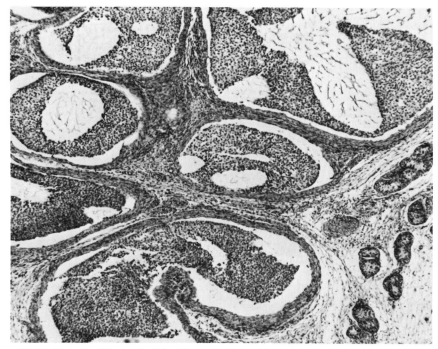

Figure 12–17. Granulosal tumor in infantile testis. Teratoid structures are present elsewhere. (× 80)

and transitional forms are frequent. Rare carcinomatous metastasizing variants are encountered.[119] Calcification and annular tubules have been encountered in variants of the sex cord tumors[99] but are hardly separate entities.[97] An extragonadal androblastic tumor has been reported.[73]

GYNOBLASTOMA

This term should be employed for those testicular tumors in which "female" structures such as the thecoid stroma of the secondary neogenic ovarian cortex or granulosal structures (Fig. 12–17) are manifest. Such neoplasms have been called thecagranulosa tumors. They are the female homologue of the tubulointerstitial androblastomas and are included in the gonadal stromal tumor group. However, although the seminiferous tubules and granulosal epithelium are derived from the sex cords, the thecoid stroma is related to the secondary oophoroid gonadal cortex and not to the primary interstitial stroma from which the Leydig cells derive. The only possible homologue of the secondary cortex of the ovary might be the tunica albuginea of the testis. The ovarian homologues can also lead to an understanding of the similarity of certain mesotheliomas to thecomas.[84]

There are gradations in the spectrum that these lesions form that sometimes make it difficult to determine whether one is dealing with an androblastoma or a gynoblastoma.[131] This is particularly the case when abortive epithelial strands emerge from a stromal background and could be considered the beginnings of either granulosal complexes or Sertoli tubules. The background tissue is helpful in that thecoid stroma is definitely müllerian and differs from ordinary fibrous stroma. The appearance of cells resembling Leydig cells in such a stroma cannot be assumed to be androblastic since "interstitial" cells of the adrenogenital type are also seen in hyperplastic ovarian stroma, as in Stein-Leventhal syndrome.

GONADOBLASTOMA

This tumor appears in undescended testes or dysgenetic gonads. In it both somatic and germinal cell lines find expression with variegated combinations of the differing elements. Most commonly tubular or granulosal groupings are intermingled with germinomatous cells against a stromal background with interstitial cells. Some may secrete hormones.[110, 119] The basement membrane aggregates seen in the tubular tumors are conspicuous here and can undergo calcification, sometimes demonstrable radiologically. The gonadoblastic tumor described by Bolen[6] differed only in that the germ line showed evidence of spermatocytic differentiation.

The gonadoblastoma recapitulates both the embryogenesis of the gonad and the histogenesis of testicular tumors, and is a fitting neoplastic type with which to conclude this consideration of the pathology of neoplasia of the testis from the embryologic viewpoint.

References

1. Aguirre P, Scully RE: Primitive neuroectodermal tumor of the testis. Report of a case. Arch Pathol Lab Med 107:643–645, 1983.
2. Anderson KC, Li FP, Marchetto DJ: Dizygotic twinning, cryptorchidism, and seminoma in a sibship. Cancer 53:374–376, 1984.
3. Askin FB, Land VJ, Sullivan MP, et al: Occult testicular leukemia: testicular biopsy at three years continuous complete remission of childhood leukemia: a Southwest Oncology Group Study. Cancer 47:470–475, 1981.
4. Berdjis CC, Mostofi FK: Carcinoid tumors of the testis. J Urol 118:777–783, 1977.
5. Berthelsen JG, Skakkebaek NE, von der Maase H, et al: Screening for carcinoma in situ of the contralateral testis in patients with germinal testicular cancer. Br Med J 285:1683–1686, 1982.
6. Bolen JW: Mixed germ cell–sex cord stromal tumor. A gonadal tumor distinct from gonadoblastoma. Am J Clin Pathol 75:565–573, 1981.
7. Bosman FT, Louwerens JW: APUD cells in teratomas. Am J Pathol 104:174–180, 1981.
8. Boudreaux D, Waisman J, Skinner DG, Low R: Giant adrenal myelolipoma and testicular interstitial cell tumor in a man with congenital 21-hydroxylase deficiency. Am J Surg Pathol 3:109–123, 1979.
9. Braunstein GD, Friedman NB, Sacks SA, et al: Germ cell tumors of the testes. West J Med 12:362, 1977.
10. Brodner OG, Grube D, Helmstaedter V, et al: Endocrine GEP-cells in primary testicular teratoma. Virchows Arch (A) 388:251–263, 1980.
11. Brown NJ: Teratomas and yolk-sac tumors. J Clin Pathol 29:1021, 1976.
12. Cardoso de Almeida PC, Scully RE: Diffuse embryoma of the testis. A distinctive form of mixed germ cell tumor. Am J Surg Pathol 7:633–642, 1983.
13. Carleton RL, Friedman NB, Bomze EJ: Experimental teratomas of the testis. Cancer 6:464, 1953.
14. Carr BI, Gilchrist KW, Carbone PP: The variable transformation in metastases from testicular germ

cell tumors: the need for selective biopsy. J Urol 126:52–54, 1981.

15. Chen KT, Arhelger RB, Flam MS, Hanson JH: Malignant mesothelioma of tunica vaginalis testis. Urology 10:316–319, 1982.

16. Coffin CM, Ewing S, Dehner LP: Frequency of intratubular germ cell neoplasia with invasive testicular germ cell tumors. Arch Pathol Lab Med 109:555, 1985.

17. Cohnheim J: Lectures on General Pathology: A Handbook for Practitioners and Students. (Translated from the 2nd German edition by AB McKee). London, The New Sydenham Society, 1889, p 750.

18. Collins DH, Pugh RCB: The pathology of testicular tumors. Br J Urol 36(Suppl):1, 1964.

19. Damjanov I: Immunohistochemical localization of murine stage-specific embryonic antigens in human testicular germ cell tumors. Am J Pathol 108:225, 1982.

20. Davis S, Di Martino NA, Schneider G: Malignant interstitial cell carcinoma of the testis: report of two cases with steroid synthetic profiles, response to therapy, and review of the literature. Cancer 47:425–431, 1981.

21. Debre B, Steg A: Tumours of the undescended testis. Nouv Presse Med 8:3341–3343, 1979.

22. Depue RH, Pike MC, Henderson BE: Estrogen exposure during gestation and risk of testicular cancer. JNCI 71:1151–1155, 1983.

23. Dixon FJ, Moore RA: Tumors of the male sex organs. In Atlas of Tumor Pathology. Washington DC, Armed Forces Institute of Pathology, 1952, Fascicles 31b and 32.

24. Donohue JP: Testis Tumors. Baltimore, Williams & Wilkins, 1983.

25. Duncan PR, Checa F, Gowing NF, et al: Extranodal non-Hodgkin's lymphoma presenting in the testicle: a clinical and pathologic study of 24 cases. Cancer 45:1578–1584, 1980.

26. Elbadawi A, Batchvarov MM, Linke CA: Intratesticular papillary mucinous cystadenocarcinoma. Urology 14:280–284, 1979.

27. Erickson RP, Gondos B: Alternative explanations of the differing behavior of ovarian and testicular teratomas. Lancet 1:407, 1976.

28. Feek JD, Hunter WC: Papillary carcinoma arising from rete testis. Arch Pathol 40:399–402, 1945.

29. Frable WJ: Thin-Needle Aspiration Biopsy. Philadelphia, WB Saunders, 1983.

30. Fram RJ, Garnick MB, Retik A: The spectrum of genitourinary abnormalities in patients with cryptorchidism, with emphasis on testicular carcinoma. Cancer 50:2243–2246, 1982.

31. Friedman NB: The comparative morphogenesis of extragenital and gonadal teratoid tumors. Cancer 4:265, 1951.

32. Friedman NB: Choriocarcinoma of the testis and extragenital choriocarcinoma in men. Ann NY Acad Sci 80:161, 1959.

33. Friedman NB: Comparison of British and American classifications of testicular tumors. Sixth Congress European Soc Pathol, London, September, 1977.

34. Friedman NB: Mesothelioma of tunica testis and carcinoma of rete. Thirteenth Int Congress Int Acad Pathol, Paris, September, 1980.

35. Friedman NB: Pathogenesis and histogenetic classification of testicular germ cell tumors. In DG

Skinner (ed), Urological Cancer. New York, Grune & Stratton, 1983.

36. Friedman NB, Moore RA: Tumors of the testis: a report on 922 cases. Milit Surg 99:573, 1946.

37. Friedman NB, Van de Velde RL: Germ cell tumors in man, pleiotropic mice, and continuity of germplasm and somatoplasm. Hum Pathol 12:772–776, 1981.

38. Fujime M, Chang H, Lin CW, Prout GR Jr: Correlation of vascular invasion and metastasis in germ cell tumors of the testis—a preliminary report. J Urol 131:1237–1241, 1984.

39. Gabrilove JL, Nicolis GL, Mitty HA, Sohval AR: Feminizing interstitial cell tumor of the testis: personal observations and a review of the literature. Cancer 35:1184, 1975.

40. Gedde-Dahl T, Hannisdal E, Klepp OH, et al: Testicular neoplasms occurring in four brothers. A search for a genetic predisposition. Cancer 55:2005–2009, 1985.

41. Gill WB, Schumacher GF, Bibbo M, et al: Association of diethylstilbestrol exposure in utero with cryptorchidism, testicular hypoplasia and semen abnormalities. J Urol 122:36–39, 1979.

42. Gisser SD, Nayak S, Kaneko M, Tchertkoff V: Adenocarcinoma of the rete testis: a review of the literature and presentation of a case with associated asbestosis. Hum Pathol 8:219–224, 1977.

43. Goldman RL: A Brenner tumor of the testis. Cancer 26:853, 1970.

44. Hamlin JA, Kagan RA, Friedman NB: Lymphomas of the testicle. Cancer 29:1352, 1972.

45. Hedinger C, von Hochstetter AR, Egloff B: Seminoma with syncytiotrophoblastic giant cells. A special form of seminoma. Virchows Arch (A) 383:59–67, 1979.

46. Heyderman E: Multiple tissue markers in human malignant testicular tumors. Scand J Immunol 8(Suppl):119, 1978.

47. Hirsch EF: Extragenital choriocarcinoma: with comments on the male origin of trophoblastic tissues. Arch Pathol 48:516, 1949.

48. Hoekstra HJ, Mehta DM, Koops HS: Synchronous bilateral primary germ cell tumors of the testis: a case report and review of the literature. J Surg Oncol 22:59–61, 1983.

49. Hong WK, Wittes RE, Hajdu ST, et al: The evolution of mature teratoma from malignant testicular tumors. Cancer 40:2987–2992, 1977.

50. Iyengar B: The germ cell: oncogenic and embryogenic correlates. Experientia 38:1239–1240, 1982.

51. Jacobsen GK, Jacobsen M: Immunohistochemical demonstration of hemoglobin F (HbF) in testicular germ cell tumors. Oncodev Biol Med 4:C45–51, 1983.

52. Jacobsen GK, Jacobsen M: Possible liver cell differentiation in testicular germ cell tumors. Histopathology 7:537, 1983.

53. Japko L, Horta AA, Schreiber K, et al: Malignant mesothelioma of the tunica vaginalis testis: report of first case with preoperative diagnosis. Cancer 49:119–127, 1982.

54. Javadpour N: (Discussion.) Int J Androl Suppl 4:91, 1981.

55. Johnson RE, Scheithauer B: Massive hyperplasia of testicular adrenal rests in a patient with Nelson's syndrome. Am J Clin Pathol 77:501–507, 1982.

56. Kadar RG, Block MB, Katz FH, Hofeldt ED: "Masked" 21-hydroxylase deficiency of the adrenal presenting with gynecomastia and bilateral testicular masses. Am J Med 62:278, 1977.

57. Kay S, Fu Y, Koontz WW, Chen ATL: Interstitial cell tumor of the testis: tissue culture and ultrastructural studies. Am J Clin Pathol 63:366, 1975.

58. Kirkland RT, Kirkland JL, Keenan BS, et al: Bilateral testicular tumors in congenital adrenal hyperplasia. J Clin Endocrinol Metab 44:369–378, 1977.

59. Krabbe S, Skakkebaek NE, Berthelsen JG, et al: High incidence of undetected neoplasia in maldescended testes. Lancet 1:999–1000, 1979.

60. Kula K, Romer TE, Wlodarczyk WP: Somatic and germinal cells' interrelationship in the course of seminiferous tubule maturation in man. Arch Androl 4:9–16, 1980.

61. Kurman RJ, Scardino PT, McIntyre KR, et al: Cellular localization of alpha-fetoprotein and human chorionic gonadotropin in germ cell tumors of the testis using an indirect immunoperoxidase technique. A new approach to classification utilizing tumor markers. Cancer 40:2136–2151, 1977.

62. Kurman RJ, Andrade D, Goebelsmann U, Taylor CR: An immunohistological study of steroid localization in Sertoli-Leydig tumors of the ovary and testis. Cancer 42:1772–1783, 1978.

63. Lange PH: Serum and tissue markers of testicular tumors. Int J Androl 4(Suppl):191, 1981.

64. Linder D, McCaw BK, Hecht F: Parthenogenic origin of benign ovarian teratomas. N Engl J Med 292:63, 1975.

65. London MZ, Grossman SN: Secondary testicular tumor resembling Krukenberg tumor: a case report. J Urol 62:713, 1949.

66. Lykkesfeldt G, Høyer H, Lykkesfeldt AE, Skakkebaek NE: Steroid sulphatase deficiency associated with testis cancer. Lancet 2:1456, 1983.

67. Maatman T, Bukowski RM, Montie JE: Retroperitoneal malignancies several years after initial treatment of germ cell cancer of the testis. Cancer 54:1962–1965, 1984.

68. Madden M, Goldstraw P, Corrin B: Effects of chemotherapy on the histological appearances of testicular teratoma metastatic to the lung: correlation with patient survival. J Clin Pathol 37:1212, 1984.

69. Marin-Padilla M: Histopathology of the embryonal carcinoma of the testes: embryological evaluation. Arch Pathol 85:614, 1968.

70. Marshall AHE, Dayan AD: An immune reaction in man against seminomas, dysgerminomas, pinealomas and the mediastinal tumors of similar histological appearance? Lancet 2:1102, 1964.

71. Martin DC: Germinal cell tumors of the testis after orchiopexy. J Urol 121:422–424, 1979.

72. Masson P: Human Tumors. Histology, Diagnosis and Technique, 2nd ed (Revised and translated by SD Kobernick). Detroit, Wayne State University Press, 1970.

73. Maurer R, Taylor CR, Schmucki O, Hedinger CE: Extratesticular gonadal stromal tumor in the pelvis. A case report with immunoperoxidase findings. Cancer 45:985–990, 1980.

74. Melicow MD: Embryoma of testis: report of a case and a classification of neoplasms of the testis. J Urol 44:333, 1940.

75. Melicow MD: Classification of tumors of testis: a clinical and pathological study based on 105 primary and 13 secondary cases in adults, and 3 primary and 4 secondary cases in children. J Urol 73:547, 1955.

76. Meyer R: The pathology of some special ovarian tumors and their relation to sex characteristics. Am J Obstet Gynecol 33:697, 1931.

77. Mintz B, Illmensee K: Normal genetically mosaic mice produced from malignant teratocarcinoma cells. Proc Nat Acad Sci 72:3585, 1975.

78. Monaghan P, Raghavan D, Neville AM: Ultrastructural studies of xenografted germ cell tumors. Cancer 49:683–697, 1982.

79. Mostofi FK: Testicular tumors: epidemiologic, etiologic and pathologic features. Cancer 32:1186, 1973.

80. Mostofi FK: Pathology of germ cell tumors of testis: a progress report. Cancer 45(Suppl):1735–1754, 1980.

81. Mostofi FK: Tumor markers and pathology of testicular tumors. Prog Clin Biol Res 153:69–87, 1984.

82. Mostofi FK, Price EB Jr: Tumors of the male genital system. In HI Firminger (ed), Atlas of Tumor Pathology. Washington, DC, Armed Forces Institute of Pathology, 1973, Fascicle 8, 2nd series.

83. Müller J, Skakkebaek NE, Nielsen OH, Graem N: Cryptorchidism and testis cancer. Atypical infantile germ cells followed by carcinoma in situ and invasive carcinoma in adulthood. Cancer 54:629–634, 1984.

84. Nevius DB, Friedman NB: Mesotheliomas and extraovarian thecomas with hypoglycemic and nephrotic syndromes. Cancer 12:1263–1269, 1959.

85. Newbold RR, Bullock BC, Melachlan JA: Carcinoma of the rete testis in mice exposed prenatally to diethylstilbestrol: the male counterpart of vaginal adenocarcinoma? Proc Am Assoc Ca Res 26:196, 1985.

86. Nochomovitz LE, Orenstein JM: Adenocarcinoma of the rete testis. Case report, ultrastructural observations, and clinicopathologic correlates. Am J Surg Pathol 8:625–634, 1984.

87. Nocks BN, Dann JA: Primitive neuroectodermal tumor (immature teratoma) of testis. Urology 22:543–544, 1983.

88. Neunsch-Bachmann IH, Hedinger C: Atypische Spermatogonien als Präkanzerose. Schweiz med Wschr 107:795, 1977.

89. Ober WB, Kabakow B, Hecht H: Malignant interstitial cell tumor of the testis: a problem in endocrine oncology. Bull NY Acad Med 52:561, 1976.

90. Oosterhuis JW, Suurmeyer AJ, Sleyfer DT, et al: Effects of multiple-drug chemotherapy (cis-diammine-dichloroplatinum, bleomycin and vinblastine) on the maturation of retroperitoneal lymph node metastases of nonseminomatous germ cell tumors of the testis. No evidence for De Novo induction of differentiation. Cancer 51:408–416, 1983.

91. Parkinson C, Beilby JO: Testicular germ cell tumours: should current classification be revised? Invest Cell Pathol 3:135–140, 1980.

92. Peyron A: Faits nouveaux relatifs à l'origine et à l'histogénèse des embryomes. Bull Assoc Franc, p. l'étude de Cancer 28:658, 1939.

93. Pierce BG, Abell MR: Embryonal carcinoma of the testis. In SC Sommers (ed), Genital and Mammary

Pathology Decennial. New York, Appleton-Century-Crofts, 1975.

94. Pierce GB, Bullock WK, Huntington RW Jr: Yolk sac tumors of the testis. Cancer 25:644, 1970.

95. Pierce GB, Pantazis CG, Caldwell JE, Wells RS: Embryologic control of malignancy. J Supramol Struct 15(Suppl):156, 1981.

96. Price EB Jr: Epidermoid cysts of the testis: a clinical and pathologic analysis of 69 cases from the testicular registry. J Urol 102:708, 1969.

97. Proppe KH, Scully RE: Large-cell calcifying Sertoli cell tumor of the testis. Am J Clin Pathol 74:607–619, 1980.

98. Pugh RCB: Pathology of the Testis. Oxford, Blackwell Scientific Publications, 1976.

98a. Pugh RCB: Pathology of testicular tumors—a British perspective. In JP Donohue (ed), Testis Tumors. Baltimore, Williams & Wilkins, 1983, pp 1–22.

99. Ramaswamy G, Jagadha V, Tchertkoff V: A testicular tumor resembling the sex cord with annular tubules in a case of androgen insensitivity syndrome. Cancer 55:1607–1611, 1985.

100. Rather LJ, Gardiner WR, Frerichs JB: Regression and maturation of primary testicular tumors with progressive growth of metastases: a report of six new cases and a review of the literature. Stanford Med Bull 12:12, 1954.

101. Raghavan D, Heyderman E, Monaghan P, et al: Hypothesis: when is a seminoma not a seminoma? J Clin Pathol 34:123–128, 1981.

102. Raghavan D, Sullivan AL, Peckham MJ, Neville AM: Elevated serum alphafetoprotein and seminoma. Clinical evidence for a histologic continuum? Cancer 50:982–989, 1982.

103. Riley PA, Sutton PM: Why are ovarian teratomas benign whilst teratomas of the testis are malignant? Lancet 1:1360, 1975.

104. Riley PA, Sutton PM: Origin of teratomas. Lancet 1:642, 1976.

105. Rosai J, Khodakoust K, Silber I: Spermatocytic seminoma, II: ultrastructural study. Cancer 24:103, 1969.

106. Roth LM, Panganiban WG: Gonadal and extragonadal yolk sac carcinomas. Cancer 37:812, 1976.

107. Russell DS: The pinealoma: its relationship to teratoma. J Pathol Bacteriol 56:145, 1944.

108. Schoborg TW, Whittaker J, Lewis CW: Metastatic spermatocytic seminoma. J Urol 124:739–741, 1980.

109. Schulze C, Holstein AF: On the histology of human seminoma: development of the solid tumor from intratubular seminoma cells. Cancer 39:1090–1100, 1977.

110. Scully RE: Gonadoblastoma: a review of 74 cases. Cancer 25:1340, 1970.

111. Shah KH, Maxted WC, Chun B: Epidermoid cysts of the testis: a report of three cases and an analysis of 141 cases from the world literature. Cancer 47:577–582, 1981.

112. Skakkebaek NE: Atypical germ cells in the adjacent "normal" tissue of testicular tumors. Acta Pathol Microbiol Immunol Scand (A) 83:127, 1975.

113. Skakkebaek NE: Carcinoma-in-situ of testis in testicular feminization syndrome. Acta Pathol Microbiol Immunol Scand (A) 87:87–89, 1979.

114. Sokal M, Peckham MJ, Hendry WF: Bilateral germ cell tumours of the testis. Br J Urol 52:158–162, 1980.

115. Stevens LC: Origin of testicular teratomas from primordial germ cells in mice. J Nat Canc Inst 38:549, 1967.

116. Sussman EB, Hajdu SI, Lieberman PH, Whitmore WF: Malignant lymphoma of the testis: a clinicopathologic study of 37 cases. J Urol 118:1004–1007, 1977.

117. Talerman A: Malignant Sertoli cell tumor of the testis. Cancer 28:446, 1971.

118. Talerman A: Spermatocytic seminoma: clinicopathological study of 22 cases. Cancer 45:2169–2176, 1980.

119. Talerman A, Delemarre JF: Gonadoblastoma associated with embryonal carcinoma in an anatomically normal man. J Urol 113:355, 1975.

120. Teilum G: Homologous tumors in ovary and testis: contribution to classification of gonadal tumors. Acta Obstet Gynecol Scand 24:480, 1944.

121. Teilum G: Endodermal sinus tumors of the ovary and testis. Comparative morphogenesis of the so-called mesonephroma ovarii (Schiller) and extraembryonic (yolk sac-allantoic) structures of the rat's placenta. Cancer 12:1092, 1959.

122. Teilum G: Special Tumors of Ovary and Testis and Related Extragonadal Lesions: Comparative Pathology and Histological Identification. Philadelphia, JB Lippincott, 1971.

123. Teilum G, Albrechtsen R, Norgaard-Pedersen B: Immunofluorescent localization of alpha-fetoprotein synthesis in endodermal sinus tumor (yolk sac tumor). Acta Pathol Microbiol Immunol Scand (A) 82:586, 1974.

124. Tiltman AJ: Metastatic tumours in the testis. Histopathology 3:31–37, 1979.

125. Tollerud DJ, Blattner WA, Fraser MC, et al: Familial testicular cancer and urogenital developmental anomalies. Cancer 55:1849–1854, 1985.

126. Ulbright TM, Clark SA, Einhorn LH: Angiosarcoma associated with germ cell tumors. Hum Pathol 16:268, 1985.

127. Ulbright TM, Loehrer PJ, Roth LM, et al: The development of non-germ cell malignancies within germ cell tumors. A clinicopathologic study of 11 cases. Cancer 54:1824, 1984.

128. Von Hochstetter AR: Mitotic count in seminomas—an unreliable criterion for distinguishing between classical and anaplastic types. Virchows Arch (A) 390:63–69, 1981.

129. Walter P: Spermatocytic seminoma. Study of 8 cases and review of the literature. Virchows Arch (A) 386:175–177, 1980.

130. Warner NE, Friedman NB: Lipogranulomatous pseudosarcoid. Ann Intern Med 45:662, 1956.

131. Warner NE, Friedman NB, Bomze EJ, Masin F: Comparative pathology of experimental and spontaneous androblastomas and gynoblastomas of the gonads. Am J Obstet Gynecol 79:971, 1960.

132. Willis RA: The Borderland of Embryology and Pathology, 2nd ed. Washington DC, Butterworths, 1962.

133. Wurster K, Menges V: Microcalcifications in testicular germ cell tumors. Orientating study concerning its diagnostic utilization. Virchows Arch (A) 374:45–62, 1977.

PART IV

Diagnosis and Therapy of Genitourinary Tumors

WILLIAM D. BOSWELL, JR., M.D.

CHAPTER 13

Diagnostic Imaging in Genitourinary Cancer

All physicians are faced with an ever increasing number of available diagnostic imaging modalities. Vast changes have occurred within the fields of diagnostic radiology and uroradiology. In the 1950s, KUB, excretory urogram, and retrograde pyelography were the mainstay of urologic diagnosis. Angiography, venography, double-dose intravenous pyelography, nephrotomography, and lymphangiography were added to the armamentarium in the 1960s. Nuclear medical examinations were introduced in the late 1960s and refined in the next decade with the addition of new radionuclides and the gamma camera. In the 1970s, the accuracy, safety, and speed of diagnosis were improved with the addition of ultrasound and computerized tomography (CT) scanning. Noninvasive imaging methods to be used in the diagnosis of urologic problems were finally available. Digital subtraction angiography (DSA) and nuclear magnetic resonance imaging (NMR, MRI) are finding their places in the diagnostic evaluation of patients in the present decade. Notwithstanding all of these available modalities, it must always be kept in mind that the appropriate diagnostic examinations depend upon the information that is necessary for a timely and accurate diagnosis. Only this will lead to better care for the patient.

RENAL MASS

Today a renal mass may be found by many different imaging methods ranging from the plain film or KUB to computed tomography. Although most renal masses prove to be benign, both the urologist and the radiologist encounter problems in making a complete evaluation. For all patients, unsuspected renal masses will be found in approximately 5 to 8% of all intravenous pyelograms.[33] With patients in whom the suspicion of renal cell carcinoma is high, the incidence of renal masses may be as great as 60%. In those being evaluated for prostatic problems, unsuspected renal masses may be found in 16 to 18%. Although most of these renal masses are benign (renal cysts, inflammatory lesions, and pseudotumors), 10 to 12% will prove to be malignant. A systematic evaluation is essential in order to obtain the most cost effective and least invasive path to the diagnosis (Fig. 13–1). Despite the introduction of new and sometimes costly radiologic examinations as well as the rising cost of health care in general, there has been a 30% decrease in overall costs in evaluating a patient with a renal mass.[64] An overall diagnostic accuracy of 97 to 98% can be realized by employing the different imaging modalities in a logical manner.

Intravenous Pyelogram

Intravenous pyelogram (IVP) with tomography is the screening test of choice for the patient with a suspected renal mass. The KUB or scout film may demonstrate a mass overlying or adjacent to the kidney or the kidney may appear enlarged. Occasionally, calcifications may be recognized within or

237

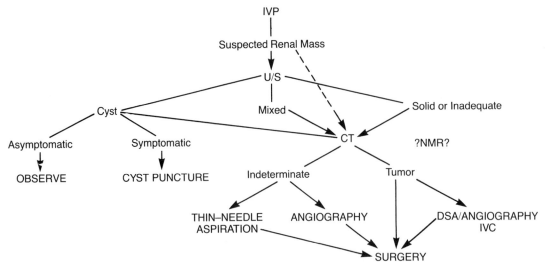

Figure 13–1. Systematic diagnostic approach to a renal mass. IVP = intravenous pyelogram; U/S = ultrasound; CT = computed tomography; MRI = magnetic resonance imaging; DSA = digital subtraction angiography; IVC = inferior venocavography.

on the periphery of the mass. Calcifications have been seen in virtually all renal masses, both benign and malignant. Approximately 10% of all renal cell carcinomas show evidence of calcifications, usually central in location.[12] However, peripheral ring-like calcification does not exclude malignancy, as 20% of these lesions will be malignant. Ninety per cent of renal masses with central, punctate, or mottled calcifications will prove to be renal cell carcinomas.

Intravenous pyelogram detects the presence or absence of a renal mass with great accuracy, although differentiating the benign lesion from the renal cell carcinoma is only 70 to 75% accurate. Rarely, the IVP will be completely normal and only another imaging modality (usually CT scanning) will demonstrate the renal cell carcinoma.[28] Incidental renal cysts occur frequently in those over the age of 50 and are commonly encountered on both ultrasound and CT examinations performed for other reasons.[30]

The benign renal cyst on IVP usually reveals a mass bulging the contour of the kidney. It is seen as a well-circumscribed, homogeneous lucent defect against the opacified renal parenchyma. With tomography, which is essential in the evaluation of any renal mass, the cyst wall that projects beyond the parenchyma is noted to be paper thin. The interface between the cyst and the renal parenchyma usually has a beak-like or claw-like deformity. Depending upon the

position and size of the cyst, there is usually calyceal displacement or splaying. On the other hand, renal cell carcinoma usually distorts the renal outline or causes renal enlargement, and there may be calcifications within the tumor. There is an irregular junction between the normal renal parenchyma and hypernephroma, and the mass appears nonuniform in density. The calyces may be stretched, elongated, obliterated, or invaded. With medial extension of the tumor into the renal pelvis, there is distortion or obliteration of the renal pelvis and irregular filling defects within it, due to blood clots or tumor. A large renal cell carcinoma may cause complete distortion and disruption of the normal renal architecture. A nonfunctioning kidney may result from either renal vein invasion or involvement of the entire renal pelvis.

Ultrasound

More accurate characterization becomes necessary when a renal mass is detected on intravenous pyelography. Ultrasound is the next step in the assessment of the renal mass. The chief advantages of ultrasound examinations are that they are easy to perform, noninvasive, relatively inexpensive, and able to reveal differences between fluid-containing lesions, such as renal cysts, and solid masses, such as renal cell carcinomas. Classic ultrasound findings for a simple renal cyst are a well-defined, anechoic renal lesion with a smooth back wall and distal sonic enhancement (Fig. 13–2). The diagnosis of a simple renal cyst can be made with confidence only when these criteria are met. Asymptomatic renal cysts generally may be observed, whereas cysts with accompanying symptoms, no matter how minor, should be punctured with a thin needle for analysis of the fluid and instillation of contrast medium into the cyst to assess the internal architecture.[46]

Fluid obtained from a benign cyst is clear and slightly straw-colored and has low levels of protein, fat, and lactic acid hydrogenase (LDH). Cytologic examination reveals no neoplastic or inflammatory cells. Cysts that are expanding, or may reform after puncture and drainage, tend to have a higher glucose content than the normal blood glucose and an opening pressure of greater than 160 mm of water. The fluid obtained from inflammatory cysts is usually cloudy and shows a mild elevation of fat and protein content. The LDH and amylase levels may be significantly elevated, and cytologic examination shows inflammatory cells. Benign hemorrhagic cysts may yield either blood or brown, cloudy aspirates with elevated levels of fat, protein, and LDH. Cytologic study shows acellular particulate debris with cholesterol clefts, hemosiderin deposits, and no neoplastic cells. Cloudy or bloody aspirates are obtained from cystic or necrotic tumors. The fluid tends to be high in fat content, protein, and LDH, and cytologic examination will demonstrate neoplastic cells. When the needle is verified to be within the center of the lesion and no fluid is obtained, a solid mass should be assumed and further study is necessary.[33]

The ultrasonographic appearance of a renal cell carcinoma is somewhat variable, but the tumor usually appears as a solid mass lesion with a varying complex echo pattern, frequently hyperechoic (Fig. 13–3). The more vascular the tumor, the more echogenic the lesion tends to be. When a renal cell carcinoma is suspected, further assessment of the renal vein and inferior vena cava with ultrasound can be extremely helpful.

The combination of intravenous pyelography and ultrasound increases the diagnostic accuracy of differentiating cyst from tumor to greater than 90%. Indeterminate lesions (i.e., those not meeting the full criteria for cysts), complex or mixed lesions, and solid lesions should be evaluated with CT scanning.

Computerized Tomography (CT)

The role of CT in the diagnostic evaluation of a suspected renal mass is firmly established.[41, 49] The patient with a mass demonstrating characteristics of a renal cell carcinoma on intravenous pyelogram can be examined directly with CT. Patients with nonclassic renal cysts, indeterminate lesions, or solid lesions on ultrasound should be studied with CT. Also, those patients with inadequate ultrasound examinations should be studied with CT. By applying rigid criteria to the CT appearance of renal masses, the accuracy of cyst versus tumor differen-

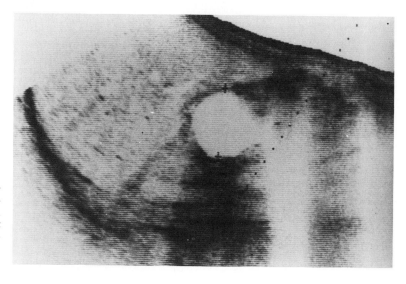

Figure 13–2. Benign simple renal cyst. An anechoic, well-circumscribed renal mass with a smooth back wall and excellent through transmission is characteristic of a renal cyst on ultrasound.

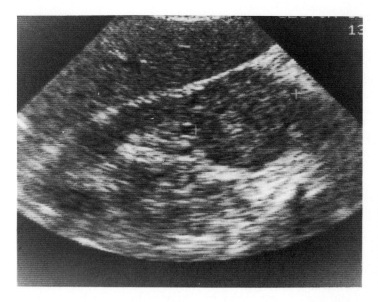

Figure 13–3. Renal cell carcinoma. Renal mass in the lower pole of the right kidney shows deformity of the outline of the kidney as well as echogenic abnormality. Echoes are seen within the mass and there is no enhancement of through transmission, as is seen with renal cysts.

tiation can be increased even further to 97 to 99%, which is better than angiography.[45]

The cross-sectional images of CT scanning provide excellent demonstration of the kidneys and adjacent structures. Renal masses are identified when they alter the normal contour or architecture of the kidney or when the density of the mass is significantly different from that of the surrounding renal parenchyma on either unenhanced or enhanced scans. The specific diagnosis of a renal mass depends on the careful evaluation of the CT numbers, interface with the surrounding tissue, presence or absence and location of any calcification, response to intravenous contrast administration, and appearance relative to the adjacent renal parenchyma.

The incidental, unsuspected benign renal cyst probably is the most common abnormality seen on CT scans of the abdomen. Up to 50% of patients over the age of 50 will have one or more cysts, often 1 cm in size or smaller. Larger incidental cysts occasionally are seen. CT scanning tends to demonstrate more renal cysts than any other imaging technique.

The CT appearance of a benign renal cyst is that of a well-defined, uniformly dense renal mass with CT number values very near that of water (i.e., zero) (Fig. 13–4).[46] The outline of the cyst is smooth, and there is a

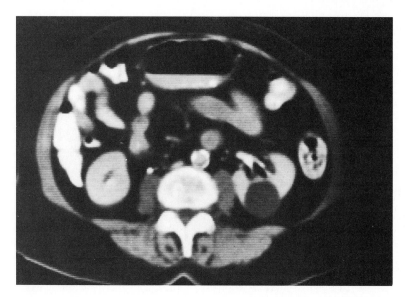

Figure 13–4. Benign simple renal cyst. CT characteristics of a renal cyst are noted with this well-circumscribed, uniformly low density, sharply marginated left renal cyst.

sharp interface with the surrounding normal renal parenchyma, especially after contrast administation. No measurable thickness of the cyst wall is noted, and no enhancement or significant change in CT numbers is seen after intravenous administration of contrast medium. Single or multiple cysts may be found in one or both kidneys (Fig. 13–5).

The appearance of a renal cell carcinoma on CT scans is, in most cases, easily distinguished from that of a renal cyst.[39, 62] Its characteristics on either noncontrast or contrast scans may be similar to other renal masses, such as abscess, hematoma, some benign tumors, and other malignant lesions involving the kidney. Clinical information and laboratory data are occasionally necessary as diagnostic aids. On noncontrast scans, renal cell carcinoma appears as an ill-defined, irregular mass lesion in the kidney whose CT numbers are close to those for normal renal parenchyma (Fig. 13–6). The hypernephroma is usually heterogeneous in density (Fig. 13–7). After the administration of intravenous contrast medium, there is definite enhancement of the tumor mass; however, its CT numbers remain less than those for the surrounding normal kidney. With a bolus injection of contrast material and rapid scanning through the mass, there may be transient marked increase in CT numbers, especially in very vascular lesions. The interface with the normal kidney becomes better defined after contrast enhancement but remains irregular and poorly marginated. More cystic or necrotic lesions will have a thick and irregular wall in contrast to the imperceptible wall of a renal cyst. Calcification within the tumor may be noted. CT is more sensitive in detecting calcifications (Fig. 13–8). Secondary signs of renal cell carcinoma may be noted; these include invasion of the renal vein or inferior vena cava, extension into Gerota's fascia, or enlargement of renal hilar lymph nodes.

Owing to the excellent cross-sectional imaging characteristics of CT scanning, the kidneys, perinephric space, renal hilum, inferior vena cava, adrenals, and adjacent organs are all well delineated with CT. These traits alone make CT the modality of choice for the staging of renal cell carcinomas. Not only may an accurate diagnosis be made with CT, but also preoperative noninvasive staging can be accomplished. Accuracy of staging with CT is reported to be approximately 90%.[41, 45, 49] Correct preoperative staging is important in assessing the prognosis and operative approach.

Stage I lesions will have a mass confined within the capsule of the kidney (Figs. 13–6 and 13–7). In Stage II renal cell carcinoma, the neoplasm has extended beyond the renal capsule to invade the perinephric fat but is still within Gerota's fascia (Figs. 13–8 and 13–9). This may be identified on CT as mass within the perinephric space but bounded peripherally by Gerota's fascia.

Stage III lesions have involvement of the renal vein or regional hilar lymph nodes with or without extension into the inferior vena cava. The renal vein is involved in 28

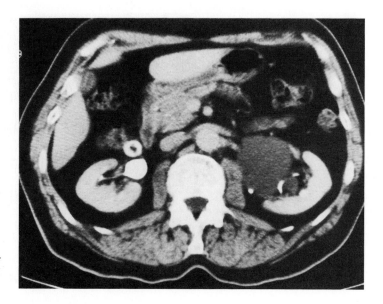

Figure 13–5. Left peripelvic renal cyst. Low-density, well-defined left peripelvic renal cyst extends from the area of the renal pelvis. Note there is no perceptible wall visualized on CT.

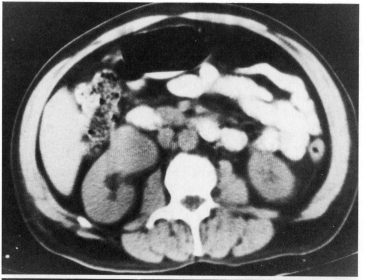

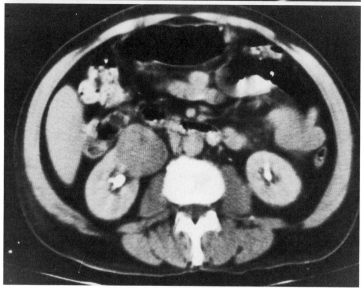

Figure 13–6. Renal cell carcinoma (top). Noncontrast CT scan shows a mass projecting off the superior and medial aspect of the right kidney. Its CT numbers are similar to those for the remainder of the kidney (bottom). Post-enhanced CT scan demonstrates enhancement of the normal renal parenchyma with the renal cell carcinoma remaining less dense than the kidney itself.

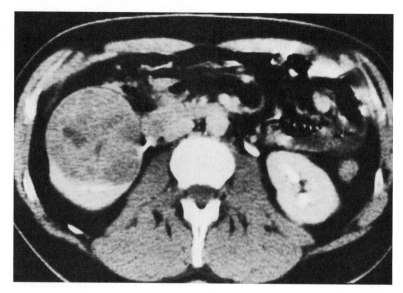

Figure 13–7. Renal cell carcinoma. Rather large renal cell carcinoma of the right kidney shows the heterogeneous nature of the tumor seen on CT. Note the normally enhanced renal parenchyma posterior to the tumor. This is a Stage I lesion.

242

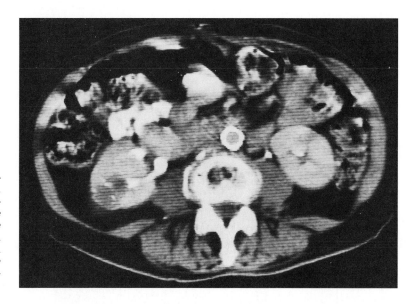

Figure 13–8. Renal cell carcinoma, Stage II with calcification. Primarily intraparenchymal tumor shows extension into the perinephric fat posteriorly. Note the small flecks of calcification within the more central portion of the low-density tumor. These were not visible on the intravenous pyelogram.

to 30% of cases, and the inferior vena cava in 5%.[58] Extension into the renal vein or inferior vena cava is more commonly found with right-sided tumors (Figs. 13–10 and 13–11). The major problem encountered in identifying Stage III lesions is the short, oblique course of the right renal vein, which makes detection of involvement sometimes difficult. Lymph nodes that are enlarged may contain no tumor, and normal-sized nodes may contain only histologic evidence of microscopic invasion. Paracaval masses may be difficult to distinguish from inferior vena caval involvement. The distal extension of the inferior vena cava thrombus or tumor is sometimes difficult to assess with CT but is extremely important in planning the surgical resection. Differentiation between Stage II and Stage III has obvious surgical implications.[13]

Stage IV renal cell carcinoma is defined as progression of tumor outside of Gerota's fascia, involvement of adjacent organs other than the ipsilateral adrenal, and distal metastases (Fig. 13–12).

The CT technique provides a method for rapid and easy assessment of these extensive tumors in giving a global picture of the abdominal and retroperitoneal contents. Scanning for involvement of the liver, op-

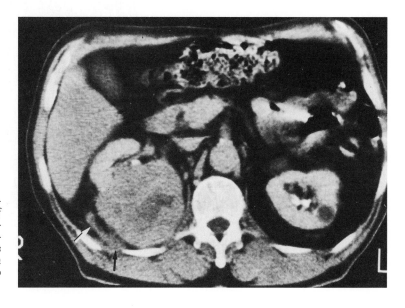

Figure 13–9. Renal cell carcinoma, Stage II. Note extension of this right-sided renal cell carcinoma posteriorly into the perinephric fat (arrows). There is thickening of Gerota's fascia. An incidental left renal cyst is also visible.

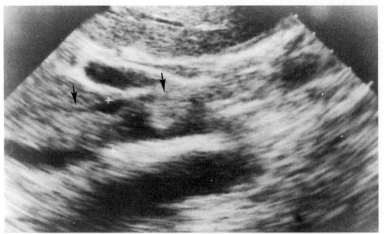

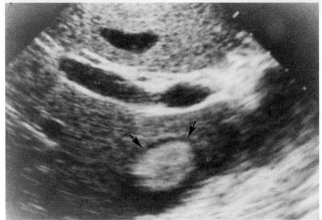

Figure 13–10. Renal cell carcinoma, Stage III. Longitudinal (top) and transverse (bottom) ultrasound views demonstrate tumor thrombus within the inferior vena cava in a patient with right-sided renal cell carcinoma (arrows).

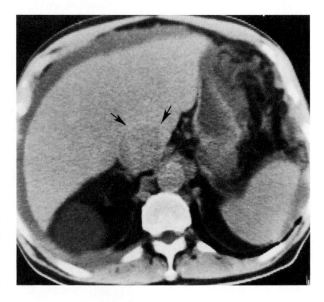

Figure 13–11. Renal cell carcinoma, Stage III. Section through the midportion of the liver demonstrates a low-density region where the inferior vena cava (IVC) is expected (arrows). This represents tumor thrombus extending superiorly within the IVC. Note the top of an incidental right cyst. Patient had right-sided renal cell carcinoma. Ascites is present around the liver due to involvement of the hepatic veins by the tumor thrombus.

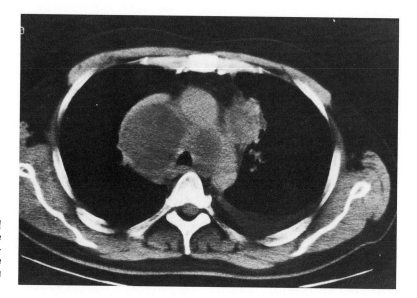

Figure 13–12. Metastatic renal cell carcinoma. CT scan of the chest demonstrates multiple enlarged lymph nodes within the mediastinum, metastatic from a renal cell carcinoma.

posite kidney, bowel, and lungs is accomplished at one time.

Large renal cell carcinomas sometimes are difficult to evaluate for extension beyond the renal capsule into Gerota's fascia. This is especially true on the right side, where it may not be possible to assess direct extension into the liver accurately (Fig. 13–13). Even with very large tumors, extension directly into the liver is uncommon. In this situation ultrasound may be very useful to delineate a plane between the renal mass and the adjacent normal liver.

With five-year survival rates for Stages I, II, and III renal cell carcinomas at greater than 50%, and 10-year survival at greater

than 40%, a larger number of patients develop tumor recurrence even after successful nephrectomy.[57] Prior to the advent of CT scanning, there was no adequate or reliable means to determine local recurrence of tumor in these patients. Normally, after a nephrectomy, the right renal bed will be filled with the hepatic flexure of the colon, second and third portions of the duodenum, small bowel, and, occasionally, the liver. On the left, the spleen migrates posteromedially with the pancreatic tail into the renal bed, along with multiple loops of small bowel. Also, a mild degree of scarring in the retroperitoneum may be found, due to postoperative hematoma or radiation therapy. On CT

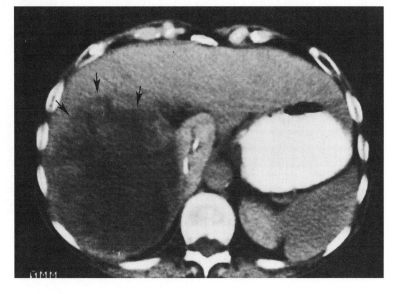

Figure 13–13. Renal cell carcinoma. Problems arise in interpretation of large right-sided renal cell carcinomas. It is difficult to determine whether or not there is extension of tumor into the liver. Note irregular interface between the renal cell carcinoma and the liver (arrows). At surgery, this proved to be a Stage II renal cell carcinoma without involvement of the liver.

scans, tumor recurrence should be suspected when a soft tissue mass is found in the renal bed, the planes between and around the aorta and inferior vena cava are not seen, or the ipsilateral psoas muscle is poorly defined, enlarged, or contains a mass. Percutaneous thin-needle biopsy under CT guidance assists in making an accurate diagnosis of tumor recurrence. With the use of CT scanning, up to 33% of patients were found in one series to have local tumor recurrence within several years of initial nephrectomy.[1] With prompt detection of local recurrence, long-term survival and prevention of distant metastasis may be improved with the more timely introduction of adjuvant chemotherapy and radiotherapy.

Angiography and Venacavography

The leading role played by angiography in the diagnosis of renal cell carcinoma has changed markedly over the past decade with the advent of ultrasound and CT. With a combined diagnostic accuracy of 97 to 98%, these modalities share the primary role in making the diagnosis of renal cell carcinoma, surpassing the accuracy of angiography (95 to 96%).[16] Originally, angiography was the preferred method of staging renal cell carcinomas, but the excellent cross-sectional images of CT and its accuracy and three-dimensional look at the kidney and surrounding structures have now made CT the imaging modality of choice in staging these neoplasms. When compared with angiography, CT scanning has been shown to be more accurate and sensitive in detecting perinephric extension of tumor and more sensitive in evaluating lymph node involvement. Angiography and CT scanning are equally accurate in detecting involvement of the renal vein and inferior vena cava.[62] Overall, staging accuracy of CT is approximately 90%. In a comparison of angiography and CT, angiography has been found to add little additional information.[45]

A small number of renal masses will prove to be within an indeterminate group even after CT scanning.[3] Almost half of these lesions cannot be classified owing to technical reasons: patient motion, inadequate slice thickness, or small size of the lesion. Repeat CT scanning with a shorter scan time, narrower slice thickness, and improved co-

operation of the patient generally leads to a resolution of these problems. In the remaining patients the indeterminate renal lesions have an appearance that combines some features of a renal cyst and also those of a renal neoplasm.

If all renal lesions identified as indeterminate by CT were studied with angiograms, most would be either hypovascular or avascular. Overall, 10 to 15% of all renal cell carcinomas are hypovascular or avascular. Because the typical features of a renal cell carcinoma are absent, namely, tumor vascularity, arteriovenous shunting, and extravasation or puddling of contrast medium, these lesions are difficult to assess by angiography (Figs. 13–14 and 13–15). Pharmacoangiographic techniques occasionally may be helpful in these cases.[26] Despite this, some lesions may remain undiagnosed. In these remaining patients, thin-needle aspiration of the renal mass has proved to be most helpful. In the renal masses judged to be indeterminate by CT, angiography was diagnostic in only 16% of cases, whereas thin-needle aspiration and cytologic examination proved to be diagnostic in 84% of

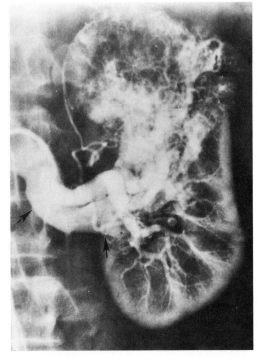

Figure 13–14. Renal cell carcinoma. Angiographically classic renal cell carcinoma demonstrates neovascularity, arteriovenous shunting with early filling of the left renal vein (arrows), and puddling of contrast medium.

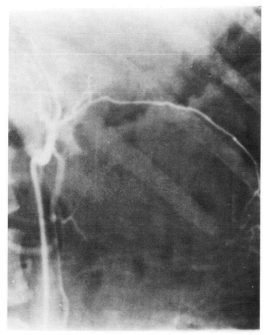

Figure 13–15. Renal cell carcinoma. "Avascular" renal cell carcinoma of lower pole of the left kidney is typical of indeterminate lesions angiographically.

cases.[3] Thus, if a technically adequate CT scan has been performed and the diagnosis is still in doubt, thin-needle aspiration of the renal mass can be the next step to be undertaken, with diagnostic angiography reserved for the last resort.

Venacavography plays a role in cases in which the inferior vena cava cannot be adequately evaluated with CT or ultrasound. This is most common with bulky right-sided tumors that compress or deviate the inferior vena cava. The CT appearance of involvement of the renal vein or inferior vena cava is that of enlargement and a filling defect or mass within the renal vein or inferior vena cava (Fig. 13–11). Flow artifacts contribute to the false-positive diagnosis when the unopacified blood from the renal vein does not mix with the opacified blood of the inferior vena cava. Some have suggested infusion of contrast medium from a vein in the foot, in order to increase the opacity of the inferior vena cava, but this has not been widely accepted nor rewarded increased overall accuracy from the more conventional infusion or bolus injection technique via the antecubital fossa.[44] Inferior venacavography via the antecubital fossa or jugular approach is the preferred method for evaluation of the infe-

rior vena cava, in that the most important piece of information is the superior (rather than the inferior) extent of involvement in the inferior vena cava (Fig. 13–16).

Angiography generally should be reserved for specific problem cases or when an arterial road map is desired by the operating surgeon. Angiography is useful in the patient with a solitary kidney and a hypernephroma in which an effort is being made to salvage an uninvolved portion of the kidney. This is also true in patients with bilateral renal cell carcinomas in whom an effort is going to be made to salvage a portion of the kidneys. Pelvic kidneys with hypernephroma may benefit from angiography owing to their aberrant blood supply and the necessity of the surgeon to be aware of this. In large, bulky, right-sided lesions with invasion or a question of invasion into the liver, angiography has proved useful in some cases. Ther-

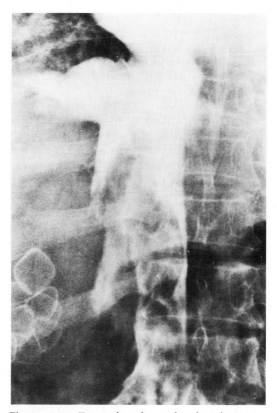

Figure 13–16. Tumor thrombus within the inferior vena cava. A large irregular filling defect is seen within the inferior vena cava, representing a tumor thrombus from a large right-sided renal cell carcinoma. Note that the right hepatic veins are not involved with tumor in this case. Incidentally noted on the right are calcified faceted gallstones.

apeutic angiography for preoperative embolization and tumor ablation still plays a role in some patients. When angiography is used, digital subtraction angiography (DSA) can be employed in both the arterial and venous evaluation of renal tumors. The DSA technique from the arterial side has the advantage of requiring much less contrast medium than conventional angiography, and small catheters can be employed, resulting in fewer complications. With the use of DSA techniques, many angiographic procedures can be performed on an outpatient basis.

Magnetic Resonance Imaging

Magnetic resonance imaging (MRI, NMR) is a newly introduced imaging modality that does not employ the use of x-rays or need intravenous iodinated contrast agents. The patient is placed in a supine position within a large-bore cylindrical magnet that has a magnetic field 1,000 to 10,000 times as intense as the earth's. Radiofrequency waves or pulses are transmitted into the area of study, and the resultant signals are received by an antenna adjacent to the patient. The collected signals are processed by a computer similar to the one used for CT. To date, more than 250,000 patients have been studied with no untoward effects or complications. However, patients with claustrophobia, cardiac pacemakers or other biostimulator devices, or ferromagnetic neurosurgical aneurysm clips in place should not undergo the study. The presence of con-

ventional surgical clips is not a contraindication to an MRI examination. Patient motion and respiratory motion may occasionally degrade the images, but this will improve with newer techniques. MRI images may be obtained directly in any imaging plane—axial, coronal, sagittal, and oblique—without the loss of resolution, as is the case with reformatted images of CT (Figs. 13–17 and 13–18).

Preliminary reports have shown that MRI differentiates solid from cystic lesions, benign simple cysts from hemorrhagic and inflammatory lesions, and also renal tumors.[23, 37] The diagnostic accuracy appears to be similar to or slightly greater than CT. In the evaluation of 27 patients with renal cell carcinoma, MRI was able to stage the lesions accurately in 26 cases (96%). The images correctly revealed the tumor mass, were able to assist in the assessment of venous patency, delineated metastatic lymph node involvement, and accurately portrayed the integrity of adjacent tissues and tissue planes.[22] Without the use of contrast agents, MRI was consistently able to reveal tumor thrombus in the renal vein and inferior vena cava and allow evaluation of the wall of the inferior vena cava. Thus, although only preliminary work has been done with MRI, the initial results appear quite promising. With adequate assessment of the renal veins and inferior vena cava with MRI, one may be able to eliminate inferior venacavography. Its exact position in the systematic evaluation of the renal

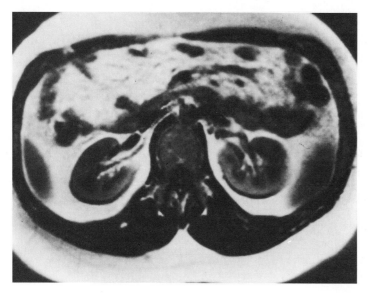

Figure 13–17. Normal magnetic resonance image of the kidneys. Transverse section through the midportion of the kidneys demonstrates the vasculature, both arterial and venous, supplying the kidneys. Also note the corticomedullary differentiation.

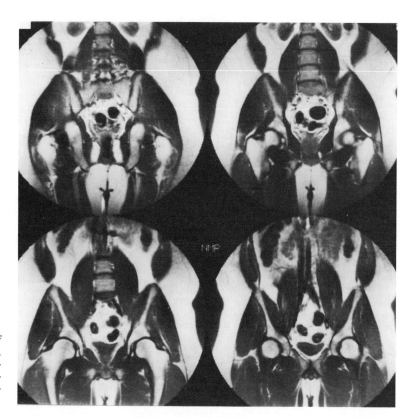

Figure 13–18. Normal MRI of the lower abdomen and pelvis. Direct coronal images demonstrate most of the retroperitoneum from the kidneys inferiorly into the pelvis.

mass remains to be shown. The next few years will undoubtedly prove its worth and establish its role.

Metastases

With a secure diagnosis of renal cell carcinoma and adequate local staging accomplished, the patient should be evaluated for distant metastases. Since the highest incidence of metastases is to the lungs from renal cell carcinoma,[5] evaluation of the lungs should generally advance beyond the routine chest x-ray. CT scanning offers higher sensitivity than whole lung tomography when the pulmonary parenchyma is evaluated, and it details the mediastinum and pleura completely (Fig. 13–12). There is lower radiation exposure to the lungs with CT than with whole lung tomograms. Although whole lung tomography is less expensive, it detects fewer nodules. Radionuclide liver and spleen scans generally are no longer necessary to detect metastases to the liver (the second most common site), since that organ is usually evaluated with the kidneys on CT scans. Radionuclide bone scanning has replaced the radiographic bone

survey as the appropriate method for assessing the skeletal system, the third most common site of distant metastases from renal cell carcinoma.

Miscellaneous Renal Lesions

In patients with von Hippel-Lindau disease, there is a very high incidence of renal mass lesions (varying from 31% to 83%).[36, 43] Benign lesions such as renal cysts, adenomas, and hemangiomas have been reported. Approximately one half of these patients develop renal cell carcinomas, frequently multiple and bilateral. All patients with known von Hippel-Lindau disease or intracranial hemangioblastomas should be examined routinely for the development of renal cell carcinomas and other renal masses. Ultrasound examinations or (preferably) CT scans, or both, should be performed on these individuals at regular intervals for early detection and evaluation of these lesions.[38]

Solid renal lesions other than cysts and renal cell carcinomas occasionally are found during the search for the cause of a renal mass. Generally these are rare, and only a

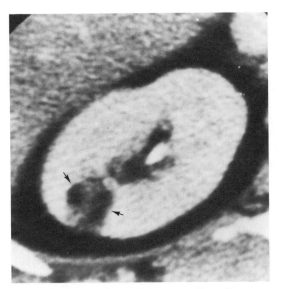

Figure 13–19. Angiomyolipoma. Small, well-circumscribed lesion in posterior aspect of the right kidney represents an angiomyolipoma. Note the low density material within the mass consistent with fat, diagnostic of angiomyolipomas (arrows).

few will be highlighted here. The angiomyolipoma (hamartoma) is a rare, benign tumor of the kidney that occurs in two forms. In patients with tuberous sclerosis, the lesions are frequently small, multiple, bilateral, and usually asymptomatic. Most symptomatic angiomyolipomas are unilateral, large, and solitary and occur in females of an older age group. Because angiomyolipomas contain varying amounts of fat, CT scanning is the

diagnostic method of choice in the evaluation of these patients; the fat-containing areas are easily detectable within the renal mass on CT (Fig. 13–19).[17, 56, 60] Excretory urography merely presents a picture similar to that of other renal masses. The angiographic findings of angiomyolipoma are remarkably similar to those for renal cell carcinoma, with more than 75% showing neovascularity identical to that of renal cell carcinomas.[11] Owing to the fat, a markedly echogenic mass that is highly suggestive of angiomyolipoma may be seen by ultrasound, but, to be certain of the diagnosis, it remains for CT scanning to demonstrate the fat within the mass.

The renal oncocytoma is considered to be a benign renal adenoma with oncocytic features. It is an uncommon lesion that usually is solitary and asymptomatic. The diagnosis may be suggested preoperatively when the information from several imaging modalities is combined.[50] A renal mass at least 3 cm in diameter, having a homogeneous appearance on CT and ultrasound, with a central stellate scar is highly suggestive of a renal oncocytoma (Fig. 13–20). These findings, combined with the angiographic features of a "spokewheel" arterial pattern and a dense homogeneous blush, are considered characteristic of a renal oncocytoma. Lesions not fulfilling these criteria should not be labelled preoperatively as oncocytoma.

Most metastases to the kidney are quite small and usually not detected before death, since they are asymptomatic. With the in-

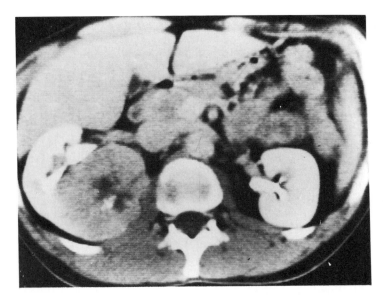

Figure 13–20. Renal oncocytoma. Contrast-enhanced CT scan shows well-circumscribed lesion that is homogeneous except for a central stellate region within the midportion of the renal mass. Focal calcification is seen centrally. Findings are relatively classic for renal oncocytomas.

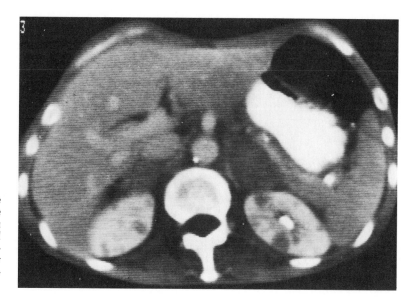

Figure 13–21. Metastases to the kidney. Patient with extensive metastatic breast carcinoma demonstrates bilateral adrenal metastases anterior to the kidneys, with multiple low-density regions within the kidneys representing metastases.

creased use of CT and ultrasound, renal metastases are detected with increasing frequency in patients with primary lesions elsewhere.

Metastatic lesions are indistinguishable from renal cell carcinoma on both CT and ultrasound. The presence of multiple bilateral lesions certainly suggests metastases in a patient with a known primary cancer (Fig. 13–21).

Lymphomatous involvement of the kidneys occurs either by direct invasion from retroperitoneal nodes or as single or multiple masses within the kidneys. Primary renal lymphoma is rare. Increased utilization of

CT and ultrasound in the staging of these patients reveals these renal abnormalities.[25] With direct extension from the retroperitoneum, the kidney is diffusely infiltrated, enlarged, and distorted. On CT scanning, the enlarged retroperitoneal nodes are found with a mass extending into the kidney. The lymphomatous tissue is less dense than the remaining kidney. When seen as single or multiple masses, retroperitoneal nodal enlargement usually is present (Figs. 13–22 and 13–23). The masses are less dense than the adjacent renal parenchyma and may appear almost as cysts, but the CT numbers are considerably higher than those for water.

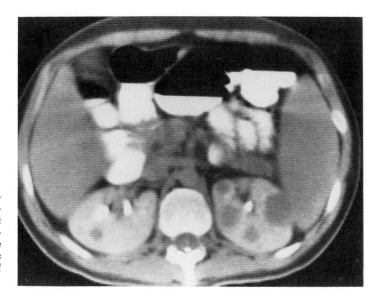

Figure 13–22. Lymphoma of the kidneys. Multiple well-circumscribed lesions are seen in both kidneys in a patient with known lymphoma. Although the lesions have an appearance similar to renal cysts, their CT numbers are much higher. No retroperitoneal adenopathy is present.

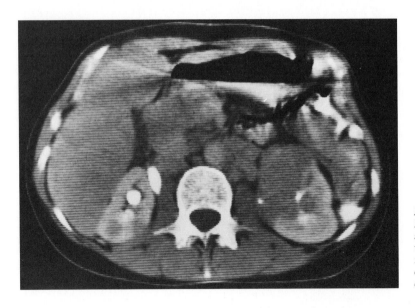

Figure 13–23. Renal lymphoma. Multiple renal masses of soft tissue density are seen in patient with renal lymphoma. Retroperitoneal adenopathy is present adjacent to the inferior vena cava and aorta.

A recently described entity of acquired renal cystic disease in patients on long-term dialysis should be commented on, as 5 to 10% of these patients may develop renal neoplasms as well. The acquired cystic disease occurs in end-stage kidneys but is not the same as congenital adult polycystic kidney disease.[15] The longer the patient undergoes dialysis, the more likely is the development of acquired cystic disease. If less than three years, the incidence may be as high as 40%, increasing to almost 80% if longer than three years. The cysts usually are 0.5 to 2.0 cm in size and are multiple and bilateral. Most are characteristically cystic on CT or ultrasound, but some may show evidence of intracystic hemorrhage.[7] Renal cell carcinomas have been found in these patients, with frequency increasing from 5 to 10%.[24] The imaging appearance of these carcinomas is similar to that of other renal cell carcinomas occurring in the general population.

The evaluation of the child with a suspected Wilms' tumor must always begin with an intravenous pyelogram. The findings are frequently characteristic, with angiography rarely necessary for diagnosis. Ultrasound or CT scanning may be employed when the diagnosis is uncertain from the IVP. The liver and adjacent organs can be evaluated with ultrasound or CT at the same time. As the lungs are the most common site of metastasis, CT of the chest should be employed.

TUMORS OF THE RENAL PELVIS AND URETER

Radiographic evaluation of the patient with a suspected tumor of the renal pelvis or ureter rests on the intravenous pyelogram and retrograde pyelogram. It is mandatory that the entire calyceal system, renal pelvis, and ureters be seen adequately during the course of any uroradiologic examination when a urothelial tumor is suspected. The most common presenting sign is painless hematuria. In any patient, especially males over the age of 50, with hematuria and hydronephrosis, the diagnosis of urothelial tumor must be excluded. An incomplete or inadequate IVP delays the proper diagnosis. With incomplete visualization of the renal pelvis or ureter, a retrograde pyelogram becomes mandatory when there is suspicion of urothelial tumor.

The pathognomonic finding of a solitary filling defect in the renal pelvis is present in only one third to one half of the cases (Fig. 13–24). Tumors of the renal pelvis may also present with multiple filling defects within the renal pelvis due to blood clots or tumor, hydronephrosis, ureteropelvic junction obstruction, or a nonfunctioning kidney. Ureteral tumors usually are seen as intraluminal lesions or diffuse strictures of the ureter. Filling defects in the renal pelvis or ureter may be smooth or irregular in contour. Rarely, faint calcifications may be identified within the lesion.

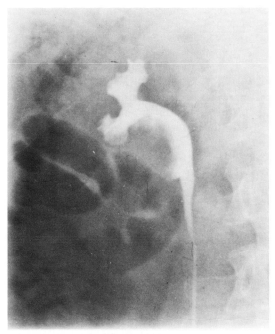

Figure 13–24. Transitional cell carcinoma of the renal pelvis. Retrograde pyelogram demonstrates a large filling defect that is somewhat irregular, involving the inferior aspect of the renal pelvis.

Benign tumors are extremely rare. They arise from the nonepithelial elements of the renal pelvis or ureteral wall. They may present as either filling defects or pedunculated polypoid defects. The vast majority of the neoplastic lesions are transitional cell carcinomas, and in 30 to 40% of patients they may be multiple.[5, 27] Squamous cell carcinoma of either the renal pelvis or ureter does occur, but only when there has been metaplasia of the uroepithelium, usually due to long-standing calculus disease, infection, or both.

When a filling defect is encountered within the renal pelvis or ureter, making a diagnosis may be a lengthy process. The most common conditions to be excluded are calculus disease, blood clot, inflammatory lesions such as pyelitis cystica or ureteritis cystica, benign or congenital obstruction of the ureteropelvic junction, external vascular imprints, and peripelvic cysts. Renal cell carcinoma, when it invades the renal pelvis, may present as a solitary filling defect and thus could be confused with a transitional cell carcinoma. When a ureteral stricture is encountered, the differential diagnosis other than urothelial tumor includes endometrio-

sis, retroperitoneal fibrosis, inflammatory strictures of the ureter, and metastases. The radiographic findings should be evaluated along with cytologic study of the urine.

The combined use of intravenous urography to identify the superior surface and retrograde pyelography to identify the inferior surface of the intraluminal mass is the radiographic method of choice for study of these patients. Antegrade pyelography may occasionally be necessary when there is poor visualization of the upper tracts and ureter during the intravenous pyelogram. Antegrade pyelography also can be used for collection of urine for cytologic study. The retrograde pyelogram has been the keystone in the evaluation of patients with suspected urothelial tumors. Bergman and co-workers,[6] in 1961, described an almost pathognomonic finding for transitional cell carcinoma of the ureter identified during retrograde examination. On retrograde pyelography as the catheter was advanced up the ureter, a coiling of the catheter occurred just beneath the intraluminal lesion. Radiographically, Bergman's sign is noted to be an intraluminal filling defect accompanied by local dilatation of the ureter distal to the mass (Fig. 13–25). This has an appearance of either a meniscus or wine goblet. In contradistinction, with calculus disease the ureter is collapsed or flattened distal to the stone.

Angiography has been uniformly unsuccessful in the diagnostic evaluation of these tumors. One exception would be the differentiation of a renal cell carcinoma that has invaded and spread into the renal pelvis from a transitional cell carcinoma that has invaded the renal parenchyma. The somewhat nonspecific angiographic findings in transitional cell carcinoma include encasement and displacement of parenchymal vessels and enlarged periureteral arteries.[32, 47]

Ultrasound and CT scanning have been helpful in some specific cases, but their routine use in tumors of the renal pelvis and ureter probably is not warranted. Ultrasonographically, a transitional cell carcinoma of the renal pelvis appears as a mass density within the central echo complex of the kidney or renal pelvis (Fig. 13–26). CT scanning is able to detect and evaluate the presence of a soft tissue mass in the renal pelvis and, occasionally, within the ureter (Fig. 13–27).[4] Ureteral wall thickening with luminal narrowing and the presence of an infiltrating mass extending into the renal parenchyma ranges on CT numbers and thus a different appearance.

The main cause of misdiagnosis or delay in diagnosis in patients with urothelial tumors of the renal pelvis and ureter is the initial finding of a "normal" intravenous pyelogram when there is incomplete visualization of the renal pelvis or ureters. For the population group at risk with painless hematuria, it is essential to persist in order to exclude or include the diagnosis of urothelial tumor.

BLADDER TUMORS

The diagnosis of urothelial tumors of the bladder is made by cystoscopy in almost all cases. It is the rare lesion that is encountered incidentally with excretory urography. Pedunculated, papillary tumors, when examined with retrograde cystography, usually are well circumscribed and smooth. They may grow to fill the entire bladder, and only a thin rim of contrast medium may be seen around the lesion (Fig. 13–28). Despite their frequently large size, these tumors tend to be noninfiltrating and nonobstructing even when in proximity to the ureteral orifice. Nonpapillary solid urothelial tumors produce flat, ill-defined defects with little if any intraluminal projection on cystography. The bladder wall appears rigid and fixed in position, since many of these lesions are infiltrating. Ureteral obstruction on excretory urography usually indicates extensive infiltration into the perivesical fat.

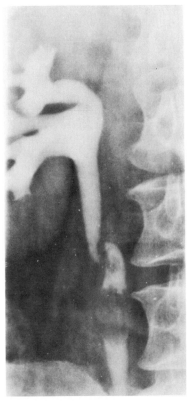

Figure 13–25. *Transitional cell carcinoma of the ureter. Large filling defect is demonstrated in the proximal right ureter, with the classic finding of dilatation of the distal as well as the proximal ureter adjacent to the tumor.*

or into the retroperitoneal fat may be determined by CT. A "nonopaque" stone may be differentiated from a blood clot or tumor with CT scanning, as they all have different

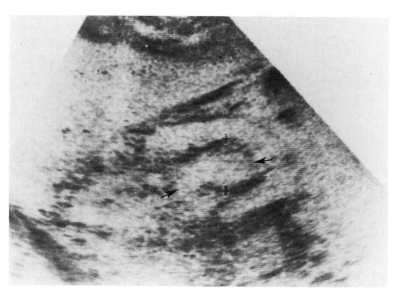

Figure 13–26. *Transitional cell carcinoma of the renal pelvis. Ultrasound demonstrates a solid mass (arrows) involving the central echo complex and renal pelvis of the right kidney.*

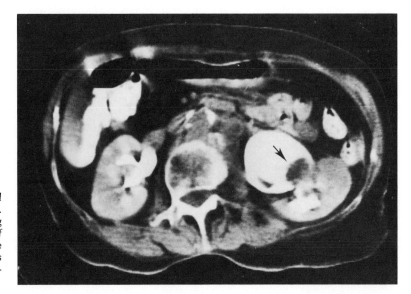

Figure 13–27. Transitional cell carcinoma of the renal pelvis. CT scan shows a mass projecting into a large extrarenal pelvis of the left kidney (arrow). Note the enlarged retroperitoneal nodes just to left of the calcified abdominal aorta.

Various methods have been used over the years in an attempt to assist in the preoperative staging of patients with bladder neoplasms. These have included air contrast cystography, perivesical insufflation of oxygen, angiography, and lymphangiography. Most have fallen quickly from favor. Lymphangiography has failed to gain wide acceptance owing to accuracy rates ranging from 50 to 90%.[59] The primary fault lies in the inability to visualize with lymphangiography the first nodal chains involved with metastatic bladder carcinoma—the obturator and internal iliac nodes.

The use of CT scanning in patients with bladder carcinoma has shown some promise. The cross-sectional imaging by CT permits assessment of the bladder wall thickness, the perivesical region, obturator and iliac nodal chains, and more distant regions. Computed tomography is unable to distinguish the stage of tumor confined to the bladder wall (Stages 0, A, B_1 and B_2). Perivesical extension in Stage C can be identified on CT scans with an accuracy of 80% (Figs. 13–29 and 13–30).[53, 55] Lymph node extension, Stage D, is identified with an accuracy range of 70 to 90% (Fig. 13–30).[31, 48] The major failing of the CT examination lies in its inability to detect microscopic ex-

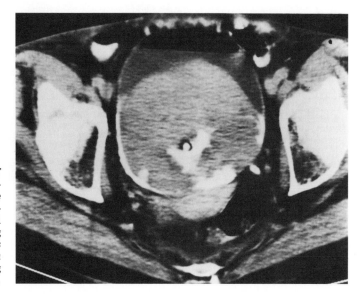

Figure 13–28. Bladder carcinoma. CT scan through the midportion of the bladder demonstrates a large papillary-type transitional cell carcinoma involving almost the entire portion of the bladder. A small amount of contrast is seen outlining the lateral aspects of the tumor. Air is within the bladder anteriorly. The tip of a Foley catheter is seen centrally, attesting to the soft, pliable nature of these lesions.

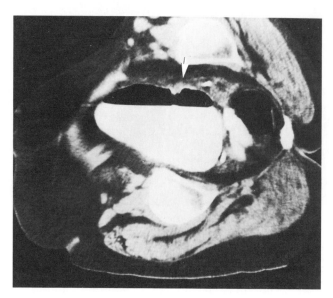

Figure 13–29. Transitional cell carcinoma of the bladder. Infiltrating nonpapillary transitional cell carcinoma is demonstrated on the lateral wall in this double-contrast CT scan through the bladder. Note extension of tumor into the perivesicular fat laterally (arrow).

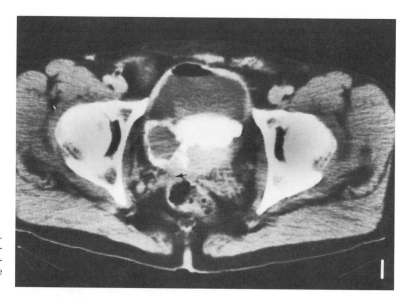

Figure 13–30. Bladder cancer. Extension of tumor into perivesicular fat (arrow) and enlargement of right obturator nodes are seen on this CT scan.

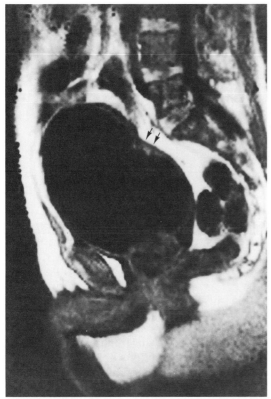

Figure 13–31. MR image of bladder carcinoma. Midline sagittal section demonstrates irregular thickening of posterior wall of bladder, representing a transitional cell carcinoma (arrows). Note inferiorly the heterogeneous prostate as well.

travesical invasion and tumor foci in normal-sized lymph nodes. The role of MRI in the detection of bladder carcinoma will probably be similar to its role in revealing other pelvic neoplasms (Fig. 13–31). This is

discussed in greater depth with regard to testicular tumors and prostatic carcinoma.

Bone scanning in patients with bladder tumors is appropriate in view of the incidence of skeletal metastases. Liver scans should be reserved for the patients with abnormal liver function tests. Chest x-ray should be performed in all patients, but the use of whole lung tomography or CT scanning does not appear to be warranted at present.

TESTICULAR TUMORS

Both diagnostic and staging information can be provided by radiographic examinations in the patient with a suspected testicular neoplasm. Testicular ultrasound is the chief method employed for radiographic analysis of the testis. The scrotum and its contents are examined either in a water bath or by direct contact scanning. The use of a high-frequency transducer, 5 MHz or higher, is mandatory in order to detect the sometimes small and subtle changes found with testicular tumors. The normal testis has a finely granular echogenic texture of medium echogenicity (Fig. 13–32). The epididymal region is more echogenic than the testis. With ultrasound, one is looking for subtle changes in the texture of the testis, solid or cystic masses, and a differentiation of extratesticular lesions from intratesticular masses.

On most occasions, testicular tumors present as masses confined to the testis. The involved testis may show focal or general-

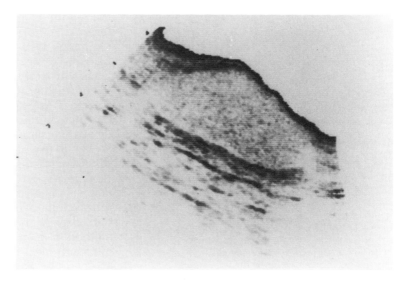

Figure 13–32. Normal testis. Sagittal ultrasound through the normal testis demonstrates its finely granular echogenicity.

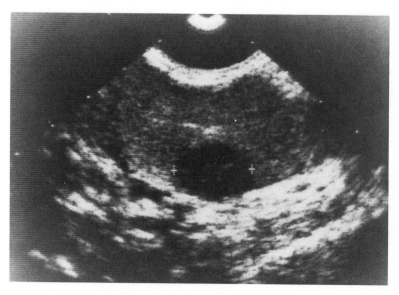

Figure 13–33. Seminoma. Relatively well circumscribed lesion is identified within the testis. A few echoes are seen within it, but there is no through transmission as would be expected with a cystic lesion. This represents a solid tumor of the testis.

ized enlargement. The key finding on ultrasound is inhomogeneity of the normal, finely granular texture and areas of decreased or increased echogenic character. The most common appearance is that of a mass with decreased echoes and attenuation of the sound distal to the lesion, signifying a solid lesion (Fig. 13–33). When the entire testis is involved, it must be compared with the normal opposite side in order to distinguish the diffusely abnormal echogenic texture (Fig. 13–34). Rarely, testicular tumors may present as cystic masses with internal sep-

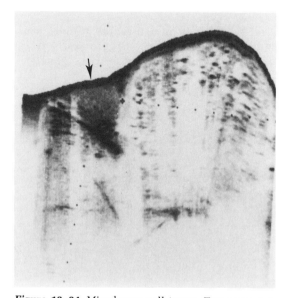

Figure 13–34. Mixed germ cell tumor. Transverse images through the scrotum demonstrate normal testicle on the right (arrow) with a markedly enlarged and heterogeneous mass involving the left testicle.

tations, solid regions, and fluid-filled areas. The differential diagnosis includes subacute or chronic torsion with mixed solid and cystic components, traumatic hematomas, chronic or granulomatous epididymitis with associated orchitis, scars due to prior trauma or inflammatory processes, and, occasionally, metastases. With careful examination and pertinent clinical information, the sensitivity of ultrasound in detecting testicular tumors approaches 100%.[54]

Ultrasound also plays a key role in the detection of occult neoplasms of the testis. In the male patient with mediastinal or retroperitoneal lymphadenopathy, or both, ultrasound of the testes should be performed even if clinical examination is normal. A small area of focal abnormal texture within the testicle may be the only finding in establishing the primary source of the metastatic lesions. A normal examination should exclude the testis as a source because false-negative ultrasound results, when the studies are properly performed, are rare.

The further assessment and radiographic staging of the patient with a testicular tumor depends upon the tumor type—seminoma versus nonseminoma. The intravenous pyelogram is useful in detecting bulky retroperitoneal adenopathy and associated obstruction to the kidneys, but in assessing lesser degrees of retroperitoneal involvement, the intravenous pyelogram has limited application. Bipedal lymphangiography is a useful method to detect the presence or absence of retroperitoneal nodal involvement. Lymphangiography has had its greatest success in

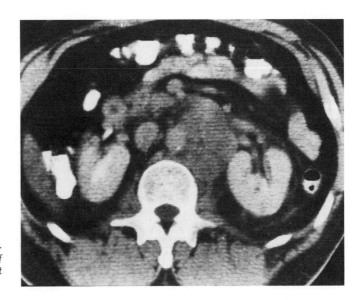

Figure 13–35. *Testicular carcinoma. Moderately enlarged nodes are noted to left of the aorta and adjacent to the left kidney at the level of the renal hilum.*

evaluating the retroperitoneal nodes in patients with pure seminomas. The major failing of lymphangiography is that the nodes that are not filled or visualized with contrast material cannot be evaluated. The primary site of lymphatic spread to testicular lesions is to renal hilar lymph nodes, which are not routinely identified with lymphangiography. Also, high abdominal and retrocrural nodes may not be seen and thus cannot be evaluated. This leads to errors in staging, particularly understaging of the pure seminoma. Despite this, accuracy rates of 70 to 90% are reported.[8] False-positive and false-negative results at rates as high as 30% have also been reported.[31, 54] In the patient with a nonseminomatous lesion, lymphangiogra-phy causes a diffuse inflammatory lymphangiitis due to the oil-based contrast material employed, which makes lymphadenectomy, the treatment of choice, more difficult technically. Occasionally, in patients with extensive retroperitoneal involvement prior to lymphadenectomy, angiography or venography, or both, have been useful in planning the surgical resection. Their routine use, however, is certainly not warranted.

The use of CT scanning in assessment of patients with metastatic retroperitoneal involvement by testicular tumors reveals an accuracy of greater than 90% (Figs. 13–35 and 13–36).[40] The advantage of CT scanning over lymphangiography rests on the ability of CT to detect metastases to the primary

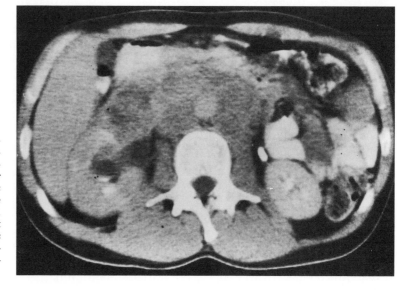

Figure 13–36. *Testicular carcinoma. Bulky retroperitoneal adenopathy is identified in this patient with a right-sided testicular neoplasm. Adenopathy extends to the left of the aorta and to the right of the inferior vena cava. Mild hydronephrosis of the right kidney is also identified. This was caused by the bulky retroperitoneal adenopathy more inferiorly.*

sites of nodal involvement. Also, CT displays high abdominal and retrocrural nodes easily. The major errors in CT interpretation occur when metastatic deposits are present in normal-sized nodes. Planning radiation therapy with CT assistance has led to greater accuracy in delivering the necessary treatment dose to the full extent of disease.[2] In patients with nonseminomatous testicular tumors, CT is the method of choice for noninvasive staging prior to lymphadenectomy. It is also replacing lymphangiography in the evaluation of patients with pure seminomas.

Preliminary studies in imaging lymph nodes with MRI show results at least equal to those for CT scanning.[14, 34] The excellent soft tissue contrast provided with MRI may lead to results better than those for CT once the optimal pulse sequences and imaging planes are established. Metastatic tumor spread to normal-sized nodes may also be identified. The great advantage of MRI may come in evaluating the postlymphadenectomy patient with multiple metallic clips in the retroperitoneum. The marked stellate artifacts caused by the metallic clips on CT are not present on MR images, because these clips give no signal. This will lead to better images of the retroperitoneum and, possibly, earlier detection of recurrent disease (Fig. 13–18).

Chest x-rays should be performed in all patients. Additionally, CT scans of the chest should be used for accurate evaluation of the pulmonary parenchyma as well as the mediastinum. The sensitivity of chest CT is higher than that for whole lung tomography, and therefore all possible lesions should be found in these potentially curable patients. Radionuclide liver and spleen scans are not necessary if the patient has had a CT scan of the abdomen as part of the staging work-up. Bone scans are necessary only when a tumor is disseminated and a bone scan is needed to document the extent of involvement. CT scans of the head are reserved for those patients with diffuse metastatic disease or focal neurologic signs.

PROSTATIC CARCINOMA

The radiographic evaluation of the patient with prostatic carcinoma is primarily directed at staging and the effects of the tumor mass on the bladder, ureters, and upper urinary tract. Only occasionally is the initial diagnosis suggested from excretory urography—for instance, when sclerotic metastatic bone lesions are identified. The intravenous pyelogram is used to assess the degree of upper urinary tract obstruction caused by the tumor. The position of the ureters may be deviated by pelvic or retroperitoneal lymph node enlargement or by the tumor mass itself. Although cystoscopic visualization is a much better method for detecting extension to the bladder floor, intravenous pyelogram or cystogram may suggest involvement. Retrograde cystourethrography has not been used widely in establishing the diagnosis of prostatic carcinoma. It has proved useful in planning radiation therapy, however, by determining the caudal limits of the gland when external beam therapy is used.[21]

The use of ultrasound in the evaluation of the prostate has met with variable success and interest.[20] As complete evaluation of the area of the prostate is technically difficult with ultrasound, consistent understaging of the tumor generally occurs. Limited work employing a transrectal ultrasonic probe for evaluation of the prostate has shown promising results.[51]

Bipedal lymphangiography has been used to assist in staging prostatic carcinoma, as it has been for other genitourinary carcinomas. Accurate diagnosis of lymph node metastasis has been variably successful, with overall accuracy in the 50 to 90% range.[59, 63] As is also true with carcinoma of the bladder, the lymphangiographic contrast medium does not fill and thus reveal the obturator and internal iliac nodes, the initial site of lymphangitic metastases. This results in errors in understaging the metastatic extension of prostatic carcinoma. In addition, as with all lymphangiograms, false-positive and false-negative results also occur.

In patients with carcinoma of the prostate, CT scanning has generally met with better success than lymphangiography. The tumor itself within the prostate cannot be seen with CT. Extension out of the gland into the adjacent fat, seminal vesicles, and side walls of the pelvis is frequently identified. Nodal enlargement of the obturator and internal iliac nodes also can be seen on CT. The overall accuracy of CT scanning approaches 90% with both high specificity and sensitivity (Fig. 13–37).[18, 35, 61] Understaging of prostatic carcinoma due to microscopic extension into the soft tissues or normal-sized

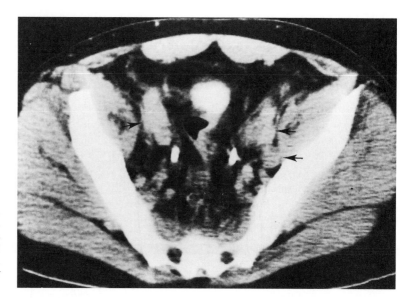

Figure 13–37. Prostatic carcinoma. CT scan through the middle level of the pelvis shows bilateral internal and external iliac nodal adenopathy (arrows). Ureters are displaced medially by the enlarged nodes.

nodes with metastatic involvement remains the most significant problem with CT scanning. It appears to be warranted, however, to use CT scanning with patients in whom there is much clinical and pathologic suspicion of advanced disease (Stages C and D). Fine-needle aspiration with either CT or lymphangiographic guidance in suspect nodes may avoid more invasive procedures, if the result is positive.[19, 29]

Initial results with MR imaging of the prostate have been mixed.[9, 10] The normal prostate has a homogeneous signal and is seen on images in any plane through the pelvis, owing to the excellent soft tissue contrast of MRI. Preliminary work suggested a specific pattern and signal intensity in patients with carcinoma of the prostate. Further evaluation showed these findings to be nonspecific and nondiagnostic. Additional work needs to be done in order to determine the optimal imaging sequences to be used in these patients. With these data, possibly a specific diagnosis can be rendered (Fig. 13–38).

Radionuclide bone scans and chest x-rays are necessary in all patients with carcinoma of the prostate. Further radiographic studies are rarely needed unless specific biochemical evidence is present. With abnormal liver function tests, either a CT scan or radionuclide liver and spleen scan should be performed.

Acknowledgment

The author wishes to thank Barbara Silletto for her assistance in the preparation of this manuscript.

References

1. Alter AJ, Uehling DT, Zweibel WJ: Computed tomography of the retroperitoneum following nephrectomy. Radiology 133:663–668, 1979.

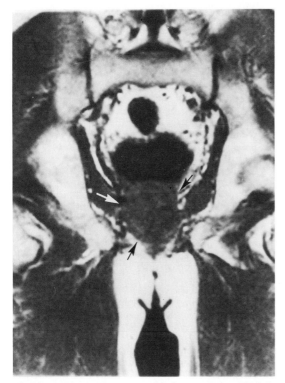

Figure 13–38. MR images of the prostate. Slightly heterogeneous prostate (arrows) is identified inferior to the bladder. The fat planes around the prostate are well maintained.

2. Badcock PC: The role of computed tomography in the planning of radiotherapy fields. Radiology 147:241–244, 1983.

3. Balfe DM, McClennan BL, Stanley RJ, et al: Evaluation of renal masses considered indeterminate on computed tomography. Radiology 142:421–428, 1982.

4. Baron RL, McClennan BL, Lee JKT, Lawson TL: Computed tomography of transitional cell carcinoma of the renal pelvis and ureter. Radiology 144:125–130, 1982.

5. Bennington JL, Beckwith JB: Tumors of the Kidney, Renal Pelvis, and Ureter. Washington DC, Armed Forces Institute of Pathology (AFIP), 1975, p 163.

6. Bergman H, Friedenberg RM, Sayegh V: New roentgenologic signs of carcinoma of the ureter. AJR 86:707–717, 1961.

7. Bommer J, Waldherr R, van Kaick G, et al: Acquired renal cysts in uremic patients—in vivo demonstration by computed tomography. Clin Nephrol 14:299–303, 1980.

8. Borski AA: Proceedings: Diagnosis, staging and natural history of testicular tumors. Cancer 32:1202–1205, 1973.

9. Bryan PJ, Butler HE, LiPuma JP, et al: NMR scanning of the pelvis: initial experience with a 0.3 T system. AJR 141:1111–1118, 1983.

10. Buonocore E, Hesemann C, Pavlicek W, Montie JE: Clinical and in vitro magnetic resonance imaging of prostatic carcinoma. AJR 143:1267–1272, 1984.

11. Clark RE, Palubinskas AJ: The angiographic spectrum of renal hamartoma. AJR 114:715–721, 1972.

12. Daniel WW Jr, Hartman GW, Witten DM, et al: Calcified renal masses. A review of ten years experience at the Mayo Clinic. Radiology 103:503–508, 1972.

13. deKernion JB, Berry D: The diagnosis and treatment of renal cell carcinoma. Cancer 45 (Suppl 7):1947–1956, 1980.

14. Dooms GC, Hricak H, Crooks LE, Higgins CB: Magnetic resonance imaging of the lymph nodes: comparison with CT. Radiology 153:719–728, 1984.

15. Dunnill MS, Millard PR, Oliver D: Acquired cystic disease of the kidneys: a hazard of long-term intermittent maintenance haemodialysis. J Clin Pathol 30:868–877, 1977.

16. Fulton RE: Techniques and applications of renal angiography. In DM Witten, GH Myers, DC Utz (eds), Emmett's Clinical Urography. 4th ed. Philadelphia, WB Saunders, 1977, pp 94–149.

17. Gentry LR, Gould HR, Alter AJ, et al: Hemorrhagic angiomyolipoma: demonstration by computed tomography. J Comput Assis Tomogr 5:861–865, 1981.

18. Golimbu M, Morales P, Al-Askari S, Shulman Y: CAT scanning in staging prostatic carcinoma. Urology 18:305–308, 1981.

19. Gothlin JH, Hoiem L: Percutaneous fine-needle biopsy of radiographically normal lymph nodes in the staging of prostatic carcinoma. Radiology 114:351–354, 1981.

20. Greenberg M, Neiman HL, Brandt TD, et al: Ultrasound of the prostate. Radiology 141:757–762, 1981.

21. Hafermann MD: Cancer of the prostate—external radiotherapy. Clin Oncol 2:371–405, 1983.

22. Hricak H, Demas BE, Williams RD, et al: Magnetic resonance imaging in the diagnosis and staging of renal and perirenal neoplasms. Radiology 154:709–715, 1985.

23. Hricak H, Williams RD, Moon KL Jr, et al: Nuclear magnetic resonance imaging of the kidney: renal masses. Radiology 147:765–772, 1983.

24. Ishikawa I, Saito Y, Onouchi Z, et al: Development of acquired cystic disease and adenocarcinoma of the kidney in glomerulonephritic chronic hemodialysis patients. Clin Nephrol 14:1–6, 1980.

25. Jafri SZH, Bree RL, Amendola MA, et al: CT of renal and perirenal non-Hodgkin lymphoma. AJR 138:1101–1105, 1982.

26. Kahn PC, Wise HM Jr: The use of epinephrine in selective angiography of renal masses. J Urol 99:133–138, 1968.

27. Kaplan JH, McDonald JR, Thompson GJ: Multicentric origin of papillary tumors of the urinary tract. J Urol 66:792–804, 1951.

28. Kass DA, Hricak H, Davidson AJ: Renal malignancies with normal excretory urograms. AJR 141:731–734, 1983.

29. Kidd R, Crane RD, Dail DH: Lymphangiography and fine-needle aspiration biopsy: ineffective for staging early prostate cancer. AJR 142:1007–1012, 1984.

30. Kissane JM: The morphology of renal cystic disease. Perspect Nephrol Hypertens 4:31–63, 1976.

31. Koss JC, Arger PH, Coleman BG, et al: CT staging of bladder carcinoma. AJR 137:359–362, 1981.

32. Lang EK: The arteriographic diagnosis of primary and secondary tumors of the ureter or ureter and renal pelvis. Radiology 92:799–805, 1969.

33. Lang EK: Roentgenographic assessment of asymptomatic renal lesions. Radiology 109:257–269, 1973.

34. Lee JK, Heiken JP, Ling D, et al: Magnetic resonance imaging of abdominal and pelvic lymphadenopathy. Radiology 153:181–188, 1984.

35. Lee JKT, Stanley RJ, Sagel SS, McClennan BL: Accuracy of CT in detecting intraabdominal and pelvic lymph node metastases from pelvic cancers. AJR 131:675–679, 1978.

36. Lee KR, Wulfsberg E, Kepes JJ: Some important radiological aspects of the kidney in Hippel-Lindau syndrome: the value of prospective study in an affected family. Radiology 122:649–653, 1977.

37. Leung AWL, Bydder GM, Steiner RE, et al: Magnetic resonance imaging of the kidneys. AJR 143:1215–1227, 1984.

38. Levine E, Lee KR, Weigel JW, Farber B: Computed tomography in the diagnosis of renal carcinoma complicating Hippel-Lindau syndrome. Radiology 130:703–706, 1979.

39. Levine E, Lee KR, Weigel J: Preoperative determination of abdominal extent of renal cell carcinoma by computed tomography. Radiology 132:395–398, 1979.

40. Lien HH, Kolbenstvedt A, Talle K, et al: Comparison of computed tomography, lymphography and phlebography in 200 consecutive patients with regard to retroperitoneal metastases from testicular tumor. Radiology 146:129–132, 1983.

41. Love L, Churchill R, Reynes C, et al: Computed tomography staging of renal carcinoma. Urol Radiol 1:3–10, 1979.

42. Maier JG, Schamber DT: The role of lymphangiography in the diagnosis and treatment of malignant testicular tumors. AJR 114:482–491, 1972.

43. Malek RS, Greene LF: Urologic aspects of Hippel-Lindau syndrome. J Urol 106:800–801, 1971.

44. Marks WM, Korobkin M, Callen PW, Kaiser JA: CT diagnosis of tumor thrombosis of the renal vein and inferior vena cava. AJR 131:843–846, 1978.

45. Mauro MA, Wadsworth DE, Stanley RJ, McClennan BL: Renal cell carcinoma: angiography in the CT era. AJR 139:1135–1138, 1982.

46. McClennan BL, Stanley RJ, Melson GL, et al: CT of the renal cyst: is cyst aspiration necessary? AJR 133:671–675, 1979.

47. Mitty HA, Baron MG, Feller M: Infiltrating carcinoma of the renal pelvis. Radiology 92:994–998, 1969.

48. Morgan CL, Calkins RF, Cavalcanti EJ: Computed tomography in the evaluation, staging, and therapy of carcinoma of the bladder and prostate. Radiology 140:751–761, 1981.

49. Probst P, Hoogewoud HM, Haertel M, et al: Computerized tomography versus angiography in the staging of malignant renal neoplasm. Br J Radiol 54:744–753, 1981.

50. Quinn MJ, Hartman DS, Friedman AC, et al: Renal oncocytoma: new observations. Radiology 153:49–53, 1984.

51. Rifkin WD: Sonourethrography: technique for evaluation of prostatic urethra. Radiology 153:791–792, 1984.

52. Safer ML, Green JP, Crews QE Jr, Hill DR: Lymphangiographic accuracy in the staging of testicular tumors. Cancer 35:1603–1605, 1975.

53. Sager EM, Talle K, Fosså S, et al: The role of CT in demonstrating perivesical tumor growth in the preoperative staging of carcinoma of the urinary bladder. Radiology 146:443–446, 1983.

54. Sample WF, Gottesman JE, Skinner DG, Ehrlich RM: Gray scale ultrasound of the scrotum. Radiology 127:225–228, 1978.

55. Seidelmann FE, Cohen WN, Bryan PJ, et al: Accuracy of CT staging of bladder neoplasms using the gas-filled method: report of 21 patients with surgical confirmation. AJR 130:735–739, 1978.

56. Sherman JL, Hartman DS, Friedman AC, et al: Angiomyolipoma: computed tomographic-pathologic correlation of 17 cases. AJR 137:1221–1226, 1981.

57. Skinner DG, Colvin RB, Vermillion CD, et al: Diagnosis and management of renal cell carcinoma: a clinical and pathologic study of 309 cases. Cancer 28:1165–1177, 1971.

58. Skinner DG, Pfister RF, Colvin R: Extension of renal cell carcinoma into the vena cava: the rationale for aggressive surgical management. J Urol 107:711–716, 1972.

59. Strijk SP, Debruyne FM, Herman CJ: Lymphography in the management of urologic tumors: radiological-pathological correlation. Radiology 146:39–45, 1983.

60. Totty WG, McClennan BL, Melson GL, et al: Relative value of computed tomography and ultrasonography in the assessment of renal angiomyolipoma. J Comput Assist Tomogr 5:173–178, 1981.

61. Walsch JW, Amendola MA, Konerding KF, et al: Computed tomographic detection of pelvic and inguinal lymph-node metastases from primary and recurrent pelvic malignant disease. Radiology 137:157–166, 1980.

62. Weyman PJ, McClennan BL, Stanley RJ, et al: Comparison of computed tomography and angiography in the evaluation of renal cell carcinoma. Radiology 137:417–424, 1980.

63. Wilson CS, Dahl DS, Middleton RG: Pelvic lymphadenectomy for the staging of apparently localized prostatic cancer. J Urol 117:197–198, 1977.

64. Zimmer WD, Williamson B Jr, Hartman GW, et al: Changing patterns in the evaluation of renal masses: economic implications. AJR 143:285–289, 1984.

GARY LIESKOVSKY, M.D.
THOMAS AHLERING, M.D.
DONALD G. SKINNER, M.D.

Diagnosis and Staging of Bladder Cancer

CHAPTER 14

The current systems for staging bladder cancer evolved from dual origins. Almost 40 years ago, at about the same time, Denoix[12] and Jewett and Strong[30] independently described systems for the classification of bladder cancer. In 1950, following Denoix's description, the Union Internationale Contre le Cancer (UICC) recommended adopting the TNM system, which permits classification of tumors based on the assessment of the extent of the primary tumor (T), the condition of the regional nodes (N), and the presence or absence of metastases (M).

The other system began in 1943 when Hugh Hampton Young, professor of urology at Johns Hopkins University, approached Hugh Jewett, then a resident, with the suggestion that he analyze more than 1400 cases to determine management guidelines for the treatment of bladder cancer. In an excellent historical review, Jewett presents his personal reminiscences about that task, which was the root of the present American classification system for bladder cancer.[28]

Jewett and George Strong, then a resident pathologist, first analyzed 100 autopsy cases of patients with bladder cancer.[30] Jewett suggested that the primary tumors be segregated into three pathologic stages and the incidence of concomitant lymph node or hematogenous metastases studied for each group (Table 14–1). No patient with a Stage A tumor (confined to the mucosa) was found to have evidence of metastases, compared with 13% of patients with Stage B tumors (involving the muscularis) and 74% of those with Stage C tumors (involving the perivesical fat). Subsequently, in 1951, based on a study of 80 clinical cases, Jewett suggested dividing Stage B into superficial and deep categories, indicating that tumors in B_1 behaved much like Stage A tumors, whereas those in B_2 resembled Stage C tumors.[27] In his report, 14 of 19 patients (74%) with tumors in Stages A or B_1 survived five years, compared with only two of 61 patients (3%) in whom the lesion had invaded the deep muscle or perivesical fat. Unfortunately, the separation of Stage B into B_1 and B_2 was based on only 18 patients, of whom four of the five with B_1 disease survived five years, compared with only one of 13 with deep muscle invasion.

In a recent editorial entitled "Comments on the Staging of Invasive Bladder Can-

Table 14–1. BLADDER CANCER STAGING*

Group	Invasion	Metastases (%)	Potentially Curable (%)
A	Submucosa	0	100
B	Muscular	13	87
C	Perivesical	74	26

*Data from Jewett HJ, Strong GH: Infiltrating carcinoma of the bladder: relation of depth of penetration of the bladder wall to incidence of local extension and metastasis. J Urol 55:366, 1946.

264

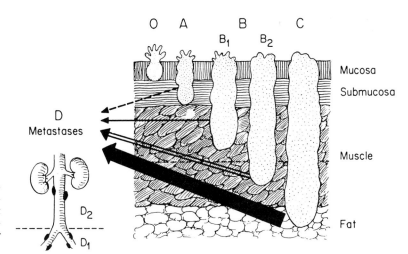

Figure 14–1. Marshall modification of Jewett and Strong system. From Skinner DG: Current state of classification and staging of bladder cancer. Cancer Res 37:2838–2842, 1977.

cer—Two B's or Not Two B's: That Is the Question," Jewett stated, "It seems probable that our arbitrary dividing line drawn 30 years ago at the halfway level to separate B_1 from B_2 tumors was too superficial. If placed at a deeper level, many of the currently reported B_2 cases would fall into Stage B_1, which they often resemble," suggesting that penetration of the muscle rather than the depth of infiltration is the most important determinant for the treatment of patients with bladder cancer.[29]

In 1952, Marshall presented a modification of the Jewett and Strong staging schema, adding Stage 0 to include tumors not infiltrating the lamina propria, patients without tumor in the definitive cystectomy specimen, and patients with carcinoma in situ.[42] In addition, Stage D was defined to include tumors with evidence of metastatic disease and was further divided into two categories: Stage D_1, lesions still confined to the pelvis (including invasion of the pelvic walls or rectus muscle below the sacral promontory), and Stage D_2, lesions beyond the limits of the pelvis, including distant metastases or lesions above the sacral promontory. Subsequently, the aortic bifurcation was chosen arbitrarily instead of the sacral promontory to separate Stage D_1 from D_2 lesions in which lymph node involvement was evident (Fig. 14–1). In 1968, following considerable discussion, the UICC published its first booklet on the classification and staging of 23 tumor sites.[76] The system was subsequently amended and revised, and the second edition in 1974 included the classification of urologic tumors.[77] Further modifications led in 1978 to the third edition, in which the

UICC recommended that the classification should remain unchanged for at least 10 years (Table 14–2).[78]

In accordance with the UICC classification system for bladder cancer, the extent of the primary tumor, designated T, is to be assessed by clinical examination, urography, cystoscopy, and bimanual examination under anesthesia, in addition to biopsy of the tumor. The condition of the regional nodes, designated N, is assessed by clinical examination with or without radiography, including lymphography and urography, and computerized tomography. Extent of metastases (M) is determined by clinical examination, radiography, or isotope studies.

A comparison of the historic and current American systems of staging with the clinical and pathological TNM system of 1978 is presented in Figure 14–2. Currently, Marshall's Stage 0 corresponds to T0 (no evidence of primary tumor), TIS (preinvasive carcinoma), or Ta (papillary tumor without invasion of the lamina propria). Stage A tumors invading the lamina propria correspond to T1. Stage B_1 tumors, invading the superficial muscle, are classified as T2 tumors. Stage B_2 tumors, invading the deep muscle, or Stage C tumors, invading the perivesical fat, correspond to T3 tumors in the TNM system. T4 tumors, which invade the prostate, vagina, uterus, or abdominal wall, correspond to tumors in Stage D_1 in the Marshall classification.

As pointed out by Skinner, the main intention of the TNM system was to assist the clinician in planning treatment for patients with bladder cancer and to provide valuable prognostic information by allowing the eval-

Table 14-2. TNM FOR BLADDER CANCER, UICC

Rules for Classification

The classification applies only to epithelial tumors. Papilloma is excluded but such cases should be listed under the category "G0." Papillary noninvasive carcinoma should be listed under the category Ta.

There should be histologic or cytologic verification of the disease. Any unconfirmed cases must be reported separately.

The following are the minimum requirements for assessment of the T, N, and M categories. If these cannot be met, the symbol TX, NX, or MX will be used.

T categories: Clinical examination, urography, cystoscopy, bimanual examination under anesthesia, and biopsy or transurethral resection of the tumor (if indicated) prior to definitive treatment.

N categories: Clinical examination and radiography, including lymphography and urography.

M categories: Clinical examination and radiograph. In the more advanced primary radiography. In the more advanced primary tumors or when clinical suspicion tumors or when clinical suspicion warrants, radiographic or isotope studies are recommended.

Regional and Juxtaregional Lymph Nodes

The regional lymph nodes are the pelvic nodes below the bifurcation of the common iliac arteries.

The juxtaregional lymph nodes are the inguinal nodes, the common iliac nodes, and the para-aortic nodes.

TNM Pretreatment Clinical Classification

T—Primary

TIS Preinvasive carcinoma (carcinoma in situ): "Flat tumor."

Ta Papillary noninvasive carcinoma.

T0 No evidence of primary tumor.

T1 On bimanual examination a freely mobile mass may be felt: this should not be felt after complete transurethral resection of the lesion and/or
Microscopically, the tumor does not invade beyond the lamina propria.

T2 On bimanual examination there is induration of the bladder wall that is mobile. There is no residual induration after complete transurethral resection of the lesion and/or
There is microscopic invasion of superficial muscle.

T3 On bimanual examination induration or a nodular mobile mass is palpable in the bladder wall, which persists after transurethral resection of the exophytic portion of the lesion and/or
There is microscopic invasion of deep muscle or extension through the bladder wall.
T3a—Invasion of deep muscle.
T3b—Invasion through the bladder wall.

T4 Tumor fixed or extending to neighboring structures and/or
There is microscopic evidence of such involvement.
T4a—Tumor infiltrating the prostate, uterus, or vagina.
T4b—Tumor fixed to the pelvic wall and/or abdominal wall.

TX The minimum requirements to assess the primary tumor cannot be met.

N—Regional and Juxtaregional Lymph Nodes

N0 No evidence of regional node involvement.

N1 Evidence of involvement of a single homolateral regional lymph node.

N2 Evidence of involvement of contralateral or bilateral or multiple regional lymph nodes.

N3 Evidence of involvement of fixed regional lymph nodes (there is a fixed mass on the pelvic wall with a free space between this and the tumor).

N4 Evidence of involvement of juxtaregional lymph nodes.

NX The minimum requirements to assess the regional and/or juxtaregional lymph nodes cannot be met.

M—Distant Metastases

M0 No evidence of distant metastases.

M1 Evidence of distant metastases.

MX The minimum requirements to assess the presence of distant metastases cannot be met.

pTNM Postsurgical Histopathological Classification

pT—Primary Tumor

pTIS Preinvasive carcinoma (carcinoma in situ)

pTa Papillary noninvasive carcinoma.

pT0 No evidence of tumor found on histologic examination of specimen.

pT1 Tumor not extending beyond the lamina propria.

pT2 Tumor with invasion of superficial muscle (not more than half-way through muscle coat).

pT3 Tumor with invasion of superficial muscle (pT3a—more than half-way through muscle coat) or with invasion of perivesical tissue (pT3b).

pT4 Tumor with invasion of prostate or other extravesical structures.

pTX The extent of invasion cannot be assessed.

G—Histopathologic Grading

"G0" Papilloma—i.e., no evidence of anaplasia.

G1 High degree of differentiation.

G2 Medium degree of differentiation.

G3 Low degree of differentiation or undifferentiated.

GX Grade cannot be assessed.

L—Invasion of Lymphatics

L0 No lymphatic invasion.

L1 Evidence of invasion of superficial lymphatics.

L2 Evidence of invasion of deep lymphatics.

LX Lymphatic invasion cannot be assessed.

pN—Regional and Juxtaregional Lymph Nodes

The pN categories correspond to the N categories.

pM—Distant Metastases

The pM categories correspond to the M categories.

Stage Grouping

No stage grouping is at present recommended.

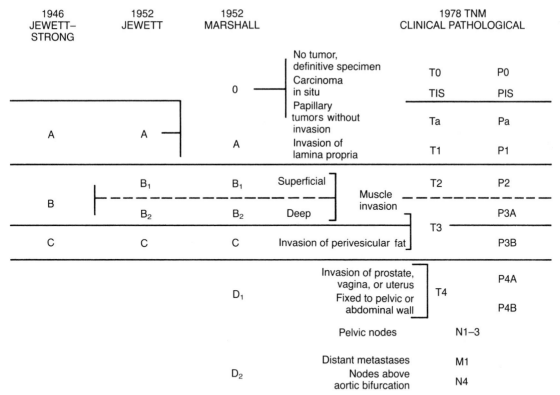

Figure 14–2. *Comparisons of American and TNM staging systems for bladder cancer. From Skinner DG: Current state of classification and staging of bladder cancer. Cancer Res 37:2838–2842, 1977.*

uation of treatment results based on a universally accepted system.[66] However, it appears that the TNM system has not met its main objective of aiding the clinician in treatment planning but, in most instances, has merely substituted numbers for the letters of the Marshall modification (with the exception of Marshall's Stage 0).

Part of the problem is that staging systems are only as good as the techniques available to assess the extent of the disease. In 1976, the National Cooperative Bladder Cancer Study revealed an error rate as high as 50% between the clinical and pathologic stages

for patients with disease in Stages B and C (Table 14–3). Understaging for all patients with Stage B disease ranged from 31 to 46%, whereas overstaging varied between 20 and 50%. This significant error reflects our inability to detect accurately the clinical stage of the tumor preoperatively. The staging error does not appear much better with the TNM system. In 1982, Skinner and associates reviewed their experience with 130 patients undergoing high-dose, short-course preoperative radiation followed by radical cystectomy and pelvic node dissection, and they found a significant staging error when

Table 14–3. BLADDER CANCER STAGING ERROR (PERCENTAGE):
CLINICAL (T) VERSUS PATHOLOGICAL (P)*

Preoperative Stage	Understage, T < P		Overstage, T > P	
	Surgery Only	Preoperative Radiotherapy	Surgery Only	Preoperative Radiotherapy
B₁	44	35	23	49
B₂	48	26	18	51
All B	46	31	20	50
C	20	0	24	74
B₂ to C	40	18	20	58
Total error	42	26	21	54

*From Skinner DG: Current state of classification and staging of bladder cancer. Cancer Res 37:2838–2842, 1977.

Table 14–4. BLADDER CANCER STAGING ERROR OF THE PRIMARY TUMOR:
CLINICAL (T) VERSUS PATHOLOGICAL (P)*

Clinical Stage (Preop)	Number of Patients	Staging Error (%)		Agreement (%) $T = P$
		Understaged, $T < P$	Overstaged, $T > P$	
T1 + T1S	55	33	15	53
T2	48	58	29	13
T3	12	8.5	42	50
Not assessable	15			
Total	130	41	23	36

*All patients were treated by 1600 rads of preoperative radiation in addition to radical cystectomy and pelvic lymph node dissection. Data from Skinner DG, et al: High dose, short course preoperative radiation therapy and immediate single stage radical cystectomy with pelvic node dissection in the management of bladder cancer. J Urol 127:671–674, 1982.

comparing the preoperative clinical stage (T) with the histopathologic stage (P) of the definitive specimen.[69] Agreement was achieved in only 53% of patients with T1 or TIS tumors, 13% of patients with T2 tumors, and 50% of patients with T3 tumors (Table 14–4). The overall rate of agreement was only 36%, with 41% of patients understaged and 23% overstaged, further emphasizing the inaccuracy of preoperative assessment of the clinical stage.

More recently, Chisholm and co-workers reviewed their records for patients with bladder cancer in 1979 by using the 1978 TNM system.[7] They concluded that it was impossible clinically to distinguish Ta from T1 tumors and proposed a single category. Furthermore, attempts to differentiate T2 from T3 tumors were frustrating and yielded little practical information, so a single T2-T3a category was recommended. These suggestions parallel our belief that the most important factor to consider in planning the therapeutic management of patients with bladder cancer is the presence or absence of muscle invasion. These authors also believe that, since the biologic behavior of clinical T2 and T3 tumors was similar, a single invasive P category (P2-P3) would be more practical.

It is our belief that, although the TNM system is useful for the accurate pathologic staging of the definitive cystectomy specimen, it offers very little to the clinical management of the patient. We believe that a more simplified clinical staging system is warranted, and any staging that cannot be accurately determined by existing techniques should be eliminated. We also encourage increased emphasis on obtaining histopathologic information at biopsy: the degree of invasion, the grade of the tumor,

and the presence or absence of carcinoma in situ. This information can eliminate expensive tests that add little to the accuracy of staging and management guidelines. We support efforts to search for improved cytologic and biochemical criteria that could predict the invasive potential of tumors, so that early and aggressive therapy can be planned for high-grade or muscle-invading tumors.

In a recent editorial Jewett states, "There is no use in agonizing over one's inability to match the clinical stage with the pathologic until one knows that pathologic segregation is significant."[29] Based on Skinner's results relating the depth of bladder wall invasion at the time of cystectomy to the incidence of positive nodes, one can readily appreciate the significance of pathologic segregation.[67] There is increased incidence of lymph nodes that have signs of disease as the pathologic stage increases: 5% in patients with P1 and PIS tumors, 30% in patients with P2 and P3a tumors, and 64% and 50% in patients with P3b and P4 tumors, respectively (Table 14–5). The results also indicate that muscle penetration is far more important and easier to determine than the depth of infiltration. In an analysis of 140 patients treated by preoperative radiation therapy and radical cystectomy, reported by Richie and associates, the five-year survival rates of patients with tumors in Stages B_1 and B_2 were identical, approaching 40% (Table 14–6).[55] In another study, Skinner and colleagues used the P designation of the TNM system to determine five-year survival in relation to the depth of bladder wall invasion at the time of cystectomy (Table 14–7).[69] In this report, the five-year survival of patients with P2 and P3a tumors (i.e., Stages B_1 and B_2) was not statistically different either when

Table 14–5. RELATION OF DEPTH OF BLADDER WALL INVASION AT TIME OF CYSTECTOMY (PATHOLOGIC STAGE) TO LYMPH NODE INVOLVEMENT*

Pathologic Stage	Number of Patients	Percentage of Positive Nodes
P1 and P1S	41	5
P2	20	30
P3A	13	31
P3B	28	64
P4	8	50

*All patients received 1600 rads of preoperative radiation in addition to radical cystectomy and pelvic lymph node dissection. From Skinner DG, Tift JP, Kaufman JJ: High dose, short course preoperative radiation therapy and immediate single stage radical cystectomy with pelvic node dissection in the management of bladder cancer. J Urol 127:671, 1982.

Table 14–7. FIVE-YEAR SURVIVAL IN RELATION TO DEPTH OF BLADDER WALL INVASION AT THE TIME OF CYSTECTOMY (PATHOLOGIC STAGE)*

Pathologic Stage	Number of Patients	Five-Year Survival (%)
P0, P1, P1S	61	81
P2	20	53
P3A	13	39
P3B	28	39
P4	8	25
P2 + 3A	33	50
P3A + P3B	41	41
N+	34	36

*All patients received 1600 rads of preoperative radiation in addition to radical cystectomy and pelvic lymph node dissection.

analyzed separately or when combined, implying that the presence or absence of muscle invasion is the significant factor in dictating therapy.

One of the major deficiencies in reporting survival data according to the Marshall modification of the Jewett and Strong system is that nodal involvement implies Stage D disease. In contrast, the P stage designation in the TNM system allows one to determine the independent influence of the extent of the primary tumor on survival, since the P stage remains the same regardless of nodal disease. As demonstrated previously, lymph node involvement does not imply incurability; in one report the five-year survival rate of 34 patients with positive nodes was 36%.[67]

Based upon our experience and the findings of others, we strongly endorse the use of the pathologic staging schema of the TNM

Table 14–6. PATHOLOGICAL STAGE AND FIVE-YEAR SURVIVAL FOR 140 PATIENTS TREATED BY CYSTECTOMY*

Stage	Five-Year Survival (%)	
0 to A	78.6	
B_1	39.9	} All B, 40.0†
B_2	40.4	
C	19.7	
D	6.2	

*From Richie JP, Skinner DG, Kaufman JJ: Radical cystectomy for carcinoma of the bladder: 16 years of experience. J Urol 113:186–189, 1975.

†Note the nearly identical survival for patients in Stage B_1 and Stage B_2 and the statistical significance between survival of those patients with tumor confined to the mucosa compared with those with muscle invasion ($p < 0.01$).

system to provide valuable prognostic information and to evaluate treatment results based on the P stage of the definitive specimen. However, we must re-emphasize our reservations about the *clinical* value of the TNM system. In its place we would recommend a simplified clinical staging system. This is based on the fact that the most important determinant of clinical staging and subsequent therapy includes a properly performed biopsy indicating the presence or absence of muscle invasion, in conjunction with the grade of the tumor and the presence or absence of carcinoma in situ.

DIAGNOSTIC PROCEDURES

Cystoscopy and Bimanual Examination

All patients suspected of having urothelial carcinoma need complete cystoscopic evaluation under anesthesia. It is helpful to obtain an intravenous urogram (IVU) so that if needed, the upper tracts may be evaluated concomitantly. Initially, bimanual examination should be performed with good pelvic relaxation. Cystoscopic examination begins with careful inspection of the urethra and prostate because of the risk of metachronous carcinoma. Examination of the bladder should be comprehensive and methodical, beginning at the bladder neck and systematically including the trigone, the ureteral orifices, and the posterior, lateral, and anterior walls. Mapping the entire bladder should be completed prior to resection or biopsy. The number, size, and configuration of all tumors should be accurately recorded or drawn. The mucosa must be evaluated for areas of erythema or irregularity consistent with carcinoma in situ. When abnormalities are present on the IVU, retrograde pyelography with cytologic examination or brush biopsies (or ureteroscopic visualization) should be performed. After the entire urothelium has been inspected, biopsy or transurethral resection may begin.

Complete transurethral resection should be carried out on small papillary lesions. A ureteral orifice may be resected for low-grade papillary lesions, but ureteral obstruction (usually mild) should be expected about 10% of the time and, in patients with a history of irradiation or interstitial cystitis, it should be expected to be greater.[4] Reflux can be expected to occur about 20% of the time after transurethral resection of bladder tumors[54] and 70% of the time following resection of a ureteral orifice.[19] Reflux in this situation has not been shown to impair renal function; however, recurrent pyelonephritis (occasionally producing infection or stones) has been noted in up to 20% of cases.[1] More importantly, one must be aware of the potential risk of systemic side effects due to reflux of intravesical agents employed in patients with superficial bladder cancer.

Selected mucosal biopsy of the bladder urothelium is an important adjunct that influences the management of superficial disease. In the presence of a low-grade tumor, adjacent mucosal atypia or in situ carcinoma is associated with increased recurrence rates (Fig. 14–3).[70] Also, Schade and Swinney

reported the 10-year follow-up of 65 patients with T1/T2 tumors; 12 of 24 with CIS were not controlled endoscopically, compared with none of the 41 patients without CIS.[59] Patients with superficial disease and associated CIS generally warrant early institution of intravesical chemotherapy. Selected mucosal biopsies also play a role in the initial evaluation or follow-up of patients with positive urine cytologic results without visible intravesical tumor.

Mucosal biopsies are best performed using cold cup biopsy forceps. An isotonic solution should be used, because water can distort histologic findings due to hypotonicity. Biopsy should include, in addition to suspicious areas, four uniform sites: lateral to both ureteral orifices, the trigone, and the dome (Fig. 14–4). Material from the prostatic urethra should also be removed in suspicious cases, particularly those with diffuse CIS of the bladder. Biopsies need not be deep, since only the mucosa is under evaluation.

Complete resection of broad-based ulcerating tumors that are highly suggestive of invasion is unnecessary. Biopsy near the center usually establishes the presence or absence of muscle invasion since the depth (superficial or deep muscle) is irrelevant in selection of subsequent therapy.[55, 68] In support of this, Dretler and associates have reported increased survival in patients who underwent total cystectomy after biopsy only, compared with those undergoing complete transurethral resection.[13] Furthermore, transurethral resection of flat tumors is tech-

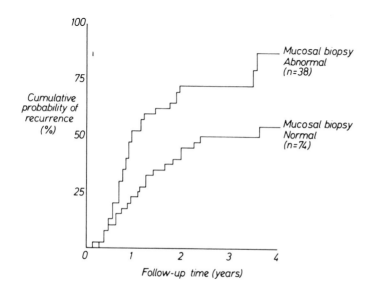

Figure 14–3. Cumulative probability of tumor recurrence in patients initially presenting with superficial bladder tumors (Ta/T1), with or without mucosal abnormalities (dysplasia or carcinoma in situ). In this prospective study, patients were treated endoscopically only, and those found to have abnormal biopsy material had a significantly higher probability of recurrence (p < 0.01). From Smith G, et al: Prognostic significance of biopsy results of normal-looking mucosa in cases of superficial bladder cancer. Br J Urol 55:665–669, 1983.

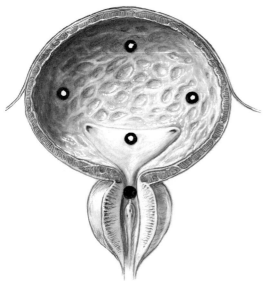

Figure 14–4. Suggested location of biopsy sites: trigone, dome, and lateral to both ureteral orifices.

nically at increased risk for perforation and possible tumor dissemination.

Urine Cytology and Flow Cytometry

Urine Cytology. In 1945 Papanicolaou reported a technique by which microscopic examination of urinary sediment could detect exfoliated cancer cells.[50] Since then, urine cytologic testing has established itself in the urologic armamentarium for the diagnosis and follow-up of urothelial malignancy.

Urine for cytologic examination should be collected early in the evaluation of patients suspected of having malignancy and those who have hematuria. The first voided urine in the morning has considerable artifact due to degeneration of cells from prolonged exposure to concentrated urine. Daytime voided urines collected randomly in the office or hospital have been shown to yield reliable results.[20, 45] Bladder washings produce the most representative and best preserved collection of exfoliated urothelial cells but, obviously, are not as easy to collect as voided urines. Cells collected from chronic indwelling catheters have a tendency to form papillary aggregates, which confuse the issue and should be avoided. In general, urine samples for cytologic testing should be sent immediately for analysis, but, if not feasible, then the urine should be

refrigerated or fixed in 95% alcohol. Murphy reported the diagnostic criteria necessary to establish the diagnosis of malignancy; they are listed in Table 14–8.

The results of urine cytologic examinations are most reliable for tumors of Grades 2 and 3 and for carcinoma in situ. The overall accuracy for detecting urothelial cancer in these high-grade lesions varies between 70 and 100%. In contrast, the accuracy is significantly less for tumors in Grade 1 and for some in Grade 2; this varies between 30 and 90%.[14, 20, 40, 47, 56, 60] For patients who have received intravesical chemotherapy, an experienced cytopathologist can usually differentiate the cytologic characteristics secondary to intravesical chemotherapy from those of carcinoma.[11, 46]

Flow Cytometry. The development of automated machines to detect malignant cells shed in the urine has been gaining considerable momentum over the last decade. This has been stimulated by the fact that urine cytologic specimens must be prepared by hand and individually evaluated; in addition, with experienced cytopathologists, the results are not consistently reproducible. Flow cytometry offers advantages because of its ability to analyze large numbers of urine samples by machine, avoiding extra cost,

Table 14–8. CYTOLOGIC CRITERIA FOR LOW- AND HIGH-GRADE UROTHELIAL CARCINOMAS*

Cytologic Constituent	Low-Grade Carcinoma	High-Grade Carcinoma
Cells		
Arrangement	Papillary and loose clusters	Isolated and loose clusters
Size	Increased, uniform	Increased, pleomorphic
Number	Often numerous	Numerous
Cytoplasm	Homogeneous	Variable
Nuclear: cytoplasmic (N:C) ratio	Increased	Increased
Nuclei		
Position	Eccentric	Eccentric
Size	Enlarged	Variable
Morphology	Variable within aggregates	Variable
Borders	Irregular, notched (creased)	Irregular, notched (creased)
Chromatin	Fine, regular	Coarse, irregular
Nucleoli	Small or absent	Variable

*According to Murphy WM: et al: Urinary cytology and bladder cancer: the cellular features of transitional cell neoplasms. Cancer 53:1555–1565, 1984.

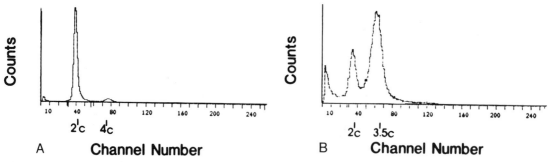

Figure 14–5. A, Normal (nontumor) DNA histogram of nuclear counts versus fluorescence intensity. The DNA content is predominantly diploid (2c) with no aneuploid peaks. B, DNA histogram of a patient with Grade 2 transitional cell cancer. Note the large aneuploid peak at 3.5c, characteristic of malignancy.

time, and subjectivity implicit in the handling of urine cytologic material. A flow cytometer can sort urine cells by size and then indirectly measure DNA content, nuclear-cytoplasmic ratio, and RNA content.

Briefly, in this procedure cells from bladder washings or voided urine have their nuclear DNA stained with fluorescent dye. The cells are sorted according to size to reduce contamination from leukocytes and other material, and a single cell suspension is passed by an argon ion laser. The nuclear size is determined and the DNA content can be measured by the amount of light emitted from the fluorescent-stained DNA that is excited by the argon laser. A DNA histogram is generated, and the content of nuclear DNA is standardized against normal 2n diploid nuclear content (Fig. 14–5A and B). Malignancy is inferred by the presence of aneuploid or hyperdiploid cell populations or an increase in S-phase population.[17, 18, 52, 74, 75] Aneuploidy has been shown to be present in 0% of Grade 1 tumors, 33% of Grade 2, and 100% of Grade 3 tumors.[75] Flow cytometry has been correlated in patients with cystoscopic and histologic evidence of bladder cancer. Generally, it has an overall false-negative rate of 10 to 45% and a rate of 0 to 25% for high-grade lesions.[8, 33, 74, 75] False-positive findings are quite unusual.

Role of Flow Cytometry Versus Cytology. Will flow cytometry replace urine cytologic examination? Currently, flow cytometry is limited in its general application because of problems that range from specimen collection and cell fixation to cellular contaminants to distinguishing DNA from RNA. With time it is expected that many of these flaws will be corrected. Urine cytologic examination has little potential as a screening

test, whereas, in theory, flow cytometry may eventually develop widespread application similar to that experienced with the cervical Pap smear. In the evaluation of patients with suspected urothelial cancer and in the follow-up of patients known to have bladder cancer, cytologic testing is currently more reliable. However, recent work suggests that flow cytometry may be complementary to cytology in the assessment of bladder cancer.[11]

Tumor Markers

The search for tumor markers and their clinical application in patients with bladder cancer has focused attention on invasive tumors and on predicting which noninvasive tumors are at risk for progression. Three broad categories of markers have thus far been identified and include cell surface antigens (ABO), chromosomal markers, and, most recently, oncogene products.

The blood group antigens (types A, B, and O), which were proved by Coombs and coworkers in 1956 to be ubiquitous on the surface of normal epithelium, have provided the prototype for antigenic cell surface markers.[9] In 1961, Kay and Wallace reported the loss of these antigens from exfoliated bladder cancer cells,[32] and, in 1968, Kovarik and associates described a technique using tissue from paraffin blocks to determine retrospectively the presence of the antigens from pathologic archives.[35]

The method for detecting cell surface blood group antigens was deftly illustrated by Coombs in 1956.[9] Simply, the tumor of interest is exposed to anti-A antibody (or B or O, depending on the patient's blood type), which will bind if the antigen is present.

The cells are washed to rid any adhering nonspecific protein. Then the specimen is exposed to a small suspension of type A red blood cells, which will adhere to the tumor only if the antigen is present on the cell surface (Fig. 14–6). Widespread use of this test is limited because of technical problems. The technician must be skillful and experienced in performing the test and in interpreting which results are truly positive. Furthermore, there is some evidence that indicates loss of antigenicity due to the effects of paraffin.[38] In addition, the H antigen, which is responsible for the O blood group, characteristically has weak reactivity and is probably responsible for some false-negative results. Radiotherapy is also known for its capacity to change antigen-negative tumors to antigen-positive ones.[10] However, centers with considerable experience should be able to mitigate these shortcomings.

The clinical applicability of these tumor markers is yet unproven. An excellent review published by Catalona in 1981 found that approximately 90% of patients whose specific red cell adherence (SRCA) results were negative suffered tumor recurrence, as compared with only 45% recurrence in SRCA-positive patients. Further, 66% of SRCA-negative patients developed invasion, compared with only 4% for SRCA-positive patients. The conclusion was that cystectomy would be unnecessary in as many as 33% of all SRCA-negative patients if they were subjected to bladder resection.[6] However, Catalona divided high-grade, low-stage lesions into SRCA-positive and -negative classes and developed the schema in Figure 14–7. Catalona astutely pointed out that high-grade, low-stage SRCA-positive patients might benefit significantly from careful observation, avoiding exenterative surgery. Conversely, high-grade, low-stage SRCA-negative tumors become invasive in 83% of cases, supporting a more aggressive initial treatment plan. No specific data have accumulated since 1981 to either support or negate such an approach.

Chromosomal Markers

During the mid-1960s, attention was focused on chromosomal abnormalities found to be present in malignant neoplasms.[72] The cells of normal tissue as well as nonmalignant entities (e.g., cystitis cystica or cystitis

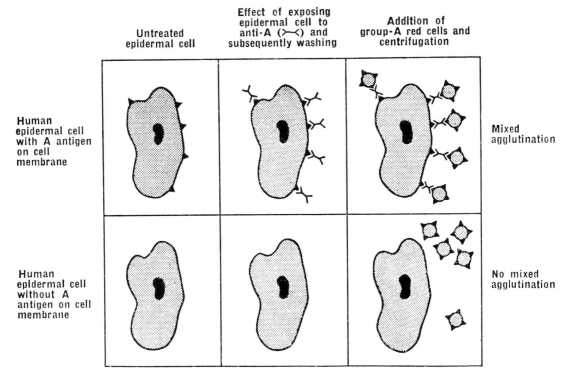

Figure 14–6. Schematic representation of the mixed red cell agglutination reaction. From Coombs RRA, et al: A and B blood-group antigens on human epidermal cells. Lancet 1:461–463, 1956.

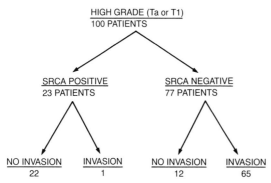

Figure 14–7. *Potential scheme for the management of high-grade, low-stage lesions, based on the results of specific red cell adherence (SRCA) test. From Catalona WJ: Practical utility of specific red cell adherence test in bladder cancer. Urology 18:113–117, 1981.*

glandularis) have 46 chromosomes, and it was discovered that solid tumors almost without exception are aneuploid.[15, 73] Falor and Ward reported on the chromosomal make-up of noninvasive bladder cancer and identified aneuploidy and chromosomal markers in well-differentiated tumors to be an ominous finding.[16] Aneuploidy is demonstrated when cells have too few or too many chromosomes; hyperdiploidy is two or three times the normal number of chromosomes. A chromosomal marker is defined as an abnormal chromosome that appears in metaphase and does not conform to any normal karyotypic pattern of the Denver classification system. Using this technique, Falor and others have demonstrated that low-grade, low-stage papillary tumors with abnormal marker chromosomes (which are histologically identical to low-grade, low-stage tumors) have a high tendency to recur and invade (Table 14–9).[58]

Oncogene Products

Modern molecular biology continues to explore and discover the genetic mechanisms responsible for malignancy. An important component believed to play a role

Table 14–9. INCIDENCE OF RECURRENCE OF PAPILLARY BLADDER TUMORS IN PATIENTS WITH OR WITHOUT ABNORMAL MARKER CHROMOSOMES

First Author	Reference	Chromosome Marker	
		Positive	Negative
Summers	73	2/20	18/20
Sandberg	58	1/18	11/32

in malignant transformation of normal cells is the "oncogene." Oncogenes are normal growth maintenance genes that are susceptible to a number of modifications (such as rearrangement, amplification, and deletion) that have been shown to be tumorigenic. Indeed, the prototype of altered oncogenes was discovered in the ras oncogene in a human bladder cancer cell line.[53] The oncogene of potential marker value in human bladder cancer is epidermal growth factor (EGF). A recent publication suggests that bladder tumors with increased EGF receptors are at increased risk for invasion and metastasis.[49] There is theoretical value in these findings (see Chapter 1), but more data are needed to substantiate any clinical role for EGF receptor as a tumor marker.

RADIOGRAPHIC EVALUATION OF THE BLADDER CANCER PATIENT

Intravenous Urography

Intravenous urograms (IVU) remain the cornerstone of roentenographic procedures in the initial evaluation of urothelial malignancy. In general, the IVU gives valuable information about the upper tracts regarding renal function and anatomy of the kidney and the collecting system, and it is the best study to screen for upper urinary tract urothelial tumors. Complete cystoscopic evaluation should not proceed without the IVU because of the potential need for retrograde pyelography and pyeloureteral cytologic examination. The coincident occurrence of upper tract transitional cell cancer with bladder tumors is 5 to 10%.[83]

The cystogram phase of the intravenous urogram is neither sensitive nor specific for bladder tumors. It also has little precision in the staging of bladder tumors. However, if a bladder tumor obstructs a ureteral orifice, muscle invasion will be present 70 to 90% of the time and may be associated with nodal metastases in up to 55% of cases.[22, 36]

Cystography

A number of methods have been advocated to evaluate the bladder radiographically. These range from simple cystography to fractionated cystograms and multiple phase contrast. Such studies cannot replace appropriate cystoscopic evaluation and biopsy and are not recommended in either the diagnosis or staging of bladder cancer.

Cystography remains the examination of choice in the evaluation of patients suspected of having a tumorigenic vesicovaginal or vesicorectal fistula. It is also recommended for recognition of ureteral reflux prior to the institution of intravesical therapy. Similarly, reflux would contraindicate the use of formaldehyde in patients with refractory hematuria.

Lymphangiography

Prior to CT scanning, bilateral pedal lymphangiography was the principal method for evaluating the pelvic lymph nodes for metastases in patients with pelvic malignancy. Several studies have reported significant discrepancy in accuracy (48 to 94%), sensitivity (57 to 100%), and specificity (29 to 100%) for such patients.[31, 41, 51, 71, 80] Limitations of the procedure historically have yielded rates for false-negative results of 15 to 40% due to the inability to detect micrometastases. Conversely, the incidence of false-positive lymphograms varied between 5 and 10%. Recently Gibod and associates advocated combining lymphography and percutaneous fine-needle aspiration biopsy of normal and abnormal nodes to determine the preoperative status of the pelvic nodes.[21] In their experience, only 11 of 35 (32%) patients with a positive lymphangiogram had a confirmatory node aspiration biopsy, whereas in the remaining patients lymphadenopathy was attributed to inflammatory changes from recent bladder tumor surgery. In this series, 28 patients with negative results from aspiration biopsy subsequently underwent a radical cystectomy and pelvic lymphadenectomy. Seven patients in this group (25%) were found to have pelvic nodes with signs of disease, a false-negative rate similar to previous reports using lymphangiography alone. Contrary to our belief, these authors justify this combined approach since they feel that any positive result from node aspiration biopsy precludes patients from any form of local radical treatment, thus sparing the patient an unnecessary surgical procedure. It is our contention, however, that the patients who benefit the most from a meticulous pelvic node dissection are those with unsuspected nodal metastases, especially when the spread is microscopic or limited to a few lymph nodes.[37]

Others have advocated bilateral selective hypogastric arteriography alone or combined with lymphangiography for preoperative staging of bladder cancer.[84] Staging accuracy rates using arteriography alone varied from 29% for pathologic Stage A tumors to 53% for Stage B lesions, but in these patients it did not improve the staging accuracy determined by using conventional diagnostic techniques. On the other hand, the arteriographic staging accuracy rates in patients with Stage C (89%) and Stage D (92%) disease was substantially improved, compared with the prearteriographic rates of 11% and 71% for Stage C and Stage D disease, respectively. When lymphography was added to arteriography and the results compared with those for patients staged using arteriography alone, no added benefit was seen except for a 10% increase in accuracy for patients with Stage D disease. Lymphography, when added to arteriography, did not increase the accuracy in patients with disease in Stages A, B, or C. It is our opinion that the results of lymphography alone, or when combined with arteriography or percutaneous needle aspiration biopsy, fail to adequately provide unquestionable evidence for the presence or absence of subclinical metastases. Currently, it is our policy not to employ these tests for the routine staging of bladder cancer since, in most circumstances, they add little to the treatment plan.

Computerized Tomography (CT) Scanning

Since its development by Hounsfield in 1972, CT scanning has provided valuable assistance in diagnosis and staging of many malignant neoplasms.[24] Advocates in favor of utilizing this modality in staging patients with bladder cancer feel that it provides reliable information regarding the local extent of the primary tumor and the identification of pelvic lymphadenopathy, which may represent metastatic disease.

Various techniques have been recommended to produce optimal visualization of the bladder wall and the intra- and extravesical extensions of bladder tumors. These methods include single contrast assessment with retrograde injection of the bladder with gas,[63] the use of dilute iodinated material alone or in combination (double contrast),[44] or, alternatively, the instillation of contrast media such as peanut oil[23] or a fat emulsion.[57] Some, however, feel that complicated investigative methods using renal contrast material or gas-filling techniques are unnecessary for routine staging of bladder cancer, since the density difference between the bladder wall (30–40 Hounsfield) and urine (10–20 Hounsfield) is sufficiently discriminating.[26, 79] Generally, most patients receive simultaneous oral and intravenous contrast, which improves the interpretational accuracy of the CT scan.

Various authors have evaluated the reliability of CT scanning in predicting the pathologic stage of bladder cancer.[26, 34, 44, 57, 62, 63, 79, 82] Since previous efforts at determining the depth of muscle infiltration have added little to the overall management of patients with muscle-infiltrating tumors, as previously discussed, it is not surprising that similar efforts incorporating CT scanning have been very difficult, discouraging, and of limited clinical value. This provided the major impetus for separating the CT stage of bladder cancer into intramural (TIS, Ta, T1, T2, and T3a) and extramural (T3b and T4) lesions. Differentiation between the two rests on the ability of the radiologist to visualize an intact margin of intervening fat without presence of soft tissue penetration or tumor extension into the adjacent pelvic organs. Interpretational errors are therefore expected, especially in patients who have received prior pelvic radiation or undergone recent bladder tumor surgery, owing to loss of definition of the surrounding fat from radiation fibrosis or extravesical edema and inflammation.

For intramural lesions the accuracy of CT in predicting the pathologic (P) stage ranges between 65 and 100% (Table 14–10). The major error in this group is overstaging, which is reported to occur in 33 to 35% of patients.[34, 82] For those with extramural extension, the accuracy of predicting the P stage varied between 25 and 61% for tumors infiltrating the perivesical fat (P3b) and, as expected, from 83 to 100% when tumor involved the adjacent pelvic organs (P4) (Table 14–11). Although overstaging by CT was uncommon in P4 tumors (three of 27 patients), it varied between 44[62] and 48%[79] in P3b tumors. When the groups were combined, Sager and associates reported 39% overstaging.[57] Similarly, understaging in patients with P3b tumors is common and varied between 66 and 75% in the small number of patients evaluated.[34, 82]

Table 14–10. ACCURACY OF CT SCANNING IN PREDICTING HISTOPATHOLOGIC STAGE (P3a OR LOWER) IN PATIENTS WITH BLADDER CANCER

First Author	Reference	Number of Patients	Accuracy Rate (%)
Weinerman	82	20	65
Koss	34	15	67
Vock	79	39	99
Seidelmann	63	8	100
Sager	57	14	100

With respect to the reliability of CT scanning in accurately predicting the status of the pelvic lymph nodes, various authors have reported overall accuracy rates between 69 and 92% (Table 14–12).[34, 44, 79, 81] Sensitivity, defined as the ability to clinically predict positive nodes in patients with pathologic nodal involvement, varied between 60 and 80%. In contrast, specificity, defined as the ability to clinically predict the absence of lymph node metastasis in patients with pathologically proven negative nodes, varied from 75 to 100%. Corresponding false-negative rates (CT negative, nodes positive) and false-positive rates (CT positive, nodes negative) varied between 6 and 40%, and up to 15%, respectively. Since evidence of muscle invasion is the hallmark of aggressive therapy (Chapter 16), attempts to differentiate between the various intramural lesions, including information provided by CT, have rarely modified the treatment plan predetermined by conventional diagnostic techniques, especially the histopathologic information obtained from a properly performed biopsy. Because of the marginal accuracy of CT staging, particularly in patients with P3b disease, we feel it is premature to endorse pretreatment programs incorporating radiation, chemotherapy, or combinations of both, since almost half of those patients thought initially to have perivesical fat involvement could have been spared the morbidity associated with these new adjuvants. In addition, the results of such pretreatment protocols would be biased in favor of those patients felt by clinical staging to have locally extensive disease. Since the best accuracy of CT staging occurs in patients with P4 or N-positive disease, pretreatment programs may have a potential role for such patients, with adjunctive surgery reserved for those tumors that have demonstrated

Table 14–11. ACCURACY OF CT SCANNING IN PREDICTING HISTOPATHOLOGIC (P) STAGE IN PATIENTS WITH BLADDER CANCER

Pathologic Stage	First Author	Reference	Number of Patients	Accuracy Rate (%)
C(P3b)	Koss	34	4	25
	Weinerman	82	6	33
Extramural Vock	79	27	52
	Seidelman	63	9	56
	Sager*	57	18	61
			Total: 64	
D(P4)	Koss	34	6	83
	Weinerman	82	7	86
	Vock	79	11	91
	Seidelman	62	3	100
			Total: 27	

*P3b and P4 combined.

significant downstaging by serial CT assessment and are felt to be surgically resectable.

Radionucleotide Scanning

In an effort to exclude metastases to liver or bone, radionucleotide scanning of these potential sites has been accepted historically as a routine part of the preoperative assessment of patients with invasive bladder cancer. However, the results of such scans have seldom influenced or significantly altered subsequent treatment. In 1982, Lindner and deKernion reported on a group of 114 patients with invasive transitional cell carcinoma of the bladder who underwent preoperative bone scanning.[39] One hundred and four of the bone scan results were essentially normal, whereas only two revealed definite metastasis. The remaining eight were interpreted as suspicious; however, site-selected plain radiographs ruled out bony involvement in five. Eighteen and 32 months following cystectomy, two of the remaining three patients developed metastasis; one remains disease-free. Alkaline phosphatase levels were increased in 13 patients, yet only one

had a positive result on the bone scan and a subsequent metastasis. In the same report, 54 of 100 patients considered candidates for cystectomy also underwent preoperative scanning of the liver and spleen. Fifty-one (94%) of 54 scans showed normal results, whereas only three revealed filling defects at surgery; one proved to be a hemangioma, but in the other two the liver was palpably normal at the time of cystectomy. Based on their experience, these authors concluded that "routine use of isotope scans is not warranted for the preoperative evaluation of bladder cancer patients." In support of this view, Belville and associates evaluated the predictive value of liver function tests and liver and spleen scans for detecting hepatic metastasis in a group of 104 patients with various genitourinary malignancies, including 27 with bladder cancer.[2] Only one positive result in the liver and spleen scan was found—in a patient with prostatic carcinomatosis and elevated results on liver function tests. Of the 27 patients with bladder cancer, no scan gave a positive result, and only one patient had elevated values on liver function tests. Interestingly, of the entire

Table 14–12. HISTOPATHOLOGIC CORRELATION OF CT SCANNING FOR DETECTING LYMPH NODE METASTASES IN BLADDER CANCER PATIENTS

First Author	Reference	Number of Patients	Sensitivity (%)	Specificity (%)	False-Positive Results (%)	False-Negative Results (%)	Accuracy (%)
Vock	79	44	80	99	15	6	90
Koss	34	25	60	100	0	40	92
Morgan	44	18	75	86	11	6	83
Walsh	81	13	60	75	15	15	69

group, 11 patients had an elevation of serum lactic dehydrogenase levels. In 10 of these, results from the liver function tests and scans were normal, yet eight were subsequently found to have nonhepatic metastases. These authors concluded that "the combination of low predictive value and high cost/benefit ratio indicates that the liver scan has no significant role in urologic oncologic staging, and their routine use should be discontinued." Finally, Berger and colleagues, in an attempt to increase clinical staging accuracy, evaluated preoperative bone or liver scans, or both, in 58 patients considered candidates for cystectomy.[3] Fifty-one of 52 (98%) bone scans had normal or apparently false-positive results. Only one patient (2%) had an abnormal result in the bone scan, indicative of metastasis and possibly predicted by his elevated serum alkaline phosphatase level. These and other authors, including ourselves, feel that liver and bone scans should not be performed routinely in patients with invasive bladder cancer; they should be specifically reserved for those circumstances in which metastases are clinically suspected by history and physical examination or predicted by elevated enzyme levels.

Ultrasound

Like CT scanning, ultrasonography also has been advocated as a means of detecting tumor extension in patients with bladder cancer.[5, 25, 43, 61, 65] However, significant limitations of transabdominal techniques that are posed by the size and location of intravesical lesions, and attempts to increase the sensitivity of the procedure, have recently led to the development and utilization of alternative approaches such as transrectal or transurethral ultrasonic scanning. The best results were obtained in one study by Nakamura and Niijima, who reported excellent correlation between the ultrasonic findings and the pathologic stage in 19 of 20 bladder tumors studied using a sophisticated transurethral intravesical scanning device.[48] Since this technique eliminates artifacts from intervening tumor or other organs, the delineation of the tumor margin, bladder surface, and depth of infiltration into the bladder wall could be accurately defined. However, these authors admit certain limitations of this device, including unidirec-

tional propagation of the beam and inability to obtain longitudinal cross-sectional images. Further refinements of sonography will undoubtedly eliminate some of these limitations, but the exact role of sonography, like that of CT scanning, has yet to be clearly defined.

References

1. Amar AD, Das S: Vesicoureteric reflux in patients with bladder tumours. Br J Urol 55:483–487, 1983.
2. Belville WD, McLeod DG, Prall RH, et al: The liver scan in urologic oncology. J Urol 123:901–903, 1980.
3. Berger GL, Sadlowski RW, Sharpe JR, Finney RP: Lack of value of routine preoperative bone and liver scans in cystectomy candidates. J Urol 125:637–639, 1981.
4. Booth CM, Kellett MJ: Intravenous urography in the follow-up of carcinoma of the bladder. Br J Urol 53:246–249, 1981.
5. Brun B, Gammelgaard J, Christoffersen J: Transabdominal dynamic ultrasonography in detection of bladder tumors. J Urol 132:19–20, 1984.
6. Catalona WJ: Practical utility of specific red cell adherence test in bladder cancer. Urology 18:113–117, 1981.
7. Chisholm GD, Hindmarsh JR, Howatson AG, et al: TNM (1978) in bladder cancer: use and abuse. Br J Urol 52:500–505, 1980.
8. Collste LG, DeVonec M, Darzynkiewicz Z, et al: Bladder cancer diagnosis by flow cytometry: correlation between cell samples from biopsy and bladder irrigation fluid. Cancer 45:2389–2394, 1980.
9. Coombs RRA, Bedford D, Rouillard LM: A and B blood-group antigens on human epidermal cells. Lancet 1:461–463, 1956.
10. Cummings KB: Carcinoma of the bladder: predictors. Cancer 45:1849–1855, 1980.
11. Dean PJ, Murphy WM: Importance of urinary cytology and future role of flow cytometry. Urology 26(Suppl):13, 1985.
12. Denoix PF: TNM Classification of Malignant Tumors, 3rd ed. Geneva, International Union Against Cancer, 1978.
13. Dretler SP, Ragsdale BD, Leadbetter WF: The value of pelvic lymphadenectomy in the surgical treatment of bladder cancer. J Urol 109:414–418, 1973.
14. Esposti PL, Zajicek J: Grading of transitional cell neoplasms of the urinary bladder from smears of bladder washings. A critical review of 326 tumors. Acta Cytol 16:529–537, 1972.
15. Falor WH: Chromosomes in noninvasive papillary carcinoma of the bladder. JAMA 216:791–794, 1971.
16. Falor WH, Ward RM: Prognosis in early carcinoma of the bladder based on chromosomal analysis. J Urol 119:44–48, 1978.
17. Farsund T: Selective sampling of cells for morphological and quantitative cytology of bladder epithelium. J Urol 128:267–271, 1982.
18. Farsund T, Laerum OP, Høstmark J: Ploidy disturbance of normal-appearing bladder mucosa in patients with urothelial cancer: relationship to morphology. J Urol 130:1076–1082, 1983.

19. Freed SZ: Vesicoureteral reflux following transurethral resection of bladder tumors. J Urol 116:184–187, 1976.

20. Friedell GH, Soto EA, Nagy GK: Cytologic and histopathologic study of bladder cancer patients. Urol Clin North Am 3:71–78, 1976.

21. Gibod LB, Katz M, Cochand B, et al: Lymphography and percutaneous fine needle node aspiration biopsy in the staging of bladder carcinoma. J Urol 132:24–26, 1984.

22. Hatch TR, Barry JM: The value of excretory urography in staging bladder cancer. J Urol 135:49, 1986.

23. Hildell JG, Nyman UR, Norlindh ST, et al: New intravesical contrast medium for CT: preliminary studies with arachis (peanut) oil. AJR 137:777–780, 1981.

24. Hounsfield GN: Computerized transverse axial scanning (tomography). I. Description of system. Br J Radiol 46:1016–1022, 1973.

25. Itzchak Y, Singer D, Fischelovitch Y: Ultrasonographic assessment of bladder tumors. I. Tumor detection. J Urol 126:31–33, 1981.

26. Jeffrey RB, Palubinskas AJ, Federle MP: CT evaluation of invasive lesions of the bladder. J Comput Assist Tomogr 5:22–26, 1981.

27. Jewett HJ: Carcinoma of bladder: influence of depth of infiltration on 5-year results following complete extirpation of primary growth. J Urol 67:672–680, 1952.

28. Jewett HJ: The historical development of the staging of bladder tumors: personal reminiscences. Urol Surv 27:37–40, 1977.

29. Jewett HJ: Comments on the staging of invasive bladder cancer—two B's or not two B's: that is the question (apologies to Shakespeare, Hamlet, Act iii, sc. I, 1. 56) (editorial). J Urol 119:39, 1978.

30. Jewett HJ, Strong GH: Infiltrating carcinoma of bladder: relation of depth of penetration of bladder wall to incidence of local extension and metastases. J Urol 55:366–372, 1946.

31. Johnson DE, Kaesler KE, Kaminsky S, et al: Lymphangiography as an aid in staging bladder carcinoma. South Med J 69:28–30, 1976.

32. Kay HE, Wallace DM: A and B antigens of tumors arising from urinary epithelium. JNCI 26:1349–1365, 1961.

33. Klein FA, Herr HW, Sogani PC, et al: Detection and follow-up of carcinoma of the urinary bladder by flow cytometry. Cancer 50:389–395, 1982.

34. Koss JC, Arger PH, Coleman BG, et al: CT staging of bladder carcinoma. AJR 137:359–362, 1981.

35. Kovarik S, Davidsohn I, Stejskal R: ABO antigens in cancer. Detection with the mixed cell agglutination reaction. Arch Pathol 86:12–21, 1968.

36. Lang EK: The roentgenographic assessment of bladder tumors. A comparison of the diagnostic accuracy of roentgenographic techniques. Cancer 23:717–724, 1969.

37. Lieskovsky G, Skinner DG: Role of lymphadenectomy in the treatment of bladder cancer. Urol Clin North Am 11(4):709–716, 1984.

38. Limas C, Lange P: A, B, H antigen detectability in normal and neoplastic urothelium. Influence of methodologic factors. Cancer 49:2476–2484, 1982.

39. Lindner A, deKernion JB: Cost-effective analysis of pre-cystectomy radioisotope scans. J Urol 128:1181–1182, 1982.

40. Loening S, Narayana A, Yoder L, et al: Longitudinal study of bladder cancer with cytology and biopsy. Br J Urol 50:496–501, 1978.

41. Loening SA, Schmidt JD, Brown RC, et al: A comparison between lymphangiography and pelvic node dissection in the staging of prostatic cancer. J Urol 117:752–756, 1977.

42. Marshall VF: Relation of preoperative estimate to pathologic demonstration of extent of vesical neoplasms. J Urol 68:714–723, 1952.

43. McLaughlin IS, Morley P, Deane RF, et al: Ultrasound in the staging of bladder tumours. Br J Urol 47:51–56, 1975.

44. Morgan CL, Calkins RF, Cavalcanti EJ: Computed tomography in the evaluation, staging and therapy of carcinoma of the bladder and prostate. Radiology 140:751–761, 1981.

45. Murphy WM, Crabtree WN, Jukkola AF, Soloway MS: The diagnostic value of urine versus bladder washing in patients with bladder cancer. J Urol 126:320–322, 1981.

46. Murphy WM, Soloway MS: The effect of thio-TEPA on developing and established mammalian bladder tumors. Cancer 45:870–875, 1980.

47. Murphy WM, Soloway MS, Jukkola AF, et al: Urinary cytology and bladder cancer: the cellular features of transitional cell neoplasms. Cancer 53:1555–1565, 1984.

48. Nakamura S, Niijima T: Staging of bladder cancer by ultrasonography: a new technique by transurethral intravesical scanning. J Urol 124:341–344, 1980.

49. Neal DE, Bennett MK, Hall RR, et al: Epidermal-growth-factor receptors in human bladder cancer: comparisons of invasive and superficial tumours. Lancet 1:366–368, 1985.

50. Papanicolaou GN, Marshall VF: Urine sediment smears as a diagnostic procedure in cancers of urinary tract. Science 101:519–520, 1945.

51. Prando A, Wallace S, Von Eschenbach AC, et al: Lymphangiography in staging of carcinoma of the prostate: the potential value of percutaneous lymph node biopsy. Radiology 131:641–645, 1979.

52. Pritchett TR, Kanzler AW, Nichols PW, et al: A simple and practical technic for detecting cancer cells in urine and urinary bladder washings by flow cytometry. Am J Clin Pathol 84:191–196, 1985.

53. Reddy EP, Reynolds RK, Santos E, Barbacid M: A point mutation is responsible for the acquisition of transforming properties by the T24 human bladder carcinoma oncogene. Nature 300:149–152, 1982.

54. Rees RW: The effect of transurethral resection of the intravesical ureter during the removal of bladder tumours. Br J Urol 41:2–5, 1969.

55. Richie JP, Skinner DG, Kaufman JJ: Radical cystectomy for carcinoma of the bladder: 16 years of experience. J Urol 113:186–189, 1975.

56. Rife CC, Farrow GM, Utz DC: Urine cytology of transitional cell neoplasms. Urol Clin North Am 6(3):599–612, 1979.

57. Sager EM, Talle K, Fosså S, et al: The role of CT in demonstrating perivesical tumor growth in the preoperative staging of carcinoma of the urinary bladder. Radiology 146:443–446, 1983.

58. Sandberg AA: Chromosome markers and progression in bladder cancer. Cancer Res 37:2950–2956, 1977.

59. Schade RO, Swinney J: The association of urothelial abnormalities with neoplasia: a 10-year followup. J Urol 129:1125–1126, 1983.

60. Schoonees R, Gamarra MG, Moore RH, Murphy GP: The diagnostic value of urinary cytology in patients with bladder carcinoma. J Urol 106:693–696, 1971.

61. Schüller J, Walther V, Schmiedt E, et al: Intravesical ultrasound tomography in staging bladder carcinoma. J Urol 128:264–266, 1982.

62. Seidelmann FE, Cohen WN, Bryan PJ, et al: Accuracy of CT staging of bladder neoplasms using the gas-filled method: report of 21 patients with surgical confirmation. AJR 130:735–739, 1978.

63. Seidelmann FE, Temes SP, Cohen WN, et al: Computed tomography of gas-filled bladder: method of staging bladder neoplasms. Urology 9:337–344, 1977.

64. Sherry UH, Colry TV, Schumann GB: Reliability of urinary cytodiagnosis. Am J Clin Pathol 83:393, 1985.

65. Singer D, Itzchak Y, Fischelovitch Y: Ultrasonographic assessment of bladder tumors. II. Clinical staging. J Urol 126:34–36, 1981.

66. Skinner DG: Current state of classification and staging of bladder cancer. Cancer Res 37:2838–2842, 1977.

67. Skinner DG: Management of invasive bladder cancer: a meticulous pelvic node dissection can make a difference. J Urol 128:34–36, 1982.

68. Skinner DG, Kaufman JJ: Management of invasive and high grade bladder cancer. In DG Skinner, JB deKernion (eds), Genitourinary Cancer. Philadelphia, WB Saunders, 1978, pp 269–283.

69. Skinner DG, Tift JP, Kaufman JJ: High dose, short course preoperative radiation therapy and immediate single stage radical cystectomy with pelvic node dissection in the management of bladder cancer. J Urol 127:671–674, 1982.

70. Smith G, Elton RA, Beynon LL, et al: Prognostic significance of biopsy results of normal-looking mucosa in cases of superficial bladder cancer. Br J Urol 55:665–669, 1983.

71. Spellman MC, Castellino RA, Ray GR, et al: An evaluation of lymphography in localized carcinoma of the prostate. Radiology 125:637–644, 1977.

72. Spriggs AI: Karyotype changes in human tumor cells. Br J Radiol 37:210–212, 1964.

73. Summers JL, Falor WH, Ward R: A 10-year analysis of chromosomes in non-invasive papillary carcinoma of the bladder. J Urol 125:177–178, 1981.

74. Tribukait B, Gustafson H, Esposti P: Ploidy and proliferation in human bladder tumors as measured by flow-cytofluorometric DNA-analysis and its relations to histopathology and cytology. Cancer 43:1742–1751, 1979.

75. Tribukait B, Gustafson H, Esposti PL: The significance of ploidy and proliferation in the clinical and biological evaluation of bladder tumours: a study of 100 untreated cases. Br J Urol 54:130–135, 1982.

76. Union Internationale Contre le Cancer. TNM Classification of Malignant Tumors, 1st ed. Geneva, 1968.

77. Union Internationale Contre le Cancer. TNM Classification of Malignant Tumors, 2nd ed. Geneva, 1974.

78. Union Internationale Contre le Cancer. TNM Classification of Malignant Tumors, 3rd ed. Geneva, 1978.

79. Vock P, Haertel M, Fuchs WA, et al: Computed tomography in staging of carcinoma of the urinary bladder. Br J Urol 54:158–163, 1982.

80. Wajsman Z, Baumgartner G, Murphy GP, Merrin C: Evaluation of lymphangiography for clinical staging of bladder tumors. J Urol 114:712–714, 1975.

81. Walsh JW, Amendola MA, Konerding KF, et al: Computed tomographic detection of pelvic and inguinal lymph node metastases from primary and recurrent pelvic malignant disease. Radiology 137:157–166, 1980.

82. Weinerman PM, Arger PH, Pollack HM: CT evaluation of bladder and prostate neoplasms. Urol Radiol 4:105–114, 1982.

83. Whitmore WF Jr: Management of urothelial tumors of the upper collecting system. In DG Skinner (ed), Urological Cancer. New York, Grune & Stratton, 1983, p 181–197.

84. Winterberger AR, Wajsman Z, Merrin C, Murphy GP: Eight years of experience with preoperative angiographic and lymphographic staging of bladder cancer. J Urol 119:208–212, 1978.

WILLIAM J. CATALONA, M.D.
STEVEN M. DRESNER, M.D.
ERIC O. HAAFF, M.D.

CHAPTER 15

Management of Superficial Bladder Cancer

Superficial bladder cancer is defined as transitional cell carcinoma that is limited to the mucosa and submucosa of the bladder. Superficial bladder tumors are categorized in the Jewett-Strong-Marshall system as clinical Stages 0 and A and in the Union Internationale Contra le Cancer (UICC) system as TIS, Ta, or T1. Tumors that fall into this classification include noninvasive papillary transitional cell carcinomas that are confined to the bladder mucosa (Stage 0 or Ta), flat carcinoma in situ (Stage 0 or TIS), and papillary transitional cell carcinoma that invades through the lamina propria into the submucosa but not into the bladder muscle (Stage A or T1).

A detailed discussion of the epidemiology and etiology of superficial bladder cancer is discussed in Chapter 2. Superficial transitional cell carcinomas account for approximately 75 to 85% of all newly diagnosed bladder cancers, which, it is estimated, will affect more than 40,000 patients in the United States in 1985.[5]

The histopathologic features of superficial bladder cancer are discussed in Chapter 6 and are addressed here only to the extent that the histologic appearance of the tumor and associated changes in the urothelium influence the natural history and treatment of the tumor. In this regard, it is important to emphasize that an entire spectrum of preneoplastic urothelial changes are found in association with transitional cell carci-

noma of the bladder. These changes are postulated to be responses to inflammation, irritation, carcinogenic influences, or any combination of these. Included among the changes are atypical epithelial hyperplasia, von Brunn's nests (Fig. 15–1), cystitis cystica (Fig. 15–2), cystitis glandularis (Fig. 15–3), severe urothelial atypia or dysplasia, and carcinoma in situ (Fig. 15–4). Other reactive lesions, including inverted papilloma and nephrogenic adenoma, are treated in a fashion identical to the treatment of superficial bladder cancer but are not discussed in detail in this chapter.

Carcinoma in situ is a poorly differentiated transitional cell carcinoma confined to the urothelium; it may be focal or diffuse. Histologically, there is loss of cellular cohesiveness and of the superficial umbrella cell layer. The usual presentation of carcinoma in situ is with diffuse urothelial involvement in association with one or more tumors. Between 30 and 70% of bladder cancers are associated with carcinoma in situ, and a higher incidence occurs in association with high-grade tumors. Carcinoma in situ occurs in the bladder in a pattern similar to that of papillary tumors. Primary carcinoma in situ is rarely seen without associated primary tumors, making up only about 3% of all bladder cancers.

Transitional cell carcinoma also may express a spectrum of malignant potentials from benign papilloma to highly anaplastic,

281

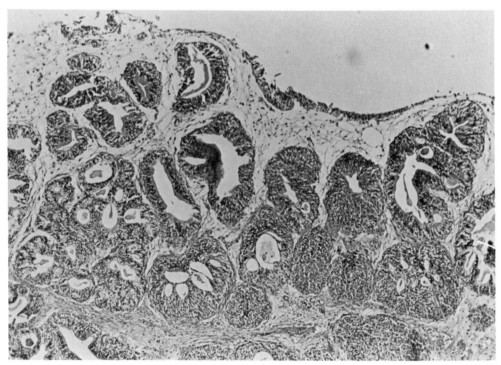

Figure 15–1. Von Brunn's nests. From Mostofi FK, et al: Histological typing of urinary bladder tumors. In International Histological Classification of Tumors, No 10. Geneva, World Health Organization, 1973. With permission.

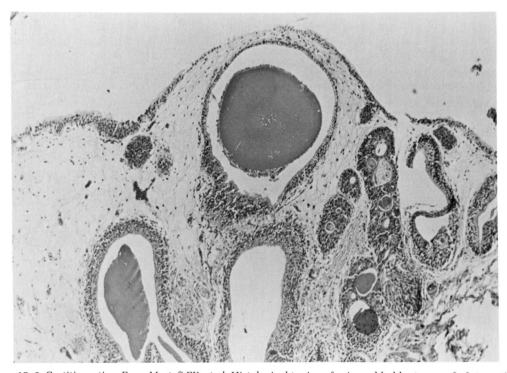

Figure 15–2. Cystitis cystica. From Mostofi FK, et al: Histological typing of urinary bladder tumors. In International Histological Classification of Tumors, No 10. Geneva, World Health Organization, 1973. With permission.

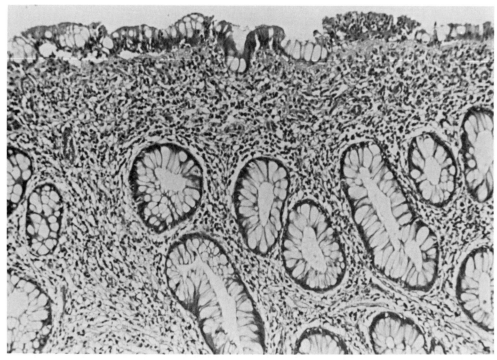

Figure 15–3. Cystitis glandularis. From Mostofi FK, et al: Histological typing of urinary bladder tumors. In International Histological Classification of Tumors, No 10. Geneva, World Health Organization, 1973. With permission.

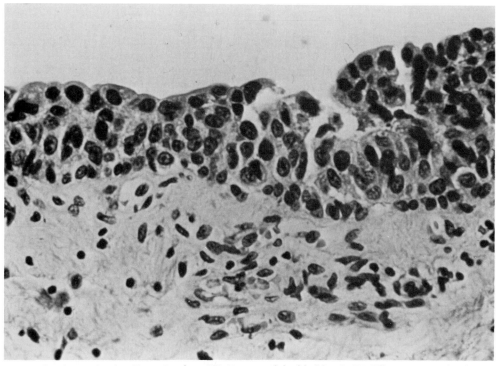

Figure 15–4. Carcinoma in situ. From Catalona WJ: Tumors of the bladder. In JY Gillenwater, et al (eds), Chicago, Year Book Medical Publishers, in press. With permission.

undifferentiated carcinoma. Diverse patterns of tumor growth may be exhibited by transitional cell carcinoma. These include papillary, sessile, infiltrating, nodular, mixed, and flat intraepithelial growth.

NATURAL HISTORY OF BLADDER CANCER

In general, well-differentiated superficial bladder cancer poses little threat to patient survival. Only 10 to 15% of patients with superficial bladder cancer subsequently develop invasive or metastatic disease;[3, 29] however, approximately 70% of patients have one or more tumor recurrences,[24] which express a higher histologic grade in approximately 25%. Some recurrences are new tumors arising from other areas of dysplastic urothelium, whereas others result from inadequate treatment or tumor cell implantation.[60] The onus is on the urologist caring for patients with superficial bladder cancer to monitor them closely for progressive disease and also to select therapy that may minimize tumor recurrences.

The natural history of diffuse carcinoma in situ of the bladder is somewhat controversial. One view is that it represents a highly aggressive neoplasm that should be treated in a fashion similar to that used for an invasive tumor. Supporting this theory are the observations that many patients with diffuse carcinoma in situ develop invasive cancer in a relatively short period of time and, despite radical surgery or radiation therapy, metastases and death from cancer occur in many patients.[76] An alternative belief concerning carcinoma in situ is that it has a limited biologic capacity to invade and metastasize despite its impressive morphologic features. This latter view is supported by clinical observations documenting conservative management of patients who had the disease for long periods of time but did not develop invasive cancer.[6, 65] No unified theory of carcinoma in situ explains all of the clinical observations; however, the available data suggest that it may run a relatively protracted course, characterized by an initial asymptomatic phase followed by a later period in which irritative voiding symptoms are prominent. Carcinoma in situ, when associated with irritative voiding symptoms or when present in patients having other papillary tumors, is an unfavorable prognostic sign. The majority of such patients develop invasive bladder cancer in a short period of time.

A variety of clinical and laboratory tests have been evaluated as potential means for predicting the clinical course of patients with superficial bladder cancer, but most have proved to be unreliable as the basis for treatment decisions. There is a large body of evidence suggesting that tumor recurrence and cancer progression rates are significantly higher among patients having (1) high-grade tumors,[29] (2) tumors that have penetrated the lamina propria,[16] (3) tumors that have invaded into vascular or lymphatic spaces,[4] and (4) those that grow with a nonpapillary configuration. Patients having frequent tumor recurrences or recurrences with multiple tumors, large tumors, solid tumors, or tumors associated with urothelial dysplasia or carcinoma in situ also have higher cancer progression rates (83%).[3] Some of these correlations (i.e., morphology, size) have not been confirmed in all studies. It is well established that patients under the age of 40 tend to have more indolent tumors.[8] Cancer progression rates and recurrences also are more frequent among patients with tumors that lack blood group antigens,[34] tumors that have marker chromosomes,[23] and those that have aneuploid tumor cell clones.[23] As discussed above, an important prognostic factor in patients with diffuse carcinoma in situ is the presence of irritative voiding symptoms. Another important factor with carcinoma in situ is the extent of involvement of the urothelium.

DIAGNOSIS AND STAGING

The signs and symptoms and the diagnostic techniques for superficial bladder cancer are discussed in Chapters 13 and 14 and are addressed here only to the extent that they influence treatment. Urinary cytologic results are often interpreted as normal in patients with superficial bladder cancer because the vast majority of these patients have low-grade tumors composed of cells that appear cytologically normal. However, routine cytologic studies should be performed because a positive cytologic result may indicate the presence of associated carcinoma in situ or other areas of high-grade cancer that have escaped clinical detection.

TREATMENT OF ONE OR MORE PRIMARY TUMORS

Transurethral Resection of Superficial Bladder Tumors

The mainstay of treatment for patients with superficial bladder tumors is transurethral resection of the tumor. There are conflicting opinions about the proper technique for performing transurethral resection. The classic teaching is that the superficial portion of the tumor should be resected first and sent as a separate specimen. This should be followed by resection of the deep portion of the tumor, including underlying muscles that have been invaded. After the tumor has been resected, the base of the resected area is fulgurated. Soloway[72] has suggested that resecting down to muscle for a superficial tumor may be unwise because, if there is a tumor recurrence resulting from implantation of tumor cells, it will occur directly on bladder muscle, which would mandate aggressive therapy for the "recurrence."

Most authors recommend the routine performance of selected site, cold cup mucosal biopsies from areas adjacent to the tumor as well as from the opposite bladder wall, the dome of the bladder, the trigone, and, in males, the prostatic urethra. Selected site biopsies, when positive for tumor cells, provide important prognostic information about the likelihood of tumor recurrence. Early studies reported that selected site biopsies showed positive evidence of severe dysplasia or carcinoma in situ in 30 to 65% of cases.[3, 79] Many recent studies, however, have shown that the overall incidence of significant abnormalities in selected site biopsies is less than 15% in normal-appearing mucosa,[72, 73] and some authors have expressed concern that selected site biopsies may denude the urothelium and unnecessarily create areas for tumor cell implantation. To obviate this problem, it has been recommended that staining the bladder mucosa with vital stains, including tetracycline, hematoporphyrin derivative, methylene blue, and acridine orange, may provide a means of detecting subclinical areas of tumor or dysplastic changes. These methods have not become generally accepted.

Some believe it is not always necessary to perform a formal transurethral resection of very small, low-grade papillary tumors. Such tumors are treated by many urologists with simple fulguration as an outpatient procedure. This approach, however, does not provide adequate tissue for histologic diagnosis.

Tumors that encroach upon a ureteral orifice may require resection of the mucosa overlying the orifice. It has been advocated that passing a ureteral catheter before tumor resection and resecting around the catheter may be helpful, but at times the catheter may prevent adequate resection of the tumor. Cauterization around the ureteral orifice should be avoided.

Tumors on the lateral bladder walls must be excised with care, because the cutting current may induce stimulation of the obturator nerve, resulting in contraction of the adductor muscles of the leg, possibly causing inadvertent bladder perforation. In tumors overlying the obturator nerve, resection should be performed with the patient under general anesthesia with simultaneous intravenous administration of pancuronium.

Patients having superficial tumors arising in vesical diverticula should be treated with partial or total cystectomy rather than with transurethral resection.

The overall survival rates of patients with superficial bladder cancer treated with transurethral resection alone are excellent, and approximately 70% survive for five years.[7]

Laser Therapy

Laser beams also have been used in the treatment of small superficial bladder tumors, since the energy is selectively absorbed by vascular tissues such as transitional cell carcinoma. Several lasers have been evaluated for treatment of bladder tumors.[71] Carbon dioxide laser energy is absorbed by water and produces minimal tissue penetration; therefore, carbon dioxide lasers cannot be used for endoscopic treatment of bladder tumors. The argon laser provides a depth of penetration of only 1 mm; therefore, it is safe in the treatment of small bladder tumors but cannot be used in the treatment of larger tumors. Perhaps the most useful laser is the neodymium yttrium-aluminum-garnet laser (Nd:YAG laser), which has a depth of penetration of 4 to 5 mm, but it is somewhat less safe.

While the patient is under local anesthesia, laser therapy can be performed through a small cystoscope without producing bleeding or stimulation of the obturator nerve. The disadvantage is that the tumor tissue is destroyed by the laser and is not obtained for histologic examination.

Photoradiation Therapy

Photoradiation therapy using hematoporphyrin derivative has recently been evaluated in the treatment of superficial bladder cancer. Hematoporphyrin derivative is a mixture of porphyrins that appear to be preferentially concentrated in neoplastic and dysplastic tissues. If these tissues are irradiated with light of an appropriate wavelength, tumor cells containing the porphyrins are killed by the formation of oxygen singlets. It has been shown that hematoporphyrin derivative can be used both to localize and to destroy areas of neoplasia and dysplasia.

Clinical trials of hematoporphyrin derivative photoradiation therapy have produced some success in patients having small superficial tumors or diffuse carcinoma in situ, but it has had limited success in patients with larger tumors.[9] A drawback of hematoporphyrin derivative therapy is that it produces generalized cutaneous photosensitivity.

Interstitial Radiation Therapy

Interstitial radiation therapy preceded by low-dose preoperative external beam radiation therapy has been used in Europe to treat superficial bladder tumors less than 5 cm in diameter.[78] It has been reported that interstitial radiation therapy is more effective than transurethral resection in controlling small tumors and that there is a lower recurrence rate as compared with patients treated by transurethral resection alone. Radon seeds, gold (^{198}Au) seeds, and iridium (^{194}Ir) all have been used for interstitial radiation therapy. Moreover, Hewett and associates have used intracavitary radiation therapy by means of a radium capsule in a urethral catheter for the treatment of patients with superficial bladder cancer.[33] Intraoperative electron beam therapy combined with conventional fractionated external beam radiation therapy has been used to treat patients with superficial bladder cancer.[52] In general, radiation therapy has not been widely accepted in the treatment of bladder cancer in the United States, because it neither prevents recur-

rences nor destroys associated carcinoma in situ and may produce severe problems with hemorrhagic radiation cystitis.

TREATMENT OF DIFFUSE OR EXTENSIVE UNRESECTABLE SUPERFICIAL BLADDER CANCER

In patients who have diffuse superficial bladder tumors that cannot be completely resected transurethrally, other forms of therapy have been used. These include total or partial cystectomy, external beam radiation therapy, hydrostatic pressure therapy, mucosal denudation, intravesical chemotherapy, systemic chemotherapy, and immunotherapy with intravesical BCG, interferon, or other biologic response modifiers.

Total or Partial Cystectomy

Total or partial cystectomy is seldom required for the treatment of superficial bladder cancer except for patients with diffuse unresectable papillary carcinoma or carcinoma in situ that has not responded to intravesical therapy. Survival rates of patients treated with cystectomy for Ta or T1 bladder cancer are comparable to those of age-matched normal patients not having bladder cancer.[10] Preoperative radiation therapy does not enhance survival in patients with superficial bladder cancer. Some authors have advocated the use of preoperative radiation therapy, however, because of the possibility that a superficial tumor may be clinically understaged. Understaging has been reported to occur in approximately 10% of patients with tumors in clinical Stages 0 or A, as compared with approximately 40% with tumors in clinical Stages B or C.[49]

Patients selected for partial cystectomy should have tumors that cannot be managed safely with transurethral resection alone. They also should have no prior history of a bladder tumor, and random biopsies should reveal no evidence of atypia or carcinoma in situ elsewhere in the bladder or prostatic urethra. (At operation the surgeon should secure a 2-cm margin around the tumor.) It is advisable to administer preoperative radiation therapy in doses of 1000 to 1200 rads to prevent wound implantation, which may occur as a result of opening the bladder.[50, 78] The bladder should be closed primarily and drained with a urethral catheter. In general, ureteral reimplantation is inappropriate except when the tumor is located above and lateral to the ureteral orifice. Ureteral reimplantation should not be performed for tumors located between the ureteral orifice and the bladder neck. The principal shortcoming of partial cystectomy is a high tumor recurrence rate, which may occur in approximately 70% of patients, particularly those having high-grade tumors.[20, 68]

External Beam Radiation Therapy

External beam radiation therapy generally has proved to be ineffective in treating patients with superficial bladder cancer. It does not prevent the occurrence of new tumors.[25] Moreover, as discussed above, external beam radiation therapy is associated with a high incidence of morbidity, particularly radiation cystitis.

Hydrostatic Pressure Therapy

In 1972, Helmstein[28] reported on the treatment of superficial bladder cancer with hydrostatic pressure. This treatment is administered either by filling the bladder with saline under pressure or inserting a balloon in the bladder and inflating it to a pressure above the diastolic blood pressure for five to seven hours, a procedure performed under regional or general anesthesia. Hydrostatic pressure therapy results in selective necrosis of bladder tumors; however, bladder perforation is a significant complication of this form of treatment.

Mucosal Denudation

Complete surgical stripping of the bladder mucosa has been performed by several authors, with mixed results, in the treatment of patients having diffuse papillomatosis of the bladder. In general, the results are favorable in the early postoperative period, but with longer follow-up there is a higher incidence of morbidity with bladder contractures and ureteral obstruction.[27] In general, mucosal denudation has been supplanted by intravesical chemotherapy and BCG therapy.

Intravesical Chemotherapy

Intravesical chemotherapy has been used in the treatment of patients who have multiple unresectable tumors or diffuse carcinoma in situ, as well as for prophylaxis against tumor recurrence. Several agents have demonstrated efficacy in the treatment of unresectable superficial bladder cancer. These include triethylenethiophosphoramide (thiotepa), etoglucid (in Britain, ethoglucid, Epodyl), mitomycin C, and doxorubicin (Adriamycin). Other agents have been used but have been found to be less effective. In general, the individual chemotherapeutic agents are nearly equally effective. Patients who fail to respond to one intravesical agent may be successfully treated with another agent. Thiotepa is the least expensive of the available agents, and doxorubicin and mitomycin C are the most expensive. At present, it appears that intravesical BCG therapy is more effective than intravesical chemotherapy and is also less expensive.

Thiotepa. The modern era of intravesical chemotherapy for superficial bladder cancer began with the use of thiotepa in the early 1960s.[37] Earlier studies had attempted, with little success, to use intravesical silver nitrate, trichloroacetic acid, and podophyllin for the treatment of superficial bladder cancer. Thiotepa is an alkylating agent that exerts its therapeutic effects by producing cross-linking of nucleic acids and proteins. In general, it is used in dosages of 1 mg/ml (30 mg in 30 ml or 60 mg in 60 ml) instilled directly into the bladder and retained for two hours. Treatment schedules have varied considerably. Most regimens call for six to eight weekly treatments, followed by monthly treatments for two years.

Thiotepa induces complete tumor regression in approximately one third of patients producing some objective responses,[41] but a prospective randomized clinical trial has shown that thiotepa is generally less effective than BCG in the treatment of patients with superficial bladder cancer.[11]

The major toxicity of thiotepa is myelosuppression, which occurs in 15 to 20% of patients. This results from transurothelial absorption of thiotepa because of its relatively low molecular weight (189).

Etoglucid (Ethoglucid, Epodyl). This alkylating agent has a higher molecular weight (262) than that of thiotepa. It is used primarily in England and in Europe. It is not as readily absorbed through the urothelium because of its higher molecular weight and therefore causes less myelosuppression. The dose schedules that have been used for eto-glucid treatment have varied. In most studies, it is administered in a 1% solution weekly for 12 weeks, followed by monthly treatments as indicated. Etoglucid causes more chemical cystitis than does thiotepa. Complete tumor responses reported using etoglucid have been observed in approximately 45% of patients, and partial responses have occurred in approximately one third of patients.[43, 66]

Mitomycin C. This antitumor antibiotic has a higher molecular weight (334) than either thiotepa or etoglucid. Mitomycin C acts primarily by inhibiting DNA synthesis. Because of its high molecular weight, mitomycin C causes little myelosuppression, but its major toxic effects are chemical cystitis and skin rashes that occur from contact of drug with the skin of the hands and genitalia. It has been demonstrated to be effective as primary therapy in patients who have failed prior thiotepa therapy.[36, 73] Mitomycin C is given in doses of approximately 40 mg weekly for eight weeks, followed by monthly maintenance therapy for one year. Complete tumor response has occurred in approximately 40% of patients, and partial response has occurred in up to another 40%.[36, 43, 73] Mitomycin C has been reported to be more effective in patients with high-grade tumors.[73]

Doxorubicin (Adriamycin). Another antitumor antibiotic with a high molecular weight (580), doxorubicin is administered with a variety of dose schedules and response rates. Most studies suggest that at least 50 mg should be used for intravesical chemotherapy. The treatment schedules have ranged from once a month to as frequently as three times per week. Complete tumor regression has been reported in less than 50% of patients; partial response occurs in about one third of patients. Most response figures have been based upon a relatively short follow-up. The major adverse side effects of doxorubicin include relatively marked chemical cystitis that in some patients has progressed to permanent bladder contractures.

Other agents, including cisplatin[53] and VM-26,[61] a semisynthetic derivative of podophyllotoxin, have been used but usually not as successfully as with the agents discussed previously.

Intravesical chemotherapeutic agents generally have produced equivalent complete response rates ranging from 33 to 57% for patients with residual papillary tumors and complete regression rates of carcinoma in situ of 55 to 66%.

Systemic Chemotherapy

Systemic chemotherapy has received very limited evaluation as a potential means of controlling superficial bladder cancer. Studies have been performed using methotrexate, cyclophosphamide, and cisplatin. Although all of these agents exhibit some activity against bladder cancer, the potential attendant side effects of systemic chemotherapy have discouraged its widespread acceptance for treatment of superficial disease. Systemic cyclophosphamide has been used in combination with intravesical BCG but has provided no additional antitumor effect.[1]

Intravesical Bacille Calmette-Guérin (BCG) Therapy

Intravesical BCG therapy was introduced by Morales and associates in 1976 as a means of prophylaxis against tumor recurrence in patients with superficial bladder cancer.[56] Studies have demonstrated that BCG also is effective in inducing the regression of residual papillary tumors and perhaps is the most effective agent for inducing the regression of diffuse carcinoma in situ. Most studies suggest that intravesical BCG is more effective than intravesical chemotherapy in this regard. BCG has been reported to be superior to both thiotepa and doxorubicin in direct comparisons.[11, 44]

A variety of different BCG strains have been used; these include Pasteur, Tice, Connaught, Glaxo, Tokyo, and Moreau strains. Recent studies have demonstrated that the viability and density of the bacilli per milligram of vaccine may vary considerably from strain to strain and even from lot to lot within the same strain.[39] The Glaxo strain has been reported to be ineffective.[54] In addition, various routes of administration have been used for BCG therapy, including combined intravesical and intradermal, intravesical alone, and oral. Although all have been reported to be successful in some patients, it is unknown which method gives optimal results. Direct intralesional injection of BCG has been evaluated in Europe but was abandoned due to severe toxic side effects.[51] Studies of BCG as prophylaxis against recurrent tumors are discussed under the section on adjunctive therapy (see later).

Several series reporting on the results of BCG therapy for residual tumor have demonstrated complete response rates of approximately 58%.[12, 17, 19, 55, 67] In some studies,[55] the response rates were reported to be higher among patients with low-grade tumors. Morales has advocated initiating BCG therapy within 10 days of tumor resection to take advantage of the increased adherence of the BCG to the disrupted bladder mucosa.[54]

Intravesical BCG therapy also has been extensively evaluated in the treatment of patients with diffuse carcinoma in situ.[12, 17, 19, 31, 32, 47, 55] Collectively, these studies reveal a complete response rate of 72%, usually associated with resolution of urinary irritative symptoms.

The principal side effect of intravesical BCG therapy is vesical irritability, which occurs in most patients. Other adverse side effects include hematuria, fever, malaise, nausea, chills, arthralgias, and pruritis, all occurring in a small fraction of patients. In general, BCG is very well tolerated. Approximately 6% of patients have symptoms severe enough to require treatment with isoniazid.[45]

The toxicity as well as the therapeutic success associated with BCG therapy is related to the intensity of the therapy. Brosman[11] reported a greater toxicity with an intensive protocol employing Tice BCG than was reported by Morales[55] using a milder regimen with Pasteur BCG. Toxicity of BCG therapy also is related to the route of administration. Severe anaphylactic reactions have been reported with intralesional injections, whereas intravesical and oral administration have not produced severe complications.

The mechanism of action of intravesical BCG therapy is not clearly understood. Clinical data currently available suggest that the development of an immune response to BCG may be involved in the antitumor effect. There is a significant correlation between the delayed cutaneous hypersensitivity response to purified protein derivative (PPD) and a favorable tumor response to BCG ther-

apy.[11, 19, 47] The correlations between skin test reactivity and granulomatous response in the bladder are imperfect. It has been reported that skin tests have converted to positive results and patients have had granulomas in the bladder yet have not responded favorably to BCG therapy.[11, 47, 56, 67] Meanwhile, granulomas have not developed and skin tests have not converted in others, yet they have had favorable response to the treatment. Thus, these findings are not sufficiently specific or accurate to be used as a basis for determining the adequacy of therapy.

Recent studies have demonstrated that patients who fail to respond to an initial six-week course of BCG therapy may improve with a more intensive regimen, probably because of differences in patient immunologic competence, differences in vaccine potency, or both.[39] In summary, intravesical BCG appears to be more efficacious than intravesical chemotherapy. Furthermore, the cost of BCG is comparable to that of thiotepa, which is significantly less costly than most of the other chemotherapeutic agents.

Intravesical Interferon

Interferons are proteins that have antiproliferative properties. Recombinant DNA techniques have produced large quantities of purified human interferons that have been used in clinical trials in the treatment of superficial bladder cancer, with an overall complete response rate of approximately 44%.[69] Toxicity of intravesical interferon therapy is negligible. Further studies are under way comparing intravesical interferon with other treatments for superficial bladder cancer.

Other Immunotherapeutic Agents

Limited trials have been conducted with other immunotherapeutic agents, including a streptococcal OK-432 bacterial preparation that has demonstrated some beneficial effects.[38] Recent studies suggest that interleukin 2 also may be effective against superficial bladder tumors,[63] and limited studies by Herr[30] and Kemeny[40] suggest that the interferon inducer, poly I:C, may improve the survival of patients with carcinoma in situ.

CARCINOMA IN SITU

As discussed above, there is considerable controversy over the appropriate management of patients with diffuse carcinoma in situ. The current data suggest that most patients deserve a trial of conservative intravesical therapy with either BCG or topical chemotherapeutic agents. Those patients failing an adequate trial of conservative therapy should be treated with cystectomy. Approximately 20% of patients treated with cystectomy for carcinoma in situ are found to have foci of microscopic invasion or pelvic lymph node metastases.[70] It is important to emphasize that although the response rates to intravesical chemotherapy and BCG for patients with carcinoma in situ are quite favorable, treatment is not successful in all patients, and some have progression to invasive or metastatic disease, or both. This is of concern, since some patients require repeated courses of intravesical chemotherapy or BCG therapy before a beneficial effect can be obtained. The danger of repeated courses of therapy in patients who do not respond initially is that the tumor may become invasive and metastasize during the attempts at conservative therapy. Accordingly, there is an urgent need to determine the optimal strain and dose schedule of BCG for intravesical therapy as well as the end point at which therapeutic failure can be declared and more aggressive therapy implemented.

Patients with carcinoma in situ involving the prostatic urethra may respond to intravesical BCG after transurethral resection of the prostate. Biopsies of the prostatic urethra should be performed routinely to rule out tumor invasion into the prostatic ducts or stroma and also to provide an open prostatic fossa for intravesical therapy.

INDICATIONS FOR ADJUNCTIVE TREATMENT

Adjunctive intravesical chemotherapy or immunotherapy is generally reserved for patients who are at high risk for tumor recurrence. At increased risk are those who have high-grade tumors, recurrent tumors, multiple tumors, tumors associated with urothelial atypia, or carcinoma in situ. Intravesical BCG therapy currently appears to be the most effective agent available for prophy-laxis against tumor recurrences, although all of the other chemotherapeutic agents discussed also appear to have some efficacy in this regard.

Prophylactic Intravesical Chemotherapy

There is evidence to suggest that prophylactic intravesical chemotherapy may exert its influence, at least to some extent, by preventing urothelial implantation of tumor cells. Several studies have shown that intravesical chemotherapy administered in the immediate postoperative period is most effective in preventing tumor recurrence,[13] whereas others have shown that a single dose given in the immediate postoperative period is as effective as multiple doses.[80] Further studies have shown that delayed intravesical therapy does not decrease tumor recurrence rates.[22]

Thiotepa. In varying dose schedules, thiotepa has been used for prophylaxis against tumor recurrence following complete transurethral resection of all visible bladder cancer. The National Bladder Cancer Collaborative Group A demonstrated that thiotepa in doses of 30 mg or 60 mg given monthly following endoscopic resection of a bladder tumor reduced the tumor recurrence rates from 73% in controls to 47% in thiotepa-treated patients at two years after resection.[41] Patients with low-grade tumors benefited significantly from thiotepa prophylaxis; however, those having tumors of higher grades did not appear to derive significant benefit.[64] Greene and associates[26] reported that patients treated prophylactically with thiotepa had a proportionately lower incidence of bladder cancer deaths than patients not treated with intravesical chemotherapy, but the difference was not statistically significant.

Etoglucid. This agent has been shown in a randomized clinical trial to be more efficacious than transurethral resection alone or doxorubicin in preventing tumor recurrence in patients having primary bladder tumors but not in those having recurrent tumors.[42]

Mitomycin C. Several studies have demonstrated the efficacy of mitomycin C for prophylaxis against recurrent tumors. Huland and associates[35] reported that mitomycin C given every two weeks for one year and then monthly for another year was effective in preventing tumor recurrence in 90% of patients and also was effective in preventing development of invasive bladder cancer. All patients in Huland's study, however, had complete tumor excision and negative cytologic test results before mitomycin C treatment was initiated. Moreover, 50% of the patients in this study were treated following resection of a solitary primary tumor, and only 29% had high-grade tumors. Other studies[18, 48] of mitomycin C prophylaxis in patients having multiple, recurrent, or high-grade tumors have not confirmed the low recurrence rate reported by Huland and associates.[35]

Doxorubicin. This agent has been used for prophylaxis against tumor recurrence in doses of 50 to 90 mg given at intervals as frequently as every three weeks to as infrequently as every three months. Garnick and associates[21] reported that 47% of patients had recurrences within 18 months and 16% subsequently developed muscle invasion. Zincke and associates[80] conducted a clinical trial in which approximately 55% of doxorubicin-treated patients were tumor-free as compared with 42% of mitomycin C–treated patients and 38% of controls. Kurth and associates[42] reported that doxorubicin was not effective in reducing recurrence rates in patients with primary bladder tumors but was effective in patients treated for recurrent tumors.

In a current trial conducted by the Southwest Oncology Group, doxorubicin was found to be significantly less effective than intravesical BCG as a prophylactic agent against tumor recurrence.[44]

In general, all chemotherapeutic agents appear to be equally effective when used as prophylaxis against tumor recurrence, and they reduce recurrence rates to 30 to 44%, as compared with a recurrence rate of approximately 70% in controls. Evidence suggesting that intravesical chemotherapy may reduce the incidence of subsequent invasive disease and ultimate cancer death is not conclusive.

Intravesical BCG. Several prospective randomized trials have evaluated BCG as a prophylactic agent against recurrent tumors.[11, 15, 43, 46, 62] Lamm[43] reported that intravesical BCG therapy reduced the tumor recurrence rate to 17%, as compared with 42% in controls treated with transurethral resection alone, with a mean follow-up of

15 months. Also, the time to recurrence was longer in the BCG-treated patients. Moreover, two prospective randomized trials[11, 57] have compared BCG with thiotepa for prophylaxis, and in both BCG was the superior agent. Recurrence rates with BCG therapy were 0% with a mean follow-up of 18 to 21 months in Brosman's study[12] and 5% with a mean follow-up of 36 to 39 months in Netto's study,[57] as compared with recurrence rates of 40% and 43%, respectively, for thiotepa in these two studies. Moreover, Pinsky and associates[62] reported data suggesting that BCG may also decrease the rate of tumor progression to muscle invasion from 36% in control patients to 9% in BCG-treated patients.

Overall, available studies have shown that intravesical BCG therapy for prophylaxis has yielded recurrence rates of 0 to 41%, with most around 10 to 20%. Control treatments have yielded recurrence rates of 40 to 80%, with most in the range of 40 to 50%. Therefore, intravesical BCG therapy appears to be more efficacious than intravesical chemotherapy for prophylaxis.

Vitamin Therapy. Several vitamins, including pyridoxine,[14, 75] ascorbic acid,[58] and vitamin A analogs (retinoids),[2, 75] have been evaluated as prophylactic agents against bladder cancer recurrence. The therapeutic efficacy of these vitamins has been modest at best and only of marginal statistical significance. Moreover, the retinoids have proved to be too toxic to be used routinely as prophylactic agents.

SUMMARY AND CONCLUSIONS

In summary, superficial bladder cancer poses more of a nuisance than a threat to the longevity of most patients afflicted with it. Therapeutic approaches generally are conservative. Solitary primary tumors are treated with transurethral resection or fulguration, and adjunctive intravesical chemotherapy or BCG therapy is generally reserved for patients having recurrent tumors, tumors that cannot be completely resected, or diffuse carcinoma in situ.

A small but significant proportion of patients who present initially with superficial bladder cancer progress to develop invasive or metastatic cancer, and the urologist must remain vigilant to identify these patients and treat them aggressively before the tumor has disseminated. In this regard, there is a need to determine accurately when conservative therapy has been given an adequate trial and more radical treatment is needed. Clinical and histologic characteristics of the tumor are helpful to some extent but do not provide accurate guidelines for timely treatment in all patients. Continuing investigations are needed to solve this problem.

References

1. Adolphs HD, Bastian HP: Chemoimmune prophylaxis of superficial bladder cancers. J Urol 129:29–32, 1983.
2. Alfthan O, Tarkkanen J, Gröhn P, et al: Tigason (etretinate) in prevention of recurrence of superficial bladder tumors. A double-blind clinical trial. Eur Urol 9:6–9, 1983.
3. Althausen AF, Prout GR Jr, Dal JJ: Non-invasive papillary carcinoma of the bladder associated with carcinoma in situ. J Urol 116:575–580, 1976.
4. Anderström C, Johansson S, Nilsson S: The significance of lamina propria invasion on the prognosis of patients with bladder tumors. J Urol 124:23–26, 1980.
5. American Cancer Society Statistics. CA 34:7–23, 1984.
6. Barlebo H, Sorensen BL, Ohlsen AS: Carcinoma in situ of the urinary bladder: flat intra-epithelial neoplasia. Scand J Urol Nephrol 6:213–223, 1972.
7. Barnes RW, Bergman RT, Hadley HL, et al: Control of bladder tumors by endoscopic surgery. J Urol 97:864–868, 1967.
8. Benson RC Jr, Tomera KM, Kelalis PP: Transitional cell carcinoma of the bladder in children and adolescents. J Urol 130:54–55, 1983.
9. Benson RC Jr: Endoscopic management of bladder cancer with hematoporphyrin derivative phototherapy. Urol Clin North Am 11(5):637–642, 1984.
10. Bracken RB, McDonald MW, Johnson DE: Cystectomy for superficial bladder cancer. Urology 18:459–463, 1981.
11. Brosman SA: Experience with bacillus Calmette-Guérin in patients with superficial bladder carcinoma. J Urol 128:27–30, 1982.
12. Brosman SA: BCG in the management of superficial bladder cancer. Urology 23(Suppl):82–87, 1984.
13. Burnand KG, Boyd PJ, Mayo ME, et al: Single dose intravesical thiotepa as an adjuvant to cystodiathermy in the treatment of transitional cell bladder cancer. Br J Urol 48:55–59, 1976.
14. Byar D, Blackard C: Comparisons of placebo, pyridoxine, and topical thiotepa in preventing recurrence of stage I bladder cancer. Urology 10:556–561, 1977.
15. Camacho F, Pinsky C, Kerr D, et al: Treatment of superficial bladder cancer with intravesical BCG. Proc Am Soc Clin Oncol 21:359, 1980.
16. Dalesio O, Schulman CC, Sylvester R, et al: Prognostic factors in superficial bladder tumors. A study of the European Organization for Research on Treatment of Cancer: Genitourinary Tract Cancer Cooperative Group. J Urol 129:730–733, 1983.

17. deKernion JB, Huang M, Linder A, et al: Management of superficial bladder tumors and urothelial atypia with intravesical bacillus Calmette-Guérin (BCG). Proc Am Urol Assoc 1984, p 139A.
18. Devonec M, Bouvier R, Sarkissian J, et al: Intravesical instillation of mitomycin C in the prophylactic treatment of recurring superficial transitional cell carcinoma of the bladder. Br J Urol 55:382–385, 1983.
19. Dresner SM, Haaff EO, Ratliff TL, et al: Bacille Calmette-Guérin intravesical therapy for superficial bladder cancer. Urology Grand Rounds, Marion Laboratories, 1984, pp 1–7.
20. Faysal MH, Freiha FS: Evaluation of partial cystectomy for carcinoma of the bladder. Urology 14:352–356, 1979.
21. Garnick MB, Schade D, Israel M, et al: Intravesical doxorubicin for prophylaxis in the management of recurrent superficial bladder carcinoma. J Urol 131:43–46, 1984.
22. Gavrell GJ, Lewis RW, Meehan WL, Leblanc GA: Intravesical thiotepa in the immediate postoperative period in patients with recurrent transitional cell carcinoma of the bladder. J Urol 120:410–411, 1978.
23. Gibas Z, Sandberg AA: Chromosomal rearrangements in bladder cancer. Urology 23(3 Suppl):3–9, 1984.
24. Gilbert HA, Logan JL, Kagan AR, et al: The natural history of papillary transitional cell carcinoma of the bladder and its treatment in an unselected population on the basis of histologic grading. J Urol 119:488–492, 1978.
25. Goffinet DR, Schneider MJ, Glatstein EJ, et al: Bladder cancer: results of radiation therapy in 384 patients. Radiology 117:149–153, 1975.
26. Greene DF, Robinson MRG, Glashan R, et al: Does intravesical chemotherapy prevent invasive bladder cancer? J Urol 131:33–35, 1984.
27. Hansen RI, Nerstrom B, Djurhuus JC, et al: Late results from mucosal denudation for urinary bladder papillomatosis. Acta Chir Scand 472:73–76, 1976.
28. Helmstein K: Treatment of bladder carcinoma by a hydrostatic pressure technique. Report on 43 cases. Br J Urol 44:434–450, 1972.
29. Heney NM, Ahmed S, Flanagan MJ, et al: Superficial bladder cancer: progression and recurrence. J Urol 130:1083–1086, 1983.
30. Herr HW, Kemery N, Yagoda A, et al: Poly I:C immunotherapy in patients with papillomas or superficial carcinomas of the bladder. Natl Cancer Inst Monogr 49:325, 1978.
31. Herr HW, Pinsky CM, Melamed MR, Whitmore WF Jr: Long term effect of intravesical BCG on flat carcinoma in situ (CIS) of the bladder. Proc Am Urol Assoc 1984, p 139A.
32. Herr HW, Pinsky CM, Whitmore WF Jr, et al: Effect of intravesical bacillus Calmette-Guérin (BCG) on carcinoma in situ of the bladder. Cancer 51:1323–1326, 1983.
33. Hewett CB, Babiszewski JF, Antunez AR: Update on intracavitary radiation in the treatment of bladder tumors. J Urol 126:323–325, 1981.
34. Huben RP: Tumor markers in bladder cancer. Urology 23(3 Suppl):10–14, 1984.
35. Huland H, Otto U, Droese M, Kloppel G: Long-term mitomycin C instillation after transurethral resection of superficial bladder carcinoma: influence on

recurrence, progression, and survival. J Urol 132:27–29, 1984.

36. Issell BF, Prout GR Jr, Soloway MS, et al: Mitomycin C intravesical therapy in noninvasive bladder cancer after failure on thiotepa. Cancer 53:1025–1028, 1984.

37. Jones HC, Swinney J: Thiotepa in the treatment of tumours of the bladder. Lancet 2:615–618, 1961.

38. Kagawa S, Ogura K, Kurokawa K, Uyama K: Immunological evaluation of a streptococcal preparation (OK-432) in treatment of bladder carcinoma. J Urol 122:467–470, 1979.

39. Kelley DR, Ratliff TR, Catalona WJ, et al: Intravesical bacillus Calmette-Guérin therapy for superficial bladder cancer: effect of BCG viability on treatment results. J Urol 134:48–53, 1985.

40. Kemeny N, Yagoda A, Wang Y, et al: Randomized trial of standard therapy with or without poly I:C in patients with superficial bladder cancer. Cancer 48:2154–2157, 1981.

41. Koontz WW Jr, Prout GR Jr, Smith W, et al: The use of intravesical thio-tepa in the management of non-invasive carcinoma of the bladder. J Urol 125:307–312, 1981.

42. Kurth KH, Schröder FH, Tunn U, et al: Adjuvant chemotherapy of superficial transitional cell bladder carcinoma: preliminary results of a European organization for research on treatment of cancer. Randomized trial comparing doxorubicin hydrochloride, ethoglucid and transurethral resection alone. J Urol 132:258–262, 1984.

43. Lamm DL: Intravesical therapy of superficial bladder cancer. AUA Update, Series 2, 1983, pp 2–7.

44. Lamm DL, Crawford ED, Montie JE, et al: BCG vs. Adriamycin in the treatment of transitional cell carcinoma in situ: a Southwest Oncology Group Study. Am Urol Assoc Meeting, Abstract 283, 1985.

45. Lamm DL, Stogdill VD, Stogdill BJ: Complications of BCG immunotherapy in patients with bladder cancer. Proc Am Urol Assoc 1984, p 140A.

46. Lamm DL, Thor DE, Harris SC, et al: Bacillus Calmette-Guérin immunotherapy of superficial bladder cancer. J Urol 124:38–42, 1980.

47. Lamm DL, Thor DE, Stogdill VD, Radwin HM: Bladder cancer immunotherapy. J Urol 128:931–935, 1982.

48. Lockhart JL, Chaikin L, Bondhus MJ, Politano VA: Prostatic recurrences in the management of superficial bladder tumors. J Urol 130:256–257, 1983.

49. Lutzeyer W, Rubben H, Dahm H: Prognostic parameters in superficial bladder cancer: an analysis of 315 cases. J Urol 127:250–252, 1982.

50. Magri J: Partial cystectomy: review of 104 cases. Br J Urol 34:74–86, 1962.

51. Martinez-Pineiro JA, Muntanola P: Nonspecific immunotherapy with BCG vaccine in bladder tumors: a preliminary report. Eur Urol 3:11–22, 1977.

52. Matsumoto K, Kakizoe T, Mikuriya S, et al: Clinical evaluation of intraoperative radiotherapy for carcinoma of the urinary bladder. Cancer 47:509–513, 1981.

53. Merrin CE: Treatment of genitourinary tumors with cis-dichlorodiammineplatinum (II): experience in 250 patients. Cancer Treat Rep 63:1579–1584, 1979.

54. Morales A: Long-term results and complications of intracavitary bacillus Calmette-Guérin therapy for bladder cancer. J Urol 132:457–459, 1984.

55. Morales A: Long term results and complications of intravesical BCG therapy for cancer. Proc Am Urol Assoc 1983, p 177.

56. Morales A, Eidinger D, Bruce AW: Intracavitary bacillus Calmette-Guérin in the treatment of superficial tumors. J Urol 116:180, 1976.

57. Netto NR Jr, Lemos GC: A comparison of treatment methods for the prophylaxis of recurrent superficial bladder tumors. J Urol 129:33–34, 1983.

58. Newling D, Robinson MRG, Lockwood R, et al: Tryptophan metabolites in superficial bladder cancer: the background to and preliminary report on EORTC Trial 30781. In L Denis, GP Murphy, GR Prout, F Schrader (eds), Controlled Clinical Trials in Urologic Oncology. New York, Raven Press, 1984, pp 307–309.

59. Niijima T, Koiso K, Akaza H: Randomized clinical trial on chemoprophylaxis of recurrence in cases of superficial bladder cancer. Cancer Chemother Pharmacol 11(Suppl):79–82, 1983.

60. Page BH, Levison VB, Curwen MP: The site of recurrence of non-infiltrating bladder tumours. Br J Urol 50:237–242, 1978.

61. Paulson DF: Treatment of superficial carcinoma of the bladder. In R Kuss, S Khoury, LJ Denis, et al (eds), Bladder Cancer, Part B: Radiation, Local and Systemic Chemotherapy, and New Treatment Modalities. New York, Alan R. Liss, 1984, pp 193–209.

62. Pinsky CM, Camacho FJ, Kerr D, et al: Treatment of superficial bladder cancer with intravesical BCG. In WD Terry, SA Rosenberg (eds), Immunotherapy of Human Cancer. New York, Elsevier North Holland, 1982, pp 309–313.

63. Pizza G, Severini G, Menniti D, et al: Tumour regression after intralesional injection of interleukin-2 (IL-2) in bladder cancer. Preliminary report. Int J Cancer 34:359–367, 1984.

64. Prout GR Jr, Koontz WW Jr, Coombs LJ, et al: Long-term fate of 90 patients with superficial bladder cancer randomly assigned to receive or not to receive thiotepa. J Urol 130:677–680, 1983.

65. Riddle PR, Chisholm GD, Trott PA, et al: Flat carcinoma in situ of bladder. Br J Urol 47:829–833, 1976.

66. Robinson MRG, Shetty MB, Richards B, et al: Intravesical epodyl in the management of bladder tumors: combined experience of the Yorkshire Urological Cancer Research Group. J Urol 118:972–973, 1977.

67. Schellhammer PF, Warden SS, Ladaga LE: Bacillus Calmette-Guérin (BCG) in the treatment of transitional cell carcinoma (TCC) of the bladder. Proc Am Urol Assoc 1984, p 139A.

68. Schoborg TW, Sapolsky JL, Lewis CW Jr: Carcinoma of the bladder treated by segmental resection. J Urol 122:473–475, 1979.

69. Shortliffe L, et al: Intravesical alpha-2 interferon therapy for superficial bladder cancer. Eur Assoc Urol, Abstract 203, Copenhagen, 1984.

70. Skinner DG, Tift JP, Kaufmann JJ: High dose, short course preoperative radiation therapy and immediate single stage radical cystectomy with pelvic node dissection in the management of bladder cancer. J Urol 127(4):671–674, 1982.

71. Smith JA Jr, Dixon JA: Laser photoradiation in urologic surgery. J Urol 131:631–635, 1984.

72. Soloway MS: The management of superficial bladder cancer. In N Javadpour (ed), Principles and

Management of Urologic Cancer. Baltimore, Williams & Wilkins, 1983, pp 446–466.

73. Soloway MS: Intravesical and systemic chemotherapy in the management of superficial bladder cancer. Urol Clin North Am 11:623–635, 1984.

74. Soloway MS, Murphy W, Rao MK, et al: Serial multiple-site biopsies in patients with bladder cancer. J Urol 120:575, 1976.

75. Studer UE, Biedermann C, Chollet D, et al: Prevention of recurrent superficial bladder tumors by oral etretinate: preliminary results of a randomized double-blind multicenter trial in Switzerland. J Urol 131:47–49, 1984.

76. Utz DC, Hanash KA, Farrow GM: The plight of the patient with carcinoma in situ of the bladder. J Urol 103:160–164, 1970.

77. van der Werf-Messing BHP: Carcinoma of the blad-

der treated by suprapubic radium implants. The value of additional external irradiation. Eur J Urol 5:277, 1969.

78. van der Werf-Messing BHP: Carcinoma of the urinary bladder treated by interstitial radiotherapy. Urol Clin North Am 11:659–669, 1984.

79. Wallace DM: Hindmarsh JR, Webb JN, et al: The role of multiple mucosal biopsies in the management of patients with bladder cancer. Br J Urol 51:535, 1979.

80. Zincke H, Utz DC, Taylor WF, Myers RP, Leary FJ: Influence of thiotepa and doxorubicin instillation at time of transurethral surgical treatment of bladder cancer or tumor recurrence: a prospective, randomized, double-blind, controlled trial. J Urol 129:505–509, 1983.

DONALD G. SKINNER, M.D.
GARY LIESKOVSKY, M.D.

CHAPTER 16

Management of Invasive and High-Grade Bladder Cancer

The successful management of carcinoma of the bladder depends upon a number of factors, chiefly the grade and stage of the initial tumor, evidence of multicentricity, and, in particular, the proper and timely selection of treatment from a wide range of therapeutic modalities.

Bladder cancer produces symptoms, the first of which usually remains fixed as a definite episode in the life of a patient, and medical consultation is usually sought promptly. Asymptomatic incidental bladder cancer is rarely encountered either in life or as an autopsy finding. Not one incidental bladder cancer was found in 2805 consecutive autopsies on male patients, and Kretschmer[18] reported that in none of 902 patients with bladder cancer was a tumor found before symptoms occurred.

It is difficult, however, to determine the relative incidence of various grades and stages of the first tumor in any consecutive series of patients managed by any of the various therapeutic options. For instance, of almost 500 consecutive new patients with bladder cancer presenting without evidence of metastatic disease to the New York Hospital and the Sloan-Kettering Memorial Hospital, 34% initially had low-grade, low-stage tumors; 18% had high-grade, low-stage tumors; and 48% had high-stage tumors, 92% of which were high-grade.[4, 22, 29, 59] This sample may not be representative, inasmuch as the New York Hospital and the Memorial Hospital are referral centers specializing in

cancer and would naturally attract patients with more advanced disease. At the Bowman Gray Medical Center, 71% of 294 consecutive new patients with bladder cancer without evidence of metastases presented with low-grade, low-stage tumors; only 3% had high-grade superficial tumors, and 26% were found to have high-grade, high-stage tumors.[8] In a review of a multi-institutional study of 457 patients with bladder tumors registered under the auspices of the Clinical Collaborative Group A of the National Bladder Cancer Project, Friedell[14] reported that nearly half of the patients presented with moderate- to high-grade invasive cancer.

Although the true incidence in the United States is not known, it can be inferred that approximately two thirds or more of all new patients with bladder cancer will present with disease that is not deeply invasive. Jewett and Strong's[17] classic article in 1946 disclosed a relationship between the depth of infiltration of the bladder wall and the potential curability of bladder cancer. Based on their autopsy study of 107 cases, 100% of patients with superficial tumors confined to the mucosa should be curable, and 80% of those whose tumors were confined to the muscularis had localized disease, whereas only 26% of patients whose tumors had penetrated into the perivesical fat were thought to be potentially curable when first seen. Five-year survival reports for patients with all stages of bladder cancer indicate, however, that the potential curability indicated by Jewett and Strong is seldom realized; in reality, nearly 50% of patients with invasive bladder cancer die within 18 months of their initial presentation.[5]

Much of this problem results from poor understanding of the malignant potential of various grades and stages of bladder tumors when first seen and the strong desire on the part of both patient and physician to avoid early aggressive therapy that requires some form of urinary diversion (and which, additionally, renders the male patient impotent). Also, many urologists either have not been trained to perform radical cystectomy and urinary diversion or they fear the substantial morbidity and risk inherent in the procedure. This fear is not without some justification.

Historically, reports of the operative mortality for radical cystectomy and urinary diversion ranged from 10 to 20%, with major postoperative complications ranging substantially higher.[21, 31, 56, 58, 59] Because of this, patients with invasive bladder cancer often are temporarily and unsuccessfully managed by conservative measures such as transurethral resection beyond the time of potential curability, or they may be subjected to segmental resection, even though the procedure is not indicated. When failure occurs, these patients are often referred for radiation therapy, with cystectomy considered only as a possible salvage procedure usually late in the course of the disease when cure is seldom possible. Further confusion exists because of a poor understanding of classification and staging, as well as the inability of even highly skilled clinicians to assess accurately the depth of muscle invasion. What seems needed, as was indicated in Chapter 14, is a simplification of the staging system, an amplification of what is known concerning histologic features and their relationship to the natural history of bladder cancer, and clear guidelines as to when aggressive therapy should be initiated.

ASSESSMENT OF PRESENT STAGING SYSTEMS

Several points mentioned in Chapter 14 should be emphasized. In the 1956 Symposium on Bladder Cancer, Marshall[21] demonstrated a clinical relationship between the histologic grade of the malignant tumor and its depth of invasion. He noted that, in general, low-grade tumors were encountered in superficial stages and high-grade tumors were associated with deep invasion; deviation from this observation was observed in only seven of 104 consecutive cystectomy specimens. Thus the grade as well as the stage of the tumor became important considerations in the classification of bladder carcinoma.

One important observation by Marshall,[21] however, has not received appropriate consideration. He observed that grade reflected or related to not only the depth of invasion but also, independently, the potential curability, inasmuch as the five-year survival rate from first symptom for patients presenting with high-grade superficial tumors was only half that enjoyed by patients with low-grade superficial tumors (37% versus 71%) and is almost as grave as that noted for patients presenting with high-grade, high-stage tumors (20%) (Fig. 16–1).

In 1975, Richie and associates[37] pointed out in a group of 141 patients that any degree of muscle infiltration significantly influenced survival (Table 16–1). In 573 consecutive patients with bladder cancer managed by transurethral resection, Barnes found that is was impossible to distinguish superficial from deep muscle penetration with any degree of accuracy, and the five-year survival rate in his hands directly related to whether the tumor was confined to the mucosa or had penetrated the muscularis.[1, 2] Similar findings can be found in the published reports of other investigators (Table 16–2).[1, 7, 13, 27, 30, 31, 33, 36, 37, 50]

The depth of muscle invasion thus becomes far less significant than the presence

Table 16–1. PATHOLOGIC STAGE AND FIVE-YEAR SURVIVAL RATES IN 140 PATIENTS TREATED BY CYSTECTOMY*

Stage	Five-Year Survival (%)	
0 and A	78.6	
B_1	39.9	All B:40.0%
B_2	40.4	
C	19.7	
D	6.2	

*Note the nearly identical survival for patients with tumors in Stage B_1 or Stage B_2 and the statistical significance between survival in those patients with tumor confined to the mucosa compared with those with muscle invasion (p < 0.01). From Richie JP et al.: Radical cystectomy for carcinoma of the bladder: 16 years' experience. J Urol 113:186, 1975.

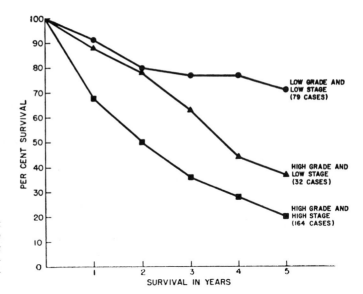

Figure 16–1. Survival rates from first symptoms according to grade and stage for 275 patients. From Marshall VF, et al: Survival of patients with bladder carcinoma treated by simple segmental resection. Cancer 9:568–571, 1956.

of infiltration, a feature that can be determined with far greater accuracy than the clinician's ability to assess depth. Therefore, if the major goals of a classification system are to aid the clinician in the planning of treatment as well as to give indications of prognosis, current evidence supports the contention that a properly performed biopsy revealing the presence or absence of muscle invasion, as well as the grade of the tumor, remains the most important determinant of clinical assessment. Further efforts to ascertain depth of penetration of the primary tumor have resulted in increasing error and confusion over management.

Although accurate pathologic staging is important in assessing the results of therapy, the accuracy of clinical staging is probably not as important to the patient as the ability of the clinician to differentiate those tumors that require aggressive therapy from those that can be satisfactorily managed by more conservative methods. In this area there has been progress, and it is hoped that the cytopathologist will offer further advances.

The presence and natural history of carcinoma in situ has become an extremely important contribution to our understanding of bladder cancer.[11, 15, 24, 25, 44, 49] Current evidence suggests that the presence of carcinoma in situ in association with overt bladder cancer is ominous and should encourage the urologist to use aggressive therapy. Carcinoma in situ is usually associated with (or

Table 16–2. REPORTED FIVE-YEAR SURVIVAL RATES ACCORDING TO STAGE*

Treatment	Authors	Reference	0 and A		B_1		B_2		All B		C	
								Stages†				
TUR	Flocks	13	130/168	(77)					68/142	(47)		
TUR	Barnes	1	146/233	(63)					46/114	(40)		
SR	Utz et al.	50	17/25	(68)	18/38	(47)	14/35	(40)	32/72	(44)	11/38	(29)
SR	Riches	36	7/12	(58)					16/44	(36)	0/6	(0)
SR	Novick and Stewart	30	10/15	(67)					8/15	(53)	1/6	(17)
RAD	Miller	27			10/39	(26)	12/40	(30)	22/79	(28)	5/32	(16)
CYST	Cordonnier	7	31/67	(46)	24/46	(52)	12/30	(40)	36/76	(47)	11/36	(31)
CYST	Richie et al.	37	43/54	(79)	14/36	(40)	9/22	(40)	23/58	(40)	4/21	(20)
CYST	Pearse et al.	31			7/14	(50)	5/12	(42)	12/26	(42)	2/15	(13)
CYST	Prout et al.	33			16/51	(31)	19/61	(31)	35/112	(31)	5/24	(21)
	Total		348/574	(67)	89/224	(40)	71/200	(36)	298/738	(40)	42/235	(18)

*Note the similarity in survival rates between patients with tumors in Stages B_1 and B_2. Both of these rates are substantially different from those for patients with tumors in Stages 0 and A or in Stage C.

†Numbers represent the ratio of surviving patients to the total in the study and the percentage (in parentheses).

KEY: CYST = cystectomy; RAD = radiation; SR = partial cystectomy; TUR = transurethral resection.

may precede) a high-grade overt tumor, which implies an ominous prognosis unless aggressive therapy is initiated.[24, 44] Thus it appears that the clinician needs simplification of staging rather than further confusion and fragmentation as offered by the TNM system. Jewett and Strong's original proposal for an A-B-C system, combined with histologic grade and the presence or absence of carcinoma in situ, would increase the accuracy of clinical staging, provide definite criteria for treatment, and closely correlate with prognosis.[39]

Several important points should be emphasized. Clinical staging of localized bladder cancer should depend primarily on the histopathologic material obtained at biopsy. Important observations are grade, presence or absence of muscle invasion, and presence or absence of carcinoma in situ. Carcinoma in situ is determined by properly obtained random biopsies (described in Chapter 14) as well as by examination of the mucosa immediately adjacent to the primary tumor. If muscle invasion is obvious at the time of biopsy, based on endoscopic appearance or bimanual examination, a biopsy sufficient to document invasion and determine grade may be all that is required to justify aggressive therapy; complete resection is not necessary and may, in fact, be detrimental. Dretler and associates[10] reported that survival in those patients with extensive localized lesions was better if only a biopsy was made for diagnosis, rather than an attempt at resection, and they suggested that resection may play a detrimental role by causing tumor dissemination.

Once the diagnosis of a high-grade or muscle-invading tumor has been established, efforts should be made to rule out metastatic disease (described in Chapter 14). Appropriate studies should include chest x-rays, bone scans correlated with bone x-rays of any suspicious areas, and liver function studies; radioisotope liver scans should be performed only if liver function studies are abnormal.[12] If there is no evidence of metastatic disease, aggressive therapy should be planned. Computerized tomography (CT) is commonly obtained in patients with invasive bladder cancer but in reality offers little to the decision-making process. Thickness implying bladder wall invasion may hasten the decision toward aggressive therapy, but the clinician should realize that there is nearly a 40% error rate in CT scan interpretation in efforts to stage the primary tumor in terms of direct invasion or metastases to regional pelvic nodes. Hence the performance of a CT scan becomes merely an elective procedure based on physician preference. Other diagnostic efforts to stage the localized primary tumor, including pelvic arteriography, bilateral pedal lymphangiography, and triple contrast cystography, offer little that might alter the treatment plan while greatly increasing the cost of management.

TREATMENT

An occasional patient with a high-grade or infiltrating tumor may be a suitable candidate for segmental resection, and in properly chosen patients, results are as good as with any more aggressive operation. The advantages of segmental resection are obvious. Patients are able to micturate in a normal manner and to maintain their potency. The key to success with this operation is proper patient selection. In the authors' experience, patients most suitable for segmental resection are those with a low-grade, unifocal, invasive tumor without evidence of prior tumor whose lesion is more than 2 cm from the bladder neck and in whom random biopsy specimens are normal. Unfortunately, these rigid criteria are seldom adhered to, and all too often the potential for cure is lost owing to an ill-chosen attempt at segmental resection.

It should be emphasized that few patients in reality are suitable candidates. Over a 20-year period at the Mayo Clinic, only 199 of 3454 patients (6%) who presented with a primary bladder tumor were considered candidates for that procedure.[49] At the Cleveland Clinic over a 10-year period, only 50 out of more than 2000 new patients with bladder cancer (2.5%) met similar criteria for the operation.[30]

If segmental resection is contemplated, it is essential to obtain random cold cup biopsies from the mucosa elsewhere in the bladder. Any evidence of atypia or, in particular, carcinoma in situ is, in our opinion, a contraindication to segmental resection. However, if these biopsies yield no evidence of malignancy and segmental resection seems desirable, we recommend 1200 to 1600 rads of radiation therapy to be delivered over a three- to four-day period (400 rads per day) prior to surgery to prevent possible tumor implantation within the incision. The ability of high-dose, short-course radiation therapy to prevent tumor seeding within the incision following cystotomy has been readily demonstrated by van der Werf-Messing.[51, 52] The return to adequate bladder capacity has not been affected by radiation therapy of this total dose.

Novick and Stewart[30] have reported a very low incidence of tumor implant (1.5% in 50 patients) by careful operative technique that includes a thorough transurethral resection and fulguration prior to surgery, irrigation of the bladder and wound with distilled water, and careful packing of the wound during the time the bladder is opened. Others have reported a wound implant incidence up to 25% following cystotomy for high-grade invasive bladder cancer.[53] Because of the low incidence of complications as well as wound implantation following preoperative radiation therapy, we recommend 1200 to 1600 rads delivered to a 15 × 15 cm portal over a three- to four-day period, followed immediately by segmental resection. Perhaps even the lower dose (1000 rads) advocated by van der Werf-Messing[51] may be sufficient. Patients truly suitable for segmental resection have been encountered rarely in our experience.

In our opinion, any invasive tumor associated with mucosal atypia or carcinoma in situ, any overt high-grade tumor associated with mucosal atypia or carcinoma in situ (even though the primary tumor may not be invasive), or any recurrence following the initial conservative treatment of a unifocal high-grade tumor warrants consideration for aggressive surgical management. In our hands, optimal surgical therapy means a radical cystectomy with en bloc bilateral pelvic iliac lymph node dissection (see Chapter 42).

The role of radiation therapy in the management of invasive bladder cancer warrants discussion. Historically, definitive radiation therapy in the range of 5000 to 7000 rads delivered by conventional fractionation over a five- to eight-week period of time was thought to equal the results of radical surgery, as reported by series 20 to 30 years ago. Proponents of radiation therapy cite excessive morbidity and mortality associated with surgery, together with loss of potency and the need for urinary diversion. The survival curves of 529 patients treated at the MD Anderson Hospital by definitive radiation therapy is shown in Figure 16–2.[27] Associated with definitive radiation therapy in that series was a 5% mortality attributed directly to the radiation itself and a 15% major complication rate with regard to bladder, rectal, or small bowel injuries.[27] Although the complications of therapy have declined in contemporary reports, there has

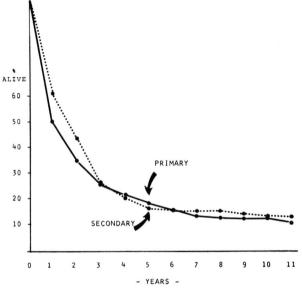

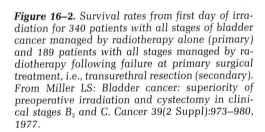

Figure 16–2. Survival rates from first day of irradiation for 340 patients with all stages of bladder cancer managed by radiotherapy alone (primary) and 189 patients with all stages managed by radiotherapy following failure at primary surgical treatment, i.e., transurethral resection (secondary). From Miller LS: Bladder cancer: superiority of preoperative irradiation and cystectomy in clinical stages B$_2$ and C. Cancer 39(2 Suppl):973–980, 1977.

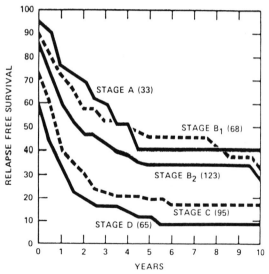

Figure 16–3. *Relapse-free survival. Most recurrences in all stages took place within three to four years of initiation of treatment. The curve is less than 100% at year 0, as some patients were never free of primary cancer. The curve is altered only by recurrence, metastasis, or persistence of bladder tumor. From Goffinet DR, et al: Bladder cancer: results of radiation therapy in 384 patients. Radiology 117:149–153, 1975.*

been little improvement in curability for patients with deeply invasive tumors (T3). In 1977, the MD Anderson group reported a randomized prospective trial in which patients with clinical Stage T3 tumors were assigned to either definitive radiation therapy or the combination of planned, preoperative radiation therapy followed by total cystectomy.[26] Those receiving radiation therapy alone enjoyed only a 16% five-year survival rate, compared with a 48% survival rate among the group receiving surgery in addition to radiation.[26] The Stanford group has reported the best results of any American radiotherapy center treating patients with invasive bladder cancer (Fig. 16–3).[16] In that series, 176 of the 384 patients had their initial recurrence of cancer in the bladder. However, only 30 of these (17%) were deemed candidates for salvage cystectomy and 15 of these have subsequently died of metastatic disease.[16]

Blandy and associates[3] have advocated a protocol of definitive radiation therapy followed by salvage cystectomy at first indication of failure. In reality, this plan is seldom followed and only a few patients ever come to subsequent surgical resection. In Blandy's series,[3] only 8% of 104 patients undergoing

definitive radiation therapy underwent salvage cystectomy, and the operative mortality of the procedure was excessive (11%) compared with an operative mortality of less than 3% for radical cystectomy without prior definitive radiation therapy. In 1976, Wallace and Bloom[53] reported another prospective trial, similar to that conducted at the MD Anderson Hospital, in which patients with deeply invasive tumors received either definitive radiation therapy or preoperative radiation therapy (4000 rads) followed by cystectomy. Patients receiving combination therapy enjoyed better than a doubled five-year survival (33%, compared with 15%).[53] Current evidence thus supports our contention that definitive radiation therapy can cure no more than 16 to 30% of patients with invasive bladder cancer, results that are neither competitive nor comparable to current therapeutic protocols in which cystectomy is the primary treatment either alone or in combination with planned preoperative radiation therapy. Thus definitive radiation therapy currently has a very limited role in the management of invasive bladder cancer.

Nonetheless, there will be some patients with invasive bladder cancer who are thought to be poor surgical candidates either because of advanced age or some underlying serious medical condition. In such patients, it is our recommendation that 4000 to 5000 rads be given by standard fractionation therapy over a four- to six-week period. After a four-week rest period, the patient undergoes cystoscopy and another biopsy. If biopsy and cytologic results are negative, the patient is either followed by periodic cystoscopy or an additional 1500 to 2000 rads are given, depending on patient tolerance. If the results of cytologic or biopsy examinations, or both, remain positive after 4000 to 5000 rads of radiation therapy, then cystectomy is recommended. Our experience has been that even in older, poor-risk patients, it is better to treat the cancer appropriately no matter what the age of the patient,[46] and there is no available evidence demonstrating that if clinical Stage T0 cannot be accomplished by 4000 to 5000 rads, an additional 1500 to 2000 will sterilize the bladder. We believe that patients with residual cancer following 4000 to 5000 rads will need cystectomy, and the morbidity and mortality of the operation is significantly less if the patients have received less than 5000 rads.

Urologic oncologists, however, still have to deal with the problem of tumor recurrence after prior definitive radiation therapy. Experience would indicate that if salvage cystectomy is contemplated, the operation should be started perineally in order to safely free the rectum off Denonvilliers' fascia and avoid rectal injury; the cystectomy could then be completed from above. Operative mortality and morbidity can be reduced significantly by this combined perineal-abdominal approach.[9] The ultimate success of salvage cystectomy depends entirely on the pathologic staging. Preoperative determination of local tumor extent is difficult owing to the dense radiation-induced desmoplastic fibrosis that occurs in the pelvis, making differentiation from tumor impossible. If tumor remains confined to the superficial portion of the bladder, more than 60% of patients may survive five years, whereas if transvesical infiltration is present, only 10 to 20% will survive.[9] Because of the good results obtained in a few highly selected patients following salvage cystectomy, some investigators recommend definitive radiation therapy followed by salvage cystectomy as soon as failure or recurrence is identified.[3] It should be emphasized again, however, that to date the number of patients who are considered candidates for salvage cystectomy and have successfully undergone the procedure represents less than 10% of the patients undergoing definitive radiation therapy.[3] Published results do not support this protocol over early cystectomy with or without planned preoperative radiation therapy. In the United States, radical cystectomy is now the accepted method of treating bladder cancer that cannot be controlled by endoscopic resection. The indications for the operation are fairly standard, and the most controversial issues are the role of adjuvant preoperative radiation therapy and the value of pelvic lymphadenectomy.

The concept of preoperative radiation therapy in an effort to reduce pelvic recurrence and lessen the possibility of tumor dissemination at the time of surgery is appealing and has been widely advocated over tha last 19 years. In 1968, Whitmore[57] reported a pilot study in which 4500 rads of planned preoperative therapy preceded radical cystectomy in patients clinically staged T3. Five-year survival figures reveal a 37% cure rate, which more than doubled the 17% cure rate achieved historically by surgery alone.[57] In addition, pelvic recurrence in the surgery-only group was historically reported to be nearly 40%, compared with a 12% recurrence in patients receiving preoperative radiation therapy.[57]

This prompted formation of the National Cooperative Bladder Cancer Group to evaluate on a prospective basis the influence of combined preoperative therapy and surgical excison as compared with surgery alone in patients with evidence of muscle invasion.[34, 47] Although this study was not without flaws and considerable protocol deviation, it represented one of the first major cooperative ventures by urologic oncologists, and several important observations were noted:

1. In the group treated without radiation therapy, the transurethral resection biopsy used to determine muscle invasion rendered the bladder tumor-free in 8% of the patients, with the pathologist unable to detect residual tumor in the cystectomy specimen. Preoperative radiation, however, rendered the bladder tumor-free in 35% of the patients and significantly downstaged the tumor, that is, the final pathologic stage was often less than that assessed clinically before operation, just the opposite to that observed in patients treated by surgery alone. This seemed to be convincing evidence that preoperative radiation therapy had a significant effect on the primary tumor.[47]

2. In those patients receiving preoperative radiation therapy, fewer pulmonary metastases were noted as first evidence of recurrence or failure than in those patients receiving cystectomy alone. This suggested that preoperative radiation therapy might alter cellular kinetics in such a way that cells were less capable, in terms of blood-borne dissemination, of establishing metastatic foci following tumor manipulation.[34]

3. In those patients undergoing segmental resection as definitive surgical therapy, preoperative radiation did not alter or reduce the incidence of new tumor development elsewhere in the bladder, when compared with patients undergoing segmental resection alone.[34]

4. Preoperative radiation therapy did not increase the operative mortality or postoperative complication rate, compared with that of patients who had only surgery; the simple exception was a slight increase in minor wound infection.[47]

Evidence from the National Cooperative Bladder Cancer Group suggested that pre-

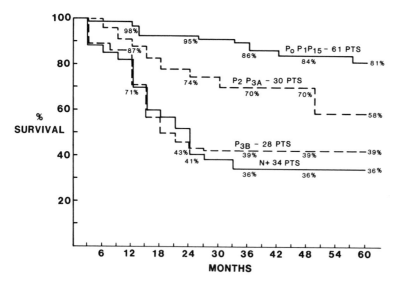

Figure 16–4. Survival according to pathologic stage of 130 patients treated by a protocol of 1600 rads preoperative radiation delivered during four days followed by immediate single-stage radical cystectomy with bilateral pelvic iliac lymph node dissection. From Skinner DG, et al: High dose, short course preoperative radiation therapy and immediate single stage radical cystectomy with pelvic node dissection in the management of bladder cancer. J Urol 127:671–674, 1982.

operative radiation therapy had a profound effect on primary invasive bladder cancer and could be safely combined with radical surgery. However, after all patients had been followed for five years, it became apparent that this randomized study failed to show a significant improvement in curability of patients receiving preoperative radiation compared with those who received surgery alone. In fact, only those patients judged clinically to be in Stage B2, whose cystectomy specimens then showed no recognizable tumor following preoperative radiation, enjoyed an improved five-year survival compared with those whose tumors remained pathologically at the same stage.[47] Of interest was the fact that pathologically, stage for stage, there was no significant difference in the five-year survival rates for those patients whose bladders still showed muscle invasion at the time of cystectomy whether they received preoperative radiation therapy or not; furthermore, those who were found to be in pathologic Stage C did worse if they received preoperative radiation therapy. Perhaps preoperative radiation therapy simply selects those tumors destined for good behavior and has no other significant effect on the natural history of bladder cancer.

During the 1970s, several centers embarked on a combination therapy protocol utilizing high-dose, short-course preoperative radiation therapy followed by immediate cystectomy.[35, 45, 56] The rationale for this protocol was based on experimental work by Perez that indicated that a single high dose of radiation therapy between 500 and

2000 rads could reduce the viable cell population of experimental tumors to 10% of their initial value.[32]

The theoretical advantage of this protocol was that as long as the bladder was removed, sterilization was not the goal of therapy, and benefits such as reduced local tumor implantation and cellular alterations decreasing metastatic dissemination with tumor manipulation could be achieved without the prolonged time interval from diagnosis to completion of therapy. In 1982, we reported our experience in 131 patients treated between 1971 and 1978 by a protocol utilizing 1600 rads of preoperative radiation delivered over a four-day period followed by immediate cystectomy.[45] The Kaplan-Meyer actuarial survival curves are illustrated in Figure 16–4, with results similar to those reported by Whitmore and associates[56] and Reid and associates[35] utilizing a similar protocol of high-dose, short-course radiation (2000 rads over five days) and immediate cystectomy.

However, most studies that support the use of preoperative radiation compare modern data on survival following combination therapy with survival figures for surgery only—procedures performed more than 20 years ago, when the mortality and morbidity of the operation were high and the patient selection criteria were different.

In 1978, we started to look at surgery alone in the management of invasive bladder cancer. By 1984 we reported a study comparing 100 patients undergoing a course of high-dose radiation therapy (1600 rads) delivered over four days, followed immediately by surgery, and 97 patients who underwent surgery without preoperative radiation.[41] All operations were performed by the authors between 1971 and 1982 and utilized a standard surgical technique in which a meticulous pelvic iliac lymph node dissection was performed en bloc with radical cystectomy. Details of the operative procedure have been recorded on film, and the technique is reported in detail in Chapter 42.[42] From August 1982 through December 1984, an additional 197 patients underwent single-stage radical cystectomy and urinary diversion without radiation. The complications occurring in the radiated group and in the surgery-only group are listed in Table 16–3. There is a slight difference in the incidence of superficial wound infection and development of prolonged ileus or partial small bowel obstruction favoring the nonirradiated group. Overall, there were nine postoperative deaths, for an operative mortality rate of 3%. It should be emphasized that patients were not excluded on the basis of age, and during this time only three patients were

excluded because of serious overriding medical problems. Ages ranged from 27 years to 87 years. Note that 250 of the 297 patients survived the operation without complication with an average postoperative stay of 11.6 days. Any complication, however, extended the postoperative stay to a mean of 25.1 days.

Stage for stage, Figures 16–5 through 16–10 compare the Kaplan-Meyer actuarial survival curves for 100 patients receiving 1600 rads of preoperative radiation therapy, followed by cystectomy, with 197 patients undergoing surgery alone. Only in pathologic Stage P3b does there appear to be a difference favoring the irradiated group. This difference, however, does not reach statistical significance, and we believe it probably represents patient selection and increased referrals of more advanced disease.

Recently, two other centers have reported similar data showing nearly identical five-year survival rates among patients with invasive bladder cancer undergoing contem-

Table 16–3. COMPLICATIONS OF SINGLE-STAGE RADICAL CYSTECTOMY WITH EN BLOC PELVIC ILIAC LYMPH NODE DISSECTION AND URINARY DIVERSION

Complication	1600 rads + Cystectomy (100 patients)		Cystectomy Alone (197 Patients)		Total Group (297 Patients)	
	Number of Patients	Average Postoperative Stay (days)	Number of Patients	Average Postoperative Stay (days)	Number of Patients	Average Postoperative Stay (days)
None	82	12.0	168	11.3	250	11.6
Wound infections	6	26	2	16	8	23.5
Ileus-partial small bowel obstruction	7	29	5	26	12	28
Sepsis with or without urine leak	1	op mort	3	op mort	4	op mort
Cirrhosis complications			3	op mort	3	op mort
Pelvic bleeding sepsis			2	op mort	2	op mort
Prolonged urine leak			4	17	4	17
Vascular			2	11.5	2	11.5
Enteric fistula	1	31	1	50	2	40
Cardiac disorder/arrhythmia			1	18	1	18
Loop infarction, reoperated			1	22	1	22
Stoma relocation			1	21	1	21
Brachial palsy (temporary)			1	9	1	9
Pancreatitis/cholecystitis	1	28	1	42	2	35
Fever of unknown cause, sepsis			2	22	2	22
Ureteral obstruction	2	30			2	30
Thrombophlebitis/pulmonary embolism	0		0		0	
Any complication	18 18%	28.1	29 15%	21.8	47 16%	26.3

The overall mortality rate was nine of 297 patients (3%). Note that 250 of 297 suffered no postoperative complication rate; the mean postoperative hospitalization stay for these patients was 11.6 days. Any complications suffered during the postoperative period, however, extended the postoperative stay to a mean of 26.3 days.

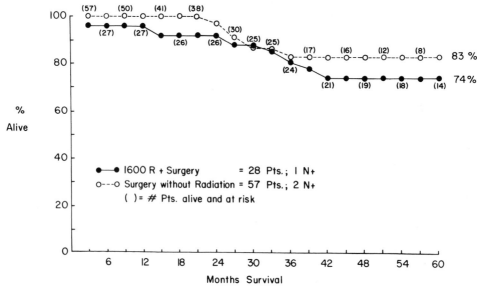

Figure 16–5. *Actuarial survival (Kaplan-Meier) of 57 patients with pathologic Stage P1 or P1S bladder cancer, or both, undergoing radical cystectomy alone, compared with 28 patients receiving 1600 rads of preoperative radiation therapy followed by immediate radical cystectomy.*

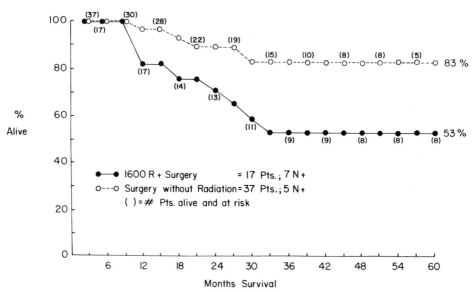

Figure 16–6. *Actuarial survival (Kaplan-Meier) of 37 patients with pathologic stage P2 bladder cancer undergoing radical cystectomy alone, compared with 17 patients receiving 1600 rads of radiation therapy followed by immediate radical cystectomy.*

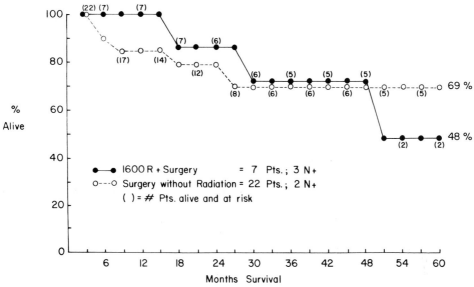

Figure 16–7. *Actuarial survival (Kaplan-Meier) of 22 patients with pathologic stage P3A bladder cancer undergoing radical cystectomy alone, compared with seven patients receiving 1600 rads of preoperative radiation therapy followed by immediate cystectomy.*

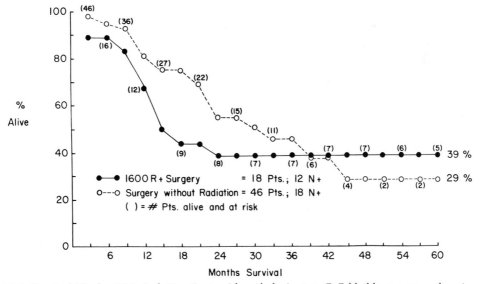

Figure 16–8. *Survival (Kaplan-Meier) of 46 patients with pathologic stage P3B bladder cancer undergoing radical cystectomy alone, compared with 18 patients receiving 1600 rads of radiation therapy followed by immediate cystectomy.*

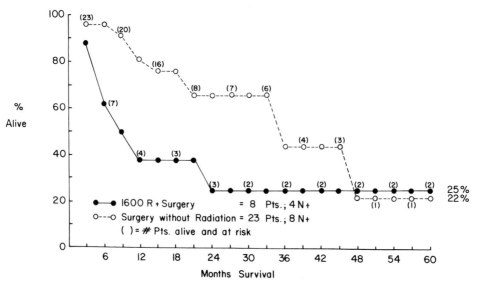

Figure 16–9. *Actuarial survival (Kaplan-Meier) of 23 patients with pathologic stage P4 bladder cancer undergoing radical cystectomy alone, compared with eight patients receiving 1600 rads preoperative radiation therapy followed by cystectomy.*

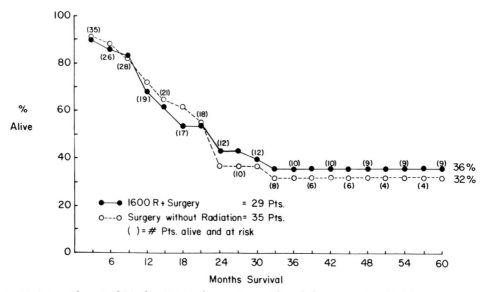

Figure 16–10. *Actuarial survival (Kaplan-Meier) of 35 patients with pathologic stage N+ bladder cancer undergoing surgery alone, compared with 29 patients receiving 1600 rads preoperative radiation. Note that 13 of the 64 patients are alive and have been followed beyond five years.*

porary surgery without radiation.[23, 28] In addition, Montie and associates[28] have shown that the decade in which patients with a given clinical stage of bladder cancer underwent surgery was more important to the chance of survival free of tumor than whether they received radiation therapy.

It seems more plausible that contemporary factors other than radiation are responsible for the significantly improved survival rates currently reported. Improved preoperative and postoperative surgical care and surgical technique have reduced the mortality and morbidity of the operation. Operative mortality rates now range from 1 to 5%, compared with the 12 to 22% mortality rates reported historically. Also, current postoperative complication rates of 14 to 20% have shown substantial improvement. In addition, a meticulous pelvic lymph node dissection facilitates performance of the operation as well as proves curative in up to one third of the patients in whom only a few nodes are positive for disease.[40, 41] In our study these factors have been standardized during the last 14 years, and an analysis of available data indicates no apparent benefit to a high-dose, short-course of preoperative radiation therapy in addition to surgery. Patient selection also may contribute to better contemporary results inasmuch as the lower morbidity of the operation and better appliances for stomal care, as well as the development of the continent form of urinary diversion (Kock pouch), may result in the patient with invasive disease being referred earlier for cystectomy. However, only three patients were excluded from our study because they were deemed poor medical risks for surgery, and all other patients without clinical evidence of disseminated disease were operated upon and included for analysis.

Perhaps the area in which preoperative radiation therapy may benefit patients the most is in reducing the incidence of pelvic recurrence as the first site of tumor failure. We observed no difference in the rate of pelvic failure (9% among those receiving preoperative radiation therapy and 7% among those undergoing surgery only) (Table 16–4). Our pelvic recurrence rate is similar to that reported by Montie and associates[28] among their surgery-only patients and parallels that reported by Whitmore and associates[48, 56] in patients receiving

Table 16–4. INCIDENCE OF RECURRENCE THROUGH MARCH 1985 ACCORDING TO SITE FOR 288 PATIENTS UNDERGOING PELVIC LYMPH NODE DISSECTION AND RADICAL CYSTECTOMY

Site	Preoperative Therapy	
	1600 Rads*	None†
Pelvis ± other	5%	4%
Wound	1%	1%
Urethra	3%	2%
Total failure, local control	9%	7%
Liver	4%	1%
Lung	3%	4%
Widespread	16%	10%
Total	31/99	42/189

*Total patients = 99.
†Total patients = 189

2000 rads for five days preoperatively or 4000 rads standard fractionation during four to six weeks, followed by a rest period before surgery. A low pelvic recurrence rate in patients not receiving preoperative radiation therapy is dependent upon meticulous surgical technique without surgical bladder injury or tumor spill. It has been shown by van der Werf-Messing[51] that when tumor spill occurs, preoperative radiation therapy can reduce significantly the incidence of wound implantation. It may be argued that in lieu of the low morbidity of high-dose, short-course preoperative radiation therapy its use might protect the patient from less than optimal surgery. If the operation results in any tumor spill or is not meticulous in terms of the node dissection, then the results may not be as good as when radiation therapy is used. It seems questionable that this is a valid argument to promote routine use of radiation.

THE ROLE OF PELVIC LYMPHADENECTOMY

In our own series of more than 290 patients undergoing radical cystectomy with en bloc pelvic lymph node dissection for bladder cancer, nodes were positive in 5% of those patients who had only carcinoma in situ or whose primary overt tumor invaded only the lamina propria, in 30% of patients whose tumor invaded the muscularis regardless of depth, and in more than half when the tumor involved perivesical fat or invaded the stroma of the prostate. A comparison of the preoperative clinical stage to the presence or absence of positive pelvic nodes reveals that 17% of those who were thought to have superficial tumor (T1) and 42% of those having histologic evidence of muscle invasion in the biopsy before cystectomy (T2) harbored nodal metastases.[45] This finding supports our belief that the pelvic lymph nodes must be included whenever aggressive therapy is planned. We and others have demonstrated that a meticulous pelvic lymph node dissection can be performed with cystectomy without adding to the operative mortality or morbidity, when compared with the results of simple or total cystectomy without node dissection.[40]

Leadbetter and Cooper[20] were early proponents of a meticulous pelvic iliac lymph node dissection in association with radical cystectomy. In 1973, Dretler and associates[10] reported on 35 patients with nodes positive for cancer who underwent the operation for cure and who were followed more than five years. These investigators indicated that some patients with a few positive nodes could be cured by lymph node dissection without increasing the morbidity or mortality associated with the operation. Of their 35 patients, six (17%) survived more than five years, and 33% of the patients with involvement of only one or two nodes survived.[10] Whitmore and Marshall[59] reported survival for more than five years in two of 13 patients (16%) who had metastases to only one or two pelvic nodes and who also had no invasion of adjacent organs. LaPlante and Brice[19] reported a 13% survival rate among 39 patients with positive lymph nodes at or below the iliac bifurcation but without invasion of adjacent pelvic structures. This was a cure rate similar to that reported in patients with Stage C disease without node involvement.

Reid and associates,[35] utilizing the protocol of high-dose, short-course preoperative radiation therapy with immediate single-stage radical cystectomy and node dissection, reported that five of 24 patients (21%) with positive nodes survived more than five years. Others have reported anecdotal long-term survival of patients with nodal metastases treated aggressively, and our own experience in 64 patients undergoing cystectomy who had positive nodes at the time of surgery reveals a 33% five-year survival (Fig. 16–10).[40]

The increased cure rate reported for patients with nodes positive for disease may reflect an important trend in the management of bladder cancer—that of patient selection and earlier treatment of invasive disease. Our overall incidence of positive nodes (20%) in patients operated on for cure is not dissimilar to other contemporary reports, such as those by Reid and associates (19%)[35] and Smith and Whitmore (19%)[48] who treated similar groups of patients with comparable protocols of preoperative radiation therapy. It seems probable that the incidence of positive nodes found at the time of cystectomy has decreased when compared with previous reports in which patients often were referred late and surgical treatment was withheld until later in the natural course of the disease. In 1968, Whitmore and associates[57] reported that the incidence of invasion of adjacent organs by the primary tumor or positive nodes was 35% in 128 patients treated with 4000 rads of preoperative radiation followed by cystectomy four to six weeks later. Another factor responsible for improved survival may be a more critical pathologic assessment of the resected pelvic nodes with better and more standard fixation techniques, including bladder inflation with formalin before sectioning. In addition, development of a technique for en bloc meticulous pelvic node dissection performed by the same surgeon on a frequent basis may be another factor leading to improved survival.

Available data reveals that approximately 20 to 35% of patients believed to be candidates for radical cystectomy for management of bladder cancer will have metastases to the pelvic nodes. The incidence of positive pelvic nodes relates directly to the pathologic stage of the primary tumor, and the most critical factors associated with nodal metastases are muscle invasion and penetration into the perivesical fat. The inaccuracy of preoperative clinical staging implies the need to treat the nodes whenever cystectomy is indicated. Patients who benefit most from a meticulous dissection are those with clinically undetectable micrometastases to a few nodes. Nearly one third of these patients can be cured, whereas it is rare for patients with multiple or macroscopic nodal involvement to survive beyond two years, regardless of current therapy.

The addition of a meticulous pelvic node

dissection with or without preoperative radiation has resulted in a low incidence of local pelvic recurrence (5 to 22%), compared with results for simple total cystectomy without node dissection or radiation therapy (38%).[6, 41, 56] This data, along with our inability to predict nodal metastases either grossly at the time of cystectomy or based on the primary tumor extent, indicates that lymph node dissection should be performed whenever cystectomy is deemed necessary either as single therapeutic modality or combined with a high-dose, short-course of preoperative radiation, since 1600 to 2000 rads appears insufficient to sterilize nodal metastases. If the surgeon performing the cystectomy is not inclined to perform lymphadenectomy, standard fractionation of higher-dose, preoperative radiation (4500 rads) would seem preferable to simple cystectomy alone or the combination of high-dose, short-course radiation with simple cystectomy.[38]

Direct extension of transitional cell carcinoma into the stroma of the prostate, or the finding of macroscopic nodal metastases, usually indicates systemic disease and a poor long-term prognosis regardless of the extent of local disease. The value of pelvic node dissection is primarily limited to those patients with a few microscopic metastases in whom a five-year survival of 15 to 33% can be anticipated.

The effect of nodal involvement, in addition to primary stage, is depicted in Figure 16–11 and illustrates a major difficulty in trying to compare results of therapy reported according to the TNM staging system with those for the Marshall modification of the Jewett-Strong system. Although pathologic Stage P3b is equivalent to Stage C in terms of the primary tumor, patients with positive nodes remain P3b in the TNM system, whereas in the Marshall-Jewett-Strong staging system, they are classified Stage D. Hence, results reported according to Stage C would be more favorable than those reported as Stage P3b (five-year survival of 49% versus 33%). Nevertheless, the great majority of patients with deep penetration of their primary tumor (P3b or Stage C) or direct extension into the stroma of the prostate (P4 or D_1) or involvement of the pelvic nodes (N+ or D_1) develop metastases usually within two years. Most of these treatment failures represent continued growth of initially unrecognized systemic micrometastases. Therefore, further improvement in survival rates requires the addition of therapy directed to systemic microscopic disease. Adjuvant chemotherapy following cystectomy would seem ideally suited for this purpose.

Randomized protocols designed to determine the possible benefits of adjuvant chemotherapy utilizing a variety of cytotoxic

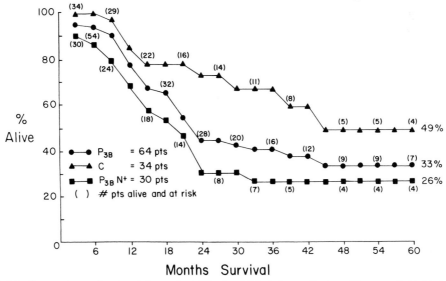

Figure 16–11. Comparison of actuarial survival (Kaplan-Meier) for patients with stage P3B bladder cancer, according to TNM classification system versus pathologic Stage C (Marshall-Jewett-Strong Classification), and patients whose primary tumors are in stage P3B and who also have pelvic nodal extension (P3BN+). The figure illustrates the difficulty of comparing results of therapy according to the TNM versus the Marshall modification of the Jewett-Strong with survival clearly favoring reporting according to Marshall-Jewett-Strong system.

agents are in progress.[43] Follow-up at the present time, however, is too short to determine possible long-term benefits of adjuvant chemotherapy. Currently cisplatin would appear to be a drug superior to any other single agent or combination not utilizing platinum in the treatment of known metastatic disease, and it seems preferable in the adjuvant setting. Preliminary studies have shown that adjuvant chemotherapy following cystectomy is feasible and acceptable to patients at a high risk for recurrence.[43] However, we eagerly await the results of a prospective randomized study to determine whether adjuvant chemotherapy will significantly improve the cure rate for invasive bladder cancer over the rate for surgery only or whether it merely prolongs the disease-free interval. If the latter is true, careful assessment of toxicity will be necessary to determine its realistic use in invasive bladder cancer (Chapter 17).

In summary, a review of current data suggests that appropriate therapy for bladder cancer should be based on histologic information derived from a properly performed biopsy of the primary tumor and assessment of remote urothelium by cold cup biopsy.[40] Aggressive therapy should be started promptly after documentation of a high-grade tumor associated with carcinoma in situ or a muscle-invading tumor of any grade not amenable to segmental resection. Current optimal therapy for such tumors appears to be the combination of preoperative radiation followed by radical cystectomy and urinary diversion or a meticulous pelvic lymph node dissection with en bloc radical cystectomy and urinary diversion without preoperative radiation therapy.[38] Definitive radiation therapy is no longer an equal alternative as far as tumor-free survival is concerned. It should be reserved for patients deemed unsuitable for operation because of medical risks or overriding personal reasons. We have demonstrated that contemporary surgery using meticulous pelvic lymph node dissection and en bloc radical cystectomy yields actuarial tumor-free five-year survival rates of 83% for patients with superficial disease (P1 and P1S), 75% when a cystectomy specimen demonstrates varying depths of muscle infiltration (P2 to P3a), 44% when the tumor penetrates deeply into muscle or involves the perivesical fat (P3a to P3b), 33% for positive pelvic nodes (N+), and 22% for direct invasion of the stroma of the prostate (P4) (Fig. 16–12). These results compare favorably with contemporary reports using any combination of radiation therapy before surgery and are significantly better than those reported historically. We have been unable to demonstrate any significant benefit from the use of preoperative radiation therapy, nor have we observed any major disadvantage to its use. The incidence of positive pelvic nodes, ranging from 3% in patients with superficial tumors to more than 50% for deeply penetrating tumors, implies the need to treat the nodes either by

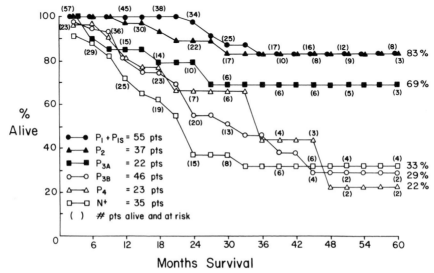

Figure 16–12. Actuarial survival (Kaplan-Meier) of 189 patients undergoing bilateral iliac pelvic lymph node dissection and en bloc radical cystectomy without preoperative radiation therapy.

meticulous node dissection at the time of cystectomy or by preoperative radiation therapy of sufficient dose to sterilize the microscopic metastases (4000 to 5000 rads). Current five-year survival data indicate that the high-dose, short-course method of preoperative radiation therapy (1600 to 2000 rads over four to five days), followed by immediate single-stage cystectomy with pelvic lymph node dissection, is just as good as standard fractionation radiation therapy (4000 to 5000 rads over four to six weeks) followed by radical or total cystectomy four to six weeks later, with or without pelvic node dissection. If patients undergo surgery alone or are treated with the high-dose, short-course of preoperative radiation therapy, pelvic lymph node dissection should be performed.

Despite improved survival, between 50 and 65% of patients with tumor penetration of the perivesical fat or with metastases to the pelvic lymph nodes have widespread metastatic disease within 30 months (90% within 24 months). This implies the need for development of adjuvant systemic therapy protocols as well as methods for early detection of patients with invasive disease. This latter point is emphasized by the fact that two thirds of our patients with pathologic Stage P2 disease or greater had symptoms or the diagnosis of bladder cancer established less than four months from the time of surgery.

References

1. Barnes RW: Endoscopic surgical management of bladder tumors. Urol Digest 6:13, 1967.
2. Barnes RW, Dick AL, Hadley HL, Johnston OL: Survival following transurethral resection of bladder carcinoma. Cancer Res 37:2895–2897, 1977.
3. Blandy JP, England HR, Evans SJ, et al: T3 bladder cancer—the case for salvage cystectomy. Br J Urol 52:506–510, 1980.
4. Brice M II, Marshall VF, Green JL, Whitmore WF Jr: Symposium of bladder tumors; simple total cystectomy for carcinoma of the urinary bladder; 156 consecutive cases 5 years later. Cancer 9:576–584, 1956.
5. Caldwell WL: Carcinoma of the urinary bladder. JAMA 229:1643–1645, 1974.
6. Chan RC, Johnson DE: Integrated therapy for invasive bladder carcinoma: experience with 108 patients. Urology 12:549–552, 1978.
7. Cordonnier JJ: Simple cystectomy in the management of bladder carcinoma. Arch Surg 108:190–191, 1974.
8. Cox CE, Cass AS, Boyce WH: Bladder cancer: a 26-year review. J Urol 101:550–558, 1969.
9. Crawford ED, Skinner DG: Salvage cystectomy after irradiation failure. J Urol 123:32–34, 1980.
10. Dretler SP, Ragsdale BD, Leadbetter WF: The value of pelvic lymphadenectomy in the surgical treatment of bladder cancer. J Urol 109:414–416, 1973.
11. Eisenberg RB, Roth RB, Schweinsberg MH: Bladder tumors and associated proliferative mucosal lesions. J Urol 83:544–550, 1960.
12. Felix EL, Bagley DH, Sindelar WF, et al: The value of the liver scan in preoperative screening of patients with malignancies. Cancer 38:1137–1141, 1976.
13. Flocks RH: Treatment of patients with carcinoma of the bladder. JAMA 145:295–301, 1951.
14. Friedell GH: Pathology. Bladder Cancer Update, presented by the American Urological Association, Office of Education, Los Angeles, April 22–24, 1982.
15. Gibbons RP, Mandler JI, Hartmann WH: The significance of epithelial atypia seen in non-invasive transitional cell papillary tumors of the bladder. J Urol 102:195, 1969.
16. Goffinet DR, Schneider MJ, Glatstein EJ, et al: Bladder cancer: results of radiation therapy in 384 patients. Radiology 117:149–153, 1975.
17. Jewett HJ, Strong GH: Infiltrating carcinoma of bladder: relation of depth of penetration of bladder wall to incidence of local extension and metastases. J Urol 55:366–372, 1946.
18. Kretschmer HL: Cancer of the bladder: a study based on 902 epithelial tumors of the bladder in the Carcinoma Registry of the American Urological Association. J Urol 31:423, 1934.
19. LaPlante M, Brice N 2nd: The upper limits of hopeful application of radical cystectomy for vesical carcinoma: does nodal metastasis always indicate incurability? J Urol 109:261–264, 1973.
20. Leadbetter WF, Cooper JF: Regional gland dissection for carcinoma of bladder: technique for one-stage cystectomy, gland dissection, and bilateral uretero-enterostomy. J Urol 63:242–260, 1950.
21. Marshall VF: Relation of preoperative estimate to pathologic demonstration of extent of vesical neoplasms. J Urol 68:714–723, 1952.
22. Marshall VF, Holden J, Ma KT: Symposium on bladder tumors; survival of patients with bladder carcinoma treated by simple segmental resection; 123 consecutive cases 5 years later. Cancer 9:568–571, 1956.
23. Mathur VK, Krahn HP, Ramsey EW: Total cystectomy for bladder cancer. J Urol 125:784–786, 1981.
24. Melicow MM: Histological study of vesical urothelium intervening between gross neoplasms in total cystectomy. J Urol 68:261–279, 1952.
25. Melicow MM, Hollowell JW: Intra-urothelial cancer: carcinoma in situ, Bowen's disease of urinary system: discussion of 30 cases. J Urol 68:763–772, 1952.
26. Miller LS: Bladder cancer: superiority of preoperative irradiation and cystectomy in clinical stages B_2 and C. Cancer 39(2 suppl):973–980, 1977.
27. Miller LS: Clinical evaluation and therapy for urinary bladder: radiotherapy. In RL Clark (ed), Oncology 1970, Vol 4. Chicago, Year Book Medical Publishers, 1971, p 283.
28. Montie JE, Straffon RA, Stewart BH: Radical cystectomy without radiation therapy for carcinoma of the bladder. J Urol 131:477–482, 1984.
29. Nichols JA, Marshall VF: Symposium on bladder

tumors; treatment of bladder carcinoma by local excision and fulguration. Cancer 9:559–565, 1956.

30. Novick AC, Stewart BH: Partial cystectomy in the treatment of primary and secondary carcinoma of the bladder. J Urol 116:570–574, 1976.

31. Pearse HD, Reed RR, Hodges CV: Radical cystectomy for bladder cancer. J Urol 119:216–218, 1978.

32. Perez CA: Preoperative irradiation in the treatment of cancer. Experimental observation and clinical implications. In JM Vaeth (ed), Frontiers of Radiation, Therapy and Oncology: The Interrelationship of Surgery and Radiation Therapy in the Treatment of Cancer. Brussels, Karger Publishers, 1970, p 1.

33. Prout GR Jr: The surgical management of bladder carcinoma. Urol Clin North Am 3:149, 1976.

34. Prout GR Jr, Slack NH, Bross ID: Preoperative irradiation as an adjuvant in the surgical management of invasive bladder carcinoma. Trans Am Assoc Genitourinary Surg 62:160, 1970.

35. Reid EC, Oliver JA, Fishman IJ: Preoperative irradiation and cystectomy in 135 cases of bladder cancer. Urology 8:247–250, 1976.

36. Riches E: Choice of treatment in carcinoma of the bladder. J Urol 84:472–480, 1960.

37. Richie JP, Skinner DG: Complications of urinary conduit diversion. In DG Skinner, RB Smith (eds), Complications of Urologic Surgery: Prevention and Management. Philadelphia, WB Saunders, 1976, p 209.

38. Skinner DG: Current perspectives in the management of high grade invasive bladder cancer. Cancer 45:1866–1874, 1980.

39. Skinner DG: Current state of classification and staging of bladder cancer. Cancer Res 37:2838–2842, 1977.

40. Skinner DG: Management of invasive bladder cancer: a meticulous pelvic node dissection can make a difference. J Urol 128:34–36, 1982.

41. Skinner DG, Lieskovsky G: Contemporary cystectomy with pelvic node dissection compared to preoperative radiation therapy plus cystectomy in management of invasive bladder cancer. J Urol 131:1069–1072, 1984.

42. Skinner DG, Lieskovsky G: Motion picture: Technique of anterior exenteration. Presented at annual meeting of American Urological Association, Las Vegas, April 17–21, 1983, and at annual meeting of American College of Surgeons, Film Library of American College of Surgeons, 1983.

43. Skinner DG, Lieskovsky G, Daniels JR: Adjuvant chemotherapy following cystectomy for deeply invasive bladder cancer: Current status. Urology 24:46–52, 1984.

44. Skinner DG, Richie JP, Cooper PH, et al: The clinical significance of carcinoma in situ of the bladder

and its association with overt carcinoma. J Urol 112:68–71, 1974.

45. Skinner DG, Tift JP, Kaufman JJ: High dose, short course preoperative radiation therapy and immediate single stage radical cystectomy with pelvic node dissection in the management of bladder cancer. J Urol 127:671–674, 1982.

46. Skinner EC, Lieskovsky G, Skinner DG: Radical cystectomy in the elderly patient. J Urol 131:1065–1068, 1984.

47. Slack NH, Bross IDJ, Prout GR Jr: Five-year followup results of a collaborative study of therapies for carcinoma of the bladder. J Surg Oncol 9:393, 1977.

48. Smith JA Jr, Whitmore WF Jr: Regional lymph node metastasis from bladder cancer. J Urol 126:591–593, 1981.

49. Utz DC, Hanash KA, Farrow GM: The plight of the patient with carcinoma in situ of the bladder. J Urol 103:160–164, 1970.

50. Utz DC, Schmitz SE, Fugelso PD, Farrow GM: A clinicopathologic evaluation of partial cystectomy for carcinoma of the urinary bladder. Cancer 32:1075–1077, 1973.

51. van der Werf-Messing B: Carcinoma of the bladder treated by suprapubic radium implants. Eur J Cancer 5:277, 1969.

52. van der Werf-Messing B: Personal communication, 1975.

53. Wallace DM, Bloom HJG: The management of deeply infiltrating (T3) bladder carcinoma: controlled trial of radical radiotherapy vs. preoperative radiotherapy and radical cystectomy. Br J Urol 48:587–594, 1973.

54. Whitmore WF Jr: The treatment of bladder tumors. Surg Clin North Am 49:349–370, 1969.

55. Whitmore WF Jr, Batata MA, Ghoneim MA, et al: Radical cystectomy with or without prior irradiation in the treatment of bladder cancer. J Urol 118:184–187, 1977.

56. Whitmore WF Jr, Batata MA, Hilaris BS, et al: A comparative study of two preoperative radiation regimes with cystectomy for bladder cancer. Cancer 40:1077–1086, 1977.

57. Whitmore WF Jr, Grabstald H, MacKenzie AR, et al: Preoperative irradiation with cystectomy in the management of bladder cancer. Am J Roentgenol 102:570–576, 1968.

58. Whitmore WF Jr, Marshall VF: Symposium on bladder tumors; radical surgery for carcinoma of urinary bladder; 100 consecutive cases 4 years later. Cancer 9:596–608, 1956.

59. Whitmore WF Jr, Marshall VF: Radical total cystectomy for cancer of the bladder: 230 consecutive cases 5 years later. J Urol 87:853–868, 1962.

JOHN R. DANIELS, M.D.
DONALD G. SKINNER, M.D.
GARY LIESKOVSKY, M.D.

CHAPTER 17   *Chemotherapy of Carcinoma of Bladder*

Despite substantial improvement in the surgical treatment of regional disease, 50% of patients with carcinoma of the bladder in Stages P3, P4, or N+ will eventually relapse with disseminated disease. There is a need for effective systemic therapy as a component of initial treatment to increase the chance for cure. Recent advances in the chemotherapy for advanced carcinoma of the bladder suggest that we may now have the ability to develop effective adjuvant chemotherapy programs.

Contemporary chemotherapy of advanced carcinoma of the bladder may be expected to achieve complete response in 40 to 50% of patients, with median duration of response in excess of one year.[39, 59] We shall review the information available regarding the design of drug programs for advanced disease as well as for the adjuvant setting, including selection of drugs, drug doses, and details of administration.

CHEMOTHERAPY OF ADVANCED DISEASE

Single-Agent Chemotherapy

Most generally accepted cytotoxic chemotherapeutic agents have been shown to have some activity in advanced bladder cancer.[5, 6, 11, 70, 72] Based on literature available

prior to 1976, cyclophosphamide, 5-fluorouracil, methotrexate, and perhaps mitomycin C have been demonstrated to have single-agent activity. More recent experience extends this list to include cisplatin, doxorubicin, and vinblastine.

Sufficient information is not available to rank the relative merits of individual drugs. Much of the literature fails to list important prognostic factors or to detail response parameters. Prognostic factors for drug response include performance status, tumor burden, sites of involvement, drug dose and schedule, and prior treatment with drug or radiation. Response parameters should include response criteria, proportions of patients who are complete and partial responders, duration of response, survival times of responders and nonresponders, and toxicity. Recognizing these limitations, review of more recent single-agent experience in Table 17–1 suggests the following:

1. In general, single-agent treatment results in partial responses of short duration.

2. Observable dose response may be apparent for several agents, including doxorubicin (Adriamycin), cisplatin, and methotrexate. Trials utilizing higher doses tend to report higher response rates.

3. Cisplatin responses are among the most durable reported for single agents. The best reported series is in patients with local regional disease who receive cisplatin as initial treatment.[46]

Table 17–1. CHEMOTHERAPY IN CARCINOMA OF BLADDER—SINGLE-AGENT EXPERIENCE

Drug*	Dose (mg/m²)	Frequency (weeks)	Number of Patients	Complete Response (%)	Partial Response (%)	Duration (months)	Reference
ADR	25	3	21		2 (10)		64
BLEO	5	Biweekly	23		2 (9)		64
ADR	45/60/75	3	37	1 (3)	5 (14)	3	70
ADR	75	3	15	0	6 (40)	2–5	12
ETOP	100 (d 1–3)	3	15		2 (13)		44
MTX	50	2	25		3 (12)		65
	100	2	23	3 (13)	9 (39)		
	200 (FA)	2	16	1 (6)	7 (44)		
MTX	100 (FA)		25		7 (28)		41
MTX	50–100	2	60		9 (43)		42
MTX	250 (FA)	2–3	9		1 (11)		37
	0.5–1	1	37		11 (30)		
PLAT	120	4	14	2 (14)	3 (21)		19
PLAT	100	3	50	8 (13)	22 (37)		46
PLAT	50	3	27		7 (26)	4	43
PLAT	50–70	3–4	28		10 (36)	5	71
PLAT	1 mg/kg	1 × 6	51	1 (2)	18 (35)	5	31
VBL	0.1–0.15	1	28		5 (18)	2–5	3
VCR	1	1	37	1 (3)	2 (5)		49

*Drug abbreviations: ADR, Adriamycin (doxorubicin); BLEO, bleomycin; ETOP, etoposide; FA, folinic acid; MTX; methotrexate; PLAT, cisplatin; VBL, vinblastine; VCR, vincristine.

4. Methotrexate is an active agent. With respect to response, there is no apparent benefit in the use of high dose followed by folinic acid. Folinic acid does not block activity, however, and reduced effect on bone marrow and mucous membranes could be of value in aggressive combination programs.

5. Vinblastine is an active agent and deserves further study in combination programs.

Combination Chemotherapy

Data from recent trials are presented in Table 17–2. The complete response rate for the most effective contemporary programs exceeds 40%, and the duration of remission for complete responders may be in excess of one year. These first-line programs contain cisplatin and two or three additional agents.

There appears to be a clear effect of drug dose. This is most explicitly demonstrated in the cisplatin, doxorubicin, and cyclophosphamide (PAC) regimen. Programs with higher doses result in higher complete response rates and longer durations of control.

Methotrexate and vinblastine were first introduced into combination programs at Memorial Sloan-Kettering Hospital (MSKH). Investigators noted that both drugs were effective as single agents, and they then confirmed significant activity for the two together.[1] An apparent independence from cross-resistance for vinblastine is supported by experience in breast and ovarian cancer, documented both clinically and by in vitro chemosensitivity testing.[34, 50]

The subsequent MSKH study combined methotrexate and vinblastine (MV) with cisplatin and doxorubicin.[59] The Northern California Oncology Group (NCOG) combined MV with cisplatin alone.[39] Both may have achieved more favorable outcomes with less toxicity than previously seen, although a formal, randomized comparison with PAC would be of interest.

Intra-arterial Chemotherapy

A limited published experience documents the use of intra-arterial infusion for advanced regional disease. There is a theoretic advantage in intra-arterial chemotherapy for drugs with high first-pass extraction and a short plasma half-life. Several studies are presented in Table 17–3. It is possible that in selected cases drug delivery by regional infusion may permit delayed cystectomy in otherwise inoperable disease. This approach must be viewed as experimental, since there are no studies that compare outcome with systemic chemotherapy, and pharmacokinetic data are not provided.

Typically, bilateral catheters are placed in the hypogastric arteries. Limiting toxicity is often cutaneous or neural. Adriamycin may cause arterial thrombosis. Technical considerations at the time of catheter placement should include specific measures to reduce skin and neural toxicity and to minimize dilutional effects of collateral arterial supply. These techniques include placement of multiple catheters and the selective proximal occlusion of collaterals (such as the inferior sacral and external pudendal) and vessels with important cutaneous branches (such as the superior gluteal). Restriction of drug to the pelvis may be enhanced by temporary femoral artery occlusion. Limited data are now available for methotrexate,[4, 62] doxorubicin,[21, 24, 28, 66] mitomycin,[40] cisplatin,[60, 68] and combination therapy with cisplatin, doxorubicin, and cyclophosphamide.[30]

COMBINED MODALITIES

Chemotherapy may be used in conjunction with surgery or radiation therapy in an attempt to enhance local control or to contribute to cure by early treatment of occult distant metastases.

Radiation and Chemotherapy

There are three reports of using cisplatin concurrently with pelvic radiation as initial therapy. Patients included in these trials have had locally advanced inoperable disease, had metastatic disease at the time of presentation, or were not considered surgical candidates. Regional treatment was radiation alone[23, 53] or planned cystectomy following initial chemotherapy and radiation.[20] Cisplatin at 70 mg/m^2 or 1.6 mg/kg may be given without apparent increase in regional toxicity and without interfering with completion of planned radiation therapy. It re-

mains to be determined, however, whether concurrent radiation and chemotherapy are as effective as the sequential administration of the most effective chemotherapy programs followed by radiation.

A single report of sequential surgery, doxorubicin, and radiation therapy for disease in Stage D was associated with significant regional morbidity.[51]

Surgical Adjuvant Chemotherapy

Recent theoretical discussions of the evolution of drug resistance have focused upon somatic mutations during tumor stem cell proliferation.[15, 16] There are several important implications for the rational design of curative adjunctive chemotherapeutic programs as well as certain principles that have been validated by experience in several diseases:

1. Chemotherapy should be begun as soon as possible in the natural history of the cancer. The probability that a tumor mass will contain at least one resistant cell lineage increases with the number of stem cell divisions required to achieve the initial tumor mass.

2. Multiple agents should be used to eradicate cells resistant to one or more drugs. Multiple drugs should be introduced as rapidly as possible into the treatment programs and should have independent mechanisms of resistance. There is growing appreciation that drugs that appear chemically quite distinct and that may have different mechanisms of action may share one or more mechanisms of resistance.

3. Adjuvant chemotherapy dose intensity should approach the maximally tolerated dose. In breast cancer, attempts to reduce toxicity by dose reduction have resulted in ineffective programs.

4. Effective adjuvant treatment may not have to exceed four to six months of intensive therapy. This has been true in cancer of the testis and of breast and in lymphomas.

Published adjunctive trials in bladder cancer are quite limited and are nonrandomized demonstrations or reports of small numbers of patients. These are summarized in Table 17–4. There are insufficient data to conclude that adjunctive chemotherapy is useful.

At the University of Southern California, we have been conducting a randomized trial

Table 17–2. CHEMOTHERAPY IN CARCINOMA OF BLADDER—COMBINATION EXPERIENCE

Drug*	Dose (mg/M, mg/kg)	Frequency (weeks)	Number of Patients	Complete Response (%)	Partial Response (%)	Mean Survival Time (mo)†	Reference
ADR + CTX	45, 60 450, 600	3	18	0	3 (17)		70
CTX ADR ADR + CTX	1000 75 40 200 × 4	3 3 3 3	21 10 18	8 (38) 1 (10) 5 (28)	3 (14) 0 4 (22)	(Stage A–D)	32
ADR + 5-FU	50 500	3 3	20	3 (15)	4 (20)	9 +	7
ADR + 5-FU	40 400 × 2	3 3	20	1 (5)	6 (30)	20 4	67
ADR + PLAT	30–60 70	3 3	6		3 (50)		71
ADR ADR + PLAT	50 50 50	3 3 3	41 37	1 (2)	8 (19) 16 (43)	4 4.8	13
PLAT CTX + PLAT	70 750 + 70	 3 3	50 59	5 (10) 3 (5)	5 (10) 4 (7)		57
CTX + PLAT	250–1000 70	3 3	35		11 (43)		71
CTX + PLAT	1000 1.6	4 4	10		2 (20)	3.5	36
VM-26 + PLAT	100 (d 1, 2) 70	3 3	41	4 (10)	17 (41)	12	61
ADR + 5-FU + PLAT	50 500 20 × 5	4 4 4	17		11 (65)		69
ADR + BLEO + 5-FU + MTX (FA)	50 (total dose) 45 500 (d 2) 100	3 3 3	9		5 (56)		17
ADR + 5-FU + MITO + VM-26	40 500 (d 4, 5) 10 (d 4) 60 (d 2, 3)	4 4 4 4	30	1 (3)	13 (45)	10	14
MTX + PLAT	50 50	2 4	5		2 (40)		25
MTX + VBL	30–40 3–4	1 1	50		21 (42)	14 8	1
ADR + CTX + 5-FU	30 (d 1, 4) 300 (d 1, 4) 250 (d 1, 4)	1 1 1	3		2 (67)		63
ADR + CTX + 5-FU 5-FU	50 500 500 600	3 3 3 1	17 15		11 (65) 4 (27)	10	55
BLEO + CTX + 5-FU + MTX + MITO + VCR	15 (d 2) 200 (d 3) 200 (d 1–7) 10 (d 1, 2) 4 (d 4) 2 (d 2)		22	2 (9)	5 (23)		29

Table continued on opposite page

Table 17–2. CHEMOTHERAPY IN CARCINOMA OF BLADDER—
COMBINATION EXPERIENCE *Continued*

Drug*	Dose (mg/M, mg/kg)	Frequency (weeks)	Number of Patients	Complete Response (%)	Partial Response (%)	Mean Survival Time (mo)†	Reference
ADR +	60	4	7	3 (43)	2 (28)	9	8
CTX +	600	4					
PLAT	100	4					
ADR +	50	3	12	1 (8)	9 (75)		58
CTX +	650	3					
PLAT	100	3					
ADR +	40	3	42	5 (12)	12 (29)	11 3	35
CTX +	400	3					
PLAT	40						
ADR +	40	3	23	5 (22)	14 (61)	8+ 3	27
CTX +	400	3					
PLAT	60	3					
ADR +	40	3	45	(22)	(11)	7.3	26
CTX +	400	3					
PLAT	60	3					
PLAT	60	3	48	(2)	(15)	6.0	
ADR +	45	3	6		3 (50)		71
CTX +	250	3					
PLAT	70	3					
ADR +	45	3	28	2 (7)	11 (38)	20 8.4	52
CTX +	250	3					
PLAT	70	3					
ADR +	30	4	24	12 (50)	17 (70)	9.5 +	59
VBL +	3 (d 2, 15, 22)	4					
MTX +	30 (d 1, 15, 22)	4					
PLAT	70	4					
VBL +	4 (d 1, 8)	4	70	21 (30)		12 +	39
MTX +	30 (d 1, 8)	4					
PLAT	100 (d 2)	4					

*Drug abbreviations: ADR, Adriamycin (doxorubicin); BLEO, bleomycin; CTX, cyclophosphamide; FA, folinic acid; 5-FU, 5-fluorouracil; MITO, mitomycin C; MTX, methotrexate; PLAT, cisplatin; VBL, vinblastine; VCR, vincristine.
†Responders and nonresponders.

Table 17–3. CHEMOTHERAPY IN CARCINOMA OF BLADDER—INTRA-ARTERIAL INFUSION

Drug Administration*	Number of Patients	Complete Response (%)	Partial Response (%)	Reference
ADR 0.4 mg/kg/d × 5, continuous	9	1 (11)	4 (44)	28
ADR 10 mg 1–2/wk × 3–16 wks	13		9 (69)	24
ADR 20–30 mg × 3, then q 3 wks	9	2 (22)	2 (22)	66
ADR + femoral artery occlusion	9	3 (33)	4 (44)	
ADR 40–75 mg/m² × 48 hr, continuous, plus intravesical heat to 45° C	9	1 (11)	8 (72)	21, 22
5-FU 15 mg/kg/d × 10 (internal iliac)	10		6 (60)	38
MTX	6		2 (33)	4
MTX (internal iliac)	3		3	62
MITO 5 mg/d × 3, then 2 mg/d × 3 wks	33		17 (32)	40
PLAT 50–100 mg/m² over 2–4 hr	4	3 (75)	1 (25)	60
PLAT 80–120 mg/m² over 24 hr	15	6 (40)	3 (20)	68
ADR 50–60 mg/m² d 1 +	28	11 (39)	7 (25)	30
CTX 650 mg/m² d 1 +				
PLAT 100 mg/m² over 24 hr d 2 q 3 wks × 3 then iv q 3 wks × 3				

*Drug abbreviations: ADR, Adriamycin (doxorubicin); CTX, cyclophosphamide; 5-FU, 5-fluorouracil; MITO, mitomycin C; MTX, methotrexate; PLAT, cisplatin.

Table 17–4. CHEMOTHERAPY IN CARCINOMA OF BLADDER—ADJUVANT EXPERIENCE

Drug*	Dose (mg/m²)	Frequency (weeks)	Number of Patients	Stage	Regional Treatment	Disease-free Period (months)	Reference
CTX or	1000	4	10	P3, P4, or	Cystectomy	At 36 mo:	54
PLAT or	100	4	10	N+		chem,	
ADR +	60	4	18			0.42; obs,	
CTX +	600	4				0.50	
PLAT	100	4					
Control (not randomized)			36				
ADR +	40	3	2	A	Cystectomy, with	2 (12+)	33
CTX	200	3	3	B	or without	3 (25)	
			3	C	radiation	2/3 (26+)	
			17	D		10/17 (13+)	
ADR +	50	3	18	T3	Radiation	15/18 (12)	47
5-FU	500						
ADR +	50	3	9	T3	Radiation plus	5/13	17
BLEO +	45	3			cystectomy		
5-FU +	500 (d 2)						
MTX	100 (FA)						
MTX	1000–2000 (FA)	3	37	T3/T4 T3a	Cystectomy Partial cystectomy	31/33 (12) 18/20 (24) 6/10 (36)	56
MTX	2000 (FA)	3	57	T3/T4	54, Transurethral resection only; 3, Partial cystectomy	45/57 (12) 23/39 (24) 6/13 (36)	18

*Drug abbreviations: ADR, Adriamycin (doxorubicin); BLEO, bleomycin; CTX, cyclophosphamide; 5-FU, 5-fluorouracil; MTX, methotrexate; PLAT, cisplatin.

of adjuvant chemotherapy following radical cystectomy and pelvic lymph node dissection.[10, 54] Eligible patients have disease Stages P3, P4, or N+, but without metastases (M0). Randomization is to observation or to chemotherapy with cisplatin 100 mg/m², doxorubicin 60 mg/m², and cyclophosphamide 600 mg/m² (CAP) every four weeks for four treatment cycles. Early in the study some patients had substitutions for doxorubicin and cyclophosphamide based upon in vitro chemosensitivity testing of tumor within the surgical specimen.[9, 34] Although the principal study objectives have not yet achieved significance, analysis after 65 patients reveals several strong trends:

1. The degree of nodal involvement is the dominant prognostic factor independent of treatment (Fig. 17–1).

2. Patients with no involvement of lymph nodes and patients with minimal lymph node involvement (less than 10% of sampled nodes) who are treated with postoperative adjuvant chemotherapy appear to have an extension of time to relapse and increased duration of survival (Fig. 17–2). There is no apparent benefit of chemotherapy for patients with extensive lymph node involvement (not shown).

3. Survival of patients over the age of 65 with no lymph node involvement was superior to that of younger cohorts. Thus older age per se should not be a contraindication to definitive surgical intervention.

Neoadjuvant Chemotherapy

Initiation of adjuvant chemotherapy prior to definitive regional surgery or radiation therapy has been called neoadjuvant chemotherapy.[46] This approach is theoretically advantageous: chemotherapy may be carried out in a setting free from postoperative catabolic effects and is initiated without delay. A pilot study using pretreatment with two doses of cisplatin at 100 mg/m² at three-week intervals has been completed. Evaluating such programs will be difficult because staging information, particularly nodal status, is compromised and will require multi-

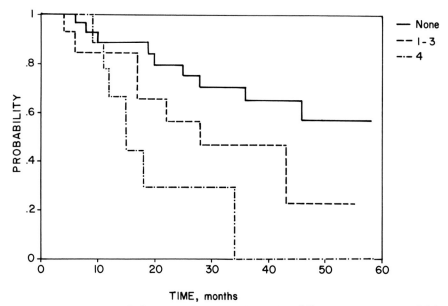

Figure 17–1. Survival of patients with disease in Stages P3, P4, or N+, following cystectomy and bilateral pelvic iliac lymph node dissection. Note the influence of nodal status. Shown are actuarial curves for patients with no involvement of lymph nodes, one to three nodes positive for disease, and four or more nodes positive for disease.

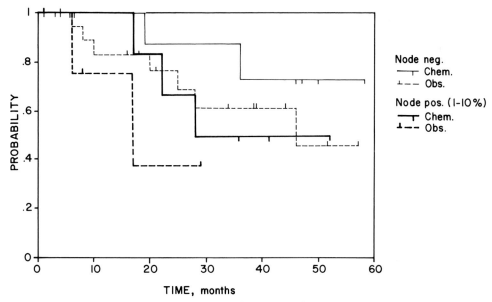

Figure 17–2. Influence of adjuvant chemotherapy with cisplatin, doxorubicin, and cyclophosphamide (PAC) on survival of patients with disease Stages P3, P4, or N+, following cystectomy and bilateral pelvic iliac lymph node dissection. Plotted separately are outcomes for patients with no involvement of lymph nodes and for those who have 1 to 10% of their lymph nodes showing presence of disease. Patients receiving chemotherapy appear to have a delay in time to death. No benefit has been seen for patients with more than 10% of their lymph nodes involved. These trends are not yet statistically significant, and the trial is continuing.

center trials involving large numbers of patients.

CONCLUSIONS

One can be cautiously optimistic that there will be continued progress in the usefulness of chemotherapy in the treatment of patients with invasive bladder cancer. In the past decade there has been the development of intensive multiagent, cisplatin-based programs, which in advanced disease are reliably associated with response and extend life. As these programs improve, there is increasing chance that they will be successful in the adjuvant setting as well. These improvements will emerge only from a broad commitment to controlled clinical trials.

References

1. Ahmed T, Yagoda A, Needles B, et al: Vinblastine and methotrexate for advanced bladder cancer. J Urol 133:602–604, 1985.
2. Blum RH, Carter SK: Adriamycin, a new anticancer drug with significant clinical activity. Ann Intern Med 80:249–259, 1974.
3. Blumenreich MS, Yagoda A, Natale RB, Watson RC: Phase II trial of vinblastine sulfate for metastatic urothelial tract tumors. Cancer 50:435–438, 1982.
4. Burn JI: Intra-arterial infusion in malignant disease of the pelvis. In PM Worrall, HJ Espiner (eds), Second Symposium on Methotrexate in the Treatment of Cancer. Bristol, Wright, 1966, pp 58–73.
5. Bush H, Thatcher N, Barnard R: Chemotherapy in the management of invasive bladder cancer. A review. Cancer Chemother Pharmacol 3:87–96, 1979.
6. Carter SK, Wasserman TH: The chemotherapy of urologic cancer. Cancer 36:729–747, 1975.
7. Cross RJ, Glashan RW, Humphrey CS, et al: Treatment of advanced bladder cancer with Adriamycin and 5-fluorouracil. Br J Urol 48:609–615, 1976.
8. Daniels JR: Unpublished data.
9. Daniels JR, Daniels AM, Luck EE, et al: Chemosensitivity testing of human neoplasms with in vitro clone formation. Cancer Chemother Pharmacol 6:245–251, 1981.
10. Daniels JR, Skinner DG, Lieskovsky G, et al: Carcinoma of bladder. Chemotherapy of advanced disease and rational design of adjuvant programs. In DG Skinner (ed), Urological Cancer. New York, Grune & Stratton, 1983.
11. deKernion JB: The chemotherapy of advanced bladder carcinoma. Cancer Res 37:2771–2774, 1977.
12. Fossa SD, Gudmundsen TE: Single-drug chemotherapy with 5-FU and Adriamycin in metastatic bladder carcinoma. Br J Urol 53:320–323, 1981.
13. Gagliano R, Levin H, El-Bolkainy MN, et al: Adriamycin versus Adriamycin plus cis-diamminedichloroplatinum (DDP) in advanced transitional cell bladder carcinoma. A Southwest Oncology Group study. Am J Clin Oncol 6:215–218, 1983.
14. Garcia-Giralt E, Auvert J, Lachand AT, et al: Combined chemotherapy in the management of metastatic bladder cancer. Br J Urol 53:318–319, 1981.
15. Goldie JH, Coldman AJ: A mathematical model for relating the drug sensitivity of tumors to their spontaneous mutation rate. Cancer Treat Rep 63:1727–1733, 1979.
16. Goldie JH, Coldman AJ, Gudauskas GA: Rationale for the use of alternating non-cross-resistant chemotherapy. Cancer Treat Rep 66:439–449, 1982.
17. Hall RR, Evans RGB, Pritchett CJ, Price DA: Combination chemotherapy for advanced bladder cancer. Br J Urol 54:16–19, 1982.
18. Hall RR, Newling DWW, Ramsden PD, et al: Treatment of invasive bladder cancer by local resection and high dose methotrexate. Br J Urol 56:668–672, 1984.
19. Harewood LM, Nunn I, Johnson W, et al: Treatment of advanced bladder cancer using cis-platinum. Aust NZ J Surg 53:333–337, 1983.
20. Herr HW, Yagoda A, Batata M, et al: Planned preoperative cisplatin and radiation therapy for locally advanced bladder cancer. Cancer 52:2205–2208, 1983.
21. Jacobs SC, Lawson RK: Pathologic effects of precystectomy therapy with combination intra-arterial doxorubicin hydrochloride and local bladder hyperthermia for bladder cancer. J Urol 127:43–47, 1982.
22. Jacobs SC, McCellan SL, Maher C, Lawson RK: Precystectomy intra-arterial cis-diamminedichloroplatinum II with local bladder hyperthermia for bladder cancer. J Urol 131:473–476, 1984.
23. Jakse G, Frommhold H: Combined radiation and chemotherapy for locally advanced bladder cancer. In KH Kurth, et al (eds), Progress and Controversies in Oncological Urology. New York, Alan R Liss, 1983, pp 365–372.
24. Kanoh S, Umeyama T, Nemoto S, et al: Long-term intra-arterial infusion chemotherapy with Adriamycin for advanced bladder cancer. Can Chem Pharm 11(Suppl):s51–s58, 1983.
25. Kaye SB, McWhinnie D, Hart A, et al: The treatment of advanced bladder cancer with methotrexate and cis-platinum—a pharmacokinetic study. Eur J Cancer Clin Oncol 20:249–252, 1984.
26. Khandekar JD, Elson PJ, DeWys WD, et al: Comparative activity and toxicity of cis-diamminedichloroplatinum (DDP) and a combination of doxorubicin, cyclophosphamide, and DDP in disseminated transitional cell carcinomas of the urinary tract. J Clin Oncol 3:539–545, 1985.
27. Kedia KR, Gibbons C, Persky L: The management of advanced bladder carcinoma. J Urol 125:655–658, 1981.
28. Kraybill WG, Harrison M, Sasaki T, Fletcher WS: Regional intra-arterial infusion of Adriamycin in the treatment of cancer. Surg Gynecol Obstet 144:335–338, 1977.
29. Kubota Y, Shuin T, Miura T, et al: Combination chemotherapy for metastatic urinary bladder cancer with 5-FU, vincristine, bleomycin, cyclophosphamide, mitomycin, and methotrexate. Cancer Treat Rep 68:1167–1168, 1984.
30. Logothetis CJ, Samuels ML, Selig DE, et al: Combined intravenous and intra-arterial cyclophosphamide, doxorubicin, and cisplatin (CISCA) in the management of select patients with invasive urothelial tumors. Cancer Treat Rep 69:33–38, 1985.

31. Merrin CE: Treatment of genitourinary tumors with cis-dichlorodiammineplatinum(II): experience in 250 patients. Cancer Treat Rep 63:1579–1584, 1979.

32. Merrin C, Cartagena R, Wajsman Z, et al: Chemotherapy of bladder carcinoma with cyclophosphamide and Adriamycin. J Urol 114:884–887, 1975.

33. Merrin C, Beckley S: Adjuvant chemotherapy for bladder cancer with doxorubicin hydrochloride and cyclophosphamide: preliminary report. J Urol 119:62–63, 1978.

34. Moon TE, Salmon SE, White CS, et al: Quantitative association between the in vitro human tumor stem cell assay and clinical response to cancer chemotherapy. Cancer Chemother Pharmacol 6:211–218, 1982.

35. Mulder JH, Fossa DS, De Pauw M, Van Oosterom AT: Cyclophosphamide, Adriamycin and cisplatin combination chemotherapy in advanced bladder carcinoma: an EORTC phase II study. Eur J Cancer Clin Oncol 18:111–112, 1982.

36. Narayana AS, Loening SA, Culp DA: Chemotherapy for advanced carcinoma of the bladder. J Urol 126:594–595, 1981.

37. Natale RB, Yagoda A, Watson RC, et al: Methotrexate: an active drug in bladder cancer. Cancer 47:1246–1250, 1981.

38. Nevin JE, Melnick I, Baggerly JT Jr, et al: The continuous arterial infusion of 5-fluorouracil as a therapeutic adjunct in the treatment of advanced carcinoma of the bladder. A preliminary report. Cancer 31:138–144, 1973.

39. Northern California Oncology Group: unpublished observations.

40. Ogata J, Migita N, Nakamura T: Treatment of carcinoma of the bladder by infusion of the anticancer agent (mitomycin C) via the internal iliac artery. J Urol 10:667–670, 1973.

41. Oliver RTD: Methotrexate as salvage or adjunctive therapy for primary invasive carcinoma of the bladder. Cancer Treat Rep 65(Suppl. 1):179–181, 1981.

42. Oliver RTD, England HR, Risdon RA, Blandy JP: Methotrexate in the treatment of metastatic and recurrent primary transitional cell carcinoma. J Urol 131:483–485, 1984.

43. Oliver RTD, Newlands ES, Wiltshaw E, Malpas JS: A phase 2 study of cis-platinum in patients with recurrent bladder carcinoma. Br J Urol 53:444–447, 1981.

44. Ponder BAJ, Oliver RTD: Phase II study of VP 16-213 (etoposide) in metastatic transitional cell urothelial cancer. Cancer Chemother Pharmacol 12:64–65, 1984.

45. Prout GR Jr, Slack NH, Bross IDJ: Irradiation and 5-fluorouracil as adjuvants in the management of invasive bladder carcinoma. A cooperative group report after 4 years. J Urol 104:116–129, 1970.

46. Raghaven D, Pearson B, Duval P, et al: Initial intravenous cis-platinum therapy: improved management for invasive high risk bladder cancer? J Urol 133:399–402, 1985.

47. Richards B, Akdas A, Corbett P, et al: Adjuvant chemotherapy following radical radiotherapy in T3 bladder carcinoma. Recent Results Cancer Res 68:334–337, 1978.

48. Richards B, Bastable JRG, Freedman L, et al: Adjuvant chemotherapy with doxorubicin (Adriamycin) and 5-fluorouracil in T3, Nx, M0 bladder cancer treated with radiotherapy. Br J Urol 55:386–391, 1983.

49. Richards B, Newling D, Fossa S, et al: Vincristine in advanced bladder cancer: a European Organization for Research on Treatment of Cancer (EORTC) phase II study. Cancer Treat Rep 67:575–577, 1983.

50. Salmon SE, Hamburger AW, Soehnlen B, et al: Quantitation of differential sensitivity of human-tumor stem cells to anticancer drugs. N Engl J Med 298:1321–1327, 1978.

51. Schaeffer AJ, Grayhack JT, Merrill JM, et al: Adjuvant doxorubicin hydrochloride and radiation in stage D bladder cancer: a preliminary report. J Urol 131:1073–1076, 1984.

52. Schwartz S, Yagoda A, Natale RB, et al: Phase II trial of sequentially administered cisplatin, cyclophosphamide and doxorubicin for urothelial tract tumors. J Urol 130:681–684, 1983.

53. Shipley WU, Coombs LJ, Einstein AB Jr, et al: Cisplatin and full dose irradiation for patients with invasive bladder carcinoma: a preliminary report of tolerance and local response. J Urol 132:899–903, 1984.

54. Skinner DG, Daniels JR, Lieskovsky G: Current status of adjuvant chemotherapy after radical cystectomy for deeply invasive bladder cancer. Urology 24:46–52, 1984.

55. Smalley RV, Bartolucci AA, Hemstreet G, Hester M: A phase II evaluation of a 3-drug combination of cyclophosphamide, doxorubicin and 5-fluorouracil in patients with advanced bladder carcinoma or stage D prostatic carcinoma. J Urol 125:191–195, 1981.

56. Socquet Y: Surgery and adjuvant chemotherapy with high-dose methotrexate and folinic acid rescue for infiltrating tumors of the bladder. Cancer Treat Rep 65(Suppl 1):187–189, 1981.

57. Soloway MS, Einstein A, Corder MP, et al: A comparison of cisplatin and the combination of cisplatin and cyclophosphamide in advanced urothelial cancer. Cancer 52:767–772, 1983.

58. Sternberg JJ, Bracken RB, Handel PB, Johnson DE: Combination chemotherapy (CISCA) for advanced urinary tract carcinoma. A preliminary report. JAMA 238:2282–2287, 1977.

59. Sternberg CN, Yagoda A, Scher HI, et al: Preliminary results of M-VAC (methotrexate, vinblastine, doxorubicin and cisplatin) for transitional cell carcinoma of the urothelium. J Urol 133:403–407, 1985.

60. Stewart DJ, Futter N, Maroun JA, et al: Intra-arterial cisplatin treatment of unresectable or medically inoperable invasive carcinoma of the bladder. J Urol 131:258–261, 1984.

61. Stoter G, Van Oosterom AT, Mulder JH, et al: Combination chemotherapy with cisplatin and VM-26 in advanced transitional cell carcinoma of the bladder. Eur J Cancer Clin Oncol 20:315–317, 1984.

62. Sullivan RD: Intra-arterial methotrexate therapy. The dose, duration and route of administration. Studies of methotrexate in clinical cancer chemotherapy. In R Porter, E Wiltshaw (eds), First Symposium on the Treatment of Cancer. Bristol, Wright, 1962, pp 50–55.

63. Tashiro K, Machida T, Masuda F, Ohishi Y: Combination chemotherapy for advanced bladder cancer with Adriamycin, cyclophosphamide, and 5-fluorouracil. Cancer Chemother Pharmacol 11(Suppl):s43–s46, 1983.

64. Turner AG, Durrant KR, Malpas JS: A trial of bleomycin versus Adriamycin in advanced carcinoma of the bladder. Br J Urol 51:121–124, 1979.

65. Turner AG: Methotrexate in advanced bladder cancer. Cancer Treat Rep 65(Suppl 1):183–186, 1981.

66. Uyama T, Moriwaki S, Yonezawa M, Fujita J: Intra-arterial Adriamycin chemotherapy for bladder cancer. Semiselective intra-arterial chemotherapy with compression of the femoral arteries at the time of injection. Cancer Chemother Pharmacol 11(Suppl):s59–s63, 1983.

67. Veronesi A, Magri MD, Figoli F, et al: Combination chemotherapy with Adriamycin and 5-fluorouracil in advanced bladder carcinoma. Clin Oncology 8:103–106, 1982.

68. Wallace S, Chuang VP, Samuels M, Johnson D: Transcatheter intraarterial infusion of chemotherapy in advanced bladder cancer. Cancer 49:640–645, 1982.

69. Williams SD, Donohue JP, Einhorn LH: Advanced bladder cancer: therapy with cis-dichlorodiammineplatinum(II), Adriamycin, and 5-fluorouracil. Cancer Treat Rep 63:1573–1576, 1979.

70. Yagoda A: Future implications of phase 2 chemotherapy trials in ninety-five patients with measurable advanced bladder cancer. Cancer Res 37:2775–2780, 1977.

71. Yagoda A: Phase II trials with cis-dichlorodiammineplatinum(II) in the treatment of urothelial cancer. Cancer Treat Rep 63:1565–1572, 1979.

72. Yagoda A: Chemotherapy of metastatic bladder cancer. Cancer 45:1879–1888, 1980.

JEROME P. RICHIE, M.D.

CHAPTER 18

Carcinoma of the Renal Pelvis and Ureter

Carcinoma of the renal pelvis is a relatively rare tumor, composing approximately 7% of all renal neoplasms and less than 1% of all genitourinary tumors. The incidence of renal tumors is often expressed in relation to the number of tumors in the urinary bladder. In a 20-year study, the ratio of tumors of the bladder, renal pelvis, and ureter was 51:3:1.[57] In other series, the ratio of renal pelvic tumors to bladder tumors has varied from 1:10 to 1:64. The only exception seems to be in regions of Balkan endemic family nephropathy, in which renal pelvic tumors account for nearly one half of all renal neoplasms.

Tumors of the renal pelvis are more frequent in men than in women by a ratio of 2:1, and the peak incidence is in the fifth and sixth decades of life, with a progressive increase in incidence with advancing age. Ureteral tumors have a propensity for the lower third of the ureter, and there is no predilection for laterality for either renal pelvic or ureteral tumors. Bilateral tumors are distinctly uncommon.

The number of reported cases of renal pelvic carcinoma has increased in the past 10 years, and there is some debate as to whether this represents a true increase or rather improvements in diagnosis and frequency of published reports. Associations of upper tract carcinomas with analgesic nephropathy and with Balkan nephropathy represent additional factors that may be relating to an increased interest in neoplasms of the upper collecting system.

The majority of these neoplasms are of urothelial origin, and most represent transitional cell tumors. Squamous cell carcinoma and adenocarcinoma, usually associated with chronic infection or stones, represent relatively uncommon occurrences. Squamous cell cancer constitutes about 10% of all tumors of the upper collecting system, and adenocarcinoma is extremely rare. The simultaneous occurrence of renal adenocarcinoma and transitional cell carcinoma of the renal pelvis has been reported but only in a few instances to date.[55]

ETIOLOGIC FACTORS

The mucosal surface of the collecting tubules, calyces, renal pelvis, ureter, bladder, and urethra has the same embryologic origin; hence, the term *urothelium* has been coined to delineate this mucosal system.[44] Because of this common transitional epithelial surface, tumors of the renal pelvis and ureter will be considered together. Many of the etiologic factors discussed herein apply to tumors of the urinary bladder as well.

Transitional epithelium lining the calyceal system and renal pelvis is exposed to various potential carcinogens via excretion in the urinary tract. Carcinogens that are excreted may be activated in the urine by hydrolyzing enzymes and would be expected to promote oncogenesis throughout the urinary system, resulting in an even higher ratio of bladder to urothelial tumors

323

of the upper tract than would be predicted on the basis of surface area alone.

Because of the paucity of animal models for renal pelvic or ureteral tumors, clinical observations have directed the research effort into etiologic factors. Specific chemicals have been associated with epidemiologic observation of transitional cell carcinoma of the upper urinary tract. A putative link between environmental factors and transitional cell carcinoma was suggested first by the observation of an increased incidence of transitional cell carcinoma in industrialized societies and in persons living in the cities rather than in rural areas. The reports of chronic exposure in the aniline dye industry, resulting in carcinoma of the bladder, heralded reports that workers in a variety of industries have a higher incidence of transitional cell carcinoma of the upper urinary tract and bladder.[46]

It has been known for a long time that compounds with structures resembling those of aminophenols can produce cancer of the bladder in both humans and animals. Specific examples of chemicals that are known to be potent carcinogens for the urothelium are benzidine, β-naphthylamine, p-aminobiphenyl, p-nitrobiphenyl, and 4,4'-diaminobiphenyl, but not aniline itself. Therefore, it is interesting that only when the amino group is attached to the benzene ring at certain points is the chemical a potent carcinogen. It is also of interest that chronic ingestion of these compounds causes mainly tumors of the bladder and not tumors of the proximal urinary tract, at least in animals, for reasons that are not understood.

The incidence of renal pelvic carcinomas in animals can be enhanced by the direct implantation into the renal pelvis of crystalline carcinogens or of carcinogen-impregnated foreign bodies. In addition, Guerin and associates produced renal pelvic cancers in mice by feeding them chemical carcinogens.[34] Also, as shown by Butler and Barnes, aflatoxin B can induce cancers of the renal pelvis in animals.[17] Finally, the chronic consumption of lead compounds can produce cancer of the renal pelvis in experimental animals.[14, 49, 50]

Several studies have shown that smoking increases the incidence of transitional cell cancer of the urinary tract, particularly of the bladder. Although the exact mechanism is not known, it has been postulated that smoking interferes with the metabolism of tryptophan and that heavy smokers excrete large quantities of intermediary metabolites of tryptophan in the urine, many of which have structures resembling the orthoaminophenols.[38] There are no properly conducted studies of whether smoking contributes specifically to the pathogenesis of cancer of the renal pelvis, although there have been claims that the incidence of renal pelvic cancer also is increased in heavy smokers.[9]

One concept that has emerged recently relative to chemical carcinogenesis in the urinary tract is that a cocarcinogen or an initiator often needs to be present. An example of an initiator that has been used in experimental animals is the wax pellet that is implanted into the bladder to enhance tumor formation in animals being fed various carcinogens. It has been postulated that the initiator causes hyperplasia of the urothelium and that the hyperplastic urothelium is then more subject to malignant transformation when brought in contact with chemicals.[18] Oncogenes may exert their effects as initiators. In the clinical setting, it is well known that long-standing irritation of the renal pelvis by stones is associated with an increased incidence of cancer of the renal pelvis, more specifically, squamous cell carcinoma. In this example, the stone would be the initiator, causing hyperplasia, but whether the chronic irritation alone can cause cancer or whether there is some other chemical potentiator in the urine or in the uroepithelium is unknown.

There are two clinical situations in which chemical carcinogens may play a direct role in the causation of cancer of the renal pelvis. The first is the renal pelvic cancer associated with chronic phenacetin ingestion. The first suggestion of an association between phenacetin abuse and uroepithelial cancer came from the small town of Huskvarna in Sweden. It has been the custom of the townsfolk there, since the influenza epidemic of 1918, to consume large quantities of Hjorton's powder, which contains, among other things, phenacetin, phenazone, and caffeine. Patients taking analgesics for long periods often develop papillary necrosis and, of those who have "analgesic nephropathy," as many as two thirds also develop cancer of the renal pelvis. In fact, it is rare for patients who have overused analgesics containing phenacetin to develop renal pelvic tumors without papillary necrosis being present. It is therefore possible that chronic inflammation localized the carcinogenic effect of the phenacetin or of one of its metabolites in the proximal urinary tract. Because of the structural resemblance of the metabolites of phenacetin to compounds known to produce cancer of the bladder, it is suspected that they are the carcinogens in these patients. For example, it has been shown experimentally that, with increasing ingestion of phenacetin, the concentration of the N-hydroxylated metabolites in the urine increases. The main metabolite of phenacetin in 11 species studied to date is 4-acetoaminophenol (NAPA), and this compound structurally resembles known urothelial carcinogens.[37] It is also feasible that the carcinogenic metabolite is secreted in active form and then inactivated in the presence of acid urine, thereby localizing the effects to the upper urinary tract.

There is also an association between cancer of the renal pelvis and Danubian endemic familial nephropathy (Balkan nephropathy). Although the etiology of both the nephropathy and the tumor is unknown, it is suspected that some environmental factor is causative. However, a variety of factors, including viruses, silicates, heavy metals, genetic factors, and even autoimmune mechanisms have been blamed.[4, 20, 41, 42] The tumors in patients having Danubian endemic familial nephropathy are, for the most part, rather typical transitional cell cancers, usually located in the proximal urinary tract.

HISTOPATHOLOGY

Metaplasia

Chronic noxious stimulation of the uroepithelium of the proximal urinary tract consistently produces a variety of proliferative changes, including cystic or papillary changes, squamous or glandular metaplasia, or all of these. There has been much speculation that the various forms of metaplasia are precancerous lesions, because cancer frequently is associated with these histologic abnormalities.

One of the most common forms of nonmalignant proliferative change seen in the epithelium of the upper urinary tract is squamous metaplasia, which usually is brought about by long-standing infection and inflammation, especially that associated with calculous disease. If the irritation is severe and of long duration, the patient may form a cholesteatoma from the desquamated cells, or the upper urinary tract may develop white, plaque-like lesions which, on the basis of their gross appearance, can be given the appellation leukoplakia.

Squamous metaplasia is characterized histologically by large, clear, polygonal cells with darkly staining, pyknotic nuclei. Also, an increase in intracellular bridges is evident, especially by electron microscopy. In long-standing squamous metaplasia, superficial keratinization and even hyperkeratosis may be present.

On histologic examination glandular metaplasia is characterized by hyperplastic islets of cells invading the subepithelial connective tissues (lamina propria) and, sometimes, nests of epithelium that lose their connection with the surface epithelium and eventually form cysts. The exact mechanism whereby cysts are formed is not known, but it has been postulated that the metaplastic columnar cells of the glands create cysts by secreting mucus. In the proximal urinary tract, this type of epithelial proliferation with cyst formation gives rise to ureteritis or pyelitis cystica, which shows up radiographically as multiple small filling defects. A similar picture is seen in the bladder mucosa, especially when there has been long-standing chronic irritation, such as in exstrophy. Gordon suggested that the reason that the transitional cell epithelium of the urinary tract may show glandular metaplasia that resembles the mucosa of the large intestine is because of the close embryologic relation between the cloaca and the lower urinary tract, especially the bladder.[30] Glandular metaplasia is seen clinically in cases of long-standing irritation of the urinary tract, and glandular metaplasia also occurs in experimentally induced animal cancers and in laboratory animals with vitamin A deficiency.[25, 27, 30, 49-51]

Cancer

Malignant lesions of the renal pelvis and ureter can be segregated into transitional cell carcinomas, squamous cell carcinomas, adenocarcinomas, and connective tissue tumors. There are also a few tumors that are so anaplastic that the cell origin cannot be identified. Tumors may be of more than one cell type on rare occasions.

Transitional cell carcinoma accounts for approximately 90% of all cancers of the renal pelvis and 99% of all cancers of the ureter. The distinction between papillary transitional cell carcinoma and papilloma is not entirely clear. Transitional cell papillomas may be at one end of the spectrum of malignant transitional cell disease, although they behave in a relatively benign fashion, just as they do in the bladder. Nonetheless, their significance lies in what they portend for the rest of the urinary tract. Approximately 25% of patients with a solitary papilloma will develop transitional cell carcinoma elsewhere in the urinary tract. Patients with multiple papillomas have a 50% chance of developing invasive cancer at some time.[9]

Transitional cell carcinomas may spread both by direct extension and via blood and lymphatics. The majority (85%) of transitional cell carcinomas of the renal pelvis are papillary; only 15% are sessile. Approximately one half of the papillary tumors will demonstrate muscle invasion at the time of resection, whereas 80% of sessile tumors will show muscle invasion at the time of resection. Squamous cell carcinomas, accounting for only 7% of renal pelvic tumors, are usually sessile and more commonly associated with inflammation. This disease is most common in the fifth and sixth decades of life and occurs with equal frequency in men and women. The tumors are usually flat, ulcerated, and quite extensive. These tumors are often seen in association with chronic inflammation, squamous metaplasia, and, possibly, renal calculus. Squamous carcinomas seldom produce obstruction and thus are often identified late in the course of the disease. Metastases are often present when the primary tumor is diagnosed; the liver, lungs, lymph nodes, and bones are the most common sites for spread. Long-standing debate exists as to whether transitional cell carcinoma of the upper urinary tract can seed the lower tract. As more information has been gathered, however, it seems reasonably certain that these cancers arise from independent multifocal origins. This may well be the effect of a promoting carcinogen within the urinary tract that produces multifocal areas of disease. In patients with carcinoma of the renal pelvis, 30 to 50% will have other urinary tract cancers, and approximately 3 to 4% have malignant disease in the contralateral renal pelvis or ureter.

DIAGNOSIS

Clinical Presentation

Hematuria, either gross or microscopic, is the most common symptom in patients with renal pelvic or ureteral tumors (70 to 95% occurrence). The appearance of pain is precipitated by ureteral or ureteropelvic junction obstruction secondary to a tumor mass and is seen in 8 to 40% of patients. Symptoms of bladder irritation are seen in 5 to 10% of patients, and constitutional symptoms are seen in an additional 5%.

The physical examination is usually not revealing. However, in 10 to 20% of patients, a flank mass secondary to tumor or associated hydronephrosis has been reported.[26]

Cytology

The value of exfoliative cytologic examination has been well documented in tumors of the bladder, but little has been reported on its use in upper urinary tract neoplasms. Cullen and associates, with use of filter preparation, reported positive cytologic evidence in 80% of their patients with tumors of the pelvis or ureter.[21]

Voided specimens for urinary cytologic testing were noted by numerous investigators to be of questionable value because of the poor yield in low-grade tumors, and the presence of concomitant bladder tumors.[23, 32, 33] Zincke and co-workers found that retrograde collections aided by furosemide diuresis yielded much better results; in 18 patients who underwent both tests, 11 (61%) were noted to have positive cytologic evidence of tumor on retrograde collections, compared with six (33%) on voided cytologic specimens.[59] Critical to the reliance on cytologic findings is the presence of a well-trained pathologist with a geniune interest in cytology.

Nuclear cytologic characteristics indicate the histologic grade of the tumor, but a direct correlation of cytologic grade with invasiveness is lacking. Eriksson and Johansson studied 43 patients with upper-tract urothelial neoplasms; positive cytologic evidence was found in two of five patients with Grade 2 invasive tumors and in 17 of 24 patients with invasive tumors in Grades 3 or 4.[24] Although no cytologic examinations were falsely positive, 35% of the patients with a negative or atypical cytologic result were found to have invasive tumors. In another series, positive cytologic evidence of tumor was demonstrated in only 29% of the patients with proven invasive ureteral carcinoma.[7]

One drawback to urinary cytologic examination is that it is a labor-intensive procedure. Flow cytometry holds promise as a precise technique to quantify the presence or absence of abnormal (malignant) cells in the bladder. The basis for this diagnostic test is staining of DNA and mechanical depiction of abnormal cellular DNA content, representing aneuploid stem lines. With the advent of flow cytometry, automated screening procedures may be more feasible in order to detect tumors of the lower and upper urinary tracts. However, at the current time, a catheterized urine specimen, rather than voided urine, must be utilized, a significant drawback to the use of flow cytometry for screening.

Excretory Urography

The diagnosis of a renal pelvic or ureteral tumor is usually suspected on the basis of an excretory urogram; almost all patients with renal pelvic carcinoma will have an abnormal result on a urogram. The most common finding is a filling defect in the renal pelvis, observed in 50 to 75% of pyelograms (Fig. 18–1).[6] In addition to a solitary filling defect, cancer of the renal pelvis may present with multiple filling defects, ureteral pelvic junction obstruction with hydronephrosis, infundibular stenosis, splaying of the calyces (suggesting a renal mass), and occasionally nonvisualization of the renal collecting system.

In patients with a ureteral tumor, radiography has also been the mainstay of diagnosis but also leads frequently to misdiagnosis. Improved techniques of radiographic procedures, including tomography, abdominal compression, and better contrast agents, have improved the accuracy of diagnosis with excretory urography.

Williams and Mitchell found intravenous pyelograms to be of value in 28 of 30 patients examined, in whom disease was found that required urgent further investigation.[57] Almgärd and associates reported abnormal intravenous pyelogram findings in all 41 patients with ureteric tumor in whom nephrectomy had not been previously performed.[3] In 20 of their patients a tumor or stricture was suspected, and in the other 21 patients the ureter could not be evaluated owing to the

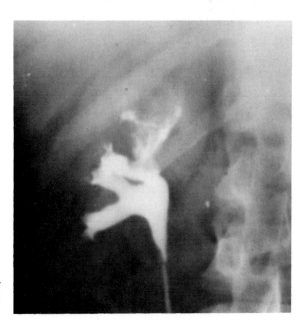

Figure 18–1. Excretory urogram reveals distortion of the upper pole collecting system and intrinsic filling defects, proven to be carcinoma of the renal pelvis.

decreased excretion of contrast material. Batata and co-workers reported findings of unilateral nonvisualization in 46% of their patients, hydronephrosis with or without hydroureter in 34%, and ureteral filling defect without obstruction in 19%.[8]

Retrograde Pyelography

The appearance of the collecting system and ureter on intravenous pyelography may be suggestive of ureteral tumor, but a firm diagnosis frequently cannot be established on the basis of the intravenous pyelogram alone. Retrograde urography is much more likely to demonstrate the presence of a lesion and to accurately define the lower margin (Fig. 18–2). The radiographic appearance of the ureteral lesion may be one of two types: an intraluminal lesion or a diffuse stricture-like, obstructive lesion.

The filling defect of an intraluminal lesion is accompanied by local dilatation of the

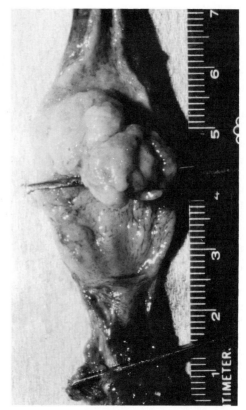

Figure 18–3. Pathologic findings of a low-grade ureteral tumor, demonstrating dilatation of the ureter distal to the tumor (Bergman sign).

ureter distal to the growth, with the characteristic contour of the lower margin of the tumor variously described as a wine-goblet or meniscus shape (Fig. 18–3). Bergman and associates have described this shape as an important diagnostic sign in distinguishing ureteral papillary tumor from a nonopaque calculus; in the latter case the ureter is flattened or collapsed distal to the stone.[10] The tendency of the ureteral catheter to coil in the dilated space below a ureteral tumor, so-called Bergman's sign, is considered almost pathognomonic for ureteral tumor. The differential diagnosis of ureteral filling defect includes nonopaque calculi, blood clots, ureteritis cystica, or seedling metastases from a renal pelvic or bladder tumor.

Endoscopy

Prior to the 1980s, endoscopy was of limited value in patients with transitional cell carcinoma of the renal pelvis or ureter. With the advent of the rigid ureteroscope, however, direct visualization of the ureter and

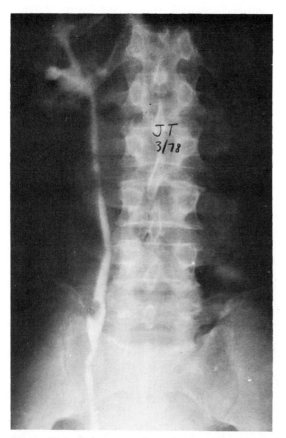

Figure 18–2. Right retrograde pyelogram demonstrates filling defect in the midureter region. This abnormality was missed on the standard intravenous pyelogram.

of the collecting system is feasible.[36] The development of flexible instruments with smaller fiberoptic bundles may allow visualization of the entire upper collecting system in the near future. Ureteroscopy does have potential complications, including perforation of the ureter. Nonetheless, this procedure can be utilized as a diagnostic aid in patients with filling defects in whom the results of cytologic examination have not given a definitive diagnosis.

Brush Biopsy

An alternate approach to ureteroscopy is the use of retrograde brushing of the upper urinary tract, as described by Gill and associates in 1973.[28] An angiographic catheter is passed transurethrally up the affected ureter and positioned adjacent to a suspicious lesion. A small nylon or steel bristle brush is passed inside its lumen and material entrapped by the bristles is sent for histologic and cytologic examination. This technique allows diagnosis of moderately differentiated transitional cell carcinoma but still has false-negative results in patients with low-grade lesions. Urine should be collected for cytologic and cell block preparation after the brush has been removed, as the diagnosis may be made more readily in this fashion. A recent survey involving 32 patients has found brush biopsy to be accurate and confirmed by operative intervention in 84% of patients.[13]

Other Diagnostic Tests

Renal arteriography usually is not helpful in diagnosing transitional cell carcinoma of the upper urinary tract, although it may be useful in differentiating tumors arising in the collecting system from renal adenocarcinoma. In advanced tumors of the renal pelvis, arteriographic findings distinct from renal cell carcinoma may be noted.[39] Other diagnostic tests, such as ultrasonography, may occasionally be helpful in defining the nature of a lesion. Ultrasonography in patients with renal pelvic tumors has shown the central renal echo complex to be separated by some low-intensity echoes, thereby excluding the diagnosis of renal calculi, which usually cause shadowing.[5] Blood clots may be difficult to distinguish from tumors on an ultrasonographic basis.

The computerized tomography (CT) scan has had major impact in the diagnosis and treatment of renal cell carcinoma; however, it has had little influence on the treatment of renal pelvic or ureteral tumors. One advantage of the CT scan is the ability to exclude or diagnose extension outside the urinary tract per se.

Staging

Careful evaluation must be carried out in patients with a diagnosis of renal pelvic or ureteral tumor to exclude both multiplicity of tumors as well as distant metastases. Grabstald and associates reported that approximately half the patients with renal tumors had associated tumor in the bladder or ureter or both.[32] In view of the likelihood of multiplicity, it is essential that the entire urinary tract, including the urethra and bladder mucosa, be visualized either by radiographic or endoscopic procedures. If the intravenous pyelogram is not adequate to reveal the entire surface, retrograde pyelograms should be used.

Staging procedures, in addition to assessment of the urothelium, should include chest radiograph, radionuclide bone scan, and a serum multichannel analysis. Liver scans or CT scans of the liver should not be utilized in the absence of abnormal liver profile studies. Ultrasonography or CT scan may be of some benefit in assessing presence or absence of retroperitoneal lymphadenopathy.

The difficulty in establishing the diagnosis, as well as the limited accuracy of available staging procedures, has precluded the development of a clinical staging system. Instead, classification of renal pelvic tumors is based upon pathologic findings. Grabstald and associates, after studying 70 patients with renal pelvic tumors, proposed a classification based on tumor stage and grade.[32] A modification of this system, proposed by Batata and associates, is illustrated in Figure 18–4. This system, similar to the Jewett-Marshall-Strong system for bladder cancer, utilizes letters to indicate depth of invasion. Stage 0 neoplasms are confined to the mucosa, Stage A tumors invade the lamina propria, Stage B tumors invade the muscle, Stage C tumors have extended into the peripelvic fat or renal parenchyma, and Stage D represents metastatic disease. Ureteral tu-

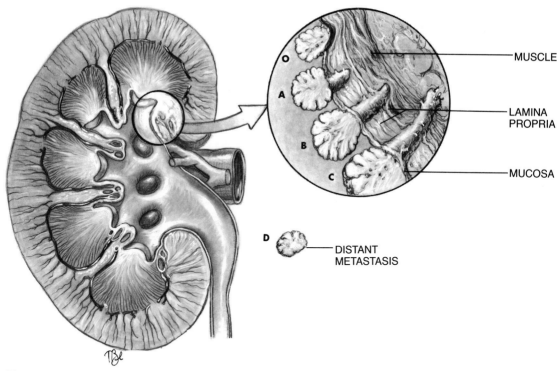

MUSCLE

LAMINA
PROPRIA

MUCOSA

DISTANT
METASTASIS

Figure 18–4. Staging system for renal pelvic tumors. Modified from Batata MA, et al: Primary carcinoma of the ureter: A prognostic study. Cancer 35:1626–1632, 1975.

mors have been given a similar staging system. However, since the wall of the ureter is comparatively thin, invasion through the wall tends to occur earlier in ureteral tumors than in bladder tumors. Bloom and associates reported a close correlation between degree of cellular metaplasia and invasion; 100% of Grade 1 and 85% of Grade 2 tumors were noninvasive, compared with 30% of Grade 3 and 8% of Grade 4 tumors.

Transitional cell carcinoma may spread by direct extension or by metastasis via hematogenous or lymphatic routes. Regional lymph nodes are commonly involved before other sites of metastasis. Therefore, surgical therapy should include regional lymphadenectomy. Almost any organ may receive metastases from transitional cell tumors of the upper urinary tract.

TREATMENT

Surgical

The classic management of renal pelvic or ureteral tumors is nephroureterectomy with excision of cuff of bladder and bladder mucosa. The removal of the entire ureter is recommended, because approximately 20% of patients with residual ureteral stumps will develop tumors within them. Although nephroureterectomy has traditionally been considered the treatment of choice, advocates of less radical procedures have continued to increase in numbers and represent a strong minority opinion. The issue is clouded with emotionalism. Proponents of radical nephroureterectomy with removal of a cuff of bladder emphasize the difficulty in distinguishing histologic grade of the tumor as well as difficulty in accurate preoperative estimation of stage. Half of all cases of ureteral tumor involve at least the musculature and may have lymphatic involvement as well. The high incidence of multiple ipsilateral lesions, both overt and in situ, makes removal of the entire ureteral segment in general preferable to partial ureterectomy for adequate tumor surgery. The well-known phenomenon of recurrence of tumor in the remaining ureteral stump has been reported in more than 30% of patients treated by nephrectomy and partial ureterectomy.[54]

Advocates of conservative surgical intervention for renal pelvic or ureteral tumors stress the poor prognosis associated with advanced lesions, regardless of the form of surgical therapy, and the higher mortality rate occurring with more radical procedures. Recent articles by Cummings,[22] Gittes,[29] and McCarron and associates[43] illustrate the difficulties in choosing radical versus conservative therapy for patients with tumors of the upper urinary collecting system. In order to derive a rational recommendation for kidney-sparing versus kidney-sacrificing treatment, several factors should be taken into consideration.

Recent advances in anesthesia and in pre- and postoperative methods of management have lowered the operative mortality rates substantially, so there is very little difference between kidney-conserving and kidney-sacrificing procedures in terms of overall risk. In fact, nephroureterectomy may often be performed more quickly and easily than some of the alternative methods of treatment. Therefore, consideration of the risks of morbidity and mortality from conservative versus radical procedures should not be a major issue.

The likelihood of implantation, especially with tumors of higher grades, must be considered an increased risk for kidney-sparing procedures as opposed to kidney-sacrificing procedures. Analogous experiences with open bladder surgery would indicate a higher likelihood of implantation unless preoperative radiation therapy is utilized.

Difficulties will still exist as to the clinical estimation of histologic grade and pathologic stage of upper tract tumors. Staging systems for upper tract tumors are not as sophisticated or as reliable as methods for staging bladder tumors, yet bladder tumor understaging continues to remain a significant problem. It is more difficult to obtain information regarding multicentricity, grade, and extent of the primary tumor in upper tract tumors than it is in bladder tumors.

Considerations of local recurrence and problems of follow-up remain a major problem for patients with kidney-sparing procedures. Since the major site of recurrence in patients with kidney-sparing procedures is in the ipsilateral system, nephroureterectomy obviates the need for follow-up of the initially involved upper system, which is the main thrust of follow-up for patients with a conservative procedure. Nocks and associates reported a high incidence of associated severe dysplasia or carcinoma in situ associated with high-grade, high-stage tumors.[45] They concluded that nephroureterectomy was preferable to conservative procedures in patients with carcinoma of the renal pelvis.

Based upon these considerations, my personal preference remains, in general, nephroureterectomy with excision of a cuff of bladder for most patients with renal pelvic or ureteral tumors. However, several exceptions are readily apparent. In the patient with a solitary kidney, compromised renal function, bilateral lesions, or endemic nephropathy, conservation is essential, and preferred treatment would be local excision of a renal pelvic lesion with or without partial nephrectomy or, in the case of ureteral tumor, ureteral excision or ureterectomy with replacement by ileum. Local excision and reanastomosis should be limited to patients with a localized filling defect, preferably polypoid, and preferably a low-grade and presumably low-stage tumor. In such a patient, local excision with adequate margins may be the preferred treatment.

For patients with apparent solitary tumors of the lower third of the ureter, especially low-grade tumors, distal ureterectomy with regional lymphadenectomy and reimplantation of the ureter with a psoas hitch represents a reasonable alternative. In the patient with a lesion of higher grade or higher stage, the likelihood of coexistent upper tract lesions or compromise to the renal parenchyma would still cause the surgeon to favor nephroureterectomy. Tumors of the middle or upper third of the ureter are generally best treated by nephroureterectomy unless cytologic and brush biopsy specimens demonstrate a low-grade and presumably low-stage tumor. In such an instance, excisional biopsy with ureteroureterostomy can be considered.

Selected lesions in the renal pelvis and calyceal system may also be considered for conservative treatment, provided that the cytologic results show less than a high-grade lesion and brushing specimens demonstrate a low-grade transitional cell tumor. In such an incidence, nephroscopy is helpful to be certain the tumor is not of a more extensive nature and that the offending collecting system can be walled off and then removed by partial nephrectomy.

Technique

This author prefers a one-incision technique with the patient positioned in a torque or semi-flank position and the table flexed,

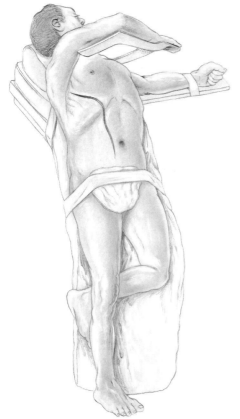

Figure 18–5. Proper positioning of the patient for thoracoabdominal single-incision approach to nephroureterectomy. The pelvis is nearly supine and the ipsilateral shoulder is angulated approximately 50°. The abdominal portion of the incision extends inferiorly as a paramedian incision.

similar to the positioning for radical retroperitoneal lymphadenectomy for testicular tumor (Fig. 18–5). The distal aspect of the incision is continued as a paramedian incision down to the symphysis pubis, allowing adequate exposure for removal of the distal ureter and cuff of bladder. The peritoneal envelope is mobilized completely across the midline, allowing complete exposure of the entire course of the ureter for resection and for lymphadenectomy. With this approach, the disadvantages of the two-incision technique are eliminated.

The addition of lymphadenectomy allows for more accurate staging and may have therapeutic implications, since the regional nodes appear to be the first and most common site of metastatic spread. Batata and associates reported that 22 of their 29 patients had initial or subsequent metastases, 17 involving the regional nodes and five

occurring in distant sites.[8] Lymphatic metastases were ipsilateral in 90% of the cases with involved pelvic nodes and 60% of cases with involved para-aortic nodes. This high incidence of predominantly ipsilateral regional lymphatic involvement in invasive tumors makes extensive lymphadenectomy a logical extension of the therapeutic surgical approach.

Regardless of the choice of incision, the bladder should be opened and the ureter removed intravesically as well as extravesically (Fig. 18–6). Attempts to extricate the distal ureter extravesically are fraught with failure. Strong and Pearse reported nine cases in which the surgical procedure was described by the surgeon as a "complete nephroureterectomy" by tenting up the distal ureter; on subsequent cystoscopy and retrograde ureterogram, all nine patients were noted to have a ureteral orifice and intramural ureter remaining on that side.[54] In two of the nine patients, there was subsequent recurrence of tumor in the ureteral stump. The cuff of bladder should include a 1-cm circumferential margin around the ureteral orifice. An anterior cystotomy allows visualization of the trigone and contralateral ureteral orifice (Fig. 18–6). A two-layer closure of the bladder is effected after dissection.

Techniques for partial nephrectomy are covered separately (Chapter 50).

Results

The rate of survival is influenced by the grade and stage of the tumor. Overall survival rates are approximately 40%, with a 5-year survival rate for a well-differentiated malignancy of 56%, as opposed to 16% for poorly differentiated lesions (Table 18–1). Sixty per cent of patients with noninvasive disease survive five years, compared with a 25% rate for those with invasive tumors.[8, 12]

ADJUVANT THERAPY

Radiation therapy remains an unproven adjunct for the control of residual tumor, unresectable disease, or local recurrence. Brady and associates reported six cases of postoperative radiation therapy, two for each of the previously mentioned indications.[15] All six patients survived free of disease for

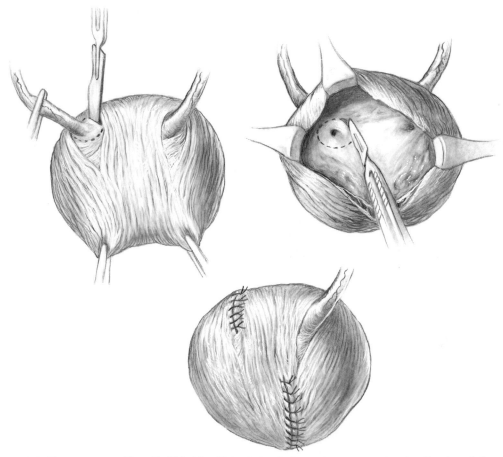

Figure 18–6. Ureterectomy with cuff of bladder. Note that anterior cystotomy permits visualization of the trigone and contralateral ureter and minimizes the chance of injury. This portion of the procedure can be approached through the thoracoabdominal incision described in Figure 18–5.

one year, and of those followed for five years, three of five survived that period without evidence of disease. Holtz reported favorably on the use of postoperative radiotherapy.[35]

Table 18–1. CORRELATION OF FIVE-YEAR SURVIVAL RATE (%) WITH PATHOLOGIC CHARACTERISTICS

	Bloom and Associates[12] 1970 (54 Patients)	Batata and Associates[8] 1975 (41 Patients)
Histologic Grade		
I	83.0	78.0
II	52.0	50.0
III	18.0	0
IV	12.0	0
Pathologic Stage		
O, A	62.0	91.0
B	50.0	43.0
C	33.3	23.0
D	0	0

Batata and associates recommended postoperative elective irradiation with 6000 rads to tumors in Stage B, C, or D.[8] A split dose of radiation therapy may render excision possible in some previously unresectable tumors, with the second course of radiotherapy to control residual disease.

A recent study evaluating postoperative irradiation therapy in 41 patients concluded that local recurrence was less, although distant failure is about the same with postoperative radiation therapy.[16] Anecdotal reports of long-term survival continue to surface.[40]

Other investigators have questioned the place of radiotherapy in the management of ureteral carcinoma. Scott[52] and Bergman and co-workers[11] recommended radiation therapy only in dealing with symptoms relative to metastatic disease. Preoperative radiotherapy has no proven place in the management of ureteral carcinoma, although Abeshouse and associates have conducted a trial of preoperative radiotherapy.[2] The difficulty in establishing an accurate diagnosis, much less accurate staging of the ureteral tumor, is a major deterrent to preoperative treatment. Moreover, the potential for abdominal complications with the amount of radiation therapy required is high. Postoperative radiation therapy in invasive disease is, however, a logical extension of combination therapy in bladder tumors. Radiotherapy should have a place in the eradication of subclinical disease and in the control of known residual tumor and will, it is hoped, improve the overall prognosis.

Chemotherapy

Until recently, adjunctive chemotherapy for renal pelvic or ureteral tumors appeared to offer no optimism for benefit. Batata and associates reported on one patient who received postoperative therapy with actinomycin D and on another who received thiophosphamide irrigation of the bladder and ureter; both patients died of disease within two years. In the last several years, however, strides have been made in systemic chemotherapy for bladder cancer. Yagoda reported on promising results with methotrexate, vinblastine, Adriamycin, and cis-platinum (MVAC).[58] Since upper tract urothelial tumors probably respond to chemotherapy in a fashion identical to that of bladder tumors, the use of several or all of these agents in combination may represent a useful program for the management of advanced upper tract collecting systems and possibly as an adjunct in patients with poor prognosis following surgical excision.

SECONDARY TUMORS OF THE URETER

These uncommon tumors may originate in the upper urinary tract and disperse by seedling metastases from a distant site and spread by blood or lymphatic channels; when the primary tumor is in proximity to the ureter, spread may be by direct extension. With the exception of the first group, signs and symptoms of urinary tract involvement occur quite late in the course of the disease and may be recognized only preterminally or at autopsy.

Drop Metastases

These tumors may be difficult to segregate from those arising as separate primary lesions owing to exposure of the entire urothelium to various carcinogens. Because ureteral tumors can be seen frequently in conjunction with bladder or renal pelvic tumors, the likelihood that cells can flow down from the renal pelvis or reflux up the ureter and implant with subsequent growth is quite real. Weldon and associates have demonstrated implantation of tumor cells in the bladder, especially in previously traumatized areas.[56] The observation of recurrent bladder tumor clustered around the ureteral orifice of an affected ureter provides strong support for the theory of seedling metastases. The diagnostic features are the same as those for primary carcinoma of the ureter, and the treatment of choice is total nephroureterectomy with a cuff of bladder.

Metastatic Ureteral Tumors

Carcinoma metastatic to the ureter is rare; only 151 cases have been reported to date. Stow[53] reported the first documented case, and Presman and Ehrlich[47] summarized 35 cases from the literature and established criteria for the diagnosis of metastatic disease to the ureter. Symptoms referable to the genitourinary tract were lacking in most patients. Abeloff and Lenhard[1] demonstrated that less than 50% of the patients with metastatic tumor were symptomatic, and Cohen and associates[19] found 85% of such patients to be asymptomatic, with tumors discovered only at autopsy.

Richie and associates listed the sites of primary tumors that later involved the ureter in the following order of frequency: breast (10 patients), colon/rectum (7), cervix (6), prostate (6), bladder (6), retroperitoneal lymphoma (5), and miscellaneous (6).[48] Predilection for the lower third of the ureter was evident, and the longest time interval from primary tumor to diagnosis of ureteral obstruction ranged from eight months (carcinoma of the cervix) to nine years (bladder carcinoma). Grabstald and Kaufman described 24 women with periureteral metastases and hydronephrosis from primary breast carcinoma.[31] In their autopsy series of 215 patients with breast carcinoma, 42 (18.3%) were found to have genitourinary metastases: kidney, 9.8%; ureter, 6.4%; and bladder, 2.1%. Less than 5% of these patients had symptoms of urinary involvement.

The therapy of ureteral obstruction secondary to metastatic tumor must incorporate ethical and moral as well as medical considerations. The relief of ureteral obstruction by indwelling tubes, exteriorized tubes, or ureterolysis, with consequent prevention of terminal uremia, may serve only to prolong suffering and should be weighed carefully against the patient's prognosis and the availability of effective alternative treatment for the primary tumor.

Tumor from Direct Extension

Ureteral involvement occurs most commonly with carcinoma of the cervix, carcinoma of the colon, or retroperitoneal lymphoma. The majority of tumors compress rather than invade the ureter. Treatment is directed mainly toward the primary tumor and toward the relief of bilateral ureteral obstruction, as noted previously.

References

1. Abeloff MD, Lenhard RE Jr: Clinical management of ureteral obstruction secondary to malignant lymphoma. Johns Hopkins Med J 134:34–42, 1974.
2. Abeshouse BS: Primary benign and malignant tumors of the ureter. A review of the literature and report of one benign and twelve malignant tumors. Am J Surg 91:237–271, 1956.
3. Almgärd LE, Freedman D, Ljungqvist A: Carcinoma of the ureter with special reference to malignancy grading and prognosis. Scand J Urol Nephrol 7:165–167, 1973.
4. Apostolov K, Spasic P: Evidence of a viral aetiology in endemic (Balkan) nephropathy. Lancet 2:1271–1273, 1975.
5. Arger PH, Mulhern CB, Pollack HM, et al: Ultrasonic assessment of renal transitional cell carcinoma: preliminary report. Am J Roentgenol 132:407–411, 1979.
6. Babaian RJ, Johnson DE: Carcinoma of the renal pelvis. Cancer Bulletin 31:21, 1979.
7. Batata M, Grabstald H: Upper urinary tract urothelial tumors. Urol Clin North Am 3:79–86, 1976.
8. Batata MA, Whitmore WF Jr, Hilaris BS, et al: Primary carcinoma of the ureter: a prognostic study. Cancer 35:1626–1632, 1975.
9. Bennington JL, Beckwith JB: Tumors of the kidney, renal pelvis and ureter. In Atlas of Tumor Pathology. Washington, DC, Armed Forces Institute of Pathology, 1975, Fasc. 12.
10. Bergman H, Friedenberg RM, Sayegh V: New roentgenologic signs of carcinoma of the ureter. Am J Roentgen 86:707–717, 1961.
11. Bergman H, Hotchkiss RS: Ureteral tumors. In H Bergman (ed), The Ureter, 2nd ed. New York, Springer Verlag, 1981, p 271.
12. Bloom NA, Vidone RA, Lytton B: Primary carcinoma of the ureter: a report of 102 new cases. J Urol 103:590–598, 1970.
13. Blute RD Jr, Gittes RR, Gittes RF: Renal brush biopsy: survey of indications, techniques and results. J Urol 126:146–149, 1981.
14. Boyland E, Dukes CE, Grover PL, Mitchley BC: The induction of renal tumours by feeding lead acetate to rats. Br J Cancer 16:283–288, 1962.
15. Brady LW, Gislason GJ, Faust DS, et al: Radiation therapy. A valuable adjunct in the management of carcinoma of the ureter. JAMA 206:2871–2874, 1968.
16. Brookland RK, Richter MP: The postoperative irradiation of transitional cell carcinoma of the renal pelvis and ureter. J Urol 133:952–955, 1985.
17. Butler WH, Barnes JM: Carcinogenic action of groundnut meal containing aflatoxin in rats. Food Cosmet Toxicol 6:135–141, 1968.
18. Clayson DB, Lawson TA, Pringle JA: The carcinogenic action of 2-aminodiphenylene oxide and 4-aminodiphenyl on the bladder and liver of the C57 × IF mouse. Br J Cancer 21:755–762, 1967.
19. Cohen WM, Freed SZ, Hasson J: Metastatic cancer to the ureter: a review of the literature and case presentations. J Urol 112:188–189, 1974.
20. Craciun EC, Rosculescu I: On Danubian endemic familial nephropathy (Balkan nephropathy). Some problems. Am J Med 49:774–779, 1970.
21. Cullen TH, Popham RR, Voss HJ: Urine cytology and primary carcinoma of the renal pelvis and ureter. Aust NZ J Surg 41:230–236, 1972.
22. Cummings KB: Nephroureterectomy: rationale in the management of transitional cell carcinoma of the upper urinary tract. Urol Clin North Am 7:569–578, 1980.
23. Cummings KB, Correa RJ Jr, Gibbons RP, et al: Renal pelvic tumors. J Urol 113:158–162, 1975.
24. Eriksson O, Johansson S: Urothelial neoplasms of the upper urinary tract. A correlation between cytologic and histologic findings in 43 patients with urothelial neoplasms of the renal pelvis or ureter. Acta Cytol 20:20–25, 1976.
25. Evans RW: Histological Appearances of Tumors. With a Consideration of their Histogenesis and Certain Aspects of Their Clinical Features and Behavior, 2nd ed. Baltimore, Williams & Wilkins, 1966, p 1170.
26. Geerdsen J: Tumours of the renal pelvis and ureter. Symptomatology, diagnosis, treatment and prognosis. Scand J Urol Nephrol 13:287–290, 1979.
27. Ghidoni JJ, Campbell MM: Fine structure of metaplastic cornified squamous epithelium in the urinary bladder of rats. J Pathol 97:665–670, 1969.
28. Gill WB, Lu CT, Thomsen S: Retrograde brushing: a new technique for obtaining histologic and cytologic material from ureteral, renal pelvic and renal caliceal lesions. J Urol 109:573–578, 1973.
29. Gittes RF: Management of transitional cell carcinoma of the upper tract: case for conservative local excision. Urol Clin North Am 7:559–568, 1980.
30. Gordon A: Intestinal metaplasia of the urinary tract epithelium. J Pathol 85:441–444, 1963.
31. Grabstald H, Kaufman R: Hydronephrosis secondary to ureteral obstruction by metastatic breast cancer. J Urol 102:569–576, 1969.
32. Grabstald H, Whitmore WF Jr, Melamed MR: Renal pelvic tumors, JAMA 281:845–854, 1971.

33. Grace DA, Taylor WN, Taylor JN, Winter CC: Carcinoma of the renal pelvis: a 15-year review. J Urol 98:566–569, 1967.
34. Guerin M, Chouroulinkor I, Riviere MR: Experimental kidney tumors. *In* C Rouiller, AF Muller (eds), The Kidney: Morphology, Biochemistry, Physiology, Vol 2. New York, Academic Press, 1969, p 199.
35. Holtz F: Papillomas and primary carcinoma of the ureter: report of 20 cases. J Urol 88:380–385, 1962.
36. Huffman JL, Bagley DH, Lyon ES: Extending cytoscopic techniques into the ureter and renal pelvis. Experience with ureteroscopy and pyeloscopy. JAMA 250:2002–2005, 1983.
37. Johansson S, Angervall L, Bengtsson U, et al: Uroepithelial tumors of the renal pelvis associated with abuse of phenacetin-containing analgesics. Cancer 33:743–753, 1974.
38. Kerr WK, Barkin M: Aetiology and biochemistry of cancer of the bladder. In E Riches (ed), Modern Trends in Urology, 3rd ed. New York, Appleton-Century-Crofts, 1970, p 163.
39. Lang EK: The arteriographic diagnosis of primary and secondary tumors of the ureter or ureter and renal pelvis. Radiology 93:799–805, 1969.
40. Leiber MM, Lupu AN: High-grade invasive ureteral transitional cell carcinoma with a congenital solitary kidney: long-term survival after ureterectomy and radiation therapy. J Urol 120:368–369, 1978.
41. Marković B: Endemic nephritis and urinary tract cancer in Yugoslavia, Bulgaria and Rumania. J Urol 107:212–219, 1972.
42. Marković B: Endemic nephropathy and cancer of the upper urinary tract urothelium in Yugoslavia. Isr J Med Sci 8:540, 1972.
43. McCarron JP, Mills C, Vaughn ED Jr: Tumors of the renal pelvis and ureter: current concepts and management. Semin Urol 1:75–81, 1983.
44. Melicow MM: Tumors of urinary drainage tract; urothelial tumors. J Urol 54:186–193, 1945.
45. Nocks BN, Heney NM, Daly JJ, et al: Transitional cell carcinoma of renal pelvis. Urology 19:472–477, 1982.
46. Oyasu R, Hopp ML: The etiology of cancer of the bladder. Surg Gynecol Obstet 138:97–108, 1974.
47. Presman D, Ehrlich L: Metastatic tumors of ureter. J Urol 59:312–325, 1948.
48. Richie JP, Withers G, Ehrlich RM: Ureteral obstruction secondary to metastatic tumors. Surg Gynecol Obstet 148:355–357, 1979.
49. Roe FJ: An illustrated classification of the proliferative and neoplastic changes in mouse bladder epithelium in response to prolonged irritation. Br J Urol 36:238–253, 1964.
50. Roe FJ, Boyland E, Dukes CE, et al: Failure of testosterone or xanthopterin to influence the induction of renal neoplasms by lead in rats. Br J Cancer 19:860–866, 1965.
51. Salm R: Combined intestinal and squamous metaplasia of the renal pelvis. J Clin Pathol 22:187–191, 1969.
52. Scott WW: Review of primary carcinoma of ureter, presenting 2 cases. J Urol 50:45–64, 1943.
53. Stow B: Fibrolymphosarcomata of both ureters, metastatic to a primary lymphosarcoma of the anterior mediastinum of the thymus origin. Ann Surg 50:901, 1909.
54. Strong DW, Pearse HD: Recurrent urothelial tumors following surgery for transitional cell carcinoma of the upper urinary tract. Cancer 38:2173–2183, 1976.
55. Von Eschenbach AC, Johnson DE, Ayala AG: Simultaneous occurrence of renal adenocarcinoma and transitional cell carcinoma of the renal pelvis. J Urol 118:105–106, 1977.
56. Weldon TE, Soloway MS, Persky L: Urothelial susceptibility to neoplastic cellular implantation. Surg Forum 25:547–549, 1974.
57. Williams CB, Mitchell JP: Carcinoma of the ureter—a review of 54 cases. Br J Urol 45:377–387, 1973.
58. Yagoda A: Chemotherapy for advanced urothelial cancer. Semin Urol 1:60–74, 1983.
59. Zincke H, Aguilo JJ, Farrow GM, et al: Significance of urinary cytology in the early detection of transitional cell cancer of the upper urinary tract. J Urol 116:781–783, 1976.

T. RAND PRITCHETT, M.D.
GARY LIESKOVSKY, M.D.
DONALD G. SKINNER, M.D.

Clinical Manifestations and Treatment of Renal Parenchymal Tumors

CHAPTER 19

Renal neoplasms may be classified into two broad categories: those that are primary of the kidney and those that are metastatic to the kidney. Although the incidence of metastatic tumors to the kidney may be much higher than that of primary renal tumors, the secondary lesions are usually silent clinically, and thus will be discussed only briefly in this chapter. Our main focus of attention is directed to the clinical manifestations and treatment of primary parenchymal lesions. Malignant renal tumors arise from renal parenchyma, renal pelvis, and renal capsule. Renal cell carcinomas (hypernephroma, Grawitz's tumor) constitute approximately 85% of all primary malignant renal tumors; renal pelvic transitional cell and squamous cell carcinomas compose about 10%; and the remaining 5% include renal sarcomas and nephroblastomas (Wilms' tumor).[11] Although most primary renal tumors are malignant, some benign tumors are worthy of mention.

TUMORS OF THE KIDNEY

Hamartoma

Renal angiomyolipoma (hamartoma), a benign tumor of the kidney, occurs rarely in the general population but is common in patients with tuberous sclerosis.[100] Its microscopic appearance is described in Chapter 8; it is generally composed of vascular, fat, and smooth muscle components responsible for the radiographic characteristics illustrated in Chapter 13. Histologically, this tumor may appear to the novice as a liposarcoma, but neither sarcomatous change nor the development of distant metastases has been clearly demonstrated with this lesion, and it should be considered a benign process.[41, 126, 161] Busch reported two patients with infiltration of regional nodes by angiomyolipoma who were successfully treated by local resection without evidence of distant metastases, although results of long-term follow-up are not available.[23]

In patients without tuberous sclerosis, angiomyolipoma characteristically is more common in women than in men, produces symptoms between the third and fifth decades of life, is typically unilateral, and, for unknown reasons, involves the right side 80% of the time.[161] Symptoms usually relate to hemorrhage into or around the tumor, resulting in pain, an enlarging flank mass, and occasionally shock.[6] Tan and associates reported that almost one third of angiomyolipomas in patients without stigmata of tuberous sclerosis initially present as acute abdominal emergencies because of spontaneous bleeding.[155]

Nearly half the reported cases of renal angiomyolipoma have been associated with

337

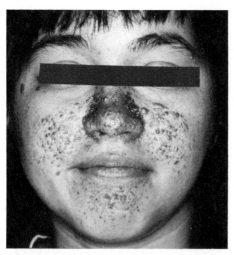

Figure 19–1. Characteristic "butterfly" distribution of adenoma sebaceum on the face of a patient with tuberous sclerosis. Courtesy of Dr. Ronald Reisner. Reprinted from Brenner BM, Rector FC Jr (eds), The Kidney, 2nd ed. Philadelphia, WB Saunders, 1981, p 2110.

tuberous sclerosis, a disease characterized by lesions of the cerebral cortex that produce epilepsy and mental retardation. A "butterfly" distribution of adenoma sebaceum on the face occurs in 80% of the patients with tuberous sclerosis (Fig. 19–1), and a variety of other organs may be involved as well, including the eyes, bones, lungs, and heart.[90, 100] Hamartoma of the kidney occurs in as many as 80% of the patients with tuberous sclerosis, and the lesions are often bilateral and multiple.[90]

Management depends on establishment of a preoperative diagnosis. In patients with stigmata of tuberous sclerosis, careful investigation of the contralateral kidney is mandatory since, in most instances, multiplicity and bilaterality of renal involvement will be detected. Conservative management is encouraged, although an occasional partial nephrectomy may be necessary. In the rare patient with tuberous sclerosis and unilateral involvement, flank exploration and biopsy are generally indicated to rule out the possibility of renal cell carcinoma. When a diagnosis of angiomyolipoma is established by frozen section, conservative surgical resection with partial nephrectomy is indicated. The role of arterial occlusion in the treatment of these tumors has not been clearly established but may have increasing importance.

The discovery of a renal tumor in a patient with tuberous sclerosis does not automatically indicate angiomyolipoma. Renal cell carcinoma has been present in as many as 26% of tumors associated with tuberous sclerosis,[58] and other authors have noted its occurrence bilaterally.[65, 142]

Renal masses in patients with tuberous sclerosis are most commonly angiomyolipomas but may be caused by cystic disease or renal cell carcinoma. In evaluation of these patients, the presence of persistent hematuria, calcification, or an enlarging mass should warrant treatment with a renal conserving operation.

In patients without evidence of tuberous sclerosis, radiographic differentiation between hamartoma and renal cell carcinoma is often impossible. The recommended treatment in these patients usually is radical nephrectomy.

Lipoma

Intrarenal lipomas are not uncommon but rarely are large enough to be of surgical significance. Dineen and associates have found only 17 cases of pure intrarenal lipoma in the literature.[38] Usually they are found in middle-aged women, occur equally in left or right kidneys, and are not bilateral or associated with tuberous sclerosis. There has been no reported case of malignant transformation of these benign tumors.

Hemangioma

Hemangiomas are benign congenital tumors arising from the endothelium of blood and lymph vessels. The liver is most commonly involved, and the kidney ranks second among internal organs hosting these vascular tumors.[124] Hemangiomas are generally unilateral, but in 12% of the patients they may be bilateral.[59] These lesions usually arise within the medullary portion of the kidney and are often adjacent to the epithelium of the renal collecting system. Intermittent hematuria is the usual clinical symptom, associated with pain and the passage of clots. Hemangioma should be considered in the differential diagnosis of patients under the age of 40 with localized hematuria and in whom the possibilities of tumor and calculi can be excluded. Selective renal arteriography should localize the lesion.[3] Treatment depends on the severity of the symptoms and the physician's ability to exlude malignant lesions, such as renal cell carcinoma. In older patients, radical nephrectomy is the treatment of choice whenever radiologic differentiation of benign hemangioma from renal cell carcinoma is difficult or whenever profuse or threatening hemorrhage occurs. Heminephrectomy should be considered in younger patients with this lesion.

Hemangiopericytoma

Hemangiopericytoma (juxtaglomerular tumor, reninoma) is a rare primary renal tumor arising from capillary pericytes in the region of the juxtaglomerular apparatus.[74] Although more commonly arising in other areas, such as the retroperitoneum and pelvis,[148] a renal origin for this tumor was first reported by Black and Heinemann in 1977.[14] Robertson and associates reported hypertension associated with renal hemangiopericytoma,[134] and Conn and associates have documented renin secretion by the tumor.[26] Through 1976, six cases of primary renal hemangiopericytoma associated with hypertension have been reported.[74] Marked elevation and inequality of renal vein renin determinations may suggest the diagnosis of this benign solitary tumor. In such instances, segmental resection may be appropriate, but most cases have been treated by nephrectomy.

Adenoma

The classification of renal adenoma as a benign lesion or an early malignant adenocarcinoma is controversial. These lesions are frequently incidental findings at autopsy, appearing as well-circumscribed cortical lesions usually less than 3 cm in diameter. It has been reported that they are present in 7 to 22% of all kidneys examined.[167] In 1938, based on an autopsy study of 30,000 cases, Bell reported that if the diameter of the so-called adenoma was less than 3 cm, metastatic lesions were seldom encountered, but if the renal tumors exceeded 3 cm in diameter, metastases were frequent. He did *not* state that "adenomas smaller than 3 cm were benign; those more than 3 cm malignant," a misconception perpetuated for many years as "Bell's Law."[8]

Similarities between adenoma and adenocarcinoma are encountered in age and sex distribution, and there is an increased incidence of both lesions in smokers. Although so-called adenomas are rarely associated with metastases, there are no histologic, histochemical, ultrastructural, or immunologic features that clearly distinguish them from early well-differentiated renal adenocarcinomas.[9, 27, 45, 116] In the past, lesions of considerable size have been reported as benign adenomas,[40] but most data suggest that the so-called renal adenoma may represent an early structural stage in the development of a well-differentiated renal adenocarcinoma. Murphy and Mostofi[116] hypothesized that about 6% of all clinically encountered renal adenocarcinomas arose from renal adenomas. Although fewer than 70 cases of symptomatic so-called benign renal adenomas had been reported by 1968,[89] the incidence of these lesions will increase as our imaging methods improve, and urologists are encouraged to treat these lesions, when encountered clinically, as early carcinoma.

Oncocytoma

Oncocytomas are tumors composed of large epithelial cells with finely granular eosinophilic cytoplasm; they have been described in kidney and other organs.[87] The clinical spectrum of presentations can be quite similar to that of renal cell carcinoma, so most patients with this diagnosis have had a radical nephrectomy. These tumors are found in middle-aged men and women and are equally divided in occurrence between the left and right kidneys. Pathologic features of this lesion usually show a well-encapsulated parenchymal tumor of uniform mahogany-brown color that, under histologic examination, shows pure, well-differentiated (Grade 1) eosinophilic granular cells. Patients with these well-differentiated tumors have an excellent prognosis; actuarial five- and 10-year survival rates are 85% and 70%, respectively.[87]

Renal Cell Carcinoma

In the United States, renal cell carcinoma is diagnosed in about 17,000 patients per year; an estimated 8000 people die each year from this disease.[143] Its peak incidence occurs during the sixth and seventh decades of life, with a male to female ratio of 2:1.[72] The tumor rarely occurs in patients under the age of 20, although it has been reported in 155 adolescents and more than 80 children.[1, 49]

Grawitz described the tumor in 1883, observed the striking resemblance of the yellow renal tumor to the adrenal cortex, and suggested that it might be derived from an adrenal rest.[80] Birch-Hirschfield in 1892 introduced the term *hypernephroma* as an appropriate name for Grawitz's tumor.[104]

Gradually, urologists and pathologists have come to realize that the majority of these renal tumors arise from renal tubular epithelial cells, a fact supported by both light and electron microscopy.[9, 27] Thus, the terms *renal cell carcinoma* and *renal cell adenocarcinoma* seem more appropriate than *hypernephroma*. Controversy continues as to whether renal cell carcinoma arises de novo from renal tubules, by evolution through adenomatous hyperplasia, or from renal cortical adenoma.[27, 125]

Parenchymal renal cell carcinomas constitute approximately 85% of all primary malignant renal tumors. Tumors of the renal pelvis and renal capsule account for the remaining 15%. The natural history of renal cell carcinoma is not always predictable. Available data on the incidence of this tumor are dependent upon the completeness of registration in the community. It may remain clinically unrecognized during life. In a review of 16,294 autopsies in Malmö, Sweden (a town in which 99% of the population has postmortem examination), 350 cases of renal carcinoma were found.[62] Of those, 235 had been unrecognized during life. This incidence is much higher than the 3.5 cases per 100,000 per year reported in the United States.[93]

Prognosis is usually poor for patients with advanced disease. Riches[131] reported a series of 443 untreated patients with an overall survival rate of 4.4% at three years and 1.7% at five years. All these patients presented with advanced disease or had serious concomitant medical problems that precluded operation. Middleton[107] reported that none of 141 patients with renal cell carcinoma associated initially with multiple distant metastases survived more than two years, regardless of whether they underwent nephrectomy. Katz and Davis[73] reported that of 62 patients who presented with metastases when first seen, 51 (82%) died within one year, regardless of therapy, and none

survived five years. This group of patients must be distinguished from those who develop metastases at a variable time after initial diagnosis, whose survival is somewhat better.[37, 128]

The cumulative survival for 86 patients with metastatic renal cell carcinoma followed at the UCLA-affiliated hospitals between 1971 and 1976 is shown in Figure 19–2.[37] The one-year survival rate of 42% and two-year survival of 25% are higher than those in the previously mentioned reports, but it is important to note that if one considers only those patients who have metastatic disease on initial presentation, the mean

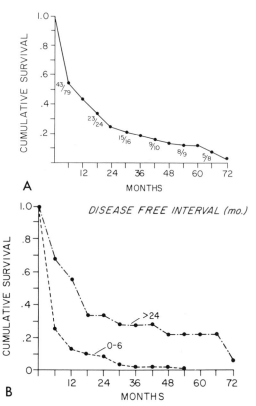

Figure 19–2. A, Cumulative survival of 86 patients with metastatic renal cell carcinoma seen at UCLA and affiliated Veterans Hospitals between 1971 and 1976. Included are patients who had metastases at the time of diagnosis, as well as those who developed metastases after nephrectomy. B, Cumulative survival based on the interval between diagnosis and appearance of metastases. Patients who had metastases at the time of diagnosis or developed them within six months had a significantly (p < 0.02) decreased survival over patients who developed metastases more than two years after nephrectomy. From deKernion JB, et al: The natural history of metastatic renal cell carcinoma: a computer analysis. J Urol 120:148–152, 1978, with permission.

survival rate for those treated at UCLA was approximately four months, and only about 10% survived one year.[37] Thus the variation in reported survival emphasizes the significant differences among patient populations at various institutions and criteria of patient selection. Nonetheless, available statistics indicate a rapid, unrelenting progression of tumor growth and spread in most patients with metastatic renal carcinoma.

Striking exceptions to this course are rare but familiar to all urologic surgeons. Reported spontaneous or idiopathic regression of renal tumors is probably out of proportion to its actual occurrence. Regression of tumors or tumor metastases has been reported in multiple studies and in over 50 cases.[4, 48, 62, 63, 168] Hellsten and associates observed regression histologically in 3.4% of 235 patients with premortem clinically unrecognized tumors.[62] Regression of primary tumors with histologic findings of fibrosis has been reported.[4, 168] Freed and co-workers reviewed 51 cases of metastatic disease in which regression was observed.[48] Pulmonary metastases regressed in 45 patients, osseous metastases in three, intestinal metastasis in one, and subcutaneous in two patients. Only 19 of the cases had histologic confirmation of regression; most were transient and not synonymous with cure. Holland reported spontaneous regression in more than 40 patients, but distant metastases may develop and become evident as long as 15 to 20 years after nephrectomy.[63] Freed's series reported only three patients with follow-up longer than 20 years after regression was observed.[48] It is evident, therefore, that the growth rate is variable and that necrosis and fibrosis within the tumor or metastatic foci is common. The unusual natural history of this disease is at present unexplained but may suggest the importance of the patient's immune mechanisms.

Renal cell carcinoma originates from the proximal renal tubules. It is a vascular tumor that tends to spread in one of two ways: by direct extension on a path of low resistance into the renal vein and occasionally further into the inferior vena cava, or by direct invasion through the renal capsule into the perinephric fat, contiguous visceral structures, or the regional lymph nodes.[144] The tumors rarely invade the renal pelvis and ureters, but malignant cells can be identified in the urine in about 7% of the patients.[138,] [157] Distant metastases occur most commonly to the lung (55%), whereas other sites of relatively common metastases include liver (33%), bone (33%), adrenal (20%), and opposite kidney (10%).[10, 79]

Direct extension into the perinephric fat or involvement of the regional nodes is a far more ominous finding than that of propagation into the renal vein or vena cava, provided that there is no evidence of distant metastases.[146]

PRESENTING SYMPTOMS AND LABORATORY ABNORMALITIES WITH RENAL TUMORS

Renal cell carcinoma may masquerade in a wide variety of symptom patterns suggestive of other illnesses, a fact that makes the final diagnosis difficult for even the most suspicious diagnostician. Patients with this tumor may have a number of complaints or physical findings ranging from the classic triad of hematuria, pain, and a palpable abdominal mass to more obscure problems such as fever of unknown origin, erythrocytosis, weight loss, anemia, symptoms from hypercalcemia, and the acute onset of a scrotal varicocele.[13, 125, 144]

Presenting symptoms, clinical abnormalities, or abnormal laboratory findings according to their incidence of presentation have been summarized in 309 patients with renal cell carcinoma treated over a 30-year period at Massachusetts General Hospital (Table 19–1).[144] Although hematuria, pain, and a palpable abdominal mass were the initial findings in only 9% of these patients, two of the three components of the triad were found in 36% of the group, and hematuria, either microscopic or gross, was noted in nearly 60%.

Ten patients (3%) in the Massachusetts General Hospital series had secondary erythrocytosis (hematocrit greater than 50% or hemoglobin greater than 15.5 gm/dl) on admission. Other series report the presence of erythrocytosis in 1 to 5% of patients.[50, 136, 139] It differs from polycythemia in that there is no elevation of the platelet or leukocyte count and there is no splenomegaly. It is due to an increase in erythropoietin, a substance known to be secreted by renal cell carcinoma—63% of patients in one series

Table 19–1. PRESENTING SYMPTOMS, LABORATORY ABNORMALITY, OR ABNORMALITY ON
PHYSICAL EXAMINATION AND ITS RELATION TO SURVIVAL RATE IN 309 CONSECUTIVE
PATIENTS UNDERGOING NEPHRECTOMY FOR RENAL CELL CARCINOMA*

Presenting Symptoms, Abnormal Laboratory Finding, or Abnormality on Physical Exam	Number of Patients, Per Cent of Total (309)	Number of Patients Surviving Five Years
Classic triad (gross hematuria, abnormal mass, pain)	29 (9%)	9 (out of 29) 31%
Hematuria	183 (59%)	74 (out of 183) 40%
Pain	127 (41%)	54 (out of 127) 44%
Abdominal mass	139 (45%)	49 (out of 139) 35%
Fever	21 (7%)	8 (out of 21) 38%
Weight loss	85 (28%)	29 (out of 85) 39%
Anemia	64 (21%)	24 (out of 64) 38%
Erythrocytosis	10 (3%)	4 (out of 10) 40%
Hypercalcemia	11 (3%)	4 (out of 11) 36%
Acute varicocele	7 (2%)	3 (out of 7) 43%
Tumor calcification on x-ray film	39 (13%)	18 (out of 39) 46%
Symptoms from metastases	31 (10%)	1 (out of 31) 3%
Cancer, an incidental finding (silent)	20 (7%)	13 (out of 20) 65%

*From Skinner DG, et al: Diagnosis and management of renal cell carcinoma. Cancer 28:1165, 1971.

showed an elevated level.[139] About 4% of patients with erythrocytosis will have renal cell carcinoma, and up to 33% of patients with hematuria and erythrocytosis will have renal cell carcinoma.[50] If no metastatic disease is present, erythrocytosis will revert to normal after nephrectomy. The late reappearance of erythrocytosis after nephrectomy implies the presence of metastases and is a bad prognostic sign.[136]

Anemia (hematocrit less than 33% or hemoglobin less than 10.0 gm/dl) was noted in 64 patients (21%) in the Massachusetts series. This is the most frequent hematologic abnormality seen with renal cell carcinoma. Ordinarily it is not secondary to hemolysis, to blood loss by hematuria, or to bone marrow replacement.[50] The anemia is usually a hypoproliferative type that creates a low total iron-binding capacity and low levels of serum iron. It is thought to be due to bone marrow depression by a toxic effect of an unknown circulating substance.[50, 136]

Fever was present in 21 patients (7%) in the Massachusetts series. Pyrexia has been noted in as many as 15 to 20% of patients in other series.[25] Caused by an endogenous pyrogen, it is frequently intermittently recurrent and usually abates with nephrectomy.[136] Renal cell carcinoma from a febrile patient will cause a fever in laboratory animals, whereas tissue from a normal kidney or from a tumor from an afebrile patient will not.[30, 50] Delayed return of fever may indicate the presence of metastases.[76]

An elevated erythrocyte sedimentation rate (ESR) is a common finding in renal

malignancy, being present in more than 75% of patients in some series.[50, 75] This finding is not specific for renal cell carcinoma, and a normal ESR does not rule one out.[50]

Seven men in the Massachusetts series were referred for sudden onset of a scrotal varicocele, six of which occurred on the left side. One patient with tumor involving the vena cava had a right varicocele. They have been reported in 0.6 to 11% of patients with renal cell carcinoma.[82] Usually this condition is due to obstruction of the testicular vein by tumor thrombus. On the left side this is due to tumor in the left renal vein, whereas on the right side the tumor is likely to have extended into the vena cava. In a review of 25 patients with vena caval extension of renal cell carcinoma, there were varicoceles in seven of 15 males (47%).[127] The presence of a varicocele should alert the clinician to the possibility of venous vascular involvement. Another patient in the Massachusetts series had a large hematoma in his right flank after the spontaneous rupture of a lower pole carcinoma.

Although 10% of these patients presented with symptoms secondary to metastases, 77 of 309 (25%) actually had radiologic or clinical evidence of metastases when first seen for therapy. In 7% of these patients, renal cell carcinoma was an incidental finding, usually discovered during the course of another surgical procedure.

With the exception of those patients who presented with symptoms from metastases and those in whom renal cell carcinoma was an incidental finding, no significant prognostic relationship could be found between various presenting symptoms or laboratory abnormalities and survival rate in the Massachusetts series.[144]

Hypertension has been associated with renal cell carcinoma, ranging from a 14 to 40% incidence for all new patients with this neoplasm.[152] Nielson[118] and Hollifield and associates[64] have reported renin secretion by the tumor. Sufrin and associates[152] have suggested that peripheral serum renin determinations might provide a useful marker for early detection of metastatic disease, and they found that elevated peripheral renin levels were associated with high-grade and high-stage lesions and thus offered a poorer prognosis. It remains unclear, however, whether renin is produced by the tumor itself as a result of relative ischemia to adjacent normal renal parenchyma due to altered blood flow, a decreased rate of degradation, or the production of renin by nonrenal sources.[152] Although nephrectomy resulted in lowering of the plasma renin level, it is not documented whether an abnormal serum renin level obtained on a routine follow-up examination heralded clinical detection of recurrence, thus indicating possible usefulness as a tumor marker.

Hypercalcemia (serum calcium greater than 10.5 mg/dl) was found on admission in 11 patients (3%) in the Massachusetts series. The presence of an elevated serum calcium level may be secondary to (1) metastatic bone disease; (2) ectopic hormone production; or (3) prostaglandin secretion by the tumor.[33, 139] In other reported series, the incidence of hypercalcemia ranged from 5 to 15%, with many of these elevations due to an ectopic production of a parathyroid hormone–like substance, which is most commonly caused by renal cell carcinoma and lung carcinoma.[82] Life-threatening hypercalcemia that is refractory to medical management has been managed by surgical debulking of primary and metastatic tumor deposits.[53]

A syndrome of reversible hepatosplenomegaly with hepatic dysfunction but without evidence of liver metastases was described by Creevy[31] in 1935 and Stauffer[150] in 1961. Often referred to as Stauffer's syndrome, this paraneoplastic syndrome has been reported and reviewed by several others.[19, 59, 130, 158, 162]

Initially this syndrome was characterized by abnormal retention of Bromsulphalein dye, elevated levels of serum alkaline phosphatase, hypoprothrombinemia, and an increased α_2-globulin fraction in the absence of hepatic metastases.[150] Hanash[59] studied 30 patients, 11 (37%) of whom had reversible hepatic dysfunction syndrome, whereas Ramos and Taylor[130] found evidence of this syndrome in 10% of patients. Although serum alkaline phosphatase is elevated in most patients, other liver function test abnormalities include increased serum bilirubin, increased γ-glutamyltransferase, and hypoalbuminemia.[59] Over a 20-year period at UCLA Hospital, only seven of 106 patients undergoing nephrectomy for renal cell carcinoma presented with hepatic dysfunction.[19] Hanash found that the histologic changes associated with the liver dysfunction included proliferation of the Kupffer's cells associated with dilated sinusoids, degenerative changes of the hepatocytes, focal lymphocytic infiltration, moderate steatosis, and focal necrosis.[59]

The presence of reversible hepatic dysfunction with a renal mass is seen not only in renal cell carcinoma but also with xanthogranulomatous pyelonephritis.[94, 139] The main feature that distinguishes xanthogranulomatous pyelonephritis from renal cell carcinoma clinically is the presence of symptoms of a urinary tract infection.[94] The exact origin of this hepatic dysfunction is unknown. Theories of metabolic hepatic damage by a tumor toxin and lymphocyte-mediated immunologic hepatic damage mechanisms have been postulated.[59]

With nephrectomy, the hepatic dysfunction should become normal unless there is metastatic disease present. The re-elevation of the results of liver function tests after normalization or the failure of normalization to occur implies the presence of recurrent or metastatic disease and is an indication of grave prognosis.[59, 136]

Increased levels of other glycoproteins and hormones and hormone-related syndromes have been associated with renal cell carcinoma. These substances and syndromes include serum human chorionic gonadotropin, prolactin, human placental lactogen, calcitonin,[139] carcinoembryonic antigen,[57] feminization, masculinization, and Cushing's syndrome.[32]

Enteropathy with protein loss has been described in a renal cell carcinoma that produced glucagon. Intestinal function and x-ray appearance became normal after nephrectomy.[51]

A reversible glomerulopathy also has been described with renal cell carcinoma that is sometimes due to immune-complex deposition.[4, 32] Secondary amyloidosis is associated with malignancy in about 15% of patients, and renal cell carcinoma is one of the most common malignancies associated with amyloidosis.[32, 50] The incidence of amyloidosis in patients with renal cell carcinoma is 1 to 3%, and most frequently it involves the kidney, liver, spleen, and adrenal.[136] The clinical presentation is one of a rapid downhill course, renal failure, and albuminuria. Renal failure and death secondary to amyloidosis without metastatic disease can occur, and resolution of the amyloidosis after the surgical removal of the renal carcinoma has not been reported.[50, 136]

DIAGNOSIS OF RENAL TUMORS

Because of the wide variety of presenting symptoms and nonspecific laboratory abnormalities and its characteristic radiographic appearance, the preoperative diagnosis of a renal cell carcinoma is primarily radiologically determined. This is discussed in greater detail in Chapter 13.

A plain abdominal film may show an irregular shape or enlargement of a kidney or evidence of intrarenal calcification. Calcifications in renal cell carcinoma are present in 2 to 35% of patients in reported series.[28, 34, 80, 141] Intravenous urography with nephrotomography is helpful in the confirmation of the presence of a renal mass. Renal cell carcinoma may cause an overall or localized enlargement of the involved kidney and, during the vascular phase of contrast injection, demonstrates a hypervascularity or avascularity of the tumefaction. Ultrasonography may be helpful in determining whether a renal mass is solid or cystic, but selective renal arteriography and more recently CT are the best methods for preoperatively detecting, diagnosing, and staging renal cell carcinomas.

The principal characteristics of renal cell carcinoma that can be demonstrated via selective renal arteriography include characteristic tumor vessels (which do not constrict upon selective administration of epinephrine angiographically), arteriovenous shunting and premature venous opacification, venous lakes within the tumor, puddling of contrast material in necrotic areas of tumor, aneurysms, and poor demarcation of the interface between the tumor and its adjacent normal renal parenchyma.[22, 39, 81, 82] CT scans have been shown to be as accurate in the diagnosis of renal cell carcinoma as arteriography and, for some surgeons, CT has replaced the latter.

With the advent of third- and fourth-generation CT scanners, the accuracy of CT in staging renal cell carcinoma is approximately 90%.[92] Although at one time angiography was the modality of choice for the staging work-up of renal cell carcinoma, as CT scanners are becoming more available they are becoming the preferred method of staging. In one review, although angiography was more accurate in determining involvement of the renal vein and inferior vena cava, CT scanning was more accurate in estimating tumor size, perinephric fat invasion, and lymph node enlargement.[54] CT scan is the procedure of choice in evaluation of a calcified renal mass seen on plain abdominal film or intravenous urogram.[77] Angiography remains useful in providing a surgical road map of the renal vasculature and should be used for solitary or congenitally abnormal kidneys. When the extent of vena caval involvement cannot be precisely defined by CT, contrast venacavography must be performed. A recent review of CT scanning of renal cell carcinoma may be consulted for further information.[54]

Once a radiographic diagnosis of renal cell carcinoma has been made, a staging work-up should be performed to determine the extent of the disease. The search for metastatic disease should include a radioisotope bone scan with radiographic films of any abnormal areas, as well as liver function studies. Hepatic dysfunction (as expressed by abnormal levels of liver enzymes) may be present with or without liver metastases. Therefore, all patients with abnormal results of liver enzyme tests should have a radioisotope liver scan or CT scan of the liver. A standard chest x-ray should be routine and CT scan of the chest included if the chest x-ray shows any abnormality. Venacavography should be performed on all patients considered for nephrectomy unless the renal vein is well visualized during the venous phase

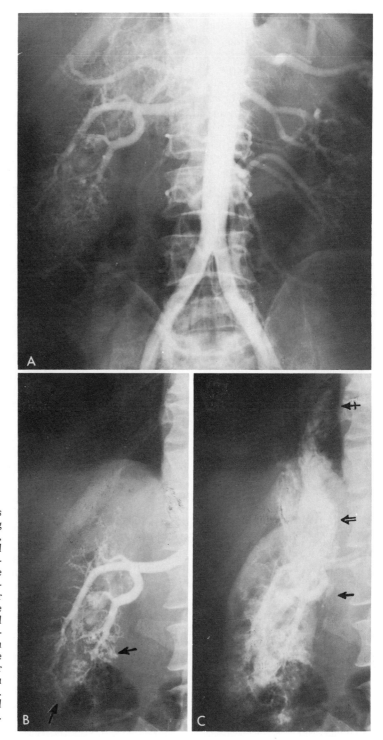

Figure 19–3. A, Aortogram reveals enlarged right renal artery supplying abnormal vessels in lower pole. B, Early arterial phase of selective renal arteriogram demonstrates tumor neovascularity (arrows). C, Intermediate arterial phase of selective renal arteriogram demonstrates profuse linear vascular pattern, extending from the level of the renal vein (arrow) and inferior vena cava (double-tailed arrow) to the level of the right atrium (crossed arrow). This represents the arterialization of an extensive tumor thrombus occluding the vena cava and extending into the right atrium. From Skinner DG, et al: The surgical management of renal cell carcinoma. J Urol 107:705–710, 1972.

of the renal arteriogram or unless the vena cava is clearly seen to be free of tumor on the CT scan.

Renal adenocarcinoma has a natural tendency to grow along venous channels, and approximately 5% of the patients undergoing nephrectomy have caval involvement.[98, 146] In half of these patients, no clinical symptoms or signs are present to suggest this involvement, although complete obstruction of the vena cava may be present.[127, 144] Intracaval extension often can be visualized on selective renal arteriography as well as by venography, since the tumor has a rich blood supply derived from the renal artery and only rarely parasitizes the vena cava (Fig. 19–3).[144] Successful removal of these neoplastic "thrombi" can produce long-term survival, but the importance of preoperative knowledge of the intracaval extension of tumor is obvious.[127, 146]

Care must be taken following diagnosis by angiography to ensure satisfactory renal function prior to surgery. Occasionally, oliguria and temporary renal shutdown may occur following extensive arteriographic studies, particularly in patients who are dehydrated at the time of arteriography. Return to normal renal function in such patients is mandatory prior to surgery to avoid significant postoperative morbidity.

TREATMENT OF RENAL TUMORS

Renal cell carcinoma is treated by surgical removal. In 1871, Walcott performed the first nephrectomy for renal cell carcinoma. By 1932, Hand and Broaders reported a 23% five-year survival rate in patients with renal parenchymal tumors treated by nephrectomy at the Mayo Clinic. Their operative mortality rate was 12%.[60]

In 1971, we reported the results of surgical treatment of 309 patients treated at the Massachusetts General Hospital between 1935 and 1965.[144] The operative mortality was 5%, with an overall survival rate of 44% at five years and 33% at 10 years. Excluding patients who had metastases when first seen for treatment, the five-year survival rate was 57% and the 10-year survival rate was 44% (Table 19–2).

Appropriate surgical treatment includes removal of Gerota's fascia (with its contents intact), together with early ligation of the renal artery and vein and regional lymph node dissection; this constitutes a radical nephrectomy.[108, 135, 137, 144]

We prefer the thoracoabdominal approach for radical nephrectomy, a technique described in Chapter 48.

PATHOLOGIC STAGING

To better evaluate the results of treatment and to better judge the prognosis in individual cases, pathologic staging of the surgical specimen has been applied to renal cell carcinoma. The staging system generally used has been proposed by Flocks and Kadesky and subsequently modified by Robson and associates.[46, 135, 137]

Stage I:　Tumor is confined to the kidney; perinephric fat, renal vein, and regional nodes show no evidence of malignancy.

Stage II:　Tumor involves the perinephric fat but is confined with Gerota's fascia; renal vein and regional nodes show no evidence of malignancy.

Stage III:　Tumor involves the renal vein or regional nodes, with or without involvement of the vena cava or perinephric fat.

Table 19–2. RENAL CELL CARCINOMA SURGICALLY TREATED AT MASSACHUSETTS GENERAL HOSPITAL FROM 1935 TO 1965*

Pathologic Stage	Number of Patients†	Operative Mortality (%)	Survival Rates 5 Years (%)	Survival Rates 10 Years (%)
Stages I through III "Potentially curable"	232	3	57	44
Stage IV Metastases on admission	77	10	8	7
All stages Total	309	5	44	33

*From Skinner DG, et al: Diagnosis and management of renal cell carcinoma. Cancer 28:1165, 1971.
†Total number of patients: 329; lost to follow-up: 20.

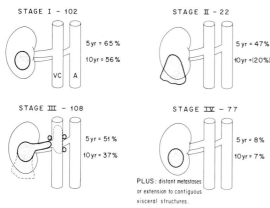

Figure 19–4. Long-term survival after nephrectomy in 309 patients with renal cell carcinoma. Results are grouped according to the pathologic stage of the lesion. From Skinner DG, et al: The surgical management of renal cell carcinoma. J Urol 107:705–710, 1972.

Stage IV: Distant metastases secondary to renal cell carcinoma are evident on presentation, or there is histologic involvement of contiguous visceral structures by tumor.

Survival according to this staging system is shown in Fig. 19–4. The limitations of this staging system, however, have become apparent after a careful analysis of patients grouped in Stage III. Renal vein involvement, or even extension into the vena cava when not associated with perinephric fat or regional lymph node involvement, does not significantly alter the prognosis, compared with that for tumors confined to the kidney (Table 19–3).[108, 119, 127, 135, 145, 156]

Robson and associates, Middleton and Presto, and Katz and Davis have documented improved survival for patients treated by radical nephrectomy, as compared with those treated by simple nephrectomy.[73, 108, 137]

By similar comparison of survival according to grade, the survival rate after a radical nephrectomy with node dissection is greater than the survival rate following simple nephrectomy by a percentage identical to the incidence of lymph node involvement for each corresponding grade (Table 19–4). This information suggests that lymph node dissection with radical nephrectomy can enhance survival in patients afflicted with renal adenocarcinoma. However, conclusive statistical data obtained in a prospective manner are not available, and thus the conclusion that radical nephrectomy with regional lymph node dissection will improve survival, compared with nephrectomy alone, remains conjecture. The operative mortality of radical nephrectomy is slightly greater (3.8%), compared with simple nephrectomy (1.4%), but in reality it is little different, since the more extensive procedures in the past have been done on patients with larger, more extensive tumors, whereas simple nephrectomy was often performed on patients with small Stage I tumors. In our hands, the addition of an en bloc regional lymph node dissection has not affected the postoperative morbidity or mortality, and it is recommended whenever radical nephrectomy is performed for cure.

VENA CAVAL INVOLVEMENT

For many years, tumor extension into the vena cava was believed to preclude surgical cure. Renal adenocarcinoma has a natural propensity to grow along venous channels, usually deriving and propagating its blood supply from the renal artery. Vena caval involvement can be found in approximately 5% of the patients with this primary tumor; it is usually noted on the right side and should be diagnosed preoperatively by the

Table 19–3. SURVIVAL RATE ACCORDING TO SPECIFIC EXTENT OF HISTOLOGIC INVOLVEMENT BY TUMOR*

Pathologic Involvement	Histologic Extent	Survival Rate	
		5 Years (%)	10 Years (%)
Stage I—kidney only	Confined	65	56
Renal vein	Alone	66	49
	+ Vena cava	55	43
	+ Perinephric fat	50	33
	+ Regional nodes	0	0
Perinephric fat	Alone	47	20
Regional nodes	Alone	33	17
Direct extension to contiguous visceral structure		0	0

*From Skinner DG, et al: Extension of renal cell carcinoma into the vena cava: the rationale for aggressive surgical management. J Urol 107:711, 1972.

Table 19–4. SURVIVAL (%) RELATING TO
GRADE AND THERAPY*

	Grade 1	Grade 2	Grade 3
Incidence of lymph node involvement	12	28	34
Five-year survival following simple nephrectomy	77	31	8
Five-year survival following radical nephrectomy	87	64	40

*From Robson CJ, et al: The results of radical nephrectomy for renal cell carcinoma. Trans Am Assoc Genitourin Surg 60:122, 1968, and Skinner DG et al: Diagnosis and management of renal cell carcinoma. Cancer 28:1165, 1971.

combination of selective renal arteriography and venacavography.

We have discovered that vena caval involvement by itself has almost the same prognosis for cure as do tumors confined to the kidney (Stage I), provided the entire thrombus is removed.[127, 145] It certainly acts far less aggressively than those tumors that extend into perinephric fat or involve regional nodes or contiguous visceral structures. An aggressive approach, therefore, seems appropriate in the patient with caval involvement and no evidence of distant metastatic disease. The management of these patients is discussed in detail in Chapter 49.

CELLULAR FEATURES RELATING TO PROGNOSIS

The histologic features of renal adenocarcinoma have been described in detail in Chapter 8. Grading on the basis of nuclear morphology has a definite predictive value and, when combined with stage, can further define the prognosis in individual patients. A retrospective review of our data and that of Robson and associates revealed an increasing incidence of lymph node involvement and a poorer survival rate with increasing nuclear grade of the tumor (Grade 1, 12% lymph node involvement; Grade 2, 28%; Grade 3, 34%).[137]

DNA flow cytometry of renal cell carcinoma has been utilized by Otto[121] and Bennington[12] and was found to correlate with clinical prognosis. An aneuploid DNA population correlated with an increased incidence of metastasis, with higher grade tumors and an expected poor prognosis.

Mancilla-Jimenez and associates[96] reported that the prognosis of patients whose renal cell carcinomas were of a papillary architecture behaved in a more benign manner than those with other histologic types. We have observed that cell type influences survival, inasmuch as 58% of patients with pure clear cell tumors survived five years, compared with only a 23% survival rate in those patients with spindle cell tumors. Colvin, however, has pointed out that most of these tumors contain a great variety of histologic patterns, cell types, and nuclear grades, and that the usual microscopic examination may not sample the most malignant portion of the tumor.[144] However, it is apparent that a careful pathologic evaluation that includes stage, grade, and cytoplasmic appearance can best define the prognosis in individual cases (Chapter 8).

MANAGEMENT OF TUMOR IN A SOLITARY KIDNEY OR BILATERAL SYNCHRONOUS TUMORS

Patients with only one kidney, or with tumors in both kidneys simultaneously, pose a special problem because they require a great deal of individualization. Conservative surgery, designed to preserve renal function, may reduce the chance of complete tumor removal and shorten survival. On the other hand, aggressive surgery may doom the patient to chronic dialysis and yet may be justified by a realistic hope of long-term survival.

Careful thought and individualization are essential in managing patients with a tumor in a solitary kidney or with bilateral synchronous tumors. Various options include (1) one or more partial nephrectomies, usually in vivo or occasionally by extracorporeal surgery and autotransplantation; (2) partial nephrectomy on one side followed by radical nephrectomy on the other; and (3) one or more radical nephrectomies with planned hemodialysis and possible later transplantation. The first step must be to assess the extent of tumor involvement completely. The operative strategy can then be chosen on an individual basis to accomplish an adequate resection, preserve renal function if possible, and at the same time offer the best chance of long-term survival.

Patients with von Hippel-Lindau disease

present special problems. Neurologic symptoms usually predominate and lead to urologic investigation. In these patients, the tumor of the central nervous system is a benign hemangioblastoma but may have associated renal cysts and multiple renal cell carcinomas. Because of early neurologic presentation, the renal cell carcinomas can be detected easily and are usually multiple and small. It is our policy to excise the renal tumors locally or, when feasible, by partial nephrectomy in order to preserve renal function. Follow-up consists of annual angiography, and subsequent reoperation is anticipated. In selected patients bilateral nephrectomy and subsequent transplantation may be considered if other manifestations of the disease appear to be controlled.

Precise assessment of tumor extent and source of blood supply allows preoperative planning that facilitates surgical excision for patients with tumors in a solitary kidney. Angiography in both the posteroanterior and oblique positions is most helpful. It provides a road map and usually allows the surgeon to determine preoperatively whether the tumor can be managed in vivo or whether ex vivo extracorporeal surgery is necessary. In most patients, complete excision can be accomplished in vivo. Care must be exercised in the amount of contrast material used at the time of angiography; surgery should not be contemplated until renal function has stabilized after angiography. CT scans may further help to localize the tumor mass but are not as helpful as angiography.

For in vivo excision we use the standard thoracoabdominal approach described in the section on the technique of partial nephrectomy. The details of this procedure are in Chapter 50.

In patients with bilateral synchronous tumors, usually one side is much more involved than the other. In these cases we like to perform partial nephrectomy first on the less involved side, followed several weeks later by radical nephrectomy on the other side. This sequence is chosen so that if the side undergoing partial nephrectomy temporarily shuts down, dialysis can usually be avoided. Once a renal scan or intravenous pyelogram (IVP) demonstrates good function on the side treated surgically, radical nephrectomy can be performed on the contralateral side. However, if function never returns to the partial nephrectomy side, a partial

nephrectomy must be considered for the remaining, more involved side or plans must be made for long-term hemodialysis.

The assessment of prognosis in patients with tumor in a solitary kidney or with bilateral synchronous tumors must be based on the management and assessment of each individual patient. Several studies have examined these issues, but different authors have reached different conclusions.

Since the report on conservative renal surgery for adenocarcinoma by Wickham[165] presented to the British Association of Urological Surgeons in 1974, there has been considerable confusion about the appropriate management of patients with tumors in a solitary kidney or bilateral synchronous tumors and about which factors might affect prognosis. Wickham's study reported that patients with a tumor in a solitary kidney, in whom the contralateral kidney was congenitally absent or was removed for benign disease, had a survival rate twice as high as that for patients whose opposite kidney was removed for renal cell carcinoma. However, his results did not take into account the fact that about two thirds of the patients (17 to 26) with a history of cancer in the opposite kidney did not undergo surgical removal of their present tumor, presumably because of advanced or unresectable disease. Management of these patients included no treatment (in eight), radiation therapy (in seven), and chemotherapy (in two). Yet of the remaining nine patients who were managed aggressively by partial nephrectomy, six (67%) were alive (range, six to 57 months; mean, 27.5 months) at the time of the report. Three had died: two at six and eight months, respectively, presumably from metastatic disease, and the other at one month from pneumonia. At postmortem examination, widespread disease was evident.

The idea that the pre-existing status of the contralateral kidney plays a significant role in patient survival was further perpetuated by Malek and associates,[95] who reported that, among operable patients, survival was half as long (3.2 vs. 6.7 years) for those who had a previous contralateral tumor as it was for those without a previous tumor. This too was misleading, because it reflected longer follow-up for the patients without a previous tumor: five of the seven surviving patients in this group had a minimum follow-up of six years (range three to 18 years), but the maximum follow-up was 3.5 years (range, two to 3.5 years) for the patients with a previous contralateral tumor.

In support of these authors, Marberger and associates[97] recently reported the results of the European Intrarenal Surgical Society (EIRSS) for 72 patients with tumor in a solitary kidney or bilateral synchronous tumors. They demonstrated that the survival of 36 patients with tumor in a solitary kidney whose contralateral kidney was removed for tumor was significantly poorer than that of 18 patients in whom the opposite kidney was without malignant disease.

Nonetheless, we believe that it is inappropriate to draw conclusions about survival rates based on the historic status of the opposite kidney without considering both the current treatment of the tumor and the adequacy of the resection. Our position is supported by the report of Schiff and associates,[140] who reviewed their own experience and the literature since 1968 concerning patients with bilateral tumors or involvement of a solitary kidney in whom the tumor was completely removed and renal function was maintained. Their results (Table 19–5) indicate that similar survival was achieved in all patients after complete surgical excision regardless of the condition of the contralateral kidney. They concluded that patient survival was directly related to the adequacy of tumor resection.

In the series reported by Malek,[95] 10 of 12 patients undergoing partial nephrectomy (seven with contralateral benign conditions and three with previous contralateral tumors) were without evidence of disease for up to 18 years (mean, 12.4 years). All of these patients had tumors confined to the kidney. Two patients died—one with Stage II disease at 1.5 years and one with Stage I disease at five years after enucleation of two tumors. In contrast, of the eight patients with advanced or locally unresectable tumors treated with biopsy, radiation, or hormonal therapy, most died within three years of follow-up. These figures further demonstrate that the stage of disease at the time of presentation and the adequacy of tumor removal are the most important factors affecting prognosis.

Recently, Topley and associates[156] from the Cleveland Clinic updated their results on partial nephrectomy in 27 patients with renal cell carcinoma. Of 23 patients who underwent complete tumor excision, seven previously had a tumor in the contralateral kidney, four had synchronous bilateral tumors, and 12 had a contralateral kidney that was either functionally impaired or congenitally absent. All these patients had either Stage I or Stage II disease, and no significant differences in survival were noted. The overall five-year disease-free rate was 70%. Of the 10 patients who died, four succumbed to disseminated disease, whereas the remainder died of other illnesses.

All of these reports, together with that presented by Smith and colleagues,[147] support the conclusion that prognosis correlates closely with adequacy of surgical excision in addition to the nuclear grade and pathologic stage at the time of surgery.

In a review of 25 patients with bilateral synchronous renal cell carcinomas, Wickham[165] reported that of the 16 patients who received no treatment, incomplete tumor excision, radiation, or chemotherapy, all were dead within five months of diagnosis. However, of the seven patients with surgically resectable tumors who were treated aggressively, 70% survived for two years. Schiff and associates[140] provide additional support for an aggressive approach, because 18 (85%) of their 20 patients with bilateral synchronous lesions who underwent complete tumor excision were free of disease, with an average follow-up of 30 months (Table 19–5). Jacobs and associates,[69] reviewing treatment results for 61 patients with synchronous bilateral renal cell carcinomas who under-

Table 19–5. RESULTS OF TREATMENT OF SOLITARY AND BILATERAL RENAL CARCINOMAS*

Status of Contralateral Kidney	Number of Patients	Number Alive and Free of Disease (%)	Average Follow-up (months)
Renal carcinoma, antecedent	16	12 (75)	31.3
Renal carcinoma, simultaneous	20	18 (85)	29.5
Benign disease	26	19 (73)†	69.3
Totals	62	49 (78)	45.7

*From Schiff MD Jr, et al: Treatment of solitary and bilateral renal carcinomas. J Urol 121:581, 1979, by permission.

†Two patients died of vascular disease after 10 years without evidence of tumor recurrence.

Table 19–6. SURVIVAL OF PATIENTS
FOLLOWING TOTAL SURGICAL EXCISION OF
SYNCHRONOUS BILATERAL RENAL
CARCINOMA*

First Author	Reference	Number of Patients	Five-Year Survival Rate (%)
Marberger	97	18	48
Zincke	169	13	61†
Jacobs	69	61	69
Topley	156	4	71
Schiff	140	20	85‡

*From Lieskovsky G, et al: Surgical management of renal cell carcinoma. In TA Stamey (ed), Monographs in Urology 5:98–125, 1984.
†Three-year survival rate.
‡Mean follow-up of 30 months.

went total excision of their tumors, similarly reported a favorable five-year tumor-free survival rate of 69% after a variety of surgical procedures. Others, including Marberger and associates,[97] Zincke and Swanson,[169] and Topley and associates[156] also reported excellent three to five-year survival rates of between 48% and 71% of their patients after surgical excision of all tumor (Table 19–6).

The concept of bilateral radical nephrectomy followed one year later by a kidney transplant may become more appealing with the availability of cyclosporin. Through 1977, Penn reported that 26 patients had received a kidney transplant after being rendered anephric for renal cell carcinoma.[123a] Of 11 patients, seven who were apparently tumor-free after at least 12 months of hemodialysis survived with functioning donor kidneys for a median follow-up of 29 months. The 12-month delay helps in patient selection: those in whom metastases develop in the interim are excluded as transplant candidates.

RADIOTHERAPY

Renal cell carcinoma is a relatively radioresistant tumor. The role of radiation therapy in the management of these tumors is unclear and at best remains controversial. Some authors have reported that preoperative or postoperative radiation therapy can improve survival over surgical treatment alone.[29, 46, 132, 159] Others have reported either no improvement or decreased survival with adjuvant radiotherapy.[18, 43, 44, 123, 135, 137]

In a prospective randomized study, van

der Werf-Messing assessed the effect of preoperative radiation therapy on survival.[159] Half of 141 patients with angiographic evidence of renal cell carcinoma received radiation therapy (3000 rads over a period of three weeks) followed by immediate nephrectomy, and the other half were treated by nephrectomy alone. The results of this study demonstrated that preoperative radiation had no influence on five-year survival, although it did reduce the incidence of residual tumor or tumor recurrence in the renal fossa.[159] The administration of 4500 rads of preoperative radiation has been shown to decrease the size of some tumors, as measured angiographically (Fig. 19–5).[7]

Transcatheter embolization with radioactive seeds has been used as treatment for locally advanced tumors.[83] Lang and de-Kernion treated eight patients with large Stage III tumors and 14 patients with Stage IV tumors by utilizing either radon or [125]iodine seeds, which were delivered at the time of diagnostic arteriogram. With a delivered range of 1600 to 14,000 rads, they documented shrinkage of primary tumor in all patients and measurable palliation in most patients. Weight gain and pain control were achieved in 75 and 80% of patients, respectively. Because of the low energy level of ^{125}I and rapid fall-off of dosage radiation, injury to adjacent organs is less likely than by external beam therapy. This method was well tolerated with minimal morbidity and should be considered for patients with locally advanced, unresectable tumors.

Some palliation of bone pain secondary to bony metastases can be achieved by radiation to the involved area. Dosages required for palliation are substantial, usually in the range of 4000 to 5000 rads delivered over four to five weeks.[21]

METASTATIC DISEASE

Approximately 25% of new patients with renal cell carcinoma will have radiographic evidence of metastases at the time of presentation.[144] In carefully selected cases, an aggressive approach to an apparently solitary metastasis seems justified, and radical nephrectomy should be performed in those patients, together with the surgical removal of their solitary metastasis.[107, 144] At the Massachusetts General Hospital, 40 patients

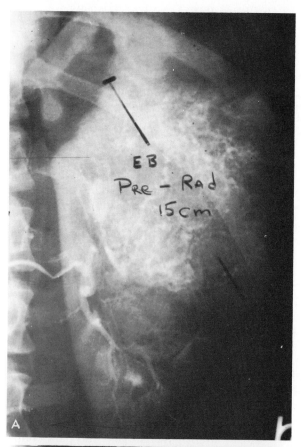

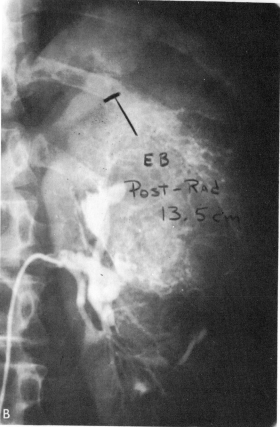

Figure 19–5. Selective left renal arteriogram demonstrates extensive neovascularity within a large renal cell carcinoma of the upper pole. The diameter of this tumor decreased from 15.0 cm (A) to 13.5 cm (B) after 4500 rads of preoperative radiation therapy. Courtesy of Dr. Edward Behnke. Reprinted from Brenner BM, Rector FC Jr (eds), The Kidney, 2nd ed. Philadelphia, WB Saunders, 1981, p 2125.

underwent 46 operations for the removal of one or two metastatic foci of renal cell carcinoma (Table 19–7). Thirteen of these patients (33%) were alive or survived more than five years following removal of their solitary lesion. From this study, it was also apparent that patients who underwent operations for an apparent solitary metastasis fared better when a significant period of time elapsed between nephrectomy and removal of the metastasis.

Considerable individualization is required in the management of patients presenting with evidence of multiple metastases from a primary renal cell carcinoma. An almost indisputable role for "adjunctive" or "palliative" nephrectomy is in the patient with disabling symptoms caused by the primary tumor. These symptoms include life-threatening blood loss secondary to gross hematuria, pain, significant compression of adjacent organs by local tumor mass, uncontrollable hypercalcemia, and heart failure secondary to arteriovenous shunting.[112] Palliative removal of vena caval tumor extension with nephrectomy may be indicated in patients with minimal metastatic tumor burden who are at imminent risk of right heart failure from atrial occlusion or massive pulmonary embolism.[127]

However, several factors should influence the decision to perform such an operation in these patients. First, relatively few patients have severe pain or hemorrhage from the primary lesion, and most of these patients have far-advanced metastases that produce equally severe and life-limiting symptoms. Secondly, the mean survival rate in patients with metastases at the time of diagnosis is approximately four months, and only about 10% survive one year.[37, 112] Nonetheless, in properly selected patients, excision of the symptomatic primary tumor can improve the quality of life.

The major debate concerns patients who have asymptomatic primary lesions and disseminated tumor, especially when such patients have extensive, nonresectable metastases. Some authors advocate nephrectomy in hopes of inducing spontaneous regression of the metastases and prolonging survival.[48, 55] The origin of this practice stems from observations on the natural history of the tumor, rather than from experimental or clinical trials. First, no effective therapy exists for the treatment of disseminated renal carcinoma. Since many patients are in the middle-aged group, the physician is frustrated by the prospect of not offering therapy, and this frustration prompts him to pursue drastic therapy that has only a remote potential for palliation. Second, the unusual natural history of the disease is well known and has been alluded to previously. Temporary waxing and waning of metastatic foci and appearance of distant metastases many years later suggest the importance of the host-immune mechanism. For poorly understood reasons, these observations have provided logic for the concept that the metastatic foci are dependent upon the primary tumor for sustained growth. Third, spontaneous regression of metastases has been reported in some cases. In a few cases, it apparently has occurred after the removal of the primary lesion.[16, 56]

Through 1973, approximately 40 acceptable cases of spontaneous regression had been

Table 19–7. RESULTS OF EXCISION OF METASTATIC LESIONS OF RENAL CELL CARCINOMA, ACCORDING TO LOCATION OF METASTASIS*

Metastatic Site	Number of Patients Treated	Number of Resections	Dead Within Two Years	Dead Within Two to Five Years	Number of Patients and Per Cent Alive after Five Years	Dead After Five Years of Metastatic Renal Cell Carcinoma
Lung	17	19	8	4	5 (29%)	1
Lung plus other site	4	8	1	0	3 (75%)	2
Opposite kidney	6	6	5	1	0 (0%)	0
Brain	1	1	0	0	1 (100%)	0
Retroperitoneum (renal fossa)	6	6	2	1	3 (50%)	0
Bone	6	6	5	0	1 (17%)	1
Total	40	46	21	6	13 (33%)	4

*From Richie JP, Skinner DG: Renal neoplasia. In BB, Brenner, FC Rector Jr (eds), The Kidney, 2nd ed. Philadelphia, WB Saunders, 1981, p. 2126.

reported.[16] All but two have involved pulmonary metastases, and 80% of the patients were male.[16] Most, but not all, instances of regression have followed nephrectomy, but in fewer than 10 cases has the diagnosis been made by roentgenogram only rather than with histologic documentation. It should be noted that the term *regression* as used by most authors does not mean complete disappearance or cure of the cancer, and it is difficult to know what role nephrectomy has in improving the quality of life for patients with disseminated metastatic disease with an asymptomatic primary lesion. Does partial or complete spontaneous regression of metastases occur with sufficient frequency to warrant nephrectomy in the patient with an asymptomatic primary tumor and evidence of multiple metastases? In a collected series of more than 1100 cases, Bloom[16] could find only three examples of spontaneous regression of metastases following nephrectomy (0.3%). In reviewing nearly 1700 cases at the Armed Forces Institute of Pathology, Mostofi noted that all but two patients with metastases at the time of admission were dead within two years, regardless of therapy.[115] In a review of 533 patients with renal cell carcinoma treated by nephrectomy at the Mayo Clinic, there was no instance in which a known metastasis disappeared following nephrectomy.[117] The mortality rate in these patients, who are often poor surgical candidates, is approximately 5%. When compared with the most optimistic and temporary response rates of 0.3%, the futility of the practice becomes obvious.

Delayed nephrectomy after renal tumor embolization has been used as a form of putative immunotherapy.[153] Swanson and associates treated 100 patients with metastatic renal cell carcinoma by angioinfarction of the primary tumor followed by radical nephrectomy.[153] Most patients were treated with progestins as well. Although no apparent statistically significant survival benefit was found from angioinfarction, they did demonstrate a 7% complete response and an 8% partial response. This 15% response rate is much higher than the reported rate of transient spontaneous regression. However, the limited response rate coupled with the estimated 2 to 6% operative mortality rate for radical nephrectomy in patients with metastatic disease precludes the widespread clinical application of this treatment modality.[56, 70] Survival of patients with metastatic disease appears to correlate with the volume and number of foci of metastatic disease. There appears to be no increased survival benefit accrued to osseous or pulmonary metastases.[153, 154]

Patients occasionally present with a limited number of metastases that are amenable to treatment by surgery or definitive radiation therapy. The five-year survival rate after excision of pulmonary metastases is between 25 and 35% (Table 19–7). Similarly, gratifying palliation can sometimes be achieved by therapy for isolated metastatic foci elsewhere. In the UCLA series, aggressive therapy of skeletal, solitary central nervous system, and skin or subcutaneous lesions produced a significant palliation interval.[36] It therefore seems reasonable to recommend adjunctive nephrectomy in patients who present with a limited number of metastases that are amenable to definitive therapy.

On the basis of the available data cited previously, nephrectomy for renal carcinoma in the presence of widespread distant metastases cannot be supported as a routine practice. Two situations, however, may be exceptions: adjunctive nephrectomy when metastases are limited to the skeletal system and nephrectomy after proven efficacy of a form of systemic therapy. In neither case has the justification for such a procedure been firmly established. Nephrectomy in the patient with a limited number of metastases that are amenable to definitive therapy may be justified in the patient who is a good surgical candidate. Finally, it is important to emphasize the only established indication for adjunctive nephrectomy is in the patient with a reasonable life expectancy who has severe symptoms from the primary tumor.

CHEMOTHERAPY

The chemotherapeutic treatment of renal cell carcinoma either as adjuvant therapy with radical nephrectomy or as treatment of unresectable or metastatic disease has not been shown to increase survival rate over that achieved by treatment without using chemotherapy. Harris reviewed retrospectively the reported activity of 38 different single-agent systemic chemotherapies in multiple series.[61] A total of only 92 objective responses were found in over 1000 treated patients. Vinblastine sulfate has been reported by Hrushesky and Murphy to be an active single agent with an objective response rate as high as 25%.[68] Carter and Wasserman reported in 1975 a 28% response rate among 25 patients treated with hydroxyurea,[24] but in a subsequent study no responses were found in 21 patients treated with this agent.[151] Most single agents have little or no activity against renal cell carcinoma.

Combinations of chemotherapeutic agents have been used in several clinical trials. Some combinations of agents used with vinblastine sulfate have occasionally shown better response rates that that of vinblastine sulfate alone, but duration of response has been short and significant morbidity has occurred from the toxicity of the agents.[36, 68, 103] Harris has reviewed the reported results of several studies of combination chemotherapy as treatment for renal cell carcinoma.[61] Response rates ranged from 0 to 30% for various trials, but none showed an objective increase in survival rate. The increase in toxicity may be greater than warranted for the small advantages in response rate that combination chemotherapy has over single-agent chemotherapy.

Intra-arterial chemotherapy has been used by Kakizoe and associates in treatment of pulmonary metastases in 12 patients.[71] By infusing various combinations of mitomycin C, carboquone, doxorubicin, and nitrosourea into bronchial arteries from one to nine times, they demonstrated a response rate of 42%. They observed no severe side effects, but mild bone marrow suppression, hair loss, nausea, vomiting, and anorexia did occur transiently in some patients. Intra-arterial chemotherapy as treatment for primary renal cell carcinoma utilizing 5-fluorouracil or actinomycin D has not been shown to be of benefit.[47, 85, 166]

In vitro clonogenic assay of human renal cell carcinomas cultured on soft agar and treated with various chemotherapeutic agents has been used to determine the in vitro chemosensitivities of these tumors.[88] Although Lieber and Kovach were able to grow 31 human renal cell carcinomas in soft agar and completed chemosensitivity testing in some of these, the overall usefulness of the assay was limited by the lack of an effective in vivo single chemotherapeutic agent.[88] Although this remains a potentially valuable research method at present, it has not been shown to be a clinically proven

method of choosing chemotherapeutic agents for treating patients with renal cell carcinoma.[86]

HORMONAL THERAPY

Hormonal manipulation utilizing progestational or androgen therapy has been used clinically for many years in hopes of improving patient survival. In 1947, Mathews and associates reported the development of kidney tumors in male Syrian golden hamsters by prolonged administration of diethylstilbestrol.[99] Bloom subsequently showed that an estrogen antagonist could inhibit growth of these tumors in the hamster.[17] Over the past 20 years, the role of androgenic or progestational agents in treating humans with renal cell carcinoma has become more clearly defined. In a review of 173 cases treated with progesterone or androgen, Bloom found that objective response rates ranged from 7 to 25%.[15] More recently, clinical trials using estrogen antagonists such as tamoxifen have been completed. At dosages ranging from 20 to 80 mg per day, an objective response rate of 0 to 16% has been reported.[2, 52, 84, 163]

Combinations of hormonal agents and chemotherapeutic agents have not shown any advantages over either group alone.[61] In conclusion, response to hormonal therapy is infrequent and responses do not improve survival to a significant degree. However, such therapy is relatively innocuous and may help a few individuals.

IMMUNOTHERAPY

The recent increase in knowledge of tumor immunotherapy may some day offer new hope for treatment response from immunotherapy. Patients may benefit from adjunctive immunotherapy of their renal cell carcinoma for two reasons: (1) renal cell carcinoma is apparently an immunogenic tumor, and (2) spontaneous regression and prolonged survival with metastases have been reported. This unusual clinical behavior of renal carcinoma indicates that innate host-immune responses may have a significant role in the natural history of the disease.

Several studies have been undertaken using bacillus Calmette-Guérin (BCG), a nonspecific immunostimulant that is injected intradermally. An occasional response to therapy has been noted, but there was no significant increase in overall survival compared with that for controls.[36, 109, 111, 113, 114]

Ramming and deKernion have described the use of xenogeneic immune ribonucleic acid (RNA) as a vaccine to supplement nephrectomy in patients with advanced disease.[129] The rationale for this approach was based on the observation that lymphocytes that have been sensitized by exposure to specific antigens will yield RNA capable of transferring specific immunologic activity to nonimmune lymphocytes. Hrushesky has also used xenogeneic immune RNA as a vaccine for adjuvant therapy.[67] Neither study has shown a significant impact on survival.

Patients also have been treated with vaccines made from special preparations of their autologous tumor cells that were processed or irradiated and treated with purified protein derivative (ppd), Candida antigen, or Corynebacterium parvum and injected intradermally.[36] McCune and associates treated 14 patients with metastatic disease with irradiated autologous tumor cells mixed with C. parvum as weekly injection.[102] An early response rate of 21% was reported. They noted that some patients under treatment had some metastases undergoing regression while others were stable or progressing. They suggested that an antigenic heterogeneity existed among renal metastases.[101] The efficacy of these vaccines has not been conclusively shown at this time.

Other forms of immunotherapy that have been used as treatment for renal cell carcinoma include transfer factor,[110, 111] serotherapy with the use of infused plasma from cured patients,[66] and interferon therapy.[36] To date, a definitive role for immunotherapy in the treatment of renal cell carcinoma has not yet been proved, but many studies are currently under way.[36, 101]

SARCOMA

Primary renal sarcomas comprise an uncommon variety of renal tumors. Overall, they constitute only about 1% of primary renal malignancies, being less common than renal cell carcinoma, Wilms' tumor, or renal pelvic tumors.[149] Collectively, they consist of leiomyosarcoma, rhabdomyosarcoma, liposarcoma, fibrosarcoma, hemangiopericytoma, and osteogenic sarcoma.[105] These tumors are usually of renal capsular origin. They exhibit rapid growth, although many tend to remain encapsulated. Invasion of the renal vein occurs in nearly 40% of patients with fibrosarcoma.[35] Leiomyosarcomas are the most common, making up about 50% of the sarcomas reported in two series.[42, 149] These tumors occur twice as often in females as in males and involve the right kidney twice as often as the left.[91] Although sarcomas are rare in children, they are usually seen at any age, ranging from 16 to 75 years. The most common presenting symptom is abdominal or flank pain; an abdominal mass, fatigue, and weight loss are less common signs, and hematuria occurs in only 17% of patients.[149] Evaluation and diagnostic workup is similar to that for renal cell carcinoma. Although no official staging classification is recognized, the one for renal cell carcinoma may be used.

Various forms of treatment have been used, including surgery, chemotherapy, and radiotherapy. Overall prognosis is poor despite therapy, with only occasional survivors among those patients who have had complete surgical removal of the tumor.[149] Metastatic disease occurs most frequently in the lung but also occurs in the liver, regional lymph nodes, peritoneum, and mesentery.[11] Combination chemotherapy with cyclophosphamide, vincristine, doxorubicin, and other agents could be considered for therapy, since various combinations of these agents have achieved response rate of 27 to 48% in soft tissue sarcomas.[149]

METASTATIC RENAL NEOPLASMS

Metastatic renal neoplasms are more common than primary renal tumors. Wagle and associates have reviewed 4413 successive autopsy records and have found 81 patients (1.8%) with secondary renal tumors.[160] Olsson estimates that lung cancer metastatic to kidney may be twice as common as primary renal cell carcinoma.[120] An autopsy record review by Bracken and colleagues of 11,328 patients who died of malignant disease found that 7.2% of patients had metastatic disease in the kidney at the time of death.[20] The most common tumor metastatic to the kidney is from the lung (27.5%). Other common primary sources include melanoma, breast, stomach, colon, pancreas, and contralateral kidney.[20, 160] In Wagle's series, microscopic hematuria was present in about 30% of patients and bilateral secondary renal tumors were seen in 50% of patients. Although these tumors are common, the symptoms are seldom severe enough to lead to clinical detection. They will, however, be detected more frequently with the increasing use of CT scans.

Renal involvement by lymphoma is also common, and Wentzell and Berkheiser reported a 53% incidence in patients with widespread disease.[164] Experience with renal arteriography in patients with lymphomas has been reported by Kursh and Persky.[78] The angiographic appearance is variable, ranging from complete avascularity in Hodgkin's disease to the orderly palisading of tumor vessels noted in more vascular lymphomas. However, only about 10% of the patients with lymphoma and renal involvement proven at autopsy will have had clinical symptoms referable to the kidney, and in less than 0.5% of these patients will renal infiltration be the main or sole cause of death.[133] Primary lymphoma arising in the kidney is extremely rare.

References

1. Abrams HJ, Buchbinder MI, Sutton AP: Renal carcinoma in adolescents. J Urol 121:92–94, 1979.
2. Al-Sarraf M, Eyre H, Bonnet J, et al: Study of tamoxifen in metastatic renal cell carcinoma and the influence of certain prognostic factors: A Southwest Oncology Group study. Cancer Treat Rep 65:447–451, 1981.
3. Anderson JB, Rasmussen T: Renal hemangioma diagnosed preoperatively by selective renal angiography. Acta Radiol [Diagn] (Stockh) 2:201, 1964.
4. Barbagelatta M, Chomette G: Renal immunopathology in renal cell carcinoma. Virchow Arch 404:87, 1984.
5. Bartley O, Hultquist GT: Spontaneous regression of hypernephromas. Acta Pathol Microbiol Scand 27:448–460, 1950.
6. Beh WP, Barnhouse DH, Johnson SH, et al: A renal cause for massive retroperitoneal hemorrhage-renal angiomyolipoma. J Urol 116:372–374, 1976.
7. Behnke E: Renal neoplasia. In BM Brenner, FC Rector Jr (eds), The Kidney, 2nd ed. Philadelphia, WB Saunders, 1981, pp 2109–2134.
8. Bell ET: Renal Disease, 2nd ed. Philadelphia, Lea & Febiger, 1950.
9. Bennington JL: Cancer of the kidney—etiology, epidemiology, and pathology. Cancer 32:1017–1029, 1973.
10. Bennington JL: Histopathology of renal adenocarcinoma. In G Sufrin, BA Beckley (eds), Renal Adenocarcinoma. A Series of Workshops on the Biology of Human Cancer, Report No 10 Vol 49.

Geneva, International Union Against Cancer, 1980.
11. Bennington JL, Beckwith JB: Tumors of the kidney, renal pelvis and ureter. In Atlas of Tumor Pathology. Washington, DC, Armed Forces Institute of Pathology, 1975, Fasc 12.
12. Bennington JL, Mayall BH: DNA cytometry on four-micrometer sections of paraffin-embedded human renal adenocarcinomas and adenomas. Cytometry 4:31–39, 1983.
13. Bissada NK: Renal cell adenocarcinoma. Surg Gynec Obstet 145:97–104, 1977.
14. Black HR, Heinemann S: Hemangiopericytoma: report of a case involving the kidney. J Urol 74:42–46, 1955.
15. Bloom HJ: Medroxyprogesterone acetate (Provera) in treatment of metastatic renal cancer. Br J Cancer 25:250–265, 1971.
16. Bloom HJG: Hormone-induced and spontaneous regression of metastatic renal cancer. Cancer 32:1066–1071, 1973.
17. Bloom HJG, Roe FJC, Mitchley BCV: Sex hormones and renal neoplasia: inhibition of tumor of hamster kidney by an estrogen antagonist, an agent of possible therapeutic value in man. Cancer 20:2118–2124, 1967.
18. Böttiger LE: Prognosis in renal carcinoma. Cancer 26:780–787, 1970.
19. Boxer RJ, Waisman J, Lieber MM, et al: Nonmetastatic hepatic dysfunction associated with renal cell carcinoma. J Urol 119:468–471, 1978.
20. Bracken RB, Chica G, Johnson DE, Luna M: Secondary renal neoplasms: an autopsy study. South Med J 72:806–807, 1979.
21. Brady LW Jr: Carcinoma of the kidney—the role for radiation therapy. Semin Oncol 10:417–421, 1983.
22. Brantley RE, Simson LR Jr: Angiography and histopathology of nephroblastomatosis. Radiology 120:151–154, 1976.
23. Busch FM, Bark CJ, Clyde HR: Benign renal angiomyolipoma with regional lymph node involvement. J Urol 116:715–717, 1976.
24. Carter SK, Wasserman TH: The chemotherapy of urologic cancer. Cancer 36:729–747, 1975.
25. Cherukuri SV, Johenning PW, Ram MD: Systemic effects of hypernephroma. Urology 10:93–97, 1977.
26. Conn JW, Cohen EL, McDonald WJ, et al: The syndrome of hypertension, hyperreninemia and secondary aldosteronism associated with renal juxtaglomerular cell tumor (primary reninism). J Urol 109:349–355, 1973.
27. Cooper PH, Waisman J: Tubular differentiation and basement-membrane production in a renal adenoma: ultrastructural features. J Pathol 109:113, 1971.
28. Cope V, Hackett M, Raphael MJ: Some observations on the value of excretion urography in the detection of renal tumours. Br J Urol 37:691–693, 1965.
29. Cox CD, Lacy SS, Montgomery WG, Boyce WH: Renal adenocarcinoma: 28-year review, with emphasis on rationale and feasibility of preoperative radiotherapy. J Urol 104:53–61, 1970.
30. Cranston WI, Luff RH, Owen D, Rawlins MD: Studies on the pathogenesis of fever in renal carcinoma. Clin Sci Mol Med 45:459–467, 1973.
31. Creevy CD: Confusing clinical manifestations of

malignant renal neoplasms. Arch Intern Med 55:895–916, 1935.

32. Cronin RE, Kaehny WD, Miller PD, et al: Renal cell carcinoma: unusual systemic manifestations. Medicine 55:291–311, 1976.

33. Cummings KB, Robertson RP: Prostaglandin: increased production by renal cell carcinoma. J Urol 118:720–723, 1977.

34. Daniel WW Jr, Hartman GW, Witten DM, et al: Calcified renal masses. A review of ten years experience at the Mayo Clinic. Radiology 103:503–508, 1972.

35. Deeming CL, Harvard BM: Tumors of the kidney. In MF Campbell, JH Harrison (eds), Urology. Philadelphia, WB Saunders, 1970, pp 885–976.

36. deKernion JB: Treatment of advanced renal cell carcinoma—traditional methods and innovative approaches. J Urol 130:2–7, 1983.

37. deKernion JB, Ramming KP, Smith RB: The natural history of metastatic renal cell carcinoma: a computer analysis. J Urol 120:148–152, 1978.

38. Dineen MK, Venable DD, Misra RP: Pure intrarenal lipoma—report of a case and review of the literature. J Urol 132:104–107, 1984.

39. Ekelund L, Lunderquist A: Pharmacoangiography with angiotensin. Radiology 110:533–540, 1974.

40. Ellner HJ, Bergman H, Alfonso G: Two cases of solitary giant tubular adenoma of the kidney simulating carcinoma of the renal parenchyma. J Urol 84:706–709, 1960.

41. Farrow GM, Harrison EG Jr, Utz DC, Jones DR: Renal angiomyolipoma. A clinicopathologic study of 32 cases. Cancer 22:564–575, 1968.

42. Farrow GM, Harrison EG Jr, Utz DC, ReMine WH: Sarcomas and sarcomatoid and mixed tumors of the kidney, in adults. Part I. Cancer 22:545–550, 1968.

43. Finney R: The value of radiotherapy in the treatment of hypernephroma—a clinical trial. Br J Urol 45:258–269, 1973.

44. Finney R: An evaluation of postoperative radiotherapy in hypernephroma treatment—a clinical trial. Cancer 32:1332–1340, 1973.

45. Fisher ER, Horvat B: Comparative ultrastructural study of so-called renal adenoma and carcinoma. J Urol 108:382–386, 1972.

46. Flocks RH, Kadesky MC: Malignant neoplasms of the kidney: An analysis of 353 patients followed five years or more. J Urol 79:196–201, 1958.

47. Freckman HA: Cancer chemotherapy: continuous intra-arterial infusion. Cancer Chemother Rep 28:57–66, 1963.

48. Freed SZ, Halperin JP, Gordon M: Idiopathic regression of metastases from renal cell carcinoma. J Urol 118:538–542, 1977.

49. Futrell JW, Filston HC, Reid JD: Rupture of a renal cell carcinoma in a child: five-year tumor-free survival and literature review. Cancer 41:1565–1570, 1978.

50. Gibbons RP, Montie JE, Correa RJ Jr, Mason JT: Manifestations of renal cell carcinoma. Urology 8:201–206, 1976.

51. Gleeson MH, Bloom SR, Polak JM, et al: An endocrine tumour in kidney affecting small bowel structure, motility and function. Gut 11:1060, 1970.

52. Glick HJ, Wein A, Torri S, et al: Phase II study of tamoxifen in patients with advanced renal cell carcinoma. Cancer Treat Rep 64:343–347, 1980.

53. Goldberg RS, Pilcher DB, Yates JW: The aggressive surgical management of hypercalcemia due to ectopic parathormone production. Cancer 45: 2652–2654, 1980.

54. Goldman SM, Gatewood OMB, Siegelman S: CT of renal carcinoma. In SM Goldman, OMB Gatewood, S Siegelman (eds), Computed Tomography of the Kidneys and Adrenals. New York, Churchill Livingstone, 1984.

55. Gonick P: Surgical therapy of renal adenocarcinoma. Semin Oncol 10:413–416, 1983.

56. Goodwin WE, Mims MM, Kaufman JJ, et al: Under what circumstances does regression of "hypernephroma" occur? In JS King Jr (ed), Renal Neoplasia. Boston, Little, Brown, 1967.

57. Guinan PD, Ablin RJ, Dubin A, et al: Carcinoembryonic antigen test in renal cell carcinoma. Urology 5:185–187, 1975.

58. Hajdu SI, Foote FW Jr: Angiomyolipoma of the kidney: report of 27 cases and review of the literature. J Urol 102:396–401, 1969.

59. Hanash KA: The nonmetastatic hepatic dysfunction syndrome associated with renal cell carcinoma (hypernephroma): Stauffer's syndrome. Prog Clin Biol Res 100:301–316, 1982.

60. Hand JR, Broaders AC: Carcinoma of the kidney: the degree of malignancy in relation to factors bearing on prognosis. J Urol 28:199, 1932.

61. Harris DT: Hormonal therapy and chemotherapy of renal-cell carcinoma. Semin Oncol 10:422–430, 1983.

62. Hellsten S, Berge T, Wehlin L: Unrecognized renal cell carcinoma: clinical and pathological aspects. Scand J Urol Nephrol 15:273–278, 1981.

63. Holland JM: Cancer of the kidney—natural history and staging. Cancer 32:1030–1042, 1973.

64. Hollifield JW, Page DL, Smith C, et al: Reninsecreting clear cell carcinoma of the kidney. Arch Intern Med 135:859–864, 1975.

65. Honey RJ, Honey RM: Tuberose sclerosis and bilateral renal carcinoma. Br J Urol 49:441–446, 1977.

66. Horn L, Horn HL: An immunological approach to the therapy of cancer. Lancet 2:466–469, 1971.

67. Hrushesky WJ: What's old and new in advanced renal cell carcinoma. Proc Am Soc Clin Oncol 18:318, 1977.

68. Hrushesky WJ, Murphy GP: Current status of the therapy of advanced renal carcinoma. J Surg Oncol 9:277–288, 1977.

69. Jacobs SC, Berg SI, Lawson RK: Synchronous bilateral renal cell carcinoma: total surgical excision. Cancer 46:2341–2345, 1980.

70. Johnson DE, Kaesler KE, Samuels ML: Is nephrectomy justified in patients with metastatic renal carcinoma? J Urol 114:27–29, 1975.

71. Kakizoe T, Matsumoto K, Nishio Y, et al: Chemotherapy by bronchial arterial infusion for pulmonary metastases of renal cell carcinoma. J Urol 131:1053–1055, 1984.

72. Kantor AF: Current concepts in the epidemiology and etiology of primary renal cell carcinoma. J Urol 117:415–417, 1977.

73. Katz SA, Davis JE: Renal adenocarcinoma: prognostics and treatment reflected by survival. Urology 10:10–11, 1977.

74. Kaufman JJ, Fay R: Renal hypertension in children. *In* J Johnston, WE Goodwin (eds), Reviews in Pediatric Urology. Amsterdam, Excerpta Medica Foundation, 1974, p 201.

75. Kaufman JJ, Mims MM: Tumors of the kidney. *In* MM Ravitch (ed): Current Problems in Surgery. Chicago, Year Book Medical Publishers, 1966, pp 1–14.

76. Keily JM: Hypernephroma—the internist's tumor. Med Clin North Am 50:1067–1083, 1966.

77. Kim WS, Goldman SM, Gatewood OMB, et al: Computed tomography in calcified renal masses. J Comput Assis Tomogr 5:855–860, 1981.

78. Kursh ED, Persky L: Selective renal arteriography in renal lymphoma. J Urol 105:772–775, 1971.

79. Kutty K, Varkey B: Incidence and distribution of intrathoracic metastases from renal cell carcinoma. Arch Intern Med 144:273–276, 1984.

80. Lang EK: The Roentgenographic Diagnosis of Renal Mass Lesions. St Louis, Green, 1971.

81. Lang EK: Arteriography in the diagnosis and staging of hypernephromas. Cancer 32:1043–1052, 1973.

82. Lang EK: Arteriographic assessment staging of renal cell carcinoma. Panminerva Medica 18:117–120, 1976.

83. Lang EK, deKernion JB: Transcatheter embolization of advanced renal cell carcinoma with radioactive seeds. J Urol 126:581–586, 1981.

84. Lanteri VJ, Dragone N, Choudhury M, et al: High-dose tamoxifen in metastatic renal cell carcinoma. Urology 19:623–625, 1982.

85. Leiter E, Edelman S, Brendler H: Continuous preoperative intra-arterial perfusion of renal tumors with chemotherapeutic agents. J Urol 95:169–175, 1966.

86. Lieber MM: Soft agar colony formation assay for in vitro chemotherapy sensitivity testing of human renal cell carcinoma: Mayo Clinic experience. J Urol 131:391–393, 1984.

87. Lieber MM, Tomera KM, Farrow GM: Renal oncocytoma. J Urol 125:481–485, 1981.

88. Lieber MM, Kovach JS: Soft agar clonogenic assay for primary human renal carcinoma: in vitro chemotherapeutic drug sensitivity testing. Invest Urol 19:111–114, 1981.

89. Loening S, Richardson JR Jr: Papillary cystadenoma of kidney. Urology 1:593–595, 1973.

90. Long WW Jr, Lynch KM Jr: Angiolipomas: a case report. J Urol 106:177–179, 1971.

91. Loomis RC: Primary leiomyosarcoma of the kidney: report of a case and review of the literature. J Urol 107:557–560, 1972.

92. Love L, Churchill R, Reynes C, et al: Computed tomographic staging of renal carcinomas. Urol Radiol 1:3–10, 1979.

93. MacDonald EJ: The present incidence and survival picture in cancer and the promise of improved prognosis. Bull Am Coll Surgeons 33:75–93, 1948.

94. Malek RS, Elder JS: Xanthogranulomatous pyelonephritis: a critical analysis of 26 cases and of the literature. J Urol 119:589–593, 1978.

95. Malek RS, Utz DC, Culp OS: Hypernephroma in the solitary kidney: experience with 20 cases and review of the literature. J Urol 116:553–556, 1976.

96. Mancilla-Jimenez R, Stanley RJ, Blath RA: Papillary renal cell carcinoma: a clinical, radiologic, and pathologic study of 34 cases. Cancer 38:2469–2480, 1976.

97. Marberger M, Pugh RCB, Auvert J, et al: Conservative surgery of renal carcinoma: the EIRSS experience. Br J Urol 53:528–532, 1981.

98. Marshall VF, Middleton RG, Holswade GR, Goldsmith EI: Surgery for renal cell carcinoma in the vena cava. J Urol 103:414–420, 1970.

99. Mathews VS, Kirkman H, Bacon RL: Kidney damage in golden hamster following chronic administration of diethylstilbestrol and sesame oil. Proc Soc Exp Biol 66:195, 1947.

100. McCullough DL, Scott R Jr, Seybold HM: Renal angiomyolipoma (hamartoma): review of the literature and report of 7 cases. J Urol 105:32–44, 1971.

101. McCune CS: Immunologic therapies of kidney carcinoma. Semin Oncol 10:431–436, 1983.

102. McCune CS, Schapira DV, Henshaw EC: Specific immunotherapy of advanced renal carcinoma: evidence for the polyclonality of metastases. Cancer 47:1984–1987, 1981.

103. McDonald MW: Current therapy for renal cell carcinoma. J Urol 127:211–217, 1982.

104. Melicow MM: Classification of renal neoplasms: a clinical and pathological study based on 199 cases. J Urol 51:333–385, 1944.

105. Micolonghi TS, Liang D, Schwartz S: Primary osteogenic sarcoma of the kidney. J Urol 131:1164–1166, 1984.

106. Middleton AW Jr: Indications for and results of nephrectomy for metastatic renal cell carcinoma. Urol Clin North Am 7:711–717, 1980.

107. Middleton RG: Surgery for metastatic renal cell carcinoma. J Urol 97:973–977, 1967.

108. Middleton RG, Presto AJ III: Radical thoracoabdominal nephrectomy for renal cell carcinoma. J Urol 110:36–37, 1973.

109. Minton JP, Pennline K, Nawrocki JF, et al: Immunotherapy of human kidney cancer. Proc Am Assoc Cancer Res Amer Soc Clin Oncol (Abst. C-258) 17:301, 1976.

110. Montie JE, Bukowski RM, Deodhar SD, et al: Immunotherapy of disseminated renal cell carcinoma with transfer factor. J Urol 117:553–556, 1977.

111. Montie JE, Bukowski RM, James RE, et al: A critical review of immunotherapy of disseminated renal adenocarcinoma. J Surg Oncol 21:5–8, 1982.

112. Montie JE, Stewart BH, Straffon RA, et al: The role of adjunctive nephrectomy in patients with metastatic renal cell carcinoma. J Urol 117:272–275, 1977.

113. Morales A, Eidinger D: Bacillus Calmette-Guerin in the treatment of adenocarcinoma of the kidney. J Urol 115:377–380, 1976.

114. Morales A, Wilson JL, Pater JL, Loeb M: Cytoreductive surgery and systemic bacillus Calmette-Guerin therapy in metastatic renal cancer: a phase II trial. J Urol 127:230–235, 1982.

115. Mostofi FK: Pathology and spread of renal cell carcinoma. *In* JS King Jr (ed), Renal Neoplasia. Boston, Little, Brown, 1967, pp 41–85.

116. Murphy GP, Mostofi FK,: Histologic assessment and clinical prognosis of renal adenoma. J Urol 103:31–36, 1970.

117. Myers GH Jr, Fehrenbaker LG, Kelalis PP: Prog-

nostic significance of renal vein invasion by hypernephroma. J Urol 100:420–423, 1968.

118. Nielson HO: Arterial hypertension due to a renin-producing renal carcinoma. Scand J Urol Nephrol 9:293, 1973.

119. Ochsner MG, Brannan W, Pond HS III, Goodier EH: Renal cell carcinoma: review of 26 years experience at the Ochsner Clinic. J Urol 110:643–646, 1973.

120. Olsson CA, Moyer JD, LaFerte RO: Pulmonary cancer metastatic to the kidney—a common renal neoplasm. J Urol 105:492–496, 1971.

121. Otto U, Baisch H, Huland H, Kloppel G: Tumor cell deoxyribonucleic acid content and prognosis in human renal cell carcinoma. J Urol 132:237–239, 1984.

122. Palma G: Paraneoplastic syndromes of the nervous system. West J Med 142:787, 1985.

123. Peeling WB, Mantell BS, Shepheard BG: Postoperative irradiation in the treatment of renal cell carcinoma. Br J Urol 41:23–31, 1969.

123a. Penn I: Transplantation in patients with primary renal malignancies. Transplantation 24:424, 1977.

124. Peterson NE, Thompson HT: Renal hemangioma. J Urol 105:27–31, 1971.

125. Pinals RS, Krane SM: Medical aspects of renal carcinoma. Postgrad Med J 38:507–519, 1962.

126. Price EB Jr, Mostofi FK: Symptomatic angiomyolipoma of the kidney. Cancer 18:761–774, 1965.

127. Pritchett TR, Lieskovsky G, Skinner DG: Extension of renal cell carcinoma into the vena cava; clinical review and surgical approach. Submitted for publication, 1984.

128. Rafla S: Renal cell carcinoma: natural history and results of treatment. Cancer 25:26–40, 1970.

129. Ramming KP, deKernion JB: Immune RNA therapy for renal cell carcinoma: survival and immunologic monitoring. Ann Surg 186:459–467, 1977.

130. Ramos CV, Taylor HB: Hepatic dysfunction associated with renal carcinoma. Cancer 29:1287–1292, 1972.

131. Riches EW: The natural history of renal tumors. In Tumors of the Kidney and Ureter. Edinburgh, Livingstone, 1964, pp 124–134.

132. Riches EW: The place of radiotherapy in the management of parenchymal carcinoma of the kidney. J Urol 95:313–317, 1966.

133. Richmond J, Sherman RS, Diamond HD, Craver LF: Renal lesions associated with malignant lymphomas. Am J Med 32:184–207, 1962.

134. Robertson PW, Klidjian A, Hardiny LK, Walters G: Hypertension due to a renin-secreting renal tumor. Am J Med 43:963–976, 1967.

135. Robson CJ: Radical nephrectomy for renal cell carcinoma. J Urol 89:37–42, 1963.

136. Robson CJ: The natural history of renal cell carcinoma. Prog Clin Biol Res 100:447–452, 1982.

137. Robson CJ, Churchill BM, Anderson W: The results of radical nephrectomy for renal cell carcinoma. Trans Am Assoc Genitourin Surg 60:122–129, 1968.

138. Roller MF, Stuppler SA, Kandzari SJ, Milan DF: Hypernephroma and associated ureteral involvement. Urology 8:575–578, 1976.

139. Samaan NA: Paraneoplastic syndromes associated with renal carcinoma. In DE Johnson, ML Samuels (eds), Clinical Conference on Cancer—Cancer of

the Genitourinary Tract. New York, Raven Press, 1979, pp 73–78.

140. Schiff MD Jr, Bagley DH, Lytton B: Treatment of solitary and bilateral renal carcinomas. J Urol 121:581, 1979.

141. Schrieber MH, Rea VE: The resectability of carcinoma of the kidney. Analysis of roentgen signs in 63 histologically verified cases. AJR 104:343–349, 1968.

142. Shapiro RA, Skinner DG, Stanley P, Edelbrock HH: Renal tumors associated with tuberous sclerosis: the case for aggressive surgical management. J Urol 132:1170–1174, 1984.

143. Silverberg E: Cancer statistics, CA 34:7–23, 1984.

144. Skinner DG, Colvin RB, Vermillion CD, et al: Diagnosis and management of renal cell carcinoma: a clinical and pathologic study of 309 cases. Cancer 28:1165–1177, 1971.

145. Skinner DG, Pfister RF, Colvin RB: Extension of renal cell carcinoma into the vena cava: the rationale for aggressive surgical management. J Urol 107:711–716, 1972.

146. Skinner DG, Vermillion CD, Colvin RB: The surgical management of renal cell carcinoma. J Urol 107:705–710, 1972.

147. Smith RB, deKernion JB, Ehrlich RM, et al: Bilateral renal cell carcinoma and renal cell carcinoma in the solitary kidney. Presented at Western Section AUA meeting. Vancouver, BC, July, 1983.

148. Smith RB, Machleder HI, Rand RW, Bentson J, Touba SP: Preoperative vascular embolization as an adjunct to successful resection of large retroperitoneal hemangiopericytoma. J Urol 115:206–208, 1976.

149. Srinivas V, Sogani PC, Hajdu SI, Whitmore WF Jr: Sarcomas of the kidney. J Urol 132:13–16, 1984.

150. Stauffer MH: Nephrogenic hepatosplenomegaly (Abstract). Gastroenterology 40:694, 1961.

151. Stolbach LL, Begg CB, Hall T, Horton J: Treatment of renal carcinoma: a phase III randomized trial of oral medroxyprogesterone (Provera), hydroxyurea, and nafoxidine. Cancer Treat Rep 65:689–692, 1981.

152. Sufrin G, Mirand EA, Moore RH, et al: Hormones in renal cancer. J Urol 117:433–438, 1977.

153. Swanson DA, Johnson DE, von Eschenbach AC, et al: Angioinfarction plus nephrectomy for metastatic renal cell carcinoma—an update. J Urol 130:449–452, 1983.

154. Swanson DA, Orovan WL, Johnson DE, Giacco G: Osseous metastases secondary to renal cell carcinoma. Urology 18:556–561, 1981.

155. Tan GC, England EJ, Low AI: Angiomyolipoma: a rare and interesting tumour of the kidney. Aust NZ J Surg 42:75–79, 1972.

156. Topley M, Novick AC, Montie JE: Long-term results following partial nephrectomy for localized renal adenocarcinoma. Presented at AUA meeting. Las Vegas, NV, April, 1983.

157. Umliker W: Accuracy of cytologic diagnosis of cancer of the urinary tract. Acta Cytol 8:186, 1964.

158. Utz DC, Warren MM, Gregg JA, et al: Reversible hepatic dysfunction associated with hypernephroma. Mayo Clinic Proc 45:161–169, 1970.

159. van der Werf-Messing B: Carcinoma of the kidney. Cancer 32:1056–1061, 1973.

160. Wagle DG, Moore RH, Murphy GP: Secondary carcinomas of the kidney. J Urol 114:30–32, 1975.

161. Walker DE, Barry JM, Hodges CV: Angiomyoli-poma: diagnosis and treatment. J Urol 116:712–717, 1976.
162. Walsh PN, Kissane JM: Nonmetastatic hyperne-phroma with reversible hepatic dysfunction. Arch Intern Med 122:214–222, 1968.
163. Weiselberg L, Budman D, Vinciguerra V, et al: Tamoxifen in unresectable hypernephroma: a phase II trial and review of the literature. Cancer Clin Trials 4:195–198, 1981.
164. Wentzell RA, Berkheiser SW: Malignant lym-phomatosis of the kidneys. J Urol 74:177–185, 1955.
165. Wickham JE: Conservative renal surgery for ade-nocarcinoma: the place of bench surgery. Br J Urol 47:25–36, 1975.
166. Wiley AL Jr, Wirtanen GW, Ansfield FJ, Ramirez G: Combined intra-arterial actinomycin D and radiation therapy for surgically unresectable hy-pernephroma. J Urol 114:198–201, 1975.
167. Xipell JM: The incidence of benign renal nodules (a clinicopathologic study). J Urol 106:503–506, 1971.
168. Zak FG: Self-healing hypernephromas. J Mt Sinai Hospital NY 24:1352, 1957.
169. Zincke H, Swanson SK: Bilateral renal cell carci-noma: influence of synchronous and asynchro-nous occurrence on patient survival. J Urol 128:913–915, 1982.

BRIAN E. HARDY, M.D.

Wilms' Tumor

In 1899, when the German surgeon Max Wilms wrote a classic monograph on mixed tumors of the kidney, he immortalized himself.[40] The tumor named after him was considered to have an almost hopeless prognosis until Ladd showed that aggressive and meticulous surgery could produce more than sporadic cures.[29] Gross furthered this work and, together with Neuhauser, demonstrated the susceptibility of the tumor to radiation therapy.[21] When Faber proved the value of adjuvant chemotherapy,[18] all three modern treatment modalities had been established. Although there have been numerous subsequent heroes in this field, most of the more recent progress can be fairly ascribed to corroborative effort, particularly to the National Wilms' Tumor Study (NWTS).

EPIDEMIOLOGY AND ASSOCIATED ANOMALIES

With an incidence among children in the United States of 7.8 per million per year, approximately 500 new cases of Wilms' tumor occur in this country annually.[41] This tumor affects males and females equally and shows no marked variation in incidence according to ethnic background or geographic location. The peak age for presentation is the third year of life. In the NWTS the mean age of onset for unilateral unicentric tumors has been 45.1 months.[10]

Wilms' tumor occurs in heritable and non-heritable forms.[10, 34] The generally accepted mode of inheritance is autosomal dominant. A review of the reported instances in which Wilms' tumor developed in two or more family members showed that the transmission pattern of familial Wilms' tumor was in keeping with an autosomal dominant gene with variable penetrance and expressivity.[34] It also has been suggested that the two-step mutational model of carcinogenesis is valid for Wilms' tumor.[28] According to this model, the nonhereditary form results from two postzygotic mutations in a single cell, whereas hereditary tumors arise as a consequence of one prezygotic mutation with a subsequent additional mutation in a cell of the target tissue, resulting in malignant transformation. All familial and bilateral Wilms' tumors are believed to have been hereditary, as are a minority (unknown percentage) of the sporadic cases. Although the risk that children of survivors of hereditary unilateral or bilateral Wilms' tumor have for developing the disease may be as high as 40%, the risk that survivors of sporadic unilateral Wilms' tumor have in transmitting the disease to children may be as low as 2 to 4%.[34]

This tumor occurs in association with a wide variety of congenital anomalies; aniridia, hemihypertrophy, and assorted genitourinary abnormalities are among the most frequently documented.[10, 35, 37] Among genitourinary anomalies, cryptorchidism and hypospadias are the most often documented lesions in addition to double collecting systems; fused kidneys are the most common urinary variants.[10] The difficulty with many of the other genitourinary anomalies that occur concomitantly with Wilms' tumor is that they also occur frequently in the population of patients without Wilms' tumor. The association of Wilms' tumor and gonadal dysgenesis is noteworthy because this association can possibly be explained by a common defect in the embryonic urogenital ridge.[38] Aniridia has been found in 0.8 to 1.4% of children who have Wilms' tumor of the sporadic type.[10, 35, 37] It has been established that a specific chromosomal deletion (11p13) occurs in those persons with the aniridia–Wilms' tumor complex.[20] Hemihypertrophy occurs in 2.5 to 2.9% of people with Wilms' tumor, and there is no indication that the laterality of the tumor and the hemihypertrophy are related.[10, 37] The predisposition of patients with hemihypertrophy to develop Wilms' tumor appears to be postzygotic in nature, but beyond this, a relationship has not yet been delineated.

DIAGNOSIS

The majority of children who have Wilms' tumor present to pediatricians for evaluation of abdominal distention or an abdominal mass. Other common symptoms at presentation are fever, abdominal pain, and hematuria. Rarely, those children with advanced disease may present with weight loss or gastrointestinal upsets. A significant percentage have hypertension, possibly due to renin production by the tumor but probably due to relative ischemia in the compressed non-neoplastic portion of the involved organ.

In addition to urinalysis, blood count, and baseline serum electrolyte and chemistry estimation, which should be routine in the evaluation of any child suspected of having a serious pathologic disorder, the following investigations play a part in the diagnosis and management of a patient with Wilms' tumor.

Ultrasound

Ultrasound should now be the first form of imaging invoked in the evaluation of a child with, or suspected of having, an abdominal mass. If a Wilms' tumor appears to be the diagnosis, careful attention should be paid to the renal vein, inferior vena cava, and right atrium during this study, which should detect a tumor thrombus when such is present.

Once the mass has been determined to be renal in origin, the investigative effort should be directed toward: (1) establishing the nature of the mass; (2) establishing the normality or abnormality of the contralateral kidney; (3) if a Wilms' tumor seems likely, determining the patency of the inferior vena cava and the presence or absence of pulmonary or hepatic metastases; and (4) establishing that there are no contraindications to surgery.

Intravenous Urography (IVU)

Prior to the advent of ultrasonography, IVU had a much more significant role to play than it does now. This study shows that a Wilms' tumor distorts the collecting system from within rather than from without (as with neuroblastoma). In comparison with neuroblastoma, there is less likely to be calcification and less likelihood of the mass crossing the midline.

Computer Axial Tomography (CAT Scanning)

Nowadays CAT scanning is essential to aid in the diagnosis of Wilms' tumor. This investigation will give the most information about the nature of the mass, its extent, and the presence or absence of disease in the other kidney. An enhanced CAT scan will also outline the collecting system of both kidneys and will show the presence or absence of renal function on either side. (It must be understood that this is a qualitative rather than a quantitative test of renal function.) At the same examination, the liver and lungs can be visualized for metastases. Usually, no other pulmonary evaluation is indicated.[12, 36] Patient cooperation is essential during CAT scanning; children between three months and four years of age require sedation. General anesthesia to attain the same ends is very rarely necessary.

Venacavogram

Cavography is rarely indicated in Wilms' tumor patients who are in large children's hospitals with excellent imaging equipment and personnel experienced in using it.[32] However, cavography is sometimes indicated to show the presence of a tumor thrombus in the inferior vena cava, particularly if the kidney is nonfunctional or if there is suspicion about the renal vein or vena cava on ultrasound or CAT scanning.

Liver and Spleen Isotope Scan

This study is still included in the evaluation protocol of many institutions to demonstrate the presence or absence of hepatic metastases. It should be recognized that such a study will very rarely show positive evidence of disease if results of the liver CAT scan are negative.

Renal Arteriogram

Renal arteriogram is not necessary in the presence of unilateral disease. However, it is indicated in bilateral Wilms' tumor, with Wilms' tumor in a solitary kidney, or with Wilms' tumor in a horseshoe kidney. The purpose of this imaging is to guide the surgeon in the planned excisional surgery.

Bone scanning is not routinely indicated in Wilms' tumor patients. We believe the only essential imaging needed for most Wilms' tumor patients is renal ultrasound and abdominal and chest CAT scanning.

Immediately prior to any surgery, the blood count should be rechecked in order to detect anemia and the possibility of platelet depletion. Renal function should be carefully evaluated in patients with bilateral disease and those with disease in a solitary kidney. Chromosome studies should be done in children with the aniridia–Wilms' tumor complex and should be considered in all patients with familial or bilateral disease.

PROGNOSTIC FACTORS

Because so few new relapses of Wilms' tumor occur after two years, a two-year disease-free interval is considered almost synonymous with cure.[8]

Pathology

Wilms' tumor arises from the multipotential cells of the metanephric cell mass. Classically, the tumors are composed of blastemal, epithelial, and stromal elements, but the ratio of these elements and the lines of differentiation of each element must be expected to vary from one tumor to another.[5]

Correlation of clinical data with pathologic specimens by the NWTS has shown that the histologic features of any given tumor can be classified as favorable or unfavorable with respect to clinical prognosis.[2, 3] The unfavorable variants of Wilms' tumor are those with anaplasia, clear cell sarcoma of kidney, and malignant rhabdoid tumor of kidney. All other histologic variants are currently regarded as favorable.

Anaplasia, or extreme cellular pleomorphism, was the major histopathologic criterion of poor prognosis in the first NWTS (NWTS I).[2] In NWTS I and II there were 769 cases without metastatic disease and without clear cell sarcoma or malignant rhabdoid tumor. The vast majority of this group who had no anaplasia had a death rate from tumor of 5%. Among 49 patients who had anaplasia, the death rate from tumor was almost 50%.[3] A more recent analysis of the same clinical material has shown an association between anaplasia and older age at diagnosis, non-white race, and advanced stage at diagnosis.[7] Anaplasia was associated with a very poor salvage rate if relapse did occur.

Clear cell sarcoma and malignant rhabdoid tumor of the kidney were originally considered to be sarcomatous variants of Wilms' tumor.[2] Subsequently, a plea has been made to consider them as distinct tumors in their own right.[3] Clear cell sarcoma of the kidney, unlike Wilms' tumor, frequently metastasizes to bone. Macroscopically, its cut surface is tan, in contrast to the gray appearance of Wilms' tumor. Its microscopic appearance is quite variable, but cytoplasm tends to be scanty and optically clear. The nuclei are round to oval and do not show frequent mitotic figures. There are fibrovascular septa forming vascular arcades that divide this tumor into cords or columns. There may be striking palisading of spindle cells around the vessels.[22] Clear cell sarcoma of the kidney is at least as malignant as anaplastic Wilms' tumor; 15 of 31 patients in the NWTS I and II died of tumor.[3] Malignant rhabdoid tumor of the kidney occurs mainly in very young children. This tumor has sheets, cords, and nests of cells that resemble rhabdomyoblasts because of their abundant eosinophilic cytoplasm and eccentric nuclei. The cytoplasm often shows a large hyaline, globular inclusion body. The nuclei frequently contain large "owl eye" nucleoli.[23] Malignant rhabdoid tumor of the kidney is extremely lethal; 19 of 21 patients with this tumor died in NWTS I and II.[3]

Staging

If a staging system categorizing patients with respect to extent of disease is to be clinically useful, it must have prognostic significance. The NWTS II showed two-year survival rates for Stages I, II, III, and IV of 95%, 90%, 84%, and 54%, respectively (without reference to the treatment given or other factors).[13] Although these figures clearly showed the overall prognostic value of the system, the differences between Stages II and III were not statistically significant. Consequently, there have been some alterations made to the staging originally used by the NWTS Group:[19] (1) lymph node involvement of hilus, periaortic chains, or site beyond has been upgraded to Stage III (previously hilus or para-aortic lymph node involvement was included in Stage II) and (2) tumor biopsied or local spillage of tumor confined to the flank has been downgraded

Table 20–1. CURRENT STAGING IN THE NATIONAL WILMS' TUMOR STUDY

Stage 1
Tumor limited to kidney; complete excision
Capsular surface intact
No tumor rupture
No residual tumor apparent beyond margins of resection

Stage II
Tumor extends beyond kidney but is completely excised
Regional extension of tumor
Vessel infiltration
Tumor biopsied or local spillage of tumor confined to the flank
No residual tumor apparent at or beyond margins of excision

Stage III
Residual nonhematogenous tumor confined to the abdomen
Lymph node involvement of hilus, periaortic chains, or site beyond
Diffuse peritoneal contamination by tumor spillage or peritoneal implants of tumor
Tumor extends beyond surgical margins either microscopically or macroscopically
Tumor not completely removable because of local infiltration into vital structures

Stage IV
Depositions beyond those of Stage III (i.e., to lung, liver, bone, brain)

Stage V
Bilateral renal involvement at diagnosis

to Stage II (tumor biopsy or any spillage was previously in Stage III, and gross spillage of tumor was and remains Stage III).

The current staging system for the NWTS is outlined in Table 20–1. Further modifications and refinements must be expected as the data base expands.

Regional Lymph Node Involvement

For those patients with Wilms' tumor who present without metastases, regional lymph nodes that show positive evidence of disease have long been known to be one of the most significant prognosticators of relapse.[8] This observation was confirmed by the results of the NWTS II.[9] In this study the mortality rate was 9.9% in patients with nodes negative for disease (or those not examined microscopically) versus 20% for those with diseased hilar nodes and 40% for those with affected aortic nodes. When regional lymph node involvement was examined as a single variable (negative versus positive), the results were 9.9% versus 32.2%, representing a threefold increase in mortality rates for those with involved nodes. A significantly decreased actuarial survival rate for patients with metastatic lymph node invasion has been confirmed by an entirely independent study group.[25]

Operative Spillage

The latest report on this subject from the NWTS shows significantly increased abdominal recurrence, relapse, and mortality rate associated with operatively spilled tumor.[9] Whether the degree of spill (local versus diffuse) is a variable is still to be determined.

Tumor Thrombus

The presence of tumor thrombus in the inferior vena cava or renal vein has been shown to have a very significant correlation to relapse.[9] The significance of intrarenal vascular invasion in the absence of extrarenal vascular involvement is not so certain.

Abdominal Spread

The surgeon's impression of regional spread of disease appears to be strongly linked to abdominal recurrence and mortality.[9] It far outweighs the pathologist's recording on the adequacy of surgical resection.

It is now thought that tumor weight as an independent variable does not affect prognosis. Likewise, age at presentation does not itself predict outcome, but it is associated with more critical factors that have led to the conclusion that children under two years of age tend to have a more favorable course.[9]

TREATMENT

The therapy for all Wilms' tumor patients at any stage should be planned with the intent to cure. Although adjuvant chemotherapy and radiation therapy have dramatically changed the prognosis of Wilms' tumor, it is significant that the term *adjuvant surgery* has not gained widespread acceptance. Surgery to extirpate tumor or, in rare instances, to prove that tumor has been eradicated remains the paramount therapeutic modality in the management of Wilms' tumor.

Surgery

There is much debate as to the best incision through which to perform a nephrectomy for this tumor. Two things should be borne in mind. First, as with any form of renal neoplasm, is the ability to adequately expose the upper pole of the kidney or tumor mass. This will determine how safely and efficiently the nephrectomy can be performed; hence the absolute necessity of placing the abdominal incision so that it can readily be extended into the thorax. Second, it is apparent from published surveys that up to one third of children with bilateral disease are thought to have unilateral disease prior to surgical exploration.[1, 6] Although CAT scanning will reduce this figure considerably, some contralateral tumors are so small and so peripherally placed as to be missed by any preoperative investigation. This makes full mobilization and visual inspection of all surfaces of the contralateral kidney mandatory. To achieve this, a transverse incision to (and often over) the abdominal midline is required. These twin objectives are beautifully summarized by the author who wrote that "surgeons who are experienced in the treatment of Wilms' tumor tend to use generous transverse incisions, with thoracic extensions if necessary."[30]

Once it is established that the disease is unilateral, the goal is to extirpate all tumor without causing spillage or embolism. A Wilms' tumor is frequently very fragile, and gentle technique is essential to prevent rupture. (Massive rupture clearly has an adverse effect on prognosis,[9] and local spill is currently under evaluation). Although all are agreed that the tumor must be removed intact if possible, there is evidence that radical nephrectomy does not offer an advantage over simple nephrectomy.[30] With accurate staging now playing a vital part in directing appropriate adjuvant therapy, any suspicious nonrenal intra-abdominal areas must be examined by biopsy. These areas include any abnormal lymph nodes, although formal lymph node dissection has not been advocated.[30] Local caval thrombi can be excised by venacavotomy after proximal and distal caval control is achieved. High caval thrombi and those involving the right atrium require coordination with a cardiac surgery team so that extracorporeal circulation is available. If the tumor involves vital intra-abdominal structures, no heroic resection should be performed. If accurate staging is performed and adequate biopsy material is obtained, appropriate adjuvant therapy can be instituted prior to a subsequent attempt at surgical excision with the high probability that the tumor will have regressed to a lower stage in the interval.[31]

Although it is always taught that the renal vasculature should be controlled first to prevent tumor embolus, this is only possible with smaller tumors. With larger tumors, not only the colon and its mesentery must be mobilized, but frequently most of the tumor mass must be gently dissected free from its surroundings and the operative specimen retracted laterally before the main vessels can be isolated. The artery and vein should be ligated separately to avoid arteriovenous fistulae. If possible, the artery should be clamped first, because interrupting the vein before the artery results in tumor engorgement with much increased bleeding from the tumor surface and an increased risk of tumor rupture.

Chemotherapy

In the treatment of Wilms' tumor it is now widely accepted that multiple-agent chemotherapy has significant advantages over single-agent therapy. The NWTS I clearly showed that the double-drug regimen of actinomycin D and vincristine reduced relapses, in comparison with results for either drug used alone.[14] The NWTS II corroborated this by demonstrating that patients with tumors in Stage II or III have a significantly higher relapse-free survival rate if treated with these agents in combination than they do if treated with either solitary actinomycin D or solitary vincristine.[13]

Stage I tumors treated with the combination of actinomycin D and vincristine for six months did equally as well as tumors of the same stage treated with the same drug regimen for 15 months.[13] Thus it was established that a six-month course of this combination of agents gives good results for Stage I tumors. Whether or not the treatment period can safely be reduced further is currently under evaluation.[15]

Patients with tumors in Stage II or Stage III, all of whom had postoperative chemotherapy, did significantly better if treated with 15 months of actinomycin D, vincristine, and doxorubicin (Adriamycin) than they did if treated for the same period with actinomycin D and vincristine without doxorubicin.[13] Thus this triple-agent therapy appears to offer advantages over double-agent therapy at this time. The possibility that the improvement recorded may have been due to more intensive chemotherapy overall rather than purely due to the addition of the extra drug is currently under evaluation.[15]

With the drug regimens mentioned above, it is clear that Stage IV disease does not respond as well as disease of a lower stage.[13] It is also clear that patients with unfavorable histologic results do not respond as well as those with favorable results of histologic examination.[7, 9] Hence, in children with Stage IV disease and in those with unfavorable histologic findings of any stage, the use of more aggressive and potentially dangerous chemotherapy is clearly justified. The NWTS is currently evaluating what advantage, if any, accrues from adding cyclophosphamide to actinomycin D, vincristine, and doxorubicin.[15]

Radiation Therapy

Initially, it appeared that patients in the NWTS who had Stage I disease, were more than two years of age, and were not treated with postoperative radiation therapy had a higher incidence of infradiaphragmatic relapse than those who were so treated.[14] However, this group of children had actinomycin D as their sole chemotherapeutic agent. Subsequently, a group of children with Stage I disease treated with a combination of actinomycin D and vincristine, but no postoperative radiation therapy, achieved relapse-free survival figures that exceeded those achieved with actinomycin D and radiation therapy. This result was independent of patient age.[13] Consequently, radiation therapy is not indicated for Stage I disease with favorable histologic results, providing the patients receive postoperative combination of actinomycin D and vincristine.

Following an analysis of the results achieved in patients with residual local disease (Stage III patients), it was suggested that local irradiation to the renal fossa was sufficient for those with disease limited to that area, but that gross peritoneal contamination required complete abdominal irradiation.[39] The earlier dosage recommendations have been modified. It has become apparent that 2000 rads are adequate for children under two years of age and that maximum response in older children is reached at 2400 rads.[15]

Currently in the NWTS, patients with Stage II disease of favorable histologic findings are receiving either 2000 rads postoperatively or no radiation therapy in an attempt to determine whether radiation therapy has any advantageous role. In this type of Stage III disease either 2000 rads or 1000 rads are administered postoperatively to determine if the higher dosage confers any advantage. All those with Stage IV tumors, and all with unfavorable histologic results regardless of stage, are receiving postoperative radiation therapy at dosages graduated according to age.[15] Liver, lung, brain, and bone metastases are irradiated at dosages determined by the site of disease and the size of the metastasis.[13]

For NWTS III protocol see Figure 20–1.

TUMOR IN A SOLITARY KIDNEY

Initial nephrectomy is contraindicated in a patient with Wilms' tumor in a solitary kidney. The principles of management are similar to those invoked with bilateral Wilms' tumor. The prognosis is likely to be

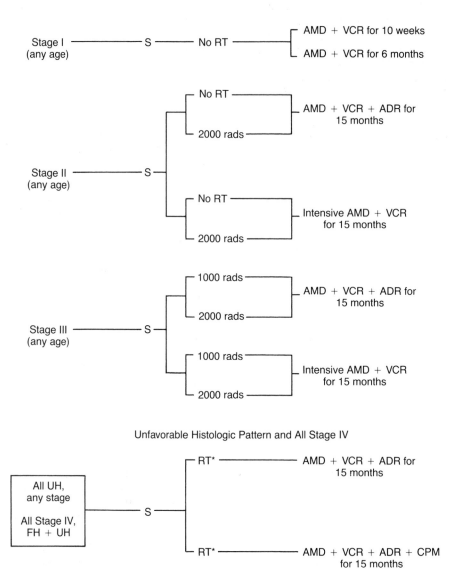

Figure 20–1. *Treatment protocol developed from the Third National Wilms' Tumor Study. Key: ADR = doxorubicin (Adriamycin); AMD = actinomycin D; CPM = cyclophosphamide; VCR = vincristine; RT = radiation therapy; S = surgery; UH = unfavorable histologic pattern; FH = favorable histologic pattern. Asterisk (*) denotes radiation therapy as follows: All patients with favorable histologic patterns, Stage IV, receive 2000 rads to flank and appropriate radiation therapy to other sites; those with unfavorable histologic patterns, in all stages, receive age-adjusted radiation therapy to the flank and appropriate radiation therapy to other sites.*

worse with a tumor in a solitary kidney than it is with bilateral Wilms' tumor, because the stage at diagnosis is likely to be higher.

BILATERAL WILMS' TUMOR

Bilateral disease at presentation is found in 4% of Wilms' tumor patients. In a further 1% the contralateral kidney will subse-quently develop a tumor.[10] Although it is commonly assumed that these bilateral tumors are the result of an inherited mutation, it has been pointed out that this is not necessarily so. They could be the result of the first oncogenic event occurring so early postzygotically as to affect embryogenesis on both sides of the midline.[10] Either cause would explain the marked association with anomalies such as hypospadias and with the earlier age of presentation than is seen for unilateral tumors.

It has long been clear that different therapeutic approaches must be employed for bilateral tumors and tumors involving a solitary kidney.[16] Even though tumor cure must always be the paramount consideration and must override all other concerns, it is also very important to avoid the anephric state if this can be accomplished simultaneously. Initial nephrectomy is contraindicated. It is well established that nephron-sparing surgery combined with the other therapeutic modalities provides excellent patient survival for synchronous bilateral tumors. An 87% two-year survival rate was reported for such patients in the NWTS I, including 19 survivors out of 22 patients left with residual disease after initial and subsequent surgery.[6] However, a more recent report on 18 children who also had synchronous bilateral disease showed four deaths occurring two years or more after diagnosis, indicating that the cure rate may not be as good as was initially hoped.[1] The prognosis for metachronous (asynchronous) bilateral tumors is currently under debate. Some claim a prognosis almost identical to that for bilateral synchronous disease,[11] whereas others show that it is worse.[1, 26, 33] As D'Angio pointed out in commentary on the article by Casale and associates,[11] the subsequent appearance of contralateral tumors is probably aborted nowadays by adjuvant therapy. Those that do break through such therapy can be predicted to be the more aggressive varieties of tumors, and a more ominous prognosis should be expected.

Two factors dictate the prognosis of bilateral Wilms' tumor. First, the vast majority of these tumors have favorable rather than unfavorable histologic features.[1, 11] However, this is not universal,[1, 17] and unfavorable histologic results here have the same significance that they do in unilateral disease. The second and possibly more cogent point was made recently. Many patients with bilateral Wilms' tumor will be found to have more than one tumor in each kidney, with the result that an apparently large tumor will be composed of multiple tumors, each of which is at an earlier stage than expected.[4] Multiple Stage I or II tumors have the same prognosis as individual tumors that have progressed to the same clinicopathologic extent. The stage of the most advanced tumor determines survival.[1, 11, 33]

The first step in treating a child with bilateral Wilms' tumor should be bilateral renal biopsy. The only exception to this should be those rare instances in which it is certain that all tumor can be excised and more than two thirds of the renal parenchyma can be left intact by bilateral partial nephrectomy. Stage is now so important in guiding appropriate chemotherapy that staging and obtaining tissue for accurate histologic diagnosis constitute the primary responsibilities of the surgeon. In addition to bilateral tumor biopsy material, any suspicious nonrenal areas, including lymph nodes, must be excised for biopsy. It will be obvious that needle biopsy cannot satisfy these needs.

Chemotherapy is mandatory in all cases and is continued for 15 months.

For those patients with favorable histologic results, the NWTS protocol calls for actinomycin D and vincristine for Stages I and II, with doxorubicin added for Stages III and IV.[27] CAT scanning is repeated every six to eight weeks, with the timing of repeat surgery dictated by the tumor response. If there is tumor growth, surgery is indicated at six weeks; if there is less than 50% shrinkage, it is indicated at three months; if there is good tumor response, surgery is deferred until that response ceases, but not beyond six months. The objective at re-explorative surgery is to conserve renal parenchyma while excising all tumor by biopsy excision or partial nephrectomy. If surgical clearance of tumor is achieved, no radiation therapy is indicated. If at the second operation it is not feasible to remove all tumor surgically without jeopardizing renal function, then excisional surgery is again deferred and radiation therapy is added, with 1500 rads given to the flank. A third operation is then undertaken, not more than six months from the second, at which time surgical excision of tumor must be achieved irrespective of the cost to renal function.

With unfavorable histologic findings, all tumor therapy must be more aggressive with less consideration given to preserving renal function than it is with favorable histologic results. Chemotherapy is again given for 15 months with the NWTS protocol (actinomycin D, vincristine, and doxorubicin for all patients, irrespective of stage),[27] and with 1500 rads administered to each flank. At the second operation all tumor must be removed even if radical surgery is necessary to achieve this. If a child diagnosed as having unilateral Wilms' tumor is found at surgery to have bilateral disease, then the planned nephrectomy should be abandoned and the treatment should proceed as outlined above.

Metachronous tumors should be treated similarly to synchronous tumors. They will, of course, be arising in solitary kidneys, making the clinician's job to preserve renal function more difficult. Clinicians should also suspect that patients in the metachronous tumor group are more likely to show unfavorable histologic signs (whether detected by pathologic examination or not) than are patients in the synchronous tumor group.

END-STAGE RENAL DISEASE

If a child develops end-stage renal disease in the course of Wilms' tumor therapy, then one should wait at least one year between the completion of chemotherapy and the commencement of the immunosuppression necessary to ensure a successful renal allograft.[16, 24] Peritoneal dialysis has been a major advance in making the achievement of this time interval feasible. An interval of at least this length is desirable to establish that the tumor has been cured and to allow the immune system to recover from the effects of the tumor therapy. If the immune system has not recovered, then it will be overwhelmed by the immunosuppressive agents, greatly increasing the risks of death from sepsis.

CONCLUSIONS

There is an ongoing attempt to improve cure rates by devising more intense therapy for high-risk groups while at the same time reducing overall morbidity by appropriately lessening therapy for low-risk groups. The unraveling of the epidemiologic and pathologic spectra of this tumor will make further refinement of treatment protocols possible. With the results of NWTS III released ahead of schedule, modification of what has been advocated up until now is certain.

Pretreatment after adequate biopsy and accurate staging is clearly indicated for bilateral tumors and for a tumor in a solitary kidney. Pretreatment is not indicated without biopsy or staging, because such a prac-

tice in the context of current knowledge is very likely to result in either undertreatment or overtreatment of the patient. Whether or not pretreatment is ever going to play a part in Wilms' tumor management with a normal contralateral kidney is not clear. The advocates of such behavior have not been able to show any survival advantage to date.

References

1. Asch MJ, Siegel S, White L, et al: Prognostic factors and outcome in bilateral Wilms' tumor. Cancer 56:2524–2529, 1985.
2. Beckwith JB, Palmer NF: Histopathology and prognosis of Wilms' tumor. Results from the first National Wilms' Tumor Study. Cancer 41:1937–1948, 1978.
3. Beckwith JB: Wilms' tumor and other renal tumors of childhood: a selective review from the National Wilms' Tumor Study Pathology Center. Hum Pathol 14:481–492, 1983.
4. Beckwith JB: Bilateral Wilms' tumor. Dial Ped Urol 10:4–5, 1985.
5. Bennington JL, Beckwith JB: Tumors of the kidney, renal pelvis and ureter. *In* Atlas of Tumor Pathology, 2nd ser. Washington, DC, Armed Forces Institute of Pathology, 1975, Fasc 12.
6. Bishop HC, Tefft M, Evans AE, D'Angio GJ: Survival in bilateral Wilms' tumor—review of 30 National Wilms' Tumor Study cases. J Pediatr Surg 12:631–638, 1977.
7. Bonadio JF, Storer B, Norkool P, et al: Anaplastic Wilms' tumor: clinical and pathologic studies. J Clin Oncol 3:513–520, 1985.
8. Breslow NE, Palmer NF, Hill LR, et al: Wilms' tumor: prognostic factors for patients without metastases at diagnosis. Results of the National Wilms' Tumor Study. Cancer 41:1577–1589, 1978.
9. Breslow NE, Churchill G, Beckwith JB, et al: Prognosis for Wilms' tumor patients with nonmetastatic disease at diagnosis—results of the Second National Wilms' Tumor Study. J Clin Oncol 3:521–531, 1985.
10. Breslow NE, Beckwith JB: Epidemiological features of Wilms' tumor: results of the National Wilms' Tumor Study. JNCI 68:429–436, 1982.
11. Casale AJ, Flanigan RC, Moore PJ, McRoberts JW: Survival in bilateral metachronous (asynchronous) Wilms' tumors. J Urol 128:766–769, 1982.
12. Cohen M, Provisor A, Smith WL, Weetman R: Efficacy of whole lung tomography in diagnosing metastases from solid tumors in children. Radiology 141:375–378, 1981.
13. D'Angio GJ, Evans A, Breslow N, et al: The treatment of Wilms' tumor: results of the Second National Wilms' Tumor Study. Cancer 47:2302–2311, 1981.
14. D'Angio GJ, Evans AE, Breslow N, et al: The treatment of Wilms' tumor. Results of the National Wilms' Tumor Study. Cancer 38:633–646, 1976.
15. D'Angio GJ, Beckwith JB, Breslow NE, et al: Wilms' tumor: an update. Cancer 45:1791–1798, 1980.
16. DeMaria JE, Hardy BE, Brezinski A, Churchill BM: Renal transplantation in patients with bilateral Wilms' tumor. J Pediatr Surg 14:577–579, 1979.
17. Ehrlich RM: Bilateral Wilms' tumor. Dial Ped Urol 10:8, 1985.

18. Faber S, Toch R, Sears EM, Pinkel D: Advances in chemotherapy of cancer in man. Adv Cancer Res 4:1, 1956.

19. Farewell VT, D'Angio GJ, Breslow N, Norkool P: Retrospective validation of a new staging system for Wilms' tumor. Cancer Clin Trials 4:167–171, 1981.

20. Francke U, Holmes LB, Atkins L, Riccardi VM: Aniridia–Wilms' tumor association: evidence for specific deletion of 11p13. Cytogenet Cell Genet 24:185–192, 1979.

21. Gross RE, Neuhauser EBD: Treatment of mixed tumors of the kidney in childhood. Pediatrics 6:843–852, 1950.

22. Haas JE, Bonadio JF, Beckwith JB: Clear cell sarcoma of the kidney with emphasis on ultrastructural studies. Cancer 54:2978–2987, 1984.

23. Haas JE, Palmer NF, Weinberg AG, Beckwith JB: Ultrastructure of malignant rhabdoid tumor of the kidney. Hum Pathol 12:646–657. 1981.

24. Hardy BE: Bilateral Wilms' tumor. Dial Ped Urol 10:7–8, 1985.

25. Jereb B, Tournade MF, Lemerle J, et al: Lymph node invasion and prognosis in nephroblastoma. Cancer 45:1632–1636, 1980.

26. Jones B, Hrabovsky E, Kiviat N, Breslow N: Metachronous bilateral Wilms' tumor, National Wilms' Tumor Study. Am J Clin Oncol 5:545–550, 1982.

27. Kelalis PP: Bilateral Wilms' Tumor. Dial Ped Urol 10:6–7, 1985.

28. Knudson AG Jr, Strong LC: Mutation and cancer; a model for Wilms' tumor of the kidney. JNCI 48:313–324, 1972.

29. Ladd WE: Embryoma of the kidney (Wilms' tumor). Ann Surg 108:885–902, 1938.

30. Leape LL, Breslow NE, Bishop HC: The surgical treatment of Wilms' tumor: results of the National Wilms' Tumor Study. Ann Surg 197:352–356, 1978.

31. Lemerle J, Voute PA, Tournade MF, et al: Preoperative versus postoperative radiotherapy, single versus multiple courses of actinomycin D, in the treatment of Wilms' tumor. Cancer 38:647–654, 1976.

32. Mahboubi S, Rosenberg HK, D'Angio GJ: Should inferior venacavography be performed in management of children with Wilms' tumors? Clin Pediatr 21:690–692, 1982.

33. Malcolm AW, Jaffe N, Folkman MJ, Cassady JR: Bilateral Wilms' tumor. Int J Radiat Oncol Biol Phys 6:167–174, 1980.

34. Matsunaga E: Genetics of Wilms' tumor. In F Vogel, AG Motulsky (eds), Human Genetics. New York, Springer-Verlag, 1981, pp 231–246.

35. Miller RW, Fraumeni JF Jr, Manning MD: Association of Wilms' tumor with aniridia, hemihypertrophy, and other congenital malformations. N Engl J Med 270:922–927, 1964.

36. Muhm JR, Brown LR, Crowe JK, et al.: Comparison of whole lung tomography and computed tomography for detecting pulmonary nodules. AJR 131:981–984, 1978.

37. Pendergrass TW: Congenital anomalies in children with Wilms' tumor: a new survey. Cancer 37:403–408, 1976.

38. Rajfer J: Association between Wilms' tumor and gonadal dysgenesis. J Urol 125:388–390, 1981.

39. Tefft DM, D'Angio GJ, Grant W III: Postoperative radiation therapy for residual Wilms' tumor. Cancer 37:2768–2772, 1976.

40. Wilms M: Die Mischgeschwülste der Nieren. Leipzig, Arthur Georgi, 1899, pp 1–90.

41. Young JL Jr, Miller RW: Incidence of malignant tumors in U.S. children. J Pediatr 86:254–258, 1975.

JOHN P. DONOHUE, M.D.

Diagnosis and Management of Adrenal Tumors

Adrenal tumors comprise a wide spectrum of benign and malignant tumors, including bilateral adrenal hyperplasia, benign adenoma, pheochromocytoma, adrenal carcinoma, and tumors causing primary hyperaldosteronism. The variability of clinical presentations of each of these makes differentiation on the basis of symptoms and physical examination both difficult and unreliable. The employment of biochemical assays and, more recently, radiologic imaging techniques is therefore of paramount importance in the investigation of adrenal disease. To complicate matters further, there are several extra-adrenal disease states (e.g., basophilic pituitary adenoma and ectopic ACTH-producing tumors) that mimic primary adrenal disease, thus making a careful preoperative evaluation essential. Perhaps for these reasons, adrenal pathology has fascinated both internists and surgeons over the centuries.

To gain access to the adrenal, numerous surgical approaches have been used, with the choice dictated by and tailored to the specific adrenal disease requiring surgery. The proper selection of the most appropriate surgical incision makes a definitive preoperative diagnosis essential.

PHEOCHROMOCYTOMA

Pheochromocytomas have been found anywhere along the distribution of chromaffin tissue, which is laid down during fetal development and has mostly disappeared by late childhood. The largest accumulations of chromaffin tissue are in the adrenal medulla and in the organs of Zuckerkandl, at the origin of the inferior mesenteric artery. Most pheochromocytomas are located between the diaphragm and the pelvic floor. In the sporadic, nonfamilial pheochromocytoma, about 80% of tumors involve a single adrenal, 10% are extra-adrenal, and 10% are malignant. For this reason they are sometimes referred to as the "10% tumors." In children, they may be called the "30% tumors."[9]

The catecholamines norepinephrine (NE) and epinephrine (E) are synthesized from the precursor amino acid tyrosine. Almost exclusively a property of the adrenal medulla, NE is converted to E by the action of the enzyme phenylethylamine N-methyltransferase (PNMT). Epinephrine constitutes 85% of adrenal catecholamine. Even though most pheochromocytomas arise in the adrenal medulla, the majority of tumors secrete primarily NE. However, if it is determined that there is predominant secretion of E, then the tumor almost invariably is located in the adrenal. A purely E-secreting tumor is extremely uncommon and difficult to diagnose since hypertension is minimal; in fact, some patients may present with shock.

The variable complex of symptoms experienced by a patient with a pheochromocytoma probably reflects the proportion of NE to E secreted. More symptoms result from secretion of E, whereas NE determines the level of hypertension. Nearly all patients have troublesome headaches, and excessive perspiration is almost as common. Other symptoms are palpitation, episodes of uneasiness or anxiety, pallor, flushing, weakness, nausea, tremor, chest pain, shortness of breath, and abdominal cramps.

As is well known, any one patient's combination of symptoms occurs in "spells" that may or may not appear related to precipitating events such as smoking, sexual intercourse, pressure on the abdomen, and defecation. Symptoms precipitated by micturition denote a location for the pheochromocytoma in the urinary bladder. Although paroxysmal hypertension is notable,[5-7] probably more than 50% of patients have sustained hypertension.[4] An orthostatic decrease in blood pressure in an untreated hypertensive patient suggests the diagnosis of pheochromocytoma, a finding also suggestive of primary aldosteronism. In some patients the single clue to the existence of a pheochromocytoma is a hypertensive crisis associated with pregnancy, the administration of a general anesthetic, surgery, or use of certain drugs. Such drugs as morphine, ACTH, parenteral guanethidine, and parenteral methyldopa may release catecholamines from the tumor, whereas propranolol may increase the pressor response to circulating E.

The diagnosis of pheochromocytoma is made from biochemical tests that can be performed on an outpatient basis. There are basically three measurements that are made of urine: vanillylmandelic acid (VMA), total metanephrines (normetanephrine and metanephrine), and free catecholamines. These tests provide important information and are nearly equal in their sensitivity and specificity. If all three are carried out simultaneously, 95% of pheochromocytomas will be detected. The urine must be kept acidic by prior addition of hydrochloric or acetic acid to the collection container.

The quantitation of catecholamines in plasma was previously carried out by fluorometric methods, procedures that required meticulous technique and large plasma samples and that frequently provided inaccurate results. A major advancement in this area was the development of the radioenzymatic assay for measurement of catecholamines. For this assay, plasma is incubated with an enzyme that transfers an ^{3}H-containing methyl group from S-adenosyl-L-methionine (SAM) to the catecholamine; the radiolabeled catecholamine is isolated and the radioactivity counted. The radioenzymatic assay used at Indiana University School of Medicine (developed by D. P. Henry) utilizes the enzyme PNMT to transfer an ^{3}H-methyl group from SAM to NE to produce ^{3}H-E. With this assay, measurements of plasma NE and urinary excretion of NE, including excretion measured in an easily collected morning urine sample ("sleep NE"), have clearly differentiated patients with pheochromocytoma from other hypertensive patients.[3] The measurement of NE can be made in plasma samples from multiple sites of venous drainage in order to find a tumor whose location has been elusive.

The radioenzymatic assay is making an important impact in investigative studies of the sympathoadrenal system, and it appears that it may in part revise our approach to the diagnosis of pheochromocytoma. Similar assays for important metabolites of catecholamines in plasma are under evaluation, and these may further increase our diagnostic accuracy.

The clonidine suppression test is another useful aid in the diagnosis of pheochromocytoma.[1] Plasma catecholamines are normally increased through the activation of the sympathetic nervous system. In pheochromocytoma, however, they arise through synthesis by the tumor itself, and the excess diffusion into the plasma bypasses normal storage and release mechanisms. Clonidine decreases resting plasma catecholamines by inhibiting centrally mediated adrenergic influences, and therefore it does not suppress catecholamine release in pheochromocytoma. This fact is useful in diagnosis of patients with essential hypertension whose catecholamine levels are thought to be neurogenically controlled and not mediated by tumor. Clonidine should suppress catecholamine release in essential hypertensives by blocking the central neurogenic release mechanisms. This is particularly helpful because clonidine suppression does not occur (i.e., plasma epinephrine and norepinephrine values are not suppressed) in patients with pheochromocytoma (Fig. 21–1A and B).[1] This test is fairly specific (i.e., few false-positive results). It is an adjunctive test that is useful in patients whose elevated catecholamines need to be distinguished from the subset with essential hypertension.

When the diagnosis of pheochromocytoma

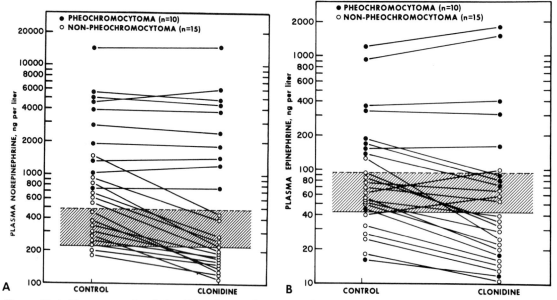

Figure 21–1. Plasma norepinephrine (A) and epinephrine (B) values in individual patients before and three hours after a single oral dose of clonidine (0.3 mg). The hatched area represents the mean of values obtained from 60 adult healthy subjects (+3 SD). To convert the norepinephrine and epinephrine values to nanomoles per liter, multiply by 0.006. (From Donohue JP: Surgical management of adrenal tumors. In EA Crawford, TA Borden (eds), Genitourinary Cancer Surgery. Philadelphia, Lea & Febiger, 1982, pp 9–19. Reprinted with permission.)

is firmly established, it has been our policy to attempt to localize it. Occasionally an intravenous pyelogram will show the tumor and, in our experience, computerized tomography can delineate most adrenal pheochromocytomas. In the past, our standard practice was to locate the tumor by arteriography; this has now been replaced by safer isotopic scanning with ^{131}I-MIBG, referred to later.[10] Knowing where the tumor resides and the anatomy of its blood supply allows the surgeon to better plan an approach.

Is arteriography dangerous? Not when carried out by an experienced radiologist and when patients are pretreated with phenoxybenzamine (Dibenzyline), an α-adrenergic receptor–blocking drug that has contributed greatly to the management of the pheochromocytoma patient. The dosage of phenoxybenzamine is determined by the antihypertensive response, and treatment should continue for a period of at least one week before adequate receptor blockade is achieved. Total protection against spikes in blood pressure is not attainable. During arteriography and surgery, preparation should be made for the administration of intravenous phenoxybenzamine (and propranolol if problematic tachycardia or arrhythmias occur). Use of propranolol should be limited

to situations in which α-blockade has already been established.

Improved techniques of computerized tomography (CT) have greatly simplified the diagnosis (i.e., localization) of pheochromocytoma. Despite these improvements, multiple, asymptomatic, or metastatic pheochromocytomas remained difficult to locate because prior imaging techniques were nonspecific. The advent of the radiopharmaceutical agent ^{131}I-MIBG permits scintigraphic localization based on functional principles.[10] This agent resembles norepinephrine in molecular structure and it is thought to enter adrenergic tissue by the same mechanism as the hormone itself. Incorporation in medullary tissue metabolic pathways localizes the isotope effectively for scanning. It has special value in localizing multiple, metastatic, or asymptomatic tumors.

Finally, a word is necessary about familial pheochromocytomas, since their characteristics differ in some ways from the more common sporadic type. Fifty per cent of familial tumors are bilateral, yet extra-adrenal locations almost never occur. The familial pheochromocytoma is more likely to secrete epinephrine, and in some instances this may be the only biochemical abnormality, which can make it difficult to diagnose. These tumors usually occur as part of well-recognized syndromes.

Multiple endocrine neoplasia (adenomatosis) type II (MEN II), or Sipple's syndrome, consists of pheochromocytoma, medullary thyroid carcinoma, and primary hyperparathyroidism. Pheochromocytoma is not associated with MEN I (pituitary, pancreatic, and parathyroid tumors); only hyperparathyroidism is common to MEN I and MEN II. A small percentage of patients with Recklinghausen's neurofibromatosis and von Hippel-Lindau's cerebellar hemangioblastomatosis will have pheochromocytomas.

In summary, routine biochemical tests can detect the presence of most pheochromocytomas. Once the diagnosis is established, subsequent interventions (localization and surgery) are best carried out by an experienced medical team after achieving adrenergic blockade with phenoxybenzamine.

Surgical Treatment

Preparation for Surgery. A team approach is required within the operating room—the team consists of internist as well as surgeon and anesthesiologist.

Preoperative treatment with phenoxybenzamine dampens or may even abolish the hypertensive episodes that can be associated primarily with induction of anesthesia and with handling of the tumor.

The adrenergic blockade created by phenoxybenzamine relieves the vasoconstrictor state produced by the excessive secretion of catecholamines and provides time prior to surgery for expansion of the vascular space. Thus, the profound hypotension that may immediately follow removal of the pheochromocytoma is for the most part prevented.

The management of the pheochromocytoma patient from the time of tumor localization and throughout the perioperative period is no simple matter. We emphatically recommend that these procedures be performed in hospitals that handle several such cases annually.

Transabdominal Approach. The author's preference is a high abdominal transverse incision, the so-called chevron incision, extending from the tip of the twelfth rib bilaterally up along the costal margins. Most bilateral adrenal exposures, together with paravertebral examination, will be obtained with this approach (Fig. 21–2).

To expose the right adrenal, the liver and gallbladder are retracted cephalad and the stomach and duodenum are drawn medially, after incision of the posterior peritoneum and development of the Kocher maneuver (Fig. 21–3). It is important to gently draw

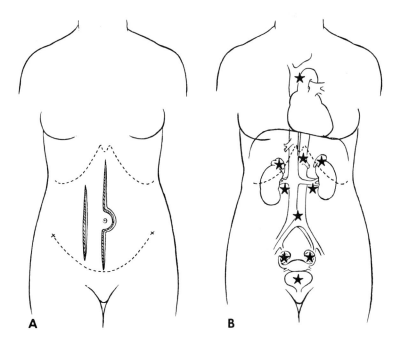

Figure 21–2. Schematic approach for pheochromocytoma. The stars represent areas of special interest. Anterior approach is required for checking contralateral glands as well as the ganglia in the paravertebral area. A thoracic aspect of this incision is very useful in large tumors, but, in smaller tumors, the incision can be basically transabdominal and transverse, with the approaches noted earlier. From Glenn JF: Adrenal surgery. In JF Glenn (ed), Urologic Surgery. New York, Harper & Row, 1975, pp 1–30.

A   **B**

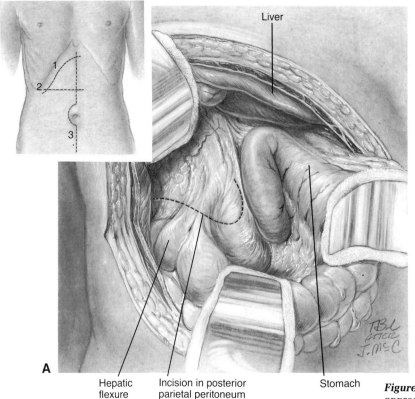

A

Liver

Hepatic flexure

Incision in posterior parietal peritoneum

Stomach

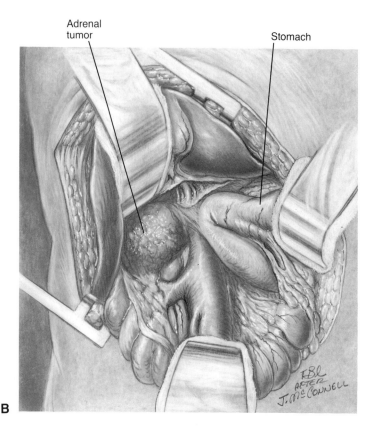

B

Adrenal tumor

Stomach

Figure 21–3. A, The right-sided approach is shown. Division of the colonic mesentery and right hepatocolic attachments allows the Kocher maneuver to expose the vena cava below the duodenum and head of the pancreas, which are placed in laparotomy pads. Retraction is medial and cephalad. B, Hepatic retraction with deep Harrington retractors is often useful with larger tumors. The coronary and triangular ligaments can be divided in unusual cases when high caval exposure is needed. Under such circumstances, the thoracoabdominal approach is necessary for control of the proximal vena cava within the pericardial sac. Here, also, hepatic arterial inflow needs to be secured by clamping the aorta above the celiac artery or cross-clamping the base of the celiac and superior mesenteric arteries. Usually, however, this approach (i.e., mobilizing caudate lobe from the rest of the liver, dividing small attachments between the two, then retracting the liver) will suffice to obtain proximal control of the vena cava and exposure above the large adrenal tumors. From Graham JB: Renal malignancies. In JF Glenn (ed), Urologic Surgery. New York, Harper & Row, 1975, pp 73–85.

the kidney caudad and develop and retract the inferior vena cava medially so as to obtain control of the right adrenal vein. It is also useful to identify and clip the small right adrenal arterial vessels as they arise from the origin of the right renal artery below the vena cava or directly from the aorta in this area.

The left adrenal gland may be exposed in the event of a small tumor by incising the posterior peritoneum and ligament of Treitz and dividing the inferior mesenteric vein. This allows cephalad retraction of the body of the pancreas in a deep Harrington retractor. The adrenal will be easily visualized just lateral to the superior mesenteric artery and medial to the upper pole of the left kidney. The left adrenal vein is easily secured, in most instances, through this approach (Fig. 21–4). If the left adrenal tumor is large, most prefer to incise the mesocolon and divide the lienocolic and lienorenal attachments and again mobilize the pancreas cephalad (Fig. 21–5). If the left adrenal tumor is quite large, it is sometimes best to continue the incision of the mesocolon cephalad to include the lienophrenic attachments. Furthermore, exposure is facilitated by continuing the posterior peritoneal incision above the spleen to the gastroesophageal hiatus. Then the spleen and pancreas can be mobilized in continuity cephalad and medially, thus exposing the entire upper retroperitoneal space. Occasionally, division of the short gastric vessels may be necessary to mobilize the adrenal completely out of the left upper quadrant (Fig. 21–6).

Once exposed, the tumor is removed with great care devoted to minimal manual pressure on the tumor itself. Ligatures and clips are preferred if at all possible, with gentle traction on proximal ligatures providing elevation of the tumor mass. With preoperative alpha blockade using phenoxybenzamine, this is somewhat less critical than it was formerly; nonetheless, it is still a very important consideration that will ensure stable blood pressure throughout the operation. Every effort is made to tie the adrenal vein first. Early opportunities to clip and divide small adrenal artery branches in the angle between the crus of the diaphragm and the renal artery should be encouraged. Once the essential vascular tributaries are divided and ligated, the tumor is gently elevated out of the wound. Every effort is made to dissect as widely as possible around the tumor capsule, even taking adjacent nodes and fat to a moderate degree. Because 10% of these lesions are malignant, we feel wide excision is better than capsular or subcapsular enucleation.

Closure of the wound is generally with size 0 nonabsorbable suture material. The authors prefer running suture to the peritoneum, transverse muscle, and the sheath of the posterior rectus abdominis. Several interrupted 0 sutures are placed at the midline in figure-of-eight fashion. The anterior rectus sheath is closed with interrupted 0 nonabsorbable suture, as are the internal and external oblique muscles. The subcutaneous tissue is closed with interrupted 3–0 chromic catgut, and the skin is closed with vertical interrupted skin staples.

Postoperative considerations include careful monitoring of the central venous pressure. We prefer a Swan-Ganz catheter for optimal central wedge pressure. We also use intra-arterial lines from the moment of surgical induction to one or two days postoperatively. Hypotension is an exceedingly rare occurrence, because these patients are generally treated for two weeks preoperatively with phenoxybenzamine. Some workers avoid preoperative adrenergic blockade, preferring to transfuse patients perioperatively following tumor removal with whole blood and colloid to manage the drops in pressure in these patients. Their rationale is that the palpation for other tumors is more effective in the patient who has not undergone adrenergic blockade. Because multiple tumors occur only 10% of the time and CAT scanning is highly effective in localizing retroperitoneal tumors, we have avoided the uncertainties of this approach with its attendant risk of hepatitis and pressure swings.

Finally, a team approach cannot be overemphasized. Internists, anesthesiologists, and urologic surgeons, all with an endocrine background and experience, make up the ideal combination for managing a patient both preoperatively and postoperatively.

ADRENAL CORTEX

Aldosteronism

Primary aldosteronism is characterized by hypertension secondary to inappropriate,

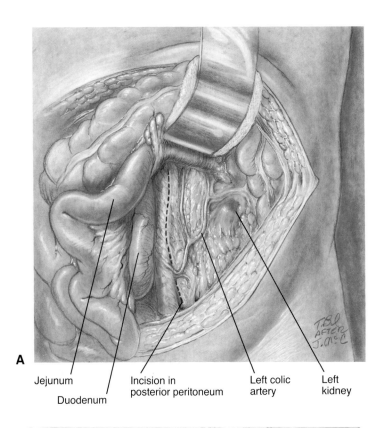

A

Jejunum   Incision in   Left colic   Left
          posterior peritoneum   artery   kidney
     Duodenum

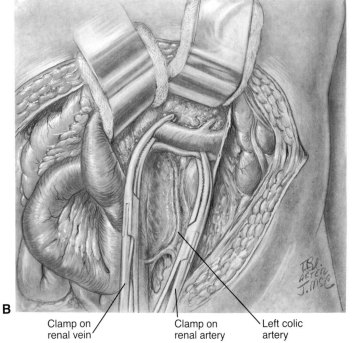

B

Clamp on   Clamp on   Left colic
renal vein   renal artery   artery

Figure 21–4. A, The transmesenteric approach to the adrenal is here shown for left-sided lesions. The root of the small bowel is divided, and the inferior mesenteric vein is divided between silk ligatures. B, An incision below the pancreas, of the posterior peritoneum and of the left colonic mesentery, is done so as to elevate the pancreas and expose the left renal vein and adrenal vein. This is a practical approach, particularly for small adrenal tumors on the left that can be approached transabdominally. From Graham JB: Renal malignancies. In JF Glenn (ed), Urologic Surgery. New York, Harper & Row, 1975, pp 73–85.

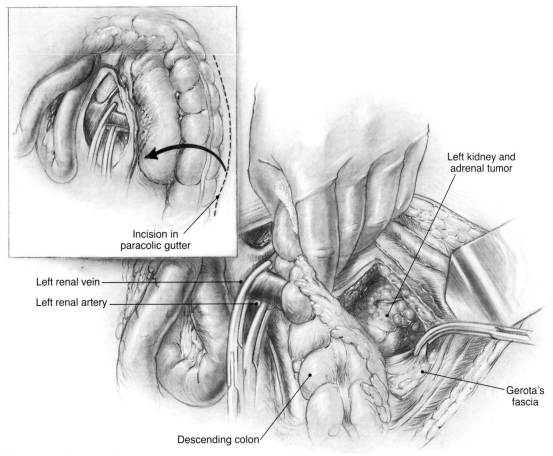

Incision in
paracolic gutter

Left kidney and
adrenal tumor

Left renal vein

Left renal artery

Gerota's
fascia

Descending colon

Figure 21–5. For left-sided tumors, the colon is reflected medially by dividing the left mesocolon and the lienocolic attachments. This standard anterior approach to both the kidney and adrenal is useful, for example, on donor nephrectomy.

excessive production of aldosterone by the zona glomerulosa of the adrenal cortex. As a result, it is associated with suppression of plasma renin activity, hypokalemia in most patients, and often metabolic alkalosis. Although primary aldosteronism here refers to the effect of a functional adrenal adenoma, it can also be caused by bilateral micronodular hyperplasia of zona glomerulosa cells in both adrenal glands. This is thought to occur in about 20% of the patients with chemical aldosteronism.

Major clinical features are benign elevation of arterial blood pressure, usually in the absence of severe vascular disease. Urinary aldosterone and potassium excretion are elevated; likewise, plasma aldosterone is elevated, but serum potassium levels are reduced. Although relative hypervolemia exists (secondary to increased sodium resorption at the proximal tubular level in

exchange for potassium), hypernatremia is only mild, and metabolic alkalosis is often not severe. Both normokalemic and nonalkalotic forms have also been recognized. This usually occurs in patients between 30 and 60 years of age; there are few reports in children. The most common symptom is relative muscle weakness, and the most common sign is hypertension.

The key to establishing the diagnosis is finding elevated levels of urinary and plasma aldosterone together with unprovoked hypokalemia. The other major criterion required for diagnosis is suppression of renal renin production. The two most reliable tests for primary aldosteronism are (1) failure to suppress aldosterone output during sodium loading (saline suppression test, i.e., 2 L per 2 to 3 hours) and (2) a failure to stimulate plasma renin activity, even in the face of sodium deprivation (negative furosemide

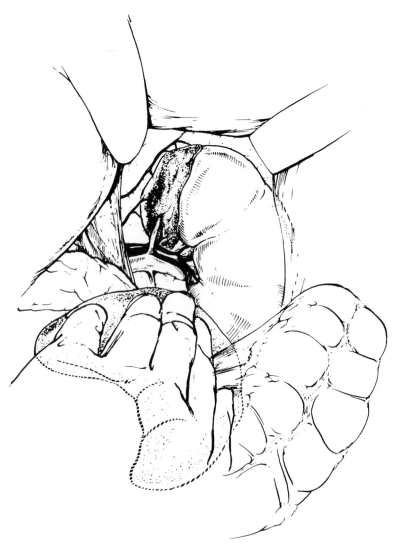

Figure 21–6. *Enlarged left-sided lesions require special exposure, with visualization of the celiac axis, superior mesenteric artery, and upper aorta. Additional incision beyond the mesocolon to include the lienophrenic attachments, extending even to the gastroesophageal hiatus in the diaphragm, will allow mobilization of the stomach, spleen, and pancreas medially (indeed, placement in the right side). Separation of the posterior peritoneum from the anterior aspect of Gerota's fascia will provide superb exposure of the upper aorta and crural aspect of the diaphragm. This is not often needed, except in large tumors or special situations in which control is needed in the area of the superior mesenteric artery and celiac axis. From Glenn JF, Peterson RE, Mannix H Jr: Surgery of the Adrenal Gland. New York, Macmillan, 1968, p 158.*

[Lasix] stimulation test) (Fig. 21–7). Therefore, the sine qua non of the diagnosis of primary aldosteronism is failure to suppress plasma aldosterone after saline loading (2 L per 3 hours) and failure of plasma renin activity to be stimulated by salt and volume depletion (40 mg furosemide every 8 hours, 10 mEq sodium diet for 24 hours, and 2 hours of ambulation). These rigid criteria positively identified some 55 patients with primary aldosteronism, and adrenal adenomas were proved by surgical removal (Fig. 21–8).

Once the diagnosis of aldosteronism is confirmed by negative results for both the saline (aldosterone) suppression test and the furosemide (renin) stimulation test, the next major step is localization of the disease. The two best localizing techniques in our experience are adrenal venous blood collections for aldosterone (with cortisol levels as a check on the accuracy of the sample) and adrenal venography.

Medical Treatment

Surgical treatment is best reserved for those patients diagnosed as having unilateral disease. As noted, the differential adrenal venous sampling and venography can provide diagnostic accuracy in more than 90% of the patients. Those with bilateral hyperplasia (excessive aldosterone production from both adrenals in the absence of any adenoma noted on venography) are best

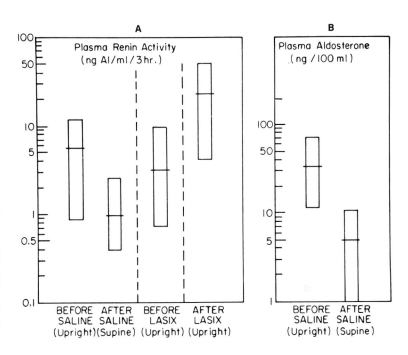

Figure 21-7. Values of renin and aldosterone in homeostatic, stimulated, and suppressed states *(Lasix stimulation and saline suppression).* Ranges are normal ± 1 SD, and values have been established in over 350 normal subjects. Ranges for these subjects allow discrimination of abnormal responses in those who might otherwise fall within the range of normal under homeostatic or unchallenged conditions. From Donohue JP: Surgical management of adrenal tumors. In ED Crawford and TA Borden (eds), *Genitourinary Cancer Surgery.* Philadelphia, Lea & Febiger, 1982, pp 9–19.

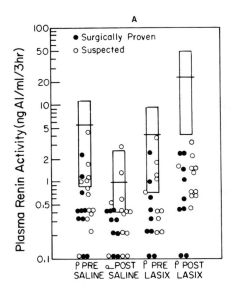

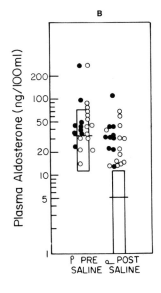

Figure 21-8. Normal values for plasma renin and plasma aldosterone activities in normal subjects and in patients with proven primary aldosteronism. Note the overlap of values within the normal range in the unstimulated or unsuppressed state with the patient under homeostatic conditions. Also note the failure of patients with primary aldosteronism to respond normally to Lasix stimulation of the renin system and to the saline suppression of plasma aldosterone. These stimulation and suppression maneuvers accurately identify those patients with primary aldosteronism. From Donohue JP: Surgical management of adrenal tumors. In ED Crawford and TA Borden (eds), *Genitourinary Cancer Surgery.* Philadelphia, Lea & Febiger, 1982, pp 9–19.

treated medically with spironolactone orally, ranging from 100 to 400 mg/day.

Surgical Treatment

In the usual case, the approach is dorsal. With the patient in the prone position, the pyelograms are reviewed and the suitable rib is chosen for subperiosteal excision. Usually, this is the twelfth rib, or the eleventh rib in a large patient, particularly on the left. The rib is removed as proximal as possible near its articulation to facilitate exposure (Figs. 21–9 to 21–11).

A key point in exposure of the adrenal through the dorsal route is the caudal mobilization of the kidney and adrenal without entering Gerota's fascia. With a hand or sponge stick placed medial and caudad in the apex of the wound, the kidney and other contents within Gerota's fascia can be drawn posteriorly and laterally. Such posterolateral retraction of the kidney will allow separation of the superior aspect of the adrenal from the diaphragm and hepatic structures

on the right and from the pancreas on the left. Very gentle dissection with forceps is satisfactory before Harrington or malleable retractors are placed on the liver or pancreas. Narrow or broad Deaver retractors are sometimes useful medially. Vascular clips and silk ligatures are used for proximal traction on the adrenal. The structures are tied in continuity by passing a right-angle clamp below the tissue to be tied and ligating with 2–0 black silk on the proximal or gland side. Vascular clips are used on the body wall or renal side. This allows meticulous dissection without blood loss. Every effort must be made not to manipulate the gland itself. Any rough movements may cause swelling within the gland and subsequent difficulty in identifying adenomas. Even slight spillage of blood into tissue planes may obscure the edges of the gland. If spillage occurs, copious irrigations may be used to clean off tissue planes.

The common adrenal vein is often the last portion of the dissection, particularly when the right adrenal is mobilized. Once the

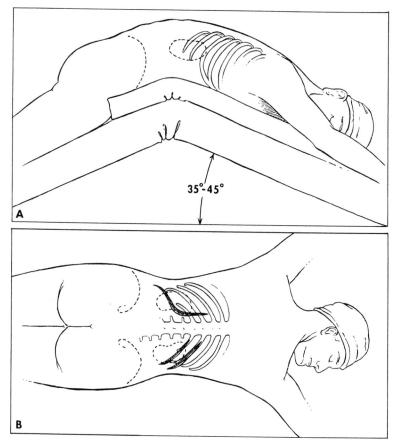

Figure 21–9. The dorsal approach to the adrenals. The patient is in the prone position. The incision is over the eleventh or twelfth rib, which is excised subperiosteally. From Glenn JF: Adrenal Surgery. In JF Glenn (ed), Urologic Surgery. New York, Harper & Row, 1975, pp 1–30.

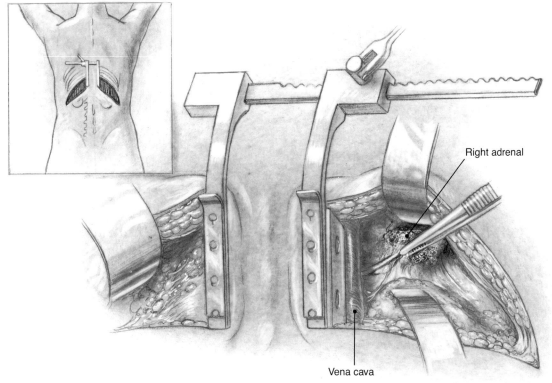

Figure 21–10. *Via the dorsal approach, the adrenal is exposed by caudad retraction of the kidney with either a sponge stick or the surgeon's hands, with care being taken not to separate the adrenal from the kidney initially. The first separations are from the cephalad and medial attachments of the adrenal.*

gland has been fully mobilized, the common right adrenal vein is secured between 2–0 silk ligatures. When the vein is more apical, its early division and removal provide better glandular mobilization. Should venous length be a problem, one can doubly clip the venous structures on either side and divide between them. Usually, with gentle elevation one can achieve enough length for double ligatures.

If the pleural cavity has been entered, both the parietal and diaphragmatic closures are made with nonabsorbable sutures. Air in the pleural space is evacuated through a small red-rubber catheter. During positive-pressure lung inflation, the tube is removed. Normally, a chest tube is not necessary postoperatively. The only special consideration postoperatively is the need to obtain serum potassium determinations twice a day for the first several days. Hyperkalemia secondary to suppression of the contralateral zona glomerulosa is rare. For the same reason, replacement therapy with mineralocorticoids has not been necessary. Over 80% of patients become normotensive within sev-

eral weeks postoperatively. When a unilateral adenoma is clearly localized, a good result can be expected from surgery.

Cushing's Syndrome

Cushing's syndrome is a general term referring to the clinical presentation of corticosteroid excess. This can be produced by administration of glucocorticoid, or it may occur naturally from several pathologic dysfunctional states. A basophilic pituitary adenoma was described by Harvey Cushing as the cause of the syndrome he originally reported, and this tumor is responsible for about two thirds of the patients presenting with this process. Other natural causes can be adrenal tumors producing excess cortisol or other benign or malignant tumors producing ACTH.

The clinical presentation is classic. Prominent findings are truncal obesity with muscle wasting of the peripheral extremities, out of keeping with the central obesity. Plethora, hypertension, and increased bruising and striae are also prominent features. In the

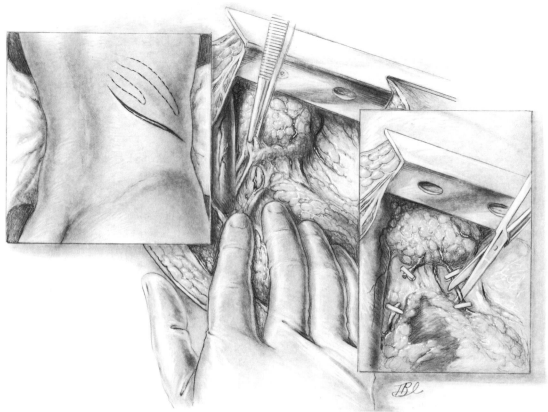

Figure 21–11. *The technique of clipping small vessels and neurovascular attachments is an excellent one for use with the dorsal approach. The limitations of space and wound depth make the use of small vascular clips the most practical means of securing hemostasis, which must be meticulous throughout the dissection. The adrenal gland is best elevated by ligatures placed on the proximal side in the fatty and neurovascular tissue. It is better to avoid touching the gland with forceps or manually, to avoid intraglandular hemorrhage. This technique allows mobilization, using the "no-touch" technique.*

female, hirsutism and amenorrhea may also be present. The classic findings on physical examination, the moon facies and buffalo hump, are well known. The moon facies is caused by an increased size of cheek fat pads. The changes are often subtle, and, therefore, old photographs are sometimes helpful in recognizing these changes. Blood pressure elevation is almost always present. Renin profiles are generally low because vascular volume is expanded. Major problems with long-term corticosteroid excess are infections and cardiovascular accidents from chronic hypertension.

Laboratory findings vary with the origin of the syndrome. Cushing's syndrome, caused by pituitary adenoma, is associated with elevated plasma ACTH (normal, 95 pg/ml ± 12 pg/ml). In Cushing's disease, these are roughly doubled, with values of 164 pg/ml ± 19 pg/ml. Elevated fasting blood sugar levels are seen late in the disease, but a diabetic-type glucose tolerance curve is very often present owing to excess production of glucocorticoids. Adrenal CAT scans reveal symmetrical bilateral adrenal enlargement. Confirmation of pituitary Cushing's syndrome requires demonstration of increased production of corticosteroids by both adrenals and increased production of ACTH from the anterior pituitary. This can be proved by demonstration of increased urinary cortisol and plasma cortisol, increased plasma ACTH, and corticosteroid suppression with synthetic corticosteroids, such as dexamethasone, and with blockers of corticosteroid synthesis, such as metyrapone. Failure to suppress with low doses of dexamethasone (1 mg), but suppression with high doses (4 mg) can be taken as evidence for pituitary-dependent Cushing's disease. The ability of metyrapone to inhibit the synthesis of corticosteroid by blocking 11-hydroxylation also makes it a useful diagnostic tool. As 11-hydroxylation is blocked, compound S (11-deoxycortisol) instead of cortisol is produced. Patients with Cushing's disease of pituitary origin have an increased production of compound S because of their hyperplastic glands, and they also have an increased ability to produce corticosteroids when stimulated by ACTH. This metyrapone stimulation test is useful in discriminating the pituitary-dependent Cushing's disease (in which there is a hyperactive response) from adrenal tumors (in which there is a failure to respond). Patients with ectopic ACTH production also fail to respond to metyrapone stimulation. A single-dose test is carried out by administering 30 mg/kg at midnight and measuring plasma levels of compound S, cortisol, and ACTH at 8:00 the following morning.

Cushing's syndrome due to benign adenomas is best proved by measurement of elevated plasma cortisol with loss of the diurnal curve (i.e., persistently elevated plasma values), even in the afternoon and evening. In patients with a primary adrenal disorder (i.e., glucocorticoid excess secondary to tumor) ACTH is suppressed. Furthermore, failure of plasma cortisol to suppress with both the 1- and 4-mg doses of dexamethasone is a characteristic feature of the adrenal tumor. Once these chemical values are confirmed, further diagnostic studies should include arteriography (for many of these tumors can be quite large and with massive and variable blood supply), administration of radioactive cholesterol (^{131}I-C19), ultrasonograms, and CAT scans. Usually, differential venous collections and venography are not necessary to localize these tumors. CAT scans are very helpful in localizing small adrenal adenomas in the 2-cm range. It should be noted that most secretory adrenal cortical adenomas are associated with hyperaldosteronism. Of 85 cases reviewed, 13 were associated with Cushing's syndrome, 65 with aldosteronism, and seven with inappropriate virilization. In one series, 149 patients with Cushing's syndrome were analyzed; 121 had bilateral hyperplasia and presumably extra-adrenal pituitary stimulation, 13 had primary adrenal adenoma, and 15 had adrenal carcinoma.[13] Therefore, about 20% of patients with Cushing's syndrome will have primary adrenal tumors, either adenoma or carcinoma.

Treatment

The treatment of Cushing's syndrome is directed toward the primary dysfunction. Adrenalectomy is indicated in the 20% of patients in whom the syndrome is caused by primary adrenal tumors; the rest have disease caused by pituitary or ACTH-producing tumors. It is of great importance to identify and localize the source of excess corticosteroid production. Localization techniques that are most practical are the CAT scan, radioisotopic study with ^{131}I-C19, and, in the event of a large tumor, arteriography.

It must be emphasized that preoperative preparation requires tissue fixation of corticosteroids. Therefore, cortisone acetate (50 mg q.i.d.) is recommended for at least one if not two days preoperatively. The rate of return of adrenal secretion by the contralateral suppressed adrenal cortex is variable. Therefore, intraoperative administration of corticosteroids is essential, with gradual tapering over the course of a week to a base level of 30 mg of cortisol per day maintenance for a reasonable therapeutic trial. Then, gradual tapering to levels as low as 10 to 15 mg/day can be attempted. Weakness, fatigue, hypotension, and hyponatremia are clues that replacement is inadequate.

Surgical Technique

The small adrenal adenoma producing Cushing's syndrome can be treated by the dorsal approach, as described earlier for primary aldosteronism. However, larger tumors, if localized to one side, are best approached through a transverse upper abdominal or thoracoabdominal incision.

Transabdominal Approach. A transverse incision is generally preferred, extending across both rectus muscles to the tip of the twelfth rib. To expose the right adrenal, the liver and gallbladder are retracted cephalad. The distal stomach, duodenum, and hepatic flexure of the colon are retracted medially. Occasionally, hepatic and colonic adhesions must be divided. The posterior peritoneum can be reflected medially after the mesocolon is incised and separated from the anterior aspect of Gerota's fascia (Fig. 21–13). Retraction of the duodenum and head of the pancreas medially (Kocher maneuver) is very helpful in gaining exposure of the right adrenal. Gentle caudad retraction of the upper pole of the kidney aids in the dissection of the right adrenal gland. The key to the dissection is thorough mobilization of the inferior vena cava and right renal venous structures so that the adrenal gland can be mobilized from the vena cava to obtain superior exposure. The vena cava can be retracted medially in this area by means of vein retractors. Clips and silk ligatures are quite useful in dividing fatty, neural, or small arterial structures surrounding the gland. Ligatures on the proximal glandular side assist in gentle traction, and the cava can be retracted medially to expose the common right adrenal vein. In larger tumors, exposure of the common right adrenal vein may require dissection of the caudate lobe of the liver. Deep Harrington retractors are useful in this hepatic retraction (Fig. 21–3B).

The left adrenal is more accessible when approached through the abdomen. One approach is to incise the mesentery of the transverse colon to the left of the middle colic artery and then expose the left renal vein just below this (Fig. 21–12). This is quite useful if the patient is thin and the tumor not large. However, in larger patients or in those with big tumors, if approaching transabdominally it is better either to reflect the colon, spleen, and pancreas medially (Fig. 21–6) or to incise the gastrocolic ligament and enter the lesser peritoneal sac (Fig. 21–13). The posterior peritoneum is then incised, exposing the adrenal directly below and allowing division of the adrenal vasculature between clips or ligatures as the adrenal is displaced laterally and medially. If the gastrocolic approach is used, the stomach and pancreas must be retracted medially and cephalad, the duodenum medially, and the colon laterally and inferiorly. For larger tumors it is much safer if the mesocolon and lienophrenic ligaments are divided all the way around, sometimes even as high and medial as the gastroesophageal hiatus. In so doing, the spleen, colon, and pancreas can be reflected medially and anteriorly off Gerota's fascia to expose any large tumor below.

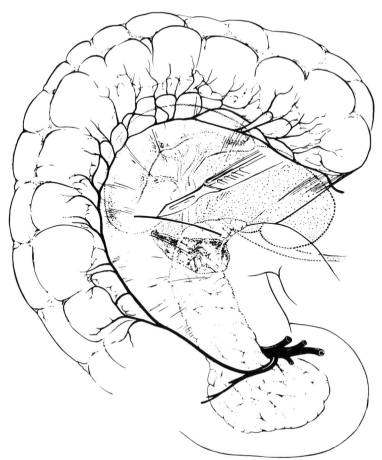

Figure 21–12. The approach to the left adrenal (advocated by Brady and Flandreau) is through an incision in the transverse mesocolon just to the left of the middle colic artery. From Glenn JF, Peterson RE, Mannix H Jr: Surgery of the Adrenal Gland. New York, Macmillan, 1968, p 157.

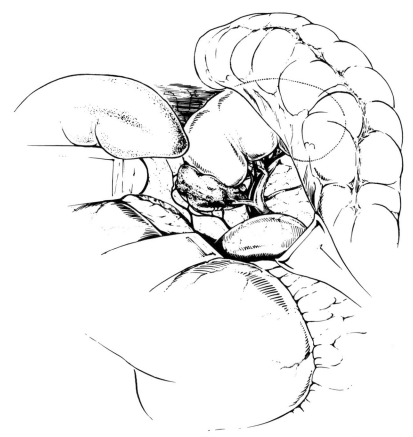

Figure 21–13. *An approach to the adrenal through the lesser sac is another option. The gastrocolic attachments are divided between clamps and ligatures, and the posterior peritoneum at the floor of the lesser sac is divided cephalad to the pancreas, which then is retracted medially and caudad. This will expose the adrenal below it. From Glenn JF, Peterson RE, Mannix H Jr: Surgery of the Adrenal Gland. New York, Macmillan, 1968, p 156.*

This also gives excellent exposure of the upper abdominal aorta, the medial diaphragm, the celiac and superior mesenteric vessels, and the crus of the diaphragm. Vascular control is much more secure with this technique (Fig. 21–6).

Another approach to the adrenal tumor is the lumbar extraperitoneal thoracoabdominal incision (Fig. 21–14). Basically, a subperiosteal incision is made in T-11 or T-12 and the diaphragm and pleura are incised. On the left side, the spleen and colon are mobilized medially in their peritoneal envelope, by means of blunt and sharp dissection. Then Gerota's fascia is exposed and the renal vein identified. On the left, the common adrenal vein can usually be secured early and the tumor mobilized between clips or ligatures off the kidney and medial aspect of the diaphragm. Various crural attachments and the inferior phrenic vascular supply are easily mobilized and divided. Some

direct aortic or renal arterial communications are also encountered, but these are usually small and well visualized in advance, provided the usual care is taken with exposure. After the tumor is removed, the area is irrigated thoroughly and the peritoneal sac is simply dropped over the kidney, which has been allowed to resume its normal position. The wound is usually closed in layers with interrupted nonabsorbable suture material. On the right side, the same principles apply. However, retraction of the liver off the anterior aspect of Gerota's fascia below may require more careful sharp and blunt dissection. Usually we prefer to enter the abdomen rather than stay outside the peritoneum in right adrenal surgery simply because it facilitates the exposure of the high vena cava and posterior venous vascular contributions of the adrenal gland itself.

The location of the adrenal on each side is more central than lateral. Therefore, there

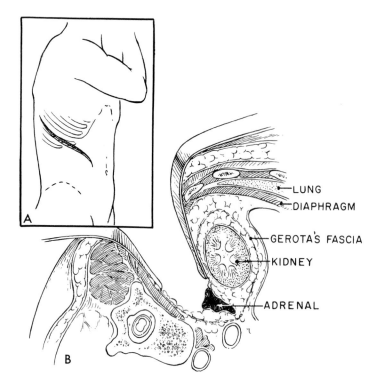

LUNG

DIAPHRAGM

GEROTA'S FASCIA

KIDNEY

ADRENAL

A

B

Figure 21-14. *The standard extraperitoneal thoracoabdominal lumbar approach is still used at times. With adrenal surgery, this is not quite as useful as it is with renal surgery. Nonetheless, this can be done by retracting the peritoneal sac medially and cephalad. From Glenn JF: Adrenal surgery. In JF Glenn (ed), Urologic Surgery. New York, Harper & Row, 1975, pp. 1–30.*

is little reason to try to stay outside the peritoneum, particularly on the right side.

Virilizing Tumors

Adrenal hirsutism and virilization may come from a variety of causes, such as congenital deficiencies in steroid production (congenital adrenal hyperplasia), adrenal tumors, Cushing's syndrome secondary to increased ACTH production by the pituitary, ovarian tumors or polycystic ovaries, or ill-defined variants thereof. The most common cause of hirsutism is idiopathic. Comments will be restricted to virilizing adrenal tumors.

Virilizing adrenal tumors in the female are characterized by amenorrhea, hirsutism, deep voice, increased muscle mass, enlargement of the clitoris, and, sometimes, decrease in breast size. In the male, such tumors may produce precocious puberty, early onset of prostatic enlargement, pubic and axillary hair, and beard growth. Testes in these cases remain small. In the more adult male, tumors may be recognized only as a space-occupying lesion or by their metastases. As noted, these tumors must be differentiated from congenital adrenal hyper-

plasia, idiopathic hirsutism, Cushing's syndrome, and other ovarian components. Generally, adrenal tumors do not produce much testosterone but ovarian tumors will. Measurement of elevations in levels of ketosteroids and dehydroepiandrosterone elevations will aid in diagnosis. As noted, elevations in testosterone levels are more likely to be gonadal in origin. Also, levels of other major androgen precursors, such as pregnenolone, progesterone, and 17-hydroxyprogesterone, may be elevated. Most virilizing adrenal tumors are not suppressable by administration of dexamethasone. They also will fail to increase secretion in response to ACTH administration. Localization by adrenal radioisotope scanning, CAT scans, and, sometimes, venography, arteriography, and ultrasonography are sometimes useful. Usually, if a solitary benign tumor can be located and removed, the prognosis is good. Large tumors are often malignant, and prognostic advice to the patient should be guarded.

The surgical approach to these tumors is the same as for the adrenal tumor causing Cushing's disease. Smaller tumors can be approached dorsally or by the lumbar routes. Larger tumors are best approached through large upper transverse incisions, and care should be taken to obtain central vascular exposure by utilizing the transabdominal techniques noted earlier.

References

1. Bravo EL, Tarazi RC, Fouad FM, et al: Clonidine-suppression test: a useful aid in the diagnosis of pheochromocytoma. N Engl J Med 305:623–626, 1981.
2. Cushing H: The Pituitary Body and Its Disorders. Philadelphia, JB Lippincott, 1912.
3. Donohue JP: Primary Aldosteronism. Urologic Therapy. Philadelphia, WB Saunders, 1980.
4. Egdahl RH: Surgery of the adrenal gland. N Engl J Med 278:939–949, 1968.
5. Frankel F: Ein fall von Doppelseitigem, vollig latent verlaufenen Nebennieren-tumor und gleichzeitiger Nephritis mit veranderungen und Circulations apparat und retinitis. Arch Pathol Anat Phys 103:244, 1886.
6. Freitas JE, Beierwaltes WH, Nishiyama RH: Adrenal hyperandrogenism: detection by adrenal scintigraphy. J Endocrinol Invest 1:59–64, 1978.
7. Ganguly A, Henry DP, Yune HY, et al: Diagnosis and localization of pheochromocytoma. Detection by measurement of urinary norepinephrine excretion during sleep, plasma norepinephrine concentration and computerized axial tomography (CT-scan). Am J Med 67:21–26, 1979.
8. Givens JR: Hirsutism and hyperandrogenism. Adv Intern Med 21:221–247, 1976.
9. Glenn JF, Boyce WH: Urologic Surgery. Philadelphia, Holber, 1969, pp 9–36.
10. Glenn JF, Peterson RE, Mannix H Jr: Surgery of the Adrenal Gland. New York, Macmillan, 1968.
11. Hume DM: Pheochromocytoma and hypertension: an analysis of 207 cases. Int Abstr Surg 99:458, 1960.
12. Hunt TK, Schambelan M, Biglieri EG: Selection of patients and operative approach in primary aldosteronism. Ann Surg 182:353–361, 1975.
13. Hutter AM Jr, Kayhoe DE: Adrenal cortical carcinoma. Clinical features of 138 patients. Am J Med 41:572–580, 1966.
14. Jubiz W, Meikle AW, West CD, et al: Single-dose metyrapone test. Arch Intern Med 125:472–474, 1970.
15. Lewinsky BS, Grigor KM, Symington T, et al: The clinical and pathologic features of "non-hormonal" adrenocortical tumors. Report of twenty new cases and review of the literature. Cancer 33:778–790, 1974.
16. Liddle GW: Tests of pituitary-adrenal suppressibility in the diagnosis of Cushing's syndrome. J Clin Endocrin 20:1539–1560, 1960.
17. Mayo CH: Paroxysmal hypertension with tumor of retroperitoneal nerve: report of case. JAMA 89:1047–1050, 1927.
18. Nelson DH: The Adrenal Cortex: Physiological Function and Disease. Philadelphia, WB Saunders, 1980.
19. Neville AM: The nodular adrenal. Invest Cell Pathol 1:99–111, 1978.
20. Neville AM, Mackay AM: The structure of the human adrenal cortex in health and disease. Clin Endocrinol Metab 1:361–395, 1972.
21. Pincoffs MC: A case of paroxysmal hypertension associated with suprarenal tumor. Trans Assn Am Physicians 44:295, 1929.
22. Scott HW Jr, Liddle GW, Mulherin JL Jr, et al: Surgical experience with Cushing's disease. Ann Surg 185:524–534, 1977.
23. Shipley AM: Paroxysmal hypertension associated with tumor of suprarenal. Ann Surg 90:742–749, 1929.
24. Singer W, Kovacs K, Ryan N, Horvath E: Ectopic ACTH syndrome: clinicopathological correlations. J Clin Pathol 31:591–598, 1978.
25. Sisson JC, Frager MS, Valk TW, et al: Scintigraphic localization of pheochromocytoma. N Engl J Med 305:12–17, 1981.
26. Stackpole RH, Melicow MM, Uson AC: Pheochromocytoma in children. Report of 9 cases and review of the first 100 published cases with follow-up studies. J Pediatr 66:314–330, 1963.
27. Weinberger MH, Grim CE, Hollifield JW, Donohue JP: Primary aldosteronism: diagnosis, localization and treatment. Ann Intern Med 90:386–395, 1979.
28. Yazaki T, Uchida K, Kaneko S, et al: Usefulness of scintigraphic imaging using ^{131}iodine-metaiodobenzylguanidine in localization of asymptomatic pheochromocytoma. J Urol 134:107–109, 1985.

DONALD G. SKINNER, M.D.

Primary Retroperitoneal Tumors

CHAPTER 22

The term *primary retroperitoneal tumors* includes a diverse group of rare tumors that originate from the wide variety of structures inhabiting or passing through the retroperitoneal space. Various types of tumors may thus arise from lymphatic tissue, fibroareolar tissue, arterial or venous blood vessels, fat, muscle, or vestigial prenatal remnants. Although primary tumors of the kidney, adrenal, and ureter are well known to urologic oncologists and are described in detail in other chapters, guidelines for the successful recognition and management of other retroperitoneal tumors (excluding those of gastrointestinal origin) are not available, although a review of the literature portends a dismal prognosis for those patients treated by the usual methods of surgical resection or radiation therapy.[4, 6, 8, 12, 13, 20, 25, 26, 29, 38, 40]

Eighty-five per cent or more of primary retroperitoneal tumors are malignant, and survival in those patients with malignant tumors other than lymphomas is dependent on complete surgical resection.[20, 28] However, inasmuch as these tumors usually are discovered late and often involve major blood vessels as well as extend into adjacent organs, complete resectability has historically been low, and the operative mortality rate has been reported as high as 36%.[4, 12, 29, 40] This morbidity stems chiefly from inadequate preoperative evaluation, insufficient preoperative diagnostic efforts, and the inexperience of most surgeons in extensive retroperitoneal operations.

BENIGN PRIMARY RETROPERITONEAL TUMORS

Benign lesions represent less than 15% of all primary retroperitoneal tumors. Included in this group are cysts representing persistent remnants of early urogenital embryonic structures. These are encountered more frequently on the left side near the kidney or tail of the pancreas. They are more common in females than in males because, in males, all the wolffian body is utilized to form the epididymis and vas deferens, whereas in the female the major portion undergoes atrophy or remains in the usual vestigial state.[26] Benign tumors derived from nerves include ganglioneuromas, neurofibromas, and extra-adrenal pheochromocytomas. Leiomyomas may arise from muscle, and xanthogranulomas and lipomas may be derived from retroperitoneal fatty tissue. Some lipomas can attain tremendous size, and it is often difficult to differentiate between a benign lipoma and a malignant liposarcoma, inasmuch as many recur following resection or may subsequently undergo sarcomatous degeneration.[6]

MALIGNANT PRIMARY RETROPERITONEAL TUMORS

Malignant tumors of lymphatic origin represent approximately one third of all primary retroperitoneal malignant neoplasms

390

and are the most common group encountered clinically. Lymphosarcomas account for about half of these tumors, and the remainder are divided between Hodgkin's disease originating in the retroperitoneum and reticulum cell sarcoma.[6]

Treatment for both Hodgkin's and non-Hodgkin's lymphomas is based primarily on staging as well as histologic type. Urinary tract involvement, usually indicated by lateral displacement of the proximal third of the ureter, is usually associated with disseminated disease and therefore with a poor prognosis. Lymphoma confined to the retroperitoneum is rare; several excellent reviews are available.[19, 40]

The most common primary retroperitoneal tumor not of lymphatic origin is liposarcoma, which is followed in frequency by leiomyosarcoma, fibrosarcoma, rhabdomyosarcoma, extra-adrenal neuroblastoma, other neurogenic sarcomas, and a wide variety of rare, miscellaneous malignant tumors, including malignant hemangiopericytoma, extragonadal primary germinal tumors, undifferentiated tumors, carcinomas, and other sarcomas. The mean age at presentation is approximately 50 years, except for those patients with embryonal rhabdomyosar-

coma, whose mean age was 11.7 years in the Memorial Sloan-Kettering Series.[8] Male patients predominate in a ratio 1.3:1.[8]

PRESENTING SYMPTOMS AND DIAGNOSIS

Characteristically, patients with primary retroperitoneal tumors are diagnosed late in the course of their disease and often have had symptoms for three to six months before they sought medical attention.[13] Nonspecific abdominal or back pain is the most common presenting symptom, followed by weight loss and abdominal swelling. Nonspecific gastrointestinal complaints such as nausea, a feeling of fullness, or changes in bowel habits occur in about 20% of the patients, and these symptoms are a result of the expansive nature of the tumor. Surprisingly, early complaints referable to the genitourinary tract are rare, despite the proximity of the kidney and ureter to many of these tumors.[6, 13, 30] Abdominal swelling or protuberance associated with peripheral muscle wasting may be observed and should alert the clinician to the possible presence of a primary retroperitoneal tumor (Fig. 22–1).

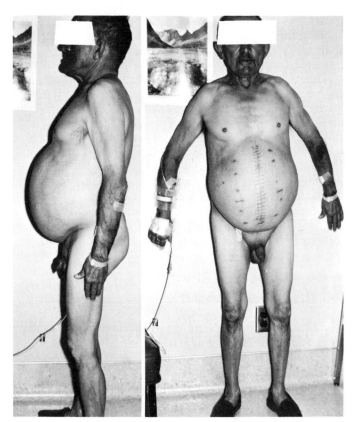

Figure 22–1. Patient with massive primary retroperitoneal tumor (myelolipoma) without metastatic disease. Note wasting of peripheral extremities.

Other less common presenting symptoms may include leg edema due to vena caval or lymphatic obstruction, lower extremity paresthesias due to nerve root compression, and fever; one patient presented with hypoglycemia due to an insulin-secreting retroperitoneal sarcoma.[27]

A physical examination nearly always reveals a palpable abdominal mass or at least abdominal fullness that does not move on respiration.[6, 13] Wasting of the muscles of the peripheral extremities may be striking (Fig. 22–1), or signs of metastatic disease may be present, such as groin or supraclavicular lymphadenopathy. Dilated, tortuous, and visible subcutaneous abdominal veins, with or without concurrent leg edema, may be observed as an indication of vena caval obstruction. Obviously, careful palpation of the testicle is essential, and an ultrasound study may permit the detection of an occult primary germinal tumor responsible for the extensive retroperitoneal disease.[18]

Laboratory data in patients with primary retroperitoneal tumors are nonspecific, simply reflecting the state of chronic illness.

Preoperative assessment and extensive efforts to secure a diagnosis are essential, inasmuch as combined modalities of therapy and often pretreatment by chemotherapy or radiation therapy may be necessary to achieve the successful surgical resection essential to the cure of nonlymphogenous malignant retroperitoneal tumors.

Although primary retroperitoneal tumors are rare, the urologic oncologist is often confronted with young, potentially curable male patients who present with massive retroperitoneal metastatic lesions owing to primary nonseminomatous tumors of the testis. The successful salvage of many of these patients, together with recent advances in the treatment of various sarcomas by using combined modalities of therapy, has led to the formulation of a plan of management to improve survival in patients afflicted by these tumors.

INITIAL EVALUATION

Computerized tomography (CT) has assumed the role of the single most important study in the diagnosis of retroperitoneal disorders. The characteristic appearance of liposarcoma originating within Gerota's fascia is illustrated in Figure 22–2. Note the low density of fat and the numerous irregular septa running within the tumors, which helps distinguish a liposarcoma from a benign lipoma. Massive retroperitoneal metastatic disease from a primary germ cell tumor of the testis is shown in Figure 22–3. Note anterior displacement of the aorta and obliteration of the vena cava. Additional studies of importance may include excretory urography, barium contrast studies of the gastrointestinal tract, abdominal ultrasound, lymphangiography and gallium scanning for lymphoma and Hodgkin's disease, aortography for neovascularity or lumbar arterial hypertrophy, venacavography, and urine vanillylmandelic acid (VMA) studies for neuroblastoma, ganglioneuroma, or pheochromocytoma. Liver function studies should be followed by liver scans if any values are abnormal, and serum determinations of the β-subunit of human chorionic gonadotropin and α-fetoprotein may be helpful.

Schulte and Emmett[32] reported displacement of the kidneys or upper third of the ureter in 73% of patients with primary retroperitoneal tumors, and Gondos[17] noted the diagnostic value of anterior rotation of the kidney or medial displacement beyond the psoas margin as indicative of a primary retroperitoneal tumor.

Barium studies of the gastrointestinal tract tend to rule out primary gastrointestinal neoplasms and usually show displacement of the bowel or stomach by tumor. Occasionally, they may show areas of invasion, alerting the surgeon to the need for possible bowel resection at the time of attempted surgical resection. Intramural infiltration by lymphomas may also be sometimes noted.[13]

In our hands, ultrasound and CT scans have been extremely helpful in defining the extent of tumor involvement and in further assessing the response to preoperative adjuvant modalities of therapy. Nuclear magnetic resonance scans (NMR) may supplant CT in this evaluation as refinement in technique and experience in interpretation are obtained. Early studies with this expensive diagnostic test have, however, been disappointing.

Lymphangiography and gallium scanning are often diagnostic for lymphomas or Hodgkin's disease, and subsequent treatment by surgical staging followed by combination

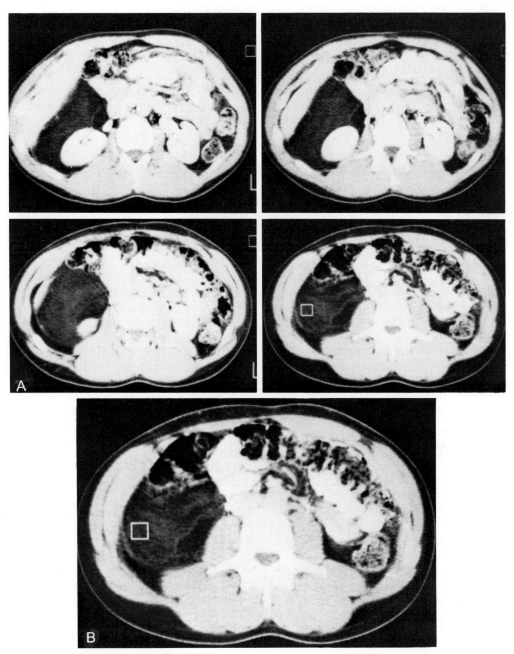

Figure 22–2. Computerized tomographic example of a primary retroperitoneal liposarcoma originating within Gerota's fascia around the right kidney. Various retroperitoneal cuts are seen in A, and B demonstrates in detail the low density of fat and the numerous irregular septa remaining within the tumor, which help distinguish a liposarcoma from a benign lipoma.

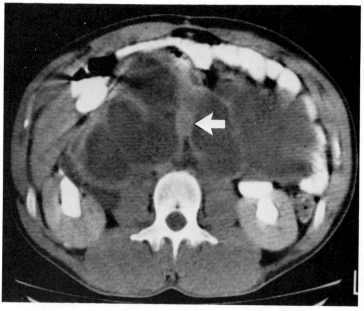

Figure 22–3. Computerized tomographic examples of massive retroperitoneal metastatic disease from a primary germ cell tumor of the testis. Note anterior displacement of the aorta (arrow) and obliteration of the vena cava.

radiation therapy and chemotherapy has been well defined, with marked improvement in survival rates.[19]

Urinary vanillylmandelic acid (VMA) or homovanillic acid (HVA) levels are elevated in nearly 95% of the patients with neuroblastomas or ganglioneuromas,[30] and almost all patients with pheochromocytomas will have an elevated level of vanillylmandelic acid.[38]

Aortography may show neovascularity with vascular pooling in patients with rhabdomyosarcomas, malignant hemangiopericytomas (Fig. 22–4), or metastatic nonseminomatous tumors of the testis (Fig. 22–5). Many primary retroperitoneal tumors, however, are hypovascular but might demonstrate hypertrophy of the lumbar artery as a clue to diagnosis.[21, 24] Venacavography is an important study to detect the possible occlusion of the vena cava or its displacement, and it may alert the clinician to the possible presence of a leiomyosarcoma.[7] Leiomyosarcomas arising in large veins are approximately five times more common than those arising in arteries, and more than half of the 48 reported cases have occurred in the vena cava.[7]

Several of these studies, including VMA determinations, barium studies, and usually lymphangiography, can be omitted if the diagnosis of nonseminomatous testicular tumor has been established by orchiectomy.

CT scans before and after preoperative chemotherapy in patients with extensive nonseminomatous testicular tumors have been helpful in determining the response to chemotherapy, as well as in planning subsequent surgical management as described in Chapter 54. It is important to scrutinize the retrocrural space, best seen on CT scans, to make sure the retrocrural, lower mediastinal nodes are not also involved by tumor.

The establishment of a tissue diagnosis of other primary retroperitoneal tumors is important, inasmuch as selection of appropriate chemotherapy for treatment with or without radiation therapy is an essential prerequisite to successful surgical resection. The use of peritoneoscopy with needle biopsy under direct vision provided the necessary histologic diagnosis of lymphoma in a patient of ours with a large abdominal mass obstructing both ureters, and this modality should be considered in those patients with hypovascularity on aortography.[10] CT-guided needle biopsy may provide the diagnosis of a malignant process, but adequate tissue for accurate histologic diagnosis may not be achieved through a needle. Sarcomas are notoriously difficult to diagnose by needle biopsy. Such patients will require a minilaparostomy and incisional biopsy if other less invasive studies have not provided an adequate diagnosis. It should be emphasized that in patients with large primary

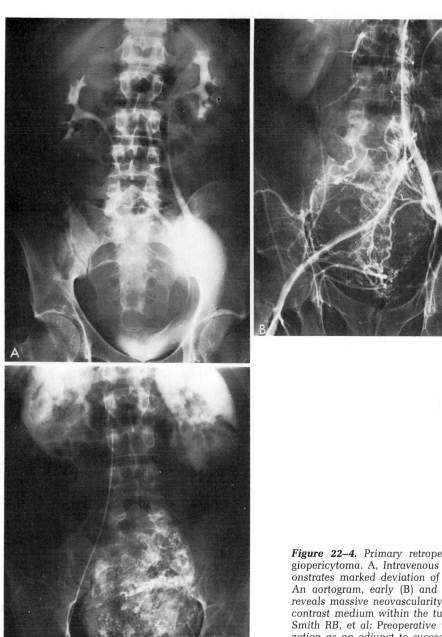

Figure 22–4. Primary retroperitoneal hemangiopericytoma. A, Intravenous pyelogram demonstrates marked deviation of the right ureter.
An aortogram, early (B) and late (C) phases,
reveals massive neovascularity with pooling of
contrast medium within the tumor mass. From
Smith RB, et al: Preoperative vascular embolization as an adjunct to successful resection of
large retroperitoneal hemangiopericytoma. J Urol
115:206, 1976.

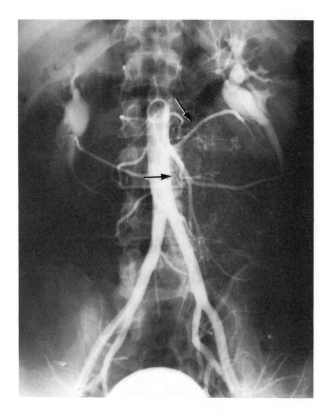

Figure 22–5. *Aortogram in a patient with a large abdominal mass proven by biopsy to be a choriocarcinoma metastatic from the left testis. Note extensive neovascularity (arrows) and lateral displacement of the left kidney.*

retroperitoneal tumors, an incisional biopsy for accurate diagnosis is often preferable to attempting excisional biopsy, since complete resection is seldom possible unless shrinkage can be achieved by preoperative chemotherapy.

TREATMENT

Chemotherapy

Once the diagnosis has been established, initial treatment depends on the histologic type of the tumor. In patients with malignant disease, every effort should be made to pretreat with appropriate chemotherapy or radiation therapy prior to embarking on extensive surgical resection, since complete surgical resection is the most important factor in prognosis.

Patients with bulky retroperitoneal metastases from nonseminomatous testicular tumors, even those patients with extensive pulmonary metastases, are treated initially by combination platinum-based chemotherapy as described in Chapter 35. Pretreatment of large, bulky retroperitoneal tumors has made surgical resection possible in all cases,

even though some of our patients had been explored previously and were thought to have unresectable tumors.[35] Considerable central necrosis may result from the initial chemotherapy, but a thick, fibrous capsule develops around the neoplasm, and this enhances surgical resection and lessens the possibility of tumor rupture.

Patients with nonlymphogenous retroperitoneal sarcomas should probably be considered for combination chemotherapy, surgery, and possibly radiation therapy. If the initial CT assessment suggests that complete surgical resection will be possible, surgery is performed first and the grade of the tumor and surgical findings then dictate the need for additional therapy. For low-grade tumors with adequate surgical margins, prophylactic therapy does not seem warranted.[3, 31] For low-grade tumors incompletely resected, adjuvant chemotherapy utilizing doxorubicin as a single agent or in combination is recommended. Potential benefits from the adjuvant use of doxorubicin, however, must be carefully weighed against toxicity, since 10 to 14% of patients receiving more than 450 mg/m² cumulative drug can expect to develop clinical cardiomyopathy manifested by signs and symptoms of congestive heart failure.[3, 31] All patients with high-grade tumors should probably receive adjuvant doxorubicin as a single agent or in combination, since pulmonary metastasis can be anticipated in a ˉsubstantial percentage of such patients treated solely by surgery.[28, 31] In addition, those patients with high-grade tumors incompletely resected may benefit from postoperative radiation therapy to the tumor bed. The major problem involves the dosage of radiation, since 5000 to 6000 rads required for tumor eradication may cause considerable morbidity. Consideration should be given for the intraoperative placement of ^{125}I seeds or a catheter placement for postoperative iridium loading if the surgeon finds that complete resection is not possible.

If initial assessment suggests that safe, complete surgical resection will probably not be feasible, then preoperative chemotherapy and possibly radiation therapy should be considered. Wiley and associates[41] have reported a protocol in which patients received 2 to 6 μg/kg/day of intra-arterial infused actinomycin D and 2000 to 3000 rads of concomitant radiation therapy delivered over a two- to three-week period. This was followed two to four weeks later by surgical resection, depending on leukocyte recovery. Doxorubicin may be substituted for actinomycin D, and if no specific vessel or vessels feeding the primary tumor can be identified on aortography, the chemotherapeutic agents may be administered through a peripheral venous site. Wiley and associates reported encouraging results in a pilot study of eight patients with massive disease.[41] More recently, Eilber and Morton[14] have reported an overall survival rate of 70% for patients with high-grade, extremity soft tissue sarcomas treated by intravenous doxorubicin, concomitant radiation therapy, and limb-sparing surgical excision. This result can be compared with an expected 40% survival rate for similar patients treated by amputation only. In addition, the local recurrence rate was reduced to less than 10%.

Experience in the preoperative treatment of soft tissue sarcoma in children indicates that the combination of vincristine, doxorubicin, actinomycin D, and cyclophosphamide (VAC plus doxorubicin) is extremely active against these tumors, often making more conservative surgical resection possible. However, when the standard VAC regimen is applied to adult soft tissue sarcomas, the results are not nearly as encouraging. Considerable individualization obviously is necessary in the treatment planning for each patient, and it is hoped that new drugs will enhance our abilities to treat these tumors effectively.

Surgery

Surgical Principles

It is imperative that the surgeon be prepared at operation for a case that may require the resection of an ipsilateral kidney or kidney en bloc with the vena cava, or even aortic replacement. All patients should have satisfactory bowel preparation in the event that a bowel resection is necessary. In a review of Memorial Sloan-Kettering experience with retroperitoneal sarcomas treated over a six-year period, adjuvant organ resection was required in 73% of patients in order to avoid leaving gross residual disease (kidney and adrenal, 25%; colon, 20%; and pancreas, 8%.[8]

The modified thoracoabdominal approach is ideally suited to the successful resection of these tumors, inasmuch as it allows access to and control of the ipsilateral great vessel above the diaphragm and provides maximum exposure to the posterior retroperitoneum, where the greatest technical difficulties in resection exist. The position of the tumor determines whether the procedure is done through the right or left side of the thorax, but it should be emphasized that this approach provides excellent exposure to the contralateral retroperitoneal region as well.

Preoperative Preparation

Preoperative preparation is fairly routine. In older patients (over 50 years), prophylactic preoperative digitalization is a usual practice unless there is a specific contraindication. Our procedure is to give 0.5 mg of digoxin early the day before the operation followed by 0.25 mg that afternoon and 0.125 mg the evening before the operation. Bowel preparation utilizing a castor oil emulsion (Neoloid), neomycin sulfate, and erythromycin is started following breakfast the day before surgery, as described in Chapter 42. Clear liquids are given thereafter until midnight before surgery, and overnight hydration with Ringer's lactate is routine.

Anesthesia and Patient Position

For a number of years, we have utilized controlled hypotensive anesthesia for patients undergoing retroperitoneal or major intra-abdominal extirpative operations. We reviewed a group of patients in whom this technique was utilized and compared them with a similar group operated on by the same surgeon in whom standard normotensive anesthesia was used. This study revealed a significant advantage to the hypotensive group in terms of blood loss and the need for replacement. The average blood loss in 25 patients undergoing the thoracoabdominal retroperitoneal node dissection utilizing controlled hypotensive anesthesia was 920 ml, compared with an average blood loss of 1341 ml in patients undergoing the same operation by the same surgeon under normotensive conditions (p < 0.001). Results concerning blood replacement, intraoperative and total (intraoperative plus postoperative requirements), also significantly favored the hypotensive group. Patients were matched stage for stage to eliminate bias due to extensive disease. A continuous epidural catheter delivering intraoperative lidocaine facilitates this technique and can be further used during the postoperative period for more effective pain control by the epidural administration of morphine sulfate. Chapters 40 and 41 discuss in detail the anesthesia that facilitates this type of surgery.

Patient positioning is extremely important, and attention to detail facilitates all phases of the operation (Fig. 22–6). The patient should be positioned on the ipsilateral side of the operating table with the break of the table located immediately above the iliac crest. The contralateral leg is flexed 90° and the hip approximately 30°. The ipsilateral shoulder is then torqued approximately 20° off the horizontal, and the ipsilateral arm is brought across the chest and placed in an adjustable arm rest. The pelvis remains nearly supine, perhaps rotated approximately 10° off the horizontal. A sheet roll is then placed longitudinally under the ipsilateral back, and a similar roll is positioned under the contralateral abdomen. The table is fully hyperextended, and the patient is secured with wide adhesive tape at the shoulders, hips, and leg. The ipsilateral leg remains extended along the ipsilateral edge of the table and is supported by a pillow.

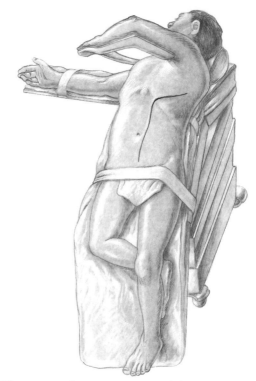

Figure 22–6. *Proper positioning of the patient for the modified thoracoabdominal approach. Note that the pelvis is nearly supine and that the shoulders are angled approximately 30°, with the patient placed as close to the ipsilateral side of the table as possible. The abdominal portion of the incision extends high into the epigastrium and then is directed inferiorly as a paramedian incision. From Skinner DG: Considerations for management of large retroperitoneal tumors: use of the modified thoracoabdominal approach. J Urol 117:605, 1977.*

Surgical Technique

The incision begins at the mid-axillary line over the eighth, ninth, or tenth rib, depending on the extent of the retroperitoneal disease—the larger the mass, the higher the incision. The incision extends over the rib and across the costochondral junction into the epigastrium, where it courses inferiorly as a midline incision toward the pelvis. The incision may also be extended across the epigastrium to improve exposure to the contralateral retroperitoneum. A subperiosteal resection of the appropriate rib is performed, and the costochondral junction is divided. The rectus muscle should be divided in the epigastrium and retracted laterally.

If a large retroperitoneal mass is present, the peritoneum is entered and the entire

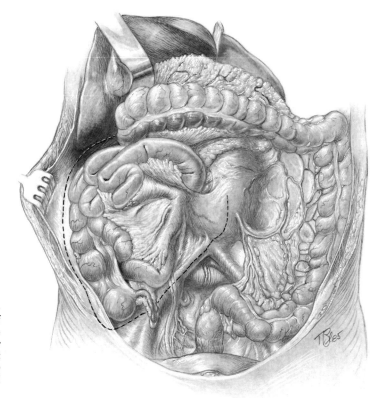

Figure 22–7. Peritoneal incision necessary for complete mobilization of small bowel, ascending colon, duodenum, and pancreas. From Skinner DG: Considerations for management of large retroperitoneal tumors: use of the modified thoracoabdominal approach. J Urol 117:605, 1977.

small bowel, ascending and transverse colon, duodenum, pancreas, and (on the left side) spleen must be mobilized completely on the superior mesenteric artery pedicle and placed in a Lahey bag on the anterior chest wall (Figs. 22–7 through 22–10). It is essential that the superior mesenteric artery be identified at the point where it crosses over the left renal vein. This artery must not be injured, since it serves as a vascular pedicle for the small and large bowel. Care must also be taken to keep from placing excessive tension on this artery and to prevent injuring it with a retractor.

The inferior mesenteric artery should be ligated to free the descending colonic mesentery, much of which may have to be sacrificed. This is a safe procedure if the marginal artery remains intact. In the author's experience, it rarely has been necessary to resect bowel in those cases in which large areas of the descending colonic mesentery have been resected en bloc with the tumor. If a portion of the colon does not appear viable at the end of the procedure, it should be resected. Occasionally, diarrhea or intermittent abdominal pain, usually associated with oral intake of food, may result from ischemia to the large bowel after ligation of the inferior mesenteric artery, but this is a rare occurrence in young patients and is usually managed successfully and conservatively without long-term sequelae.

Generally, it has been possible to mobilize the aorta and dissect it out of the large retroperitoneal mass. Ligation and division of the lumbar arteries distal to the renal pedicle facilitates aortic mobilization, and on rare occasions the aorta may be replaced with a Dacron bypass graft. Troublesome bleeding from avulsed lumbar vessels may occur, but this can be avoided by individual ligation and division of each pair of vessels distal to the renal pedicle. The placement of hemoclips on the distal portion of the vessel facilitates this part of the operation, but it is best to ligate the origin from the aorta and vena cava because the clips may be dislodged later in the procedure, causing bleeding behind the great vessels. Occasionally, troublesome bleeding from a torn lumbar vein or artery will develop despite all pre-

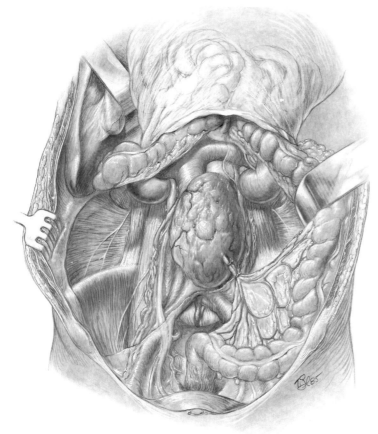

Figure 22–8. Once the peritoneal attachments to the colon and small bowel mesentery have been incised, the entire retroperitoneum can be exposed through the right side of the chest by placing the intra-abdominal contents in a Lahey bag on the anterior chest wall. Care must be taken not to put too much tension on the superior mesenteric pedicle. From Skinner DG: Considerations for management of large retroperitoneal tumors: use of the modified thoracoabdominal approach. J Urol 117:605, 1977.

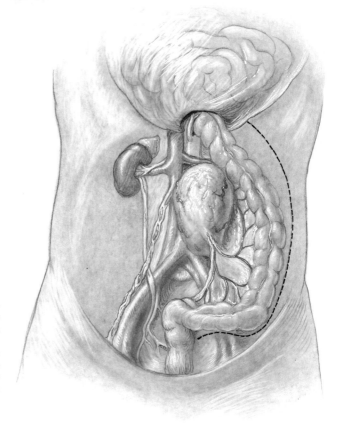

Figure 22–9. Mobilization of the spleen, transverse colon, and descending colon for exposure of predominantly left-sided lesions. For extensive tumors, the right colon and small bowel should be mobilized as illustrated in Figure 22–7 and placed in a Lahey bag on the chest wall. From Skinner DG: Considerations for management of large retroperitoneal tumors: use of the modified thoracoabdominal approach. J Urol 117:605, 1977.

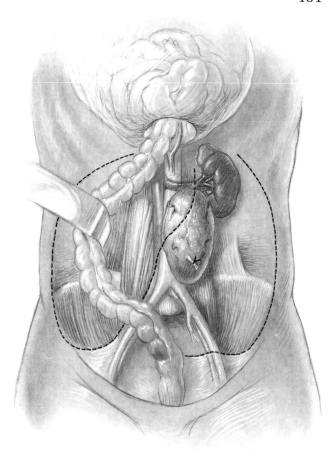

Figure 22–10. Retroperitoneal exposure obtained through the left side of the chest following mobilization of the intra-abdominal contents. Note ligation of the inferior mesenteric artery, necessary for mobilization of the descending colon. Care must be taken to protect the superior mesenteric artery. From Skinner DG: Considerations for management of large retroperitoneal tumors: use of the modified thoracoabdominal approach. J Urol 117:605, 1977.

cautions. The use of an Allis clamp is helpful, and 4–0 arterial silk should be available in all cases.

Frequently, tumors of this type will obstruct the vena cava and be associated intimately with it anatomically. In such cases, it is best to resect the vena cava en bloc with the tumor, and it may be necessary to remove the ipsilateral kidney en bloc. If the right kidney and vena cava are resected en bloc with the tumor, it is important to try to maintain the connection between the vena cava and the left renal vein, even though preoperatively the vena cava had been obstructed completely. Our experience indicates significant morbidity, in half the patients, after ligation of the left renal vein at the time of right nephrectomy and vena cava resection. Postoperative hospitalization was significantly prolonged, and temporary postoperative hemodialysis was required for up to six weeks as a result of either high renal venous pressure or renal vein thrombosis.

The cisterna chyli should be identified behind the right renal artery, medial to the right crus of the diaphragm and between the aorta and vena cava. The cisterna should be ligated or secured with a large hemoclip to prevent chylous ascites or the significant loss of protein in the postoperative period.

Results of Surgery

Experience in more than 300 consecutive patients with all stages of nonseminomatous testicular cancer, numerous patients with massive renal cell carcinomas, and a few patients with other primary retroperitoneal tumors has indicated that surgical resection of even the most extensive mass is usually possible through the modified thoracoabdominal approach, provided every effort is made preoperatively to determine the extent of the lesion and to reduce its bulk as much as possible with chemotherapy and, in the case of sarcomas, with concomitant radiation therapy.[41]

Postoperative Complications

Postoperative complications, although minimal in our experience, may occur and are similar to those of any major surgical procedure. However, two points should be emphasized. Concern over possible devascularization of the spinal cord is not warranted, provided that no lumbar arteries are ligated above the renal pedicle. The spinal cord ends at the level of the first lumbar vertebral body. The nutrient arteries to the spinal cord and cauda equina are the longitudinal anterior and posterior spinal arteries, which arise from the vertebral arteries and receive additional blood supply from the intercostal and high lumbar arteries through radicular branches.[33]

The main lower anterior radicular artery providing collateral blood supply to the anterior spinal artery is called the arteria radicularis magna (artery of Adamkiewicz).[14] This artery orginates from the thoracic aorta in 50% of patients and from the lumbar region in the other 50%.[3, 9] However, it has been demonstrated that in those patients in whom the arteria radicularis magna originates in the lumbar region, there is an important radicular artery from the lower thoracic aorta that is constantly present and provides adequate collateral circulation to the anterior spinal artery.[3, 9]

Although paraplegia after aortic replacement procedures for abdominal aortic aneurysms was not reported before 1960, and DeBakey's group[11] has reported no neurologic deficits in 1432 consecutive abdominal aortic aneurysm resections, 28 cases of paraplegia after abdominal aortic operations were reported in the world literature through March, 1975.[15, 22, 26, 34] However, a review of these 28 cases reveals that 18 were associated with ruptured aneurysms and prolonged hypotension. Permanent paraplegia occurred in only one of the 10 patients who had undergone elective abdominal aortic aneurysm resection. The remaining nine patients recovered function, and all 28 patients showed evidence of extensive atherosclerosis. Therefore, we believe that the evidence supports our contention that extensive aortic mobilization with ligation of the lumbar arteries or aortic replacement is a safe and necessary part of the surgical resection of large retroperitoneal tumors.

Ejaculatory failure or retrograde ejaculation commonly results from extensive retroperitoneal lymph node dissection due to sympathectomy (described in Chapter 34). The possibility of this complication must be discussed with the patient preoperatively, but it also must be placed in proper perspective relative to the overall merits of the retroperitoneal dissection. We suggest that young patients of reproductive age visit a sperm bank on several occasions preoperatively and have ejaculatory fluid frozen and stored in the event that subsequent artificial insemination becomes desirable.

However, there should be no doubt that the surgical resection is massive, requires great expertise, and should be attempted only by those thoroughly trained in modern retroperitoneal operations and by those who see a sufficient volume of such patients to maintain their expertise. For example, the early complication rate for patients undergoing the thoracoabdominal approach to retroperitoneal lymph node dissection for testicular cancer was only 3% in those with disease in an early stage but rose to 17% in those with bulky disease.[35] Reported operative mortality for patients undergoing resection of primary retroperitoneal tumor has ranged from 2.2 to 36%, depending largely on the era in which the surgery was performed, the expertise of the surgeon, and the available pre- and postoperative support.

Five-year survival depends almost entirely on two factors; completeness of resection and the histologic grade of the tumor. Cody and associates reported a 40% five-year survival rate among 47 patients undergoing complete resection, compared with a 3% survival rate among 62 patients whose tumors were incompletely excised.[8] Among those who had complete resection, the five-year survival rate was 80% if the tumor was of a low grade. This compared with a survival of less than 10% if the tumor was of high grade, despite complete resection.[8]

The need for adjuvant radiotherapy has been advocated by some, especially if the surgical margins are positive for residual tumor. Brachytherapy afterloading techniques utilizing ^{125}I or ^{192}Ir provides a high dose of radiation to a limited volume and may prolong the disease-free interval. Intraoperative external beam radiotherapy is currently being studied in a wide variety of intra-abdominal malignancies and may play an important future role in the management of these tumors.[1] However, if complete surgical resection is possible, there appears to be no added gain from adjuvant radiotherapy.

The use of prophylactic chemotherapy remains undefined except for embryonal rhabdomyosarcoma. Doxorubicin has been shown to produce a 35 to 40% objective response for soft tissue sarcoma, but its contribution in an adjuvant setting remains unproven.[14] Nonetheless, the known dismal results of surgical excision alone for high-grade tumors stimulate trials of adjuvant chemotherapy prophylaxis.

SUMMARY

A review of patients with primary retroperitoneal tumors of nonlymphogenous origin indicates that complete surgical excision must be accomplished to achieve success,[8, 20, 28] and recent reports suggest that pretreatment with chemotherapy or radiation therapy may increase the prospects for safe surgical resection and, thus, cure.[14, 41]

Benign tumors can obviously be managed more conservatively. Cysts respond well to simple excision or marsupialization into the peritoneal cavity. Lipomas, however, may be deceptive inasmuch as it may be impossible to distinguish them from low-grade liposarcomas; DeWeerd and Dockerty[12] reported that 60% of the retroperitoneal lipomas that they thought to be benign recurred and were followed by the death of the patient within five years. Complete surgical resection with adequate margins thus seems more appropriate treatment than simple enucleation of a so-called benign lipoma.[6, 12]

Meaningful survival statistics of patients afflicted by sarcomatous nonlymphogenous primary retroperitoneal tumors are not available, but recent reports indicate that if complete resection is possible, long-term survival can be achieved.[7, 8, 20, 28, 39, 41]

We have demonstrated that large retroperitoneal tumors can be resected safely by means of a modified thoracoabdominal approach.[35, 36] Maximum preoperative preparation, however, is essential, and the use of combined therapeutic modalities, particularly intensive treatment with chemotherapy, has achieved increased resectability and marked improvement in the long-term survival rates for patients afflicted with these tumors.

References

1. Abe M, Takahashi M, Yabumoto E, et al: Clinical experiences with intraoperative radiotherapy of locally advanced cancers. Cancer 45:40–48, 1980.
2. Adams HD, van Geertruyden HH: Neurologic complications of aortic surgery. Ann Surg 144:574–610, 1956.
3. Antman K, Suit H, Amato D, et al: Preliminary results of a randomized trial of adjuvant doxorubicin for sarcomas: lack of apparent difference between treatment groups. J Clin Oncol 2:601–608, 1984.
4. Bek V: Primary retroperitoneal tumours. Neoplasma (Bratislava) 17:253–263, 1970.
5. Boudreaux D, Waisman J, Skinner DG, Low R: Giant adrenal myelolipoma and testicular interstitial cell tumors in a mass with congenital 21-hydroxylate deficiency. Am J Surg Pathol 3:109–123, 1979.
6. Braasch JW, Mon AB: Primary retroperitoneal tumors. Surg Clin North Am 47:663–678, 1967.
7. Brewster DC, Athanasoulis CA, Darling RC: Leiomyosarcoma of the inferior vena cava. Arch Surg 111:1081–1085, 1976.
8. Cody HS III, Turnbull AD, Fortner JG, Hajdu SI: The continuing challenge of retroperitoneal sarcoma. Cancer 47:2147–2152, 1981.
9. Coupland GA, Reeve TS: Paraplegia: a complication of excision of abdominal aortic aneurysm. Surgery 64:878–881, 1968.
10. Coupland GA, Townend DM, Martin CJ: Peritoneoscopy—use in assessment of intra-abdominal malignancy. Surgery 89:645–649, 1981.
11. DeBakey ME, Crawford ES, Cooley DA, et al: Aneurysm of abdominal aorta: analysis of results of graft replacement therapy one to eleven years after operation. Ann Surg 160:622–639, 1964.
12. DeWeerd JH, Dockerty MB: Lipomatous retroperitoneal tumors. Am J Surg 84:397–407, 1952.
13. Duncan RE, Evans AT: Diagnosis of primary retroperitoneal tumors. J Urol 117:19–23, 1977.
14. Eilber FR, Morton DL: Soft tissue sarcomas. Contemp Surg 22:17–25, 1983.
15. Ferguson LRJ, Bergan JJ, Conn J Jr, Yao JST: Spinal ischemia following abdominal aortic surgery. Ann Surg 181:267–272, 1975.
16. Golden GT, Sears HF, Wellons HA Jr, Muller WH Jr: Paraplegia complicating resection of aneurysms of the infrarenal abdominal aorta. Surgery 73:91–96, 1973.
17. Gondos B: Urographic studies in abdominal masses. The diagnostic value of kidney rotation. Radiology 78:180–186, 1962.
18. Gottesman JE, Sample WF, Skinner DG, Ehrlich RM: Diagnostic ultrasound in evaluation of scrotal masses. J Urol 118:601–603, 1977.
19. Kaplan HS: Hodgkin's disease: unfolding concepts concerning its nature, management and prognosis. Cancer 45:2439–2474, 1980.
20. Kinne DW, Chu FCH, Huvos AG, et al: Treatment of primary recurrent retroperitoneal liposarcomas: 25 years' experience at Memorial Hospital. Cancer 31:53–64, 1973.
21. Lowman RM, Grnja V, Peck DR, et al: Angiographic patterns of the primary retroperitoneal tumors: the role of the lumbar arteries. Radiology 104:259–268, 1972.
22. McCullough DL, Gittes RF: Ligation of the renal vein in the solitary kidney: effects on renal function. J Urol 113:295–298, 1975.
23. Mehrez IO, Nabseth DC, Hogan EL, Deterling RA Jr: Paraplegia following resection of abdominal aortic aneurysm. Ann Surg 156:890–898, 1962.
24. Monro JL: The value of angiography in the surgical

treatment of large retroperitoneal tumors. Br J Clin Pract 24:235–238, 1970.

25. Pack GT, Tabah EJ: Collective review; primary retroperitoneal tumors; a study of 120 cases. Int Abstr Surg 99:209–231, 313–341, 1954.

26. Pack GT, Tabah EJ: Collective review; primary retroperitoneal tumors; a study of 120 cases (continued). Surg Gynecol Obstet 99:313–341, 1954.

27. Papaioannou AN: Tumors other than insulinomas associated with hypoglycemia. Surg Gynecol Obstet 123:1093, 1966.

28. Potter DA, Glenn J, Kinsella T, et al: Patterns of recurrence in patients with high-grade soft tissue sarcomas. J Clin Oncol 3:353–366, 1985.

29. Pritchett TR, Lieskovsky G, Skinner DG: Extension of renal cell carcinoma into the vena cava; clinical review and surgical approach. J Urol 135:460–464, 1986.

30. Rhamy RK: Retroperitoneal tumors. In J Glenn (ed), Urological Surgery, 2nd ed. Hagerstown, Maryland, Harper & Row, 1975, p 859.

31. Rosenberg SA: Prospective randomized trials demonstrating the efficacy of adjuvant chemotherapy in adult patients with soft tissue sarcomas. Cancer Treat Rep 68:1067–1078, 1984.

32. Schulte TL, Emmett JL: Urography in the differential diagnosis of retroperitoneal tumors. J Urol 42:215–219, 1939.

33. Sher MH, Healy EH: Paraplegia following infrarenal aneurysmorrhaphy. Vasc Surg 5:171–176, 1971.

34. Skillman JJ, Zervas NT, Weintraub RM, Mayman CI: Paraplegia after resection of aneurysms of the abdominal aorta. N Engl J Med 281:422–425, 1969.

35. Skinner DG: Considerations for management of large retroperitoneal tumors: use of the modified thoracoabdominal approach. J Urol 117:605–609, 1977.

36. Skinner DG, Melamud A, Lieskovsky G: Complications of thoracoabdominal retroperitoneal lymph node dissection. J Urol 127:1107–1110, 1982.

37. Smith RB, Machleder HI, Rand RW, et al: Preoperative vascular embolization as an adjunct to successful resection of large retroperitoneal hemangiopericytoma. J Urol 115:206–208, 1976.

38. Sunderman FW Jr: Measurements of vanillylmandelic acid for the diagnosis of pheochromocytoma and neuroblastoma. Am J Clin Pathol 42:481–497, 1964.

39. Tidrick RT, Goldstein MS: Surgical treatment of retroperitoneal tumors. Arch Surg 70:203–206, 1955.

40. Weimer G, Culp DA, Loening S, Narayana A: Urogenital involvement by malignant lymphoma. J Urol 125:230–231, 1981.

41. Wiley AL, Wirtanen GW, Joo P, et al: Clinical and theoretical aspects of the treatment of surgically unresectable retroperitoneal malignancy with combined intra-arterial actinomycin D and radiotherapy. Cancer 36:107–122, 1975.

DAVID L. McCULLOUGH, M.D.

Diagnosis and Staging of Prostatic Cancer

CHAPTER 23

Cancer of the prostate (CaP) is often diagnosed at an advanced stage, although in recent years the percentage of patients in lower stages at the time of diagnosis has increased.[51] Early diagnosis is a notable goal because the cure rate is much better in the lower stages. The key to early diagnosis is still the well-performed rectal examination, the "gold standard" of diagnostic examinations that has stood the test of time. One of the key points for courses in physical diagnosis of male patients should be that medical students learn the technique of rectal examination as a routine procedure, especially in men over 50 years of age. Thompson and associates found no prostate nodules in routine screening of 365 men, aged 40 to 49 years.[72]

STAGING DEFINITIONS

A variety of staging schemes have evolved over the years (Table 23–1).[57] However, most urologists in the United States use the A-B-C-D staging system. The scheme proposed by the American Joint Commission on Cancer (the TNM classification) is slowly gaining usage.

Stage A (also I, T0, N0) can be defined as malignant disease detected on pathologic examination of glands removed for clinically benign disease. Stage A_1 (IA, T0, N0, or focal) generally refers to cases in which three or fewer microscopic fields can be found to have well-differentiated carcinoma in biopsied material. Others would quantify this stage as less than 5% involvement of the specimen. Stage A_2 (IA, T0, N0, or diffuse) refers to the clinical situation in which more of the gland is involved than stated in A_1 or when cells show dedifferentiation. (Stage A_2 has many of the same characteristics as Stage C and often behaves in the same fashion as Stage C biologically.)

Stage B (II, T1, T2, N0, or intracapsular) refers to clinically detected disease that is intracapsular. There are no symptoms. This is the prototype of the earliest lesion thought to be detectable by clinical examination. Stage B_1 (II, T1–2, N0) generally refers to disease involving less than one lobe (often 2 cm or less, often a discrete nodule). Stage B_2 (II, T1–2) refers to lesions occupying more than one lobe. The serum acid phosphatase (SAP) level is not elevated in Stages A and B.

Stage C (III, T3, N0) refers to invasion through the prostatic capsule and often extending into the seminal vesicles. It is frequently associated with obstructive symptoms. Occasionally, it is subdivided into Stage C_1, for limited extension through the capsule, and Stage C_2, for larger lesions, often weighing more than 70 gm, that invade the rectum or bladder and become affixed to one or both pelvic walls.[36] The SAP level is sometimes mildly elevated in Stage C disease, although some would argue that if it is elevated the stage should be classified as Stage D.

In the TNM system, any of the above stages

405

Table 23–1. SURGICAL MANAGEMENT OF PROSTATIC CARCINOMA

Stage	Stage	TNM Classification	State of Local Lesion	Level of Prostatic Acid Phosphatase	Bone Metastases Detectable by Bone X-ray
A, focal	IA	T0, NX, M0	Not palpable, focal	Not elevated	No
A, diffuse	IB	T0, NX, M0	Not palpable, diffuse	Not elevated	No
B	II	T1 or T2, NX, M0	Confined to prostate	Not elevated	No
C	III	T3, NX, M0	Local extension	Not elevated	No
D	IVA	Any T, NX, M0	Any	Elevated	No
D	IVB	Any T, N1 to N4, ¨M0	Any	Any	No
D	IVC	Any T, Any N, M1	Any	Any	Yes

can have nodal involvement (N). NX is used when the nodes are not assessed. Tumors in Stages N0 through N3 require histologic examination. N0 applies when nodes are free of disease; N1 denotes one positive homolateral node; N2 indicates bilateral, contralateral, or multiple positive nodes; and N3 denotes a fixed pelvic mass with free space between it and the tumor.

Stage D (IV, any T and N stage, M0 or M1) refers to metastatic disease. This metastatic spread may be as minimal as one pelvic lymph node micrometastasis and it may be as extensive as multiple nodal involvement or bone metastasis. Stage D_1 (IVA, any T stage, N1–3, M0) refers to local nodal involvement, whereas Stage D_2 (IVB or IVC, any T or N stage, M1) refers to distant nodal, bony, or visceral metastases. Cancer of the prostate in Stage D is often associated with an elevated SAP level.

In the TNM system, distant metastasis is denoted by M. MX indicates that the assessment of distant metastasis was not met. M0 denotes no known distant metastasis, and M1 indicates that such a metastasis is present.

Grading is equally important in prognosis and is related to the probability of metastases. As the lesions become less differentiated, the rate of nodal involvement increases regardless of stage.[17] Poorly differentiated CaP has a very grim prognosis regardless of the type of therapy.

The approximate percentages of patients in the various stages are classically in the following ranges: Stage A, 5 to 10%; Stage B, 5 to 10%; Stage C, 45%; Stage D, 30 to 35%.[3, 22, 35] However, in the data from the American College of Surgeons, the percentages for their series were Stage A, 23%; Stage

B, 34%; Stage C, 20%; Stage D, 23%.[51] There is considerable disparity between the "classical" data and the ACS data. The true incidence probably lies somewhere in between. The author leans toward the "classical" percentages. Stage A percentages can be increased by compulsive and thorough examination of the entire pathologic specimen. Newman and associates found that the incidence of Stage A increased from 8 to 14% when all chips from the transurethral resection were examined. Stage A_2 was more common than Stage A_1.[52]

DIAGNOSIS

The classic example of the elderly man with back pain, weight loss, anemia, and prostatism represents an all-too-common clinical occurrence, and he is to be considered to have CaP until it is proved otherwise. Frequency and nocturia, especially of recent onset, are two of the more common presenting symptoms of clinically manifest CaP.[6, 63] Other commonly occurring symptoms incude dysuria, slow stream, urinary retention, dribbling, back pain, and hematuria.[6]

The patient with Stage A CaP often has symptoms of prostatism resulting from benign prostatic hypertrophy or hyperplasia. Cancer is unsuspected clinically and is a surprise when the pathology report is received. In the Stage B patient, the induration or nodule is often discovered on routine physical examination. Stage C patients often present clinically with symptoms of prostatism but disease is occasionally detected on routine physical examination of asymptomatic patients. Stage D patients often have significant symptoms of prostatism as well as other symptoms related to metastases, especially to bone.

Upon examination by a pathologist, a firm, palpable nodule is found to be CaP in about 50% of the cases.[68] Catalona found an incidence of 45% CaP when marked induration material was taken for biopsy.[14] The differential diagnosis of such lesions includes prostatic calculi, tuberculosis, granulomatous prostatitis, a spheroid of benign prostatic hypertrophy, rectal wall phlebolith, or perhaps localized prostatitis. Occasionally, a nodular projection of the pubic bone can fool the examiner into thinking it represents a firm prostatic nodule. It is interesting that prostatic lesions often feel comparatively different in awake and anesthetized patients, as well as different when the bladder is empty or full. Also, the position of the patient (bending over, lying on the side, or the lithotomy position) can affect the tactile representation of the lesion.

A biopsy should be performed whenever a suspicious or indurated lesion is found unless one suspects that a recent inflammatory process has caused the changes in the gland. A short trial of antibiotics and repeat examination within a month may be indicated in such cases. In more advanced lesions, the prostate may be diffusely indurated with extension through the capsule, seminal vesicle, lateral pelvic wall, and rarely into the rectum. Occasionally, it may be confused with a primary cancer of the rectum. Histologic examination, determination of SAP levels, and special acid phosphatase stains usually enable one to make the correct diagnosis.

At times, the first manifestation of CaP is a pathologic fracture, bone pain (often attributed to "arthritis"), sudden development of paresis or paraplegia (a neurosurgical emergency), a palpable inguinal or supraclavicular lymph node, disseminated intravascular coagulation, chronic renal failure, edema, hypertension, anemia, cachexia, and a myriad of other seemingly unrelated signs and symptoms. Histochemical techniques exist for the detection of acid phosphatase and the subsequent identification of CaP found in unusual sites such as fractures, lymph nodes (often supraclavicular nodes that contain "adenocarcinoma, origin undetermined"), and the rectal wall.[9, 39] Immunoperoxidase stains are helpful in identifying prostatic acid phosphatase in malignant epithelial cells of uncertain origin.[42, 61]

Biopsy Techniques

Transrectal and Transperineal Biopsy. These biopsy routes are the most commonly used in the United States. Often, a large-bore needle with a cutting device is the instrument used[63]; popular examples include the Franklin modification of the Vim-Silverman needle and new disposable biopsy needles.

These techniques may be performed under local anesthesia or mild sedation in tolerant patients. In some centers, they are performed as outpatient procedures. There is considerable pressure exerted on urologists by third-party payers to perform these biopsies in outpatient facilities. However, the patient may have complications, and extremely close follow-up is mandatory.

It is desirable to prepare the patient for a transrectal biopsy by emptying the rectum with an enema or laxatives timed in such a way as to have the fecal discharge prior to and not at the time of biopsy. A broad-spectrum antibiotic is administered a day before and several days following the procedure. Rinsing out the rectum or swabbing it with an iodine-containing preparatory solution may be helpful in reducing the infection and sepsis rates. Utilizing these techniques, it is possible to obtain an accurate diagnosis in a high percentage of cases with little danger of drastic sequelae such as impotence, rectal injury, or incontinence.[24, 50] The author's personal opinion is that transrectal biopsy is perhaps a little more accurate than the transperineal technique in sampling the lesion that can be felt rectally, but the price for this enhanced accuracy is more infections and septic problems. Fever, hematuria and sepsis may occur with either technique,[18, 56] although Kaufman and associates cited a 7% incidence of complications by the transperineal route and 15 to 33% with the transrectal route.[37]

Seeding of carcinoma along the needle track by way of either the transrectal or the transperineal route is a serious complication but is, fortunately, quite rare.[1]

Needle Aspiration. Fine-needle aspiration of prostatic lesions appears to be slowly gaining favor in the United States. The technique consists of inserting a fine aspiration needle (Franzen) either transrectally (usually with no preparation) or transperineally and aspirating "tissue juice" from the lesion; this liquid is immediately fixed on a glass slide. Fine-needle aspiration has enjoyed more popularity in Europe than in the United States for years.[76] Several authors have reported equivalent results from transrectal aspiration and transrectal needle biopsy.[2]

In 1976, Kelsey and associates studied transrectal and transperineal needle biopsies in 38 patients.[38] In 22 who had a positive evidence of cancer of the prostate upon needle biopsy, 18 had positive results from aspiration studies and another had a suspicious result from fine-needle aspiration sampling. There were no false-positive results from aspiration studies.

Chodak reported good results with needle aspiration, indicating a slightly higher accuracy for needle aspiration than for needle biopsy in the determination of CaP, and cited five other United States papers that affirmed the utility of aspiration biopsy.[15]

A review of the literature on aspiration reveals very low to nonexistent complication rates and overall high accuracy.[19] Well-differentiated cells in the aspirate can be a problem and the surgeon is dependent on the cytopathologist for accuracy in the evaluation, assuming that cells were sent from the prostatic area in question.

Open Biopsy. There is little disagreement that open biopsy (i.e., open perineal biopsy) is the most accurate way to diagnosis CaP. In Hudson's series of open perineal biopsies, the accuracy rate was 96%[32]; however, complications include impotence, rectal injury, and incontinence. Obviously, it is neither an economical nor an acceptable procedure for screening. It is most suitable for the patient who is suspected of harboring CaP and in whom other biopsy techniques have given negative results. The utility of open retropubic biopsy for CaP is limited because of the tumor's anatomic peculiarities within the gland. Some authorities think that CaP develops in the horseshoe-shaped area that lies along the posterolateral aspect of the prostate,[48] and this area is difficult to expose retropubically without mobilizing the gland.

Transurethral Biopsy. In a sense, transurethral resection of the prostate for benign prostatic hypertrophy (BPH) is a pathologic screening test for CaP that gives a positive result about 10% of the time. Prout stated that over 90% of patients with neoplasms sufficiently advanced to cause symptoms of prostatism will yield positive evidence of CaP from a transurethral resection (TURP).[63]

It is common knowledge that the yield of CaP in TURP specimens increases substantially when all of the chips are examined.[52]

Generally, TURP biopsy of a peripherally located lesion is not recommended, but Denton showed that it compared favorably with perineal biopsy.[16] Grayhack and Bockrath think transurethral samples have provided sufficient evidence of diagnostic usefulness to warrant further exploration of their use in all stages of CaP.[29] The author has had some success on several occasions in performing a successful biopsy of a peripheral lesion by elevating the lesion with a gloved finger in the rectum, thus elevating the nodule against the resecting loop. One should obviously take care not to take a deep bite through the prostate into the rectal wall when attempting a TURP biopsy.

There are also modifications of the Vim-Silverman needle that will reach through the end of a panendoscope to biopsy lesions through the urethra, but this procedure is often cumbersome. Whether such needles are still available commercially is not known.

Cytologic Studies of Urine and Prostatic Fluid

Scott and Schirmer reviewed a number of papers on cytopathologic diagnosis of CaP that used urine and prostatic fluid.[68] In one older series, abnormal cells were found in 77% of patients with CaP.[49] The consensus of the review was that results of Papanicolaou smears of expressed prostatic fluid were of merit except in patients receiving estrogen therapy.

In a more recent paper, Garrett and Jassie reported results of cytologic examination of postmassage prostatic secretions and postmassage urine in patients with and without urinary tract symptoms.[25] Urine examinations provided superior detection results. Of asymptomatic patients, about 1% had a positive result on urine cytologic examination. Of those with positive or suspicious urine cytologic findings who underwent histologic examination, the detection rate was 71%. In the symptomatic group, 10% had positive urine cytologic results. In this group, when the patients with positive, suspicious urine cytologic findings underwent histologic examination, the detection rate was 64%.

At present, urine cytologic examination does not enjoy wide usage for CaP. It would seem to be very little more trouble to perform transrectal needle aspiration biopsy with cytologic examination than to massage the prostate and collect cytologic specimens, since aspiration biopsy has good accuracy and is attended by minimal morbidity. Recently, Sharifi and associates compared cytologic results of voided urine, prostate massage, aspiration, and postmassage urine from 248 male patients with urinary complaints but without known CaP.[69] All underwent transrectal needle biopsy of the prostate, and 23% had histologic evidence of cancer. Results of the cytologic examinations were as follows: aspiration was 83% efficient; massage, 81%; postmassage urine, 80%; and voided urine, 79% accurate. The most sensitive test was aspiration cytology.

Biochemical Fluid Studies

Grayhack and Bockrath cited results in several studies of expressed prostatic fluid for detection of CaP.[29] The ratio of LDH-5 to LDH-1 (isoenzymes of lactic dehydrogenase) was found to be over 2 in 80% of those with CaP, whereas less than 15% of those with BPH had a ratio over 2. However, in men with prostatitis, the majority had a ratio over 2.

Grayhack and associates also reported that they had performed experiments analyzing prostatic fluid for complement C3 and transferrin.[29] They found that 95% of patients with a clinically normal prostate, BPH, or prostatitis had a level of complement C3 that was less than 10 mg/dl and a transferrin level of less than 30 mg/dl. However, 85% of patients with CaP had a complement C3 level of 10 mg/dl or more, and 77% had a transferrin concentration of 30 mg/dl or greater.

General Laboratory Studies

Several studies are commonly performed to screen the patient with suspected CaP. The complete blood count (CBC) will detect anemia if present. Widely metastatic CaP to bone often produces an anemia due to marrow replacement by tumor. A serum biochemical profile (SMAC) is relatively inexpensive and can detect elevations in creatinine due to obstruction of the ureter or bladder neck. Elevated levels of alkaline phosphatase are found in 80 to 90% of patients with bony or liver metastases, or

both.[74] When the serum alkaline phosphatase is elevated, the site of origin can be detected by isoenzyme fractionation of the alkaline phosphatase. Serum calcium levels may be elevated owing to bony metastases or lowered owing to uptake of calcium by blastic metastases. Hypocalcemia is more common than hypercalcemia.[34]

Determination of the serum acid phosphatase (SAP) is the "gold standard" biochemical test used to detect and stage CaP. This utilizes tartrate inhibition and specific biochemical substrates such as thymolphthalein to isolate a fraction of serum acid phosphatase produced by prostatic epithelial cells, so-called prostatic acid phosphatase. Elevation of SAP occurs in over 80% of patients with Stage D disease and in about 25% of those with Stage C disease.[62] In general, elevation of the SAP level indicates metastatic disease even though disease cannot be identified by bone scan. About 60% of patients with elevated SAP levels and negative results from bone scans will have nodes with positive evidence of disease.[57]

A false-positive SAP result is not rare, and, when levels are elevated, tests should be repeated. Various types of prostatic manipulations, such as prostate massage or transurethral resection, may elevate the SAP level transiently, but it usually returns to normal within 48 hours.[8, 60] Ejaculation does not elevate the level of SAP. Prostatic infarction may cause an elevated level of SAP. Recent episodes of fever may result in spuriously low levels of SAP in patients with CaP.[50]

Other nonprostatic causes of an elevated SAP level include myeloma, osteogenic sarcoma, thrombocytopenia, Gaucher's disease, nonprostatic malignant tumors with bony metastases, Paget's disease of bone, hyperparathyroidism, osteoporosis, diseases of erythrocytes, hematologic neoplasms, hyperparathyroidism, and others.[80]

The prostate normally contains 1000 times more acid phosphatase than any other organ, and the enzyme is concentrated in the glandular epithelium. In prostatic carcinoma, the epithelium is often poorly developed; therefore, the enzyme activity per unit of prostatic malignant tissue is often less than that of the normal prostate or in benign prostatic hypertrophy. The elevation of the SAP level is probably secondary to increased bulk of tissue in the prostate (Stages C and D) and in metastatic foci and is also probably because of the involvement of blood and lymphatic vessels with resultant leakage of the enzyme into the general circulation. Yam reviewed the literature and found that SAP levels were elevated in 65 to 92% of the patients with bony metastases, in 30% of those without radiographic evidence of bony metastases, and in 5 to 10% of those with no identifiable metastases.[80]

There are several theories to explain why not all patients with bony metastases have an elevated SAP level. Among these are (1) lack of production of acid phosphatase by the metastases (especially the poorly differentiated ones), (2) slightly elevated levels that are present but not detected, and (3) inactivation of the elevated enzyme levels that occurred prior to assay.

When antiandrogen therapy is given, elevated SAP levels often fall, paralleling the clinical response in a majority of cases.[33]

Immunologic assays have been developed to measure prostatic acid phosphatase. Counterimmunoelectrophoresis (CIEP) and radioimmunoassay (RIA) are two of these tests.

Foti and associates showed that the assay gave positive results in a higher percentage of cases in all stages than were found by the enzymatic methods.[23] However, the RIA was also positive in 5% of those with nonprostatic cancer, 4% of those who had undergone total prostatectomy, and even 6% of patients with benign prostatic hypertrophy. Positive results from the biochemical test were not elevated in such BPH patients. However, Guinan found that RIA was no more effective than the standard enzymatic method in detecting CaP,[31] as did Fair.[20] Both RIA and enzymatic tests are limited in their usefulness for early detection of CaP, and this makes RIA not as cost-effective as a general screening test. Gittes also questioned the value of RIA as a screening test for occult carcinoma, citing an unacceptable false-positive rate of over 6% in patients with BPH.[27]

Conventional SAP and RIA determinations, or CIEP, are useful in following patients with CaP who are undergoing therapy for various types, such as hormonal manipulation or chemotherapy, or simply in screening for recurrent disease after surgical or radiation therapy. A recent study by Carson and associates found no differences in diagnostic accuracy between RIA, CIEP, catalytic acid phosphatase determinations, and immunoenzymatic assays for prostatic examinations in patients with all stages of CaP or benign conditions of the prostate.[12]

Serum Alkaline Phosphatase (SAKP). As mentioned earlier, SAKP levels are usually elevated in CaP metastatic to bone. Liver disease, including metastases, intestinal obstruction, Paget's disease of bone, primary bone tumors, and neoplasms (other than CaP) may result in elevated levels. In patients with metastatic disease to bone, the highest levels of SAKP seen are associated with blastic lesions.[70]

As indicated, isoenzyme fractionation may help identify the site of origin of the neoplasm, and alkaline phosphatase will be elevated in bony metastases. Following this enzyme level in patients with CaP and bone metastases while they are under hormonal manipulation or chemotherapy is sometimes helpful. After an initial rise following institution of therapy, the level of this enzyme begins to fall, as does the SAKP level in many patients.

Other Chemical Studies

Fibrinolysis. Twelve per cent of patients with metastatic CaP demonstrate fibrinolytic activity in the serum. Patients who have this disease have a fibrinogen deficiency and prolongation of the prothrombin time. The enzyme responsible for the fibrinolysis originates in the malignant tissue and is released into the blood stream.[71]

Cystoscopy

Cystoscopy is generally unrewarding in helping to diagnose CaP, especially in the lower stages. In the advanced stages, CaP is evident on rectal examination. It would be extremely rare to find involvement of the bladder neck or membranous urethra at cystourethroscopy without having suspicious findings when the rectum was palpated.

Radiologic Studies

Retrograde urethrocystography of CaP reveals urethral defects consisting of interrupted, irregular, "moth-eaten" and granular areas. In BPH the mode of compression is regular and continuous.[79] The normal motility of the lower urinary tract may be altered with CaP, although this study has not gained much popularity.

A *chest x-ray* may reveal metastases to ribs, lungs, or hilar nodes or lymphangitic spread. A *plain radiograph of the abdomen* (kidney, ureter, and bladder) may reveal typical osteoblastic metastases in the vertebrae (71%), femoral heads, ilium (83%), or pubic bones (78%). Paget's disease may resemble metastatic CaP, but the dense areas of Paget's disease are trabeculated and do not have the nodular consistency of blastic metastases from CaP.[68]

The *intravenous urogram* may reveal filling defects in the bladder neck area, hydroureteronephrosis, or nonfunction of either or both kidneys.

Bone surveys (skeletal) have been supplanted for the most part by isotopic bone scans ([99m]technetium). Such scans have demonstrated bony metastases in approximately 35% of all patients judged to be free of disease on routine bone surveys and have shown positive evidence of disease in 75 to 85% of patients with advanced disease.[57, 74] In fact, SAP may be a more sensitive indicator of bony metastases than a bone survey.[57] Skeletal surveys are helpful in patients who have positive results of isotopic scans if there is some question about the findings (i.e., the results of arthritis, old fractures, or other bone disorders).

There are several reasons why skeletal surveys are not helpful in detecting early bone metastases: there must be a loss of at least 30 to 50% of the normal bone mineral to show an early metastatic lesion,[10] in the vertebrae a loss of 50 to 70% must be noted before a lesion may be visible,[26] a lesion in the vertebrae may need to be over 1.5 cm before one can detect it radiographically,[5] and an area testing positive on an isotopic bone scan may antedate a lesion seen radiographically by three to six months.[55]

Isotopic bone scans have become an integral part of the staging work-up of patients with CaP. As has been mentioned, [99m]technetium scans are quite popular and enjoy wide usage. Alterations in bone physiology and pathologic condition produce abnormal results on scans. Processes that cause increased blood flow or blood supply to an area result in more radionuclide reaching that area. Repair mechanisms include altered exchange processes in new bone formation and increased turnover as osteoid is formed. All of these conditions result in increased radioisotopic activity on a bone scan.

Total body scanning is the method of choice for bone scanning. No preparation of the patient is necessary; the process requires approximately an hour or less and is performed two to three hours after an injection of the isotope. The kidneys are the main route of excretion of the isotope.[55] A good view of the kidneys, ureters, and bladder is provided. Occasionally, when the scan results are positive, a confirmatory bone biopsy is necessary to verify the presence of a metastasis. As most bones are within biopsy range, this technique has proved useful in screening patients who are candidates for radical surgery.[7] Causes of false-positive results include arthritis, fractures, osteomyelitis, previous surgery, and migratory osteoporosis. Occasionally, "false-negative" results are reported, especially if the metastases are symmetrical in the bones. Areas of decreased uptake may occur with osteolytic metastases.[73]

Pedal Lymphangiography

This invasive procedure requires local anesthesia in both feet and considerable expertise in performance and interpretation. A running debate continues as to whether the obturator nodes are visualized routinely on this study (these nodes are the first echelon of metastases to nodes). The external iliac, common iliac, and para-aortic nodes are well seen. Lymphangiography does not demonstrate metastases unless they are 5 mm or larger.[40] Many early metastases in CaP are micrometastases that are unable to be seen on lymphangiography. Pulmonary disease of a moderate degree or greater is a contraindication to the study because the oily compound that contains the iodine is briefly disseminated into the lungs.

Criteria used to evaluate metastases to the lymphatics include obstruction of lymphatic channels, collateral lymphatic vessels, filling defects in nodes, and failure of opacification of nodes. Tomography may assist in delineating lesions.

Some authors are utilizing lymphangiography, computerized tomography (CT), and fine-needle aspiration of suspicious nodes as a staging procedure, which, if results are positive, saves the patient from undergoing a staging lymphadenectomy. Flanigan and associates found an overall accuracy of 90% utilizing the studies and identified 50% of patients ultimately found to have lymphatic metastases.[21] A negative result from needle biopsy does not rule out disease either in a specific node or in nodes that appear normal and harbor micrometastases, so only positive results make the study helpful.

Lymphangiography is not a routine study in patients with CaP in most centers, but it may gain more popularity in combination with needle aspiration of suspicious nodes in CaP.

Computerized Tomography (CT), Utrasonography, and Magnetic Resonance Imaging (MRI) in Evaluating the Prostate

Ultrasonography was reported to be fairly accurate in detecting CaP in 100 consecutive patients.[11] Braeckman and Denis reported no false-negative ultrasonographic results among 27 patients with CaP and four false-positive results in diagnoses of carcinoma among patients who had a pathologic diagnosis of adenoma.

Rifkin says that transrectal ultrasound diagnosis of malignancy overlaps with benign disease, and biopsy of a focal lesion will provide the answer.[64] Cancer often demonstrates acoustic alterations of the normal homogenous echogenicity of the gland, as most such lesions are hyperechoic. He also states that the diagnosis of clinically non-palpable CaP is dependent on ultrasound evaluation and biopsy of tissue.[64] Invasive malignancy can be diagnosed when extension of the tumor from the prostatic capsule can be defined.

Peeling and Griffiths found that ultrasonography is also helpful in monitoring size and changes of the prostate following external radiation or administration of hormones.[59]

Relative to lymph node involvement, CT is complementary to lymphangiography[74] and is not invasive. It does not reveal intra-nodal architecture but is helpful in evaluating enlarged nodes that are replaced by tumor. Its sensitivity is about 40 to 50% in detecting nodal metastases. It can be used in combination with thin-needle aspiration of enlarged lymph nodes.

CT is unable to discriminate intracapsular CaP from BPH and is useful only for evaluating large tumors.[74] MRI reveals soft tissues well and can give views in sagittal, coronal, and axial orientations. It may become the modality of choice for staging malignancy and defining lymph node abnormalities. Further work is needed to better define the benefits and weaknesses of CT versus MRI.[64] MRI can demonstrate involvement of the seminal vesicles, distortion of the prostatic contour, and disruption of the lower intensity surgical capsule in patients with Stage C CaP.[77]

Obviously, further refining of the above imaging techniques to detect intra- and extracapsular disease and extent of local invasion as well as nodal involvement is eagerly anticipated.

Surgical Staging by Pelvic Lymphadenectomy

This method of staging is widely utilized and, combined with isotopic bone scans, will reveal higher stages of tumor in about 50% of patients who present with CaP.[57] Mentioned earlier were techniques for detection of suspicious nodal metastases by CT and lymphangiography with biopsy confirmation by thin-needle aspiration. This is utilized at some centers, and, when results are positive, may obviate the need for the open surgical procedure, saving considerable money and patient risk.[21] If the results of the studies are negative, then surgical staging is indicated. More centers will probably attempt the CT and needle aspiration in the future.

Surgical staging for A_1 lesions is not indicated because the yield of nodes positive for disease is near 0. Patients with small B_1 lesions that are well differentiated will have an incidence of less than 10%. On the other end of the scale, patients in Stage C with elevated SAP levels and poorly differentiated cells will have nearly 90% of their nodes positive for disease.[24]

Those falling between the last two groups mentioned above are candidates for node dissection. In any stage, the poorly differentiated lesions have a much higher incidence of positive nodes. However, well-differentiated lesions above Stage B_1 metastasize frequently enough to warrant node dissection, in the author's opinion.

There is considerable debate about whether one can predict (on the basis of the Gleason grading score system) whether a given patient will have diseased nodes based on that score. Paulson stated that only 14% of patients with Gleason's score of 2 to 5 will have positive nodes, whereas 100% of those with Gleason's score of 9 or 10 had positive nodes.[58] These data have created considerable discussion about omitting the node dissection in these two groups. Olsson has disagreed with this approach because he found affected nodes in 20% of patients with Gleason's score of 2 to 4, and in only 62% of those with scores of 8 to 10.[54] From Olsson's data, it is apparent that as the stage increased, the percentage of patients with positive nodes in Gleason's score of 2 to 4 increased markedly. A significant percentage (40%) of patients with CaP in low Stage A_2 or B and Gleason's score of 8 to 10 had diseased nodes, and 100% of patients in Stage C had positive nodes. Sagalowsky found only 44% of patients with positive nodes who were in Gleason's scores of 7 to 9.[66] The other issue debated is whether one should decide to perform a lymphadenectomy on the basis of Gleason's score on the needle biopsy or on the needle aspiration. In several series, the initial Gleason's score in the low range was significantly lower than the final score on the radical specimen.[4, 43, 54] The interested reader may peruse the literature in regard to these issues.

Formulation of treatment plans and evaluation of treatment results are aided if the presence and extent of nodal involvement are known. An occasional patient with one positive node may be cured, in the author's opinion.

Clinical understaging is common and related to whether CaP has extended into or through the capsule. Also, the amount of intracapsular disease is often underestimated. Whitmore and MacKenzie reported 45% of the patients thought to have CaP in clinical Stage B actually had disease through the capsule and in Stage C.[75] Saltzstein and McLaughlin reported no metastases in patients with less than 35% of the gland involved at pathologic examination, although many of the patients were thought to have small Stage B_1 lesions prior to prostatectomy.[67] Nicholson and Richie reported that their clinical Stage B estimation was low in 35% of the patients in their series.[53] Wilson and associates were more accurate in their clinical staging, and their estimate of clinical Stage B was accurate 85% of the time.[78] One can readily see that in the best of hands, clinical understaging by rectal examination is common, and, if one obtains SAP levels and results of bone scans, performs pelvic lymphadenectomy, and removes the prostate, one or more of these tests will frequently change the patient's condition to a higher stage than the one that was clinically suspected.

As a general rule, the operation is performed extraperitoneally from pubis to umbilicus, an approach the author prefers. Nodal tissue is removed from the medial aspect of the external iliac artery, but lymphatics along the lateral aspect of the artery are preserved to prevent lymphedema. The nodal tissue from the area by the circumflex iliac vein proximal to the common iliac artery, the tissue from the obturator fossa around the obturator nerve, and the area around the hypogastric artery are all removed. This node dissection, less radical than formerly performed, has resulted in less lymphedema and little difference in the incidence of positive nodes.[57] However, the author often performs a more radical lymphadenectomy than described if a radical prostatectomy rather than radiation therapy is planned. An extensive node dissection plus external radiation therapy results in an increased incidence of lymphedema. Von Eschenbach states that removing the hypogastric obturator group of nodes will identify almost all patients with nodal metastases, although the extent of nodal disease will be underestimated in 55 to 80% of patients having this limited surgery.[74]

There are some data to support the contention that the prognosis is much better with one positive node than with more than one. Generally, the disease is considered systemic when nodes are involved. If the nodes are not grossly enlarged and feel normal, it is impossible to predict whether micrometastases are present. Examination of frozen sections will help, but the false-negative rate is around 11 to 16%.[41, 65] This one-stage procedure of node dissection and radical prostatectomy is weighed against two separate operations and greater expense if node dissection and radical prostatectomy are performed on different occasions. Most false-negative results from frozen section errors involve micrometastases. If one believes that radiation therapy offers no survival benefit to patients with diseased nodes, then no great harm is done by proceeding with the surgery, because no other form of therapy that the author is aware of is better for micrometastases. However, this is an individual decision and regards philosophy of treatment of micrometastatic nodal disease. Most authors agree that obturator nodes are involved earliest;[13, 46, 47] therefore, an involved common iliac node is a more ominous sign and indicates further spread.

Complications of lymphadenectomy occur, but the mortality rate is extremely low. An operative morbidity of 20 to 34% is reported by von Eschenbach, including wound infection (5 to 10%), atelectasis, ileus, sepsis, pulmonary embolus (5 to 10%), thrombophlebitis, lymphoceles, and edema of the penis and lower extremities (5 to 10%). McCullough also has reported on complications of lymphadenectomy.[45] It is difficult to determine the cause of morbidity when one performs a combined node dissection and radical retropubic prostatectomy.

The incidence of positive nodes in patients in Stage A_1 is less than 5% and approaches 0. Stage A_2 is associated with approximately 25 to 30% of patients with affected nodes; in those in Stage B_1, 15% have positive nodes; Stage B_2, 40%; and Stage C, approximately 50%. As mentioned earlier, moderately differentiated or poorly differentiated CaP (medium to higher Gleason's scores) results in an increased incidence of positive nodes.[17, 46] In the series reported by McLaughlin and associates, only 10% of patients with CaP in clinical Stage B or C had positive nodes and well-differentiated tumors, whereas 56% of those with undifferentiated tumors had positive nodes.[47] In another series of 149 patients, Liebner and co-workers found that those with high-grade lesions had a twofold greater increase in positive results of nodal biopsies and lymphangiograms than did patients with low-grade lesions.[44] Grossman reported on a series of 91 patients undergoing staging node dissection.[30] Twenty-two per cent of 45 patients with Grade I lesions

Table 23–2. PELVIC LYMPHADENECTOMY— STAGES A_1, A_2, B_1, B_2, and C

Stage	Number of Patients	Patients with Affected Nodes	Percentage
A_1	44	1	2
A_2	212	56	26
B_1	504	52	10
B_2	420	106	25
B	332	73	22
C	946	438	46
Total	2458	726	30

Table 23–3. PELVIC LYMPHADENECTOMY— STAGE AND GRADE

Stage and Grade	Number of Patients	Patients with Affected Nodes	Percentage
Stage A_1			
w/d	44	1	2
Stage A_2			
w/d	19	1	5
m/d	13	3	23
p/d	12	6	50
Stage B_1			
w/d	37	2	5
m/d	39	8	20
p/d	11	3	27
Stage B_2			
w/d	25	7	28
m/d	51	14	27
p/d	21	8	38
Stage C			
w/d	11	2	18
m/d	55	22	42
p/d	32	22	68

*Key: w/d = well-differentiated; m/d = moderately differentiated; p/d = poorly differentiated.

had positive nodes, as did 54% of 37 patients with Grade II lesions and 77% of 7 patients with Grade III lesions. Tables 23–2 and 23–3 demonstrate some of the statistics relative to grade and stage affecting nodal metastases.[17]

Further improvement in staging and diagnosis will probably evolve from improved histologic and immunochemical tests of serum, urine, and prostatic fluid as well as improved imaging techniques and minimally invasive biopsy procedures. Much has been learned in the past decade, and the future looks bright for improved diagnosis and staging of prostate cancer.

References

1. Addonizio JC, Kapoor SN: Perineal seeding of prostatic carcinoma after needle biopsy. Urology 8:513–515, 1976.
2. Alfthan B, Klintrup HE, Koivuniemi A, et al: Cytological aspiration biopsy and Vim-Silverman biopsy in the diagnosis of prostatic carcinoma. Ann Chir Gynaecol Fenn 59:226–229, 1970.
3. Arduino LJ: Carcinoma of the prostate: treatment comparisons. J Urol 98:516–522, 1967.
4. Babaian RJ, Grunow WA: Reliability of Gleason grading system in comparing prostate biopsies with total prostatectomy specimens. Urology 25:564–567, 1985.
5. Bachman AL, Sproul EE: Correlation of radiographic and autopsy findings in suspected metastases in the spine. Bull NY Acad Med 31:146–148, 1955.

6. Barnes RW: Carcinoma of the prostate: a comparative study of modes of treatment. J Urol 44:169–176, 1940.

7. Basinger GT, McCullough DL, McLaughlin AP: "Positive" bone scan—a contraindication to surgery? Urology 6:547–553, 1975.

8. Belville WD, Mahan DE, Clements JC, et al: Prostatic trauma and release of acid phosphatase. Urology 16:168–171, 1980.

9. Blennerhassett JB, Cohen RB, Vickery AL Jr: Carcinoma of the prostate: enzyme histochemistry. Cancer 20:2133–2138, 1967.

10. Borak J: Relationship between clinical and roentgenological findings in bone metastases. Surg Gynecol Obstet 75:599–604, 1942.

11. Braeckman J, Denis L: The practice and pitfalls of ultrasonography in the lower urinary tract. Eur Urol 9:193–201, 1983.

12. Carson JL, Eisenberg JM, Shaw LM, et al: Diagnostic accuracy of four assays of prostatic acid phosphatase. Comparison using receiver operating characteristic curve analysis. JAMA 253:665–669, 1985.

13. Castellino RA, Ray G, Blank N, et al: Lymphangiography in prostatic carcinoma: preliminary observations. JAMA 223:877–881, 1973.

14. Catalona WJ: Yield from routine prostatic needle biopsy in patients more than 50 years old referred for urologic evaluation: a preliminary report. J Urol 124:844–846, 1980.

15. Chodak GW, Bibbo M, Straus FH, et al: Transrectal aspiration biopsy versus transperineal core biopsy for the diagnosis of carcinoma of the prostate. J Urol 132:480–482, 1984.

16. Denton SE, Valk WL, Jacobson JM, et al: Comparison of the perineal needle biopsy and the transurethral prostatectomy in the diagnosis of prostate carcinoma: an analysis of 300 cases. J Urol 97:127–129, 1967.

17. Donohue RE, Mani JH, Whitesel JA, et al: Pelvic lymph node dissection, guide to patient management in clinically locally confined adenocarcinoma of prostate. Urology 20:559–565, 1982.

18. Dowlen LW, Block NL, Politano VA: Complications of transrectal biopsy examination of the prostate. South Med J 67:1453–1456, 1974.

19. Esposti PL, Elman A, Norlen H: Complications of transrectal aspiration biopsy of the prostate. Scand J Urol Nephrol 9:208–213, 1975.

20. Fair WR, Heston WDW, Kadmon D, et al: Prostatic cancer, acid phosphatase, creatine kinase-BB and race: a prospective study. J Urol 128:735–738, 1982.

21. Flanigan RC, Mohler JL, King CT, et al: Preoperative lymph node evaluation in prostatic cancer patients who are surgical candidates: the role of lymphangiography and computerized tomography scanning with directed fine needle aspiration. J Urol 134:84–87, 1985.

22. Flocks RH: Present status of interstitial irradiation in managing prostate cancer. JAMA 210:328–330, 1969.

23. Foti AG, Cooper JF, Herschman H, et al: Detection of prostatic cancer by solid-phase radioimmunoassay of serum prostatic acid phosphatase. N Engl J Med 297:1357–1361, 1977.

24. Freiha FS, Pistenma DA, Bagshaw MA: Pelvic lymphadenectomy for staging prostatic carcinoma: is it always necessary? J Urol 122:176–177, 1979.

25. Garrett M, Jassie M: Cytologic examinations of post prostatic massage specimens as an aid in diagnosis of carcinoma of the prostate. Acta Cytol 20:126–131, 1976.

26. Gillespie GA, Grebell FS: The radiological demonstration of osseous metastasis—experimental observations. Clin Radiol 18:158, 1967.

27. Gittes RF: Prostate Cancer (Guest Editorial). J Urol 129:330, 1983.

28. Grabstald H: Cancer of the prostate. CA 15:1, 1965.

29. Grayhack JT, Bockrath JM: Diagnosis of carcinoma of prostate. Urology (Suppl)17:54–60, 1981.

30. Grossman IC, et al: Staging pelvic lymphadenectomy for carcinoma of the prostate: review of 91 cases. J Urol 124:632–634, 1980.

31. Guinan P, Bush I, Ray V, et al: The accuracy of the rectal examination in the diagnosis of prostate carcinoma. N Engl J Med 303:499–503, 1980.

32. Hudson PB: Prostatic cancer. XIV. Its incidence and behavior in 686 men studied by prostatic biopsy. J Am Geriatr Soc 5:338–350, 1957.

33. Huggins C, Hodges CV: Studies on prostatic cancer. I. The effect of castration, of estrogen, and of androgen injection on serum phosphatases in metastatic carcinoma of the prostate. Cancer Res 1:293–297, 1941.

34. Jacobs SC: Spread of prostatic carcinoma to bone. Urology 21:337–344, 1983.

35. Jewett HJ: Prostatic cancer: a personal view of the problem. J Urol 131:845–849, 1984.

36. Johnson DE, Boileau MA: Genitourinary tumors—fundamental principles and surgical techniques. In DE Johnson (ed), Cancer of the Prostate: Overview. New York, Grune & Stratton, 1982, pp 1–32.

37. Kaufman JJ, Ljung BM, Walther P, et al: Aspiration biopsy of the prostate. Urology 19:587–591, 1982.

38. Kelsey DM, Kohler FP, MacKinney CC, et al: Outpatient needle aspiration biopsy of prostate. J Urol 116:327–328, 1976.

39. Kirchheim D, Györkey F, Brandes D, et al: Histochemistry of the normal, hyperplastic, and neoplastic prostate gland. Invest Urol 1:403–421, 1964.

40. Koehler PR: Current status of lymphography in patients with cancer. Cancer 37:503–516, 1976.

41. Kramolowsky EV, Narayana AS, Platz CE, et al: The frozen section in lymphadenectomy for carcinoma of the prostate. J Urol 131:899–900, 1984.

42. Kuriyama M, Wang MC, Lee CL, et al: Multiple marker evaluation in human prostate cancer with the use of tissue-specific antigen. JNCI 68:99–105, 1982.

43. Lange PH, Narayan P: Understaging and undergrading of prostate cancer. Argument for postoperative radiation as adjuvant therapy. Urology 21:113–118, 1983.

44. Liebner EJ, Stefani S: An evaluation of lymphography with nodal biopsy in localized carcinoma of the prostate. URO-Oncology Research Group. Cancer 45:728–734, 1980.

45. McCullough DL, McLaughlin AP, Gittes RF: Morbidity of pelvic lymphadenectomy and radical prostatectomy for prostatic cancer. J Urol 117:206–207, 1977.

46. McCullough DL, Prout GR Jr, Daly JJ: Carcinoma of the prostate and lymphatic metastases. J Urol 111:65–71, 1974.

47. McLaughlin AP, Saltzstein SL, McCullough DL, et al: Prostatic carcinoma: incidence and location of unsuspected lymphatic metastases. J Urol 115:89–94, 1976.

48. Mostofi FK, Price EB: Tumors of the male genital system. *In* Atlas of Tumor Pathology. Washington, DC, Armed Forces Institute of Pathology, 1973, Fasc. 8.

49. Mulholland SW: A study of prostatic secretion and its relation to malignancy. Proc Staff Meet Mayo Clinic 6:733–735, 1931.

50. Murphy GP: The diagnosis of prostatic cancer. Cancer 37:589–596, 1976.

51. Murphy GP, Natararagan N, Pontes JE, et al: The national survey of prostate cancer in the United States by the American College of Surgeons. J Urol 127:928–934, 1982.

52. Newman AJ Jr, Graham MA, Carlton CE Jr, et al: Incidental carcinoma of the prostate at the time of transurethral resection: importance of evaluating every chip. J Urol 128:948–950, 1982.

53. Nicholson TC, Richie JP: Pelvic lymphadenectomy for Stage B adenocarcinoma of the prostate: justified or not? J Urol 117:199–201, 1977.

54. Olsson CA: Staging lymphadenectomy should be an antecedent to treatment in localized prostatic carcinoma. Urology (Suppl) 25:4–6, 1985.

55. O'Mara RE: Skeletal scanning in neoplastic disease. Cancer 37:480–486, 1976.

56. Ostroff EB, Almario J, Kramer H: Transrectal needle method for biopsy of the prostate: review of 90 cases. Am Surg 41:659–661, 1975.

57. Paulson DF: Surgical management of prostatic carcinoma. *In* DG Skinner (ed), Urological Cancer. New York, Grune & Stratton, 1983, pp 21–33.

58. Paulson DF: Staging lymphadenectomy should not be an antecedent to treatment in localized prostatic carcinoma. Urology (Suppl) 25:7–14, 1985.

59. Peeling WB, Griffiths GJ: Imaging of the prostate by ultrasound. J Urol 132:217–224, 1984.

60. Phatak PS, James N: Acid phosphatase after examination of the prostate. Ann Clin Biochem 19:195–196, 1982.

61. Pontes JE: Biological markers in prostate cancer. J Urol 130:1037–1047, 1983.

62. Prout GR Jr: Chemical tests in the diagnosis of prostatic carcinoma. JAMA 209:1699–1700, 1969.

63. Prout GR Jr: Diagnosis and staging of prostatic carcinoma. Cancer 32:1096–1103, 1973.

64. Rifkin MD: The prostate and seminal vesicles. *In* MD Rifkin (ed), Diagnostic Imaging of the Lower Urinary Tract. New York, Raven Press, 1985, pp 121–208.

65. Sadlowski RW, Donahue DJ, Richman AV, et al: Accuracy of frozen section diagnosis in pelvic lymph node staging biopsies for adenocarcinoma of the prostate. J Urol 129:324–326, 1983.

66. Sagalowsky AL, Milam H, et al: Prediction of lymphatic metastases by Gleason histologic grading in prostatic cancer. J Urol 128:951–952, 1982.

67. Saltzstein SL, McLaughlin AP III: Clinicopathologic features of unsuspected regional lymph node metastases in prostatic adenocarcinoma. Cancer 40:1212–1221, 1977.

68. Scott WW, Schirmer HKA: Carcinoma of the prostate. *In* MF Campbell and JH Harrison (eds), Urology. 3rd ed. Philadelphia, WB Saunders, 1970, pp 1143–1189.

69. Sharifi R, Shaw MS, Ray V, et al: Evaluation of cytologic techniques for diagnosis of prostate cancer. Urology 21:417–420, 1983.

70. Swartz MK: Laboratory aids to diagnosis. Enzymes. Cancer 37:542–548, 1976.

71. Tagnon HJ, Whitmore WF Jr, Schulman P, et al: The significance of fibrinolysis occurring in patients with metastatic cancer of the prostate. Cancer 6:63–67, 1953.

72. Thompson IM, Ernst JJ, Gangai MP, et al: Adenocarcinoma of the prostate: results of routine urological screening. J Urol 132:690–692, 1984.

73. Vieras F, Herzberg DL: Focal decreased skeletal uptake secondary to metastatic disease. Radiology 118:121–122, 1976.

74. von Eschenbach AC: Monograph on Carcinoma of the Prostate, Home Study Course Series VII, Course #4. American Urological Association, Office of Education, Houston, Texas, 1985.

75. Whitmore WF Jr, MacKenzie AR: Experiences with various operative procedures for the total excision of prostatic cancer. Cancer 12:396–405, 1959.

76. Williams JP, Still BM, Pugh RCB: The diagnosis of prostatic cancer: cytological and biochemical studies using the Franzen biopsy needle. Br J Urol 39:549–554, 1967.

77. Williams RD, Hricak H: Magnetic resonance imaging in urology. J Urol 132:641–649, 1984.

78. Wilson CS, Dahl DS, Middleton RG: Pelvic lymphadenectomy for the staging of apparently localized prostatic cancer. J Urol 117:197–198, 1977.

79. Wong W, Saito W, Ogawa H: Radiologic detection of prostatic carcinoma by double contrast retrograde urethrocystography. J Urol 114:746–751, 1975.

80. Yam LT: Clinical significance of the human acid phosphatases: a review. Am J Med 56:604–616, 1974.

DAVID F. PAULSON, M.D.

CHAPTER 24

Surgical Therapy for Cancer of the Prostate

Prostatic adenocarcinoma presents a major health risk to the aging male population. It is anticipated that over 70,000 new cases of prostatic carcinoma will be diagnosed in 1987; half that number of patients will die of prostatic carcinoma and an equal number of aging males will die with, but not of, prostatic malignancy. With the increasing ability of the medical community to prevent death due to other disease processes that compete in the aging male, the health care risk posed by prostatic malignancy will increase. Recent studies have identified the perplexing nature of this malignant disease process and provided an understanding as to why our therapeutic strategies have been confused with respect to this specific disease process. The control concepts of malignant disease that have been identified from the study of prostatic adenocarcinoma are presently applicable to most of the solid tumors in humans. Recognition of these concepts allows the surgical oncologist to understand why certain treatments are ineffective and permits the development of new concepts for the control of this malignant disease. In order to understand current thinking regarding the management of prostatic malignancy, the urologic oncologist must be aware of the necessity to assess accurately the anatomic extent of disease in the patient under treatment and the necessity to examine treatment response data as a function of the therapy and the anatomic distribution of the disease. Current data would indicate that surgery plays a major role in determining the ana-

tomic extent of disease, in establishing control of the disease that is confined to the organ, in initiating androgen deprivation in patients who have symptomatic metastatic disease, and in the rehabilitation of patients who are unable to function as intact males either as a result of the primary malignant disease process or of an applied treatment.

EVALUATION OF THE ANATOMIC EXTENT OF DISEASE

In the patient with newly diagnosed prostatic malignancy, the malignancy can be widely disseminated throughout the tumor-bearing host, regionally disseminated, or confined to the organ. As the surgical oncologist approaches the patient with newly diagnosed prostatic adenocarcinoma, his initial studies should be those that are most global in nature and have the potential for identifying widely disseminated disease. These staging maneuvers are designed to focus with increasing intensity on the prostate itself until finally the physician has excluded disease outside the anatomic limits of the prostate. Prostatic adenocarcinoma is one of the few human solid tumors that, when disseminated, signifies its dissemination by an elevation of a marker protein within the serum.[1, 2, 7–9, 13–15, 17, 21, 27–29] This serum marker protein is prostatic acid phosphatase. In the normal anatomic situation, prostatic acid phosphatase is released by

417

epithelial cells lining the acini of the prostate into a ductal system that has no direct contact with interstitial body fluids. Therefore, the process is not reflected by an elevation of the serum prostatic acid phosphatase. However, when metastatic deposits of prostatic cancer cells occur at sites in the body that do not have access to this prostatic ductal system, prostatic acid phosphatase released by epithelial cells has direct access to body fluids, and an acid phosphatase elevation may be noted in the serum. A normal level of serum prostatic acid phosphatase may not signify that the patient with prostatic carcinoma is free of metastatic disease, as not all malignant prostatic epithelial cells release acid phosphatase. However, elevation of the serum prostatic acid phosphatase level revealed by colorimetric or enzymatic assay in a patient with prostatic malignancy should be taken as an indicator of metastatic disease even though subsequent staging studies may fail to identify a metastatic deposit. Thus, when confronted with a patient with histologically proven prostatic adenocarcinoma, the oncologist's first global staging study to determine the anatomic extent of disease should be an assay of serum acid phosphatase. Current methods that employ radioimmunoassay for the detection of serum prostatic acid phosphatase elevations may be no more accurate than the colorimetric assay in detecting disease that has spread to distant metastatic sites.[7, 15]

Prostatic adenocarcinoma has the propensity to metastasize to bone. Classically, the radiographic lesion produced by prostatic carcinoma is characterized by an electron-dense area in bone that has lost the trabecular pattern. However, in patients who do not show osteoblastic lesions by routine bone x-rays, the next study should be the radioisotopic bone scan. In a large multicenter study, patients with newly diagnosed biopsy-proven prostatic adenocarcinoma who, by routine bone survey, had no detectable bony metastasis were subjected to isotopic bone scans using technetium-99m medronate. Approximately 25% of all patients found to have no bony disease on the basis of skeletal radiographs had metastatic disease on the basis of isotopic bone scanning, and the incidence of bony disease increased as the volume of local disease increased (Fig. 24–1).

When the urologic oncologist determines that there is no evidence of bony extension, the physician may then direct careful attention to the pelvis and the periprostatic area. Prostatic carcinoma, like other human solid tumors, has a propensity to metastasize to the regional lymphatics. Metastatic disease in the regional lymphatics that parallel the hypogastric, obturator, and external iliac vasculature are poorly identified by either bipedal lymphangiography or pelvic computerized axial tomography. Accumulated experience has indicated that staging pelvic lymphadenectomy is the most accurate method to determine the presence or absence of pelvic lymph node extension. The limits of the dissection are those that will encompass the primary and secondary areas of nodal drainage to the prostate but will leave undisturbed the tertiary lymphatics

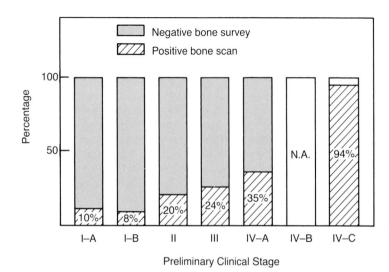

Figure 24–1. Incidence and comparison of positive results of bone scans and negative results from bone surveys.

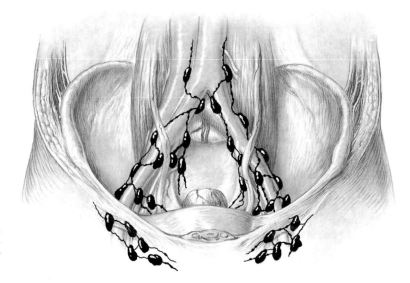

Figure 24–2. The triangular area represents the limits for the dissection of lymph nodes in pelvic lymphadenectomy.

that are lateral to the external iliac artery and vein. Therefore, the limits of the dissection are the triangle subtended by the external iliac artery laterally, the pelvic floor inferiorly, and the hypogastric vasculature medially (Fig. 24–2). All lymphatic tissue within this triangle should be removed, including the lymphatics surrounding the obturator nerve. When pelvic lymphadenectomy is performed in patients who have no detectable disease in their axial and appendicular skeleton by isotopic bone scan and who have no elevation of acid phosphatase levels, it is seen that the incidence of pelvic nodes positive for disease increases as the volume of the local disease increases (Fig. 24–3).[24] Expanding the area of dissection may increase the number of nodes removed

but does not change the incidence of node-positive disease in a given population of patients.

By sequential application of these staging maneuvers, the clinician can determine the anatomic extent of malignancy in the patient under treatment prior to proceeding with treatment selection.

TREATMENT SELECTION BASED UPON THE ANATOMIC EXTENT OF DISEASE: THE ROLE OF SURGERY

Much of the confusion regarding the effect of the various applied treatments in patients

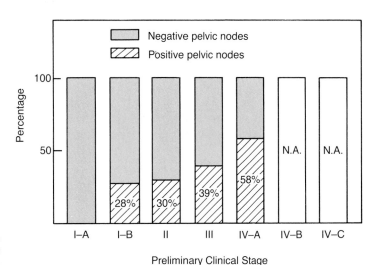

Figure 24–3. Incidence of pelvic nodes showing presence of disease in patients with varying stages of prostatic cancer.

with prostatic carcinoma has been based upon the failure of previous studies to determine accurately the anatomic extent of disease prior to treatment application. Local treatments, such as surgery, are effective only when they encompass the total anatomic extent of disease; failure of the applied treatment to do this leaves residual portions of the disease untreated. Thus, many of the earlier studies that failed to use radioisotopic bone scanning and pelvic nodal dissection to determine the anatomic extent of disease had failure rates that placed the selected treatment modality in disrepute.[3, 11, 20] Only approximately 50% of patients will not be upstaged after radioisotopic bone scanning and pelvic node dissection (Fig. 24–4). Thus, a local treatment to ablate or neutralize cancer in a patient who did not have this appropriate sequence of staging maneuvers would have a 50% chance of failure, since half of the patients could be expected to have distant disease at the time of the initial treatment. It now seems reasonable to examine the effect of surgery or alternative treatments in patients with accurately defined disease.

In a large multi-institutional trial, all patients with prostatic cancer, and in whom the following circumstances applied, were randomly assigned in balanced groups of four either to radical prostatectomy or to megavoltage radiation therapy:[26]

1. Carcinoma was confined to the anatomic boundaries of the prostate by rectal examination
2. The patients were in clinical Stage A or B (B_1 or B_2, N0, M0)

3. There was no elevation of serum prostatic acid phosphatase levels (King-Armstrong units)
4. There was no detectable metastatic disease involving either the appendicular or axial skeleton
5. No lymph node extension could be identified after staging pelvic lymphadenectomy.

Patients with occult focal carcinoma were excluded from the randomization schema, as were any patients who had clinical Stage C disease. Prostatectomy could be accomplished either via a perineal or retropubic approach; however, the anatomic limits of dissection had to include the apex of the prostate and the seminal vesicles. Patients assigned to radiation therapy were treated only with megavoltage equipment and with the highest available energy, a minimum source to axis distance of 80 cm. Initial treatment was either through a four-quadrant or rotational technique. The field size had to include the prostate gland, the periprostatic region, and the pelvic lymph nodes, as determined by the aid of lymphograms and localization films. Otherwise, the field was at the level of the iliac crest, with the lateral margins extending 1 cm below the iliac nodes and the lower margin at least 1 cm below the inferior extent of the prostate. All fields were treated using currently applied schema with an appropriate tumor dose of 4500 to 5000 rads in approximately 40 days total elapsed time. The isodose is specified from the appropriate isodose curves as the minimum dose for the volume of the prostate gland. Additional treatment with 2000 rads

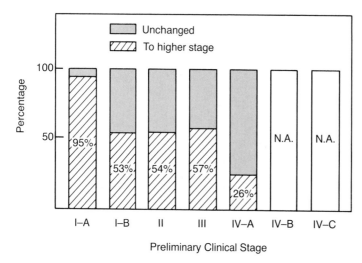

Figure 24–4. Percentage of patients with prostatic cancer whose disease remains in its preliminary clinical stage after the patient undergoes bone scan and biopsy of the lymph nodes.

was delivered to a reduced volume, which had to include the prostate gland.

Patients were followed at two-month intervals for the first year and at three-month intervals thereafter. Complete serum biochemical profiles with acid phosphatase determinations and Karnofsky's performance ratings of physical examination were obtained at each follow-up; chest x-rays and isotopic bone scans were obtained at six-month intervals. The ability of the assigned treatment to control the disease was assessed by using first evidence of treatment failure as the end point. Treatment failure was identified by elevation of acid phosphatase levels evident on two consecutive follow-ups or by the concomitant appearance of bony or parenchymal disease with or without concomitant acid phosphatase elevation. The identification of cancer in the prostate on follow-up biopsy after radiation did not signify treatment failure for purposes of assessing the relative treatment efficacy. Curves representing nonparametric estimates of time to first evidence of treatment failure were generated using the Kaplan-Meier method.[21] Censored values representing patients without evidence of treatment failure at the time of last follow-up were represented by single vertical ticks on the graph. Treatment efficacy of pairs of subgroups were tested for differences by the Cox-Mantel test.[10] The use of time to first evidence of treatment failure as the end point of treatment efficacy was chosen and seems reasonable, as the patient population is aged and at risk for death from intercurrent competing nonmalignant disease. This method of analysis also addressed the problem of treatment evaluation in a disease in which survival may be altered by the subsequent or sequen-

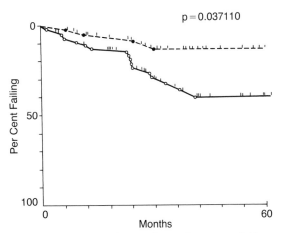

Figure 24–5. Time to first evidence of treatment failure for patients with cancer of the prostate. The solid line represents those patients who received radiation therapy (n = 56); the dashed line represents those who had radical surgery (n = 41).

tial application of additional treatments such as androgen ablation, radiation, or chemotherapy.

An analysis of the time to failure curves in the two treatment groups with localized prostatic carcinoma indicated that radical surgery possessed a distinct advantage over radiation therapy in controlling disease, significant at the 0.037 level (Fig. 24–5). The relative impact of the two treatments initially observed at 60 months continued to be evident at 80 months (Fig. 24–6). Furthermore, had biopsy-persistent disease after radiation been used as an indicator of treatment failure, the difference in disease control would have been even more dramatic. Patients with affected nodes upon biopsy were not initially counted as treatment failures in the radiotherapy group, as the adverse biologic impact of a positive result of biopsy was initially controversial. However,

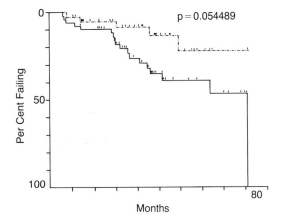

Figure 24–6. Continued study of time to first evidence of treatment failure for patients with cancer of the prostate. The solid line denotes those who received radiation (n = 55), and the dashed line represents those who underwent surgery (n = 41).

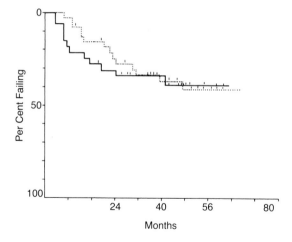

Figure 24–7. Time to first evidence of treatment failure for patients with cancer of the prostate. Those represented by the solid line received delayed hormonal therapy, whereas those patients denoted by the dashed line received radiation therapy.

current data[30] would indicate that a positive node found on biopsy after radiation is an adverse prognostic sign and identifies patients likely to fail with metastatic disease.

A recent modification of the technique of radical prostatectomy permits preservation of the neural innervation for spontaneous erectile control. Although unproven, there is concern that modification of the limits of the surgical dissection necessary to preserve these nerves may compromise the cancer procedure. Therefore, the clinician who recommends this form of operative intervention to his patients should provide caution regarding the potential reduction in the surgical control of malignant disease.

Although it is highly likely that some prostatic carcinomas will respond to radiation therapy, the dilemma that exists is the selection of patients whose malignancy is radiosensitive. It is worrisome that recently derived data suggest that the apparent observed effect of radiation therapy may be only a phenomenon of the natural progression of the disease. A series of patients who had normal serum acid phosphatase levels, no evidence of bony extension by isotopic scanning, and no lymph node extension were randomly assigned to either external beam radiation therapy with portal fields

and a dosage similar to that used for the Stage T1 or T2, N0, M0 disease, or to delayed androgen deprivation therapy, with treatment being withheld until disease spread was identified (Fig. 24–7).[25] Time to first evidence of treatment failure was again used as the end point. The data strongly suggest that radiotherapy does not alter the subsequent appearance of parenchymal or bony spread of this disease and that the incidence of disseminated disease occurs with equal frequency in patients treated with external beam radiation therapy and those who receive delayed androgen deprivation. This raises considerable doubt as to the potential impact of external beam radiation therapy in the management of patients with large-volume, localized prostatic carcinoma. One must question whether the apparent effect of radiation is nothing other than an observation of the natural history of the disease.

CONCLUSION

No randomized data exist to examine the effect of the alternative forms of therapy for disease that is either confined to the organ or demonstrates local extension without regional metastases. However, there are three

Table 24–1. STANFORD EXPERIENCE WITH EXTERNAL BEAM RADIATION*

| Clinical Stage | Number of Patients | 5-Year | Survival Rates (%) | |
			10-Year	15-Year
A or B	458	80 ± 4	59 ± 5	37 ± 8
C	385	60 ± 5	36 ± 6	22 ± 7

*Results are given as the actuarial survival rates by clinical stage at each interval.

Table 24–2. BAYLOR EXPERIENCE WITH ^{198}Au SEEDS AND EXTERNAL BEAM IRRADIATION*

Clinical Stage	Number of Patients	Survival Rates		
		5-Year (NED)	10-Year (NED)	Median (months)
A or B	353	58 ± 4	35 ± 5	72
A$_2$	(103)	57 ± 6	46 ± 8	82
B	250	58 ± 4	32 ± 5	72
B$_1$N	(26)	81 ± 8	60 ± 8	155+
B$_1$	(126)	62 ± 5	42 ± 8	89
B$_2$	(98)	45 ± 6	15 ± 6	53
C$_1$	99	41 ± 6	7 ± 5	53
Total	452	53 ± 6	27 ± 7	64

*Disease-free survivors (NED) are indicated only if they have been continuously free of local or recurrent disease and have received no hormonal therapy.

large single institutional clinical trials that examine a single treatment modality.

Radiation therapy may be applied to the prostate by using either external beam radiation, combination gold seed implantation with external beam radiation, or radioactive iodine implants. External beam therapy utilizes at least 6500 to 7000 rads. Multiple delivery techniques are available in order to spare normal tissues any adverse effects of the radiation therapy. For gold seed implantation with external beam radiation, between six and 10 high-energy radioactive gold seeds are implanted in the prostate at the time of pelvic lymph node dissection. This provides a "booster" dose of approximately 3500 rads. The seminal vesicles may be implanted with seeds if they are involved with tumor. Radioactive gold emits a high-energy radiation and has a high half-value layer in tissue of approximately 4.5 cm. Therefore, precise localization of the seeds is not critical. Approximately three weeks after the gold implantation, a course of external beam radiotherapy is given, using a linear accelerator to deliver approximately 5000 rads through opposed anterior and posterior portals to the full pelvis and prostate, administered in a split course with a two-week rest period after the first three weeks of therapy. It is estimated that the total dose of radiation delivered to the prostate ranges between 8000 and 8900 rads.

Radioactive iodine-125 seeds may be implanted in the prostate at the time of staging pelvic lymphadenectomy. In this form of therapy, multiple implant needles are placed at regular intervals. The total dosage is calculated to be 16,000 to 30,000 rads delivered over approximately one year. A dose level of 16,000 rads utilizing this technique appears to be biologically equivalent to 7000 rads delivered by external beam or combined gold seed–external beam radiotherapy.

The results of therapy are given in Tables 24–1, 24–2, and 24–3. Assuming the patient selection was equivalent among the institutions and among the patients randomized in the Veterans Administration Cooperative Urology Research Group (VACURG), one would have to believe that the five-year disease-free percentage for the various treatments would differ as indicated in Table 24–4.

In conclusion, one must believe that surgical removal of confined disease provides the best possible disease control.

Table 24–3. MEMORIAL SLOAN-KETTERING EXPERIENCE WITH ^{125}I IMPLANTATION*

Clinical Stage	Five-Year Survival (NED)
B	60
B$_1$	79
B$_2$	53
C$_1$	45
C$_2$	19

*Results are reported as disease-free survival; however, hormonal therapy was provided to some of these patients.

Table 24–4. DISEASE-FREE RATES FOR VARIOUS TREATMENTS FOR PATIENTS IN STAGE B PROSTATIC CANCER*

Treatment	Five-Year Disease-Free Survival Rate (%)
Radical Surgery	85–88
External Beam Radiation	62–66
^{198}Au Pelvic Seeding + External Beam	50–58
^{125}I	50–58

*Data from Paulson DF, Scardino PT, personal communication.

References

1. Babson AL, Read PA: A new assay for prostatic acid phosphatase in serum. Am J Clin Pathol 32:88–91, 1959.
2. Babson AL, Read PA, Phillips GE: The importance of substrate in assays of acid phosphatase in serum. Am J Clin Pathol 32:83–87, 1959.
3. Belt E: Radical perineal prostatectomy in early carcinoma of the prostate. J Urol 48:287–297, 1942.
4. Birke G, Franksson C, Planton LO: Estrogen therapy in carcinoma of prostate. Acta Chir Scand 109:1, 1955.
5. Blackard CE, Byar DP, Jordan WP Jr: Orchiectomy for advanced prostatic carcinoma: a reevaluation. Urology 1:553–560, 1973.
6. Brendler H: Therapy with orchiectomy or estrogens or both. JAMA 210:1074–1075, 1969.
7. Chu TM, Wang MC, Scott WW, et al: Immunological detection of serum prostatic acid phosphatase. Methodology and clinical evaluation. Invest Urol 15:319–323, 1978.
8. Coodley EL: Diagnostic Enzymology. Philadelphia, Lea & Febiger, 1970, p 156.
9. Cooper JF, Foti AG, Shank PW: Radioimmunochemical measurement of bone marrow prostatic acid phosphatase. J Urol 119:392–395, 1978.
10. Cox DR: Regression models and life tables. J R Stat Soc 34:187, 1972.
11. Dees JE: Radical perineal prostatectomy for carcinoma. J Urol 104:160–162, 1970.
12. Emmett JL, Greene LF, Papantonious A: Endocrine therapy in carcinoma of the prostate gland: 10-year survival studies. J Urol 83:471–484, 1960.
13. Fishman WH, Lerner FA: A method for estimating serum acid phosphatase of prostatic origin. J Biol Chem 200:89–94, 1953.
14. Fosså SD, Sokolowski J, Theodorsen L: The significance of bone marrow acid phosphatase in patients with prostatic carcinoma. Br J Urol 50:185–189, 1978.
15. Foti AG, Cooper JF, Herschman H, Malvaez RR: Detection of prostatic cancer by solid-phase radioimmunoassay of serum prostatic acid phosphatase. N Engl J Med 297:1357–1361, 1977.
16. Freiha FS, Bagshaw MA: Carcinoma of the prostate: results of post-irradiation biopsy. Prostate 5:19, 1984.
17. Gutman AB, Gutman EB: An "acid" phosphatase occurring in the serum of patients with metastasizing carcinoma of the prostate gland. J Clin Invest 17:473–478, 1938.
18. Huggins C: Anti-androgenic treatment of prostatic carcinoma in man. In Approaches to Tumor Chemotherapy. Washington, DC, American Association for the Advancement of Science, 1947, p 379.
19. Huggins C, Stevens RE Jr, Hodges CV: Studies on prostatic cancer: the effects of castration on advanced carcinoma of the prostate gland. Arch Surg 43:209–223, 1941.
20. Jewett HJ: The case for radical perineal prostatectomy. J Urol 103:195–199, 1970.
21. Kaplan EL, Meier P: Non-parametric estimation from incomplete observations. J Am Stat Assoc 53:457, 1958.
22. Maramba TP Jr: Histochemical differentiation of carcinoma of the prostate gland from other tumors by a modified acid phosphatase reaction. Am J Clin Pathol 43:319, 1965.
23. Nesbit RM, Baum WC: Endocrine control of prostatic carcinoma: clinical and statistical survey of 1,818 cases. JAMA 143:1317–1320, 1950.
24. Paulson DF: Carcinoma of the prostate: the therapeutic dilemma. Annu Rev Med 35:341–372, 1984.
25. Paulson DF, Hodge GB, Hinshaw W: Radiation therapy versus delayed androgen deprivation for stage C carcinoma of the prostate. J Urol 131:901–902, 1984.
26. Paulson DF, Lin GH, Hinshaw W, et al: Radical surgery versus radiotherapy for adenocarcinoma of the prostate. J Urol 128:502–504, 1982.
27. Pontes JE, Choe B, Rose N, Pierce JM Jr: Reliability of bone marrow acid phosphatase as a parameter of metastatic prostatic cancer. J Urol 122:178–179, 1979.
28. Prout GR Jr: Chemical tests in the diagnosis of prostatic carcinoma. JAMA 209:1699–1700, 1969.
29. Rutenberg AM, Seligman AM: The histochemical demonstration of acid phosphatase by a post-incubation coupling technique. J Histochem Cytochem 3:455–470, 1955.
30. Scardino PT, Carlton CE Jr: Combined interstitial and external irradiation for prostatic cancer. In N Javadpour (ed), Principles and Management of Urologic Cancer. Baltimore, Williams & Wilkins, 1983, pp 392–408.

MALCOLM A. BAGSHAW, M.D.

CHAPTER 25

Radiation Therapy for Cancer of the Prostate

Approximately 76,000 new cases of carcinoma of the prostate are diagnosed annually in the United States,[1] and the disease causes about 25,000 deaths per year. The incidence of this neoplasm is slightly greater than that of male colorectal carcinoma, and it is exceeded only by the 96,000 new cases of male lung cancer per year. Carcinoma of the prostate continues to be more common in men than the total for all cancers in the buccal cavity and pharynx, leukemia, and all the lymphomas. In the United States, there is a slightly higher incidence of prostatic carcinoma in the black population than in the white population. Although the incidence is appreciably lower in Japan, it appears to be increasing there. The highest incidence appears to be in Sweden.

HISTORY OF RADIOTHERAPY FOR PROSTATIC CANCER

In 1910, Paschkis and Tittinger first used a radium source to treat carcinoma of the prostate by incorporating it into a cystoscope.[51] Pasteau, in 1911, employed a radium source in a catheter placed in the prostatic urethra.[52] This work was reported by Pasteau and Degrais at the International Congress of Medicine in London in 1913.[53] Hugh Young of Johns Hopkins University apparently heard this presentation and soon thereafter devised special radium applicators to treat his first patient in 1915.[81–83] Young and his co-workers designed their applicators to hold the radium sources precisely positioned adjacent to the prostate when placed intravesically, intraurethrally, or transrectally.[23] These surface applications were supplemented occasionally with external x-ray treatments, by the insertion of radium needles through the perineum, or by the direct insertion of radium needles into the gland after surgical exposure. Some understanding of the principles of fractionation of radiation dose was evident in these early approaches, because patients received multiple treatments even before the unit of radiation exposure, the roentgen, was described, and only 17 years after the discovery of radium.

Through the 1920s and 1930s, many urologists treated large numbers of patients with carcinoma of the prostate by using various types of radium applications and external beam radiation therapy.[12, 15, 23, 72] This interesting early era seems to have terminated with Barringer's report from Memorial Hospital in New York in which he described a series of 352 consecutive patients treated between 1922 and 1936.[13] Most of his patients received some form of interstitial radiation, and in two cases he cited postmortem evidence of cure at six and seven years post-treatment. The closing of this pre-World War II era was foretold by Barringer himself, who wrote that there were remarkable effects of castration upon primary prostatic carcinoma, bone metastases, pain, and general health, which was also reported by Huggins at the previous meeting of the

425

American Urological Association.[34] There were occasional publications from radiotherapists.[35, 80] but little was done with radiotherapy in the treatment of prostatic cancer between the early demonstration of the hormonal dependence of prostatic cancer[34] and the megavoltage radiotherapy era, except for the introduction by Flocks of the use of radioactive gold solution injected interstitially into the prostate or regional lymph nodes.[26]

CONTEMPORARY RADIOTHERAPY

In 1964, Budhraja and Anderson reported on the treatment of 81 patients with carcinoma of the prostate, some of whom had received radiotherapy.[14] Although they recognized that the prior experience with radiotherapy had not been exceptional, they suggested that with the improvement in radiotherapeutic equipment the issue should be re-explored. Their study compared 53 patients who had advanced disease and were treated with a combination of surgery, stilbestrol, and radiotherapy (the radiotherapy group), with a group of 28 patients who were treated with stilbestrol and surgery alone (the nonradiotherapy group).

Although the study was neither randomized nor completely contemporaneous, the conclusion was that the radiotherapy was beneficial in patients who relapsed after estrogen treatment, because survival at three years for the radiotherapy group was 60% and only 43% for the nonradiotherapy group. By five years, however, there was no difference in survival.

Stanford Series

Independent of the study by Budhraja and Anderson, the treatment of prostatic carcinoma with external beam megavoltage irradiation was initiated at Stanford in 1956, and the first 45 cases so treated were reported at the International Congress of Radiology in Montreal in 1962.[8] The technique and goals of treatment in this series were different from those employed previously. The therapeutic model at Stanford was based on the work of Flocks and co-workers, who had used local injections of colloidal radioactive gold into the prostatic bed following

subtotal resection.[27] But to control the distribution of irradiation from an external source more precisely, a well-collimated 4.7 MV photon beam, generated by the new Stanford Medical Linear Accelerator, was used for treatment of the patients. Initially, they received the treatment in a standing position with a fixed horizontal beam delivered by either 360° or 120° lateral arc rotational technique with relatively small beam cross sections (6 × 6 to 8 × 8 cm). This restricted the high-dose region as tightly as possible to the prostate and the immediately surrounding periprostatic tissue. After 1970, the treatment volume was extended to include the obturator, iliac, presacral and, occasionally, the para-aortic lymph nodes. The intent of the treatment was to achieve sterilization of the neoplasm in the prostatic region and relevant lymph nodes.

The early patients were those with localized carcinoma that was too extensive for consideration of radical prostatectomy or those who might have been considered candidates for radical prostatectomy but who either rejected the operation or were rejected as poor surgical risks. The results of therapy on this group of patients have been presented.[4, 7, 9, 11, 54] An overview and current status of the Stanford experience follows.

The Stanford series is neither prospective nor retrospective but rather should be considered a contemporary and continuing study. The criteria for patient evaluation, treatment policies, and continuing followup of these patients has been stipulated and carried out by the author, with the able collaboration of a number of colleagues cited in the bibliography.

The 27-year period of study extends from October 1956 through December 1983. The case profile for the total experience is tabulated in Table 25–1. During this interval, a total of 1714 patients with prostatic cancer were referred to the Stanford Radiation Therapy Division, and approximately one half of these were excluded from the definitive evaluation for the reasons noted. Thus, 879 patients were treated definitively in the study.

"Definitive treatment" is defined as the delivery of a dose of radiation compatible with maximum normal tissue tolerance to the prostate, the primary and secondary echelons of potential lymph node involvement, or to both areas. In each patient a search for more distant spread was carried out at the

Table 25–1. PROSTATIC CANCER
REFERRALS FOR RADIATION THERAPY,
OCTOBER 1956 TO DECEMBER 1983

Total Referrals		1714
Consult only	165	
Metastatic disease	469	
Subtotal for referrals	634	
Remaining Patients		1080
Excluded for Various Reasons		
Second primary	60	
Prostatectomy	32	
Unusual primary	6	
Previous radiotherapy	14	
Palliation or incomplete radiotherapy	14	
Questionable histologic results	4	
Implants	71	
Subtotal for exclusions	201	
Patients in This Analysis		879
Disease limited to prostate (DLP)	477	
Extracapsular extension (ECE)	402	
(Total number of surgically staged patients = 146)		

dures was used in every instance as a means of case selection. However, within the patient group there is one cohort, to be discussed later, in which the status of lymph node involvement was precisely determined by surgical staging.

Unless otherwise specified, the survival curves to be presented do not take into account the presence or absence of lymph node metastases, inasmuch as the status of lymphadenopathy was often unknown. Similarly, the status of the acid phosphatase determination was not used as a staging measurement, although serial acid phosphatase determinations have been used as a matter of routine for at least the past 15 years.

The staging system that has been used in the Stanford study is the Stanford TNM system,[61] a classification similar to the TNM system adopted by the International Union Against Cancer (UICC)[76] and the American Joint Committee.[2] The Stanford series also has consistently been divided into two broad categories: those patients with disease limited to the prostate (DLP) and those with extracapsular extension (ECE). Thus, the DLP category represents the nominal Stages A and B, and ECE represents Stage C.

The age distribution of the Stanford series is depicted in Figure 25–1. The mean age

time of evaluation, consistent with contemporary standards for the detection of distant metastases. In certain subgroups of the series, lymph node metastases were detected by staging or lymphangiography or both, although neither of these diagnostic proce-

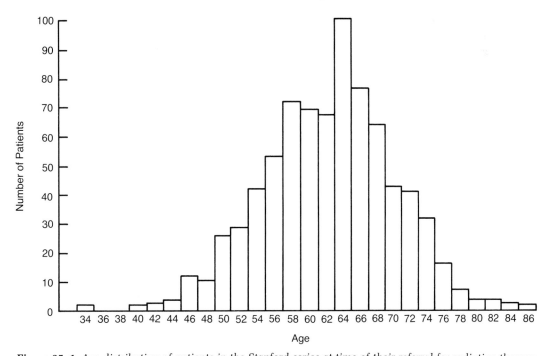

Figure 25–1. Age distribution of patients in the Stanford series at time of their referral for radiation therapy.

was slightly less than 63 years for those with DLP and slightly greater than that for those with ECE, with an overall mean age of 63 years.

RADIOTHERAPY TECHNIQUE

Current treatment at Stanford is carried out with 4 or 6 MV well-collimated x-ray beams generated by linear accelerators* and employs a four-field technique, isocentrically localized, to treat the prostate and the pelvic adenopathy. This technique was described in 1978[4] and has been further detailed by the author,[5, 10] as well as by Hafermann.[31] With the patient lying comfortably supine, the pelvic region is treated through

---

*Clinac 4: 4 MV at 80 cm SSD. Clinac 6: 6 MV at 100 cm. Produced by Varian Associates, Palo Alto, California.

parallel opposed anterior and posterior fields and isocentrically placed left and right lateral fields. All four fields have their central axes coincident at the isocenter of the linear accelerator. The beam alignment is carried out with the aid of a radiation therapy simulator, a device that precisely produces the beam geometry of the linear accelerator but utilizes low-energy, diagnostic-quality x-rays for treatment planning and beam position verification. At the medium energies (i.e., 4 to 10 MV) all four fields are treated on each treatment day, and special care is exercised to protect the posterior wall of the rectum and the anus from excessive radiation exposure.

In practice, 2600 rads are delivered through the four-field technique, which includes the prostate and the regional lymph nodes (Fig. 25–2). This is given at a rate of 200 rads per day. Then the radiation fields are reduced in cross section and changed to left and right moving beam arc therapy di-

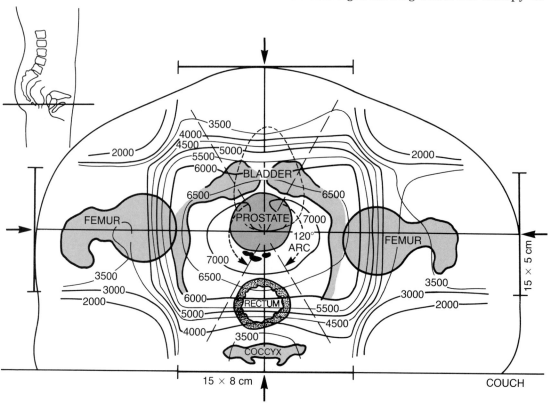

Figure 25–2. A composite treatment plan for the four-field technique as well as the 120° lateral arc rotation. The plane of the treatment plan is indicated at the level of the insert (Left). Several intercalating lymph nodes are indicated posterior to the prostate. The iliac nodes do not extend this far inferiorly. The position of the bladder is indicated, although it is anatomically superior to the level of this plane. At medium energies, in our case 4 MV photons, this technique is extremely well tolerated. For example, most patients are able to complete the course of treatment as outpatients without missing any employment. Damage to the small bowel has not been observed with this fractionation program and total dose.

rected at the prostate, periprostatic tissues, and seminal vesicles only, and an additional 2000 rads are delivered to the prostate and the immediate periprostatic tissue by this technique. Following this, the original four-field arrangement is resumed, and an additional 2400 rads are delivered in this manner. The dosage calculation is made at the isocenter point. This program delivers 7000 rads to the prostate in a period of seven weeks and 5000 rads to the regional adenopathy up to the level of L5, also in seven weeks. In patients who tolerate the treatment with essentially no side effects, two or three additional booster treatments to the prostate only may be added at the end of this sequence. In certain patients the para-aortic lymph nodes may be treated also (Fig. 25–3). Although this has not significantly improved survival, it appears to have reduced the potential of subsequent lymphatic obstruction.

RADIOTHERAPY RESULTS

According to surveys of patterns of care of prostate cancer in the American College of Surgeons Approved Cancer Programs, the use of radiotherapy for prostatic cancer increased in each stage between 1974 and 1983.[47] For example, in Stage B, use of radiation therapy was increased from about 15 to 40%, and in Stage C, from about 20 to 40% (Fig. 25–4).[47] The current overall survival status of the patients treated definitively at Stanford is illustrated in Figure 25–5. For those with disease limited to the prostate (DLP), Stages A and B, the actuarial survival is 81%, 59%, and 36% at five, 10, and 15 years, respectively. For those with extracapsular extension (ECE), Stage C, the comparable survivorship is 62%, 36%, and 18%.

During the past decade, a number of authors have described similar survival rates

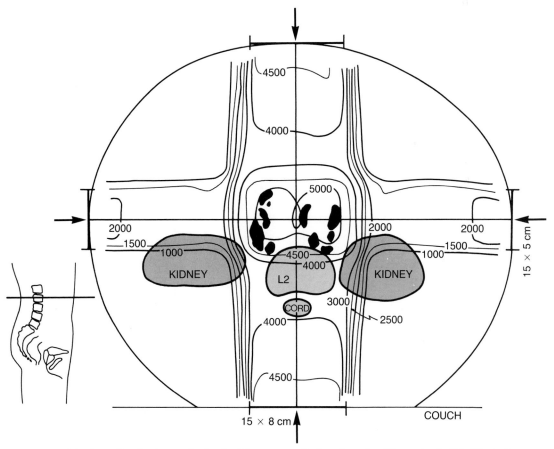

Figure 25–3. The dose distribution at the level of the para-aortic lymph nodes. The nodes in this illustration were accurately positioned relative to the kidneys and lumbar spine. It is clear from the isodose pattern that most of the dose is delivered by the anterior and posterior portals, thus ensuring the delivery of about 4000 rads to the lumbar spine. By adding the lateral portals, the dose in the region of the spinal cord does not exceed 4000 rads.

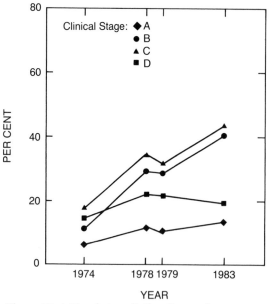

Figure 25–4. *Trends in radiation therapy from 1974 to 1983. From Mettlin C: Long-term and short-term surveys of patterns of care of prostate cancer in American College of Surgeons' approved cancer programs. Preliminary report to the American College of Surgeons' Committee on Cancer Patient Care and Research Committee. Private correspondence, October, 1984.*

study by the American College of Radiology on patterns of care outcome.[41] In this study, the records of 682 patients from 106 randomly selected radiotherapy facilities in the United States were reviewed. The study is especially important because a wide variety of radiation therapy facilities were surveyed, ranging from those employing only a part-time radiation therapist and treating fewer than 200 patients per year, to facilities with large staffs, extensive equipment, residency programs, and external funding in which more than 1100 patients per year were treated. The results, therefore, represent a true benchmark of the national status of the outcome of radiation therapy of prostatic cancer. Although the follow-up period in this study is limited, survival data are presented at five years and can be extracted from the published survival curves. Thus, for patients with tumors in Stages A and B, the survival appears to be 80%, and for Stage C, just under 60%. The concordance with the Stanford series at five years (81% for Stages A and B and 62% for Stage C) is remarkable. Agreement with the results summarized in Table 25–2 is also remarkable.

in patients who have received external beam irradiation, and some of these are summarized in Table 25–2. Further confirmation of this general experience with prostatic cancer has recently become available through the

If one restricts the case selection among the patients with disease limited to the prostate to the criteria advocated by Jewett for the ideal selection of patients for radical prostatectomy,[37] then long-term survival equal to that expected for all males at a

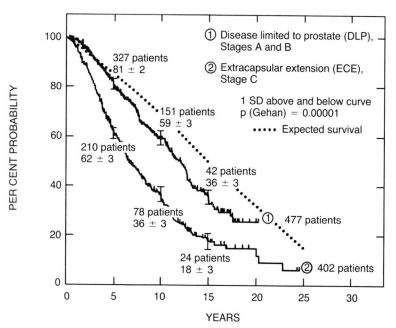

Figure 25–5. *The probability of duration of survival after external beam irradiation of carcinoma of the prostate (Kaplan-Meier). Deaths due to all causes are counted, and there is no adjustment for intercurrent death. An upward tick indicates that the patient was alive for the time interval shown on the abscissa at last observation. The total number of patients in each group and the number of patients at risk for the varying intervals are shown. For example, for patients with diseases in Stages A or B, at least 327 patients were at risk for five years; 151 for 10 years; 42 for 15 years; and three for 20 years. A downward step indicates death for any cause at the interval shown on the abscissa.*

Table 25–2. REPORTED SURVIVAL AFTER DEFINITIVE EXTERNAL BEAM RADIATION THERAPY FOR PROSTATIC CANCER IN STAGES A, B, AND C*

Institution	Reference	Stages A and B Number of Patients	Per cent Survival for years— 5	10	15	Stage C Number of Patients	Per cent Survival for Years— 5	10	15
Stanford University†		327	81			210	62		
		151		59		78		36	
		42			36	24			18
Virginia Mason Medical Center	75	46	61‡			221	58‡	30‡	
MD Anderson Hospital	36					165	61§	40§	
Columbia-Presbyterian Medical Center	32	34	87§			112	58§	35§	
Los Angeles County/USC	42	23	95§			56	55§		
Washington University	59	42 ‖	80			141	56		
Mayo Clinic	22	96 ‖	80**	58		39	75	65	
Totals		623				983			

*Modified and updated from Hafermann MD: External radiotherapy. Urology 17(Suppl):15–23, 1981.
†Kaplan-Meier survival rates (see Fig. 25–5). All survivors lived beyond stated interval (i.e., 5, 10, or 15 years).
‡Absolute cumulative survival.
§Actuarial cumulative survival.
‖ Stage B only.
**Percentages for Mayo Clinic data are interpolated from survival curves.

mean age of 63 is achieved (Fig. 25–6). Jewett and associates defined a solitary nodule in Stage B, "a palpably discrete nodule of firm or stony consistency limited to a part of one lateral lobe averaging 1 cm or a little more in diameter, with compressible prostatic tissue always on two, and sometimes on three, sides," as being the critical determinant in the selection of patients for radical prostatectomy.[37] A small subset of 40 patients in the Stanford series, included in the

group with disease limited to the prostate, fits Jewett's description precisely. His description was used for the T1a designation in the Stanford TNM staging system. The long-term survival in these patients is equal to that achieved in the highly selected surgical series of Walsh and Jewett[79] and Gibbons and associates.[29] A survival of 62% at the 15-year interval for patients with a 1-cm solitary nodule, and a 49% survival for the 134 patients with a nodule that occupies up

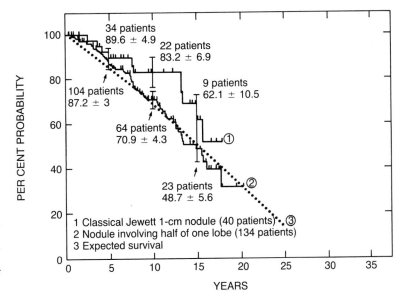

Figure 25–6. The probability of duration of survival after radiation therapy for patients with prostatic carcinoma who appear to qualify for radical prostatectomy on the basis of primary tumor stage alone. Selection did not take into account medical criteria for operability, lymph node status, or acid phosphatase levels. Curve 1 follows the strict criteria of Jewett. Curve 2 includes somewhat larger primary nodules. Curve 3 denotes the expected survival for cohort of males with mean age of 63.

34 patients 89.6 ± 4.9
22 patients 83.2 ± 6.9
104 patients 87.2 ± 3
9 patients 62.1 ± 10.5
64 patients 70.9 ± 4.3
23 patients 48.7 ± 5.6

1 Classical Jewett 1-cm nodule (40 patients)
2 Nodule involving half of one lobe (134 patients)
3 Expected survival

PER CENT PROBABILITY

YEARS

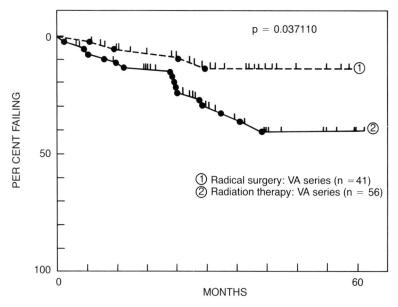

Figure 25–7. Time to first evidence of treatment failure, in a study conducted by the Veterans Administration Uro-Oncology Research Group. Patients were in Surgical Stages A_2 and B_1. From Paulson DF, et al: Radical surgery versus radiotherapy for adenocarcinoma of the prostate. J Urol 128:502–504, 1982.

to half of one lobe are demonstrated in Figure 25–6. Although these patients were carefully clinically staged from the standpoint of their T stage, *all* patients within the T1a and T1b categories are reported. No patients were excluded because of advanced age, medical status, high-grade histopathologic stage, or either proven or presumed lymph node involvement.

The Veterans Administration Uro-Oncology Research Group studied the time to first evidence of distant metastasis in two groups of patients who were assigned to either definitive radiation therapy or radical prostatectomy.[56] A significant advantage was credited to the group of patients receiving a radical prostatectomy, using first evidence to distant metastasis as the end point (Fig. 25–7). A cohort of patients is present in the Stanford series who were treated between 1970 and 1978 and who were surgically staged in a manner identical to that used for those in the Uro-Oncology Research Group study. The outcome in the group of 51 patients treated at Stanford is presented in Figure 25–8. It is superior to those treated

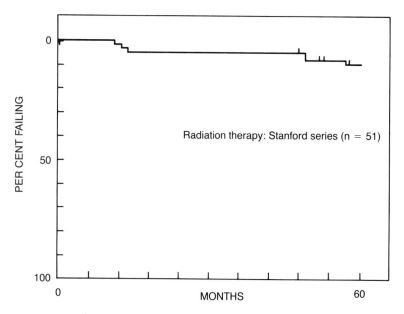

Figure 25–8. Time to first evidence of treatment failure, Stanford series. Patients were in Surgical Stages A_2 and B_1 (n = 51).

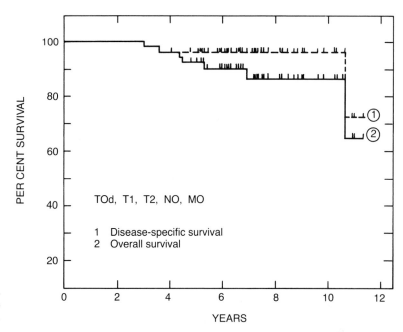

Figure 25–9. *Survival in Stanford series for patients in Surgical Stages A_2 and B_1 (n = 51).*

by irradiation, and identical to the outcome observed in the radical prostatectomy group of the VA study.[11] A strict comparison is not possible because the Stanford study was not prospectively randomized. However, it does suggest that the radiotherapy results in the VA study were unaccountably poor. The Stanford cohort has been followed for a longer period than the VA study patients, and survival rates are 80% at 10 years (Fig. 25–9). Thus, survival data demonstrated in Figures 25–6 and 25–9 indicate that a high

level of patient survival can be achieved with radiation therapy, if careful attention is given to case selection.

Unfortunately, there is no standard that would allow a stage-by-stage comparison of the survival following radiation therapy for patients who either receive no treatment or receive an alternate therapy, such as surgery or hormone deprivation. There is no doubt that patients with low-stage and low-grade disease often survive for many years, and occasionally even patients with more ad-

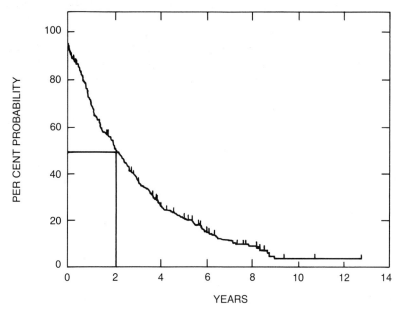

Figure 25–10. *Survival among 318 patients in the Stanford series who developed metastatic disease. The median survival was exactly two years.*

vanced disease enjoy a lengthy survival. In our experience, however, once the metastatic process has started, the course of prostatic cancer is relentless and lethal. Reference to Figure 25–10 demonstrates that the median survival following the first evidence of metastasis is two years, and the longest survivor in this series of 318 patients followed from first evidence of metastasis to death was 11 years. An occasional patient may live a longer time, creating a false sense of security regarding prostatic cancer, but extraordinarily prolonged survival with manifest disease is, in our experience, a memorable but rare event.

STAGE, GRADE, AND ADENOPATHY

Early staging data correlated clinical stage with adenopathy.[3, 26] Throughout the 1970s, additional surgical series firmly established the relationships between stage and adenopathy,[43] and these relationships were generally reflected by the results observed in 93 patients whose stages were surgically determined at Stanford at that time.[61] Thus, 10 of 52 patients (19%) with Stage B disease had proven adenopathy, and 23 of 41 (56%) in Stage C had proven adenopathy. Altogether, 33 of 93 patients (35%) with no other evidence of distant metastases had lymphadenopathy. The precise anatomic localization of the affected lymph nodes is given in Table 25–3.

The histologic pattern in the Stanford series has been categorized by both the Kempson modification of the Broders grading system and the Gleason pattern score method of grading prostatic cancer.[38, 46] In a subset of the Stanford series that was classified by the Kempson grading, only one of eight patients (12.5%) with well-differentiated tumor was in Stage C, whereas 17 of 23 patients (74%) with poorly differentiated tumor were in Stage C. Conversely, among the group of 36 patients with Stage C tumors, only one had well-differentiated tumor tissue. Thus, although there are exceptions, progressing tumor enlargement as manifest by advancing stage and advancing grade go together, as was pointed out by McNeal in 1969.[45]

Gleason described a method of identifying the glandular pattern as viewed by low-power microscopy and assigning a pattern score, which ranged from 2 to 10 for the

Table 25–3. INCIDENCE OF LYMPH NODE INVOLVEMENT BY TUMOR (93 PATIENTS)

Lymph Node Group	Number of Patients Biopsied	Number With Tumor (%)	Per cent Opacified*
Para-aortic	74	13 (18%)	93
Common iliac	76	13 (17%)	95
External iliac	74	16 (22%)	94
Internal iliac	63	15 (24%)	87
Obturator	51	16 (31%)	94

*Per cent opacified refers to histologic evidence of retained contrast material within the lymph node specimen.

observed histopathologic features.[46] Gleason noted that as the pattern score increased from 2 to 10, the survival became progressively less. The same was noted in the Stanford series. Figure 25–11 demonstrates a systematic decline in disease-specific survival as the Gleason pattern score increased from 2 through 10. Previously, a relationship was demonstrated between an increasing risk for lymph node metastases and both stage and differentiation of the primary tumor.[4] Later studies revealed a crisper association between the incidence of lymph node metastases and tissue differentiation. By using the Gleason pattern score as the quantitative measure of the histopathologic stage, one may observe a systematic increase in lymph node metastases as a function of the Gleason pattern score (Fig. 25–12).[10, 61] This can be helpful as an aid for either preoperative or preradiotherapeutic assessment of potential adenopathy.

Thus, histologic pattern, whether it be determined by a modification of the Broders classification or the more contemporary Gleason method, can be a predictor of clinical stage, the relative probability of lymph node metastases, and, ultimately, survival.

SIGNIFICANCE OF LYMPH NODE METASTASES RELATIVE TO RADIATION THERAPY

It is well known that the presence of overt lymph node metastases has a profound adverse influence on the eventual outcome of the treatment of prostatic cancer. Although it has been shown that individual lymph node metastases are radioresponsive, the radiation treatment of the regional lymph nodes in patients with adenopathy proven

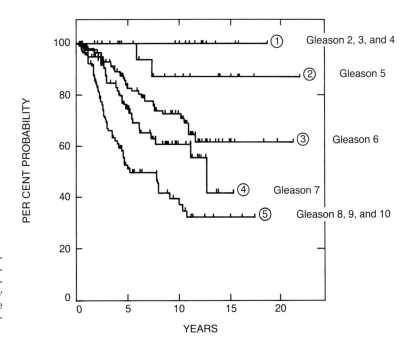

Figure 25–11. Probability of disease-specific survival as a function of the histopathologic pattern score as described by Gleason (see ref. 46). Death due to intercurrent disease is withdrawn.

by biopsy apparently has not improved the absolute survival (Fig. 25–13).[6] A study that was undertaken to determine whether irradiation of the next most likely echelon of potential lymph node metastases would improve survival did not demonstrate initially a clear survival advantage for patients who received this prophylactic treatment.[61] However, a recent update of that series shows improved, but not statistically significantly improved, survival among the patients who received lymphatic irradiation.[6]

On the other hand, one special group of patients in the Stanford series does seem to demonstrate an advantage for prophylactic lymph node irradiation. From 1970, most patients in the study have been treated with extended field irradiation—that is, a radiation program including the first-echelon lymphatics, which drain the prostate; the internal, external, and common iliac nodes; and the presacral nodes. Prior to that time the treatment volume was limited to the prostate and the immediate periprostatic tissue. In the early 1970s there was an overlap of the two treatment philosophies, and some patients received treatment to the prostate and immediate periprostatic region only, whereas others received treatment to the prostate and the pelvic adenopathy as well. If one selects the clinical stages most likely to have occult metastases only—Stanford Stages T1b, T1c, T2a, T2b (i.e., the patients with B_2 neoplasms)—then a statistically significant survival advantage is observed among those patients who received extended field or lymph node irradiation, as compared with those who received treatment to the prostatic region only (Fig. 25–14). McGowan also noted a significant survival advantage for patients who were in Stage B_2 or C and who received extended field irradiation (Fig. 25–15).[44] Conversely, the experience at the Joint Center for Radiation Therapy (JCRT)[67] showed no difference in survival for patients with tumors in Stage B or C that were treated with fields either greater or less than 150 cm^2. One might question the merit of that arbitrary distinction. A precise grouping of patients according to whether the prostate only was treated, or whether there was a specific intention to treat all of the pelvic lymph nodes, was not apparent.

Radiotherapy of macroscopic metastases in lymph nodes is capable of reducing the bulk of metastasis within the lymph nodes and often of relieving symptoms of lymphatic obstruction, but it apparently does not render the patients tumor-free.[6] Patients with overt adenopathy ultimately die of progression in other organ systems. Whether irradiation of the adenopathy slows the process is uncertain. Using time to first evidence of treatment failure as an end point, the VA Uro-Oncology Group could find no difference between patients with Stage C prostatic cancer who were irradiated and those who received no therapy.[55] However, in a com-

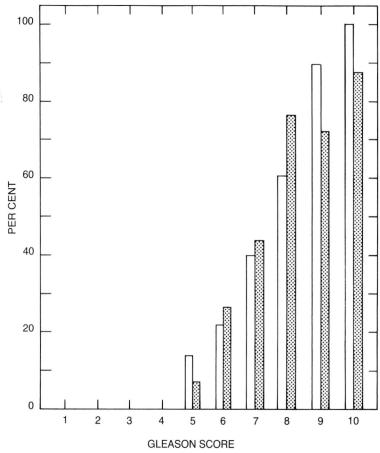

First Author	Reference	Number of Patients
Bagshaw (Stanford)*	10	93
Paulson	59	122
Kramer	39	144
Sagalowsky	68	90
TOTAL[†]		449

*Striped bar.

[†]Solid bar.

Fifty-two patients with a score less than 5 had no metastases.

Figure 25–12. Percentage of patients with lymph node metastases as a function of the Gleason pattern score.

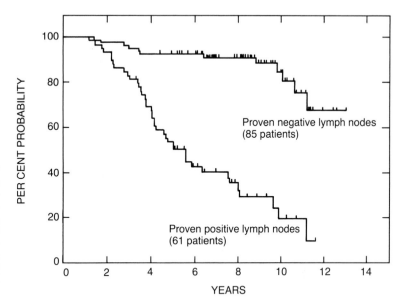

Figure 25–13. Comparison of long-term survival between patients with biopsy-proven adenopathy and those with biopsy-proven absence of disease in lymph nodes. Although there are nine survivors among the patients with proven adenopathy, all but one have either positive bone scans or elevated acid phosphatase levels.

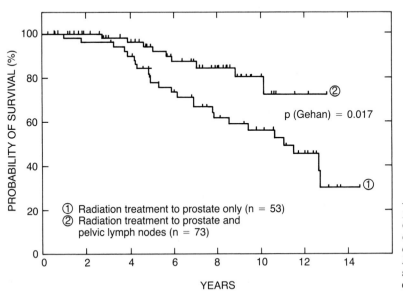

Figure 25–14. For Stage B₂ neoplasms, irradiation of the first echelon lymphatic groups—the obturator, internal, external and common iliac, and presacral lymph nodes—appears to offer a statistically significant survival advantage.

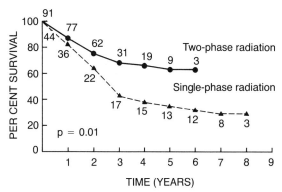

Figure 25–15. *Comparison of disease-free survival for single- and two-phase radiation (late Stage B₂ to C). From McGowan DG: The value of extended field radiation therapy in carcinoma of the prostate. Int J Radiat Oncol Biol Phys 7:1333–1339, 1981.*

panion publication based upon patients who had prostatic adenocarcinoma with metastases to lymph nodes, an advantage for patients treated with irradiation was observed.[54] In those studies, simple elevation of the level of acid phosphatase in two determinations was used as one of several indicators of failure. Other variables included conversion of negative results of a bone scan or discovery of metastases by roentgenography. Perhaps the acid phosphatase elevations were not specific indicators of failure, causing the above apparent discrepancy. Thus, although long-term survival is unaffected by lymphatic irradiation, symptoms secondary to lymphatic obstruction can be alleviated and occult or microscopic involvement may be sterilized. In view of the relatively low morbidity of extended field irradiation, it appears to be justified in patients with suspected microscopic disease, who have a reasonable probability of involvement because of moderate to high Gleason scores and negative results of lymphangiograms and in whom lymph node involvement, if present, might be assumed to be microscopic. Irradiation of overt adenopathy also appears to be justified in order to forestall symptomatic lymphatic obstruction.

COMPLICATIONS

Adverse sequelae in the Stanford series, using the technique described briefly earlier, have been minimal and, therefore, have not been surveyed recently, although they are the subject of a current review. A prior review based on 430 patients (Stages A, B, and C, inclusive) showed urethral stricture in 16, or 3.7%.[62] The incidence of stricture was related to multiple preradiotherapeutic transurethral resections. A colostomy was required in one patient with persistent tumor, and three had fecal stress incontinence and urinary stress incontinence. Erectile potency was maintained in 65 (59%) of the 110 patients available for evaluation. Pilepich detailed urethral stricture following irradiation in 5.2%, and proctitis was noted in 4.5% of irradiated patients.[60] In the patterns of care outcome studies, major complications requiring admission to the hospital following radiation therapy occurred in 28 of 619 (4.5%) of patients evaluated in Stages B and C.[41] Complications involved the urinary tract in 13, the bowel in eight, and both in three. Sixteen patients required surgical intervention, and one complication was fatal. A 60% preservation of erectile potency seems possible after x-radiation, although this probably applies to the younger patients. In the Stanford series, for example, the mean age of those who reported preservation of potency was 59 years, whereas the mean age for the group as a whole was 63 years.

HORMONE DEPRIVATION AND RADIATION THERAPY

Regression of many primary prostatic neoplasms and metastatic foci following testosterone deprivation is well known. This maneuver may be a useful adjuvant to radiation therapy. For example, obstructive symptoms may be relieved with either concomitant or preirradiation castration or estrogen administration. In patients with advanced disease, this may prevent frank obstruction during radiotherapy. Lipsett and associates found androgen deprivation useful in achieving better local control, and they even noted an 18% improvement in survival at five years for those who were treated with hormonal therapy in addition to x-radiation.[42] This degree of improvement, however, was not statistically significant. A retrospective examination of the use of hormone deprivation in the Stanford series showed no statistical improvement in survival,[64] and several other authors have confirmed this observation.[17, 31, 32, 50, 59, 77] Thus, although hormone deprivation is useful as an adjunctive treatment in the patient with obstructive symptoms, it does not appear to alter long-term survival when given concomitantly with the radiation. Whether it might alter long-term survival if given sequentially prior to irradiation is unknown and could be the subject of an interesting clinical trial.

DELAY BETWEEN DIAGNOSIS AND RADIATION TREATMENT

Any delay between diagnosis and treatment permits cell division and presumably increases the number of viable cells. It also undoubtedly presents more opportunity for the metastatic process to occur. Because cells are killed by irradiation logarithmically, a cell doubling may require an additional radiation dose of 200 to 300 rads in order to achieve sterilization. Since radiation dose is limited by the tolerance of normal tissues, a disadvantage of several hundred rads may make the difference between successful and unsuccessful sterilization of tumor cells. In addition to the adverse influence of delay, which was first noted in this series, Hafermann tabulated the same phenomenon from several other authors (Table 25–4).[31]

SIGNIFICANCE OF POSTIRRADIATION BIOPSY

The controversy concerning the significance of postirradiation biopsy started in 1972 with the report of Rhamy and coworkers, who noted apparent viability of

Table 25–4. CORRELATION OF SURVIVAL RATES WITH TIME BETWEEN DIAGNOSIS AND DEFINITIVE EXTERNAL BEAM IRRADIATION FOR PROSTATIC CANCER*

First Author	Reference	Survival Rate	
Ray	64	<1 year, 61%	>1 year, 39%
Harisiadis	32	<6 mos, 70%	>6 mos, 32%
Cantril	17	<3 mos, 50%	>3 mos, 28%
Perez	59	<3 mos, 71%	>3 mos, 35%

*From Hafermann MD: External radiotherapy. Urology 17(Suppl):15–23, 1981.

Table 25–5. INCIDENCE OF POSITIVE BIOPSY RESULTS AFTER DEFINITIVE EXTERNAL BEAM IRRADIATION (VARIABLE TIME INTERVALS)*

First Author	Reference	Number of Patients	Positive Biopsy Results (%)
Hill	33	21	24
Perez	58	11	27
Nachtsheim	49	50	27
Grout	30	11	45
Cosgrove	20	23	48
Mollenkamp	48	77	58
Sewell	70	31	74

*From Hafermann MD: External radiotherapy. Urology 17(Suppl):15–23, 1981.

prostatic neoplasm in 13 of 15 patients from whom biopsies were taken at four to 38 months following definitive irradiation.[66] Rhamy and Sewell later extended this series to 17 patients but noted that results of biopsies in six of the 17 (35%) later became negative, and eight of the 17 patients exhibited long-term survival.[70] Reports of several additional authors have been reviewed earlier.[4] Additional contributions are listed by Hafermann in Table 25–5.[31] In most of these efforts, the long-term status of the patients was not available and, indeed, it was difficult to determine whether the histopathologic specimens were biologically viable (in the sense that the cells were capable of sustained replication) or whether, in the course of time, the cells might perish, being unable to withstand the stress of the next mitotic process. This seemed to be the case for the series of Cox and Stoffel, who followed 38 consecutive patients with Stage C1 carcinoma of the prostate who were treated aggressively with the equivalent of 7000 rads in 31 fractions in 43 days.[21] One hundred thirty-nine serial biopsies were obtained; the results of 49 were considered positive and 90 negative. In that study the percentage of biopsies positive for disease appeared to correlate inversely with the interval after radiation: 60% positive at six months, 37% at one year, 30% at 18 months, and 19% at 2.5 years. The positive results did not correlate with radiation dose, previous hormone therapy, or prognosis.

More recently, this issue was examined in 64 patients selected from the Stanford series of 146 patients who had been surgically staged and in whom the lymph node status was known.[28] The 64 patients were selected on an ad hoc basis as they arrived for follow-

Table 25–6. RESULTS OF BIOPSY ACCORDING TO STAGE OF PRIMARY TUMOR

Stage	Number	Number and Percentage of Positive Biopsy Results
A_2	1	0 (0%)
B_1	2	0 (0%)
Small B_2	8	3 (38%)
Large B_2	22	13 (59%)
C	31	23 (74%)
Total	64	39 (61%)

up examinations. The biopsies were obtained transperineally by multiple cores extracted with a Tru-cut biopsy needle. Twenty-eight of the 64 patients were judged to have clinically normal prostates, and 36 had abnormal tissue. Seven of 28 normally palpable prostates were positive for disease (25%), whereas 32 of 36 abnormally palpable prostates tested positive (89%). The overall positive rate was 61%, and it bore a direct relationship to advancing clinical stage, as is shown in Table 25–6. The status of the patients relative to stable or progressive neoplasm is presented in Table 25–7. Eleven patients are living without metastases; however, seven were placed on diethylstilbestrol (DES), and two have received interstitial irradiation of the prostate and are still living after seven and five years, respectively, without further disease. Of the 25 patients with no evidence of disease on biopsy, 19 remain alive, three are alive with metastases, and three died of progressive disease. Of those

with positive results of biopsies, eight are alive with metastases, 18 died of progressive carcinoma of the prostate, and two died of other causes but had metastatic prostate cancer. It is of interest that those patients who had evidence of lymphadenopathy were especially susceptible to treatment failure even at the local site. Contrary to the findings of Cox and Stoffel, the biopsy status of the patients in the Stanford series was highly predictive of later disease status. For example, 28 of the 39 patients with positive results of postirradiation biopsy later developed overt metastatic disease, whereas only six of the 25 patients with negative results later developed metastases.

These data are quite compatible with those of Scardino and Wheeler.[69] They found that 56 of 146 patients (38%) had one or more positive results of biopsies following prostatic irradiation with a combination of external beam and gold-198 interstitial implantation. As in the Stanford series, they found a positive correlation with clinical stage, which extended from 17% in Stage B_{1N} to 59% in stage C_1 (Table 25–8). Moreover, they plotted the percentage of positive results of biopsies against those found by Cox and Stoffel (Fig. 25–16). It is of interest that the two curves are similar out to 18 months, after which the curve of Cox and Stoffel continues to decline to 20% positivity, whereas at 24 months the curve by Scardino takes a turn upward and exceeds 40%. Scardino criticized the Cox and Stoffel data because more than one half of the patients received androgen deprivation therapy. On the other hand, the technique of irradiation used in the Scardino series represents a departure from the usual technique in that it relied upon a combination of a relatively

Table 25–7. CURRENT STATUS OF 64 PATIENTS

	Patients With Positive Biopsy Results	Patients With Negative Biopsy Results
Alive without metastases or progression	11*	19
Alive with metastases	8	3†
Dead of progressive disease	18	3†
Dead of other causes, with metastases	2	0

*Seven of 11 patients are on DES for local control; two of 11 have received interstitial irradiation.

†Four of six patients had positive nodes at initial staging.

Table 25–8. BIOPSY RESULTS AMONG 146 PATIENTS AND CORRELATION WITH INITIAL CLINICAL STAGE OF TUMOR*

Clinical Stage	Number of Patients	Biopsy Results			
		Negative		Positive	
		N	%	N	%
A_2	24	16	67	8	33
B_{1N}	12	10	83	2	17
B_1	40	29	72	11	28
B_2	31	19	61	12	39
C_1	39	16	41	23	59
Totals	146	90	62	56	38

*From Scardino PT, Wheeler TM: Prostatic biopsy after irradiation therapy for prostatic cancer. Urology 25(Suppl):39, 1985.

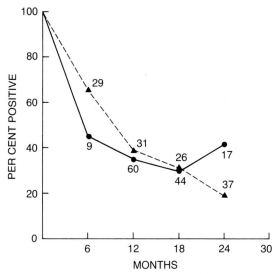

Figure 25–16. *Incidence of positive biopsy results as a function of time after radiotherapy. Triangles connected by a dashed line represent data from Cox JD, Stoffel TJ: The significance of needle biopsy after irradiation for Stage C adenocarcinoma of the prostate. Cancer 40:156–160, 1977. The circles connected by a solid line denote data points for the study report from which this figure is reproduced: Scardino PT, Wheeler TM: Prostatic biopsy after irradiation therapy for prostatic cancer. Urology 25(Suppl):39, 1985.*

modest gold seed implantation to supplement a somewhat lower external beam radiation dose.

It would seem, therefore, in light of the more recent studies that perhaps employ more aggressive biopsy techniques and a longer follow-up to assess the status of the patient, that post-therapeutic biopsy status does have predictive value in assessing disease status. From the standpoint of designing improved therapy, the correlation of positive post-treatment biopsies with advancing stage and later dissemination cannot be ignored. The radiotherapist must redefine local control in terms of the histopathologic evaluation of the status of the primary tumor and must design treatment techniques that confront the failure to sterilize the larger lesions in a significantly high proportion of cases. These techniques do exist. Examples include boosting the primary site by means of interstitial implants with removable iridium-192[73] or more extensive permanent interstitial implants, as has been advocated by Charyulu;[19] turning to adjuvant methodologies, such as radiosensitizers with electron affinity, other chemotherapeutic agents, or hyperthermia; or even using a different spe-

cies of radiation, such as negative pi mesons, heavy ions, neutrons, or protons.[40, 71]

RADIATION SALVAGE FOLLOWING RADICAL PROSTATECTOMY

Interest in radical prostatectomy has been rekindled with the trend toward earlier diagnosis in prostatic cancer[47] as well as the employment of penile prostheses and the development of an operative procedure that promises the preservation of erectile potency in some patients.[78] Unfortunately, a reliable preoperative method for ensuring containment of the prostatic cancer within the prostatic capsule has not been developed. CT scanning and ultrasonograms have not proved reliable in this regard, and, although magnetic resonance imaging (MRI) is promising, its specificity in detecting intracapsular tumor versus extracapsular extension has not been fully assessed. Thus, the greater use of surgery portends an increasing number of patients who will be candidates for irradiation salvage following incomplete resection. For example, Byar and Mostofi demonstrated that prostatic neoplasm occurred in the periphery of the gland in 97% of the cases and that in 85%, the tumor was multicentric in origin.[16] Elder and associates demonstrated that 66% of the 53 patients in clinical Stage B_2 in the Johns Hopkins series had extraprostatic extension upon examination of the resected specimen.[25] Moreover, disease-free survival at 15 years occurred in only four of the 32 patients in this group with extracapsular extension. Catalona and co-workers observed extracapsular extension or seminal vesicle invasion, or both, in 10% of 39 Stage B_1 patients and in 38% of Stage B_2 patients with negative results of lymph node biopsy.[18] Extracapsular extension increased to eight of 11 patients in Stage B_1 or B_2 who had pathologically positive lymph nodes. In 215 patients carefully selected for radical perineal prostatectomy, Gibbons found microscopic extracapsular disease in 49 of 195 (25%) in clinical Stage B.[29] In Jewett's original discourse on radical prostatectomy, a highly selected group of 103 patients were available for evaluation and at risk for 15 years.[37] In 17 (16.5%) from this group, tumor cells were found beyond the prostate, and only one survived 15 years with cancer. Ten others died with cancer.

Currently there are two situations in which radiation therapy should be considered following radical resection. In the first the patient may develop a local recurrence in the prostatic bed at some interval of time remote from the original radical prostatectomy. If there is no evidence of distant metastasis, a second attempt at definitive therapy may be carried out with external beam irradiation. Even in the face of distant metastases, symptomatic local recurrence may justify a trial of radiation therapy. Secondly, if the radical prostatectomy specimen discloses neoplasm at the margins of the resection, then an early attempt at radiation salvage should be carried out. This takes maximum advantage of a minimum number of tumor cells and permits radiation therapy to be given before the recurrence becomes firmly established. Of course, one must first await complete healing after surgery and maximum recovery of function. We prefer to wait for two or three months postoperatively before starting irradiation, unless the tumor is of especially high grade, in which case earlier radiotherapy may be required. The experience with radiation salvage has been reviewed elsewhere.[17, 24, 50, 59, 65, 74] Since then, the 1975 series by Ray has been updated.[63] It includes 13 patients treated within four months of incomplete excision and 19 who were treated after palpable local recurrence. The five-year actuarial survival free of disease in the patients treated soon after surgery was 57% but only 20% for patients treated after a frank clinical recurrence. Although in this early group of patients the radiotherapeutic technique was identical to that described earlier for patients treated by radiotherapy alone, more recently the treatment has been slightly modified for the early group because of the fear of increased complications. In the postoperative patients, a lymph node sampling was usually performed prior to prostatectomy, and prostatectomy was completed only in patients with negative results of lymph node biopsy. Therefore, in this instance whole pelvic irradiation, which would include the first echelon lymphatic drainage, is not necessary. Rather, the treatment is confined to the surgical bed of the prostate, and special care is taken to ensure that the periprostatic tissues, the site of anastomosis, and the proximal corpora are well included in the radiation volume. This usually requires radiation fields of 8 × 8 cm or 9 × 9 cm. The left and right lateral arc routine is employed, as was described previously for the prostatic booster dose. In this situation, eight to 12 weeks is allowed for full recovery from the surgical procedure, and a radiation dose of 6000 rads is delivered over six weeks, calculated at the isocenter.

In patients who have a frank recurrence, lymph node disease is more likely and full pelvic irradiation is applied as described earlier.

SUMMARY

The use of radiation therapy for the treatment of prostatic cancer has increased for patients in all clinical stages during the past decade. This is most apparent for disease Stages B and C, for which radiation treatment has increased from about 20% in 1974 to slightly over 40% in 1983. In the Stanford series reported herein, an actuarial survival of 81% at five years, 59% at 10 years, and 36% at 15 years had been achieved within a group of 477 patients in clinical Stage A or B, followed from two through 25 years. Among 402 patients in clinical Stage C, followed for the same interval, an actuarial survival of 62% at five years, 36% at 10 years, and 18% at 15 years was recorded. These data (at least at the five-year interval) are virtually identical to results of the national practice in the radiotherapy of prostatic carcinoma, reported by the American College of Radiology patterns of care outcome studies, which appear to accurately reflect the national benchmark for external beam radiation treatment of prostatic cancer. Most radiotherapists continue to advocate radiotherapy with curative intent for patients with primary tumors that are somewhat more advanced than those tumors considered for resection according to rigorous criteria but still not so advanced that palliation by hormone therapy should be considered.[4] Thus from the radiotherapeutic viewpoint, a proper sequence for the selection of treatment in prostatic carcinoma would include (1) radical resection following clearance of the regional lymph node drainage for patients with a 1-cm (or a little larger) truly localized nodular lesion (Jewett criteria) and negative results of lymph node biopsy; (2) aggressive irradiation of the prostate and potential regional adenopathy in patients with lesions in Stage B_2 or C or as an alternative to surgery in patients with solitary nodules who are considered poor surgical risks or who decline surgery.

Androgen deprivation therapy should continue to be reserved for palliative treatment in the event of radiation failure or in patients with more advanced disease, such as skeletal or parenchymal metastases. Radiotherapy also may play an important role for the relief of specific symptoms at a variety of metastatic sites, even though the patient may also be receiving androgen deprivation treatment.

The radiation treatment of overt lymphadenopathy has not improved the long-term survival in patients with known lymph node metastases. Whether a small group of patients exists in whom microscopic metastases can be sterilized by radiation therapy has not been proved, although there is retrospective data reported herein that suggests that this may be true. In any case, proof of lymphadenopathy by biopsy prior to radiation therapy is not indicated, inasmuch as it is convenient to treat the regional lymph nodes along with the primary neoplasm without undue morbidity and without compromising the treatment of the primary tumor.

Androgen deprivation therapy concomitant with external beam irradiation does not appear to improve survival; however, some evidence indicates that androgen deprivation therapy prior to irradiation as a maneuver to reduce cellular burden may be of benefit. In terms of reduced tumor cell numbers, better survival is achieved when the delay between diagnosis and treatment is kept to the very minimum. Improved survival is also achieved with early salvage by radiation therapy following incomplete resection, as compared with the results of awaiting frank tumor recurrence.

Finally, recent data suggests that the postirradiation biopsy status may have value in predicting outcome, especially when the primary tumor is of advanced stage and grade. In such instances, more aggressive radiation boost treatment to the prostate may be necessary. This may include boost by interstitial irradiation techniques or combination therapy with hyperthermia, adjuvant therapy with radiosensitizers, or boost by particle therapy, such as protons, heavy ions, pi mesons, or neutrons.

References

1. American Cancer Society: Cancer statistics, 1984. CA 34:14, 1984.
2. American Joint Committee for Cancer Staging and End Results Reporting: Classification and staging of cancer by site. Chicago, American Joint Committee, 1983.
3. Arduino LJ, Glucksman MA: Lymph node metastases in early carcinoma of the prostate. J Urol 88:91–93, 1962.
4. Bagshaw MA: Radiation therapy for cancer of the prostate. In DG Skinner, JB deKernion (eds), Genitourinary Cancer. Philadelphia, WB Saunders, 1978, p 355.
5. Bagshaw MA: A technique for external beam irradiation of carcinoma of the prostate. In SH Levitt, N Tapley (eds), Technological Basis of Radiation Therapy: Practical Clinical Applications. Philadelphia, Lea & Febiger, 1984, p 244
6. Bagshaw MA: Radiotherapeutic treatment of prostatic carcinoma with pelvic node involvement. Urol Clin North Am 11:297–304, 1984.
7. Bagshaw MA: Potential for radiotherapy alone in prostatic cancer. Cancer 55(Suppl):2079, 1985.
8. Bagshaw MA, Kaplan HS: Radical external radiation therapy of localized prostatic carcinoma. Proc Tenth Int'l Congress of Radiology. Montreal, Canada, September, 1962.
9. Bagshaw MA, Kaplan HS, Sagerman RH: Linear accelerator supervoltage radiotherapy. VII. Carcinoma of the prostate. Radiology 85:121–129, 1965.
10. Bagshaw MA, Ray GR: External beam radiation therapy of prostate carcinoma. In DG Skinner (ed), Urological Cancer. New York, Grune & Stratton, 1983, p 53.
11. Bagshaw MA, Ray GR, Cox RS: Radiotherapy of prostatic carcinoma: long- or short-term efficacy. Urology 25(Suppl):17, 1985.
12. Barringer BS: Carcinoma of prostate. Surg Gynecol Obstet 34:168–176, 1922.
13. Barringer BS: Prostatic carcinoma. J Urol 47:306–310, 1942.
14. Budhraja SN, Anderson JC: An assessment of the value of radiotherapy in the management of carcinoma of the prostate. Br J Urol 36:535–540, 1964.
15. Bumpus HC Jr: Roentgen rays and radium in diagnosis and treatment of carcinoma of prostate. AJR 9:269–287, 1922.
16. Byar DP, Mostofi FK: Carcinoma of the prostate: prognostic evaluation of certain pathologic features in 208 radical prostatectomies. Cancer 30:5–13, 1972.
17. Cantril ST, Vaeth JM, Green JP, et al: Radiation therapy for localized carcinoma of the prostate: correlation with histopathological grading. Front Rad Ther Oncol 9:274, 1974.
18. Catalona WJ, Fleischmann J, Menon M: Pelvic lymph node status as predictor of extracapsular tumor extension in clinical stage B prostatic cancer. J Urol 129:327–329, 1983.
19. Charyulu KKN: Transperineal interstitial implantation of prostate cancer: a new method. Int J Radiat Oncol Biol Phys 6:1261–1266, 1980.
20. Cosgrove MD, Kaempf MJ: Prostatic cancer revisited. J Urol 115:79–81, 1976.
21. Cox JD, Stoffel TJ: The significance of needle biopsy after irradiation for stage C adenocarcinoma of the prostate. Cancer 40:156–160, 1977.

22. Cupps RE, Utz DC, Fleming TR, et al: Definitive radiation therapy for prostatic carcinoma: Mayo Clinic experience. J Urol 124:855–859, 1980.

23. Deming CL: Cancer of prostate and seminal vesicles treated with radium. Surg Gynecol Obstet 34:99–118, 1922.

24. Dykhuizen RF, Sargent CR, George FW 3rd, et al: The use of cobalt 60 teletherapy in the treatment of prostatic carcinoma. J Urol 100:333–338, 1968.

25. Elder JS, Jewett HJ, Walsh PC: Radical perineal prostatectomy for clinical stage B2 carcinoma of the prostate. J Urol 127:704–706, 1982.

26. Flocks RH, Culp D, Porto R: Lymphatic spread from prostatic cancer. J Urol 81:194–196, 1959.

27. Flocks RH, Kerr HD, Elkins HB, Culp D: Treatment of carcinoma of the prostate by interstitial radiation with radio-active gold (Au^{198}): preliminary report. J Urol 68:510–522, 1952.

28. Freiha FS, Bagshaw MA: Carcinoma of the prostate: results of postirradiation biopsy. Prostate 5:19–25, 1984.

29. Gibbons RP, Correa RJ Jr, Brannen GE, Mason JT: Total prostatectomy for localized prostatic cancer. J Urol 131:73–76, 1984.

30. Grout DC, Grayhack JT, Moss W, Holland JM: Radiation therapy in the treatment of carcinoma of the prostate. J Urol 105:411–414, 1971.

31. Hafermann MD: External radiotherapy. Urology 17(Suppl):15–23, 1981.

32. Harisiadis L, Veenema RJ, Senyszyn JJ, et al: Carcinoma of the prostate: treatment with external radiotherapy. Cancer 41:2131–2142, 1978.

33. Hill DR, Crews QE Jr, Walsh PC: Prostate carcinoma: radiation treatment of the primary and regional lymphatics. Cancer 34:156–160, 1974.

34. Huggins C, Stevens RE Jr, Hodges CV: Studies on prostatic cancer: effect of castration on advanced carcinoma of prostate gland. Arch Surg 43:209–223, 1941.

35. Hultberg S: Results of treatment with radiotherapy in carcinoma of the prostate. Acta Radiol 27:339–349, 1946.

36. Hussey DH: Carcinoma of the prostate. In GH Fletcher (ed), Textbook of Radiotherapy, Ed 3. Philadelphia, Lea & Febiger, 1980, pp 894–914.

37. Jewett HJ, Bridge RW, Gray GF Jr, Shelley WM: The palpable nodule of prostatic cancer. Results 15 years after radical excision. JAMA 203:403–406, 1968.

38. Kempson RL, Levine G: The relationship of grade to prognosis in carcinoma of the prostate. Front Radiat Ther Oncol 9:267, 1974.

39. Kramer SA, Spahr J, Brendler CB, et al: Experience with Gleason's histopathologic grading in prostatic cancer. J Urol 124:223–225, 1980.

40. Laramore GE, Krall JM, Thomas FJ, et al: Fast neutron radiotherapy for locally advanced prostate cancer: results of an RTOG randomized study. Int J Radiat Oncol Biol Phys 11:1621, 1985.

41. Leibel SA, Hanks GE, Kramer S: Patterns of care outcome studies: results of the national practice in adenocarcinoma of the prostate. Int J Radiat Oncol Biol Phys 10:401–409, 1984.

42. Lipsett JA, Cosgrove MD, Green N, et al: Factors influencing prognosis in the radiotherapeutic management of carcinoma of the prostate. Int J Radiat Oncol Biol Phys 1:1049–1058, 1976.

43. McCullough DL: Diagnosis and staging of prostatic cancer. In DG Skinner, G Lieskovsky (eds), Diagnosis and Management of Genitourinary Cancer. Philadelphia, WB Saunders, 1987, pp 405–416.

44. McGowan DG: The value of extended field radiation therapy in carcinoma of the prostate. Int J Radiat Oncol Biol Phys 7:1333–1339, 1981.

45. McNeal JE: Origin and development of carcinoma in the prostate. Cancer 23:24–34, 1969.

46. Mellinger GT, Gleason D, Bailar J 3rd: The histology and prognosis of prostatic cancer. J Urol 97:331–337, 1967.

47. Mettlin C: Long-term and short-term surveys of patterns of care of prostate cancer in American College of Surgeons' approved cancer programs. Preliminary report to the American College of Surgeons' Commission on Cancer Patient Care and Research Committee. (Private correspondence, October, 1984).

48. Mollenkamp JS, Cooper JF, Kagan AR: Clinical experience with supervoltage-radiotherapy in carcinoma of the prostate: preliminary report. J Urol 113:374–377, 1975.

49. Nachtsheim DA Jr, McAninch JW, Stutzman RE, Goebel JL: Latent residual tumor following external radiotherapy for prostate adenocarcinoma. J Urol 120:312–314, 1978.

50. Neglia WJ, Hussey DH, Johnson DE: Megavoltage radiation therapy for carcinoma of the prostate. Int J Radiat Oncol Biol Phys 2:873–883, 1977.

51. Paschkis R, Tittinger W: Radiumbehandlung eines prostatasarkoms. Weiner klinische Wochenschrift Nr. 48, 1910.

52. Pasteau O: Traitement du cancer de la prostate par le radium. Revue des Maladies de la Nutrition, 1911, p 363.

53. Pasteau O, Degrais A: Traitement des tumeurs de la prostate par le radium. Transactions 17th Int'l Congress of Medicine. London, 1913. Section XIV, H. Frowde (ed), Urology, Part II. London, Oxford University Press, 1913, p 28.

54. Paulson DF, Cline WA Jr, Koefoot RB Jr, et al: Extended field radiation therapy versus delayed hormonal therapy in node positive prostatic adenocarcinoma. J Urol 127:935–937, 1982.

55. Paulson DF, Hodge GB Jr, Hinshaw W: The Uro-Oncology Research Group: Radiation therapy versus delayed androgen deprivation for stage C carcinoma of the prostate. J Urol 131:901–902, 1984.

56. Paulson DF, Lin GH, Hinshaw W, et al: Radical surgery versus radiotherapy for adenocarcinoma of the prostate. J Urol 128:502–504, 1982.

57. Paulson DF, Piserchia PV, Gardner W: Predictors of lymphatic spread in prostatic adenocarcinoma: Uro-Oncology Research Group Study. J Urol 123:697–699, 1980.

58. Perez CA, Ackerman LV, Silber I, Royce RK: Radiation therapy in the treatment of localized carcinoma of the prostate. Preliminary report using 22 MeV photons. Cancer 34:1059–1068, 1974.

59. Perez CA, Bauer W, Garza R, Royce RK: Radiation therapy in the definitive treatment of localized carcinoma of the prostate. Cancer 40:1425–1433, 1977.

60. Pilepich MV, Perez CA, Walz BJ, Zivnuska FR: Complications of definitive radiotherapy for carcinoma of the prostate. Int J Radiat Oncol Biol Phys 7:1341–1348, 1981.

61. Pistenma DA, Bagshaw MA, Freiha FS: Extended-field radiation therapy for prostatic adenocarcinoma: status report of a limited prospective trial.

In DE Johnson, ML Samuels (eds), Cancer of the Genitourinary Tract, New York, Raven Press, 1979, p 229.

62. Pistenma DA, Ray GR, Bagshaw MA: The role of megavoltage radiation therapy in the treatment of prostatic carcinoma. Semin Oncol 3:115–122, 1976.

63. Ray GR, Bagshaw MA, Freiha F: External beam radiation salvage for residual or recurrent local tumor following radical prostatectomy. J Urol 132:926–930, 1984.

64. Ray GR, Cassady JR, Bagshaw MA: Definitive radiation therapy of carcinoma of the prostate. A report on 15 years of experience. Radiology 106:407–418, 1973.

65. Ray GR, Cassady JR, Bagshaw MA: External-beam megavoltage radiation therapy in the treatment of post-radical prostatectomy residual or recurrent tumor: preliminary results. J Urol 114:98–101, 1975.

66. Rhamy RK, Wilson SK, Caldwell WL: Biopsy-proved tumor following definitive irradiation for resectable carcinoma of the prostate. J Urol 107:627–630, 1972.

67. Rosen E, Cassady JR, Connolly J, Chaffey JT: Radiotherapy for prostate carcinoma: the JCRT experience (1968–1978). II. Factors related to tumor control and complications. Int J Radiat Oncol Biol Phys 11:725, 1985.

68. Sagalowsky AI, Milam H, Reveley LR, Silva FG: Prediction of lymphatic metastases by Gleason histologic grading in prostatic cancer. J Urol 128:951–952, 1982.

69. Scardino PT, Wheeler TM: Prostatic biopsy after irradiation therapy for prostatic cancer. Urology 25(Suppl):39, 1985.

70. Sewell RA, Braren V, Wilson SK, Rhamy RK: Extended biopsy follow-up after full course radiation for resectable prostatic carcinoma. J Urol 113:371–373, 1975.

71. Shipley WU, Tepper JE, Prout GR Jr, et al: Proton radiation as boost therapy for localized prostatic carcinoma. JAMA 241:1912–1915, 1979.

72. Smith GG, Peirson EL: Value of high voltage x-ray therapy in carcinoma of the prostate. J Urol 23:331–342, 1930.

73. Syed AM, Puthawala A, Tansey LA, et al: Management of prostate carcinoma. Combination of pelvic lymphadenectomy, temporary Ir-192 implantation, and external irradiation. Radiology 149:829–833, 1983.

74. Taylor WJ: Radiation oncology: cancer of the prostate. Cancer 39:856–861, 1977.

75. Taylor WJ, Richardson RG, Hafermann MD: Radiation therapy for localized prostate cancer. Cancer 43:1123–1127, 1979.

76. TNM Classification of Malignant Tumors, 2nd ed. Geneva, Union International Contre le Cancer, 1974.

77. van der Werf-Messing B, Sourek-Zikova V, Blonk DI: Localized advanced carcinoma of the prostate: radiation therapy versus hormonal therapy. Int J Radiat Oncol Biol Phys 1:1043–1048, 1976.

78. Walsh PC, Donker PJ: Impotence following radical prostatectomy: insight into etiology and prevention. J Urol 128:492–497, 1982.

79. Walsh PC, Jewett HJ: Radical surgery for prostatic cancer. Cancer 45:1906–1911, 1980.

80. Widman BP: Cancer of the prostate. The results of radium and roentgen-ray treatment. Radiology 22:153–159, 1934.

81. Young HH: The diagnosis and treatment of early malignant disease of the prostate. Transactions 17th Int'l Congress of Medicine, London, 1913. Section XIV, Urology, Part I, p 1. H Frowde (ed). London, Oxford Univ Press, 1913.

82. Young HH: Technique of radium treatment of cancer of prostate and seminal vesicles. Surg Gynecol Obstet 34:93–98, 1922.

83. Young HH: Fronz WA: Some new methods in the treatment of carcinoma of the lower genitourinary tract with radium. J Urol 1:505, 1917.

C. EUGENE CARLTON, JR., M.D.

Radioactive Isotope Implantation for Cancer of the Prostate

The use of radioactive isotopes for the definitive treatment of cancer of the prostate was first reported by Flocks and his associates in 1952.[2] These authors reported the successful ablation of both primary prostatic cancer and node disease by the interstitial implantation of colloidal ^{198}Au. This experience encouraged other workers to seek isotopes that were easier to handle and more predictable than colloidal gold in dosimetry and distribution. Although a number of radionuclides have been evaluated for the treatment of cancer of the prostate, at the present time only iodine-125 and gold-198 are used to a significant extent. Our series at Baylor using ^{198}Au and supplemental external beam radiotherapy began in 1965,[1] and shortly thereafter Whitmore and associates at Memorial Sloan-Kettering Cancer Center (MSKCC) began using interstitial ^{125}I.[5] Each of these techniques has its advantages and disadvantages, and the results achieved with each modality will be discussed.

SELECTION OF PATIENTS

The patient should be in reasonably good health and have an estimated life expectancy of five or more years, though no arbitrary age limitation is stipulated. The evaluation should include a history, physical examination, serum acid and alkaline phosphatase determinations, excretory urogram, skeletal survey, technetium bone scan, and cystoscopy. Lymphangiography has been recommended as a staging procedure by some authors, but the false-negative rate of approximately 47%, the relatively high morbidity, and the failure to fill the important obturator and internal iliac nodes raise questions as to the usefulness of this procedure. If the patient is found to be free of evidence of metastatic disease and has a Stage A_2, B, or limited Stage C lesion, he is a candidate for attempted cure with interstitial implantation of radionuclide. Patients who have a more extensive Stage C lesion (greater than 6 cm in diameter) are not considered candidates for definitive treatment with interstitial irradiation because the technique of interstitial implantation requires palpably well-defined margins of tumor extension, and the likelihood of definitive control of a bulky lesion by radioisotope implantation is remote. Tumor grade has not been utilized by either Whitmore or the author in the selection of patients. Both authors have observed, however, that higher grade neoplasms tend to be larger, metastasize earlier, and have a higher incidence of lymph node involvement.

If the patient has urinary retention requiring catheter drainage, or if in the judgment of the attending physician urinary retention is imminent, consideration should be given to a preliminary transurethral resection of the prostate. This procedure will obviously delay definitive therapy for six to eight weeks, but it is felt to be preferable to a prolonged period of indwelling catheter drainage with its attendant discomfort, probability of infection, and reduced tolerance to radiotherapy. In cases in which a transurethral resection is believed to be indicated, it should be done in a limited manner with an effort made to leave sufficient tissue to support subsequent implantation. The implantation is then delayed six to eight weeks to allow healing of the prostatic fossa and resolution of any infection.

OPERATIVE EXPOSURE AND PELVIC LYMPHADENECTOMY

The patient is placed in a modified lithotomy position with the thighs flexed approximately 30° from the central axis. A No. 16 French Foley catheter is inserted and connected to closed drainage. Whitmore employs an O'Connor drape to allow digital rectal examination during the interstitial implantation of ^{125}I. Digital rectal examination is rarely required during the implantation of ^{198}Au, inasmuch as the placement is less exacting. A midline umbilicus-to-pubis incision (Whitmore) or Pfannenstiel incision (Carlton) may be employed. The incision is carried into the prevesical space in a standard manner, with care being taken to stay extraperitoneally (Fig. 26–1). The peritoneal envelope is mobilized in a medial and cephalad direction to expose the pelvic vasculature. The retraction of the peritoneal envelope is facilitated by mobilization of the spermatic cord structures at the internal ring by incising the overlying transverse fascia (Fig. 26–2). In many instances the vas deferens is divided to provide even more exposure. Medial retraction of the peritoneal envelope will expose the external iliac vessels, and the common iliac vessel will be easily exposed to the level of the ureter (Fig. 26–2).

The dissection is started at the midportion of the common iliac vessels, with care being taken to clip or ligate the lymphatics as they are transected to prevent the subsequent formation of a lymphocele. The dissection is carried inferiorly along the common and external iliac vessels to the level of the inguinal ligament, where the lymphatics are again ligated or clipped and divided. Inasmuch as the lymphadenectomy is a staging instead of a therapeutic procedure, the lymphatic tissue lateral to the common or external iliac arteries is left intact (Fig. 26–3) to decrease lymphedema of the lower extremities. The nodes around the hypogastric artery are dissected to the level of the vesical arteries. The obturator fossa is dissected free of all fat and lymphatic tissue, with care being taken to preserve the obturator nerve. This dissection is facilitated by anterior retraction of the external iliac vein with a vein retractor. The fat is cleaned from the lateral aspect of the prostate, and an incision is made in the endopelvic fascia as it reflects onto the prostate from the superior surface of the urogenital diaphragm (Fig. 26–4). The prostate can then be mobilized by blunt dissection to an extent allowing easy accessibility of the prostatic tumor to the radiotherapist for implantation. It is not necessary to separate the prostate from the rectum or to divide the puboprostatic ligaments. The dissection should be limited to the extent that is necessary for access by the radiotherapist for implantation, in that an extensive dissection will increase the incidence of complications, particularly impotence.

IMPLANTATION OF RADIOACTIVE IODINE

^{125}I has practical and theoretical advantages as a radiation source. A half-life of 60 days means that loss of activity with brief periods of storage is not a practical problem. There is also the theoretical possibility that the protracted irradiation resulting from a 60-day half-life may be advantageous in the treatment of a generally slow-growing neoplasm with a relatively long doubling time.

A disadvantage of ^{125}I is its limited zone of irradiation—it has half-value layers of 0.025 mm in lead. Since all of the radiation with this technique is delivered by the radionuclide, it is imperative that extreme care be taken with the pattern of implantation to assure homogeneity of dose. The implanted seeds consist of ^{125}I absorbed on two portions of ion exchange resin, separated by a gold marker (to obtain radiopacity), and incorporated in a titanium container that is 4.5 mm in length, 0.75 mm in diameter, and

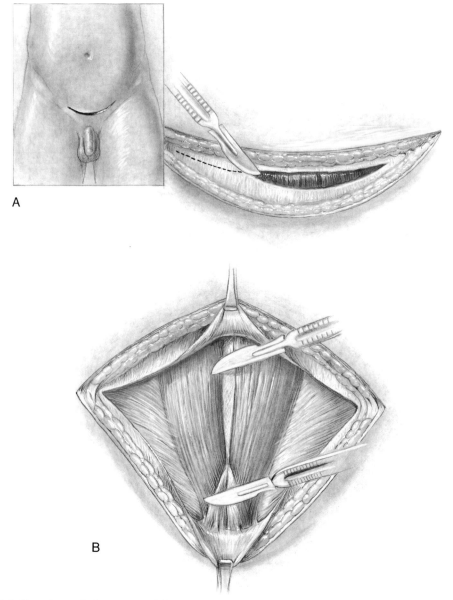

Figure 26–1. Steps in surgical exposure of the prostate for implantation of gold grains.

Illustration continued on opposite page

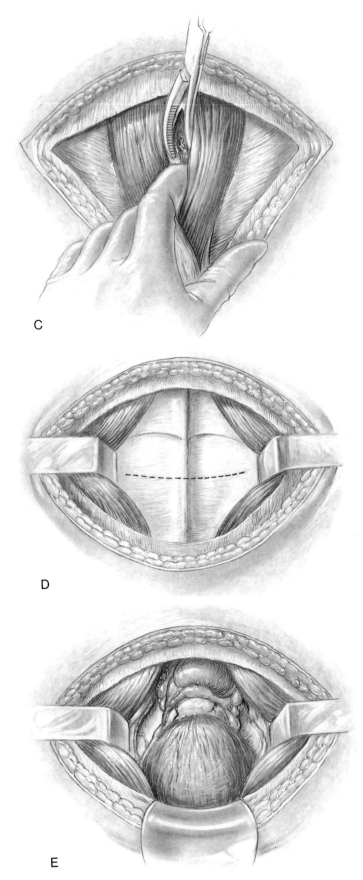

C

D

E

Figure 26–1 Continued

449

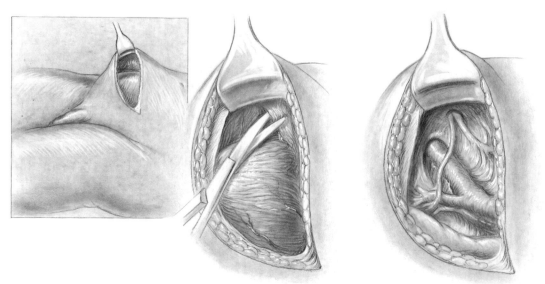

Figure 26–2. Mobilization and retraction of the peritoneal envelope is facilitated by incision of the fascial attachments at the internal inguinal ring.

capable of being implanted through a 17-gauge needle.

Hollow stainless steel needles, 17 gauge and 15 cm long, are inserted into the prostate in a more or less anterior-posterior direction parallel to one another and approximately 1 cm apart, starting from the superior margin of the gland and proceeding inferiorly. Keeping an index finger inside the rectum against the prostate during insertion of the needles permits the tip of the needle to be sensed before the rectal wall can be perforated.

Since the implanted seeds are 4.5 mm in length, it is important to withdraw the sensed needle approximately 0.5 cm so that subsequent implantation of the seeds will not result in rectal wall perforation. Although it seems inevitable that the prostatic urethra or bladder is traversed by one or more of the needles, this has not created a recognized problem. Penetration of the periprostatic veins during implantation inevitably occurs.

The dimensions of the volume of radioactive isotope to be implanted are estimated from the vertical and horizontal distances between the most peripheral needles and from the anterior-posterior diameter of the gland, indicated by the average actual depth to which the needles have been inserted.

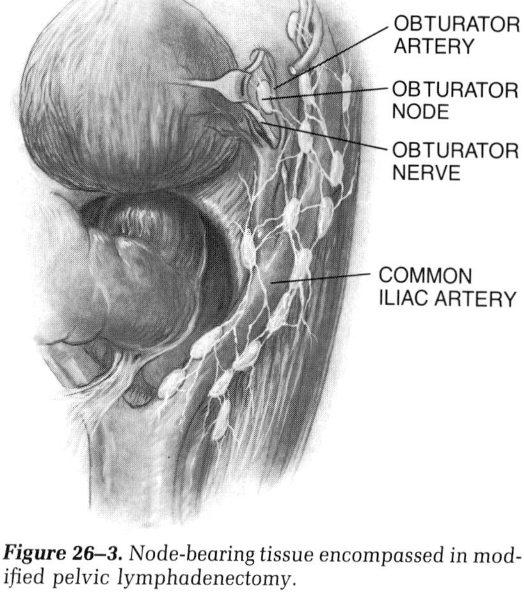

OBTURATOR ARTERY

OBTURATOR NODE

OBTURATOR NERVE

COMMON ILIAC ARTERY

Figure 26–3. Node-bearing tissue encompassed in modified pelvic lymphadenectomy.

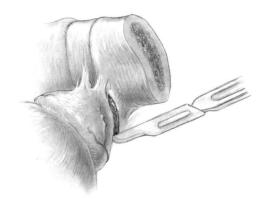

Figure 26–4. Incision of endopelvic fascia to allow more extensive exposure of prostate.

The average of these three dimensions multiplied by an empirically derived factor of 5 has been found to denote the number of millicuries of ^{125}I required to deliver the planned dose within the implanted volume. This minimum effective dose is in the range of 16,000 rads in one year or 8000 rads in two months, or an equivalent single dose of approximately 5300 rads, as calculated by the Shuttleworth and Fowler nomogram. The indicated number of millicuries divided by the average activity of the ^{125}I seeds available yields the actual number of seeds required. A semiautomatic inserter is utilized to deposit the seeds at 0.5- to 1-cm intervals as each needle is successively withdrawn.

IMPLANTATION OF RADIOACTIVE GOLD FOLLOWED BY EXTERNAL RADIOTHERAPY

This technique employs the interstitial implantation of radioactive gold grains as an initial or boost dose followed postoperatively by supplemental external beam radiotherapy. The advantages of this technique are that it requires less exactitude in implantation because of the larger zone irradiation (2.5 mm in lead) and the use of external therapy, which tends to increase the homogeneity of the dose as well as deliver radiotherapy to the periprostatic area not covered by the interstitial implantation.

The isotope employed is radioactive gold grains that have been plated with platinum and are 2 mm long by approximately 0.5 mm in diameter. The gold has a half-life of 2.7 days. The radioactive gold grains are inserted by means of a needle implanter to deliver an approximate dose of 3500 rads. Following the implantation, the wound is thoroughly irrigated and closed without drainage. When the patient has recovered from the surgical procedure, usually in two weeks, he is started on a course of external beam radiotherapy with the 8 MEV linear accelerator, receiving 4000 to 5000 rads of external beam radiotherapy to the prostate and immediate periprostatic area, usually through 4 × 4 cm opposing portals or rotational technique. This course of therapy is accomplished with 16 treatments over a 30-day period.

COMPLICATIONS OF THERAPY

With almost 1000 patients now reported,[3, 6] complications of ^{125}I implantation have been mild in the MSKCC experience, but they may not be apparent for several months after the implantation because of the long half-life of the isotope. Approximately 28% of patients experienced delayed irritative voiding symptoms, but bowel complications were rare, although rectal prostatic fistulae have been reported. Prolonged distressing proctitis, rectal ulceration or fistula, or both conditions, necessitating colostomy, occurred in 2 to 25% of patients. Potency was preserved in 93% of patients who were potent before therapy, although others state that problems with potency occur in as many as 24% of the patients, and 16.1% may experience dry ejaculation when they receive additional external beam radiotherapy. Although there were four hospital deaths in the first 400 patients in the MSKCC series, there have been no deaths in the last 500 cases.

Complications of gold seed implantation and external beam irradiation have been few and are quite comparable to those reported for ^{125}I implantation. Among 523 patients treated before 1980 with total doses of 6500 to 7500 rads, there were three deaths. With the limited area of dissection and the relatively low dosage of external irradiation required by this procedure, we have seen genital edema in only 3% and lower extremity edema in 3 to 8% of our patients. Urinary complications were rare. Rectal complications have occurred in 13.8%, but only in 1% were the symptoms persistent or disabling, requiring colostomy in 0.3% of the patients in our earlier series. Erectile potency has been preserved in over 70% of the patients potent before treatment.

LYMPHADENECTOMY

The patients with Stage B_1 lesions have been found to have involvement of the lymph nodes in 11% of the instances, whereas those with B_2 lesions are found to have nodal involvement 20% of the time. The overall incidence of nodal involvement in patients with Stage C lesions is 60%. However, when the Stage C lesions are subcategorized into those less than 6 cm in diameter (patients considered to be candidates for definitive therapy), only 31% have been found to have nodal involvement.

RESULTS

The efficacy of definitive radiotherapy for prostatic carcinoma should be judged primarily by the eradication of the local tumor and, secondarily, by the prevention of distant metastases after therapy. Metastasis may reflect only the insensitivity of the staging studies employed rather than progressive dissemination of tumor from an uncontrolled primary lesion. Both digital rectal examination of the prostate and prostatic biopsy have been used to assess local control after radiotherapy. Controversy continues to surround the meaning of histologic examination of the prostate after radiotherapy. Some investigators have chosen not to perform biopsies on their patients, claiming that the results are uninterpretable and that there are no grounds for prognosis.

Whitmore and associates have recently analyzed and reported their results with about 600 patients, including 240 followed for five or more years.[6] Routine postoperative biopsies were not performed, and local recurrence was detected either by digital rectal examination or by development of urinary obstructive symptoms. For patients followed from two to 10 years, the disease-free survival rate for Stage T1 was 84%; stage T2, 59%; Stage T3, 58%; and Stage T4, 24%. As these authors have already noted, the data address survival only, not necessarily disease-free survival, which more accurately reflects the results of the treatment; endocrine therapy was instituted after a documented recurrence of the tumor, and the five-year survival reported is a very short period of time to assess the efficacy of the therapy. Our own data support these findings.[4]

We also have recently reviewed the results

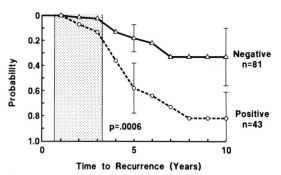

Figure 26–5. *Probability of local recurrence of prostatic cancer, based on biopsy results.*

of pelvic lymphadenectomy, combined gold seed implantation, and external irradiation in 475 patients whose disease was in clinical Stage A_2, B, or C_1 and who had no hormonal therapy before proven recurrence of tumor (local or distant). One hundred and forty-six patients (32%) underwent needle biopsy of the prostate more than six months and less than 36 months after the completion of therapy (Table 26–1). Fifty-six patients (38%) had a positive biopsy result. Figure 26–5 shows the actuarial probability of recurrence, related to biopsy results. The relapse rate was significantly greater when the biopsy result was positive ($p < 0.0005$). If the MSKCC criteria for recurrence are applied to our series, patients in clinical Stage A_2 had a disease-free survival of 46% at five years, and the respective figures for patients in Stage B_{1n}, B_1, B_2, and C_1 were 94%, 61%, 69%, and 51% at five years. We feel that these figures compare favorably with the results for any other known radiation therapy for prostatic cancer.

If the results are analyzed by surgical stage (that is, considering the survival rates only for those with unaffected nodes), they were much better. Among Stage A_2 patients, 66 (18%) were alive without tumor at ten years, and for those in Stage C_1, there were 53 survivors (10%). The median duration of survival for each stage was more than 160 months, except for 92 months for patients in

Table 26–1. BIOPSY RESULTS BY CLINICAL STAGE

Result	Number of Patients	Stage				
		A_2	B_{1n}	B_1	B_2	C_1
Negative	90	16	10	29	19	16
Positive	56 (38%)	8 (33%)	2 (17%)	11 (28%)	12 (39%)	23 (59%)
Total	146	24	12	40	31	39

Stage C_1. Patients with minimal nodal metastases achieve long-term survival free of tumor with no other systemic therapy and seem to fare as well as patients with no nodal disease. But whether such long-term cures can be attributed to the natural history of the disease, the lymphadenectomy, or the pelvic radiotherapy remains unclear.

CONCLUSIONS

There can be little question that therapy with radioisotope implantation for prostatic cancer with or without subsequent radiotherapy has the capacity to eradicate the primary lesion. Success often depends on the biologic potential of the tumor as much as on the specifics of the treatment techniques. Survival free of recurrence or residual tumor is best when the tumor is palpable and confined to the gland (Stage B), and worse for tumors in Stages A_2 and C_1, for high-grade tumors, and for those patients with affected nodes. The results of needle biopsy following treatment and the emerging data on long-term survival with no evidence of disease suggest that these forms of radiotherapy are at least as effective as radical surgery in the ablation of the primary tumor

in Stage B disease and that they offer a significant chance of cure to those patients with limited Stage C disease. As Whitmore has stated, "Whatever may be the long-term effect on the course of the prostatic cancer, the implantation of radionuclides has as few or fewer adverse effects on the quality of life of the prostate cancer patient as any currently extant form of therapy."[7]

References

1. Carlton CE Jr, Hudgins PT, Guerriero WG, Scott R Jr: Radiotherapy in the management of stage C carcinoma of the prostate. J Urol 116:206–210, 1976.
2. Flocks RH, Kerr HD, Elkins HB, Culp D: Treatment of carcinoma of the prostate by interstitial radiation with radioactive gold: preliminary report. J Urol 68:510–522, 1952.
3. Fowler JE Jr, Barzell WW, Hilaris BS, Whitmore WF Jr: Complications of ^{125}I implantation and pelvic lymphadenectomy in the treatment of prostatic cancer. J Urol 121:447–451, 1979.
4. Scardino PT: The prognostic significance of biopsies after radiotherapy for prostatic cancer. Semin Urol 1:243–251, 1983.
5. Whitmore WF Jr, Hilaris B, Grabstald H: Retropubic implantation of iodine-125 in the treatment of prostatic cancer. J Urol 108:918–920, 1972.
6. Whitmore WF Jr, Hilaris B, Batata M, et al: Interstitial radiation: short-term palliation or curative therapy? Urology 25(Suppl):24–29, 1985.
7. Whitmore WF Jr: Personal communication, 1985.

THOMAS E. AHLERING, M.D.
GARY LIESKOVSKY, M.D.
DONALD G. SKINNER, M.D.

Salvage Options Following Radiotherapy Failures

CHAPTER 27

Definitive radiotherapy for adenocarcinoma of the prostate has proven efficacy; however, not all tumors respond completely. The objective of this chapter is to examine the role of prostatic biopsy following definitive radiotherapy and outline management options in patients with evidence of treatment failure.

HISTORICAL OVERVIEW OF RADIATION THERAPY FOR PROSTATIC CANCER

The introduction of radiation to the management of prostatic cancer dates to the early 1900s. Paschikis and Tittinger (1910), Pasteau (1911), Barringer (1916), and Young (1917) were among the early contributors of this form of treatment for prostatic cancer.[49] Generally, radium was implanted into the prostate either transurethrally, transrectally, or transperineally. In the 1920s external beam orthovoltage radiation was advanced as a noninvasive method of delivering radiation to the prostate. Many patients had dramatic improvement in their symptoms and significant reduction in tumor size, attesting to the radiosensitivity of prostatic cancer, but adjacent soft tissue injury, especially to the overlying skin, became a limiting side effect. Radiation was largely abandoned in 1941 after Huggins reported the profound dependence of prostatic cancer on testosterone.[25] After World War II, technical advances bolstered efforts to cure prostatic cancer with radiation therapy as it became increasingly apparent that hormonal therapy was not curative. Methods were investigated that allowed application of higher doses of radiation to the prostate while soft tissue scatter injury was reduced. Direct implantation into the prostate of radioactive isotopes was advocated by Flocks[17] in 1952; high-energy "super" or "mega" voltage external beam therapy was instituted by Bagshaw[4] in 1956. These events initiated the modern era of radiation treatment for cancer of the prostate. Radioactive iodine (^{125}I), radioactive gold (^{198}Au) plus external beam radiotherapy, and radioactive iridium (^{191}Ir) have all been added to the radiation options available in the treatment of prostatic cancer.

Flocks felt that by directly implanting radioactive isotopes into the prostate he could limit injury to adjacent soft tissue while supplying a tumoricidal dose of radiation.[24] He used ^{198}Au, which has a half-value tissue range of 4.5 cm, emits both beta and gamma radiation, and has a half-life of 2.7 days. He also found that at least 5500 rads delivered to the prostate was necessary to be tumoricidal, but significant injury to the rectum occurred with these doses and the method was abandoned.[16] Carlton, in 1972, advocated combining smaller amounts of im-

454

planted [198]Au (to minimize rectal injuries) with an additional radiation boost via external beam therapy.[7] Because of the high tissue penetration of [198]Au, accurate placement of the gold grains is not critical and delivers 2500 to 3000 rads over three weeks. Four to six weeks after implantation the patient receives 4000 to 5000 rads of external beam radiotherapy, which amounts to a total dose of about 7000 rads in seven weeks.

Implantation of radioactive iodine for the treatment of prostatic cancer was introduced by Whitmore in 1970.[51] Relatively lower energy radiation is emitted by ^{125}I than by [198]Au and results in less tissue penetration (half-value tissue range of 1.7 cm).[24]

The half-life of ^{125}I is 60 days, so it takes about one year to deliver its total dose of 15,000 to 35,000 rads. This is equivalent to 7000 rads of external beam radiotherapy given over seven weeks. Because of the lower penetration into tissue, accurate placement of the seeds is critical to ensure adequate doses of radiation to all of the tumor-bearing regions of the prostate. Experience has shown that significant seminal vesicle involvement contraindicates the use of ^{125}I because of inadequate dosing to these structures.[29, 48]

Supervoltage external beam radiotherapy utilizes gamma radiation of 2 million to 4 million electron volts.[24] Rotational techniques have been introduced that allow the highly energized photons to pass safely through overlying skin. External beam radiotherapy supplies the most uniform distribution of radiation to the prostate but also has the highest level of scatter injury to the bladder, distal ureters, rectum, and the pelvic nerves responsible for erectile function.

RADIATION–INDUCED CELL DEATH

The mechanism of cell death due to radiation is not fully understood but is believed to be related to interruption of DNA replication. Radiation creates super oxide-free radicals in the nucleus that induce nicks in the double-stranded DNA. The DNA polymerases needed for cell replication are unable to "read" nicked DNA, and the cells are unable to replicate. The cells die during replication or mitosis, hence the term "mitotic death." In general, enzymes needed for daily maintenance of the cell are not de-

stroyed by radiation at these doses,[2, 3] and, until the cells replicate, their histologic appearance should be maintained. The doubling time for prostate cancer has been estimated to be about 60 to 120 days, and one would expect slow histologic resolution of malignant cells.[45] Several studies have documented that, following definitive radiation, serial prostatic biopsies may reveal a gradual resolution of malignant-appearing cells (Fig. 27–1).[10, 39, 46] Tumor regression typically is complete around 12 to 24 months after radiotherapy. Therefore, it appears that biopsies performed less than one year from the time of radiation treatment may be premature and should be performed after 12 months for Stage B tumors and 18 months for Stage C lesions. A positive result on a biopsy performed 18 to 24 months post-treatment is rarely followed by a later negative result.

SIGNIFICANCE OF POSTIRRADIATION PROSTATE BIOPSIES

Controversy exists over the prognostic significance of a biopsy of the prostate follow-

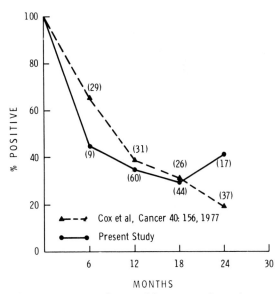

Figure 27–1. Correlation of biopsy results with time after radiotherapy. The incidence of biopsies positive for disease at Baylor College of Medicine (circles, solid line) is compared with the results of Cox and Stoffel (triangles, dashed line; see ref. 11) during the first 24 months. From Scardino PT, Wheeler TM: Prostatic biopsy after irradiation therapy for prostatic cancer. Urology 25(Suppl):39, 1985.

ing definitive radiotherapy. Many radiation oncologists and urologists feel that there is no significance to a postirradiation needle biopsy of the prostate that reveals the presence of cancer. Others maintain that a positive result on a biopsy reflects treatment failure and a poorer prognosis, manifested by disease progression. Reviewing published studies on the prognostic significance of a positive postirradiation prostatic biopsy result can be confusing. Most studies are handicapped because of incomplete or inaccurate preradiotherapy staging, uncontrolled application of adjunctive hormonal therapy, or incomplete follow-up.

Incomplete or inaccurate preradiotherapy staging is probably the most important factor biasing five-year survival results. Studies on clinical staging have shown that 20-60% of tumors in clinical Stage B and C are actually in stage D_1 when subjected to staging lymphadenectomy.[13, 32-35, 44] Many reports on the significance of postirradiation biopsies rely on clinical staging and therefore have a substantial group of patients in Stages B or C who are actually in Stage D_1. The laboratories of Bagshaw[5] Grossman,[22] Paulson,[36] and others have shown that radical radiotherapy in patients with positive evidence of disease in pelvic nodes is largely ineffective. Thus some patients with negative results on biopsy will develop metastatic disease because the radiotherapy did not control the nodal disease.[18, 40] The report by Freiha and Bagshaw[18] quantitates the effect of this bias. They revealed that 25 of ,64 patients undergoing biopsy had negative results; six of the 25 (33%) had Stage D_1 disease. Patients with affected nodes adversely biased the disease-free survival status of the group with negative results from 90% to 76% because of understaged patients with Stage D_1 disease (Table 27-1).

Many studies are biased because they lack uniformity in their use of hormonal therapy. Some studies report that irradiated patients with high-grade lesions are often concurrently treated with hormone manipulation.[10, 11, 27, 28, 37] When these patients are evaluated it is not possible to discern whether the radiotherapy or the hormonal manipulation was responsible for control of disease. Thus the survival of the group of patients who had positive results on biopsy but who were treated with both modalities would be favorably biased by the uncontrolled use of hormonal therapy.

Table 27–1. ANALYSIS OF THE INFLUENCE OF NODAL DISEASE ON DISEASE-FREE SURVIVAL FOR PATIENTS WITH NEGATIVE RESULTS OF POSTIRRADIATION PROSTATE BIOPSIES*

Negative Biopsy Group	Alive,† No Evidence of Disease
All patients	19/25 (76%)
Nodes negative only	17/19 (90%)
Nodes positive only	2/6 (33%)

*From Freiha FS, Bagshaw MD: Carcinoma of the prostate: results of postirradiation biopsy. Prostate 5:19–25, 1984.
†Mean follow-up after biopsy equals 4.5 years.

Some studies report survival statistics without reference to disease status. The study by Kiesling[27] illustrates some of the flaws caused from attaching significance to survival status only. In their group of 39 patients with positive results on biopsy, 28% had disease progression at an average of 25 months, whereas the group of 29 patients with negative results had only 14% progression at a mean time of 40 months. However, when these patients were evaluated for five-year survival, regardless of disease status, their survival rates were the same.

In order to draw meaningful conclusions from studies on the prognostic significance of postirradiation prostatic biopsies, we maintain that studies should adhere to the criteria in Table 27-2. Results from our search showed the only study to fulfill these requirements for patients treated with external beam radical radiotherapy is by Freiha and Bagshaw.[18] In their study, 146 patients had undergone staging lymphadenectomy and definitive external beam radiotherapy; 64 underwent biopsy at least 18 months following therapy. Patients were randomly selected for biopsy, and in no case had hormonal therapy been administered prior

Table 27–2. FACTORS INFLUENCING THE RESULTS OF STUDIES ON THE PROGNOSTIC SIGNIFICANCE OF POSTIRRADIATION PROSTATE BIOPSIES

1. Patients should be accurately staged with pelvic lymphadenectomy identifying patients with Stage D_1 disease
2. Hormonal therapy should be withheld until there is documentation of disease progression
3. Uniform application of postirradiation biopsy approximately 12 to 18 months after treatment
4. Accurate follow-up to assess for disease progression and disease-free survival

to biopsy. Overall, 11 of 39 (28%) patients with positive results of biopsy were alive without disease, with a mean follow-up of 4.5 years after biopsy (range of 2 to 9 years). This was compared with 19 of 25 (76%) patients with negative biopsy results who were alive with no evidence of disease, with a mean follow-up of 4.5 years after biopsy (range of 3 to 9 years). If patients with evidence of Stage D_1 disease are excluded, 38 patients remain, and 19 (50%) had positive biopsy results. Ten of the 19 (53%) patients with positive results were alive without evidence of disease, whereas 17 of 19 (89%) with negative results were alive with no evidence of disease. Also, seven of the 10 patients with positive results and no evidence of disease had hormonal manipulation after the results of the biopsy were known.

The evaluation of patients treated with radioactive gold and external beam radiotherapy in a manner meeting the criteria in Table 27–2 was reported by Scardino.[39] In that study, all patients had preradiotherapy staging lymphadenectomy, and hormonal manipulation was withheld until there was evidence of disease progression. Disease progression was defined as progressive local growth of the tumor, causing either hydronephrosis or symptomatic bladder outlet obstruction or metastatic disease. Scardino found that the five-year disease-free survival was approximately 82% in 69 patients with negative biopsy results (all biopsies were taken 6 to 30 months after treatment) and approximately 30% in 52 patients with positive results. Further, in a subgroup of patients without nodal metastases, he demonstrated that the risk of local recurrence was significantly greater for 22 patients with positive biopsy results (75%), as compared with 50 patients with negative results (22%).

Schellhammer performed biopsies at least 18 months after regional lymphadenectomy and ^{125}I implantation in 57 patients who were followed for more than three years and found that 15 (26%) had positive biopsy results and 42 (74%) had negative results.[23, 41] Hormonal manipulation commenced only after there was evidence of treatment failure manifested by local prostatic growth, two reports of elevation of serum acid phosphatase, or evidence of distant metastasis. Treatment failure occurred in nine of 15 patients (60%) with positive biopsy results and nine of 42 patients (21%) with negative results.

We were unable to find any reports adhering to these criteria that give no prognostic significance to postirradiation biopsies. Large series supporting the concept that postirradiation biopsies have no prognostic significance have been reported by the laboratories of Cox,[10] Kagan,[26] Leach,[28] and Perez.[37] Patients in these studies were not surgically staged, and hormonal manipulation was not rigorously controlled. In addition, the survival status in one series[33] was reported without reference to disease status. Currently, a positive result on postirradiation biopsy 12 to 24 months following definitive radiotherapy for prostatic cancer is indicative of treatment failure.

EVALUATION OF POSTIRRADIATION BIOPSY

Histologic findings of prostatic biopsy following irradiation have been well characterized.[6, 40] Cellular changes typical of malignancy are unreliable in irradiated prostates because radiation injury to normal cells can produce similar findings. Therefore, criteria for malignancy are essentially the same after radiation as they were before. Atypical architecture of glandular structures in relation to surrounding prostatic stroma, as described by Gleason,[20] is the finding that confirms the presence of malignancy.

There is supporting evidence that an appropriate interval allowing maximal regression of tumor is necessary for evaluation of control of local disease following the completion of radiotherapy.[10, 39, 52] The risk of having a positive result on biopsy and the appropriate interval following definitive radiotherapy is listed for the different forms of radiotherapy in Table 27–3. There is some evidence that the interval should be shortened to 12 months for smaller lesions, and for larger Stage C lesions, the interval should be at least 18 to 24 months.[37] In addition, the risk of a positive result on postirradiation biopsy is substantial in patients with normal results on prostate examination. Freiha and Bagshaw[18] reported that, of 28 patients with normal findings on examination, seven (25%) had positive biopsy results; Scardino and associates[39] similarly reported that 12 of 55 patients (22%) with normal results of examination who were treated with [198]Au and external beam radiotherapy were found to have a positive biopsy result.

Table 27–3. SUGGESTED INTERVAL TO ALLOW MAXIMAL TUMOR REGRESSION AFTER COMPLETION OF RADIOTHERAPY AND THE EXPECTED RATE OF POSITIVE BIOPSY RESULTS FOR DIFFERENT FORMS OF RADIOTHERAPY

Form of Radiotherapy	Interval to Biopsy, Post-treatment (months)	Rate of Positive Biopsy Results (% patients)
External beam	12–24	50–60
[198]Au and external beam	12–24	30
[125]I	24–36	40

Patients treated for cure with radical radiotherapy who have a positive biopsy result should be evaluated for metastatic disease. If the studies are normal and it is believed that the patient is an appropriate surgical candidate, he should undergo cystoscopy and bimanual examination under anesthesia for evaluation of tumor extension to the bladder neck or external sphincter and for assessment of the mobility of the prostate and bladder.

SALVAGE RADICAL PROSTATECTOMY

Theoretically, patients with tumor confined to the prostate can be cured while the bladder is preserved with salvage prostatectomy. Important exceptions to this group are patients with severe voiding symptoms or incontinence, who are better managed with total cystoprostatectomy.

Historically, heavily irradiated patients are at increased risk for hemorrhage, pulmonary embolism, fistula formation, and edema in the lower extremities. Following high-dose radiation, the plane between Denonvilliers' fascia and the anterior surface of the rectum is often fused. This may make it technically difficult to resect the prostate completely without injuring the rectum. In addition, the external sphincter may not be competent, even if the surgeon is able to complete the urethrovesical anastomosis. The consequences of almost certain disease progression must be weighed carefully against the risks of surgical excision.

Data regarding the morbidity or survival of patients undergoing salvage prostatectomy following failure of definitive radiotherapy are few. Small series have indicated that the procedure can be performed with "acceptable" operative and postoperative complications. The largest series, by Mador

and associates, reported successful removal of the prostate in four of five patients.[30] The remaining patient required cystoprostatectomy because of severe fibrosis at the time of surgery. Of the four, one died immediately postoperatively from fluid overload and pulmonary edema. The remaining three recovered without complication. Two had transient urinary incontinence that resolved at two and 12 months postoperatively, respectively. Carson and co-workers reported on 18 patients undergoing radical prostatectomy and pelvic lymph node resection following radiotherapy.[8] Only nine patients received definitive radiotherapy, and seven had a planned radical prostatectomy four to six weeks later; two patients underwent salvage prostatectomy at, respectively, 16 months and six years following radiation because of local progression. The planned prostatectomies did not have the attendant fibrosis that one would expect with delayed procedures, and the authors did not comment on the individual outcomes of these patients. In 1974, Gill and associates reported two successful radical prostatectomies at seven and 11 months following administration of 7500 rads.[19] The protocol entailed definitive radiotherapy for Stage C adenocarcinoma of the prostate followed by a prostatic biopsy at least six months later. Three patients with Stage C tumors and positive results of biopsy whose status was lowered to Stage B were explored. Two were found to have no evidence of nodal disease, and a radical prostatectomy was performed. Both had transient urine leaks that resolved within two months. Both patients were continent and alive with no evidence of disease 13 and 16 months following prostatectomy, respectively.

In order to determine the feasibility of resecting the prostate while sparing the bladder, we started performing salvage prostatectomies on patients with small glands that

Table 27–4. DATA FOR PATIENTS UNDERGOING SALVAGE PROSTATECTOMY

Patient	Preradiotherapy Stage	Preoperative Stage	Type of Radiation	Evidence of Disease in Margins
1	A_2	C	External beam*	−
2	A_2	B_1†	External beam*	−
3	B_1	B_1	External beam*	−
4	B_1	B_1	^{125}I	+
5	B_1	B_1	^{125}I	−
6	C	C	^{191}Ir	−

*7000 rads.
†Increased level of acid phosphatase.

had histologic evidence of persistent disease (Table 27–4). The average age was 64.7 years (range, 55 to 69 years), and the average interval from completion of therapy to biopsy was 48 months (range, 14 to 96 months). Four of the six patients were clinically assessed as being in Stage B, two were in Stage B_2/C. The prostates were successfully separated from the anterior rectal wall in all six patients. There were no postoperative complications, and the average hospital stay was 8.3 days (range, 6 to 12 days). Pathologic examination revealed one patient with a positive margin at the bladder neck (Table 27–5); to date there have been two local recurrences, both occurring in patients with seminal vesicle involvement. Patients with lesions confined to the prostate have received no adjunctive therapy. Patients with seminal vesicle invasion were treated prophylactically with hormonal and outpatient chemotherapy.

Follow-up is short, but three of six patients are alive, without evidence of disease, for an average of 17 months following surgery (range, 1 to 37 months). Three of the six patients were incontinent and needed placement of an artificial urinary sphincter. Because of the increased risk of tumor recurrence in the bladder with seminal vesicle involvement and the rate of incontinence, we believe that salvage prostatectomy is

rarely indicated and that these individuals are better off undergoing cystoprostatectomy.

RADICAL CYSTECTOMY OR PELVIC EXENTERATION

Cystoprostatectomy has been used in patients with marginal bladder capacity or debilitating voiding symptoms, or because of tumor extension to the bladder neck, seminal vesicles, or external sphincter. Radiation fibrosis frequently obliterates fascial planes, and if the bladder and prostate feel fixed on rectal examination, cystoprostatectomy should be performed. In addition, all patients undergoing salvage prostatectomy should be prepared for possible cystoprostatectomy.

Radiation fibrosis is frequently accompanied by radiation vasculitis, which can be responsible for poor wound healing. Vasculitis and ureteritis of the distal ureter is probably the factor most responsible for breakdown of the ureterointestinal anastomosis, which has been reported to carry a 50% mortality rate.[1] Historically, these patients are also at increased risk for pulmonary embolism, rectotomy, fistulae, pelvic and wound abscesses, and small bowel obstruction. However, the technical feasibility

Table 27–5. RESULTS OF PATHOLOGIC EXAMINATION OF PATIENTS UNDERGOING SALVAGE PROSTATECTOMY

Patient	Bladder Neck	Tumor Involvement Seminal Vesicle	Nodes	Apex	Margins
1	−	+/+		−	−
2	−	+/+		−	−
3	−	−/−		−	−
4	+	+/+		−	+
5	−	−/−		−	−
6	−	−/−	0/16	−	−

Table 27–6. DATA FOR PATIENTS UNDERGOING CYSTOPROSTATECTOMY

Patient	Preradiotherapy Stage	Preoperative Stage	Type of Radiation	Evidence of Disease in Margins
1	A_2	B_2/C*	[125]I	−
2	A_2	B_2/C	External beam†	−
3	B_1	B_2/C	[125]I	+
4	B_1	B_2/C	External beam‡	−
5	B_1	C	External beam†	−
6	B	B_2/C*	External beam†	−
7	B	B_2/C	External beam†	−
8	B_2	C*	External beam†	+
9	B_2	C	[198]Au	+
10	C	B_2/C	[125]I	−
11	C	C	External beam‡	−

*Increased level of phosphatase.
†7000 rads.
‡6500 rads.

of this surgery has been established in patients undergoing salvage cystectomy after definitive radiotherapy for bladder cancer. In experienced hands, salvage cystectomy can be performed with low operative morbidity (15 to 30%) and mortality (0 to 5%).[12, 15, 42, 45]

As with salvage prostatectomy, salvage cystoprostatectomy or pelvic exenteration are not often referred to as options for the management of prostatic carcinoma. Articles by Whitmore,[47, 49] McCullough and Leadbetter,[31] and others have discussed surgical procedures for extensive localized disease either as primary or palliative treatment. In 1978, Spaulding and Whitmore[43] analyzed their results of radical surgery in the management of extensive localized prostatic cancer. Before 1960, patients were treated primarily with radical excision and had a five-year disease-free survival rate of 17%. After 1960, the patients were generally treated secondarily with radical excision following failure of hormonal manipulation or radio-

therapy to control the local tumor. The five-year disease-free survival increased to 31%, but a survival rate was not specifically mentioned for the radiotherapy group.

In 1985, Mador and associates specifically referred to the use of cystoprostatectomy as a salvage option for cure after failure of definitive radiotherapy.[30] Of the three patients reported, 7000 rads of external beam radiotherapy had failed to eradicate disease in two, and ^{125}I treatment had failed to stop disease in one. All three had had at least one prior transurethral prostatectomy; at surgery two had primary closure of rectotomies healed without incident. One patient had incomplete resection of the prostate gland in order to avoid rectotomy. This patient had a long and protracted course but eventually did well. The follow-up on these patients was too short to allow comment on survival.

Since August of 1977, we have performed 11 salvage procedures after failure of definitive radiotherapy (Table 27–6). The average

Table 27–7. RESULTS OF PATHOLOGIC EXAMINATION OF PATIENTS UNDERGOING CYSTOPROSTATECTOMY

Patient	Tumor Involvement				
	Bladder	Seminal Vesicle	Nodes	Apex	Margins
1	−	−/−		−	−
2	−	−/−		−	−
3	+	+/+		+	+
4	−	+/+		−	−
5	+	+/+	1/17	−	−
6	+	+/+		−	−
7	+	+/+		−	−
8	+	+/+	7/15	+	+
9	+	+/+		+	+
10	−	−/−		−	−
11	+	+/+		−	−

age was 60.6 years (range, 54 to 69); five patients were referred because of severe voiding difficulties or incontinence, and six because of a positive result on prostatic biopsy. The average interval between radiation and surgery was 40.8 months (range, 22 to 84 months). Nine patients had salvage cystoprostatectomy; one, cystoprostatectomy and low anterior colon resection; and one, total pelvic exenteration. The colon resection was necessary because of tumor extension to the rectum, and the patient undergoing total exenteration had previously undergone permanent colostomy secondary to radiation proctitis. Urinary diversion consisted of five Bricker ileostomies and six continent Kock urinary reservoirs. Ten of the patients had concurrent bilateral orchiectomy. There were no operative complications or deaths, and the average hospital stay was 12.6 days (range, 11 to 15 days). All patients were assessed preoperatively as hving either bulky B_2 or C lesions. Three of the 11 had positive margins at the apex (Table 27–7). There have been no local recurrences, but two have developed distant metastases. To date, eight of 11 (73%) are alive with no evidence of disease (one died of disease, and two are alive with disease) with an average follow-up of 28.6 months (range, 12 to 97 months).

RADIATION AND CHEMOTHERAPY OPTIONS

An option for persistent carcinoma after full-dose external beam radiotherapy is ^{125}I implantation, which was reported by Goffinet and associates in 1980.[21] They reported on 14 patients who had been followed for six to 36 months. Eleven of the 14 had local control, but only eight (57%) were free of disease. They noted six patients with major complications (cystoproctitis, incontinence, or fistula), which were associated with high-intensity seeds (greater than 0.50 mCi). They concluded that prostatic volumes should be less than $5 \times 4 \times 3$ cm to avoid complications. They further recommended that patients chosen for this treatment have no tumor encroachment into the bladder, rectum, or external sphincter. External beam radiotherapy following ^{125}I treatment is generally considered to be contraindicated because of untoward side effects.[14, 38]

Table 27–8. PATHOLOGIC STAGE FOR PATIENTS WHOSE INTERVAL BETWEEN RADIOTHERAPY AND SURGERY IS LESS THAN 30 MONTHS (LESS THAN 36 MONTHS FOR ^{125}I)

Pathologic Stage	Number of Patients (%)
B (confined)	5 (62.5%)
C (bladder neck/seminal vesicle)	1 (12.5%)
D (bladder/nodes)	2 (25%)
Involvement of margin	0

Chemotherapy as a salvage option has been proposed by Scardino.[31] He reported conversion of prostatic biopsy results from positive to negative in 12 of 26 patients treated with intra-arterial cisplatinum to the prostate.

DISCUSSION

Evidence has accumulated that surgical excision is technically feasible. Pathologic review of our patients revealed that four of 17 had evidence of disease in the margins and four had extension to the bladder or nodal disease. However, when the interval between radiotherapy and the salvage procedure is less than 30 months (less than 36 months for ^{125}I) our results indicate that the surgical margins should be improved (Tables 27–8 and 27–9). Longer follow-up is needed to confirm the significance of thse pathologic findings. Nonetheless, it is suggestive that early biopsy and intervention are influential factors that may ultimately define the role of surgical excision in the management of patients with persistent localized disease following definitive radiotherapy.

Definitive radiotherapy has proven efficacy in the management of adenocarcinoma of the prostate. As reported by Freiha and Bagshaw[18] and Scardino,[39] 75 to 85% of pa-

Table 27–9. PATHOLOGIC STAGE FOR PATIENTS WHOSE INTERVAL BETWEEN RADIOTHERAPY AND SURGERY WAS PROLONGED (MEAN = 60 MONTHS)

Pathologic Stage	Number of Patients (%)
B (confined)	1 (11%)
C (bladder neck/seminal vesicle)	2 (22%)
D (bladder/nodes)	2 (22%)
Involvement of margin	4 (44%)

tients with a negative biopsy result (compared with 25 to 30% with a positive result) will survive more than seven years free of disease after radiotherapy. Conversely, 10 to 15% with a negative biopsy result (compared with 45 to 50% of patients with a positive result) currently managed will be dead of disease within seven years of radiotherapy.[18] We maintain that patients with radioresistant local disease warrant continued investigation of carefully planned surgical excision of all residual tumor.

References

1. Alfert HJ, Gillenwater JY: The consequences of ureteral irradiation with special reference to subsequent ureteral injury. J Urol 107:369–371, 1972.
2. Arena V: Ionizing Radiation and Life. St. Louis, CV Mosby, 1971, pp 320–321.
3. Bacq ZM, Alexander P: Fundamentals of Radiology, 2nd ed. Oxford, Pergamon Press, 1961, p 191.
4. Bagshaw MA, Kaplan HS, Sagerman RH: Linear accelerator supervoltage radiotherapy. VII. Carcinoma of the prostate. Radiology 85:121–129, 1965.
5. Bagshaw MA, Ray GR: External beam radiation therapy of prostate carcinoma. In DG Skinner (ed), Urological Cancer. New York, Grune & Stratton, 1982, p 59.
6. Bostwick DG, Egbert BM, Fajardo LF: Radiation injury of the normal and neoplastic prostate. Am J Surg Pathol 6:541–551, 1982.
7. Carlton CE Jr, Dawoud F, Hudgins P, et al: Irradiation treatment of carcinoma of the prostate: a preliminary report based on 8 years of experience. J Urol 108:924–927, 1972.
8. Carson CC 3rd, Zincke H, Utz DC, et al: Radical prostatectomy after radiotherapy for prostatic cancer. J Urol 124:237–239, 1980.
9. Cosgrove MD, Kaempf MJ: Prostatic cancer revisited. J Urol 115:79–81, 1976.
10. Cox JD, Kline RW: The lack of prognostic significance of biopsies after radiotherapy for prostatic cancer. Semin Urol 1:237–242, 1983.
11. Cox JD, Stoffel TJ: The significance of needle biopsy after irradiation for Stage C adenocarcinoma of the prostate. Cancer 40:156–160, 1977.
12. Crawford ED, Skinner DG: Salvage cystectomy after irradiation failure. J Urol 123:32–34, 1980.
13. Dahl DS, Wilson CS, Middleton RG, Bourne GG: Pelvic lymphadenectomy for staging localized prostatic cancer. J Urol 112:245–246, 1974.
14. deVere White R, Babaian RK, Feldman M, et al: Adjunctive therapy with interstitial irradiation for prostate cancer. Urology 19:395–398, 1982.
15. Droller MJ, Walsh PC: Therapeutic efficacy of salvage cystectomy. Do results reflect natural history of bladder cancer? Urology 22:118–122, 1983.
16. Flocks RH, Kerr HD, Elkins HB, Culp D: Treatment of carcinoma of prostate by interstitial radiation with radio-active gold (Au 198): a preliminary report. J Urol 68:510–522, 1952.
17. Flocks RH, Kerr HD, Elkins HB, et al: The treatment of carcinoma of the prostate by interstitial radiation with radio-active gold: follow-up report. J Urol 71:628–633, 1959.
18. Freiha FS, Bagshaw MD: Carcinoma of the prostate: results of post-irradiation biopsy. Prostate 5:19–25, 1984.
19. Gill WB, Marks JE, Straus FH, et al: Radical retropubic prostatectomy and retroperitoneal lymphadenectomy following radiotherapy conversion of stage C to stage B carcinoma of the prostate. J Urol 111:656–661, 1974.
20. Gleason DF, Mellinger GT: The Veterans Administration Cooperative Urological Research Group: Prediction of prognosis for prostatic adenocarcinoma by combined histological grading and clinical staging. J Urol 111:58–64, 1974.
21. Goffinet DR, Martinez A, Freiha F, et al: [125]Iodine prostate implants for recurrent carcinoma after external beam irradiation: preliminary results. Cancer 45:2717–2724, 1980.
22. Grossman HB, Batata M, Hilaris B, Whitmore WF Jr: [125]I implantation for carcinoma of prostate: further follow-up of first 100 cases. Urology 20:591–598, 1982.
23. Herr HW, Whitmore WF Jr: Significance of prostatic biopsies after radiation therapy for carcinoma of the prostate. Prostate 3:339–350, 1982.
24. Hilaris BS (ed): Handbook of Interstitial Brachytherapy. Acton, MA, Publishing Sciences Group, 1978.
25. Huggins C, Hodges CV: Studies on prostatic cancer: effect of castration, of estrogen and of androgen injection on serum phosphatases in metastatic carcinoma of prostate. Cancer Res 1:293–297, 1941.
26. Kagan AR, Gordon J, Cooper JF, et al: A clinical appraisal of post-irradiation biopsy in prostatic cancer. Cancer 39:637–641, 1977.
27. Kiesling VJ, McAninch JW, Goebel JL, Agee RE: External beam radiotherapy for adenocarcinoma of the prostate: a clinical followup. J Urol 124:851–854, 1980.
28. Leach GE, Cooper JF, Kagan AR, et al: Radiotherapy for prostatic carcinoma: post-irradiation prostatic biopsy and recurrence patterns with long-term follow-up. J Urol 128:505–509, 1982.
29. Lytton B, Collins JT, Weiss RM, et al: Results of biopsy after early stage prostatic cancer treatment by implantation of ^{125}I seeds. J Urol 121:306–309, 1979.
30. Mador DR, Huben RP, Wajsman Z, Pontes JE: Salvage surgery following radical radiotherapy for adenocarcinoma of the prostate. J Urol 133:58–60, 1985.
31. McCullough DL, Leadbetter WF: Radical pelvic surgery for locally extensive carcinoma of the prostate. J Urol 108:939–943, 1972.
32. McCullough DL, Prout GR, Daly JJ: Carcinoma of the prostate and lymphatic metastases. J Urol 111:65–71, 1974.
33. McLaughlin AP, Saltzstein SL, McCullough DL, Gittes RF: Prostatic carcinoma: incidence and location of unsuspected lymphatic metastases. J Urol 115:89–94, 1976.
34. Paulson DF, Uro-Oncology Research Group: The impact of current staging procedures in assessing disease extent of prostatic adenocarcinoma. J Urol 121:300–302, 1979.
35. Paulson DF: Surgical management of prostate carcinoma. In DG Skinner (ed), Urological Cancer. New York, Grune & Stratton, 1982, pp 22–27.
36. Paulson DF, Cline WA Jr, Koefoot RB Jr, et al, and The Uro-Oncology Research Group: Extended field

radiation therapy versus delayed hormonal therapy in node positive prostatic adenocarcinoma. J Urol 127:935–937, 1982.

37. Perez CA, Walz BJ, Zivnuska FR, et al: Irradiation of carcinoma of the prostate localized to the pelvis: analysis of tumor response and prognosis. Int J Radiat Oncol Biol Phys 6:555–563, 1980.

38. Ross G Jr, Borkon WD, Landry LJ, et al: Preliminary observations on the results of combined [125]iodine seed implantation and external irradiation for carcinoma of the prostate. J Urol 127:699–701, 1982.

39. Scardino PT: The prognostic significance of biopsies after radiotherapy for prostatic cancer. Semin Urol 1:243–245, 1983.

40. Schellhammer PF, Ladaga LE, El-Mahdi AE: Histological characteristics of prostatic biopsies after [125]iodine implantation. J Urol 123:700–705, 1980.

41. Schellhammer PF, El-Mahdi AE, Ladaga LE, Schultheiss T: [125]Iodine implantation for carcinoma of the prostate: 5-year survival free of disease and incidence of local failure. J Urol 134:1140–1145, 1985.

42. Smith JA, Whitmore WF Jr: Salvage cystectomy for bladder cancer after failure of definitive irradiation. J Urol 125:643–645, 1981.

43. Spaulding JT, Whitmore WF Jr: Extended total excision of prostatic adenocarcinoma. J Urol 120:188–190, 1978.

44. Spellman MC, Castellino RA, Ray GR, et al: An evaluation of lymphography in localized carcinoma of the prostate. Radiology 125:637–644, 1977.

45. Stamey, TA: Prostate cancer. Monographs in Urology 4(3):67–70, 1983.

46. Swanson DA, von Eschenbach AC, Bracken RB, Johnson DE: Salvage cystectomy for bladder carcinoma. Cancer 47:2275–2279, 1981.

47. van der Werf-Messing B: Prostatic cancer treated at the Rotterdam Radiotherapy Institute. Strahlentherapie 154:537–541, 1978.

48. Whitmore WF Jr: The rationale and results of ablative surgery for prostatic cancer. Cancer 16:1119–1132, 1963.

49. Whitmore WF Jr: Experience with [125]iodine implantation in the treatment of prostate cancer. In DG Skinner (ed), Urological Cancer. New York, Grune & Stratton, 1982, p 37.

50. Whitmore WF Jr, Mackenzie AR: Experiences with various operative procedures for the total excision of prostatic cancer. Cancer 12:396–405, 1959.

51. Whitmore WF Jr, Hilaris B, Grabstald H: Retropubic implantation of iodine 125 in the treatment of prostatic cancer. J Urol 108:918–920, 1972.

DAVID F. PAULSON, M.D.

Role of Endocrine Therapy in the Management of Prostatic Cancer

CHAPTER 28

The observation that adult prostatic epithelium atrophies when the sustaining physiologic effect of androgenic hormones is removed led to the therapeutic application of androgen ablation or suppression in the management of prostatic adenocarcinoma.[4, 5, 20, 21] The biologic effect of androgens on prostatic epithelium seems dependent on the ability of testosterone to be converted to dihydrotestosterone, the principal intracellular androgen.[1, 8, 9, 25, 49] Circulating testosterone enters the prostatic cell, where it is converted by the enzyme 5-α-reductase to dihydrotestosterone, which is then bound to a specific intracellular macromolecular receptor protein. The resulting dihydrotestosterone-receptor complex, after penetrating the cytoplasm, undergoes a conformational change that permits the intranuclear translocation of this complex. Once within the nucleus, chromatin binding occurs with initiation of transcription and subsequent messenger RNA formation. In the intact animal, androgen withdrawal disrupts this orderly progression and results in marked atrophy of the prostatic epithelium.

Testosterone production in the adult male is dependent on an intact hypothalamic-pituitary-testicular axis.[48] Decreased levels of circulating testosterone initiate the hypothalamic release of luteinizing hormone–releasing factor (LHRH). This in turn initi-

ates the pituitary release of luteinizing hormone, which subsequently prompts testosterone synthesis by the Leydig cells of the testis. The resultant enhanced levels of circulating testosterone produce feedback inhibition of LHRH at the hypothalamic level. In response to Leydig cell stimulation, the testis produces 95% of the circulating androgens.[45] The remaining androgens, androstenedione and dehydroepiandrosterone, are of adrenal origin. Ninety-five per cent of the circulating androgens are either specifically bound to steroid-binding globulin or nonspecifically bound to albumin. The unbound androgens are believed responsible for the cellular response.[32, 36]

The hormonal treatment of prostatic adenocarcinoma is based on the assumption that malignant prostatic epithelium is androgen-dependent, as is nonmalignant prostatic tissue. The reduction of androgenic support of prostatic epithelium can be accomplished therapeutically by (1) the removal of the primary source of circulating androgens; (2) the removal or suppression of hypothalamic luteinizing hormone–releasing factor, thereby reducing the release of pituitary luteinizing hormone as well as the production of testicular testosterone; (3) the direct inhibition of androgen synthesis at the cellular level; and (4) the blocking of androgens or their effect at the cellular level.

464

REMOVAL OF THE PRIMARY ANDROGEN SOURCE

Serum testosterone levels in the normal male range between 400 and 1000 ng/dl. Bilateral orchiectomy will reduce plasma testosterone levels by 90%.[24, 32, 36, 52] In the adult human male, there is no detectable increase in plasma testosterone levels from the activation of secondary androgen sources following orchiectomy. The appearance of endocrine-unresponsive symptomatic disease after bilateral orchiectomy is not associated with demonstrated increases in the level of circulating plasma androstenedione, dehydroepiandrosterone, or testosterone, indicating that symptomatic recurrence is not associated with an increase in circulating androgens or their metabolic end products.[23, 24, 45]

These studies indicate that an estrogen rescue of patients who progress after orchiectomy or low-dose estrogen therapy is unlikely. The published reports of experience with high-dose estrogen therapy trials support these observations.

HYPOTHALAMIC SUPPRESSION

Estrogens establish their major effect at the hypothalamic level by occupying the hypothalamic binding site of testosterone. They thus inhibit the release of luteinizing hormone–releasing factor, which produces subsequent suppression of luteinizing hormone release by the pituitary and a reduction in testosterone production by the testis (Figure 28–1). In the adult human male, no evidence exists to date that estrogens may directly induce regression of prostatic epithelium. Studies in the intact dog have indicated that estrogens (stilbestrol) may directly influence the secretory ability of the prostate.[18] In addition, in vitro studies have indicated that stilbestrol in high levels can directly inhibit DNA polymerase and 5-α-reductase.[37, 51] However, the level of estrogen required for in vitro enzyme inhibition is far greater than the pharmacologic levels that can be achieved in humans.[19, 37]

Plasma testosterone levels in males treated with 1 mg/day of stilbestrol or its equivalent show variation not only between subjects but also with respect to serial values obtained during longitudinal observations in a single subject. Serum testosterone levels may not reach anorchid levels. Three mg per day of stilbestrol suppresses testosterone levels to the castrate range, and doses exceeding 3 mg/day have no additional effect (Table 28–1).

Although most natural and synthetic estrogens exert their effect via a reduction in the hypothalamic release of LHRH, chlorotrianisene (Tace) apparently mediates its effect through a different mechanism. At dosages of 24 mg daily, Tace does not reduce plasma luteinizing or follicle-stimulating hormone, although it has been variously reported either to reduce serum testosterone levels by 40 to 60% or not to affect them at all.[2, 36] The clinical effectiveness of Tace in controlling symptomatic (apparent) malignant disease does not exceed that of diethylstilbestrol or the other synthetic estrogens, although there is no evidence of enhanced cardiovascular risk with this drug.[11]

Megestrol acetate, a synthetic progestin, has been used in the management of Stage D prostatic adenocarcinoma. Megestrol acetate causes regression of prostatic carcinoma by suppression of plasma testosterone production. However, patients who show an initial response to megestrol acetate and who then experience symptomatic recurrence may achieve pain relief with orchiectomy, indicating either that there is escape of testosterone suppression or that an alternative mechanism produces the initial disease response. The information accrued to date indicates that megestrol acetate is not the drug of choice for the initial treatment of prostatic carcinoma.

The recent demonstration that luteinizing hormone-releasing analogues may function at a central level to suppress testosterone synthesis has prompted examination of this alternative method to achieve disease con-

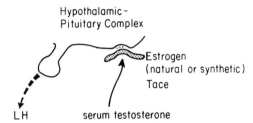

Figure 28–1. Certain exogenously administered agents block hypothalamic receptors, sequentially suppressing both luteinizing hormone–releasing factor and luteinizing hormone secretion. The activity of chlorotrianisene (Tace) at this site is debated.

Table 28–1. EFFECT OF BILATERAL ORCHIECTOMY OR TREATMENT WITH STILBESTROL ON PLASMA LEVELS OF TESTOSTERONE IN MEN WITH CARCINOMA OF THE PROSTATE*

		Mean Plasma Testosterone Levels (ng/dl ± standard deviation)					
			Bilateral	Stilbestrol (mg/day)†			
Authors	Reference	Pretreat-ment	Orchiec-tomy	0.2	1.0	3.0	5.0
Young HH 2d, Kent JR	53	560	<50				<50
Robinson MRG, Thomas BS	33	607 ± 235	30			<10a	
Mackler MA, et al	24	620 ± 260	50 ± 50		80c	46 ± 19b	190d
Kent JR, et al	23						
Stage C		620 ± 288		570 ± 335b	320 ± 220b		210 ± 246b
Stage D		640 ± 335		700 ± 276	410 ± 359		130 ± 110
Shearer RJ, et al	37	280	47 ± 23		66–86 ± 58	45 ± 20e	47 ± 25

*From Walsh PC: Physiologic basis for hormonal therapy in carcinoma of the prostate. Urol Clin North Am 2:132, 1975.

†Treatment Key: a = <6 months; b = >6 months; c = 7 days; d = 2 days; e = 6 to 24 months.

trol. Luteinizing hormone–releasing hormone (LHRH) is a hypothalamic decapeptide that induces release of luteinizing hormone (LH) and follicle-stimulating hormone (FSH) from the pituitary. Native LHRH has a short-lived effect on gonadotropin secretion and therefore is not suitable for long-term therapy. By substituting other amino acids within the decapeptide chain, LHRH analogues have been synthesized that produce a marked and prolonged effect. The mode of action of these agents is not fully understood. The current hypotheses include pituitary depletion of luteinizing hormone, pituitary desensitization to pituitary luteinizing hormone feedback, and direct extrapituitary action of the luteinizing hormone analogue on the testis. Following treatment with the LHRH analogues, there is an initial increase in serum testosterone production; however, after several days serum androgens will decrease to the castrate level. Serum prolactin will not change significantly and serum estradiol will decrease. The accumulated evidence would indicate that these agents are as effective as orchiectomy in managing previously untreated disease but that they will not permit rescue of patients who have failed alternative forms of androgen deprivation therapy. The relative cost of these agents in comparison with that for standard therapy remains to be determined. It should be recognized that treatment with these drugs requires daily administration by subcuticular injection or nasal inhalation. There is no objective evidence that combining the LHRH analogues with other therapies will induce an enhanced clinical response in previously untreated patients or permit rescue of patients who experience disease progression despite previous androgen deprivation.[6, 14, 22, 38, 43]

INHIBITORS OF ANDROGEN SYNTHESIS AT THE CELLULAR LEVEL

Selective inhibitors of androgen synthesis should produce pharmaceutical orchiectomy; however, although certain of these agents are available for clinical trial, none has yet been released with this specific indication. Aminoglutethimide blocks side-chain cleavage of cholesterol and subsequent hydroxylation, thus inhibiting the production of both cortisone and aldosterone (Fig. 28–2).[32] Cyproterone acetate blocks 17,20-desmolase and thus interferes with androgen synthesis.[17, 48] Both agents have been evaluated in the treatment of endocrine-unresponsive malignant prostatic disease, but neither

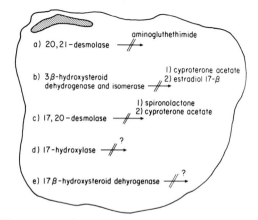

Figure 28–2. *Three of the five major enzymes involved in androgen synthesis may be selectively inhibited.*

has been found effective in reversing the clinical course of this patient population.[32, 36] Although Robinson and Thomas showed that aminoglutethimide suppressed plasma testosterone levels to below 10 ng/dl, Shearer and associates failed to demonstrate any significant suppression of plasma testosterone levels in 12 patients treated with aminoglutethimide.

Worgul and associates, in a study of 25 previously castrated men with progressive Stage D carcinoma who were treated with 1000 mg of aminoglutethimide and 40 mg hydrocortisone daily, demonstrated a complete response in one and a partial response in four patients.[50] Significant suppression of both serum testosterone and dihydrotestosterone were noted in these orchiectomized males after treatment with aminoglutethimide and hydrocortisone. The observations are of interest, but whether they imply that lowering of serum testosterone levels below castrate levels will induce a further clinical response is unproved. Nonetheless, these observations do prompt the necessity for further clinical study.

Walsh and Siiteri, using spironolactone, found that plasma testosterone levels were suppressed by 90%, and plasma androstenedione and dehydroepiandrosterone levels were suppressed by 40 to 60%.[33, 39, 48] Since it has not been demonstrated that the symptomatic reactivation of malignant prostatic disease is associated with residual androgen production either by the adrenal or by a residual testis, the theoretical lack of efficacy of these agents is confirmed in practice.

Ketoconazole is an orally administered synthetic imidazole dioxolane that has been used in the treatment of superficial and deep fungal infections. This drug has been demonstrated to reduce adrenal and testicular androgen production in both animals and humans. It is felt that ketoconazole exerts its effect by interference with cytochrome P-450–dependent 14-demethylation, thereby interfering with conversion of lanosterol to cholesterol. The predominant effect is the inhibition of the formation of androstenedione, dehydroepiandrosterone, and testosterone. When ketoconazole is administered at a dose level of 400 mg every 12 hours, serum testosterone initially will decrease to castrate levels, and previously untreated patients will demonstrate a clinical response evidenced by improvement in pain and a decrease in serum prostatic acid phosphatase levels. Preliminary data would indicate that, as an initial treatment, the drug is effective in the management of previously untreated patients, but again no advantage is achieved by combining this with alternative medication, nor will it establish rescue of previously treated patients.[29, 30, 44]

ANTIANDROGENS

Antiandrogens block the effectiveness of androgens at the target level by interfering with the intracellular events that mediate androgenic action. These agents are capable of inhibiting both endogenously secreted and exogenously administered androgens.[13, 27, 47] All effective compounds tested to date act through a common mechanism by inhibiting the formation of the receptor-dihydrotestosterone complex, interrupting the binding of a dihydrotestosterone-receptor complex to nuclear chromatin and thereby suppressing RNA formation and protein synthesis (Fig. 28–3). Cyproterone acetate is the most potent of the steroidal antiandrogens. It is well absorbed locally, and it not only produces target organ inhibition but also interferes with gonadotropin release and inhibits steroidogenesis.

The peripheral antiandrogenic action of cyproterone acetate on the adult untreated male is accompanied by a decrease in total plasma testosterone concentration and suppression of the plasma follicle-stimulating hormone concentration.[33] Cyproterone acetate has been used as the initial form of therapy in a small series of previously untreated males with malignant prostatic disease. Plasma testosterone and luteinizing hormone concentrations were determined at varying levels during therapy. The plasma testosterone concentration showed a sharp decline from control levels within the first week of therapy and was maintained at greatly reduced levels for at least 16 weeks. The plasma follicle-stimulating hormone levels were significantly suppressed during the second and fourth weeks of therapy, whereas the plasma luteinizing hormone concentration was essentially unchanged during cyproterone acetate treatment. The findings suggest that the peripheral antiandrogenic action of cyproterone acetate may be augmented by a reduction of plasma tes-

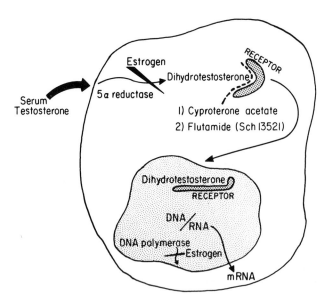

Figure 28–3. *The antiandrogens cyproterone acetate and flutamide block the formation of the dihydrotestosterone receptor complex. Estrogens in vitro will inhibit 5-α-reductase and DNA polymerase activity.*

tosterone concentration and suppression of pituitary gonadotropin secretion. No special benefit seems to be derived from the use of cyproterone acetate in the treatment of estrogen-unresponsive males.[15, 39]

Flutamide (Sch-13521) is a nonsteroidal antiandrogen that does not reduce either gonadotropin or plasma testosterone levels.[27, 40, 42] Flutamide appears no more effective than standard hormonal programs in the management of either previously untreated or estrogen-unresponsive disease.

The antiestrogen tamoxifen has been utilized in both previously untreated and in androgen-independent prostatic carcinoma. No significant response in either treatment group has been identified with tamoxifen, and it is currently felt that the accrued data do not support the continued investigation or use of tamoxifen in advanced prostatic malignancy.[16, 41]

The controversy with regard to the hormonal treatment of prostatic carcinoma has been engendered by both the clinical observation that hormonal manipulation may provide dramatic symptomatic relief and disease regression and the statistical observation that survival in the patient with prostatic cancer may not be enhanced by endocrine intervention.[4, 5, 7, 12, 28] The resulting uncertainty has focused on the form of endocrine intervention selected, the dose level of exogenous estrogen administered, and the timing of therapeutic intervention in the course of disease. The accepted clinical assumption is that survival must necessarily be prolonged as a consequence of any treatment that appears so effective in reducing the debilitating symptoms of disease progression. Historical controls published by Nesbit and Baum established an overall 6% five-year survival rate in patients with prostatic cancer who demonstrated metastases at the time of diagnosis.[28] A retrospective multi-institutional study of 1118 patients with prostatic cancer who were treated by orchiectomy, either alone or with diethylstilbestrol, demonstrated a 21% five-year survival rate. The major defect in the assessment was the failure to account for the probability of increased survival due to general medical care in patients with prostatic cancer.

The importance of recognizing this factor is evident in the report of Poole and Thompson, who showed that in the pre-endocrine era, among 349 patients with prostatic carcinoma treated between 1926 and 1936 with transurethral resection only, the survival rate was 13.8%. Among 562 patients similarly treated between 1937 and 1941, the survival rate was 21%.[31] This might indicate that improvements in general medical management, including improved techniques of transurethral resection to relieve urinary obstruction, infection, and azotemia, led to increased survival rates in this disease so that they equaled those established by endocrine therapy.

The first publication to question the role

of estrogens in promoting enhanced survival was that of Emmett and co-workers in 1960.[12] In this series, patients without metastases at presentation who were treated by orchiectomy alone experienced a 26% 10-year survival, whereas those treated with estrogens experienced a 10% 10-year survival. The 10-year survival of patients with metastases at presentation who were treated by estrogens was 8% and for those treated by orchiectomy, 3%. More importantly, the authors demonstrated that estrogen therapy in those males with Broder's Grade 1 disease produced a survival of 35%, as opposed to 50% in those who received no treatment. The data implied that estrogen therapy alone might not prolong survival in low-grade disease, although the authors did not address the specific question of cardiovascular risk in patients receiving exogenous estrogen therapy.

The wide variations in recommended estrogen dosage and disease staging in the majority of publications to date prevent a rational assessment of the relative benefits and hazards of estrogen control. The randomized study of the Veterans Administration Cooperative Urologic Research Group (VACURG) was established specifically to examine questions raised by previous publications.[5] The randomized application of four treatments (placebo; placebo plus orchiectomy; diethylstilbestrol, 5 mg/day; and orchiectomy plus diethylstilbestrol, 5 mg/day) was evaluated in 1903 patients with prostatic cancer in Stages C and D. In stage C disease, placebo and orchiectomy plus placebo were significantly more effective than orchiectomy plus estrogen with respect to overall survival. However, nine years after the initiation of treatment, a less than 10% difference could be detected between the worst and the best results. In Stage D disease, in which the competing risk from cancer was significant, no difference in overall survival in any of the four treatment groups could be detected at any one time. When disease in Stages C and D were combined and survival curves established (dependent upon death from prostatic cancer alone), diethylstilbestrol (5 mg/day) and orchiectomy plus estrogen were both more effective than orchiectomy plus placebo or placebo alone.

Subsequent studies by the same group indicated that 1 mg/day of diethylstilbestrol was as effective as 5 mg/day in controlling cancer deaths in either Stage C or Stage D disease, but that in Stage C disease in which there was less competing risk of death from malignancy, there were fewer cardiovascular deaths on the 1-mg dose than on the 5-mg dose. The results from these higher doses were both superior to those obtained with placebo or 0.2 mg of diethylstilbestrol daily in controlling death from malignant disease. Thus it would appear that there is a dose-dependent association between the negative effects of diethylstilbestrol on the cardiovascular system and the therapeutic effect in controlling malignant disease.

The minimal impact on overall survival produced by the various endocrine treatments indicates that the predictors that determine the relative cardiovascular and cancer risks within a specific patient have not yet been established. Although it is possible theoretically to select those patients with the least cardiovascular risk and thus identify those who would be optimal candidates for hormonal control of their malignant disease, a practical application of these selection processes has not yet been accomplished.

A single large retrospective analysis of patients randomly assigned to either placebo or estrogen indicates that it may be possible to develop predictors of relative risk.[10] Using a double-blind method, 441 patients with Stage C or Stage D cancer were randomly allocated into treatment with placebo; diethylstilbestrol, 0.2 mg/day; diethylstilbestrol, 1 mg/day; or diethylstilbestrol, 5 mg/day. For the purposes of analysis, the two lower doses (placebo and 0.2 mg of diethylstilbestrol) were treated as placebo and the two higher doses were treated as the hormonal arm.

The patient population was examined with respect to the presence or absence of bone metastases, their performance, the serum hemoglobin, any history of previous cardiovascular disease, the combined index of tumor stage and grade, electrocardiogram, weight, age at diagnosis, prostatic acid phosphatase level, serum 17-hydroxycorticoid concentration, and the size of the malignant lesion. The data were examined using these covariants, with the end point of analysis being death, in order to determine whether or not a subset of patients could be selected who would do best if they were untreated or who would do better if they received hormonal manipulation. Using this type of analysis, the patients could be divided into three sets: those who would benefit more from placebo, those who would benefit most from estrogen, and those in whom there was not sufficient evidence to establish one treatment preference over another.

The analysis did demonstrate that covariants of low hemoglobin, high combined index of stage and grade category, and size of the primary lesion selected those patients who would survive longer if the initial treatment was hormonal rather than placebo. The covariants of performance, low combined grade and stage index, history of cardiovascular disease, and excessive weight or age were selectors for those patients who would survive best if their initial treatment was placebo. The implication of this analysis is that those patients who are most likely to die of cardiovascular disease should not be treated initially with 1.0 or 5.0 mg/day of diethylstilbestrol, but the patients more likely to die of prostatic cancer might benefit from these treatments. Careful longitudinal studies have shown that plasma fibrinogen levels are decreased whereas plasminogen, cholesterol, and triglyceride levels are increased in response to diethylstilbestrol, so pretreatment levels or the levels achieved in response to treatment are not useful predictors in selecting patients with increased cardiovascular risks.[34, 35]

In addition to the problems that have accrued with regard to patient selection and the form of chosen treatment, there is currently much debate centered on the appropriate form of treatment evaluation. The biology of the disease in the individual under treatment may play as important a role in the apparent treatment response as the selected treatment itself. Much controversy currently exists as to the utilization of partial response or stable disease as an appropriate indicator of the response to treatment. Unless it can be determined that the disease is truly progressive at the time that androgen deprivation therapy is undertaken, the appearance of stable disease after the initiation of androgen deprivation may merely reflect the latent and indolent course of the disease and not the impact of treatment.

Therefore, to assess accurately the effect of any form of androgen deprivation, equivalent populations should be studied in a randomized fashion with criteria of disease progression defined prior to the initiation of therapy, and with the exclusion of stable disease as an indicator of treatment response. It may very well be, as demonstrated in the early VACURG studies, that survival is the best assay of treatment effect and that efforts to identify alterations in disease progression may be misleading.

It has been recommended by many students of the disease that there is little advantage in giving hormonal therapy prior to the onset of symptoms of bone pain or evidence of active progression such as weakness, anemia, and increasing symptoms of prostatism or ureteral obstruction. Considerable controversy exists as to the form that hormonal therapy should take.

It would seem ideal to select a level of hormonal intervention that both provides the least risk and establishes adequate disease control. Advocates of orchiectomy argue that this maneuver ensures the removal of the source of continuing testosterone production and negates the necessity for faithful estrogen consumption. The administration of diethylstilbestrol, 1 mg/day, does not produce uniformly anorchid levels of serum testosterone but has less cardiovascular hazard than 5 mg/day.[5] Diethylstilbestrol, 3 mg/day, does produce anorchid levels of serum testosterone; however, the relative cardiovascular hazard of this dose level has not been determined.[32, 36] Diethylstilbestrol, 5 mg/day, also produces anorchid levels of serum testosterone, but it is associated with a greater cardiovascular hazard than the 1-mg dose.[5, 36, 52]

Currently, use of the antiandrogens flutamide or cyproterone acetate, or the use of the LHRH analogues either singly or in combination with the antiandrogens, is an attractive but as yet unproven method for the management of metastatic prostate carcinoma. Theoretically attractive, these new methodologies have yet to be proved to rescue patients who fail androgen deprivation or to be more effective than standard therapies in the management of previously untreated patients.[41]

Orchiectomy seems the surest way to reduce serum testosterone while providing the least cardiovascular hazard.[5, 23, 24, 32, 36, 52] The simultaneous administration of diethylstilbestrol, 1 mg daily, or its equivalent is postulated but unproved in providing additional control at the cellular level (Table

Table 28–2. COMPARATIVE EQUIVALENCE OF ESTROGENS USED IN THE TREATMENT OF PATIENTS WITH PROSTATIC ADENOCARCINOMA

Agent	Equivalent Dose
Diethylstilbestrol	1.5 mg
Ethinylestradiol	0.05 mg
Chlorotrianisene	12.5 mg

28–2). When estrogen therapy is administered with or without orchiectomy, certain biologic effects can be anticipated. Gynecomastia uniformly occurs and may be both physiologically and psychologically painful. Radiation of the breasts (300 to 400 rads) in a single or divided dose prior to estrogenization will prevent this problem and should be considered in each male before initiation of therapy. Fluid retention and dependent edema usually can be managed with salt restriction and diuretics. Prophylactic anticoagulation either with Coumadin or aspirin to reduce the thromboembolic hazards of estrogen control are attractive treatment adjuncts but are unproved.

In summary, hormonal manipulation is important in providing symptomatic relief for the patient with prostatic adenocarcinoma. Although the form of dosing and the timing of therapy are under debate, there seems to be little disagreement that the larger doses of estrogen are associated with increased cardiovascular toxicity. Similarly, there seems to be little disagreement that the patient with disease cannot be rescued by increasing dosages of estrogen. Further progress in the hormonal control of prostatic adenocarcinoma will await the identification of those predictors that will permit pretreatment identification of the hormonally sensitive malignant lesion and the hormonally susceptible patient.

References

1. Anderson KM, Liao S: Selective retention of dihydrotestosterone by prostatic nuclei. Nature 219:277–279, 1968.
2. Baker HW, Burger HG, deKrester DM: Effects of synthetic oral oestrogens in normal men and patients with prostatic carcinoma: lack of gonadotrophin suppression by chlorotrianisene. Clin Endocrinol 2:297–306, 1973.
3. Bennett AH, Dowd JB, Harrison JH: Estrogen and survival data in carcinoma of the prostate. Surg Gynecol Obstet 130:505–508, 1970.
4. Birke G, Franksson C, Planton LO: Estrogen therapy in carcinoma of prostate. Acta Chir Scand 109:1–10, 1955.
5. Blackard CE, Byar DP, Jordan WP Jr: Orchiectomy for advanced prostatic carcinoma—a reevaluation. Urology 1:533–560, 1973.
6. Block M, Bonomi P, Anderson K, et al: Treatment of stage D prostatic carcinoma with megestrol acetate. J Surg Oncol 17:367–371, 1981.
7. Brendler H: Therapy with orchiectomy or estrogens or both. JAMA 210:1074–1075, 1969.
8. Bruchovsky N: Comparison of the metabolites formed in the rat prostate following the in vivo administration of seven natural androgens. Endocrinology 89:1212–1222, 1971.
9. Bruchovsky N, Wilson JD: The conversion of testosterone to 5-alpha-androstan-17-beta-ol-3-one by rat prostate in vivo and in vitro. J Biol Chem 243:2012–2021, 1968.
10. Byar DP, Corle DK: Selecting optimal treatment in clinical trials using covariate information. J Chronic Dis 30:445–459, 1977.
11. Carroll G, Brennan RV: Tace in prostatic cancer: clinical and biochemical considerations. J Urol 72:497–503, 1954.
12. Emmett JL, Greene LF, Papantoniou A: Endocrine therapy in carcinoma of the prostate gland: 10-year survival studies. J Urol 83:471–484, 1960.
13. Fang S, Liao S: Antagonistic action of anti-androgens on the formation of a specific dihydrotestosterone-receptor protein complex in rat ventral prostate. Molec Pharmacol 5:428–431, 1969.
14. Geller J, Albert J, Yen SSC: Treatment of advanced cancer of the prostate with megestrol acetate. Urology 12:537–541, 1978.
15. Geller J, Vazakas G, Fruchtman B, et al: The effect of cyproterone acetate on advanced carcinoma of the prostate. Surg Gynecol Obstet 127:748–758, 1968.
16. Glick JH, Wein A, Padavic K, et al: Phase II trial of tamoxifen in metastatic carcinoma of the prostate. Cancer 49:1367–1372, 1982.
17. Goldman AS: Further studies of steroidal inhibitors of delta 5,3-beta-hydroxysteroid dehydrogenase and delta 5-delta 4,3-ketosteroid isomerase in *Pseudomonas testosteroni* and in bovine adrenals. J Clin Endocrinol 28:1539–1546, 1968.
18. Goodwin DA, Rasmussen-Taxdal DS, Ferreira AA, Scott WW: Estrogen inhibition of androgen-maintained prostatic secretion in the hypophysectomized dog. J Urol 86:134–136, 1961.
19. Harper ME, Fahmy AR, Pierrepoint CG, et al: The effect of some stilbestrol compounds on DNA polymerase from human prostatic tissue. Steroids 15:89–103, 1970.
20. Huggins C: Anti-androgenic Treatment of Prostatic Carcinoma in Man; Approaches to Tumor Chemotherapy. Washington, D.C., American Association for the Advancement of Science, 1947, pp 379–383.
21. Huggins C, Stevens RE Jr, Hodges CV: Studies on prostatic cancer. The effects of castration on advanced carcinoma of the prostate gland. Arch Surg 43:209–223, 1941.
22. Johnson DE, Kaesler KE, Ayala AG: Megestrol acetate for treatment of advanced carcinoma of the prostate. J Surg Oncol 7:9–15, 1975.
23. Kent JR, Bischoff AJ, Arduino LJ, et al: Estrogen dosage and suppression of testosterone levels in patients with prostatic carcinoma. J Urol 109:858–860, 1973.

24. Mackler MA, Liberti JP, Smith MJV, et al: The effect of orchiectomy and various doses of stilbestrol on plasma testosterone levels in patients with carcinoma of the prostate. Invest Urol 9:423–425, 1972.

25. Mainwaring WIP, Irving R: The use of deoxyribonucleic acid-cellulose chromatography and isoelectric focusing for the characterization and partial purification of steroid-receptor complexes. Biochem J 134:113–127, 1973.

26. Mainwaring WIP, Managan FR, Wilce PA: Androgens. 1. A review of current research on the binding and mechanism of action of androgenic steroids, notably 5-alpha-dihydrotestosterone. Adv Exp Biol 36:197–231, 1973.

27. Neri R, Florance K, Koziol P, Van Cleave S: A biological profile of a non-steroidal antiandrogen Sch-13521 (4'-nitro-3'-trifluoromethylisobutyranilide). Endocrinology 91:427–437, 1972.

28. Nesbit RM, Baum WC: Endocrine control of prostatic carcinoma: Clinical and statistical survey of 1,818 cases. JAMA 143:1317–1320, 1950.

29. Pont A, Williams PL, Azhar S, et al: Ketoconazole blocks testosterone synthesis. Arch Intern Med 142:2137–2140, 1982.

30. Pont A, Williams PL, Loose DS, et al: Ketoconazole blocks adrenal steroid synthesis. Ann Intern Med 97:370–372, 1982.

31. Pool TL, Thompson GJ: Conservative treatment of carcinoma of the prostate. JAMA 160:833–837, 1956.

32. Robinson MRG, Thomas BS: Effect of hormonal therapy on plasma testosterone levels in prostatic carcinoma. Br Med J 4:391–394, 1971.

33. Schoonees R, Schalch DS, Murphy GP: The hormonal effects of antiandrogen (SH-714) treatment in man. Invest Urol 8:635–639, 1971.

34. Seal US, Doe RP, Byar DP, Corle MS, Veterans Administration Cooperative Urological Research Group: Response of serum cholesterol and triglycerides to hormone treatment and the relation of pretreatment values to mortality in patients with prostatic cancer. Cancer 38:1095–1107, 1976.

35. Seal US, Doe RP, Byar DP, Corle DK, Veterans Administration Cooperative Urological Research Group: Response of plasma fibrinogen and plasminogen to hormone treatment and the relation of pretreatment values to mortality in patients with prostatic cancer. Cancer 38:1108–1117, 1976.

36. Shearer RJ, Hendry WF, Sommerville IF, Fergusson JD: Plasma testosterone: an accurate monitor of hormone treatment in prostatic cancer. Br J Urol 45:668–677, 1973.

37. Shimazaki J, Horaguchi T, Oki Y, et al: Properties of testosterone 5-reductase of purified nuclear fraction from ventral prostate of rats. Endocrinol Jpn 18:179–187, 1971.

38. Smith JA Jr: Androgen suppression by a gonadotropin releasing hormone analogue in patients with metastatic carcinoma of the prostate. J Urol 131:1110–1112, 1984.

39. Smith RB, Walsh PC, Goodwin WE: Cyproterone acetate in the treatment of advanced carcinoma of the prostate. J Urol 110:106–108, 1973.

40. Sogani PC, Vagaiwala MR, Whitmore WF Jr: Experience with flutamide in patients with advanced prostatic cancer without prior endocrine therapy. Cancer 54:744–750, 1984.

41. Spremulli E, DeSimone P, Durant J: A phase II study of Nolvadex: tamoxifen citrate in the treatment of advanced prostatic adenocarcinoma. Am J Clin Oncol 5:149–153, 1982.

42. Stoliar B, Albert DJ: SCH 13521 in the treatment of advanced carcinoma of the prostate. J Urol 111:803–807, 1974.

43. Trachtenberg J: The treatment of metastatic prostatic cancer with a potent luteinizing hormone releasing hormone analogue. J Urol 129:1149–1152, 1983.

44. Trachtenberg J: Ketoconazole therapy in advanced prostatic cancer. J Urol 132:61–63, 1984.

45. Vermeulen A, Verdonck L: Studies of the binding of the testosterone to human plasma. Steroids 11:609–635, 1968.

46. Walsh PC: Physiologic basis for hormonal therapy in carcinoma of the prostate. Urol Clin North Am 2:125–140, 1975.

47. Walsh PC, Korenman SG: Mechanism of androgenic action: effect of specific intracellular inhibitors. J Urol 105:850–857, 1971.

48. Walsh PC, Siiteri PK: Suppression of plasma androgens by spironolactone in castrated men with carcinoma of the prostate. J Urol 114:254–256, 1975.

49. Wilson JD, Gloyna RE: The intranuclear metabolism of testosterone in the accessory organs of reproduction. Recent Progr Horm Res 26:309–336, 1970.

50. Worgul TJ, Santen RJ, Smojlik E, et al: Clinical and biochemical effect of aminoglutethimide in the treatment of advanced prostatic carcinoma. J Urol 129:51–55, 1983.

51. Yanaihara T, Troen P, Troen BR, et al: Studies of the human testis. 3. Effect of estrogen on testosterone formation in human testis in vitro. Clin Endocrinol Metab 34:968–973, 1972.

52. Young HH 2nd, Kent JR: Plasma testosterone levels in patients with prostatic carcinoma before and after treatment. J Urol 99:788–792, 1968.

ROBERT P. HUBEN, M.D.
GERALD P. MURPHY, M.D., D.Sc.

CHAPTER **29**

Management of Advanced Cancer of the Prostate

Some notion of the impact of prostatic cancer on the health and well-being of American males can be gathered from the fact that an estimated 25,000 men in this country will die from this disease in 1985.[34] Recent studies of prostatic cancer by the Commission on Cancer of the American College of Surgeons have shown the presence of advanced disease at diagnosis in an alarming percentage of patients.[26] Once metastatic disease has been documented, hormone therapy is the standard and appropriate form of treatment of prostatic cancer. Although hormone therapy is of unquestionable benefit in the majority of patients with symptomatic disease, duration of response is unpredictable but generally limited, and it has been suggested that the overall effect of hormone therapy may be marginal.[15] Once prostatic cancer is no longer responsive to hormonal manipulation, survival usually can be measured in months. Further hormonal approaches are still commonly proposed once hormone resistance develops, although there is little if any evidence that such treatment will be of significant benefit to the patient.[8] Studies by the National Prostatic Cancer Treatment Group (NPCTG) and others have shown that chemotherapy is generally superior to further hormone therapy in this clinical situation in both palliation of symptoms and prolongation of survival.[29, 38] Yet chemotherapy for prostatic cancer has been viewed with skepticism by many. Some of the reasons why chemotherapy has not been undertaken include reliance on hormonal ther-

apy for metastatic disease, concern about possible side effects in patients who may be elderly or debilitated, and the lack of significant clinical data on the rationale and results of chemotherapy for prostatic cancer.[3, 19, 39] Although considerably more data are available at present concerning the effects of chemotherapy for prostatic cancer, the results and interpretation of many clinical trials may be highly variable, despite efforts to standardize patient eligibility, treatment characteristics, and evaluation of response.

The purpose of the present discussion is to present an update of clinical experience with chemotherapy for metastatic prostatic cancer, with particular emphasis on the results of the NPCTG studies. Because of their critical significance in evaluating the results of chemotherapy, response criteria will also be reviewed.

DETERMINATION OF TREATMENT RESPONSE AND RESPONSE CRITERIA

Defining response to treatment of metastatic prostatic cancer is a complex and controversial issue, and this problem is a major cause of the great variability of response rates using the same or similar chemotherapy regimens.[39] Prostatic cancer has a poorly understood predilection to metastasize to bone, and 70 to 84% of patients will have or develop positive results on bone scans.[14, 36] In numerous studies, bone scans have been shown to be more accurate in demonstrating bone metastases than skeletal survey, and changes on bone scan may precede those seen on conventional radiographs by three to six months.[36] Bone scans are highly sensitive but have low specificity. Despite problems of interpretation and quantitation, serial bone scans have been shown to be highly sensitive and practical in determining the response of bone metastases to treatment.[4, 11] Other objective parameters of response that are commonly used include serum acid phosphatase measurements, serial rectal examinations, and change in size of measurable soft tissue metastases. It has been suggested that only patients with bidimensionally measurable soft tissue lesions are appropriate subjects in whom response to treatment is the end point of study.[5, 42] But such selectivity is impractical in the majority of patients with metastatic prostate cancer, since 10% or less of patients may be evaluated by these standards.[5, 41] A potential bias in treating patients with extensive soft tissue metastases, which may be associated with poorer survival and less responsiveness to chemotherapy, also has been suggested.[42]

Currently, the most widely accepted response criteria in the treatment of metastatic prostate cancer are those of the National Prostatic Cancer Project (NPCP), now known as the National Prostatic Cancer Treatment Group (NPCTG), which have been extensively described.[23] These response criteria have been modified over the years and are undergoing routine re-evaluation on a regular basis. The most recent trend in response determination is the use of progression-free survival as the major indicator of treatment efficacy, rather than response at a single point in time. Progression-free survival refers to the minimum time to progression or death, and this determination appears to be more efficient in indicating the impact of treatment on the cause of disease.

Criticism of NPCTG response criteria frequently has centered on the significance of stabilization of disease as a response category. Early NPCP trials demonstrated convincingly that both survival and duration of response in stable patients parallel those of partial objective responders, which strengthens the argument that stabilization is a valid means of tumor response.[32, 33, 39] Others have contended that stabilization of disease is more a reflection of an inherently longer

survival in those patients who have slowly growing tumors rather than a true response to therapy.[12, 41] This controversy is yet to be resolved, but it is only in large randomized studies such as those of the NPCP that the variability of the clinical cause of disease can be minimized by stratification of patients according to symptoms or extent of disease. The NPCP response criteria, however, represent a major advance in the systematic investigation of chemotherapy in the treatment of prostatic cancer through the establishment of a reasonable and reproducible method of comparing treatment results by established parameters. The current NPCTG response criteria will be reviewed briefly.

NPCTG CRITERIA FOR COMPLETE RESPONSE

All of the following must occur: (1) tumor masses, if present, totally disappear and no new lesions appear; (2) elevated acid phosphatase and prostatic antigen levels, if present, return to normal; (3) osteolytic lesions, if present, recalcify; (4) osteoblastic lesions, if present, disappear, with a negative result on bone scan; (5) hepatomegaly, if a significant indicator, must change so that there is complete return of liver size to normal and normalization of all pretreatment abnormalities of liver function; (6) no significant cancer-related deterioration in weight (more than 10%), symptoms, or performance status.

NPCTG CRITERIA FOR PARTIAL RESPONSE

Any of the following may occur: (1) recalcification of one or more of any osteolytic lesions; (2) a reduction by 50% in the number of increased uptake areas on the bone scan; (3) decrease of 50% or more in cross-sectional area of any measurable lesions; (4) hepatomegaly, if a significant indicator, must show at least a 30% reduction in liver size measurements and at least a 30% improvement of all pretreatment abnormalities of liver function.

All of the following must be present: (1) no new sites of disease; (2) acid phosphatase and prostatic antigen levels return to normal;

(3) no deterioration in weight (more than 10%), symptoms, or performance status.

NPCTG CRITERIA FOR STABLE DISEASE

All of the following must be present: (1) no new lesions occur and no measurable lesions increase more than 25% in cross-sectional area; (2) elevated acid phosphatase level, if present, decreases though need not return to normal; (3) osteolytic lesions, if present, do not appear to worsen; (4) osteoblastic lesions, if present, remain stable on bone scan; (5) hepatomegaly, if present, does not appear to worsen by more than a 30% increase in liver measurements, and symptoms of hepatic abnormalities do not become worse; (6) no significant cancer-related deterioration in weight (greater than 10%), symptoms, or performance status.

NPCTG CRITERIA FOR PROGRESSION

Any of the following may be present: (1) significant cancer-related deterioration in weight (more than 10%), symptoms, or performance status; (2) appearance of new areas of malignant disease by bone scan or x-ray, or in soft tissue by other appropriate techniques; (3) increase in any previously measurable lesion by greater than 25% in cross-sectional area; (4) development of recurring anemia secondary to prostatic cancer (not related to treatment—Protocols 500, 600, and 1300); (5) development of ureteral obstruction (Protocols 500, 600, and 1300).

NATIONAL PROSTATIC CANCER TREATMENT GROUP STUDIES

Protocol 100

The first of the National Prostatic Cancer Project (NPCP) studies of chemotherapy for metastatic prostate cancer was conducted from July 1973 through July 1975. Patients who failed to respond or had become refractory to conventional hormonal therapy were randomized through a central statistical center to receive either 1 gm/m^2 cyclophosphamide intravenously (IV) every three weeks, 600 mg/m^2 5-fluorouracil (5-FU) IV weekly, or "standard" therapy. Standard therapy consisted of further hormonal therapy, steroids, radiation, and other palliative therapies. In this and subsequent NPCP studies, stabilization of disease as well as improvement was considered a positive response. Response rates were 46% with cyclophosphamide, 36% with 5-FU, and 19% with standard therapy.[29] It was also observed that duration of survival for patients who responded to chemotherapy was greater than that of patients who failed to respond and was also greater than survival in patients receiving standard therapy. The results of this first study suggested that chemotherapy could be given safely and effectively within a large randomized clinical study, and it encouraged further studies of chemotherapy in this setting.

Protocol 200

Pelvic radiotherapy of more than 2000 rads as well as failure of conventional hormone therapy for metastatic prostatic cancer were prerequisites for entry into this and several subsequent NPCP studies. Chemotherapeutic agents were chosen in part for their lesser myelosuppressive potential, since bone marrow reserve may be seriously compromised following pelvic radiation. Patients were chosen in a randomized fashion from July 1974 through March 1976 to receive oral estramustine phosphate (Emcyt), 600 mg/m^2 daily; streptozotocin, 500 mg/m^2 IV for five days every six weeks; or standard therapy. In 105 evaluated patients, the response rate was 32% for streptozotocin, 30% for estramustine phosphate, and 19% for standard therapy, identical to the results for standard therapy in Protocol 100.[21] As in Protocol 100, survival was noted to be greater in patients who responded to chemotherapy than in patients who failed to respond. Nausea and vomiting were the predominant toxic effects for all manners of treatment. Other toxic effects or abnormalities were reported to be equal in incidence among the three treatment groups. Duration of response was also significantly longer for patients on estramustine phosphate than for patients on streptozotocin or standard therapy.

Protocol 300

Cyclophosphamide was chosen as one treatment arm in Protocol 300 because of the high response rate of this agent in Protocol 100 in patients who had failed hormone therapy. From April 1975 to June 1977, patients were randomly chosen to receive cyclophosphamide, 1 gm/m² IV every three weeks; imidazole carboxamide (DTIC), 200 mg/m² IV on days 1 and 5 every three weeks; or oral procarbazine, 100 mg/m² for three weeks of every six-week period. In 129 evaluated patients, response rates were 26% for cyclophosphamide, 27% for imidazole carboxamide, and 14% for procarbazine.[27] Because of its relatively low antitumor activity and high toxicity, procarbazine was considered an unsuitable agent for subsequent chemotherapy trials. Although the response rate to cylophosphamide in this trial was lower than in Protocol 100, it remained a reference agent in a subsequent chemotherapy trial because of its beneficial effect on performance status and survival. Imidazole carboxamide appeared to be another fairly active agent in advanced prostatic cancer on the basis of this study. Survival beyond 40 weeks was about the same for patients in all three treatment groups.

Protocol 400

This second study in patients with a history of extensive pelvic radiation was conducted from March 1976 to May 1977. Random patients received oral estramustine phosphate 600 mg/m² daily plus 30 mg oral prednimustine daily for six of every seven days, or prednimustine alone at the same dosage. Prednimustine is an ester of chlorambucil and prednisone and has shown good activity in previous human and animal studies.[22] In 116 evaluated patients the response rate was 13% for both treatments, and the combination of two agents failed to show any advantage over the single-agent therapy in this particular study.[22] Although prednimustine alone exhibited a minimal objective response rate, about one third of patients reported pain relief or improved performance status while on this agent.

Protocol 500

Patients with newly diagnosed metastatic prostatic cancer were the subjects of this study, in an effort to determine if the combination of hormone therapy and chemotherapy resulted in higher response rates and improved survival when compared with hormone therapy alone. Patients without previous chemotherapy or hormone therapy were randomly chosen from July 1976 to September 1980 to be treated by orchiectomy or diethylstilbestrol (DES) at 3 mg/day, or 3 mg/day DES plus 1 gm/m² cyclophosphamide IV every three weeks, or cyclophosphamide plus oral estramustine phosphate, 600 mg/m² daily. Objective response rates, evaluated initially at 12 weeks, were similar in all three treatment arms.[20] However, chemotherapy appeared to exhibit an improved effect on overall survival when compared with hormone therapy alone. A positive effect of chemotherapy on survival was most evident in patients with pain at presentation. There was no apparent difference in survival between patients who received DES and those who had undergone orchiectomy. Toxicity in the chemotherapy treatments was not excessive. Since nearly 50% of patients remained in remission at the time that these preliminary results were published, further follow-up is necessary to determine whether early chemotherapy is associated with a significant survival advantage.

Protocol 600

Another patient population was studied in Protocol 600, consisting of patients regarded as stable on hormone therapy. The purpose of this study was to determine if the addition of chemotherapy improved survival when compared with continued hormone therapy alone. As in Protocol 500, the agents employed were DES or orchiectomy plus cyclophosphamide, cyclophosphamide plus estramustine phosphate, and conventional hormone therapy in the form of DES or orchiectomy. Overall response rate in the DES plus cyclophosphamide group was higher (80%) than that of the hormone therapy–only group (67%), although this difference is not statistically significant.[31] Complete and partial responses were also more frequent in the DES/orchiectomy plus cyclophosphamide group (18%) than the hormone therapy–only group (6%).

Protocol 700

On the basis of the results of treatment with this agent in Protocols 100 and 300, cyclophosphamide was chosen as the reference agent in this third trial of chemotherapy in patients who had failed or never responded to hormone therapy. Hydroxyurea and methyl-CCNU were selected following reports of good activity of these agents in animal models as well as in patients with prostatic cancer.[17] Between May 1977 and April 1979, a total of 125 patients were randomly chosen to receive cyclophosphamide, 1 gm/m² IV every three weeks; methyl-CCNU, 175 mg/m² orally every six weeks; or hydroxyurea, 3 gm/m² orally every three days. Response rates were 35% for cyclophosphamide, 30% for methyl-CCNU, and 15% for hydroxyurea.[17] Both methyl-CCNU and hydroxyurea showed poor chemotherapeutic activity and significant hematologic toxicity. Regarding observed survival, there was a highly significant ($p < 0.01$) advantage for cyclophosphamide over hydroxyurea and a marginal ($p = 0.05$) advantage over methyl-CCNU in this measurement of response. After this third clinical trial, cyclophosphamide continued to be regarded as the single drug of choice for patients with advanced prostatic cancer and adequate bone marrow reserve.[28]

Protocol 800

As in Protocols 200 and 400, patients in Protocol 800 received chemotherapy following extensive pelvic irradiation and progression on hormone therapy. From May 1977 to April 1979, patients were randomly selected to receive estramustine phosphate, 600 mg/m²; vincristine, 1 mg/m² IV every two weeks; or the combination of both agents. In 90 evaluated patients, the response rate for vincristine was only 15%, for estramustine phosphate 26%, and for combination therapy 24%.[34] Almost one half of the patients receiving vincristine reported symptoms of neuropathy, particularly numbness of the extremities. Vincristine, both alone and in combination with estramustine, was regarded as relatively inactive in the treatment of metastatic prostatic cancer. Probability of survival did not differ significantly among the three treatment methods. On the basis of this and preceding NPCP studies, estramustine phosphate continued to be regarded as the most active chemotherapeutic agent in previously irradiated patients.

Protocols 900 and 1000

The potential benefit of adjuvant chemotherapy following definitive therapy for clinically localized prostatic cancer is being examined in these NPCP studies. Protocols 900 and 1000 examine the role of adjuvant chemotherapy following either surgery or radiation therapy, respectively, for Stages B_2, C, and D_1 prostatic cancer. Begun in May 1978, these studies seek to determine the effect of adjuvant chemotherapy on rate of relapse, time to relapse, and survival after definitive local therapy. In both protocols, patients undergo staging pelvic lymph node dissection or lymphangiogram and needle aspiration to determine the pathologic stage of disease. Patients in Protocol 900 undergo radical prostatectomy or cryosurgery, whereas patients in Protocol 1000 receive a radiation dosage of 6600 to 7020 rads to the prostate if nodes are negative for disease and 5040 rads to the pelvic nodal area with a cone-down dosage to the prostate if nodes are positive. Patients are randomly selected for chemotherapy with oral estramustine phosphate, 600 mg/m² daily; cyclophosphamide, 1 gm/m² IV every three weeks; or for a control group receiving no further therapy. In the absence of progression of disease, chemotherapy is generally given for a two-year period, during which patients are evaluated at 12-week intervals. A longer period of follow-up is necessary to determine the effect of adjuvant chemotherapy on survival of patients with localized prostatic cancer. However, results should be forthcoming in patients with positive nodes, since about one half of these patients show evidence of progression within three years of diagnosis.[40] Whether the promising results of adjuvant chemotherapy following definitive treatment of other tumors such as breast cancer are also possible in prostatic cancer may then be more readily answered. Preliminary data from Protocol 900 were reported recently by Schmidt.[25] Since two thirds of patients have had negative lymph nodes, the recurrence rate has been low (15 of 128 patients), and survival analyses are not yet possible, as only two patients have died. In comparison, nearly three fourths of patients receiving definitive radiation therapy in Protocol 1000 have had histologic evidence of lymph node involvement. This finding reflects selection of radiation therapy over surgery by the contributing urologists in the presence of known or suspected lymph node involvement. Since the major cause of treatment failure for localized prostatic cancer is the presence of undetectable microscopic metastases at the time of definitive treatment, further studies of "adjuvant" chemotherapy in high-risk patients with prostatic cancer are urgently needed.

Protocol 1100

This fourth study of single-agent chemotherapy of advanced, hormone-refractory prostatic cancer was conducted from April 1979 to December 1981. Patients received, by random selection, oral estramustine phosphate, 600 mg/m^2 daily; methotrexate, 40 mg/m^2 IV then 60 mg/m^2 weekly; or cisplatin, 60 mg/m^2 IV on days 1, 4, 21, 24, and then monthly. In 158 evaluated patients, response rates were 34% for estramustine phosphate, 41% for methotrexate, and 36% for cisplatin.[16] Leukopenia and stomatitis were the most common side effects of methotrexate therapy, and administration of the full dose (60 mg/m^2) at two-week intervals rather than weekly was found to be the most tolerable regimen. Nausea and vomiting were the most common complications of cisplatin therapy. There was one complete response to methotrexate, which lasted about 12 months. Due to the high activity of methotrexate in this study, it replaced cyclophosphamide as reference single agent in a subsequent NPCP clinical trial (Protocol 1500).

Protocol 1200

This fourth trial of chemotherapy in patients with prior irradiation was conducted from April 1979 to January 1982. There were 124 patients who were chosen randomly to receive oral estramustine phosphate in the usual dosage; cisplatin, 60 mg/m^2 IV monthly; or these two agents in combination. Response rates were 18% for estramustine phosphate, 21% for cisplatin, and 33% for combination therapy.[35] Nausea, vomiting, and anorexia were the most common side effects for all treatments, but they were more frequent for combination therapy. The increased response rate for combination therapy was considered an additive rather than synergistic effect. Proportionately, more patients receiving combination therapy experienced reduced pain levels or performance

status, and there was also a small survival advantage for patients on combination therapy. Unlike the results of two prior NPCP studies, combination therapy appeared clearly superior in this study to the results of single-agent therapy.

Protocol 1300

Begun in September 1980, this second study of chemotherapy in newly diagnosed and untreated prostatic cancer completed patient entry in June 1983. There were 283 patients who were randomly selected for one of three treatments: a control group that underwent conventional hormone therapy (orchiectomy or DES), one that received oral estramustine and one that received hormone therapy plus cyclophosphamide, 650 mg/m^2 IV every three weeks, plus 5-FU, 350 mg/m^2 IV weekly. Dosages of cyclophosphamide and 5-FU are lower than in other NPCP protocols in order to decrease the risk of enhanced toxicity, particularly myelosuppression. Results of this study have not yet been reported because of high response rates and the relatively limited duration of follow-up.[31]

ONGOING NPCP CHEMOTHERAPY TRIALS

Protocol 1400

Patients who have stable disease and are on hormone therapy are the subjects of this study, as in Protocol 600. Randomization is to either continued hormone therapy (orchiectomy or DES) or hormone therapy plus 5-FU, 700 mg/m^2 IV plus cyclophosphamide, 700 mg/m^2 IV, every 3 weeks.

Protocol 1500

This is the current study of the efficacy of chemotherapy in hormone refractory prostatic cancer. Because of the high response rate to methotrexate in Protocol 1100, one treatment arm consists of this agent alone at the same dosage of 60 mg/m^2 IV, but at two-week intervals rather than weekly. The other arms are the combination of doxorubicin (Adriamycin), 50 mg/m^2 IV, plus cyclophosphamide, 500 mg/m^2 IV, every three weeks; or cisplatin, 50 mg/m^2 IV, plus cyclophosphamide, 500 mg/m², plus 5-FU, 500 mg/m² IV, every three weeks.

Protocol 1600

The present clinical trial for patients with hormone refractory disease and extensive pelvic radiation, this study compares chemotherapy in the form of streptozotocin at 500 mg/m² IV daily for five days every six weeks with further hormonal therapy. There are three hormone therapy arms: fosfestrol (Stilphostrol), 1 gm IV daily for five days, then 50 mg orally three times daily; versus megastrol acetate (Megace), 40 mg orally three times daily, with or without DES, 0.1 mg orally each day.

Protocol 1700

This is the present study of treatment of newly diagnosed, metastatic prostatic cancer patients in whom the response to conventional hormone therapy is compared with that to buserelin acetate, a leutinizing hormone–releasing hormone analog, and hormone therapy plus methotrexate, 60 mg/m² IV every two weeks.

OTHER CLINICAL TRIALS OF CHEMOTHERAPY OF METASTATIC PROSTATIC CARCINOMA

In addition to the cooperative clinical trials of the NPCTG, a number of other recent reports on chemotherapy of prostatic cancer have been reported, with highly variable results and conclusions. An encouraging report of the effects of chemotherapy consisting of doxorubicin and oral cyclophosphamide was reported by Ihde and associates.[13] Thirty-two patients were treated with doxorubicin, 30 mg/m² IV on days 1 and 8, and oral cyclophosphamide, 100 mg/m² on days 1 to 14 of each 28-day cycle. Seven patients (32%) were documented to have objective partial responses, and four patients (18%) had stable disease. Similar to the results of the early NPCP studies, these results showed that patients with partial response lived significantly longer than those with no response and survival of patients with stable disease approximated that of partial responders. Although the authors

found that no single staging test identified all patients with objective tumor response or progression, worsening results of bone scans accurately indicated progressive disease in 11 of 12 patients. This regimen was fairly well tolerated except in patients with prior radiation therapy, which was associated with significant hematologic toxicity.

Another seemingly effective regimen was studied by Logothetis and associates.[18] The agents were doxorubicin, 50 mg/m² IV on day one; 5-FU, 750 mg/m² IV on days 1 and 2; and mitomycin C, 10 mg/m² IV on day one (DMF). Courses were given at increasing intervals that were determined by marrow recovery, with a mean interval of 4.5 weeks between the first and second courses. Objective partial responses were reported in 30 of 62, or 48% of patients. In patients with osseous metastases, those with only axial skeletal involvement had a higher response rate (52%) than those with axial and appendicular skeletal involvement (33%); in patients with visceral metastases the higher response rate was in patients with pulmonary parenchymal metastases only (88%), whereas patients with advanced visceral disease had the expected poorer survival and lower response rate (33%). There were three treatment-related deaths in this group of 62 patients. Responding patients in each clinical category survived longer than nonresponding patients with advanced visceral metastases. Although the authors concluded that this is an effective regimen in hormone-refractory prostatic cancer, the benefits of this treatment must be weighed against the toxicity encountered.

The results of a modified FAM regimen in patients with hormone-refractory prostatic cancer were recently reported by Babaian and Hsu.[1] This regimen consisted of 5-FU, 600 mg/m² on days 1 and 7; Adriamycin, 40 mg/m² on day 1; and mitomycin C, 10 mg/m² on day 1 (two courses), then every other course. Treatment was repeated every four weeks initially, then at increasing intervals as determined by bone marrow recovery. In 14 evaluated patients, there were no complete or partial objective responses, and five were considered stable by NPCP criteria. Two patients were also reported to have a measurable decrease in soft tissue metastases. Pain relief following initiation of chemotherapy was complete in two patients and moderate in eight, for an overall subjective response rate of 71%. Median survival of patients who achieved stabilization of disease with FAM was 330 days, compared with 199 days for those without an objective response. No treatment-related deaths were recorded. Due in part to the high rate of pain relief with this regimen, the authors felt that FAM may prove to be an effective palliative therapy in patients with advanced prostatic cancer.

The results of a prospective randomized trial of single-agent versus combination chemotherapy have recently been reported.[12] Single-drug therapy was lomustine (CCNU), 130 mg/m^2 orally every six weeks. The combination regimen consisted of methotrexate, 45 mg/m^2; and 5-FU, 500 mg/m^2 IV on days 1 and 8; and cyclophosphamide, 75 mg/m^2 orally on days 1 to 14 of each 28-day cycle. Of the 20 patients receiving combination therapy, three (15%) had partial objective response (as defined by NPCP criteria) and four (20%) had stable disease. There were no partial responses to CCNU, and six patients (30%) were stable, resulting in similar overall response rates of 35% and 30% for each treatment arm. Patients with partial regression or stabilization survived longer than patients whose disease progressed (52 weeks versus 24 weeks, respectively). Subjective improvement occurred in all seven patients who responded to the combination regimen and in three of six patients who were stable on CCNU. The author noted a significant difference in lead time (interval between diagnosis and initiation of chemotherapy) in responders versus those who progressed and suggested that these drug regimens may have selected those patients with slower growing tumors and a longer natural history of disease.

The results of a Southwest Oncology Group (SWOG) study were recently reported in which patients randomly received either a combination of doxorubicin and cyclophosphamide or hydroxyurea as a single agent.[37] There were 43 patients with measurable soft tissue lesions. Objective response was reported in six of 19 (32%) on the combination regimen and in only one of 24 (4%) who received hydroxyurea. The low activity of hydroxyurea in this study confirms the results of an early NPCP study (Protocol 700) in which significant toxicity of hydroxyurea was also reported.

Citrin and associates treated 28 patients with doxorubicin, 40 to 60 mg/m^2 IV every three weeks, for a median duration of treatment of 67 days, and reported that 25% of patients had significant reduction (greater than 50%) in bidimensionally measured tumor masses.[5] In a similarly restricted group of patients, Scher and associates[24] reported measurable partial remission in only two of 41 patients (5%) receiving doxorubicin on a similar dosage schedule to a total of 500 mg/m^2. The authors of the latter study concluded that doxorubicin has only marginal activity in soft tissue lesions in patients with prostatic cancer. Since the same response criteria were applied to similarly measurable, nonbony metastases following a similar treatment schedule, the cause of the wide variability in results in these two reports is unclear.

The role of adjuvant or prophylactic chemotherapy in patients at high risk of progression, such as those with positive but excised lymph node involvement, has received relatively little attention despite the certainty of progression of disease. There is growing acceptance of the concept that pelvic nodal involvement represents disseminated disease, and that treatment, in turn, should be systemic.[10, 39] Clinical studies of this approach are very limited, and it is the intention of NPCTG Protocols 900 and 1000 to address the problem and determine the potential benefit of early chemotherapy. DeVere White and associates[40] have reported the results of a clinical trial of adjuvant chemotherapy in a group of 37 patients with pelvic lymph node metastases. Chemotherapy consisted of cyclophosphamide, 750 mg/m^2, and doxorubicin, 50 mg/m^2 IV, every three weeks for a six-month period. Of 12 patients receiving chemotherapy, progression occurred in four, with average time to progression of 15 months, whereas in 25 control patients, 12 progressed within an average interval of 12 months. No significant toxicity was reported. Early chemotherapy following diagnosis of local nodal involvement in this report appeared to delay the emergence of bone metastases. As more effective regimens are developed for metastatic prostatic cancer, their application in patients at high risk of recurrence may prove to be of practical value to patients with advanced disease.

FUTURE DIRECTIONS

Areas of major research in treatment approaches to disseminated prostatic cancer include the development of new hormonal agents, new cytotoxic agents, and new combinations of agents based on biochemical modulation and biologic response modifiers.[7] Promising classes of agents undergoing further investigation include the lipid-soluble antifolates, anthracyclines, nitrosoureas, and platinum analogs.[6]

Immunotherapy and immune modulation of prostatic cancer is of theoretical interest but is in a very early stage. The use of biologic response modifiers such as interferon is another active research area. However, an early study by the NPCTG (Protocol 2100) of interferon-B (human fibroblast interferon) in a group of 16 patients with hormone-refractory prostatic cancer demonstrated a low response rate and moderate toxicity.[2]

SUMMARY

Although the role of chemotherapy in the management of metastatic prostate cancer remains controversial, numerous clinical studies have shown that chemotherapy has an acceptable risk-benefit ratio and may improve survival and improve the quality of life to a greater degree than secondary hormonal approaches or other available palliative measures with tolerable side effects. Treatment must be individualized according to the patient's condition, prognosis, and expectations, but further randomized clinical trials involving large numbers of patients are necessary to avoid the problems of reliability and interpretation that have limited the value of many early studies. When the impact of metastatic prostatic cancer on the health and well-being of men in this country and throughout the world is again considered, the urgent need for further carefully designed and conducted clinical trials is readily apparent.

References

1. Babaian RJ, Hsu SD: Chemotherapy of hormone-refractory carcinoma of prostate with 5-fluorouracil, Adriamycin, and mitomycin C. Urology 23:272–275, 1984.
2. Bulbul M, Huben RP, Murphy GP: Interferon-beta treatment of metastatic prostate cancer. J Surg Oncol, in press.
3. Catalona WJ (ed): Chemotherapy. In Prostate Cancer, Vol 10. Orlando, FL, Grune & Stratton, 1984, pp 172–193.
4. Chisholm GD, Stone AR, Beynon LL, Merrick MV:

The bone scan as a tumour marker in prostatic carcinoma. Eur Urol 8:257–260, 1982.
5. Citrin DL, Elson P, DeWys WD: Treatment of metastatic prostate cancer. An analysis of response criteria in patients with measurable soft tissue disease. Cancer 54:13–17, 1984.
6. Creaven PJ: Cytotoxic chemotherapeutic agents under development with a possible future role in prostate cancer. Prostate 5:485–493, 1984.
7. Creaven PJ, Madajewicz S, Mittelman A: New potential treatment modalities for disseminated prostatic cancer. Urol Clin North Am 11:343–356, 1984.
8. deKernion JB, Lindner A: Chemotherapy of hormonally unresponsive prostate carcinoma. Urol Clin North Am 11:319–326, 1984.
9. Donohue RE, Mani JH, Whitesel JA, et al: Stage D₁ adenocarcinoma of prostate. Urology 23:118–121, 1984.
10. Elder JS, Catalona WJ: Management of newly diagnosed metastatic carcinoma of the prostate. Urol Clin North Am 11:283–295, 1984.
11. Fitzpatrick JM, Constable AR, Sherwood T, et al: Serial bone scanning: the assessment of treatment response in carcinoma of the prostate. Br J Urol 50:555–561, 1978.
12. Herr HW: Cyclophosphamide, methotrexate and 5-fluorouracil combination chemotherapy versus chloroethyl-cyclohexyhyphernitrosourea in the treatment of metastatic prostate cancer. J Urol 127:462–465, 1982.
13. Ihde DC, Bunn PA, Cohen MH, et al.: Effective treatment of hormonally unresponsive metastatic carcinoma of the prostate with adriamycin and cyclophosphamide. Methods of documenting tumor response and progression. Cancer 45:1300–1310, 1980.
14. Jacobs SC: Spread of prostatic cancer to bone. Urology 21:337–344, 1983.
15. Lepor H, Ross A, Walsh PC: The influence of hormonal therapy on survival of men with advanced prostatic cancer. J Urol 128:335–340, 1982.
16. Loening SA, Beckley S, Brady MF, et al.: Comparison of estramustine phosphate, methotrexate and cis-platinum in patients with advanced, hormone refractory prostate cancer. J Urol 129:1001–1006, 1983.
17. Loening SA, Scott WW, deKernion J, et al.: A comparison of hydroxyurea, methyl-chloroethyl-cyclohexy-nitrosourea and cyclophosphamide in patients with advanced carcinoma of the prostate. J Urol 125:812–816, 1981.
18. Logothetis CJ, Samuels ML, von Eschenbach AC, et al: Doxorubicin, mitomycin-C and 5-fluorouracil (DMF) in the treatment of metastatic hormonal refractory adenocarcinoma of the prostate, with a note on the staging of metastatic prostate cancer. J Clin Oncol 1:368–379, 1983.
19. Murphy GP: Management of disseminated prostatic carcinoma. Prostatic Cancer 13:213–233, 1979.
20. Murphy GP, Beckley S, Brady MF, et al: Treatment of newly diagnosed metastatic prostate cancer patients with chemotherapy agents in combination with hormones versus hormones alone. Cancer 51:1264–1272, 1983.
21. Murphy GP, Gibbons RP, Johnson DE, et al.: A comparison of estramustine phosphate and streptozotocin in patients with advanced prostatic carcinoma who have had extensive irradiation. J Urol 118:288–291, 1977.
22. Murphy GP, Gibbons RP, Johnson DE, et al.: The

use of estramustine and prednimustine versus prednimustine alone in advanced metastatic prostatic cancer patients who have received prior irradiation. Trans Am Assoc Genitourin Surg 70:69–71, 1978.

23. Murphy GP, Slack NH: Response criteria for the prostate of the USA National Prostatic Cancer Project. Prostate 1:375–382, 1980.

24. Scher H, Yagoda A, Watson RC, et al: Phase II trial of doxorubicin in bidimensionally measurable prostatic adenocarcinoma. J Urol 131:1099–1102, 1984.

25. Schmidt JD: Cooperative clinical trials of the National Prostatic Cancer Project: Protocol 900. Prostate 5:387–399, 1984.

26. Schmidt J, Mettlin C, Natarajan N, et al: Long-term and short-term surveys of patterns of care of prostate cancer. In: American College of Surgeons Approved Cancer Program. J Urol 136:416–421, 1986.

27. Schmidt JD, Scott WW, Gibbons RP, et al: Comparison of procarbazine, imidazole-carboxamide and cyclophosphamide in relapsing patients with advanced carcinoma of the prostate. J Urol 121:185–189, 1979.

28. Schmidt JD, Scott WW, Gibbons RP, et al: Chemotherapy programs of the National Prostatic Cancer Project (NPCP). Cancer 45:1937–1946, 1980.

29. Scott WW, Gibbons RP, Johnson DE, et al.: The continued evaluation of the effects of chemotherapy in patients with advanced carcinoma of the prostate. J Urol 116:211–213, 1976.

30. Silverberg E: Cancer statistics 1985. CA 35:19–35, 1985.

31. Slack NH: Results of chemotherapy protocols of the USA National Prostatic Cancer Project (NPCP). Clin Oncol 2:441–459, 1983.

32. Slack NH, Brady MF, Murphy GP: National Prostatic Cancer Project: Stable versus partial response in advanced prostate cancer. Prostate 5:401–415, 1984.

33. Slack NH, Mittelman A, Brady MF, Murphy GP: National Prostatic Cancer Project: The importance of the stable category for chemotherapy treated patients with advanced and relapsing prostate cancer. Cancer 46:2393–2402, 1980.

34. Soloway MS, deKernion JB, Gibbons RP, et al: Comparison of estramustine phosphate and vincristine alone or in combination for patients with advanced, hormone refractory, previously irradiated carcinoma of the prostate. J Urol 125:664–667, 1981.

35. Soloway MS, Beckley S, Brady MF, et al: A comparison of estramustine phosphate versus cis-platinum alone versus estramustine phosphate plus cis-platinum in patients with advanced hormone refractory prostate cancer who had had extensive irradiation to the pelvis or lumbosacral area. J Urol 129:56–61, 1983.

36. Spirnak JP, Resnick MI: Clinical staging of prostatic cancer: new modalities. Urol Clin North Am 11:221–235, 1984.

37. Stephens RL, Vaughn C, Lane M, et al: Adriamycin and cyclophosphamide versus hydroxyurea in advanced prostatic cancer. A randomized Southwest Oncology Group Study. Cancer 53:406–410, 1984.

38. Torti FM: Prostatic cancer chemotherapy. Recent Results Cancer Res 85:58–69, 1983.

39. Torti FM, Carter SK: The chemotherapy of prostatic adenocarcinoma. Ann Intern Med 92:681–689, 1980.

40. White RD, Babayan RK, Krikorian J, et al.: Adjuvant chemotherapy for stage D$_1$ adenocarcinoma of prostate. Urology 21:270–272, 1983.

41. Yagoda A: Cytotoxic agents in prostate cancer: an enigma. Semin Urol 1:311–322, 1983.

42. Yagoda A, Watson RC, Natale RB, et al: A critical analysis of response criteria in patients with prostatic cancer treated with cis-diamminedichloride platinum II. Cancer 44:1553–1562, 1979.

BRIAN E. HARDY, M.D.

CHAPTER 30

Management of Pediatric Pelvic Sarcomas

The marked improvement in the survival rate of children with pelvic sarcomas that occurred 20 years ago can be specifically ascribed to the adoption of multidiscipline therapy.[11, 23] In more recent years this coordination of treatment disciplines has been developed and refined so that the percentage of children who can now be saved by the united efforts of chemotherapists, radiotherapists, and surgeons far exceeds the cure rates achieved with surgery alone.[1, 4, 5, 34, 38] At our present level of understanding of sarcomas, the foreseeable progress in their treatment is linked to the statistical analysis of large series of patients. Because these tumors are rare, this progress is heavily dependent on multicenter studies, examples of which are currently under way.

CURRENT THERAPY CONSIDERATIONS

With multidiscipline cancer treatment, surgery, chemotherapy, and radiotherapy all have their price with respect to the morbidity they produce. The mutilating sequelae of exenterative surgery are obvious to all. Bone marrow depression, cystitis, and pulmonary, cardiac, intestinal, renal, and gonadal dysfunction are well-recorded side effects of the other two therapeutic modalities.[9, 19] The oncogenic potential of chemotherapy and radiotherapy cannot be overlooked.[3, 36]

In addition to these factors general to all oncology patients, children present special problems. Growth (physical, intellectual, and emotional) must be allowed for and assisted. Consequently, radiotherapy has to be considered with the knowledge of its effect on bone and organ growth.[19] Chemotherapeutic agents may affect pediatric and adult tissues differently, and with tumor cure, the side effects of such agents may take far longer to become manifest in a child than in an adult.[33] Surgery has to be planned with due consideration to functions required later in life (e.g., sexual and reproductive). All three treatment disciplines must respect the need to minimize hospitalization, as even an ideal hospital is a poor environment for child development. The need for tumor cure overrides all these considerations and their interdigitation.

With survival rates of pediatric pelvic sarcomas so encouragingly improved, specific attention has become focused on the quality of life being achieved. There is a suspicion that "over-therapy" is occurring with the established treatment regimens. To explore the possibility that cure rates can be maintained or improved while at the same time total treatment and morbidity rates are reduced, several multifaceted protocols have been tested or are currently under evaluation.[24, 25, 37] Changes in recommended treatments are likely to occur as these studies continue.

Although the full range of sarcomatous lesions can be encountered in the pelvis of a child, nearly all pediatric pelvic sarcomas are rhabdomyosarcomas or undifferentiated

483

sarcomas. Both appear to have a similar therapeutic response and are currently treated by the same protocols. Consequently, the remainder of this discussion will be limited to the management of rhabdomyosarcomas.

RHABDOMYOSARCOMAS (RMS)

Incidence and Factors Influencing Prognosis

RMS is thought to be derived from unsegmented, undifferentiated, mesodermal tissue. As reported in 1975, it ranks as the seventh most common malignant tumor of childhood, with a yearly incidence of 4.5 per million white children under 15 years of age.[39] Approximately 20% of these tumors occur in the genitourinary region,[7] and it can thus be calculated that 50 or more new cases of RMS of urologic interest present in the United States each year.

Although clinical stage at the time of presentation is clearly the most significant indicator as to the likely outcome, there is no unanimity as to how this tumor should be staged. Pleas have been made to use a TNM staging system for soft tissue sarcomas,[31, 33] but this has not yet won widespread acceptance. As so much of the recent data have come from the intergroup RMS study, it is appropriate to use their grouping system (Table 30–1).

Table 30–1. GROUPING
SYSTEM—INTERGROUP
RHABDOMYOSARCOMA STUDY

Group I: Localized disease, completely resected. Regional nodes not involved.
    a. Confined to muscle or organ of origin.
    b. Contiguous involvement—infiltration outside the muscle or organ of origin, as through fascial planes.
Group II: Regional disease.
    a. Grossly resected tumor with microscopic residual tumor. No clinical or microscopic evidence of regional node involvement.
    b. Regional disease, completely resected (regional nodes involved completely resected with no microscopic residual).
    c. Regional disease with involved nodes, grossly resected, but with evidence of microscopic residual.
Group III: Incomplete resection or biopsy with gross residual disease.
Group IV: Metastatic disease present at onset.

Clinical group, as indicated above, is of major importance, but the following factors also have a bearing on prognosis.[8, 12, 32]

1. Tumor size. Large size is unfavorable and has a direct relationship to stage, as it does in adults. However, in children it is not always absolute tumor size that is relevant, but rather tumor size relative to the size of the child.

2. Tumor histology. For RMS from all sites, the incidence of histologic type has been reported: embryonal, 62%; alveolar, 16%; botryoid embryonal, 8%; pleomorphic, 1%; extraosseous Ewing's sarcoma, 7%; and undifferentiated mesenchymal sarcoma, 6%.[18] Of 115 patients with genitourinary tumors who were eligible for evaluation, 81 (70%) had embryonal and 24 (21%) had botryoid subtype tumors.[7] Both of these histologic types have a favorable prognosis. The unfavorable outlook for alveolar tumors has been substantiated by authors independent of the intergroup RMS study.[21]

3. Lymphocyte count at diagnosis. A high count is favorable; a low count is unfavorable.

4. Recurrence. Failure to achieve tumor eradication at the initial attempt has the expected unfavorable significance.

5. Age at diagnosis. Patients under two years of age and older than 10 years of age have an unfavorable prognosis.

6. Bone marrow. The presence of bone marrow metastases at diagnosis is a poor prognostic sign.

7. Gender. With pelvic tumors, gender is related to the organ of origin in many instances.

8. Primary site of origin. This affects not only prognosis but also the specific details of management. Both aspects will be discussed together.

Management

For anatomic reasons, differences in the primary site of origin are reflected in the rapidity of clinical presentation, the feasibility and desirability of radical surgery, and the hazards of radiotherapy. For biologic reasons, the response of RMS to chemotherapy varies quantitatively according to the primary site of origin. All these factors affect management and cause it to differ with each primary site. Before detailing these differences in management, there are certain aspects of treatment common to all pediatric pelvic RMS that should be discussed.

Because it has been clearly shown that chemotherapy can prevent the appearance of distant metastases with childhood RMS,[17] chemotherapy is recommended in all children with this tumor. There is no unanimity on the exact details of chemotherapy, but vincristine, actinomycin, and cyclophosphamide (VAC) administered for one to two years is the most widely used protocol. The addition of doxorubicin (Adriamycin) to pulse VAC has so far not produced any dramatic improvement in response![1] There is evidence that in certain patient groups, cyclophosphamide may be deleted from the VAC without increased mortality.[26, 27] On the other hand, some have advocated a more intense regimen than VAC.[4, 10]

Irrespective of the primary site of origin, radiotherapy is not advocated for Group I RMS patients.[26, 27] Its role in all other RMS patient groups is diminishing as the efficacy of multiagent chemotherapy becomes more apparent. The required dosage of radiotherapy is still under evaluation but appears to be between 4000 and 5500 rads, varying with the age of the child, the clinical group, and the size of the tumor.[35]

Paratesticular RMS

The very high incidence of retroperitoneal lymph node involvement at the time of diagnosis is a major consideration in the management of the paratesticular RMS patient. Raney and associates reported six of 15 (40%) retroperitoneal node dissections that were positive for disease.[29] On reviewing the published literature, these same authors found the cumulative positive incidence to be 45%. Although meaningful figures on contralateral node involvement are not available, it seems that it is nearly always the ipsilateral nodes alone that are involved. Contralateral node involvement without ipsilateral node involvement is rare in adult testicular carcinoma patients,[30] and there is nothing to suggest that it is any more common with this tumor.

All are agreed that radical orchiectomy is indicated. Suspicious scrotal masses should be explored through an inguinal incision, with early control of the spermatic cord vessels. All are likewise agreed that chemotherapy should be administered once the pathologic condition has been established. Whether or not ipsilateral retroperitoneal node dissection should be undertaken for Group I patients is somewhat debatable.

Computerized axial tomography (CAT scaning) has aided in distinguishing patients in Group I from those in Group II without retroperitoneal node dissection. One must be aware that retroperitoneal node dissection has not been proved to offer a beneficial therapeutic effect, though it will confirm the diagnosis.[28, 29] If there is indication of retroperitoneal disease, the nodes should be removed. Any suspicion that tumor has involved the scrotal wall should lead to hemiscrotectomy. Presumed spread to inguinal nodes should result in node dissection. If scrotal radiotherapy is given, the contralateral testicle should first be transplanted to the thigh.

Using the treatment principles outlined in Table 30–2, the prognosis for paratesticular RMS is good. In a group of patients with clinically advanced disease, 71% were tumor-free at greater than 15 months.[4] With a more favorable group of children, 89% were free of disease at more than eight months.[29]

RMS of the Female Genital Tract

When excision appeared to be the only effective tool against tumors from this site, a strong case was made for exenterative surgery.[2, 18] It then became clear that by adding chemotherapy and radiotherapy to treatment regimens a very high percentage of cures could be attained without violating the urinary tract.[22] More recently it has been shown that female genital tract RMS is particularly susceptible to chemotherapy.[14] In this latest series, Hays and associates re-

Table 30–2. PARATESTICULAR RMS IN CHILDREN—MULTIDISCIPLINE THERAPY

Surgery	Radical orchiectomy	All patients
	Ipsilateral retroperitoneal node dissection	If necessary to render the patient free of macroscopic tumor
	Hemiscrotectomy	
	Inguinal node dissection	
	Contralateral retroperitoneal node dissection	
Chemo-therapy	VAC for 1 to 2 years	All patients
Radiotherapy	4000 to 5500 rads	If node dissection is positive; if there is residual local tumor

ported nine patients with vaginal lesions, eight of whom presented without distant metastases. These eight with localized disease all had a two-year course of multiple-agent chemotherapy. Six of the eight had incomplete initial tumor resection (five gross and one microscopic tumor residual), and six had no or inadequate radiotherapy. All eight were alive and tumor-free at the time of reporting (36 to 84 months after commencing observation). One patient had had an inguinal node recurrence, but after node dissection and further chemotherapy was then disease-free 3.5 years after this relapse. If the natural history of tumors from this site, the therapy administered, and the success achieved are all considered together, the only conclusion that can be reached is "an exceptional response to chemotherapy." Why the response of these nine tumors should be better than with RMS from other sites is not clear, but their histologic classification is pertinent. Seven tumors were botryoid embryonal, and the two remaining were embryonal.

At present the following can be said about pediatric vaginal RMS: (1) pelvic exenteration (anterior or total) is rarely required for cure; (2) these tumors respond very well to multiple-agent chemotherapy. Whether or not this response is universal, and whether or not it is so good that postsurgical residual tumor should be treated without radiotherapy or further surgery, are points that need elucidation from further studies and even longer follow-up.

In the light of current knowledge, it is suggested that pediatric vaginal RMS be treated as in Table 30–3. Based on the data available, close to 100% tumor cure can be expected for those patients presenting without distant metastases.

Only small numbers of vulval lesions are available for review. With Group I patients, excellent results can be expected following complete local excision and two years of multiple-agent chemotherapy.[13, 14] Radiotherapy may need to be added to cure those children with microscopic residual or lymph node involvement.[4]

Bladder and Prostatic RMS

In a 1973 review of the literature, Tefft and Jaffe found that no child with bladder RMS had been saved by partial cystectomy alone.[34] This contrasts with more recent re-

Table 30–3. VAGINAL RMS IN CHILDREN PRIMARY CHEMOTHERAPY

Step 1	Biopsy	
Step 2	Chemotherapy (VAC) and reevaluate at 8 out of 52 weeks	Responders continue VAC; nonresponders require surgical excision
Step 3	Tumor excision	When response to Step 2 ceases At 8 out of 52 weeks, if no response or progression on Step 2
Step 4	Continue VAC	For 1 to 2 years
Step 5*	Irradiation or further surgery	If Step 3 is not complete

*May represent overtreatment for Group II and Group III patients but must be recommended until the extent of the chemotherapeutic response of vaginal RMS is further evaluated.

ports that showed that segmental bladder resection was not followed by tumor recurrence, providing the surgery achieved complete tumor excision and the patient stayed on chemotherapy for two years.[14, 15] This change in prognosis for Group I children treated by partial cystectomy must be attributed to the effect of chemotherapy, since the patients in the above series were randomly chosen with respect to radiotherapy and it was not administered to all. For obvious reasons, bladder RMS lesions of the dome and lateral wall were those most likely to be treated by partial cystectomy. If anterior exenteration placed a child in Group I or Group II and that patient was then treated with multiple-agent chemotherapy (plus radiotherapy for a Group II patient), such a child could be expected to do well. In 1982, Hays and associates reported on 10 children whose treatment met the above criteria. There were nine Group II patients and one in Group I, with only two recurrences at more than 30 months (both were in Group II patients). One of these relapses was distant and was fatal, whereas the other was a local recurrence that responded well to chemotherapy and radiotherapy. Of interest, this last child was the only one of the nine Group II patients not to receive radiotherapy immediately after exenteration.[15] The one child in this same report who was placed in Group III by anterior exenteration had subsequent chemotherapy and radiotherapy and was disease-free at more than 63 months.

The prognosis for prostatic RMS was hopeless until 20 years ago,[11, 23] clearly showing that the tumor cannot be cured by surgery alone. However, it has now been established that prostatic RMS is very responsive to chemotherapy and radiotherapy and has a good prognosis with multidisciplinary therapy.[15] Hays and associates have reported on two Group I, nine Group II, and three Group III patients all treated by exenterative surgery and chemotherapy with radiotherapy also administered to the Group II and Group III children. These 14 patients did not show a single relapse at 34 to 91 months of follow-up. One child had died of treatment-related causes but was tumor-free.

It can be seen from the above that excisional surgery followed by chemotherapy and radiotherapy gives very impressive cure rates of both bladder and prostatic RMS. However, the proven efficacy of multiagent chemotherapy, plus a desire to improve the quality of life by avoiding extirpative pelvic surgery whenever possible, has resulted in a considerable deviation from the traditional treatment approach to these tumors.[25] Primary intensive multiagent chemotherapy with subsequent chemotherapy, surgery, and radiation therapy, as outlined in Figure 30–1, is now the recommended management.

There is little reason to doubt that primary chemotherapy with routine secondary excision of residual tumor will give excellent survival rates. In fact, it is clear that this can be accomplished.[6, 10, 15, 20] In some the continuity of the urinary tract can be reconstructed, as by radical prostatectomy[13, 20] or by partial cystectomy.[6, 10, 20] In some the urinary tract stays in continuity because no excisional surgery appears to be necessary.[10, 20]

However, it must not be thought that exenterative surgery is a rare necessity. It currently appears that at least a third of children with RMS of the bladder, prostate, or both will be left without a functional lower urinary tract.[10, 16, 20]

CONCLUSION

In the last 20 years a dramatic improvement has been seen in the management of pediatric pelvic sarcomas. Although the initial progress resulted from localized interdisciplinary cooperation, more recent advances have come about by intercenter coordination. With multiagent chemotherapy, the role of surgery has diminished. The surgical challenge presently is to (1) attempt salvage of extremely ill children, as no RMS patient can now be considered beyond potential cure, and (2) design any excisional

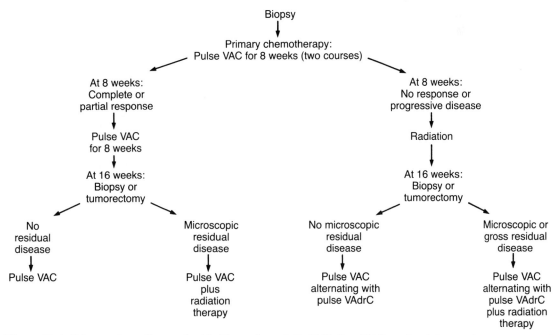

Figure 30–1. Primary chemotherapy for bladder and prostatic RMS. Key: VAC = vincristine, actinomycin D, and cyclophosphamide; VAdrC = vincristine, doxorubin (Adriamycin), and cyclophosphamide.

surgery to preserve maximum function. This surgery can involve delicate reconstruction on tissues affected by radiation and in patients debilitated by chemotherapy.

There are two main objectives of the current clinical studies: (1) to further improve patient survival rates, and (2) to attain tumor cure and at the same time achieve reduced morbidity. Unfortunately, surgery, radiotherapy, and chemotherapy all have the potential to damage normal tissue. Thus, the ultimate protocol—cure with zero morbidity—may have to await the development of new treatment modalities.

References

1. Crist WM, Raney RB, Tefft M, et al: Soft-tissue sarcomas arising in the retroperitoneal space in children: a report from the IRS Committee. Cancer 56:21–32, 1986.
2. Daniel WW, Koss LG, Brunschwig A: Sarcoma botryoides of the vagina. Cancer 12:74–84, 1959.
3. Donaldson SS: The value of adjuvant chemotherapy in the management of sarcomas in children. Cancer 55:2184–2197, 1985.
4. Exelby PR, Ghavimi F, Jereb B: Genitourinary rhabdomyosarcoma in children. J Pediatr Surg 13:746–752, 1978.
5. Flamant F, Hill CF: The improvement in survival associated with combined chemotherapy in childhood rhabdomyosarcoma. A historical comparison of 345 patients in the same center. Cancer 53:2417–2421, 1984.
6. Fleming ID, Etcubanas E, Patterson R, et al: The role of surgical resection when combined with chemotherapy and radiation in the management of pelvic rhabdomyosarcoma. Ann Surg 199:509–514, 1984.
7. Gaiger AM, Soule EH, Newton WA Jr: Pathology of rhabdomyosarcoma: experience of the Intergroup Rhabdomyosarcoma Study, 1972–78. NCI Monogr 56:19–27, 1981.
8. Gehan EA, Glover FN, Maurer HM, et al: Prognostic factors in children with rhabdomyosarcoma. NCI Monogr 56:83–92, 1981.
9. Ghavimi F, Exelby PR, Lieberman PH, et al: Multidisciplinary treatment of embryonal rhabdomyosarcoma in children: a progress report. NCI Monogr 56:111–120, 1981.
10. Ghavimi F, Herr H, Jereb B, Exelby PR: Treatment of genitourinary rhabdomyosarcoma in children. J Urol 132:313–319, 1984.
11. Goodwin WE, Mims MM, Young HH: Rhabdomyosarcoma of the prostate in a child: First 5-year survival. (Combined treatment by preoperative, local irradiation; actinomycin D; intra-arterial nitrogen mustard and hypothermia; radical surgery and ureterosigmoidostomy). J Urol 99:651–655, 1968.
12. Hammond GD: Multidisciplinary clinical investigation of the cancers of children: a model for the management of adults with cancer. Cancer 55:1215–1225, 1985.
13. Hardy, BE: (Unpublished data).
14. Hays DM, Raney RB Jr, Lawrence W Jr, et al: Rhabdomyosarcoma of the female urogenital tract. J Pediatr Surg 16:828–834, 1981.
15. Hays DM, Raney RB Jr, Lawrence W Jr, et al: Bladder and prostatic tumors in the Inter-group Rhabdomyosarcoma Study (IRS-1): results of therapy. Cancer 50:1472–1482, 1982.
16. Hays DM, Raney RB Jr, Lawrence W Jr, et al: Primary chemotherapy in the treatment of children with bladder-prostate tumors in the Intergroup Rhabdomyosarcoma Study (IRS-II). J Pediatr Surg 17:812–820, 1982.
17. Heyn RM, Holland R, Newton WA Jr, et al: The role of combined chemotherapy in the treatment of rhabdomyosarcoma in children. Cancer 34:2128–2141, 1974.
18. Hilgers RD, Malkasian GD Jr, Soule RH: Embryonal rhabdomyosarcoma (botryoid type) of the vagina: a clinicopathologic review. Am J Obstet Gynecol 107:484–502, 1970.
19. Jaffe N, McNeese M, Mayfield JK, Riseborough EJ: Childhood urologic cancer therapy related sequelae and their impact on management. Cancer 45:1815–1822, 1980.
20. Kaplan WE, Firlit CF, Berger RM: Genitourinary rhabdomyosarcoma. J Urol 130:116–119, 1983.
21. Kingston JE, McElwain TJ, Malpas JS: Childhood rhabdomyosarcoma: experience of the children's Solid Tumour Group. Br J Cancer 48:195–207, 1983.
22. Kumar APM, Wrenn EL Jr, Fleming ID, et al: Combined therapy to prevent complete pelvic exenteration for rhabdomyosarcoma of the vagina or uterus. Cancer 37:118–122, 1976.
23. Marshall VF: A five-year cure of rhabdomyosarcoma of the prostate in childhood. J Pediatr Surg 4:366–369, 1969.
24. Maurer HM: The Intergroup Rhabdomyosarcoma Study (NIH): Objectives and clinical staging classification. J Pediatr Surg 10:977–978, 1975.
25. Maurer HM: The Intergroup Rhabdomyosarcoma Study II: Objectives and study design. J Pediatr Surg 15:371–372, 1980.
26. Maurer HM: The Intergroup Rhabdomyosarcoma Study: Update, November 1978. NCI Monogr 56:61–68, 1981.
27. Maurer HM: The Intergroup Rhabdomyosarcoma Study. Cancer Bull 34:108–110, 1982.
28. Olive D, Flamant F, Zucker JM, et al: Paraaortic lymphadenectomy is not necessary in the treatment of localized paratesticular rhabdomyosarcoma. Cancer 54:1283–1287, 1984.
29. Raney RB Jr, Hays DM, Lawrence W Jr, et al: Paratesticular rhabdomyosarcoma in childhood. Cancer 42:729–736, 1978.
30. Ray B, Hajdu SI, Whitmore WF Jr: Distribution of retroperitoneal lymph node metastases in testicular germinal tumors. Cancer 33:340–348, 1974.
31. Russell WO, Cohen J, Edmonson JH, et al: Staging system for soft tissue sarcoma. Semin Oncol 8:156–159, 1981.
32. Ruymann FB, Newton WA Jr, Ragab AH, et al: Bone marrow metastases at diagnosis in children and adolescents with rhabdomyosarcoma. A report from The Intergroup Rhabdomyosarcoma Study. Cancer 53:368–373, 1984.
33. Simone JV, Cassaday JR, Filler RM: Cancers of childhood. In VT DeVita Jr, S Hellman, SA Rosenberg (eds), Cancer—Principles and Practice of Oncology. Toronto, JB Lippincott, 1982, pp 1254–1327.

34. Tefft M, Jaffe N: Sarcoma of the bladder and prostate in children: rationale for the role of radiation therapy based on a review of the literature and a report of fourteen additional patients. Cancer 32:1161–1177, 1973.

35. Tefft M, Lindberg RD, Gehan EA: Radiation therapy combined with systemic chemotherapy and rhabdomyosarcoma in children: local control in patients enrolled in the Intergroup Rhabdomyosarcoma Study. NCI Monogr 56:75–81, 1981.

36. Vance D, King DR, Boles ET Jr: Secondary thyroid neoplasms in pediatric cancer patients: increased risk with improved survival. J Pediatr Surg 19:855–860, 1984.

37. Voute PA, Vos A, deKraker J, Behrendt H: Rhabdomyosarcomas: chemotherapy and limited supplementary treatment program to avoid mutilation. NCI Monogr 56:121–125, 1981.

38. Williams DIO, Martin J: Tumors of the lower genitourinary tract. In DI Williams, JH Johnston (eds), Pediatric Urology, 2nd ed. London, Butterworth, 1982, pp 411.

39. Young JL, Miller RW: Incidence of malignant tumors in U.S. children. J Pediatr 86:254–258, 1975.

EILA C. SKINNER, M.D.
DONALD G. SKINNER, M.D.

Management of Carcinoma of the Female Urethra

CHAPTER 31

Carcinoma of the female urethra accounts for less than one out of 50,000 malignancies in women. Urethral carcinoma is the only urologic cancer more common in women than in men. Fewer than 1000 cases have been reported to date, with most series including less than 20 patients. These tumors commonly occur in the sixth and seventh decades, although several patients under 40 have been reported.[4, 9, 16] Because of the rarity of the lesion, treatment recommendations are often based on anecdotal successes. In general, the prognosis has been poor except in superficial lesions confined to the anterior or distal third of the urethra.

PATHOLOGY

The female urethra is approximately 4 cm in length, lined with transitional epithelium in its proximal third and squamous epithelium in its distal two thirds. The periurethral glands of Skene empty into the urethra primarily at the meatus but may extend along this entire length. They are lined with stratified and pseudostratified columnar epithelium. Any of these three epithelial types may undergo neoplastic change, and in general distal lesions are more likely to be squamous and proximal lesions transitional cell or adenocarcinoma. Overall, squamous cell carcinoma predominates, and the incidence of the various histologic types in 16

series of 594 patients is shown in Table 31–1.[1–8, 10, 12, 14–16, 20]

Prognosis does not appear to be related to histologic features, and for treatment purposes the different tumor types can be considered a single entity. An exception to this is primary urethral melanoma. Approximately 40 cases have been reported to date, and this is the most common site of primary melanoma of the urinary tract. Some theorize that these lesions actually represent metastases from a primary skin lesion that has spontaneously regressed. Urethral melanoma has had a much worse prognosis than other urethral cancers, with only a few long-term survivors reported. Treatment has usually been surgical, and early recurrence or metastases have been the rule.[13]

Carcinoma of the urethra may be confined

Table 31–1. INCIDENCE OF HISTOLOGIC TYPES FOR CARCINOMA OF THE FEMALE URETHRA*

Tumor Histology	Number of Patients	Percentage of Total
Squamous Cell	345	58
Transitional Cell	95	16
Adenocarcinoma	103	17
Other†	51	9
Total	594	100

*See references 1 to 8, 10, 12, 14 to 16, and 20.
†Includes melanoma, undifferentiated tumors, and patients with undocumented histologic results.

to the urethral mucosa (carcinoma in situ) or may extend through the lamina propria, invade the muscularis, and extend into the periurethral tissues. Adjacent structures including the bladder neck, vagina, vulva, and pubic rami may be involved by direct extension. Carcinoma has also been discovered arising within a urethral diverticulum. These are most often transitional cell or adenocarcinoma and appear to have a better prognosis than other urethral carcinomas, perhaps because of earlier stage at diagnosis.[15]

The lymphatic drainage of the urethra is to the inguinal nodes distally and to the external iliac and hypogastric pelvic nodes proximally. The actual incidence of nodal involvement of urethral carcinoma at the time of presentation is unknown. The reported incidence of palpable inguinal lymphadenopathy varies from 35 to 60%.[8, 10, 15] These nodes are nearly always found to be metastatic rather than reactive on biopsy.[9] However, the ability to clinically detect involvement of deep pelvic nodes with current radiologic techniques is notoriously poor. Because pelvic lymph node dissection has not routinely been done in this disease, there are no good figures available as to the expected rate of pelvic node metastases for each stage. Grabstald did report that 50% of the patients who ultimately came to pelvic node dissection had positive nodes.[8, 9]

Urethral carcinoma metastasizes primarily to lung, liver, bones, and brain, probably due to hematogenous spread. Several series have noted the lack of correlation between lymph node metastases and the appearance of distant disease.[9, 15] Less than 10% of the patients have distant metastases at the time of initial presentation. Local recurrence is the most common cause of failure after treatment and usually precedes the appearance of distant disease.[18]

The etiology of urethral carcinoma is unknown. An association with chronic infection or irritation has been suggested, as with male urethral carcinoma, but the majority of the cases have no such history. Several reports of carcinoma discovered in urethral caruncles have prompted some authors to recommend biopsy of all such lesions that do not respond quickly to treatment. No other predisposing factors have been delineated to date.[15]

DIAGNOSIS AND STAGING

The symptoms of urethral carcinoma vary somewhat depending on the location of the lesion. Urethral or vaginal spotting is most common, seen in 40 to 60% of all patients. Patients may also present with irritative voiding symptoms such as dysuria, urgency, frequency, and incontinence, and urinary obstruction may be seen especially in those with more proximal lesions. Up to 40% may present with a perineal mass, and pain and dyspareunia are also frequently noted.[2, 5, 6] Unfortunately, delay in diagnosis frequently occurs and is often due to symptoms attributed to other more common urologic and gynecologic illnesses.

Cystourethroscopy and biopsy are the cornerstones of the diagnostic work-up. Examination under anesthesia with palpation and biopsy of any suspicious inguinal lymph nodes is also necessary for staging. Radiologic studies to assess pelvic nodes, including CT scan and lymphangiogram, are of limited value because of substantial errors in interpretation with high false-negative and false-positive rates. Although pelvic nodal disease implies a poor prognosis, aggressive attempt to control pelvic disease may be warranted in light of the primarily local nature of these tumors. Further metastatic work-up should include chest x-ray, assessment of the liver (CT or liver scan), and bone scan.

Clinical stage is clearly the most important prognostic factor in urethral carcinoma. Two staging systems have evolved from Whitehouse's original division of tumors into urethral and vulvourethral (Table 31–2).[22] Grabstald's system, which arose from a basic division into "anterior" and "posterior or entire" tumors, is the most widely used today. The Prempree system, which was modified from Chau, does not provide a classification for superficial posterior lesions, which are admittedly rare. On the other hand, this system does separate vulvar from bladder neck involvement, which has a much worse prognosis. No matter which staging system is used, it is essential to differentiate lesions in the distal third from those involving either the entire or more proximal urethra. Depth of penetration or extent of the primary tumor correlates well with overall survival, regardless of type of

Table 31–2. STAGING SYSTEMS FOR CARCINOMA OF THE FEMALE URETHRA

Grabstald System*

O: Carcinoma in situ
A: Submucosal
B: Muscular (invading periurethral tissues)
C: Periurethral
    1: Invading muscular wall of vagina
    2: Invading muscle and mucosa of vagina
    3: Invading other adjacent structures (bladder, labia, clitoris)
D: Metastases
    1: Inguinal nodes
    2: Pelvic nodes
    3: Nodes above aortic bifurcation
    4: Distant metastases

Prempree System†

  I: Disease limited to distal half of urethra
 II: Entire urethra, with extension to periurethral tissues, but not involving vulva or bladder neck
III: a: Urethra and vulva
    b: Urethra and vaginal muscle
    c: Urethra and bladder neck
IV: a: Parametrium or paracolpium
    b: Metastases
        1: Inguinal nodes
        2: Pelvic nodes
        3: Para-aortic nodes
        4: Distant metastases

*From Grabstald H, et al: Cancer of the female urethra. JAMA 197:835–842, 1966.

†From Prempree T, et al: Radiation treatment of primary carcinoma of the female urethra. Cancer 42:1177–1184, 1978.

treatment. Bracken reported five-year survival rates of 45% for Stage A, 41% for Stage B, 26% for Stage C, and 18% for Stage D lesions.[5]

Fifty to 60% of patients present with lesions that are already in Stage C or D, and approximately 35 to 50% have clinically evident inguinal lymphadenopathy.[5, 10] Although there has been no published study of the accuracy of clinical staging, by analogy to other pelvic tumors there is undoubtedly a very significant degree of understaging by currently available methods.

Grading of urethral carcinoma has largely been borrowed from that developed for the various histologic types of bladder cancer. The prognostic importance of tumor grade, and therefore the impact it should have on treatment decisions, has not been adequately studied. However, Grabstald noted that low-stage lesions are more likely to be of lower grade than more extensive lesions.[9]

TREATMENT

Treatment of female urethral carcinoma has varied widely over time and from center to center. Surgery and radiation therapy have been used alone and in various combinations, with chemotherapy primarily reserved for metastatic disease and, in general, ineffective. Attempts to draw conclusions about the efficacy of any one treatment approach are severely hampered by the small number of patients in each series and by the lack of uniformity of treatment. Many authors have not reported their results in terms of the stage of presentation, and in addition, many of the larger series span 25 years or more, during which time techniques of surgery and radiation therapy have changed dramatically. Thus only broad generalizations can be made about treatment recommendations in this disease, which must still be approached on a case-to-case basis.

Surgical approaches have historically included local resection, partial or total urethrectomy, and radical anterior exenteration, with or without vulvectomy or excision of the pubic rami. Inguinal node dissection has generally been reserved for patients with palpable adenopathy. Pelvic node dissection has usually been done only as part of a radical cystourethrectomy, and then only by a few surgeons. Operative mortality from anterior exenteration has been as high as 20% in some reports but should be well under 5% with modern surgical techniques.[15] Surgical complications include wound infection, small bowel obstruction, lymphedema, and complications of urinary diversion. Excision of the inferior pubic rami can be accomplished without significant increased morbidity and does not appear to lead to pelvic girdle instability.[14]

Radiation therapy has evolved from the older methods of orthovoltage external beam and permanent gold or radon implants to modern supervoltage techniques, with radium needles or iridium wires used for brachytherapy. Vaginal intracavitary treatment has also been used to supplement interstitial therapy. Protocols are generally designed to deliver 5000 to 7000 total rads to the tumor area.[5, 17, 21] Complications from radiation therapy have been as high as 42% in some reports. Urethral strictures are most common, followed by incontinence, radiation cystitis and enteritis, mucosal ulcers, and fistulae.[5] The latter often result from recurrent pelvic carcinoma rather than the radiation therapy itself. Most modern series have noted a decrease in complication rates to as low as 5 to 10%, probably due to improved delivery techniques.[16]

In superficial distal urethral lesions, Stage A or I, interstitial radiation therapy alone has achieved excellent results. Cure rates of 60 to over 80% are consistently reported.[7, 8, 20, 21] Surgical excision with partial urethrectomy has also achieved cure in most Stage A patients. Up to two thirds of the urethra can be excised with the tumor without incontinence, allowing for good surgical margins for small superficial distal lesions.[15] Thus either wide excision or interstitial radiation therapy may be used for these low-stage tumors. Theoretically, carcinoma in situ and exophytic lesions can be treated with transurethral resection. However, there are only rare reports of the disease discovered at this early stage, and concerns about understaging might prompt a more aggressive treatment.

The approach to proximal invasive urethral carcinoma, Stages B and C, is quite controversial. Historically, these patients have done poorly regardless of the mode of therapy. Five-year survival rates of less than 20% are typical of most series of patients treated before 1975.[19] Grabstald reported on 38 patients with carcinoma of the proximal or entire urethra in 1966. Eleven of 13 treated with radiation therapy alone suffered local recurrence, as did six of 10 treated with surgery and seven of 14 treated with a combined approach.[9] Similar results were reported in 12 additional patients treated from 1966 to 1972.[8]

Recent reports suggest some improvement in outcome. Johnson described 29 patients treated at the MD Anderson Hospital since 1974. One of two patients in Stage B and four of six in Stage C were alive and disease-free from one to six years following radiation therapy alone. The other two Stage C patients died without recurrence at one and three years. Seven Stage C and D_1 patients were treated with combined radiation plus anterior exenteration. Three of these were disease-free, though with less than one year follow-up.[12] The MD Anderson group however, does not separate their results according to tumor location, and many of the patients who were successfully managed by irradiation may have had favorable, distal-third lesions.

Prempree has recently reported improved survival in a few patients treated with external beam plus interstitial radiation therapy alone. Two of four patients in Stage II and four of five in Stage III achieved five-year survival without recurrence with this approach. The latter cures included one Stage IIIc patient with bladder neck involvement. Prempree now recommends surgery only for Stage IIIc and for recurrent disease following primary radiation therapy.[16] However, survival following salvage surgery for a local recurrence has historically been very poor.[5] Based on our own experience, it would seem appropriate to perform another biopsy six weeks after completion of radiation therapy on all patients with proximal urethral tumor or any patient with residual palpable abnormality. Any patient with evidence of residual or recurrent disease should be promptly considered for aggressive ablative surgery.

Our own experience has been that lesions in the distal third of the urethra can be easily controlled and treated by local excision with or without postoperative radiation therapy regardless of histologic results. On the other hand, proximal or panurethral tumors invading the muscularis represent the most difficult and challenging urologic malignancy to cure. Of 15 proximal urethral tumors seen over a 10-year period, only one was cured by radiation therapy alone.

In order to try to improve survival, we have utilized an aggressive combined-modality approach to invasive proximal urethral carcinoma. Forty-five hundred rads of external radiation is initially delivered over a four- to six-week period, with or without a 2000-rad boost with isotope brachytherapy, followed six weeks later by anterior exenteration with en bloc removal of the inferior rim of the pubic ramus together with some form of urinary diversion. Of 11 patients, all had residual cancer at the time of surgery. This approach was effective in controlling the primary tumors, as only one recurred in the pelvis. Four of 11 (36%) survived beyond three years; the rest developed distant metastases, all within two years of treatment.

SURGICAL TECHNIQUE

The goal of any surgical approach is to achieve local control, since pelvic recurrence has been the commonest cause of ultimate failure and characteristically occurs before distant metastases are seen. Traditional ablative surgical approaches often fail to achieve adequate margins around the periurethral infrapubic region. We have utilized, since 1972, a surgical approach in which the inferior rim of the pubis can be

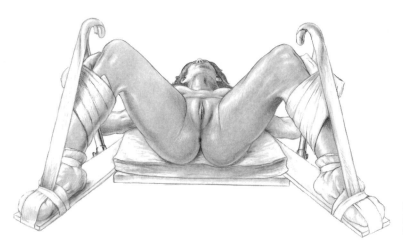

Figure 31–1. Modified frog-leg position as seen from foot of operating table.

resected en bloc with the anterior pelvic organs including the anterior vaginal wall, vulva, and clitoris.

Preoperative preparation is the same as that described in Chapter 42 on the technique of radical cystectomy. Patient positioning, however, differs in order to provide necessary exposure to the vaginal area. The patient is placed in a hyperextended frog-leg position with the feet separated to allow the surgeon direct access to the perineum (Fig. 31–1). The operation commences through a long midline incision. A pelvic lymph node dissection and the lateral and posterior pedicles are developed and divided as described in Chapter 42. Once the vagina has been opened distal to the cervix, the posterior pedicle is divided by incising the lateral vaginal wall on each side distally so that the anterior vaginal wall remains attached to the anterior pelvic organs.

After the vagina is incised approximately two thirds of the way distally, attention is directed to the perineum. The midline incision is continued over the pubis into the perineum (Figs. 31–2 and 31–3). It is then directed around the clitoris and along the vulva on either side of the vagina until the 180° point of the vaginal circumference is reached. The incision is deepened with cautery down to the inferior ischial rim of the pubic ramus on either side. A periosteal elevator with assistance of the cautery should then free the origins of the adductor muscles from the anterior ischial rim and pubic ramus laterally to the obturator foramen. Then the lateral vagina is incised proximally on each side to join up with the

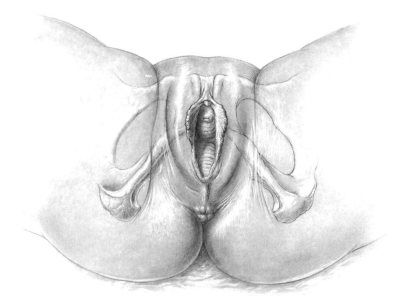

Figure 31–2. View of perineum with underlying body structures superimposed.

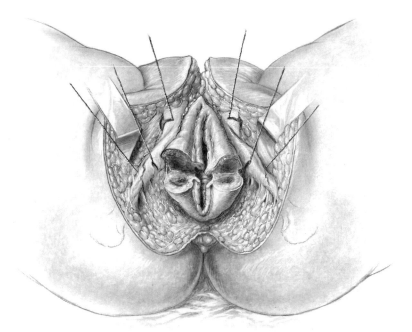

Figure 31–3. Diagram showing position of three Gigli saws that will allow en bloc removal of the anterior vaginal wall and inferior rim of the pubis with the bladder and lymph node specimen.

vaginal incision started within the abdomen (Fig. 31–3).

Next, a blunt, curved Kocher clamp is passed gently through the obturator foramen from the perineum into the pelvis. Care should be taken to make sure the clamp is medial to the obturator nerve and to avoid the obturator vessels previously ligated within the pelvis. One end of a Gigli wire saw can then be attached to the Kocher clamp and gently passed through the obturator foramen from the pelvis to the perineum. Another curved Kocher clamp is then passed medially to the ischium and the other end of the Gigli saw grasped within the pelvis and brought out to the perineum.

A second Gigli saw is then positioned around the opposite ischial rim of the pubic ramus by a similar technique. Next, curved Kocher clamps are again passed through each obturator foramen and the two ends of a third Gigli saw grasped within the pelvis, and each are gently brought out into the perineum; the two ends are joined at that location. This third saw will allow the pubis to be divided in half horizontally. The three Gigli saws have thus been placed so that once remaining soft tissue between the lateral vaginal wall and the ischial rim of the pubic ramus has been divided, three cuts in the pubis will allow all of the anterior pelvic organs to be removed en bloc with the lower rim of the pubis. This maneuver provides excellent and wide margins around the periurethral tissue (Fig. 31–3).

The perineum can be easily closed by mobilizing the posterior vaginal wall to bring it anteriorly and by sewing the lateral edges to the incised vulva. The wound can be closed primarily in the area of the resected clitoris. A polyglycolic acid mesh can be used within the pelvis to further reinforce the pelvic floor and prevent a possible enterocele. In two young patients we have utilized bilateral myocutaneous gracilis flaps for pelvic closure and to reconstruct a functional vagina. This additional procedure significantly lengthens an already long and tedious operation and would rarely seem indicated in the vast majority of patients with primary urethral carcinoma.

We have found that removal of the inferior rim of the pubis is better than an attempt to remove the entire central pubis. The anterior pubic ramus is not anatomically associated with the urethra and is an unnecessary part of a successful cancer operation. In addition, total pubectomy may lead to sacroiliac subluxation and instability, producing postoperative morbidity, which we have observed in one obese patient.

This operation carries the same postoperative complication rate as that seen following radical cystectomy, as described in Chapter 42. An additional unique late sequela may be a development of osteitis pubis with pain and adductor muscle spasm. This complication was observed in two of 11 patients. Preoperative radiation in excess of 5000 total rads may increase the risk of this complication. Conservative reassurance and analgesic support is about all one can do to relieve the problem, which is usually self-limited and refractory to heparin anticoagulation and anti-inflammatory medication.

RESULTS

Eleven patients undergoing this surgical approach ranged from 36 to 82 years, with a median age of 61 years. Nine underwent the operation as part of the combined treatment protocol, and two underwent the operation as a salvage procedure after failure of definitive radiation therapy plus interstitial radiation. Both patients undergoing the salvage procedure developed widespread metastases four and six months following surgery even though neither developed local recurrence. Neither of these patients were referred for surgery until clear evidence of significant local recurrence developed, five and six months following radiation therapy, respectively.

Of the nine patients treated with the planned combined approach, four (44%) have survived from four to 11 years following surgery without recurrence. A fifth patient is alive without disease at two years. There was one postoperative death due to pulmonary embolus. The remaining three patients all developed widespread metastases within two years, although only one had documented pelvic recurrence.

Various combinations of chemotherapy have been tried for patients with metastatic disease without any appreciable success, regardless of primary histologic findings.

COMMENTARY

Proximal invasive urethral carcinoma remains the most aggressive and virulent of all urologic cancers. Earlier diagnosis and more aggressive combined therapy will be necessary in order to improve survival. Currently, most urologic oncologists recommend a combined radiotherapy-surgical approach. We recommend 4500 rads of external beam radiation therapy with or without a brachytherapy boost followed by anterior exenteration and pelvic lymph node dissection, with resection of the inferior pubic ramus, anterior vaginal wall, and vulva as described herein. Inguinal lymph node dissection is reserved for patients in whom metastatic nodes were found on biopsy.

We look for further reports of successful therapy by definitive radiation therapy as reported by Prempree and associates. Brachytherapy would seem ideally suited for local control, but we have observed the successful treatment of only one patient by radiation alone. If radiotherapy is chosen as initial treatment, extremely close follow-up and repeated biopsies must be done if subsequent salvage surgery can offer any hope of cure.

Treatment of distant metastases has been mainly palliative. The role of various chemotherapy regimens has not been studied systematically owing to the paucity of patients. Chemotherapy may also eventually have a place in adjunctive treatment of advanced local disease, but to date no drug or combination has been reported that has achieved control or cure of known metastatic disease.

In conclusion, urethral carcinoma in women is a rare disease that is clearly curable when diagnosed early and treated aggressively. Invasive posterior lesions have historically carried a dismal prognosis, but modern techniques of surgery and radiation therapy may be improving the outlook for this disease. A high index of suspicion, accurate staging, and aggressive treatment aimed at the local disease are the cornerstones of urethral cancer management.

References

1. Allen R, Nelson RP: Primary urethral malignancy: review of 22 cases. South Med J 71:547–550, 1978.
2. Antoniades J: Radiation therapy in carcinoma of the female urethra. Cancer 24:70–76, 1969.
3. Benson RC Jr, Tunca JC, Buchler DA, Uehling DT: Primary carcinoma of the female urethra. Gynecol Oncol 14:313–318, 1982.
4. Bolduan JP, Farah RN: Primary urethral neoplasms: review of 30 cases. J Urol 125:198–200, 1981.
5. Bracken RB, Johnson DE, Miller LS, et al: Primary carcinoma of the female urethra. J Urol 116:188–192, 1976.
6. Chu A: Female urethral carcinoma. Ther Radiol 107:627–630, 1973.
7. Elkon D, Kim JA, Huddleston AL, Constable WC: Primary carcinoma of the female urethra. South Med J 73:1439–1442, 1980.
8. Grabstald H: Tumors of the urethra in men and women. Cancer 32:1236–1255, 1973.
9. Grabstald H, Hilaris B, Henschke U, Whitmore WF: Cancer of the female urethra. JAMA 197:835–842, 1966.

10. Hopkins S, Vider M, Nag SK, et al: Carcinoma of the female urethra. J Urol 106:454–457, 1976.
11. Howe GE, Prentiss RJ, Mullenix RB, Feeney MJ: Carcinoma of the urethra: diagnosis and treatment. J Urol 89:232–235, 1963.
12. Johnson DE, O'Connell JR: Primary carcinoma of the female urethra. Urology 21:42–45, 1983.
13. Katz JI, Grabstald H: Primary malignant melanoma of the female urethra. J Urol 116:454–457, 1976.
14. Klein FA, Whitmore WF Jr, Herr HW, et al: Inferior pubic rami resection with en bloc radical excision for invasive proximal urethral carcinoma. Cancer 51:1238–1242, 1983.
15. Pointon RC, Poole-Wilson DS: Primary carcinoma of the urethra. Br J Urol 40:682–693, 1968.
16. Prempree T, Amornmarn R, Patanaphan V: Radiation therapy in primary carcinoma of the female urethra: II. An update on results. Cancer 54:729–733, 1984.
17. Prempree T, Wizenberg MJ, Scott RM: Radiation treatment of primary carcinoma of the female urethra. Cancer 42:1177–1184, 1978.
18. Schellhammer PF: Urethral carcinoma. Semin Urol 1:82–89, 1983.
19. Sullivan J, Grabstald H: Management of carcinoma of the urethra. In DG Skinner, JB deKernion (eds), Genitourinary Cancer. Philadelphia, WB Saunders, 1978, pp 419–429.
20. Turner AG, Hendry WF: Primary carcinoma of the female urethra. Br J Urol 52:549–554, 1980.
21. Weghaupt K, Gerstner GJ, Kucera H: Radiation therapy for primary carcinoma of the female urethra: a survey over 25 years. Gynecol Oncol 17:58–63, 1984.
22. Whitehouse B: Primary carcinoma of the female urethra. Obstet Gynecol 20:269–276, 1911.
23. Zeigerman JH, Gordon SF: Cancer of the female urethra. A curable disease. Obstet Gynecol 36:785–789, 1970.

JEROME P. RICHIE, M.D.

Diagnosis and Staging of Testicular Tumors

CHAPTER 32

Carcinoma of the testis is a relatively rare cancer, accounting for only 2% of all cancers in men. The annual incidence in the United States is 2.5 per 100,000 males per year.[24] Nonetheless, testicular tumors are the most common malignancy in boys and men between the ages of 15 and 34 years and, until recently, represented the third leading cause of mortality in that age group.[40] The disease, occurring in a crucial evolutionary period of a young man's life, carries a profound social, economic, and emotional impact far beyond its seeming rarity.

Evidence is accumulating that the incidence of testicular cancer is increasing throughout the world. Skinner has reported a marked increase in incidence of testicular cancer in Los Angeles County, and the Dateca Series from Denmark showed an increased incidence of 1.5:1 over a 10-year period. This seems to represent a long-standing trend of increasing occurrence in young males in Europe and North America.[10, 36]

The incidence of testicular cancer varies significantly in different geographic areas. Testicular tumors are more rare in the black population than they are in the white population.[38] The continued low rate in the black population seems to be unique to that racial group, and the difference occurs regardless of the geographic origin of the group studied. A slightly lower incidence of testicular cancer exists in the Oriental race as well.

Testicular tumors have been noted at every age period of life, from newborn to the ninth decade. However, there are three peak age groups in which testicular tumors are more common. In the newborn and neonatal period, embryonal cell carcinoma and yolk sac tumor represent the most common types of testicular tumor. In the young adult, from 15 to 34, all varieties of germinal cell tumors occur. In the older age group, above 50, seminomas may occur, but the most common tumor of the testis in that age group is lymphoma.

The incidence of testicular cancer also varies with social class, with rates in the upper social classes approximately double those of the lower social classes. A similar gradient appears to exist among blacks as well.[30] Sporadic familial occurrence has been reported rarely.[39] Therefore, meaningful familial or genetic factors remain unknown.

ETIOLOGY

The etiology of testicular tumors is unknown, although such factors as age, trauma, repeated infections, familial or genetic elements, and possible endocrine abnormalities have been thought to contribute to their development. Cryptorchidism has the strongest etiologic relationship, with up to a 50-fold increase in the incidence of malignant degeneration in a patient with this condition. The risk of occurrence of testicular cancer seems to be greater in a patient with an abdominal cryptorchid testis than

498

in one with an inguinal cryptorchid testis.[34] The likelihood of malignant degeneration seems to be the same whether or not orchiopexy is performed.[2] There is some suggestion in the literature of a protective effect of orchiopexy performed prior to age 10.[23] A significant lag period exists between orchiopexy and the subsequent development of a testicular cancer; therefore, relatively recent changes in the timing of orchiopexy may not allow sufficient observation to assess a possible preventive effect. Subsequent development of a testicular cancer has been reported in a patient who underwent orchiopexy at six years of age.[11]

In patients with a history of cryptorchidism, not only the undescended testis but also the normally descended contralateral testis is at increased risk. In approximately 25% of patients with cryptorchidism who subsequently develop a testicular cancer, the tumor occurs in the normally descended contralateral testis.[15] Thus, there may be some relationship of dysgenesis as an etiologic factor in testicular tumors.

DIAGNOSTIC TECHNIQUES

Clinical

The most common symptoms related to testicular cancer are painless testicular enlargement or mass. Bosl and associates reported pain as an associated finding in 45% of their cases.[7] More commonly, however, the lack of pain, as well as the patient's fear of the diagnosis, result in significant delay in diagnosis from the time of initial recognition of the lesion until orchiectomy. This delay may be as long as 3 to 6 months in some instances. The length of delay correlates directly with an increased incidence of metastases.[25]

The most common symptom attributable to testicular cancer is painless testicular enlargement or a sensation of heaviness in the hemiscrotum. A mass or swelling is the presenting sign in 70 to 90% of individuals with testicular cancer. The testicular enlargement is usually gradual, although approximately 10% of individuals report rapid testicular involvement. Trauma may serve to call the individual's attention to the mass. Alternatively, the patient's sexual partner may identify the mass.

In approximately 10% of patients, the initial presenting symptoms are referable to metastases. These can include abdominal pain, anorexia, or back pain related to large retroperitoneal metastases. Retroperitoneal lymphadenopathy occasionally results in back pain, although testicular cancers rarely involve the bony skeleton. Patients with advanced pulmonary metastases may present with cough, hemoptysis, or dyspnea on exertion.

Gynecomastia may be seen as one of the early signs of a testicular tumor. Germ cell tumors of the testis that produce human chorionic gonadotropin may stimulate the Leydig cells to produce estradiol.[43]

The most common misdiagnosis in patients with testicular cancer is epididymitis or epididymo-orchitis. Associated inflammation, hemorrhage, or trauma may make initial examination difficult, and it may be impossible to determine whether a mass is intra- or extratesticular. Approximately 20% of patients with testicular tumor are initially thought to have epididymitis. If the patient is seen early, the enlarged epididymis can clearly be separated from the testis as a distinct entity. After several days of inflammation, however, differentiation may be impossible. In the past, if clinical circumstances have suggested epididymitis, the recommendation has been for antibiotic therapy for several weeks with reevaluation. Testicular ultrasonography can be quite helpful in allowing differentiation of intratesticular masses from extratesticular tumors or other lesions that may mimic testicular cancer.

The second most common erroneous diagnosis is hydrocele. The tumor may be cystic or somewhat soft in consistency and mimic the presentation of a hydrocele. Scrotal transillumination is important as an indicator of whether fluid is present or whether a solid mass exists. If the scrotal mass does not transmit light, exploration is mandatory. Aspiration of the "hydrocele" is contraindicated, as positive results of cytologic examination have been reported in hydroceles associated with testicular cancer.[26] Other diagnoses to be considered include hematocele, spermatocele, hematoma, and granulomatous orchitis.

Although the majority of intratesticular masses are malignant, benign tumors do exist but are extremely uncommon. The most

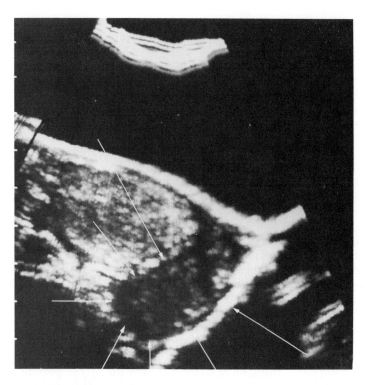

Figure 32–1. Testicular ultrasound recording revealing inflammation of the epididymis (arrows) and normal heterogeneity of the uninvolved testis.

common benign mass within the testicle is an epidermoid cyst. Usually, this represents a very small nodule just beneath the surface of the tunica albuginea, often with a history of several years' duration. Shah and associates reported a discrete mass with a mean diameter of 2 cm in 75% of his series of patients.[37] Epidermoid cysts may be difficult to differentiate histologically from teratoma, especially on frozen section. Epidermoid cysts contain keratin but lack other elements. The surgical approach for such a lesion is an inguinal incision, with orchiectomy preferred to excisional biopsy.[9]

Ultrasonography

Testicular ultrasonography has become an important diagnostic procedure and essentially is an extension of the physical examination. The development of more sophisticated equipment, including 8 and 10 megahertz (MHz) transducers, has increased the specificity and sensitivity of scrotal ultrasonography. The higher-megahertz transducers do not require a water bath. The use of high-resolution real-time scanning has improved imaging considerably. Scrotal ultrasound can now reliably distinguish extratesticular involvement, such as epididymitis (Fig. 32–1) from intratesticular lesions such as tumor (Fig. 32–2). Sample and co-workers reported on 55 patients with a diagnostic accuracy of more than 80%.[33] In 1982, Richie and associates reported on 243 ultrasound examinations, disclosing a high degree of accuracy.[27] Of 22 patients diagnosed by ultrasound to have tumor, 19 were confirmed,

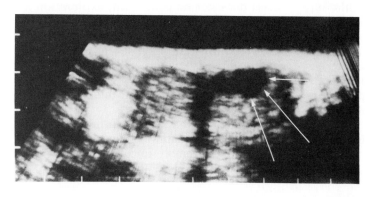

Figure 32–2. Testicular ultrasound recording revealing intratesticular echo-poor mass (arrows), histologically proven to be seminoma. Note normal contralateral side for comparison.

and there were three false-negative examination results. There were no false-positive results, confirming the importance of ultrasonography as a diagnostic adjunct. Recent studies show a sensitivity and specificity of 100% and 95%, respectively, with 5 and 8 MHz real-time scanners.[47]

Testicular CT scans and magnetic resonance imaging may represent technical advances, but experience to date has been quite limited. Magnetic resonance imaging has an advantage in a lack of radiation as well as ability to reconstruct images in multiple planes.

If a high clinical suspicion exists for the possibility of testicular tumor, inguinal exploration of the testis is mandatory. Scrotal incisions are absolutely contraindicated, as this alters the lymphatic drainage and, hence, subsequent therapeutic approaches. After division of the external oblique fascia, the spermatic cord is secured at the deep inguinal ring with a Penrose drain to prevent lymphatic spread, and the testicle is mobilized into the inguinal incision. Careful palpation of the mass through the tunica vaginalis can be performed, and radical orchiectomy completed if suspicion of tumor exists. Rarely, a wedge biopsy may be necessary prior to radical orchiectomy.

STAGING

Clinical staging serves to predict the presence or absence of residual tumor following orchiectomy as well as site and extent of remaining tumor. There is a variety of commonly applied staging systems, with varying

Table 32–2. CLASSIFICATION FOR EXTENT OF DISEASE

IIIA:	Disease confined to supraclavicular lymph nodes
IIIB-1:	Gynecomastia with or without elevation in biologic markers (AFP, hCG)
IIIB-2:	Minimal pulmonary disease (< 5 lesions in each lung field, with none > 2 cm in diameter)
IIIB-3:	Advanced pulmonary disease (any mediastinal, hilar lesion, positive pleural effusion, or pulmonary mass > 2 cm)
IIIB-4:	Visceral disease (excluding lung); liver, gastrointestinal tract, central nervous system, inferior vena caval or bone involvement fall into this category

degrees of complexity. Basically, however, all staging systems recognize three well-defined stages of tumor spread, as initially advocated by Boden and Gibb:[6] tumor confined to the testis, tumor metastases to the retroperitoneal lymphatics only, or tumor metastases to sites beyond the retroperitoneal lymphatics. Clinical staging is critically important because decisions for treatment are based upon a presumed orderly fashion of metastases, first to the retroperitoneal lymphatics and thence beyond. Furthermore, the extent and volume of metastases have important implications for treatment and prognosis. Therefore, most contemporary staging systems include subcategories to define the range of volume of metastases as well as extent.

The two most commonly utilized systems of staging, proposed by Maier[22] and Skinner,[41] are outlined in Table 32–1. A subclassification for patients with advanced disease is detailed in Table 32–2. Accurate staging

Table 32–1. STAGING OF TESTICULAR TUMORS

Walter Reed General Hospital*	Skinner†
IA: Confined to testis; no clinical or x-ray evidence of spread	A: Same, but includes no positive nodes on lymph node dissection
IB: Same as IA, but at lymph node dissection, metastases to iliac or para-aortic lymph nodes	B: Disease below diaphragm, normal mediastinum, normal chest x-ray
II: Disease below diaphragm, with no spread to visceral organs; clinical or x-ray evidence of metastases to para-aortic, femoral, inguinal, and iliac lymph nodes	B_1: < 6 positive nodes that are well encapsulated and show no extension into retroperitoneal fat
II+: Palpable abdominal mass (≥ 5 cm)	B_2: > 6 positive nodes that are capsular and may or may not show extension into retroperitoneal fat; any node > 2 cm
III: Disease above diaphragm or spread to body organs (clinical x-ray)	B_3: Bulky, palpable abdominal mass (> 5 cm)
	C: Metastases above diaphragm or liver involvement

*From Maier JG, Sulak MH: Proceedings: radiation therapy in malignant testis tumors. II. Carcinoma. Cancer 32:1212–1216, 1973.

†From Skinner DG: Non-seminomatous testis tumors: a plan of management based on 96 patients to improve survival in all stages by combined therapeutic modalities. J Urol 115:65–69, 1969.

allows for proper selection of the appropriate form of therapy.

A disadvantage of the two staging systems is a lack of information on the local extent of the primary tumor. A TNM classification proposed by the American College of Surgeons does include a detailed T stage for the evaluation of the primary tumor.[3] This classification, however, is rather cumbersome and has not met with widespread acceptance.

Clinical Evaluation for Metastases

After radical orchiectomy and histologic delineation of the neoplasm, staging procedures are used to identify potential sites of metastases. The extent of the staging procedure is dependent upon plans for therapy. With the development of newer techniques, a surfeit of diagnostic tests is available to attempt to delineate retroperitoneal or systemic involvement. With improved technology to detect small metastases, as well as improved chemotherapy to treat the patients with established metastases, controversy exists as to the appropriate diagnostic steps in the evaluation of patients with germ cell cancers. Should all available tests be used in each patient, regardless of expense? Treatment philosophy becomes an important variable as to whether retroperitoneal node dissection or chemotherapy is to be avoided. The recent development of sophisticated radiologic techniques, including ultrasound, CT scanning, and nuclear medicine and magnetic resonance imaging, allow focus of different techniques to delineate retroperitoneal or systemic involvement. The following diagnostic techniques will be evaluated critically as to their role in staging and their necessity depending upon therapeutic alternatives to be selected.

Physical Examination

Careful attention must be directed to possible sites of metastases, particularly in the supraclavicular area and in the cervical region. Eighty-five per cent of patients will have drainage to the left supraclavicular nodes, with 5% draining to the right supraclavicular region and 10% draining bilaterally.

A thorough abdominal examination should be performed, including palpation for abnormal masses or hepatomegaly. Inguinal nodes should be carefully palpated, especially in patients with prior scrotal or inguinal surgery or trans-scrotal violations. Careful examination of the breasts should be carried out for unilateral or bilateral gynecomastia, which may suggest the presence of trophoblastic elements in the primary lesion.

Chest X-Ray

The pulmonary parenchyma is involved as a site of metastases more commonly than any other location, with the exception of the retroperitoneal lymph glands. A routine chest x-ray will often detect mediastinal or pulmonary metastases; routine posteroanterior and lateral chest films will detect from 85 to 90% of patients with pulmonary metastases.[14] However, a small number of falsely positive or falsely negative chest x-ray results may occur, especially with smaller nodules. Demonstration of pulmonary tumor nodules is of critical importance in planning of therapy, as patients so identified have Stage C disease and are therefore treated initially with intensive combination chemotherapy. Without evidence of pulmonary metastases, however, most patients would undergo initial retroperitoneal lymphadenectomy or possibly be considered for some observation protocols. Pulmonary parenchymal or other intrathoracic metastases are found in 20 to 30% of patients undergoing initial staging.

Whole Lung Tomography and Chest CT Scans

Routine chest x-ray can detect chest lesions as small as 1 cm in diameter, but whole lung tomography can detect lesions as small as 5 or 6 mm in diameter, and computed tomography scanning can detect lesions down to 3 mm in diameter.[35] Nonetheless, as the window of detection becomes narrower, an appreciable lack of specificity occurs, giving rise to false-positive readings by the detection of small pulmonary granulomata. These factors have raised legitimate concerns about the use of whole lung tomography or CT scanning for routine screening in patients with testicular cancer.

Bergman and associates reported on 58 patients with testicular tumors and normal chest x-ray results, 19% of whom had lesions detected by whole lung tomography.[5] This study is in contrast with a previous study of 76 patients in whom whole lung tomography failed to detect a single metastatic lesion not previously found on routine chest films.[53]

Because of these discrepant studies, we embarked upon a large prospective study at our institution to evaluate the role of whole lung tomography versus conventional chest x-ray and to indicate how the addition of whole lung tomography would alter the therapeutic approach.[17] Both modalities were used in staging 120 patients in order to determine whether whole lung tomography provided added information that would be useful in patient management. In four patients there was a discrepancy with negative chest x-ray results and positive whole lung tomography findings. Three of the four patients had advanced abdominal disease and would be treated by chemotherapy in any event. In only one of the 120 patients was therapy altered by the addition of whole lung tomography. However, whole lung tomography did demonstrate more pulmonary parenchymal metastases than chest x-ray in 16 patients with multiple pulmonary metastases. From this prospective study we concluded that whole lung tomography was not a useful adjunct for routine staging of patients, especially those with minimal retroperitoneal involvement.

Tumor Markers

The term *tumor markers* in testicular cancer refers to several substances elaborated by various cells within testicular tumors: human chorionic gonadotropin (hCG and specifically the β sublevel), α-fetoprotein (AFP), and lactate dehydrogenase (LDH). Radioimmunoassay techniques for measuring hCG and AFP have provided dramatic improvements in monitoring patients with testicular cancer by markedly increasing the sensitivity of these assays.[50] LDH, although nonspecific, has been demonstrated to be of value, especially in delineation of the extent of metastases.[29]

Beta Human Chorionic Gonadotropin. Gonadotropins are composed of two polypeptide chains, the α and β subunits. The β subunit seems to be responsible for a majority of biologic activity of these hormones. The delineation of a specific antibody for the β subunit of hCG allows for a very sensitive and specific radioimmunoassay,

even in the presence of elevation of luteinizing hormone, which cross-reacts with the α subunit of hCG.[46] The β subunit of hCG, used in pregnancy tests in females, is not present in significant amounts in normal males and thus represents a very specific marker of tumor activity. The normal serum level of hCG is below 1 ng/ml, and its half-life in serum is approximately 18 to 24 hours. The level of hCG, shown to be elaborated by syncytiotrophoblastic cells, is elevated in 100% of patients with choriocarcinoma, 60% of patients with embryonal carcinoma, 25% of patients with yolk sac tumors, and less than 10% of patients with pure seminoma.[16] The treatment of patients with pure seminoma but elevation of the β-hCG remains controversial.

Alpha-fetoprotein. Alpha-fetoprotein is an α_1-globulin that represents the dominant serum protein in the fetal serum of many mammalian species. However, beyond the age of one year of life, it is present in only trace amounts in the serum. The normal level is less than 20 ng/ml, and the serum half-life is between five and seven days. Alpha-fetoprotein was originally described as a marker in patients with hepatocellular carcinoma. The α-fetoprotein is elevated in approximately 70% of patients with embryonal carcinoma and 75% of patients with yolk sac tumor, but it has been absent in patients with choriocarcinoma or with pure seminoma.[16]

The expense of obtaining the β subunit of hCG or α-fetoprotein preclude their use as screening for large patient populations. Their major impact has been as an adjunct to histologic staging (especially in cases of α-fetoprotein elevation in patients with seminoma) and as a means of following patients both prior to and during therapy to give some indication of response to treatment.

There may be a discordance between tumor markers, so both AFP and hCG must be measured sequentially. There are very few false-negative elevations of tumor markers; therefore consistently elevated levels of tumor markers following therapy do indicate residual active disease, assuming that the elevation does not represent appropriate reduction by the normal serum half-life. Nonetheless, there are significant limitations to the specificity of negative results from tumor marker studies. Return of marker levels to normal after therapy does not ensure that all viable tumor has been removed or obliterated. Skinner and Scardino reported that viable tumor was still present at the time of extirpative surgery in almost 80% of patients whose results of marker studies became normal after chemotherapy.[42] Likewise, Donohue reported on histologic findings of 50 patients who underwent cytoreductive surgery after chemotherapy. In 19, residual cancer was found, but only six of the 19 had elevated tumor markers at the time of exploration.[12]

Although most patients with extensive metastatic disease will have elevation of either the AFP or β-hCG after orchiectomy but prior to implementation of other therapeutic procedures, patients with less advanced disease demonstrate prelymphadenectomy marker elevation that does not correlate as well with pathologic findings. Skinner and Scardino reported that 50% of patients with Stage B_1 disease had elevated marker levels after orchiectomy alone, and 64% of patients with Stage B_2 disease had elevated marker levels prior to lymphadenectomy.[42] However, this means that 50% of patients with Stage B_1 and 36% of those with Stage B_2 disease had false-negative rates, even with documented metastases in the retroperitoneum. These data have been confirmed by Bosl and associates.[8] Thus, negative results of tumor marker studies do not preclude the presence of disease in the retroperitoneum, and caution should be the watchword when therapeutic decisions concerning lymphadenectomy are influenced by apparently normal marker values.

Computerized Tomography (CT) Scan

Germ cell tumors of the testis spread initially to the retroperitoneal lymph nodes and thence to supradiaphragmatic lymph nodes, lungs, and other sites of systemic involvement. Until recently, determination of the abdominal metastases has been based upon physical examination, excretory urography, inferior venacavography, and bipedal lymphangiography. However, all these techniques have a limited ability to delineate accurately the degree of retroperitoneal nodal involvement. CT scan has been suggested as a technique with a high degree of accuracy in the depiction of retroperitoneal lymph node involvement in patients with testicular tumors. Because of the more accurate depic-

tion of the extent of nodal metastases, CT scan has largely replaced the more invasive lymphangiography for depiction of retroperitoneal disease. CT scanning of the retroperitoneum has shown a high (more than 90%) rate of prediction of metastases in patients with lymphoma.[44] Several early series seemed to confirm the capability of CT scan to correctly predict extent of retroperitoneal involvement. Lee and associates reported that nine out of 10 patients with testicular tumor and pathologic confirmation were assessed correctly by the CT scan.[20] Other investigators confirmed the accuracy of CT scan in depicting retroperitoneal nodal involvement in patients with extensive or moderate amounts of disease in the retroperitoneum. However, the importance of the CT scan should lie not only in its ability to depict retroperitoneal involvement but in the confidence gained from a negative result (i.e., the predictive value of a negative result), especially when one considers the possibility of observation versus retroperitoneal lymph node dissection.

In 1982, Richie and associates reported on a prospective study of 30 patients with all stages of testis tumor who underwent CT scan within one week prior to retroperitoneal lymphadenectomy.[28] The sensitivity was 65% and the specificity 90%, giving an overall accuracy of 73%. Most importantly, however, of 16 CT scans interpreted as normal, seven (44%) proved to be falsely negative. Thus, the predictive value of a negative result in our series was only 56%. This high false-negative rate has been confirmed by several other centers, including Sloan Kettering and Indiana University.

Undoubtedly, improvements in CT scanning techniques invariably will result in improved accuracy and diminished false-negative rates for the depiction of retroperitoneal lymph node involvement in patients with testicular tumors. As newer scanners become available, shorter scanning times and narrower tissue slices will improve pictorial quality and, therefore, interpretation. One of the limitations of CT scanning is the difficulty in separating intraperitoneal from retroperitoneal contents in thin patients without adequate fat planes for delineation. Repetitive administration of oral contrast agents may help to reduce this problem of interpretation as well.

CT scanning appears to be a highly accu-

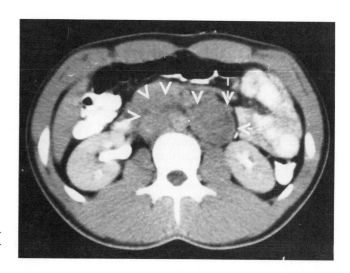

Figure 32–3. CT scan reveals large retroperitoneal nodal involvement (arrows) surrounding and encasing the great vessels.

rate method for the depiction of bulky or extensive retroperitoneal disease in Stage II+ or III (Fig. 32–3). However, the normal CT examination still does not approach the accuracy level at which retroperitoneal nodal metastases can be excluded with confidence.

Bipedal lymphangiography has been utilized to evaluate retroperitoneal lymph nodes since 1955.[19] Many centers have utilized lymphangiography as the standard technique for determining regional retroperitoneal lymph node involvement in patients with testicular tumors. Although testicular lymphangiography would probably provide better visualization of the nodes draining the testis, practical considerations have favored the bipedal lymphangiography route instead.

The major concern with lymphangiography has to do with its inability to identify small volume nodal metastases. Excellent reviews on the subject of lymphangiography in patients with testicular cancer are available.[51] Lymphography should include both a filling or lymphatic phase and a nodal phase of the lymphangiogram, with criteria for positive results being marginal filling defects, lymph vessel deviation, lymphatic blockage, or nonfilling of lymph nodes. In Wobbes's series of lymphography, pathologic examination revealed a false-negative predictive value rate of 16 out of 61 patients.[52] Thus, the accuracy rate and predictive value of a negative result from lymphangiography seems similar to, or certainly no better than, the rates reported with CT scanning. Overall accuracy of lymphangiog-

raphy has ranged from 62%[45] to a high of 89%.[18]

Because lymphangiography is an invasive technique with potential complications including fever, local pain, superficial wound infection, and more serious effects such as pulmonary dysfunction, my preference is to avoid lymphangiography and utilize CT scan as the primary method of staging the retroperitoneal lymph nodes.

When lymphography and CT scanning are combined, no significant difference among either group can be appreciated. Ultrasonography likewise does not seem to be more effective in evaluation of retroperitoneal lymph node dissections than is CT scan.

Vugrin and associates[49] from Sloan-Kettering Memorial Hospital and Rowland and coworkers[31] from Indiana University have correlated clinical staging with pathologic findings in patients with Stage B_1, B_2, and B_3 retroperitoneal metastases by utilizing various combinations of CT scan, ultrasound, tumor markers, and lymphangiography. In both of these series, pathologic stage correlated with the clinical stage in only 36 to 46% of patients with Stage B_1 disease, 67 to 73% for Stage B_2 disease, and 100% for Stage B_3 disease. Thus, all staging modalities fall far short of accurately predicting minimal or even moderate retroperitoneal lymph node involvement.

Other Staging Techniques

Excretory Urography. The excretory urogram is a simple and relatively safe method to evaluate the retroperitoneum and formerly was utilized quite frequently. With the advent of CT scanning to better delineate retroperitoneal nodal involvement, the intravenous pyelogram (IVP), or excretory urogram, represents an extraneous and unnecessary procedure. If the results of CT scan or ultrasound show hydronephrosis, an IVP may be useful to delineate the level of obstruction prior to placement of a ureteral stent. Stents should be employed to improve renal function prior to administration of cisplatin-based chemotherapy.

Inferior Venacavography. Inferior venacavography may be a useful adjunct in certain patients with bulky or extensive retroperitoneal disease, especially in those who present with lower extremity edema.

Supraclavicular Node Biopsy. Several authors have advocated the use of routine supraclavicular node biopsy as a staging modality for patients with testicular cancer in order to pick up subclinical Stage III disease.[13] Other authors have advocated supraclavicular biopsy only in patients who have palpable lymph nodes.[32] In 1980 we reported on 73 patients who had undergone supraclavicular lymph node biopsy as a staging method for testicular cancer.[21] Only four of the 73 patients had positive results on biopsy and palpable supraclavicular nodes were noted in three of those. The complication rate of 8% militated against the use of routine supraclavicular lymph node biopsy. Furthermore, most patients with palpable supraclavicular nodes have other evidence of disseminated disease, thus negating the need for supraclavicular nodal biopsy.

Nucleotide Scans. Metastatic seminoma may be visualized by the use of gallium-67 citrate scans. Presumably, the gallium localizes in lymphocytes infiltrating the seminoma rather than in the cells of the seminoma per se.[1]

Liver and spleen scans and bone scans have a relatively low yield in patients with testicular cancer and should not be utilized routinely. Liver function studies, especially determination of alkaline phosphatase levels, are much more sensitive than nucleotide scans for the detection of liver metastases.[4]

SUMMATION

Although numerous staging techniques are available to attempt to visualize the retroperitoneum and other sites of metastatic involvement, all these techniques fall short in the depiction of minimal nodal involvement. Diagnostic modalities are continually improving; nonetheless, attention should be directed to earlier elucidation of the primary disease process in order to improve survival rates and lessen morbidity. Testicular self-examination, a straightforward and reliable technique, should be introduced at the high school or college level in order to promote awareness and bring about earlier diagnosis and hence therapy. Testicular ultrasound should be utilized in questionable cases in order to expedite diagnosis and definitive therapy.

In patients with proven testicular cancer, staging procedures should be streamlined and directed at determination of bulky or extensive disease that would require initial chemotherapy. The appropriate place of expectant therapy or observation for clinical Stage I testicular cancer patients will have to be determined in terms of overall survival and reduced morbidity when contrasted with the gold standard of retroperitoneal lymphadenectomy.

References

1. Bailey TB, Pinsky SM, Mittemeyer BT, et al: A new adjuvant in testis tumor staging: gallium-67 citrate. J Urol 110:307–310, 1973.
2. Batata MA, Whitmore WF Jr, Chu FC, et al: Cryptorchidism and testicular cancer. J Urol 124:382–387, 1980.
3. Beahrs OH, Myers MH (eds): *Manual for Staging of Cancer.* Philadelphia, JB Lippincott, 1983, p 165.
4. Belville WD, McLeod DG, Prall RH, et al: The liver scan in urologic oncology. J Urol 123:901–903, 1980.
5. Bergman SM, Lippert M, Javadpour N: The value of whole lung tomography in the early detection of metastatic disease in patients with renal cell carcinoma and testicular tumors. J Urol 124:860–862, 1980.
6. Boden G, Gibb R: Radiotherapy and testicular neoplasms. Lancet 2:1195–1197, 1951.
7. Bosl GJ, Vogelzang NJ, Goldman A, et al: Impact of delay in diagnosis on clinical stage of testicular cancer. Lancet 2:970–973, 1981.
8. Bosl GJ, Lange PH, Fraley EE, et al: Human chorionic gonadotropin and alphafetoprotein in the staging of nonseminomatous testicular cancer. Cancer 47:328–332, 1981.
9. Buckspan MB, Skeldon SC, Klotz PG, Pritzker KPH: Epidermoid cysts of the testicle. J Urol 134:960–961, 1985.
10. Clemmesen J: A doubling of morbidity from testis carcinoma in Copenhagen, 1943–1962. Acta Pathol Microbiol Scand 72:348–349, 1968.
11. DeCenzo JM, Leadbetter GW Jr: Early orchiopexy and testis tumors. Urology 5:365–366, 1975.
12. Donohue JP, Roth LM, Zachary JM, et al: Cytore-

ductive surgery for metastatic testis cancer: tissue analysis of retroperitoneal masses after chemotherapy. J Urol 127:1111–1114, 1982.

13. Donohue RE, Pfister RR, Weigel JW, Stonington OG: Supraclavicular node biopsy in testicular tumors. Urology 9:546–548, 1977.

14. Fraley EE, Lange PH, Williams RD, Ortlip SA: Staging of early nonseminomatous germ-cell testicular cancer. Cancer 45:1762–1767, 1980.

15. Gehring GG, Rodriguez FR, Woodhead DM: Malignant degeneration of cryptorchid testes following orchiopexy. J Urol 112:354–356, 1974.

16. Javadpour N: The role of biologic tumor markers in testicular cancer. Cancer 45:1755–1761, 1980.

17. Jochelson MS, Garnick MB, Balikian JP, Richie JP: The efficacy of routine whole lung tomography in germ cell tumors. Cancer 54:1007–1009, 1984.

18. Kademian M, Wirtanen G: Accuracy of bipedal lymphangiography in testicular tumors. Urology 9:218–220, 1977.

19. Kinmonth JB, Taylor GW, Harper RAK: Lymphangiography: technique for its clinical use in lower limb. Br Med J 1:940–942, 1955.

20. Lee JK, McClennan BL, Stanley RJ, Sagel SS: Computed tomography in the staging of testicular neoplasms. Radiology 130:387–390, 1979.

21. Lynch DF Jr, Richie JP: Supraclavicular node biopsy in staging testis tumors. J Urol 123:39–40, 1980.

22. Maier JG, Sulak MH: Proceedings: radiation therapy in malignant testis tumors. II. Carcinoma. Cancer 32:1212–1216, 1973.

23. Martin DC: Germinal cell tumors of the testis after orchiopexy. J Urol 121:422–424, 1979.

24. Mostofi FK: Proceedings: testicular tumors. Epidemiologic, etiologic, and pathologic features. Cancer 32:1186–1201, 1973.

25. Oliver RTD: Factors contributing to delay in diagnosis of testicular tumours. Br Med J 290:356, 1985.

26. Orecklin JR: Testicular tumor. Occurring with hydrocele and positive cytologic fluid. Urology 3:232–234, 1974.

27. Richie JP, Birnholz J, Garnick MB: Ultrasonography as a diagnostic adjunct for the evaluation of masses in the scrotum. Surg Gynecol Obstet 154:695–698, 1982.

28. Richie JP, Garnick MB, Finberg H: Computerized tomography: how accurate for abdominal staging of testis tumors? J Urol 127:715–717, 1982.

29. Robertson AG, Read G: The value of lactate dehydrogenase as a nonspecific tumour marker for seminoma of the testis. Br J Cancer 46:994–998, 1982.

30. Ross RK, McCurtis JW, Henderson BE, et al: Descriptive epidemiology of testicular and prostatic cancer in Los Angeles. Br J Cancer 39:284–292, 1979.

31. Rowland RG, Weisman D, Williams SD, et al: Accuracy of preoperative staging in stages A and B nonseminomatous germ cell testis tumors. J Urol 127:718–720, 1982.

32. Sago AL, Montie JE, Novicki DE, Weber CH Jr: Accuracy of preoperative studies in staging nonseminomatous germ cell testicular tumors. Urology 12:420–422, 1978.

33. Sample WF, Gottesman JE, Skinner DG, Ehrlich RM: Gray scale ultrasound of the scrotum. Radiology 127:225–228, 1978.

34. Sauer HR, Watson EM, Burke EM: Tumors of testicle. Surg Gynecol Obstet 86:591–603, 1948.

35. Schaner EG, Chang AE, Doppman JL, et al: Comparison of computed and conventional whole lung tomography in detecting pulmonary nodules: a prospective radiologic-pathologic study. AJR 131:51–54, 1978.

36. Schottenfeld D, Warshauer ME, Sherlock S, et al: The epidemiology of testicular cancer in young adults. Am J Epidemiol 112:232–246, 1980.

37. Shah KH, Maxted WC, Chun B: Epidermoid cysts of the testis: a report of three cases and an analysis of 141 cases from the world literature. Cancer 47:577–582, 1981.

38. Sherman FP, Ciavarra VA, Cohen MJ: Testis tumors in Negroes. Urology 2:318–320, 1973.

39. Shinohara M, Komatsu H, Kawamura T, Yokoyama M: Familial testicular teratoma in 2 children: familial report and review of the literature. J Urol 123:552–555, 1980.

40. Silverberg E: Cancer Statistics, 1985. CA 35:19–35, 1985.

41. Skinner DG: Non-seminomatous testis tumors: a plan of management based on 96 patients to improve survival in all stages by combined therapeutic modalities. J Urol 115:65–69, 1969.

42. Skinner DG, Scardino PT: Relevance of biochemical tumor markers and lymphadenectomy in management of non-seminomatous testis tumors: current perspectives. J Urol 123:378–382, 1980.

43. Stepanas AV, Samaan NA, Schultz PN, Holoye PY: Endocrine studies in testicular tumor patients with and without gynecomastia: a report of 45 cases. Cancer 41:369–376, 1978.

44. Stephens DH, Williamson B Jr, Sheedy PF II, et al: Computed tomography of the retroperitoneal space. Radiol Clin North Am 15:377–390, 1977.

45. Storm PB, Kern A, Loening SA, et al: Evaluation of pedal lymphangiography in staging non-seminomatous testicular carcinoma. J Urol 118:1000–1003, 1977.

46. Vaitukaitis JL, Braunstein GD, Ross GT: A radioimmunoassay which specifically measures human chorionic gonadotropin in the presence of human luteinizing hormone. Am J Obstet Gynecol 113:751–758, 1972.

47. Vogelzang RL: Real-time scrotal ultrasound with a water bath: comparison of results using 5 and 8 MHz transducers. J Urol 134:687–690, 1985.

48. Vugrin D, Whitmore WF Jr, Golbey RB: VAB-6 combination chemotherapy without maintenance in treatment of disseminated cancer of the testis. Cancer 51:211–215, 1983.

49. Vugrin D, Whitmore WF Jr, Nisselbaum J, Watson RC: Correlation of serum tumor markers and lymphangiography with degrees of nodal involvement in surgical stage II testis cancer. J Urol 127:683–684, 1982.

50. Waldmann TA, McIntire KR: The use of a radioimmunoassay for alpha-fetoprotein in the diagnosis of malignancy. Cancer 34:1510–1515, 1974.

51. Watson RC: Lymphography of testicular carcinoma. Semin Oncol 6:31–36, 1979.

52. Wobbes T, Blom JM, Oldhoff J, et al: Lymphography in the diagnosis of non-seminoma tumours of the testis. J Surg Oncol 19:1–4, 1982.

53. Woodhead DM, Johnson DE, Pohl DR, Robison JR: Aggressive management of advanced testicular malignancy: experience with 147 patients. Milit Med 136:634, 1971.

ROBERT B. SMITH, M.D.

Testicular Seminoma

CHAPTER 33

NATURAL HISTORY

Seminoma is the most common histologic type of testicular germinal neoplasm reported, comprising from 27 to 71% of testicular tumors. We have reviewed nearly 7500 cases of testicular tumors from the literature. The incidence of pure seminoma was 47.7% (3540 of 7421 cases of tumor); seminoma mixed with other tumor occurred in 13.2% of the cases.[1, 9–13, 29–31, 34–36, 40, 41, 43, 44, 47, 51, 54, 57, 60, 62, 63, 70]

There are two variants of seminoma in addition to the classic form: anaplastic seminoma and spermatocytic seminoma. Anaplastic seminoma, the type found in 10% of seminoma patients, is diagnosed if more than three mitoses per high-power field are noted; it does not show trophoblastic elements. Although the age incidence is identical to that of typical seminoma, patients have a 70% overall survival rate, compared with nearly a 90% survival rate for those with classic seminoma.[2, 55] This decrease in survival seems to be related to the fact that anaplastic seminoma presents with a higher stage of disease when the diagnosis is made than does classic seminoma. For diseases of similar stages, the survival rates for patients with classic seminoma and those with anaplastic seminoma are identical.[21–23] Kademian and associates,[27] however, have reported eight patients with anaplastic seminoma whose survival rates suggest that the prognosis is poorer than that for typical seminoma, even when the diseases are compared stage for stage. The treatment of anaplastic seminoma should be the same as that for classic seminoma, although some workers recommend 500 to 1000 rads additional radiation therapy for those with anaplastic seminoma.[15] Others state that anaplastic seminoma should be treated with retroperitoneal lymph node dissection[31] or adjuvant chemotherapy.[15] Janssen and Johnston[22] have studied anaplastic seminoma from the ultrastructural standpoint and concluded that the features are similar to those of classic testicular seminoma. Other workers recently have recommended that the designation "anaplastic seminoma" be dropped.

Spermatocytic seminoma, the other variant, appears to be a neoplasm that is distinct from classic seminoma and has a different natural history. Weitzner,[68] in a review of 52 cases from the literature, showed that features differentiating this tumor from typical seminoma include the advanced age of onset (70% of the patients are over 50 years of age) and its tendency not to metastasize. Jackson and associates[19] however, reported four of five patients who died of spermatocytic seminoma. (A review of these cases by other workers has shown that these four patients were incorrectly diagnosed and in fact had anaplastic seminomas.) A report by Schoborg and associates[52] confirms a single case of metastatic spermatocytic seminoma. A spermatocytic seminoma in a cryptorchid testis has never been reported, nor has it been known to occur in association with nonseminomatous germinal tumors, as occurs with classic seminoma. Of all seminomas, 3.5 to 7.5% are of the spermatocytic variety. Six per cent of spermatocytic seminomas are bilateral, compared with only 2%

of the classic seminomas. Macroscopically, spermatocytic seminomas are yellow-white or gray and are softer than the typical seminoma. They often are gelatinous, with interspaced cystic areas. Rosai and associates[48] postulated that the reason for the greater degree of differentiation characteristic of spermatocytic seminomas, when compared with classic seminomas, was that the lesions originate from different cells. Rosai and associates believed that the classic seminoma was derived from an undifferentiated germ cell, whereas the spermatocytic seminoma originated from relatively mature spermatogonia. Despite the single reported case of metastatic spermatocytic seminoma,[52] the prognosis with this type of tumor is excellent. It is uncertain whether or not radiation is indicated in patients with spermatocytic seminoma. Radical orchiectomy may be the only treatment necessary unless metastatic disease is documented. It would seem that prophylactic radiation therapy might be overtreatment for this condition.

Seminoma is the most common tumor occurring in cryptorchid testes. Approximately two thirds of all cryptorchid testes that undergo malignant degeneration contain seminomas.[47, 56] This figure is compared with the overall incidence of seminomas of 47%. As mentioned previously, spermatocytic seminoma is not seen in the cryptorchid testis.

Approximately 25% of seminomas are metastatic when first seen. In an extensive review of the literature of nearly 2400 cases of seminoma, 74.7% presented as Stage I tumors, 19.5% as Stage II, and 5.8% as Stage III and IV (Table 33–1). The seminoma usually spreads early via the lymphatic system and later by the blood system. Up to 26% of patients seen with seminoma will show evidence of metastasis on lymphangiograms.[70] Spread to mediastinal or supraclavicular nodes usually occurs later, following significant retroperitoneal disease, but exceptions do exist. Seminomas cause ureteral obstruction more commonly than other germinal testicular tumors, either by bulk disease or a sheet-like growth in the retroperitoneum. Spread to organs such as lungs, liver, and the adrenal gland, or to bone, is a late manifestation of the disease. When the patient presents with a "pure" seminoma, having negative results on the lymphangiogram but with evidence of metastasis to lung or liver, one should strongly suspect that a nonsem-

Table 33–1. STAGING OF PATIENTS WITH SEMINOMAS AT THE TIME OF DIAGNOSIS*

Clinical Stage	Number of Patients	Percent
Stage A	1753	74.7
Stage B	457	19.5
Stage C	136	5.8
Total	2346	100.0

*From Smith RB: Management of testicular seminoma. In DG Skinner, JB deKernion (eds), Genitourinary Cancer. Philadelphia, WB Saunders, 1978, p 461.

inomatous tumor element is present that had been missed when the primary tumor was examined pathologically. Hepatic and pulmonary metastases are rare in pure seminoma without evidence of other disseminated disease. It is interesting to note, however, that in an autopsy series of patients dying from all types of testicular tumors, seminoma had a higher incidence of bony metastases (47%) than did any other germinal neoplasm.[24]

CLINICAL STAGING OF SEMINOMAS

For purposes of consistency in this chapter, the following staging system will be used: Stage I, disease confined to the testis; Stage IIA, retroperitoneal disease less than 2 cm in diameter; Stage IIB, retroperitoneal disease between 2 and 5 cm in diameter; Stage IIC, retroperitoneal disease greater than 5 cm in diameter; Stage III, supradiaphragmatic lymphatic disease; and Stage IV, extralymphatic disease.

The prognosis and therapy of seminomas depends on accurate clinical staging. Not only must the extent of the disease be defined, but one must be sure that no other tumor element exists in combination with a pure seminoma. Careful step sectioning of the primary lesion is mandatory.

Despite the fact that a seminoma produces hormone-like substances less commonly than do nonseminomatous tumors, markers should be followed. Wilson and Woodhead[72] reported that 12% of 50 seminoma patients had elevated levels of urinary gonadotropin. One third of these patients died, compared with a zero mortality rate in seminoma patients with normal titers. Maier and Sulak[34] noted a 100% mortality rate in five seminoma patients with positive urinary gonadotropin determinations. Serum radioimmune assay determinations of α-fetoprotein and the β subunit of human chorionic gonadotropin (β-hCG) have replaced urinary gonadotropin determinations in the evaluation of patients with testicular tumors, and it is essential to obtain results of these studies in all patients with seminomas. Braunstein and associates[5] found an elevated hCG level in 38% of patients with metastatic seminomas. An elevated level of hCG, however, does not necessarily correlate with a poor survival, as patients have been reported cured by orchiectomy and irradiation even though they present with elevated levels of β-hCG. One therefore cannot unequivocally state that an elevated hCG titer in a seminoma patient indicates that a nonseminomatous element is present. However, β-hCG levels elevated to greater than 30 IU postorchiectomy, and increasing with each determination, are cause for alarm. Low levels (less than 30 IU) that have not increased on recheck probably represent luteinizing hormone cross-reactivity and are not cause for alarm. Another cause for concern is elevation of α-fetoprotein levels. A single example of elevation of this protein in a case of atypical seminoma has been reported with positive staining by an immunoperoxidase technique.[3] (It seems possible that embryonal cell carcinoma could be confused with a very poorly differentiated anaplastic seminoma.) Thus, the presence of an elevated α-fetoprotein level or a β-hCG level above 30 IU and rising postorchiectomy, is certainly worrisome in patients with seminoma. It is our policy, therefore, to treat such patients as if they had nonseminomatous tumors—with retroperitoneal lymphadenectomy. Subsequent radiation therapy or chemotherapy, or both, is dictated by the pathologic findings in the retroperitoneal tissue.

Placental alkaline phosphatase (PLAP) is another tumor marker of use in patients with seminoma. A monoclonal antibody has been raised against PLAP. Results of this test are also positive in smokers without tumor. In the experience of Peckham,[46] of nine nonsmokers with active seminoma, eight tested positive for placental alkaline phosphatase. Of 22 nonsmokers who were considered free of disease, only one tested positive. Patients with relapse have been shown to have a rising level of PLAP, and in addition, immunoperoxidase staining for PLAP was positive in 95% of seminoma patients.[21] This marker may be useful if surveillance of Stage

I tumors becomes the recommended treatment of choice.

Bilateral pedal lymphangiography is capable of detecting the presence of retroperitoneal disease and is helpful for determination of staging. An overall accuracy rate as high as 87% has been reported,[4] but most authors report false-positive rates of 6 to 33% and false-negative rates of 15 to 31%.[16, 33, 49, 67] The value of lymphangiography in staging a patient with pure seminoma is unquestioned, however. Computerized tomography (CT) is acquiring an increasingly important role in the staging of testicular tumors. In a report by Thomas and co-workers,[61] the overall accuracy of CT was 89%, with a sensitivity of 90%. By comparison, in the same tumors, lymphangiography had an accuracy of 70%, with a sensitivity of 71%. In addition, in 48% of the cases, CT provided better delineation of tumor margins. The radiation therapy treatment plan for seminoma in most centers depends on the presence or absence of retroperitoneal disease. Thus, complete evaluation of the retroperitoneal nodes with bipedal lymphangiography and CT scan is essential for proper management in these cases.

Despite the fact that pure seminomas rarely metastasize early to the lungs, it is important to have chest x-ray films of excellent quality to rule out pulmonary or mediastinal disease. Occasionally, tomograms of the mediastinum are helpful. Other studies such as computed axial tomography scanning, gallium-67 citrate scans, and inferior venacavograms in patients with advanced disease may provide important baseline information that allows monitoring the response to therapy more accurately. It has been our experience that patients with advanced metastatic disease, including those with bulky retroperitoneal disease (Stage B_3) as well as those with metastases present above the diaphragm, respond poorly to standard therapy and require special treatment planning.

TREATMENT AND RESULTS

Stage I, IIA, and IIB

Seminomas are exquisitely radiosensitive tumors, and they generally are associated with an excellent prognosis. A radical orchiectomy followed by radiation therapy continues to be the primary treatment, although some workers have recommended retroperitoneal lymph node dissection even for classic seminoma.[31] Our outline of therapy for tumors in Stages I, IIA, and IIB parallels that found in the literature. In clinical Stage I disease, the ipsilateral inguinal-iliac and bilateral para-aortic-caval nodes are treated up to the crura of the diaphragm. A dose of 2500 rads is given over a period of three weeks. Prophylactic mediastinal or supraclavicular radiation for Stage I patients is not necessary.[17, 26, 45, 46, 51, 58, 73] If a scrotal orchiectomy was performed or if the tunica vaginalis or spermatic cord were involved with tumor, the involved hemiscrotum should be included in the treatment field.

At present, there is an increasing tendency for surveillance only in Stage I patients.[42, 45, 46] The incidence of positive nodes in clinical Stage I patients is low, and thus the vast majority of Stage I patients who receive prophylactic radiation therapy to the retroperitoneal nodes have no tumors. Maier in 1968 reported on a series of 96 patients with Stage I seminoma who underwent retroperitoneal lymph node dissection; only eight of 96 were found to have affected nodes.[32] The availability of effective chemotherapy to salvage those who relapse, and also the use of PLAP as a valid tumor marker, allows surveillance of Stage I patients to be a possible treatment option. At the present time, however, this must be considered experimental, used in tightly controlled clinical studies. Also, seminoma patients on surveillance studies must be followed closely for a longer period of time than used for similar studies of patients with nonseminoma, as relapse occurs later with patients who have seminoma.

Patients with evidence of retroperitoneal disease should receive irradiation to the same areas targeted in patients with Stage I disease, with an additional 1000 rads delivered to areas of known nodal disease. The mediastinal and both supraclavicular regions should also be included. Doses to the mediastinum and supraclavicular nodes range from 2000 to 3500 rads over two to four weeks. When this treatment regimen is followed in Stage I, IIA, and IIB patients, excellent survival is possible.

If one analyzes the failures in the treatment of Stage II disease (in those series in which this is possible), it becomes apparent that most failures occur in patients with bulky retroperitoneal disease (Stage IIC). It is our contention that routine radiation therapy is not adequate for these patients, even when whole abdominal radiation boosts are given to the area of bulky disease. In the UCLA series of seven patients with Stage IIC disease who were treated with conventional irradiation therapy, only 38.5% of patients (two out of seven) are alive without evidence of disease. Three other patients treated with some other adjuvant therapy in addition to radiation therapy survived.

Current evidence indicates that prophylactic supradiaphragmatic radiation in patients with Stage IIA disease probably is not necessary, as perhaps may be the case with Stage IIB disease. In early studies of Stage IIA patients from whom supradiaphragmatic radiation was withheld, recurrence in supradiaphragmatic areas was rare.[17, 46, 50, 58] Patients who relapse often present with extralymphatic disease. Salvage chemotherapy is much better tolerated in those patients who have been spared supradiaphragmatic radiation.

Stage IIC, III, and IV

As mentioned previously, patients with localized seminoma or those with limited retroperitoneal metastasis do well with standard therapy. The patients with advanced seminoma (Stages IIC, III, and IV) do not fare so well, however, especially when compared with those patients with "more ominous" nonseminomatous tumors, stage for stage. Standard radiation therapy is not a satisfactory treatment for such lesions. The cumulative survival rate for patients with Stage II seminoma is 69.4% (304 of 438 patients), but after careful analysis it becomes apparent that the failures in Stage II disease occur in patients with bulky retroperitoneal disease (Stage IIC). A survival rate of 22% in patients with Stage III or IV seminoma is not acceptable.[53] Although the current survival rates with modern radiation therapy are superior to these figures,[7, 20, 39, 59] the relapse-free survival rates for advanced-stage seminoma do not compare favorably with those for nonseminomatous tumors. Radiation therapy does have the potential to eradicate localized metastatic disease to the mediastinum, but local treatment failures have been reported. Most failures in advanced-stage seminoma come from systemic disease outside radiation therapy fields or are secondary to unrecognized nonseminomatous tumor elements. It is essential that adjuvant systemic chemotherapy be given to these patients.

Several chemotherapeutic regimens are available and have been used on a sufficient number of patients with advanced seminoma. Most experience is with a combination of vinblastine, bleomycin, and cisplatin (Einhorn regimen) with or without doxorubicin.[38, 71]

Mendenhall and colleagues[38] and Williams and associates[71] have been using a combination of cisplatin, vinblastine, and bleomycin as their first choice of chemotherapy in patients with disseminated seminoma. This regimen has a theoretic advantage over the combination of vincristine, cyclophosphamide, and dactinomycin, since it is more effective if a nonseminomatous tumor element is present. The development of sensitive radioimmunoassay techniques for the detection of tumor markers unquestionably has lessened the incidence of this cause of failure in treatment of advanced seminoma. Combination chemotherapy, as described by Mendenhall and co-workers,[38] consists of 20 mg/m² of cisplatin for five consecutive days every three weeks for four courses (total, 400 mg/m²), vinblastine in a dose of 0.3 mg/kg every three weeks for four courses (if the patient has received prior chemotherapy, this dose should be reduced by 25%), and 30 units of bleomycin given weekly for 12 consecutive weeks. Doxorubicin is added to the regimen in some patients. The possible renal toxicity of cisplatin is greatly reduced by prior saline hydration, with the addition of mannitol given in a dose of 12.5 gm approximately one hour before cisplatin administration. Urinary output should be in excess of 150 ml/hr before cisplatin is given, and hydration should be continued throughout the five-day drug course, utilizing saline at the rate of 100 to 125 ml/hr.

A report on the use of the Einhorn regimen, but with vincristine substituted for vinblastine, has shown results comparable with those for the original vinblastine, bleomycin, and cisplatin combination.[66] The substitution of vincristine for vinblastine results in better drug tolerance, especially in patients who have recurrent seminoma after prior radiation therapy. The combination of vincristine, cisplatin, and cyclophospha-

mide,[69] and cisplatin and cyclophosphamide alone,[64] have also been used with success.

A combination of VP-16 and cisplatin has also been used successfully. It is better tolerated in those patients who relapse after radiation therapy.[66] Cisplatin alone also is effective. VAB VI (vinblastine, cyclophosphamide, dactinomycin, bleomycin, and cisplatin) also has been used with success. Vugrin[65] reported a complete response (CR) in seven patients with Stage III and IV disease. In a parallel series at the same institution,[39] excellent results were noted in bulky retroperitoneal disease. Of 10 patients who were considered to have only partial responses (PR), with persistent retroperitoneal masses, none had viable tumor when the residual mass was removed.

A combination of vincristine, cyclophosphamide, and dactinomycin has been used as well. It appears to be as effective as cisplatin-based therapy and less toxic.[8] Vincristine, cyclophosphamide, and actinomycin D are given according to the schedule in Table 33–2, and this regimen is then repeated in three weeks. Two or three of these courses are administered prior to radiation therapy. Three to four weeks after the completion of chemotherapy, radiation therapy is given to the retroperitoneal lymph nodes in a dose of 3000 rads over a four-week period in daily fractions of 150 to 200 rads. An additional tumor boost of 1000 rads divided into five fractions may be given to areas of positive nodes, as determined by lymphangiography or CT scanning. After a three- to six-week rest period, the mediastinum and supraclavicular areas are irradiated to a dose of 2500 rads over a period of three weeks.

In order to prevent compromise of the ability to administer full-dose chemotherapy, radiation therapy should be withheld initially in patients receiving these drugs. Not only does radiation cause bone marrow toxicity, but pulmonary fibrosis is more likely to occur after prior radiation therapy, especially if bleomycin is to be one of the drugs used in combination chemotherapy. Radiation therapy can be utilized later for salvage if systemic measures fail to eradicate disease.

Carboplatin as a single agent has been used with success by Peckham.[46] Mendenhall and colleagues[38] advocate surgical debulking rather than radiation to areas of

Table 33–2. PLAN OF CHEMOTHERAPY*

Drug	Dose (mg)							
	Day 1	Day 2	Day 3	Day 4	Day 5	Day 6	Day 7	Day 8
Actinomycin D	0.5	0.5	0.5	0.5	0.5			
Vincristine	1.8							1.8
Cyclophosphamide	600		600					600

*From Smith RB: Management of testicular seminoma. *In* DG Skinner, JB deKernion (eds), Genitourinary Cancer. Philadelphia, WB Saunders, 1978, p 465.

residual bulk disease following chemotherapy. Although the survival rates with both approaches are excellent, surgical excision may be unnecessary and indeed dangerous. The removal of persistent retroperitoneal disease in seminoma patients is more difficult than in nonseminoma patients because of considerable fibrosis, and viable tumor is seldom found.[39] Peckham[46] points out that true complete response rate in patients with bulk seminoma is rare (4 out of 33). Despite this low CR rate, relapse is rare in so-called PR patients.

Patients with bulk seminoma treated with chemotherapy are left with fibrotic masses. Thus conventional scoring of response in bulk seminoma patients is a poor indication of eventual outcome. It may be that adjuvant surgical or radiation therapy in these patients with advanced seminoma is unnecessary in addition to the primary chemotherapy. Early results show a similar relapse rate in patients receiving chemotherapy only.

Treatment of Recurrent Seminoma

The treatment of recurrent tumors depends on the site of recurrence and type of prior therapy. Patients with disseminated disease should receive chemotherapy. We believe that the combination of vincristine, cyclophosphamide, and dactinomycin is the regimen best tolerated in this group of patients, especially if prior radiation therapy has been given, which is generally the case. VP-16 and cisplatin are effective and well tolerated in this difficult group of patients. Because these patients will have received prior radiation therapy, intravenous hyperalimentation and intermittent prednisone may be necessary during chemotherapy, especially if the mediastinal and supraclavicular nodes have been previously irradiated. If other tissue elements are suspected, based on elevated tumor marker levels, vinblastine sulfate, bleomycin, and cisplatin, or VP-16

and cisplatin, may be preferable chemotherapeutic agents. Dosage modification may be necessary in those patients with prior radiation therapy. Bleomycin occasionally produces pulmonary fibrosis and may be particularly hazardous in the patient who has received radiation to the lungs or mediastinal area.

Newer combinations such as VP-16 and cisplatin, cisplatin alone, and carboplatin may be better tolerated in patients who have received prior chemotherapy.

COMPLICATIONS OF THERAPY

Complications related to x-ray therapy for seminoma should be minimal unless tumor recurrence, a second primary tumor, or diffuse disease exist. Chemotherapy has potential risks and should be given prior to x-ray therapy whenever possible. Careful monitoring of the white blood cell count is essential in those patients receiving chemotherapy who have already undergone x-ray therapy. As mentioned, hyperalimentation and prednisone may improve the patient's tolerance of the therapy.

Although radiation therapy may not alter the long-term fertility of patients with seminomas, we nonetheless recommend semen cryopreservation of two or three ejaculations prior to the initiation of radiation therapy, to ensure maximum chances of fertility. We also recommend no attempt at coitus for conception until 180 days following the completion of radiation therapy, to avoid possible insemination by sperm that may have been damaged by radiation.

SUMMARY AND CONCLUSION

Seminoma is the most common germinal tumor of the testicle. A high rate of cure with orchiectomy and definitive radiation therapy can be expected in patients with disease in Stage I, IIA, or IIB. Chemotherapy is the mainstay of therapy for disease in Stage IIC, III, or IV, with or without adjuvant radiation therapy. Patients with Stage IIC disease who have persistent retroperitoneal disease after chemotherapy and radiation therapy may not need surgical excision; it is rare that viable disease is found or relapse is seen in these patients.

Ongoing studies are underway to evaluate follow-up surveillance only after orchiectomy for Stage I patients. Other surveys will assess the usefulness of supradiaphragmatic radiation for patients with Stage IIA or IIB disease.

References

1. Atkinson L, Ewing DP, DeWilde FW: The place of radiotherapy in testicular tumors. Br J Urol 44:123–124, 1972.
2. Bains MS, McCormack PM, Cvitkovic E, et al: Results of combined chemo-surgical therapy for pulmonary metastases from testicular carcinoma. Cancer 41:850–853, 1978.
3. Bombardieri E, et al: UICC Conference on Clinical Oncology, Lausanne, Switzerland, October 28–30, 1981.
4. Borski AA: Proceedings: Diagnosis, staging and natural history of testicular tumors. Cancer 32:1202–1205, 1973.
5. Braunstein GD, Vaitukaitis JL, Carbone PP, Ross GT: Ectopic production of human chorionic gonadotrophin by neoplasms. Ann Intern Med 78:39–45, 1983.
6. Cade I: The clinical picture and management of testicular tumours. Clin Radiol 24:385–391, 1973.
7. Caldwell WL, Kademian MT, Frias Z, Davis TE: The management of testicular seminomas, 1979. Cancer 45(Suppl):1768–1771, 1980.
8. Crawford ED, Smith RB, deKernion JB: Treatment of advanced seminoma with pre-radiation chemotherapy. J Urol 129:752–781, 1983.
9. Culp DA, Boatman DL, Wilson VB: Testicular tumors: 40 years' experience. J Urol 110:548–553, 1973.
10. Dean AL: Treatment of testis tumors. J Urol 76:439–446, 1956.
11. Doornbos JF, Hussey DH, Johnson DE: Radiotherapy for pure seminoma of the testis. Radiology 116:401–404, 1975.
12. Dykhuizen RF, George FW III, Kurohara S, et al: The use of cobalt 60 telecurietherapy or x-ray therapy with and without lymphadenectomy in the treatment of testis germinal tumors: a 20-year comparative study. J Urol 100:321–328, 1968.
13. Earle JD, Bagshaw MA, Kaplan HS: Supervoltage radiation therapy of the testicular tumors. Am J Roentgenol Radium Ther Nucl Med 117:653–661, 1973.
14. Friedman M: Calculated risks of radiation injury of

normal tissue in the treatment of cancer of the testis. Proceedings of the Second National Cancer Conference. Philadelphia, JB Lippincott, 1952, pp 390–400.
15. Friedman M, Purkayashtha MC: Recurrent seminoma of testis: causes and treatment of late metastasis, recurrence or second primary tumor. J Urol 84:360–368, 1960.
16. Göthlin J, Jonsson K: Lymphangiographic criteria of metastases. An evaluation of patients with malignant testicular teratoma. Acta Radiol [Diagn] 17:321–327, 1976.
17. Herman J, Stengeon J, Thomas GM: Mediastinal prophylactic irradiation in seminoma. Proc Am Soc Clin Oncol 2:C821, 1983.
18. Hope-Stone HF, Blandy JP, Dayan AD: Treatment of tumours of the testis. 282 testicular tumours seen at the London Hospital during 1926–61. Br Med J 5336:984–989, 1963.
19. Jackson JR, Magner D: Spermatocytic seminoma, a variant of seminoma with specific microscopical and clinical characteristics. Cancer 18:751–755, 1965.
20. Jackson SM, Olivotto I, McLoughlin MG, Coy P: Radiation therapy for seminoma of the testis: results in British Columbia. Can Med Assoc J 123:507–512, 1980.
21. Jacobsen GK, Nrgaard-Pederson B: Placental alkaline phosphatase in testicular germ cell tumors and in carcinoma in-situ of the testis. An immunohistochemical study. Acta Pathol Microbiol Immunol Scand 92:343, 1984.
22. Janssen M, Johnston WH: Anaplastic seminoma of the testis: ultrastructural analysis of three cases. Cancer 41:538–544, 1978.
23. Johnson DE, Gomez JJ, Ayala AG: Anaplastic seminoma. J Urol 114:80–82, 1975.
24. Johnson DE, Appelt G, Samuels ML, Luna M: Metastases from testicular carcinoma. Study of 78 autopsied cases. Urology 8:234–239, 1976.
25. John GC: Seminoma. Q.E.D. Radiology 80:539–549, 1963.
26. Jose B, Perkins LP, Kays H, et al: Is mediastinal irradiation necessary for Stage I testicular seminoma? J Surg Oncol 25:250–251, 1984.
27. Kademian M, Bosch A, Caldwell WL, Jaeschke W: Anaplastic seminoma. Cancer 40:3082–3086, 1977.
28. Kunkler PB, Farr RF, Luxton RW: Limit of renal tolerance to x-rays; investigation into renal damage occurring following treatment of tumours of the testis by abdominal baths. Br J Radiol 25:190–201, 1952.
29. Lee F, Perez CA: Radiation therapy in the management of testicular tumors. J Urol 111:201–204, 1974.
30. LeFevre RE, Stewart BH, Levin HS, Banowsky LH: Testis tumors: review of 125 cases at the Cleveland Clinic. Urology 6:588–593, 1975.
31. Lindsey CM, Glenn JF: Germinal malignancies of the testis: experience, management, and prognosis. J Urol 116:59–62, 1976.
32. Maier JG, Mittemeyer BT, Sulak MH: Treatment and prognosis in seminoma of the testis. J Urol 99:72–78, 1968.
33. Maier JG, Schamber DT: The role of lymphangiography in the diagnosis and treatment of malignant testicular tumors. Am J Roentgenol Radium Ther Nucl Med 114:482–491, 1972.

34. Maier JG, Sulak MH: Radiation therapy in malignant testis tumors. II. Carcinoma. Cancer 32:1217–1226, 1973.

35. Maier JG, Van Buskirk K: Treatment of testicular germ cell malignancies. JAMA 213:97–98, 1970.

36. Martin LS, Woodruff MW, Webster JH: Testicular seminoma. A review of 179 patients treated over a 50-year period. Arch Surg 90:306–312, 1965.

37. Medini E, Rao Y, Levitt SH: Radiation therapy for the various subtypes of testicular seminoma. Int J Radiat Oncol Biol Phys 6:297–300, 1980.

38. Mendenhall WL, Williams SD, Einhorn LH, Donohue JP: Disseminated seminoma: re-evaluation of treatment protocols. J Urol 126:493–496, 1981.

39. Morse M, Herr H, Sogani P, et al: Surgical exploration of metastatic seminoma following VAB 6 chemotherapy. Proc Am Soc Clin Oncol 2:C559, 1983.

40. Nefzger MD, Mostofi FK: Survival after surgery for germinal malignancies of the testis. I. Rates of survival in tumor groups. Cancer 30:1225–1232, 1972.

41. Notter G, Ranudd NE: Treatment of malignant testicular tumours: a report on 355 patients. Acta Radiol [Ther] 2:273–301, 1964.

42. Oliver RTD: Surveillance for Stage I seminoma and single agent cis-platinum for metastatic seminoma. Proc Ann Mtg Am Soc Clin Oncol 3:162, 1984.

43. Patton JF, Hewitt CB, Mallis N: Diagnosis and treatment of tumors of the testis. JAMA 171:2194–2198, 1959.

44. Peckham MJ, McElwain TJ: Testicular tumors. Clinics Endocrinol Metab 4:665, 1975.

45. Peckham MJ, Harwick R, Henday W: The current management of seminoma. Abstract from 3rd annual meeting of European Society for Therapeutic Radiology and Oncology, 1984, p 174.

46. Peckham MJ: Presentation at the Second Urological Cancer Symposium, USC School of Medicine, Los Angeles, CA, January 18, 1985.

47. Pugh RCB: Testicular tumors—introduction. In RCB Pugh (ed), Pathology of the Testis. London, Blackwell, 1976.

48. Rosai J, Silber I, Khodadoust K: Spermatocytic seminoma. II. Ultrastructural study. Cancer 24:103–116, 1969.

49. Safer ML, Green JP, Crews QE, et al: Lymphangiographic accuracy in the staging of testicular tumors. Cancer 35:1603–1605, 1975.

50. Sause WT: Testicular seminoma—analysis of radiation therapy for Stage II disease. J Urol 130:702–703, 1983.

51. Saxena VS: Seminoma of the testis. Am J Roentgenol Radium Ther Nucl Med 117:643–652, 1973.

52. Schoborg TW, Whittaker J, Lewis CW: Metastatic spermatocytic seminoma. J Urol 124:739–741, 1980.

53. Smith RB, deKernion JB, Skinner DG: Management of advanced testicular seminoma. J Urol 121:429–431, 1979.

54. Smithers D, Wallace EN, Wallace DM: Radiotherapy for patients with tumours of the testicle. Br J Urol 43:83–92, 1971.

55. Snyder RN: Completely mature pulmonary metastasis from testicular teratocarcinoma. Case report and review of literature. Cancer 24:810–819, 1969.

56. Sulak MH: Testicular tumors. Classification of different pathologic types. JAMA 213:91–93, 1970.

57. Thackray AC: Seminoma. In RCB Pugh (ed), Pathology of the Testis. London, Blackwell, 1976.

58. Thomas GM: Controversies in the management of testicular seminoma. Abstract, National Conference Radiation Oncology, 1984, p 41.

59. Thomas GM, Rider WD, Dembo AJ, et al: Seminoma of the testis: results of treatment and patterns of failure after radiation therapy. Int J Radiat Oncol Biol Phys 8:165–174, 1982.

60. Thomas H: Testicular tumours. Br J Urol 44:124, 1972.

61. Thomas JL, Bernardino ME, Bracken RB: Staging of testicular carcinoma: comparison of CT and lymphangiography. AJR 137:991–996, 1981.

62. Utley WF, Goldstein AM: An unselected series of patients with testicular tumours–results of treatment of 100 cases. Br J Urol 44:124, 1972.

63. Vechinski TO, Jaeschke WH, Vermund H: Testicular tumors. An analysis of 112 consecutive cases. Am J Roentgenol 95:494–514, 1965.

64. Vugrin D, Whitmore WF Jr, Batata M: Chemotherapy of disseminated seminoma with combination of cis-diamminedichloroplatinum (II) and cyclophosphamide. Cancer Clin Trials 4:423–427, 1981.

65. Vugrin D, Whitmore WF Jr: The VAB-6 regimen in the treatment of metastatic seminoma. Cancer 53:2422–2424, 1984.

66. Wajsman Z, Beckley SA, Pontes JE: Changing concepts in the treatment of advanced seminomatous tumors. J Urol 129:303–306, 1983.

67. Wallace S, Jing BS: Lymphangiography: diagnosis of nodal metastases from testicular malignancies. JAMA 213:94–116, 1970.

68. Weitzner S: Spermatocytic seminoma. Urology 7:646–648, 1976.

69. Wettlaufer JN, Finer AS: Vincristine, cisplatinum and cytoxan in the management of advanced metastatic seminoma. Presented at the annual meeting of the American Urological Association, Las Vegas, April 17–21, 1983.

70. Wilkinson DJ, MacDonald JS: A review of the role of lymphography in the management of testicular tumours. Clin Radiol 26:89–98, 1975.

71. Williams SD, et al: Treatment of advanced seminoma with cisplatinum, vinblastine, bleomycin-Adriamycin. Presented at annual meeting of the American Urological Association, Kansas City, 1982.

72. Wilson JM, Woodhead DM: Prognostic and therapeutic implications of urinary gonadotropin levels in the management of testicular neoplasia. J Urol 108:754–756, 1972.

73. Ytredal DO, Bradfield JS: Seminoma of the testicle: prophylactic mediastinal irradiation versus periaortic and pelvic irradiation alone. Cancer 30:628–633, 1972.

DONALD G. SKINNER, M.D.
GARY LIESKOVSKY, M.D.

Management of Early Stage Nonseminomatous Germ Cell Tumors of the Testis

CHAPTER 34

TREATMENT OF GERM CELL TUMORS

Tremendous advances have occurred in the treatment of testicular cancer so that today patients with germ cell tumors of the testis enjoy the highest cure rate for any solid tumor that occurs in humans.[5, 8, 15, 16, 23, 38, 41, 58] Most centers treating large numbers of such patients report three-year tumor-free survival rates of higher than 95% for patients with early stage disease (A, B_1, and B_2) and nearly 80% for patients presenting with advanced disease (B_3 to C).[5, 8, 15, 16, 23, 38, 41, 58, 59]

Several factors are largely responsible. Foremost has been the development of effective cytotoxic drugs. In the 1970s the synergistic activity of vinblastine sulfate and bleomycin and its clinical efficacy in metastatic testicular cancer was demonstrated at the MD Anderson Hospital.[33, 35] This represented a major advance over the standard treatment of the 1960s, utilizing actinomycin D with or without methotrexate and chlorambucil. Next, the striking single-agent activity of cisplatin was recognized; Einhorn and Donohue presented the initial report in 1977, in which 27 of 47 evaluated patients were rendered disease-free with the combination of platinum, vinblastine sulfate, and bleomycin (PVB).[12] This led the way to the remarkable series of reports from Indiana and a number of other institutions that cur-

rent therapy now expects to cure nearly 80% of patients presenting with advanced metastatic disease.[1, 12, 13, 32, 50, 52, 60] Chapter 35 traces this remarkable success story and details current chemotherapy strategies.

Second has been the demonstration that a meticulously performed retroperitoneal lymphadenectomy can cure patients with minimal metastatic disease and can effectively control retroperitoneal disease, regardless of its extent.[5, 14, 16, 23, 41, 42] As described in Chapters 54 and 55, modern surgical technique yields a retroperitoneal recurrence rate of less than 1% without operative mortality and with a complication rate of less than 5%. Surgical technique has undergone remarkable progress in terms of reducing morbidity and increasing efficacy, similar to the development of chemotherapy.

The third major advance was the discovery of serum biochemical markers produced by the tumor that can be used for careful monitoring of response to therapy and early detection of recurrent disease (see Chapter 32).

Not to be overlooked are the contributions of Friedman, Mostofi, Pierce, Stevens, and others who developed a classification system based on the hypothesis that the germ cell tumors arise from totipotent primordial germ cells and that there is a natural tendency toward maturation or the development of adult teratomatous tissue.[17, 24, 25, 28, 29, 37, 48, 49]

516

Thus, clinically it is not unusual to find primary tumors containing a wide variety of cell types and to observe different and often more mature histologic patterns in metastases. Germ cell tumors also exhibit extremely short tumor doubling time. We have observed the tumor doubling time of the embryonal stem cell to be as short as a few days, and this rapid growth factor may explain their extreme chemosensitivity. However, once differentiation occurs, tumor growth slows appreciably. This observation helps explain why the mixed tumors containing teratomatous elements may not respond as completely to chemotherapy as pure embryonal cell or seminoma does.

In addition, several characteristics of germ cell tumors enhance their curability. They tend to metastasize in a predictable manner, first to the retroperitoneal lymph nodes in the periaortic and vena caval region of the renal hilum and then to the lung. Approximately two thirds of all new patients with nonseminomatous germ cell tumors of the testis will have metastases at the time of presentation, compared with only 25 to 30% of patients presenting with pure seminoma. Important contributions have been made by Chiappa and associates,[2, 3] Ray and associates,[31] and more recently by Donohue,[4, 8] who have carefully analyzed the distribution of lymph node metastases in terms of both the site of primary tumor and retroperitoneal tumor stage. This information serves as the basis for the current modified surgical dissection, which is designed to preserve potential fertility, effectively treat the initial metastatic site, and do so with extremely low morbidity rates (Figs. 34–1 to 34–5).

MANAGEMENT OF EARLY STAGE DISEASE

Current treatment protocols for early stage disease consistently yield greater than 96% three-year cure rates for all patients with Stage A, B_1, and B_2 disease.[4, 6, 14, 15, 23, 38, 40] Fundamental to these protocols has been utilization of retroperitoneal lymphadenectomy for accurate staging, with use of adjuvant chemotherapy dependent on the extent of disease. We utilize a thoracoabdominal approach similar to that described in Chapter 54 and reported elsewhere as well as illustrated on film.[42, 43, 45, 46] The transperitoneal approach is equally effective and is described in Chapter 55. When performed properly, retroperitoneal lymphadenectomy is extremely effective in the treatment of regional metastatic disease, since recurrence at that location is reported to be less than

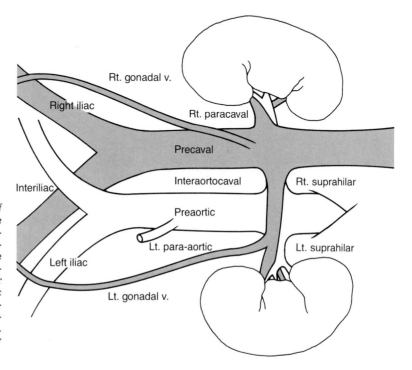

Figure 34–1. The 11 zones of possible lymphatic spread in the retroperitoneal space from testicular cancer that were analyzed by the Indiana group. The mediastinal lymphatics are continuous with the right suprahilar and left suprahilar lymphatic chains. From Donohue JP: Metastatic pathways of nonseminomatous germ cell tumors. Semin Urol 2:217–229, 1984, by permission.

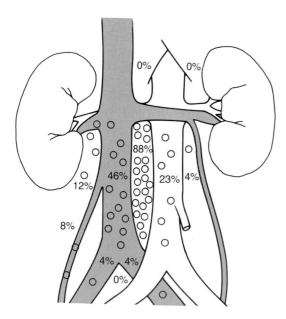

Figure 34–2. The incidence of positive nodes in patients with right-sided Stage B₁ (II-A) testicular cancer. Each dot represents a positive case. At times these dots are separated to avoid overlap on the figure. For example, most interaortocaval-positive nodes were in the upper portion of the zone. Note the absence of any suprahilar nodes in low-stage, right-sided disease. Also note the absence of contralateral para-aortic disease below the inferior mesenteric artery and bifurcation of the iliacs. From Donohue JP: Metastatic pathways of nonseminomatous germ cell tumors. Semin Urol 2:217–229, 1984, by permission.

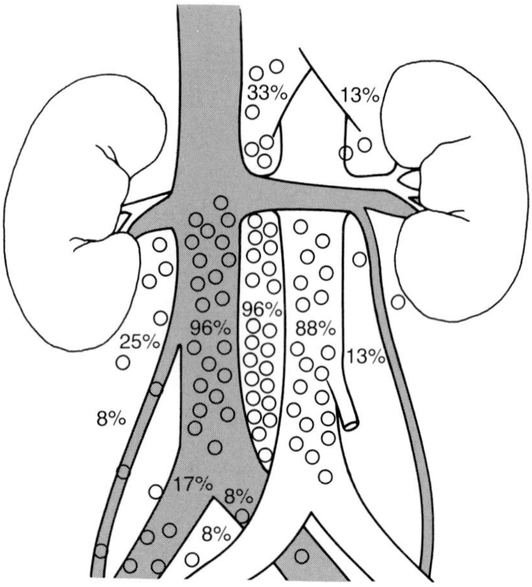

Figure 34–3. Right-sided Stage B₂ (II-B) disease contribution. Again, contralateral spread is a rarity, but an increasing incidence of suprahilar nodal involvement is seen, particularly as an extension of the interaortocaval group, which is the primary zone of spread in right-sided testicular tumors. Also note some increase in ipsilateral involvement. From Donohue JP: Metastatic pathways of nonseminomatous germ cell tumors. Semin Urol 2:217–229, 1984, by permission.

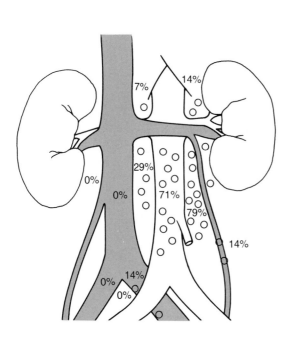

Figure 34–4. Distribution of nodal metastases from left-sided primary testicular tumors in Stage B₁ (II-A). Note that the primary zone of spread is left para-aortic and preaortic. Also note the impressive absence of any contralateral tumor in the iliac, precaval, and right paracaval zones. Occasionally, a suprahilar node is positive for disease; this is probably due to the higher insertion of the left gonadal vein. From Donohue JP: Metastatic pathways of nonseminomatous germ cell tumors. Semin Urol 2:217–229, 1984, by permission.

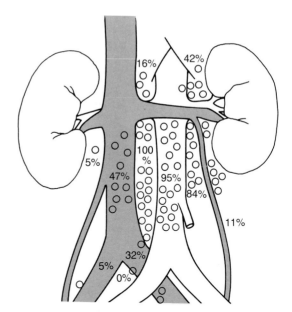

Figure 34–5. Note the increase of incidence of para-aortic, suprahilar, and, especially, interaortocaval involvement in more advanced metastatic disease (B_2) originating from left-sided primary testicular tumors. Even with this increase, contralateral paracaval or iliac tumors are a rarity. From Donohue JP: Metastatic pathways of nonseminomatous germ cell tumors. Semin Urol 2:217–229, 1984, by permission.

1% and an overall consistent three-year cure rate in excess of 95% has been achieved (Table 34–1). Controversy has centered primarily on the issue of adjuvant chemotherapy: Is it necessary? What drugs should be used? And how long should they be given? It has now emerged that if chemotherapy is not given following lymphadenectomy, pulmonary metastases will develop in 8 to 15% of patients with pathologic Stage A disease, approximately 25% of those with Stage B_1, and 66% of those with Stage B_2. With careful monthly follow-up and appropriate platinum-containing combination chemotherapy as described in Chapter 35, nearly all patients can subsequently be cured. On the other hand, prophylactic use of less toxic outpatient chemotherapy in all patients can substantially reduce the recurrence rate.[23, 34, 53, 54, 55]

Our own experience shows a recurrence rate of 5% for Stage A patients receiving two courses of actinomycin D (4.0 mg IV over five days), 12% for Stage B_1 patients after a short course of vinblastine sulfate (10 mg IV, days 1 and 2) and bleomycin (30 units IM, days 1 to 5), and less than 8% for Stage B_2 patients after more prolonged cycles of vinblastine sulfate and bleomycin.[23] The Southeastern Oncology Group has demonstrated that, after lymphadenectomy for patients with positive nodes, two cycles of combination chemotherapy using the Einhorn protocol of PVB will reduce the recurrence rate to nearly zero.[59] There is now fairly uniform opinion among urologic oncologists that patients with more advanced retroperitoneal disease (Stage B_2) need aggressive chemotherapy after lymphadenectomy. However, controversy continues over patients with Stage A and B_1 disease, for whom the choice is largely philosophical. These patients and their physicians must weigh three alternatives: no adjuvant therapy with a calculated

Table 34–1. NONSEMINOMATOUS GERM CELL TESTICULAR TUMORS, 1974 to 1983*

Stage	Number of Patients	Continuous No Evidence of Disease (%)	Relapse (%)	Survival
A	112	96	4	112/112 = 100%
B_1	32	88	12	30/32
B_2	63	87	13	60/63
Total B				90/95 = 95%
Total All Stages	207	92	8	202/207 = 98%

*Results obtained after retroperitoneal lymph node dissection and adjuvant chemotherapy in 207 consecutive patients in Stage A, B_1, or B_2 (I, IIA, or IIB). From Lieskovsky G, et al: Surgical management of early-stage nonseminomatous germ cell tumors of the testis. Semin Urol 2:208–216, 1984, by permission.

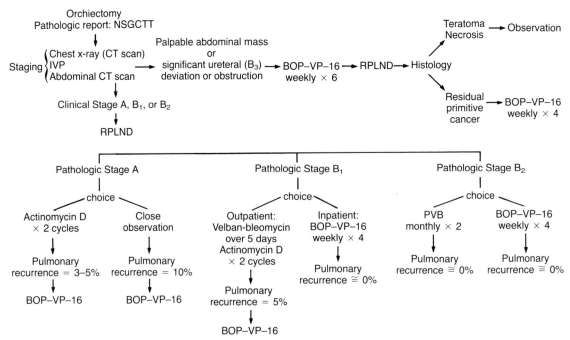

Figure 34–6. *Algorithm of current management of nonseminomatous germ cell tumors of the testis (NSGCTT) as practiced at the USC Medical Center. Key: BOP–VP-16 = Bleomycin, 20 units/m²; Oncovin (vincristine sulfate), 1.4 mg/m², not to exceed 2.0 mg; platinum diamminedichloride (cisplatin), 60 mg/m²; VP-16, 75 mg/m², day 1 and day 2. Velban-bleomycin = Velban (vinblastine sulfate), 10 mg IV, day 1 and day 2; bleomycin, 30 units IM, days 1 through 5. PVB = Platinum diamminedichloride (cisplatin), 100 mg/m²; Velban (vinblastine sulfate), 0.3 mg/m²; bleomycin, 30 units weekly × 4. RPLND = Retroperitoneal lymph node dissection.*

10% to 25% risk of recurrence; two cycles of fairly toxic PVB, which will eliminate the risk of recurrence; or a less toxic outpatient form of therapy that reduces but does not eliminate the recurrence risk. It should be emphasized that cure using platinum-based combination therapy, as described in Chapter 35, is still anticipated in those patients whose tumor recurs. The treatment plan for early stage nonseminomatous germ cell tumors of the testis that has evolved at our institution is shown in algorithmic form in Figure 34–6.

The operation as described in Chapters 54 and 55 for early stage disease is one with low morbidity and without reported mortality.[7, 15, 45] The early complication rate among 496 patients undergoing the operation at three different institutions has been reported to be 3.5%.[5, 15, 41] However, it may result in loss of semen emission at the time of climax, resulting in long-term infertility. This side effect and the finding that combination chemotherapy can cure patients with metastatic disease has led to the evolution of the non-operative "watch" or surveillance-only protocol for patients thought to have clinical

Stage A disease. Peckham was the first to advocate this approach, and to date six centers (Royal Marsden Hospital in London, MD Anderson Hospital in Houston, Memorial Sloan-Kettering Hospital in New York, the Denmark Cooperative Group, and groups in Toronto and Milan, Italy) have reported their preliminary results in the treatment of slightly over 300 patients.[18, 19, 20, 27, 30, 36, 47] Potential candidates for this nonoperative approach must have normal serum marker levels after orchiectomy, normal results of chest and abdominal computerized tomography (CT) scans, and normal findings on pedal lymphangiograms. Such patients are watched closely at monthly intervals, and aggressive combination chemotherapy and possibly surgery is begun at the first sign of recurrence. Obviously, this nonoperative approach is an attractive alternative to a young patient confronted with the prospect of undergoing a major operation, and it has stirred considerable interest. The results available through January 1985 are listed in Table 34–2.[18, 20, 27, 30, 36, 47]

Several points need to be emphasized. First, the MD Anderson and Royal Marsden

Table 34–2. PROTOCOLS OF CLINICAL SURVEILLANCE (NONOPERATIVE) FOR PATIENTS IN CLINICAL STAGE A (I)

Center	Number of Patients	Continuous No Evidence of Disease (%)	Relapse Rate (%)	Median Follow-up (months)
MD Anderson	31	84	16	10
Royal Marsden	53	83	17	12
Memorial NY	59	80	20	14
Toronto	38	60	40	17
Denmark	66	73	27	?
Milan	54	81	19	14
Total	301	77	23	10–17

hospitals have the highest accuracy rate in correctly interpreting lymphangiograms and CT scans. Most other centers that have reported their staging accuracy have a higher false-negative rate, as reported in Chapter 32. In centers in which the false-negative rate is higher, the number of patients developing widespread metastases will also be higher, and the risk of ultimate failure will be increased.

Second, the reported follow-up is short, with a median of only 10 months and recurrence rates ranging from 17% to more than 40% among the six centers. Experience indicates that patients with minimal disease have a longer time interval between diagnosis and clinical detection of metastatic disease. For example, the interval for Stage A can be as long as 24 months, with a median of 13 months, whereas in patients with known nodal disease (Stage B) the longest reported interval is only 13 months, with a median of nine months. Hence, we can expect further erosion of the tumor-free percentage. It seems likely that in time the recurrence rate for clinical Stage A patients in these protocols will be at least 25% to 30%.

Third, it may not be safe to assume that 100% of patients with recurring disease can be salvaged by PVB chemotherapy. Certainly, the salvage rate for patients with minimal pulmonary recurrence following lymphadenectomy approaches 100%, but it should not be forgotten that retroperitoneal disease has been surgically eradicated in these patients. Few data have been published to indicate that retroperitoneal nodal disease will respond as completely as pulmonary disease. Already three deaths are known to have occurred among patients following this protocol; all had been closely followed and had received appropriate platinum-containing combination chemother-

apy at the first indication of failure, and none were salvaged even by the subsequent VP-16 protocol.[11, 57] The surveillance-only protocols are obviously dependent on extremely close monthly follow-up visits. Vacations, meetings, or any schedule variance may result in a patient having a more advanced recurrence, for which the salvage rate with PVB will more likely be 70% than 100%. The clinician must not lose sight of the fact that this group of patients currently has close to a 100% cure rate when treated by lymphadenectomy. It is one thing to offer a less toxic, nonoperative alternative but quite another to substitute a treatment plan whereby potentially curable patients may die. The reader should pay close attention to the article on infertility issues by Lange and colleagues.[21] The primary reason for the evolution of the watch policy was to preserve fertility, and Lange and colleagues discuss the fallacy of this argument. It is their belief that in the best of circumstances, the watch policy may result in only a 16% increase in potential fertility. Certainly, if a patient contemplates such a therapeutic choice because of fertility, a semen analysis should be performed to determine whether he has fertility worth risking his life to preserve. At present, the watch policy should be considered preliminary, experimental, and not state of the art. We will wait for consistent three-year cure rates to be reported.

In time it may be possible to select a subset of patients for whom surveillance might be appropriate. Some recent observations by Peckham[26] suggest that the histologic features of the primary tumor may further help predict the probability of recurrence. In his series at the Royal Marsden, patients with clinical Stage A disease whose primary tumors contained pure embryonal cell carcinoma had a 47% incidence of failure, whereas those with teratocarcinoma had only a 12% failure rate. This observation, however, was not confirmed by Duncan at Edinburgh, where failure rates of 33% for patients with teratocarcinoma and only 27% for patients with embryonal cell carcinoma were observed.[10]

The extent of the primary tumor may also have predictive value. Whitmore reports that in patients with pathologic Stage A disease, pulmonary recurrence was found in only 6% if the primary tumor was confined to the testis (P1) but in 43% if it extended outside the testis (P2). If the retroperitoneal nodes were positive, pulmonary recurrence was noted in only 11% of P1 patients but in 67% of P2 patients.[56] In time, all of these factors may help identify individual patients for whom surveillance is appropriate, but currently the nonoperative approach for the management of clinical Stage A nonseminomatous germ cell tumors of the testis is still experimental and should be conducted only in a study setting.

The fertility issue deserves further comment. In the first place many patients with testicular cancer have abnormal sperm production, some due to an atrophic or abnormal contralateral testis, a condition that may have been a factor in the development of malignancy. Others may present with an abnormal semen analysis as a result of the underlying malignant process. We observed in 1980 that only five of 24 patients (21%) had semen of sufficient quantity or quality to be considered fertile after orchiectomy but before any other therapy.[39] Thachil and associates have reported that 52% of 36 patients with early Stage A or B disease had subfertile sperm density at the time of diagnosis and before treatment other than unilateral orchiectomy.[51] Lange estimates that if one takes into account the effect of orchiectomy and the underlying malignant process,

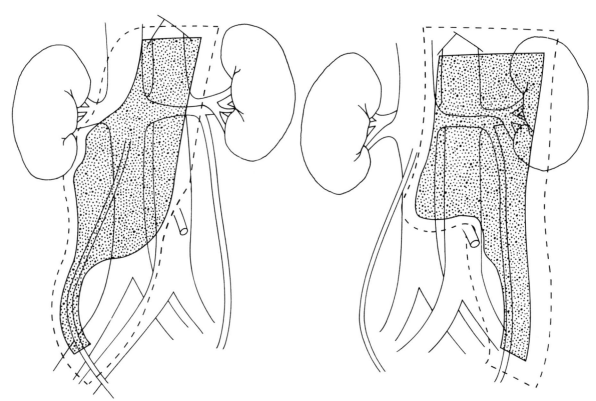

Figure 34–7. Surgical boundaries of retroperitoneal lymphadenectomy developed at the University of Minnesota for right- and left-sided nonseminomatous germ cell tumor of the testis (NSGCTT), clinical Stage A disease. Stippled areas within boundaries encompass those regions of disease in pathologic Stages B_1 and B_2 in which the prevalence of NSGCTT-containing lymph nodes is greater than 10%, according to the criteria established by Donohue and associates (Distribution of nodal metastases in nonseminomatous testis cancer. J Urol 128:315–320, 1982). From Lange P, et al: Fertility issues following therapy for testicular cancer. Semin Urol 2:264–274, 1984, by permission.

the actual potential for fertility among testicular tumor patients is probably in the neighborhood of 75%.[21] The Minnesota group has helped clarify the neuroanatomy of ejaculation and provides surgical guidelines that allow for an increased frequency of ejaculatory return following lymphadenectomy.[21, 22] They point out that emission is mediated by sympathetic fibers from the T-12 to L-3 thoracolumbar outflow that travel, via the paravertebral sympathetic ganglia and the hypogastric neuroplexus, over the anterior surface of the lower portion of the aorta close to the bifurcation. From there they go on to the hypogastric plexus, located in front of the vertebral bodies of S-2, S-3, and S-4.

Because of the careful mapping work of Donohue, it is now clear that retroperitoneal lymphadenectomy can be modified to carefully protect the sympathetic ganglia lying in the groove between the psoas and the vertebral column and to avoid resection of the sympathetic nerve fibers passing over the distal aorta and its bifurcation.[4, 8, 21] We agree with the anatomic boundaries advocated by Lange and associates as appropriate for early stage disease (Fig. 34–7).[21] In our experience nearly 75% of patients with right-sided tumors and more than 50% with left-sided tumors will continue to have ejaculatory emission following the modified dissection. Fosså and associates from Oslo, Norway, report that all 18 patients with right-sided tumors and 10 out of 18 with left-sided tumors had good return of ejaculatory function following a similar modified dissection.[16] However, if more advanced disease is encountered, a more aggressive dissection is necessary, and return of ejaculation in such patients is unlikely.

One further factor concerning fertility warrants discussion; that is, the effects of chemotherapy. Many cytotoxic drugs are known to suppress sperm production, and reports by Lange and associates indicate that virtually 100% of patients exposed to the PVB protocol will become azoospermic.[21] The long-term effects remain unclear, but it appears that by 24 months only about 50 to 60% will show evidence of recovery of spermatogenesis.[9, 21] Therefore, among the 75% of early stage testicular tumor patients with potential for fertility, it appears that at least 25% to 30% will fail the nonoperative or "watch" protocol requiring use of PVB chemotherapy. Hence, Lange and associates

have been able to calculate that in the end only 69% might be fertile.[21] By similar calculations, if the same group of patients were treated by the more established retroperitoneal lymphadenectomy approach using a modified dissection, 54% might be fertile.[21] Lange and associates conclude that the "watch" or surveillance-only policy "would be of benefit to the fertility of only 16 (out of 100) patients—a surprisingly low number considering the fact that retained fertility was the primary reason for initiating expectant therapy clinical trials."[21]

From these discussions, some conclusions about the treatment of early stage nonseminomatous germ cell tumors of the testis seem appropriate. First, numerous changes have occurred in management over the last 15 years and this group of patients currently has the highest cure rate of any solid tumor that occurs in man. This has been a natural consequence of a better understanding of (1) the natural history of the disease, its classification, and its natural maturation process; (2) improved surgical techniques; and, most importantly, (3) treatment. In the last regard, it is our continued belief that improved surgical technique of retroperitoneal lymphadenectomy should be the foundation on which a rational selection of adjuvant chemotherapy is based, leading to long-term survival approaching 100%.

Second, the fertility issue and morbidity of the operative approach to early stages of the disease has been overstated, and adoption of a "watch" or surveillance-only policy is currently not warranted by the facts. Further progress will undoubtedly include better identification of risk factors that will permit rational modification of therapy, diminishing the treatment burden for the low-risk patients and increasing it for the high-risk patient.

References

1. Bosl GJ, Kwong R, Lange PH, et al: Vinblastine, intermittent bleomycin, and single-dose cisdichlorodiammineplatinum(II) in the management of stage III testicular cancer. Oncology Overview, Oct 1984, p 23.
2. Chiappa S, Uslenghi C, Bonadonna G, et al: Combined testicular and foot lymphangiography in testicular carcinomas. Surg Gynecol Obstet 123:10–14, 1966.
3. Chiappa S, Uslenghi C, Galli G, et al: Lymphangiography and endolymphatic radiotherapy in testicular tumors. Br J Radiol 39:498–512, 1966.

4. Donohue JP: Metastatic pathways of nonseminomatous germ cell tumors. Semin Urol 2:217–229, 1984.

5. Donohue JP: Transabdominal lymphadenectomy. In JP Donohue (ed), Testis Tumors, Baltimore, Williams and Wilkins, 1983, p 178.

6. Donohue JP, Einhorn LH, Perez JM: Improved management of nonseminomatous testis tumors. Cancer 42:2903–2908, 1978.

7. Donohue JP, Rowland R: Complications of retroperitoneal lymph node dissection. J Urol 125:338–340, 1981.

8. Donohue JP, Zachary JM, Maynard BR: Distribution of nodal metastases in nonseminomatous testis cancer. J Urol 128:315–320, 1982.

9. Drasga RE, Einhorn LH, Williams SD, et al: Fertility after chemotherapy for testicular cancer. J Clin Oncol 1:179–183, 1983.

10. Duncan W: Personal communication, 1983.

11. Einhorn LH: Personal communication, 1983.

12. Einhorn LH, Donohue JP: Cis-diamminedichloroplatinum, vinblastine and bleomycin combination chemotherapy in disseminated testicular cancer. Ann Intern Med 87:293–298, 1977.

13. Einhorn LH, Williams SD: Chemotherapy of disseminated testicular cancer, a random prospective study. Oncology Overview, Oct 1984, pp 24–25.

14. Fossa SD, Klepp O, Ous J, et al: Unilateral retroperitoneal lymph node dissection in patients with nonseminomatous testicular tumor in clinical stage I. Eur Urol 10:17–23, 1984.

15. Fraley EE, Lange PH: Technical nuances of extended retroperitoneal dissection for low-stage nonseminomatous testicular germ-cell cancer. World J Urol 2:43–47, 1984.

16. Fraley EE, Markland C, Lange PH: Surgical treatment of stage I and II nonseminomatous testicular cancer in adults. Urol Clin North Am 4:453–463, 1977.

17. Friedman NB, Moore RA: Tumors of the testis: a report on 922 cases. Milit Surg 99:573–593, 1946.

18. Jewett MAS: Nonoperative approach for the management of clinical stage A nonseminomatous germ cell tumors. Semin Urol 2:204–207, 1984.

19. Jewett MAS, Herman JG, Sturgeon JFG, et al: Expectant therapy for clinical stage A nonseminomatous germ-cell testicular cancer? Maybe. World J Urol 2:57, 1984.

20. Johnson DE, Lo RK, von Eschenbach AC, et al: Surveillance alone for patients with clinical stage I nonseminomatous germ cell tumors of the testis: preliminary results. J Urol 131:491–496, 1984.

21. Lange PH, Narayan P, Fraley EE: Fertility issues following therapy for testicular cancer. Semin Urol 2:264–274, 1984.

22. Lange PH, Narayan P, Vogelzang NJ, et al: Return of fertility after treatment for nonseminomatous testicular cancer: Changing concepts. J Urol 129:1131–1135, 1983.

23. Leiskovsky G, Weinberg AC, Skinner DG: Surgical management of early-stage nonseminomatous germ cell tumors of the testis. Semin Urol 2:208–216, 1984.

24. Mostofi FK: Testicular tumors: epidemiologic, etiologic and pathologic features. Cancer 32:1186–1201, 1973.

25. Mostofi FK, Price EB Jr: Tumors of the male genital system. Atlas of Tumor Pathology. Washington, DC, Armed Forces Institute of Pathology, Fascicle 8, 2nd series, 1973.

26. Peckham MJ: Personal communication, 1985.

27. Peckham MJ, Barrett A, Husband JE, Hendry WF: Orchidectomy alone in testicular stage 1 non-seminomatous germ-cell tumours. Lancet 2:678–680, 1982.

28. Pierce GB Jr: Ultrastructure of human testicular tumors. Cancer 19:1963–1983, 1966.

29. Pierce GB, Abell MR: Embryonal carcinoma of the testis. In SC Sommers (ed), Pathology Annual, Vol 5. New York, Appleton-Century-Crofts, 1970, pp 27–60.

30. Pizzocaro G, Zanoni F, Milani A, et al: Surveillance following orchidectomy alone in clinical stage 1 nonseminomatous germ cell tumors of testis (NSGCTT). Proc Am Soc Clin Oncol 3:164, 1984 (abstr C-641).

31. Ray B, Hajdu SI, Whitmore WF Jr: Distribution of retroperitoneal lymph node metastases in testicular germinal tumors. Cancer 33:340–348, 1974.

32. Samsom MK, Fisher R, Stephens RL, et al: Vinblastine, bleomycin and cis-diamminedichloroplatinum in disseminated testicular cancer: response to treatment and prognostic correlations. A Southwest Oncology Group study. Oncology Overview, Oct 1984, p 24.

33. Samuels ML, Howe CD: Vinblastine in the management of testicular cancer. Cancer 25:1009–1017, 1970.

34. Samuels ML, Johnson DE, Bracken RB: Adjuvant chemotherapy in metastatic testicular neoplasia: results with vinblastine-bleomycin. In DE Johnson, ML Samuels (eds), Cancer of the Genitourinary Tract. New York, Raven Press, 1979, pp 173–179.

35. Samuels ML, Johnson DE: Adjuvant therapy of testis cancer: the role of vinblastine and bleomycin. Oncology Overview, Oct 1984, p 22.

36. Schultz H, Frederiksen PL, Sandberg Neilsen E, et al: Orchiectomy alone versus orchiectomy plus radiotherapy in the treatment of stage 1 non-seminomatous testicular cancer. A randomized study by the Danish Testicular Cancer Study Group. Proc Am Soc Clin Oncol 3:154, 1984 (abstr C-603).

37. Skakkeback NE: Atypical germ cells in the adjacent "normal" tissue of testicular tumors. Acta Pathol Microbiol Scand [A] 83:127–130, 1975.

38. Skinner DG: The management of germ cell tumors of the testis: an overview. Semin Urol, 2:189–193, 1984.

39. Skinner DG: Role of surgery in the management of nonseminomatous germ cell tumors of the testis. In AT van Oosterom (ed), Therapeutic Progress in Ovarian Cancer, Testicular Cancer and Sarcomas. London, Nijhoff, 1980, pp 159–172.

40. Skinner DG: Surgical management of germ cell tumors of the testis. In DG Skinner (ed), Urological Cancer. New York, Grune & Stratton, 1983, p 301–314.

41. Skinner DG: Surgical staging of testicular tumors. In JP Donohue (ed), International Perspectives in Urology, Vol 7: Testis tumors. Baltimore, Williams & Wilkins, 1983, pp 145–158.

42. Skinner DG: Technique of the thoracoabdominal approach to retroperitoneal surgery. Surgical Rounds, May:12–23, 1980.

43. Skinner DG: Thoracoabdominal approach to radical retroperitoneal lymphadenectomy: A movie. Available from Eaton Laboratories Medical Film Library, Eaton Laboratories, Norwich, New York.

44. Skinner DG: Non-seminomatous testis tumors: a plan of management based on 96 patients to improve survival in all stages by combined therapeutic modalities. J Urol 115:65–69, 1976.

45. Skinner DG, Lieskovsky G: The thoracoabdominal approach for management of nonseminomatous germ cell tumors of the testis. Film. Available from Davis & Geck Surgical Film and Video Cassette Library, American College of Surgeons, 1984.

46. Skinner DG, Melamud A, Lieskovsky G: Complications of thoracoabdominal retroperitoneal lymph node dissection. J Urol 127:1107–1110, 1982.

47. Sogani PC, Whitmore WF Jr, Herr H, et al: Orchiectomy alone in treatment of clinical Stage 1 nonseminomatous germ cell tumor of testis (NSGCTT). Proc Am Soc Clin Oncol 2:140, 1983, (abstr C-547).

48. Stevens LC: Origin of testicular teratomas from primordial germ cells in mice. JNCI 38:549–552, 1967.

49. Stevens LC: Embryonic potency of embryoid bodies derived from a transplantable testicular teratoma of the mouse. Develop Biol 2:285–297, 1960.

50. Stoter G, Vendrik CP, Struyvenberg A, et al: Combination chemotherapy with cis-diammine-dichloro-platinum, vinblastine, and bleomycin in advanced testicular non-seminoma. Oncology Overview, Oct 1984, p 22.

51. Thachil JV, Jewett MAS, Rider WD: The effects of cancer and cancer therapy on male fertility. J Urol 126:141–145, 1981.

52. Vugrin D, Cvitkovic E, Whitmore WF, et al: VAB-4 combination chemotherapy in the treatment of metastatic testis tumors. Oncology Overview, Oct 1984, p 26.

53. Vugrin D, Whitmore WF, Cvitkovic E, et al: Adjuvant chemotherapy in non-seminomatous testis cancer: "mini-VAB" regimen: long-term followup. Oncology Overview, Oct 1984, p 20.

54. Vugrin, D, Whitmore WF, Cvitkovic E, et al: Adjuvant chemotherapy with VAB-3 of stage II-B testicular cancer. Oncology Overview, Oct 1984, p 20.

55. Vugrin D, Whitmore WF, Cvitkovic E, et al: Adjuvant chemotherapy combination of vinblastine, actinomycin D, bleomycin, and chlorambucil following retroperitoneal lymph node dissection for stage II testis tumor. Oncology Overview, Oct 1984, p 21.

56. Whitmore WF: Germinal testis tumors. In DG Skinner (ed), Urological Cancer. New York, Grune & Stratton, 1983, p 335.

57. Whitmore WF: Personal communication, 1984.

58. Whitmore WF: Surgical treatment of clinical stage I nonseminomatous germ cell tumors of the testis. Oncology Overview, Oct 1984, p 19.

59. Williams SD, Loehrer PJ Sr, Einhorn LH: Chemotherapy of advanced testicular cancer. Semin Urol 2:230–237, 1984.

60. Williams SD, Turner S, Loehrer PJ, Einhorn LH: Testicular cancer: results of re-induction therapy. Proc Am Soc Clin Oncol 2:137, 1983 (abstr).

LAWRENCE H. EINHORN, M.D.

Chemotherapy of Disseminated Testicular Cancer

CHAPTER 35

Perhaps the most striking advance in oncology in the decade of the 1970s was the improvement in the results of chemotherapeutic management of disseminated testicular cancer. During the 1960s, standard treatment of advanced disease was actinomycin D with or without methotrexate and chlorambucil. Results of treatment were quite respectable, with an objective response rate of 40 to 50% and a complete remission rate of 10 to 20%. Most impressive was that around half of the complete responders never relapsed. If recurrence was destined to occur, it would do so within the first two years.

In the late 1960s and early 1970s the single-agent activity of vinblastine and bleomycin was documented. Subsequently, studies at MD Anderson Hospital provided clinical evidence of the previously postulated synergism of these two agents. Finally, the striking single-agent activity of cisplatin was recognized in the early 1970s. Later studies at Indiana University employed combinations of cisplatin, vinblastine, and bleomycin.

During the last decade, the evolution of chemotherapy regimens for advanced disease has been illustrated by sequential studies done at Indiana University. In the original group of 47 patients studied between 1974 and 1976, it was found that 27 remained disease-free for five or more years.[4] The regimen of treatment for that first study

is shown in Table 35–1. Of note, the vinblastine dose was 0.4 mg/kg, patients received a fourth course only if they had not yet attained complete remission (CR), and all patients received maintenance vinblastine. Neutropenia was the most frequent side effect of this regimen.

The second study, between 1976 and 1978, was a random prospective trial evaluating a reduced vinblastine dose (0.3 mg/kg).[5] The third series assessed the benefit of adding doxorubicin (Adriamycin) as a fourth drug. The results of therapy were identical, and 57 of 58 patients remained disease-free survivors.

More recently, a study done by Indiana University and the Southeastern Cancer Study Group further evaluated the usefulness of doxorubicin and the value of maintenance therapy for patients in CR or who are disease-free after resection of teratoma.[7] No differences were found in induction trials and no demonstrable value was seen for maintenance vinblastine. Overall, of 181 Indiana patients, 138 were disease-free throughout a minimum follow-up of three years.

During this same time period, investigators at Memorial Sloan-Kettering Hospital have evaluated various combinations of vinblastine, actinomycin D, bleomycin, cyclophosphamide, and cisplatin (VAB programs). The results of VAB I through VAB IV generally were inferior to those of plati-

Table 35-1. ORIGINAL PVB REGIMEN*

Drug	Dose
Cisplatin	20 mg/m² IV daily × 5
Vinblastine	0.2 mg/kg IV days 1 and 2
Bleomycin	30 units IV days 2, 9, 16

*Courses repeated every three weeks (total courses, three to four).

num (cisplatin), vinblastine, and bleomycin (PVB) programs, probably because cisplatin was given at infrequent intervals. Their most recent regimen (VAB VI), although used in relatively few patients, appears to give excellent results (28 of 34 patients disease-free).[13] This regimen is shown in Table 35-2. Of note, high-dose cisplatin given at frequent intervals no doubt accounts for the improved results of therapy. Although no random comparison exists, this treatment regimen is probably therapeutically equivalent to PVB. The acute toxicity is likely to be similar. However, as will be discussed in a subsequent section, the inclusion of the alkylating agent cyclophosphamide, which appears unnecessary, no doubt will increase chronic toxicity. Furthermore, a recent randomized study done at Memorial Sloan-Kettering revealed equal therapeutic results with a two-drug combination of platinum and VP-16, compared with VAB VI.

Numerous other institutions and cooperative groups, including the European Organization for Research on Treatment of Cancer (EORTC), have duplicated these results. Space does not allow discussion of all of these studies. One series of note, however, has been reported by the Southwest Oncology Group.[11] Apparently they have demonstrated a dose response curve for cisplatin. CR rate and survival for a regimen including high-dose cisplatin (120 mg/m²) was superior to that of a low-dose regimen (15 mg/m² daily for five days).

Our fourth-generation study at Indiana and the Southeastern Cancer Study Group

Table 35-2. VAB-6*

Day 1:	Cyclophosphamide, 600 mg/m² IV
	Bleomycin, 30 units IV
	Actinomycin D, 1 mg/m² IV
	Vinblastine, 4 mg/m² IV
Days 1 to 3:	Bleomycin 20 units/m²/day by continuous infusion
Day 4:	Cisplatin, 120 mg/m²

*Every three weeks for three to four total courses.

was a comparison of PVB to platinum plus VP-16 (100 mg/m² × 5) plus bleomycin. This study, completed in 1984, demonstrated equivalent therapeutic results but less neuromuscular toxicity with the VP-16 format. Therefore, future studies will employ platinum plus VP-16 plus bleomycin as standard chemotherapy.

In summary, it seems obvious that about 80% of patients with disseminated disease will achieve disease-free status with cisplatin-based chemotherapy. Relapse rate will be approximately 10%, and about 70% will be long survivors. Maintenance therapy is not required for patients in CR, and maximum benefit from initial chemotherapy will be attained in 9 to 12 weeks. The addition of other active drugs to regimens containing cisplatin, vinblastine, and bleomycin has proved of no value.

DISCUSSION

There is some disagreement in the literature regarding the independent variables affecting prognosis. However, the outcome is definitely related to tumor bulk. Germ cell tumors in general are rapidly proliferating, and chemotherapy should be instituted as soon as feasible after the diagnosis is established; chemotherapy courses should be closely spaced, and dosage should not be reduced unless necessary (i.e., granulocytopenia-induced fever). These young, comparatively healthy patients tolerate aggressive chemotherapy very well.

A special subgroup of patients are those with brain metastases. This finding occasionally will be present in newly diagnosed patients and will occur in a few others during therapy. However, brain metastasis as the sole cause of death is very unusual, occurring in only two of 276 consecutive Indiana patients. Moreover, in this same group of 276 patients, five out of 19 patients with CNS involvement are long-term disease-free survivors.[8] These five patients received cranial irradiation; craniotomy was done in only one. However, all received at least two courses of cisplatin-based therapy after CNS treatment. The numbers are small, but such patients probably should receive chemotherapy.

Postchemotherapy surgery is a complex decision. Most major centers usually have excised any masses that persist radiographically following chemotherapy. The usual procedure is retroperitoneal lymph node dissection (RPLND) with or without excision of residual pulmonary or mediastinal masses. On many occasions, a combined thoracoabdominal procedure can be accomplished. Pathologic findings of the surgical specimen will be fibrosis and necrosis in 40%, mature or immature teratoma in 40%, and carcinoma in 20%. The last two groups of patients (60%) benefit from surgery, for the majority will remain disease-free if they receive postoperative chemotherapy, whereas earlier experience had shown a high relapse rate if no chemotherapy were given.

More complex is the consideration to excise residual teratoma. It appears that at least some patients with unresected teratoma are at high risk of local growth of the residual mass, which potentially will cause compression of adjacent structures. Likewise, we have seen a few patients with recurrent carcinoma four to 10 years after initial treatment. It is possible that late recurrences arise in previously unresected teratoma.

In a recent review of the Indiana University experience, 52 patients with resected teratoma underwent blinded retrospective pathologic assessment.[9] Among them, nine patients experienced recurrent teratoma and nine had carcinoma. Some of them with recurrent teratoma (usually manifested as a slowly enlarging local mass with normal response to marker studies) were successfully treated with further surgery. Risk of recurrence of teratoma or finding of carcinoma did not correlate with histologic grade of teratoma. However, it was more frequent in patients who previously had had bulk disease resected and also in a subgroup of seven patients whose pathologic diagnosis at initial surgery was "sarcoma."

It is impossible to predict preoperatively which patients will exhibit only fibrosis and necrosis and those who have teratoma or carcinoma. Patients who are drug refractory (i.e., demonstrate rising levels of markers) do not benefit from surgery. However, those with normal marker responses and persistent teratoma or carcinoma do appear to benefit from complete excision of residual masses. There is no good evidence that exploratory surgery is required in patients who have normal results of chest and abdominal radiographic studies after completion of chemotherapy.[2, 6, 14]

Of concern in a group of patients who have the expectation for long survival are the potential long-term effects of treatment. As mentioned earlier, the most common short-term toxic effect of treatment is myelosuppression. Cisplatin nephrotoxicity and bleomycin lung disease are occasionally seen. There has, however, been no evidence that progressive dysfunction of either of these organ systems will ensue after completion of treatment.

Raynaud's phenomenon has been well described as a troublesome late effect of treatment.[12] Precise etiologic factors are unclear. It has been reported in patients treated with vinblastine plus bleomycin only, as well as with the PVB regimen; in the latter group it may be seen in as many as 30 to 35% of patients. It is more prevalent in cigarette smokers and may be only partially reversible over a long period. Management is not particularly successful but should at least include cessation of smoking as well as other therapeutic methods for this condition.

Second neoplasms have not been a major complication, although the period of observation of PVB patients may not yet be sufficient to define the ultimate risk. To date, only one nontesticular second cancer has been seen in our hospital. Pathologically, this was a widely disseminated angiosarcoma in a patient who had also had radiation therapy. More commonly, additional neoplasms may be seen in patients receiving classic alkylating agents in addition to PVB. Also, it must be remembered that there is a 1% incidence of new primary tumors in the contralateral testis in successfully treated patients.

Finally, effects of chemotherapy on gonadal function must be considered. In prospective and retrospective studies from our hospital,[3] it has been documented that the majority of patients with disseminated disease are oligospermic or azoospermic at initial diagnosis, before any treatment other than unilateral orchiectomy. Most are not suitable candidates for semen cryopreservation. Initial effects of chemotherapy are the development of azoospermia in almost all patients. However, with the passage of time a remarkable recovery ensues. Approximately 50% of patients in our series had normal semen analysis at a median follow-up of 40 months after initiation of treatment. There were no consistent effects on levels of follicle-stimulating and luteinizing hormones and testosterone. Thus, reproductive effects of PVB appear to be substantially less than those seen in patients with Hodgkin's disease and lymphoma who have been treated with regimens containing alkylating agents and procarbazine. However, although there are only minimal data available, alkylating agents contained in the VAB-type regimens will presumably have deleterious effects similar to those seen in patients treated for lymphoma. To date, there has been no information that there is risk of fetal abnormality in children fathered by treated patients. Several Indiana patients have impregnated their wives with no resulting obvious excess fetal wastage or congenital abnormality.

SALVAGE THERAPY

An additional drug with single-agent activity is VP-16 (etoposide). Several investigators have noted an objective response in drug-refractory patients (overall response rate about 25%). These responses are partial and not of major clinical benefit. However, this agent is of considerable value when combined with cisplatin in patients failing to attain CR or relapsing from complete remission but not refractory to cisplatin.

PVB combination chemotherapy will consistently produce disease-free status in 80% of patients with disseminated testicular cancer. Approximately 10% of these patients will relapse. Therefore, approximately 30% of patients become candidates for some form of secondary chemotherapy.

As previously mentioned, it is our philosophy to resect residual disease after four courses of induction therapy if marker responses are normal and if it is anatomically possible to extirpate persistent disease. If a patient has an "unresectable partial remission" (PR) and has normal levels of serum markers, he is observed monthly (either on no therapy or maintenance vinblastine) until he develops serologic or radiographic evidence of progressive disease. This practice is followed because some patients with an "unresectable PR" have no remaining carcinoma (i.e., they have persistent necrotic and fibrous tissue with or without teratoma). In fact, some such patients will become radiographic CRs or undergo enough further

Table 35–3. SALVAGE THERAPY*

Drug	Dose
Cisplatin	20 mg/m² daily × 5
VP-16	100 mg/m² daily × 4 or 5
	±
Bleomycin	30 units weekly

*Every three weeks for three to four total courses.

regression to allow surgery even with no further treatment.

Prior to 1978, when we first began using cisplatin plus VP-16 with or without bleomycin (EP or BEP) as salvage chemotherapy, no patient ever achieved CR with any form of second-line chemotherapy. Drugs such as actinomycin D, mithramycin, doxorubicin, and cyclophosphamide were essentially ineffective for later therapy.

We have utilized EP or BEP as salvage therapy since 1978.[16] This regimen is used for patients who achieve a CR with PVB and then relapse or those who progress after an initial unresectable PR. It is not used if the patient fails to respond to PVB or if the disease progresses within four weeks of the last dosage of cisplatin. Our present salvage regimen is depicted in Table 35–3.

Our experience and that of several others is that 25 to 35% of such patients will achieve durable CR with salvage therapy. The numbers of treated patients are relatively small. However, it appears that initial response and time to progression are important prognostic factors.[17] Patients who relapse several months after initial CR have about a 50% chance of attaining durable CR with EP or BEP. However, CR is distinctly unusual in patients whose disease progresses within eight weeks of previous cisplatin-chemotherapy or who did not attain initial CR (10% or less).

Another active drug in refractory patients is ifosfamide.[15] Currently we are evaluating the combination of cisplatin plus VP-16 plus ifosfamide (VIP) in patients who are not cured with first therapy and who are deemed by these criteria to have poor potential for cure with EP or BEP.

NEW STUDIES

It has been evident for many years that tumor bulk is the most important prognostic factor related to outcome of chemotherapy of disseminated testicular cancer. However, it has seemed to us that current systems used to define disease extent semiquantitatively were less than optimum. Therefore, classification was developed (Table 35–4).

A group of 181 patients treated at Indiana University between 1978 and 1981 were retrospectively classified by this scheme with the determination that 80 of 81 patients with "minimal disease" achieved CR, as did 33 of 37 (89%) "moderate disease" patients. It should be noted that the latter patients would have been classified as having advanced disease in other systems. Finally, 36 of 63 patients (57%) with advanced disease achieved CR. In this group, a series of logistic regression analyses were performed, and the only factor to improve predictive value was the level of human chorionic gonadotropin (hCG) elevation. Cell type, liver or CNS metastases, primary site (testes versus extragonadal), α-fetoprotein level, and number of metastatic sites were not independent prognostic variables.[1] These data were prospectively confirmed on a more recent protocol.

It would seem that relevant investigative efforts should focus on the patients with advanced disease in an effort to improve therapeutic results. In addition, patients with minimal and moderate disease could

Table 35–4. DISEASE EXTENT CLASSIFICATION

Minimal
1. Elevated markers only
2. Cervical ± retroperitoneal nodes
3. Unresectable, nonpalpable retroperitoneal disease (± cervical nodes)
4. Minimal pulmonary metastases: less than five per lung field and largest less than 2 cm (± nonpalpable abdominal disease; ± cervical nodes)

Moderate
1. Palpable abdominal mass with no supradiaphragmatic disease
2. Moderate pulmonary metastases: five to 10 per lung field with largest less than 3 cm; or solitary pulmonary mass of any size; or mediastinal mass less than 50% intrathoracic diameter (± nonpalpable abdominal disease; ± cervical nodes)

Advanced
1. Advanced pulmonary metastases: mediastinal mass greater than 50% intrathoracic diameter; or more than 10 pulmonary metastases per lung field; or multiple pulmonary metastases with largest metastasis greater than 3 cm (± nonpalpable retroperitoneal disease; ± cervical nodes)
2. Palpable abdominal mass + pulmonary metastases
3. Hepatic, osseous, or CNS metastases

Table 35–5. NEW STUDIES

Institution	Study
Southeastern Cancer Study Group	PVB vs BEP
EORTC	BEP vs EP
Memorial Sloan-Kettering Cancer Center	VAB-6 vs EP
Australasian Group	PVB vs platinum + vinblastine
National Cancer Institute (US)	PVB vs PVB + VP-16 (40 mg/m² × 5 high-dose platinum)

be studied on protocols designed to lessen toxicity. We are currently evaluating three courses (nine weeks) of BEP versus four courses of BEP in patients with minimal or moderately disseminated disease, and "standard" BEP versus the same chemotherapy but with double-dose platinum (40 mg/m² × 5) in advanced patients.

Several new studies that have been started in the 1980s are shown in Table 35–5. It is still too early for any definitive results from these programs. Perhaps the most intriguing is the NCI study that has randomly selected patients with advanced disease (some of whom in reality have moderate disease) to receive standard PVB or aggressive chemotherapy with double-dose cisplatin and VP-16 added to PVB. Vinblastine is given in a dosage of 0.2 mg/kg; VP-16, 100 mg/m² (days 1 to 5); and bleomycin, 30 units weekly. Courses are given every three weeks × 3. The preliminary results, although not yet statistically significant, are demonstrating a suggestion of superiority for the aggressive regimen in this 2:1 randomization. Fifteen of 18 patients have achieved CR, and 12 to 18 currently have no evidence of disease (NED), compared with six to nine patients in CR and only three to nine with NED of those receiving standard PVB.[10] If these results can be achieved in "advanced disease" (rather than "moderate disease") it will represent a significant improvement.

References

1. Birch R, Williams SD, Einhorn LH: Prognostic variable in disseminated testicular cancer. Submitted to J Clin Oncol, 1984.
2. Bracken RB, Johnson DE, Frazier OH, et al: The role of surgery following chemotherapy in stage III germ cell neoplasms. J Urol 129:39–43, 1983.
3. Drasga RE, Einhorn LH, Williams SD, et al: Fertility after chemotherapy for testicular cancer. J Clin Oncol 1:179–183, 1983.

4. Einhorn LH, Donohue J: Cis-diamminedichloroplatinum, vinblastine, and bleomycin combination chemotherapy in disseminated testicular cancer. Ann Intern Med 87:293–298, 1977.

5. Einhorn LH, Williams SD: Chemotherapy of disseminated testicular cancer. Cancer 46:1339–1344, 1980.

6. Einhorn LH, Williams SD, Mandelbaum I, Donohue JP: Surgical resection in disseminated testicular cancer following chemotherapeutic cytoreduction. Cancer 48:904–908, 1981.

7. Einhorn LH, Williams SD, Troner M, et al: The role of maintenance therapy in disseminated testicular cancer. N Engl J Med 305:727–731, 1981.

8. Lester SG, Morphis JG II, Hornback NB, et al: Brain metastases and testicular tumors: need for aggressive therapy. J Clin Oncol, 2:1397–1403, 1984.

9. Loehrer PJ, Williams SD, Clark SA, et al: Teratoma following chemotherapy for non-seminomatous germ cell tumor (NSGCT): a clinicopathologic correlation. Proc Am Soc Clin Oncol 2:139, 1983 (abstr).

10. Ozols RF, Corden BJ, Jacob J, et al: High-dose cisplatin in hypertonic saline. Ann Intern Med 100:19–24, 1984.

11. Samson MK, Stephens RL, Klugo RC: Positive dose-response of high (H) versus low (L) dose cisplatin (DDP), vinblastine (VLB) and bleomycin (BLEO) in disseminated germ cell neoplasm of the testis. Proc Am Soc Clin Oncol 22:470, 1981 (abstr).

12. Vogelzang NJ, Bosl GJ, Johnson K, Kennedy BJ: Raynaud's phenomenon: a common toxicity after combination chemotherapy for testicular cancer. Ann Intern Med 95:288–292, 1981.

13. Vugrin D, Whitmore WF Jr, Golbey RB: VAB-6 combination chemotherapy without maintenance in treatment of disseminated cancer of the testis. Cancer 51:211–215, 1983.

14. Vugrin D, Whitmore WF Jr, Sogani PC, et al: Combined chemotherapy and surgery in treatment of advanced germ-cell tumors. Cancer 47:2228–2231, 1981.

15. Wheeler B, Einhorn L, Loehrer P, Williams S: Ifosfamide (IFOS), an active agent in refractory germ cell tumors (RGCT). Proc Am Soc Clin Oncol 3:154, 1984.

16. Williams SD, Einhorn LH: Etoposide salvage therapy for refractory germ cell tumors: an update. Cancer Treat Rev 9(Suppl A):67–71, 1982.

17. Williams SD, Turner S, Loehrer PJ, Einhorn LH: Testicular cancer: results of re-induction therapy. Proc Am Soc Clin Oncol 2:137, 1983 (abstr).

DAVID A. BLOOM, M.D.

Management of Testicular Tumors in Children   CHAPTER 36

Pediatric tumors represent a small but controversial aspect of testicular lesions; of approximately 1100 testicular malignancies treated at Walter Reed Army Medical Center between 1950 and 1985, only 12 occurred in prepubertal boys. Many older reports extended the definition of the pediatric age range well beyond puberty; however, we find it appropriate to consider pediatric testicular tumors as those of the prepubertal period. In children, three quarters of testicular tumors are germ cell tumors and one quarter are non–germ cell testicular tumors, whereas in adults the ratio between germ cell and non–germ cell lesions is more than 95% to 5%.[11] The youngest "adult-type" testicular tumor among the recent Walter Reed patients was a teratocarcinoma in a well-developed 16-year-old postpubertal boy. Most postpubertal, or adult-type, testicular tumors occur in patients between 20 and 45 years of age. Muir's review of the epidemiology of testicular cancer found the incidence of these tumors for all ages to range from one to 4.5 cases per hundred thousand population, but the author did not list prepubertal lesions.[90] If the Walter Reed experience of approximately one prepubertal lesion per 100 testicular tumors is any reflection of reality, then the incidence of prepubertal testicular lesions should be 0.01 to 0.045 cases per hundred thousand. Li observed a rising frequency of testicular tumors in young adults but thought that the mortality rate for children with testicular tumors was stable, with particularly low rates in black children (Fig. 36–1). The overall death rate for boys with testicular tumors in the first four years of life was 0.95 per million per year and that for black youngsters was about one third the overall rate.[70]

Historically, reports of prepubertal testicular tumors (PPTTs) were uncommon; the *Transactions of the Pathological Society of London* in 1885 contained three consecutive reports of what were interpreted as congenital sarcomas of the testis in three-, eight-, and 11-month old boys.[17, 99, 123] Clark's report in 1899 is a typical example wherein a youngster was probably cured by simple orchiectomy (Fig. 36–2).[20] In spite of the many additional therapeutic modalities that have since been brought to bear on the various PPTTs, evidence is lacking that chances of cure are improved, and, for many lesions, orchiectomy alone is still adequate therapy.

Most PPTTs present as painless testicular masses that are generally hard and do not transilluminate, although as many as half are associated with a hydrocele. Proper diagnosis is frequently delayed because of confusion with hydrocele or hernia.[1] A hydrocele may be safely aspirated to better palpate the testis, but we prefer to examine any questionable testicle with ultrasound to best define a testicular mass. Brosman found that the duration of symptoms prior to diagnosis and treatment was as long as six months[12] (hardly any improvement over Belt's observation in 1937 that 70% of testicular tumor patients did not seek medical advice for at least four months[6]). In our recent experience,

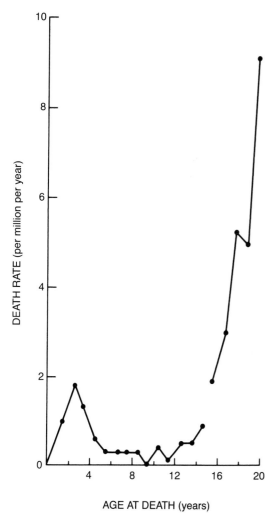

Figure 36–1. Mortality rates for testicular cancer in the United States. From Li FP, Fraumeni JF Jr: Testicular cancers in children: epidemiologic characteristics. Natl Cancer Inst Bull 48:1575–1581, 1972, by permission.

however, we find that children are brought in for evaluation more quickly. Children with PPTTs tend to be more infantile than prepubertal in age, and cases have even been reported in newborns.[31] The literature suggests that with some tumors, boys younger than two years have a better prognosis than do older boys; this difference has not been clearly proved.[11] Hormonally active interstitial cell tumors may present with gynecomastia or precocious puberty.[34] Sakashita found four of 25 patients with PPTT to have a congenital anomaly such as bladder diverticulum, retrocaval ureter, inguinal hernia, or Down's syndrome.[115] A similar finding was made by Li, noting 21% of children with testicular tumors had inguinal hernias, undescended testes, ureteral duplications, or other genitourinary problems.[70]

The Section on Urology of the American Academy of Pediatrics recently classified PPTTs in a rational system that we will discuss in sequence (Table 36–1).[11] Although rhabdomyosarcomas are extratesticular, they are so closely related to the PPTTs that they will be considered among the testicular lesions.

GERM CELL TESTICULAR TUMORS

Yolk Sac Tumor

Yolk sac tumor (YST) is the most common testicular tumor of childhood. The incidence of this lesion was nine per 1100 testicular tumors at Walter Reed Army Medical Center. YST was first distinguished from the adult

---

MALIGNANT DISEASE OF THE TESTICLE IN AN INFANT.

By H. J. CLARK, M.R.C.S. ENG., L.R.C.P. LOND.

THE following exceptionally rare case of malignant disease of the testicle in early infant life is worthy of record.

The second child of exceptionally healthy parents was born in January, 1899. At birth the testicles had descended and no abnormal condition was observed until the child was 10 weeks old, when a slight enlargement of the left testicle was observed, without, however, any apparent cause. The enlargement in the gland increased gradually until the child was 11 months old, when it had attained to the size of a small hen's egg. There was an entire absence of swelling in the inguinal or neighbouring glands. On removal the testicle weighed 29 grammes. After operation the child did well and at present looks healthy and free from any neighbouring glandular implication.

Swanage.

Figure 36–2. Clark's report of a prepubertal testicular tumor in 1899 that was cured by orchiectomy. From Clark HJ: Malignant disease of the testicle in an infant. Lancet 2:145, 1901.

Table 36–1. CLASSIFICATION OF PREPUBERTAL TESTICULAR TUMORS (AMERICAN ACADEMY OF PEDIATRICS SECTION ON UROLOGY)

1. Germ Cell Testicular Tumor
   A. Yolk sac tumor
   B. Teratoma
   C. Other germ cell testicular tumors
2. Gonadal Stromal and Interstitial Cell Tumors
   A. Leydig cell tumor
   B. Sertoli cell tumor
   C. Intermediate tumors
3. Gonadoblastoma
4. Tumors of Supporting Structures (sarcomas, fibromas, leiomyomas, hemangiomas)
5. Leukemias and Lymphomas
6. Tumor-like Lesions
7. Secondary Tumors
8. Adnexal (Paratesticular) Tumors

form of embryonal carcinoma in 1951, when Magner and Bryant reported cases in 14- and 22-month-old boys treated successfully with orchiectomy and radiation:

"While they were similar to tumors of the carcinoma pattern, they did not resemble the embryonal carcinoma of adults. ... We believe these neoplasms to have been of a morphologically distinctive type and postulate a dysontogenetic origin from rete blastema for them."[77]

Magner updated the report in 1956, with seven cases in boys younger than two years, and commented on the aggressive behavior of this tumor, which invaded the epididymis in two patients. He called the tumors adenocarcinomas with clear cells.[78] The ovarian variant of the YST was initially described by Schiller in 1939 as a tumor with a glomerulus-like formation that was called mesonephroma or extraembryonic mesoblastoma.[133] Ovarian YSTs have a worse prognosis than testicular YSTs, perhaps because of the greater difficulty in detecting early lesions. A variety of names has been used to describe YST (Table 36–2), but YST is the favored current term. Many reports still use the term YST synonymously with embryonal cell tumor even though it has been clear, since Magner and Bryant's report in 1951, that the two malignancies are distinct. The yolk sac terminology derives from the work of Teilum, who observed that the histologic pattern of the tumor mimicked the developmental pattern of rodent yolk sac endoderm. Specifically, in 1959 Teilum noted the similarity of the tumor with the endodermal sinus (Duval body) of the rat yolk sac and proposed the term *endodermal sinus tumor*.[133] Marsden suggested the term *archenteronoma* because of the assumed derivation from the archenteron—that is, the precursor of the fetal liver, yolk sac, and gastrointestinal tract.[75] Teoh introduced the term *orchioblastoma* in 1960.[134] It is important to recognize that, whatever terminology one prefers, YST is a germ cell testicular tumor and not a tumor of yolk sac origin. Talerman, in fact, suggests that the YST should not be considered a distinctive neoplasm of the infant testis but rather a germ cell testicular tumor with a characteristic pattern of differentiation. He noted that he had never seen a pure YST in an adult, although YST elements are admixed with other germ cell elements in 38% of adult-type nonseminomatous germ cell testicular tumors.[129] Logothetis found almost the same percentage of YST elements in patients with Stage III nonseminomatous germ cell testis tumors (NSGCTT) and observed that this involvement diminished prognosis.[73]

It is useful to understand some of the comparative embryology of yolk sacs. The chick yolk sac absorbs yolk for embryonic nutrition, there being no other available source. This sac additionally synthesizes serum proteins. In mammals, the primary source of nutrition is maternal and the yolk sac serves other purposes. In the rat, the yolk sac membrane encompasses the fetus and apposes maternal endoderm, although the functional purpose of this proximity is not known. The rat yolk sac also makes serum proteins. The human yolk sac is a small vesicle that becomes atretic by the end of the first trimester, but prior to this it synthesizes albumin, prealbumin, α-fetoprotein

Table 36–2. SYNONYMS FOR YOLK SAC TUMORS

Adenocarcinoma with clear cells
Adenosarcoma of rete testis
Archenteronoma
Distinctive adenocarcinoma of infant testis
Endodermal sinus tumor
Extraembryonic mesoblastoma
Infantile embryonal carcinoma
Juvenile testicular embryonal carcinoma
Mesoblastoma ovarii
Mesoblastoma vitellinum
Orchidoblastoma
Schiller's tumor
Teilum's tumor
Vitelline tumor
Yolk sac tumor

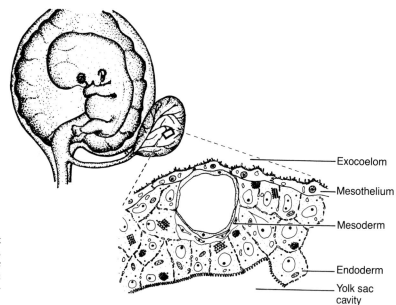

Figure 36–3. The human yolk sac. From Gonzalez-Crussi F, Roth LM: The human yolk sac and yolk sac carcinoma. Hum Pathol 7:675–691, 1976, by permission.

(AFP), α_1-antitrypsin, and transferrin.[40] Ultrastructural studies suggest that the yolk sac, by virtue of its hematopoietic, glycogenic, and protein-synthesizing capabilities may be a sort of primordial liver for the fetus (Fig. 36–3).[43]

The clinical presentation of YSTs is much like that of other PPTTs: a painless testicular enlargement is detected by chance. Huntington suggests that any prepubertal testicular enlargement that is not an obvious hydrocele should be suspected to be testicular tumor (similarly, any ovarian enlargement in a young girl that is not a simple unilocular cyst should also be suspect).[53] The mean age of diagnosis seems to be around three years and two months, although the ages in Ravich's review range between six weeks and 15 years.[107] Osborn and Jeffery reported a YST in an undescended testis of a 17-year-old patient.[97] Some authors observed a favorable prognosis for boys under two years of age. Pierce's series of 13 boys reported cures for all nine children younger than 20 months, whereas the four older boys, ages 28 to 37 months, died.[101] Young, however, had contrary findings. Among 18 children with yolk sac tumor of the testis, the three boys older than two years were alive at the time of the report (although one had recurrent tumor), but among the 15 boys under two years, there had been five deaths.[145] Overall, approximately 30% of boys with YST have died, usually within the first two years of diagnosis.[88]

The staging system for PPTTs is the same as used with adult testicular tumors, wherein Stage I lesions are limited to the testis, Stage II involves regional nodes, and Stage III consists of distant metastases that are usually above the diaphragm. Initial staging of a testicular mass in a boy should include serum AFP determination prior to orchiectomy. The orchiectomy is both diagnostic and therapeutic. Once a testicular malignancy has been identified, chest x-ray, abdominal computerized tomography, and post-orchiectomy marker studies are important means for evaluation.

YSTs disseminate lymphatically to regional nodes or hematogenously to lungs. There is debate in the literature as to the more common route but the important point is that these lesions can spread either way. The older literature seems to include many more deaths from metastatic disease than recent literature reflects; perhaps this is due to earlier detection and orchiectomy. Perhaps Scobie said it best when he commented:

"Orchioblastoma is a highly malignant testicular tumour with a poor prognosis, unless one is fortunate enough to perform orchiectomy before any metastatic spread has occurred."[116]

Macroscopically, YST is usually grayish-white, soft, and homogeneous, although there may be cystic spaces and areas of hemorrhage. The tumor tends to replace or infiltrate the testis, but the tunica remains intact. The nodule is not encapsulated within the testicular parenchyma and may appear mucinous when cut. YST has a variety of characteristic microscopic features that Mostofi and Price defined.[88] Epithelial and mesenchymal elements may coalesce. The epithelial components consist of anastomosing glandular, ductal, and papillary structures, although sometimes the tumor cells are arranged in sheets. The cytoplasm is typically vacuolated and contains glycogen (identified by positive PAS or Best's stain) and lipids. Vacuoles may vary from fine to large and may coalesce to produce a reticular pattern of tumor cells. Nuclei are large and irregular with prominent nucleoli. Perivascular glomeruloid structures are produced by mantling of tumor cells around a central vessel, and these formations are the Schiller-Duval bodies. The mesenchymal elements consist of myxoid or fibrous cellular stroma in between or merging with epithelial elements. Vascular invasion and angiogenesis are additional features of YST. On careful examination, Mostofi found occasional teratomatous elements in almost every YST.[88] Immunohistochemical staining demonstrates AFP in intracytoplasmic tumor cell vacuoles as well as in extracellular hyaline globules.[122] Kramer demonstrated additional protein markers with immunohistochemical staining in tumor from 14 children with YST but found only the AFP was of prognostic significance.[66]

Ise and associates described two patterns in the 36 patients of their series: the more common "pure type" with a predominately medullary pattern, which had a more favorable prognosis, and the mesonephroma (Schiller's) type with glomerulus-like structures.[54] There is no histologic difference in the tumors that metastasize and those that remain localized.[53]

AFP is produced by YST and is predictably found in tissue examined immunohistochemically in intracellular hyaline globules or extracellular basement membrane–like material. Serum levels are usually elevated, often to enormous amounts (normal serum AFP is less than 40 ng/ml). AFP is an albumin precursor normally synthesized in utero by structures derived from the archenteron—the yolk sac initially and later the liver and gut. Peak levels in utero are around 12 to 13 weeks.[91] Synthesis stops around the time of birth and, because of the half life of 3.5 to 5 days, elevations of AFP later in infancy are due to abnormal postnatal synthesis by a hepatoma, YST, rare GI tumors, or certain non-neoplastic hepatopathies.[40] Synthesis of AFP persists for a short time after birth in low-birth-weight infants for whom the half life of this marker is 7.7 days.[84] A specific chromosomal site has recently been identified as the source of AFP synthesis, namely bands q11 to 22 of human chromosome 4.[83] AFP levels do not correlate with tumor volume, but the persistence or resurgence of AFP after orchiectomy is clear evidence of residual tumor and grounds for further therapy. However, false-negative AFP levels have been recorded in spite of retroperitoneal nodal metastases (Homsy had two such patients, one with one positive node and another with three positive nodes at the time of retroperitoneal dissection).[49] Elevations of human chorionic gonadotropin (hCG) would not be expected in YST because the source of this marker, the syncytiotrophoblast, is not a normal component of the YST. Nonetheless, Kramer has identified production of the β subunit of this marker by immunoperoxidase staining in one patient with YST, although there was no serum elevation.[68]

YST was originally managed by orchiectomy alone. Radiation, node dissection, and chemotherapy have subsequently been applied with good results. However, there is current debate concerning the necessity of the new modalities in management of a youngster with a localized YST. Evidence has been brought to bear on all sides of the issue, but there have been some strong arguments for orchiectomy and surveillance as primary management of Stage I YSTs.[79] Exelby suggested orchiectomy alone for pure YSTs in infants and reserved node dissection for older boys with embryonal carcinomas.[33] Carroll agreed that the chance of retroperitoneal metastases is small in younger boys (6%), the lungs being more likely the primary site of disseminated disease.[16] Older boys with embryonal elements, however, may have a greater predisposition for retroperitoneal node spread. Nelson argued against isolated orchiectomy after he reviewed 103 cases in boys younger than two years and found the mortality in the orchiectomy patients to be 40%, compared with a 17% mortality in patients who underwent some form of combination therapy that included chemotherapy, node dissection, or radiation.[92] Homsy's flow chart accords node dissection a very limited role, reserving it for patients with clinically evident Stage II disease.[49]

Orchiectomy is the usual initial diagnostic and therapeutic step for a suspected prepubertal testicular tumor. The ideal approach is a high inguinal isolation of the spermatic cord, which is clamped prior to delivery and handling of the testis. A decision is then made to remove or take a biopsy of the testis, although orchiectomy is generally the proper approach. We ligate the major components of the spermatic cord with synthetic absorbable suture material. Occasionally a surgeon will be misled into exploration for hydrocele, hernia, or undescended testis and will happen upon a testicular tumor. The best approach for these conditions in children is inguinal so that high inguinal orchiectomy can be accomplished. When a testicular tumor is found unexpectedly during scrotal operations, orchiectomy should be performed as completely as possible and the wound irrigated with sterile distilled water. Further resection of cord and hemiscrotum may be dictated by the final pathologic results. Simple enucleation of a suspected benign lesion, such as teratoma, is to be avoided unless confidence in the identity of the lesion is overwhelming.

Node dissection for yolk sac tumor is a topic of considerable debate. Whereas node dissection is an important diagnostic and therapeutic cornerstone in the management of adult nonseminomatous germ cell testicular tumors, there is no such consensus of opinion in management of the PPTTs. Lewis, in 1957, was one of the early advocates of node dissection for the pediatric lesion.[69] Unilateral retroperitoneal node dissection can be performed with minimal morbidity and clearly has unequalled diagnostic capability with respect to the retroperitoneal nodes (Fig. 36–4). For left-sided lesions the primary nodal target is the left para-aortic region, whereas the primary zone for right-sided lesions is the interaortocaval zone. The major apprehension with node dissection has been ejaculatory failure, which is a more likely result in left-sided dissections. Standard bilateral node dissection impairs seminal emission in 75% of postpubertal patients,[26] and normal ejaculation may still be possible after standard retroperitoneal node dissection.[80] Ephedrine stimulation may restore ejaculation and fertility in postlymphadenectomy ejaculatory failure.[74] A uni-

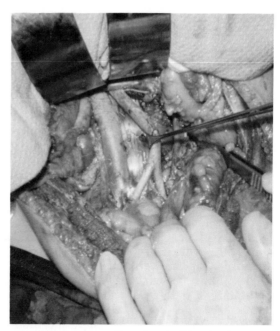

Figure 36–4. Retroperitoneal node dissection for a yolk sac tumor.

lateral node dissection with efforts to spare the sympathetic ganglia, particularly in the L-3 to L-5 area, will probably avoid ejaculatory failure. It is argued that diagnostic accuracy is not important if the patient can be followed with serum AFP and treated with rescue chemotherapy should relapse occur. In addition, the nodal route of metastasis may be no more, and perhaps less, important than the hematogenous routes in YST, so that node dissections frequently have negative findings. Node dissections were performed in four of the six recent YST patients at Walter Reed, and all had nodes that were negative. Kaplan and Firlit, however, found 33% of the nodes dissected in their series to be positive.[62] Hopkins argues convincingly for node dissection,[50] whereas Brosman,[11] Kramer,[67] and Weissbach[141] make rational cases for surveillance rather than routine lymphadenectomy. Wobbes suggested staging node dissection in patients of one to two years of age but surveillance for boys under one year of age.[144] At Walter Reed, we used unilateral staging lymph node dissection as a guide to adjuvant chemotherapy, reasoning that positive nodes would upgrade the extent of the adjuvant course. It is likely, however, that we could make the same decisions today by following serum AFP, especially in the infant boys with classic YST. Perhaps through pooled data we may learn what specific factors (e.g., boys older than two years, long intervals between presentation and orchiectomy, or embryonal elements admixed with YST) would favor node dissection for a patient.

Radiation therapy has a limited role in management of YST of the testis. Some groups have used radiation as a cornerstone of their management programs. Matsumoto successfully treated 19 patients with orchiectomy and radiation (2000 to 3000 rads) and had no deaths, but among his nine patients managed with orchiectomy alone there were four deaths.[81] Ise found 89% long-term survival in 69 boys managed with orchiectomy plus retroperitoneal radiation consisting of 3000 rads over three to four weeks.[54] Others reserve radiation for patients with positive retroperitoneal nodes.[50] Retroperitoneal YST seems to be radiosensitive to doses in the range of 3500 rads. Most centers now save radiation for specific localized tumor targets in individual recalcitrant cases. YST seems to progress from a tumor localized to the testis to a systemic disease, and blind retroperitoneal radiation is not a rational therapeutic modality. The chance of radiation injury to the spinal cord, bowel, marrow, testes, and kidneys in young children is substantial, so we have preferred to reserve it for specific localized tumor targets in instances recalcitrant to chemotherapy.

Chemotherapy is very effective against YST, and combination protocols have been curative in patients with large tumor burdens. The unresolved issue is when to treat. Some authors favor adjuvant chemotherapy for all patients.[32, 50, 104] Quintana reported fine results in 10 boys managed by orchiectomy and chemotherapy (methotrexate, actinomycin D and cyclophosphamide). Tumor recurred in two patients, but both were salvaged with chemotherapy, although one required additional radiation therapy.[104] However, Drago's patient, in spite of prophylactic actinomycin D and staging node dissection, relapsed with mediastinal disease nine months later and was salvaged with seven courses of vincristine, actinomycin D and cyclophosphamide.[32] Some groups withhold chemotherapy until there is some evidence of recurrent tumor, such as elevation of AFP levels or radiographic evidence.[49] Archson downplays the effectiveness of VAC regimens (vincristine, actinomycin D, and cyclophosphamide) and favors PVB (cis-plati-

num, vinblastine, and bleomycin) with additional doxorubicin, actinomycin D, and cyclophosphamide.[3] Kramer reported on a boy with completely normal study results after orchiectomy who developed AFP elevations eight months later and was found to have a nonresectable retroperitoneal mass. Salvage chemotherapy (vinblastine, bleomycin, cis-platinum, actinomycin D, cyclophosphamide, and doxorubicin) melted the tumor away and the boy has been free of disease five years after a negative second-look procedure.[66] All of these drugs are double-edged swords, and cytoxan in particular has some specific genitourinary complications including hemorrhagic cystitis[105] and testicular damage.[86] We believe there is a place for adjuvant chemotherapy, reasoning that it seems more logical to expect cure from treating a little disease than a lot of disease. However, any indicator of residual or systemic disease is, in our opinion, enough reason for chemotherapy. Rescue therapy can save most but not all patients. The specific agents used and duration of therapy should reflect the most current attitudes of the pediatric oncologist on the team.

A surveillance program for patients who are not managed with node dissection or chemotherapy is not without risks. Donohue argues that the "essential transaction" is deferred in these patients and that responsibility for patient compliance must be firmly determined.[29] A formal protocol is the best means of tracking patients. Surveillance must be persistent and complete; cases followed casually are easily lost. The Montreal plan for Stage I patients requires reassessment three weeks after orchiectomy, with monthly AFP studies and chest x-rays in addition to chest tomography at three-month intervals for one year.[49] Snyder's plan is appealing, calling for postorchiectomy observation of children under one year of age with Stage I disease. Children over one year receive adjuvant chemotherapy with vincristine and actinomycin for one year.[126]

Sequential physical examination, serum AFP determinations, and chest x-rays should be performed for at least a few disease-free years. At least one negative CT scan should be documented after orchiectomy. Patients who have undergone chemotherapy or radiation therapy should have lifelong follow-up because of the chance of late secondary malignancies. Follow-up must be guaranteed for all patients with PPTTs, not only for the sake of the patient but also to advance our position on the learning curve for management of PPTTs. At some point in their course, these patients should be directed to a center that can monitor them and provide all of the potential management modalities.

The Registry for patients with PPTTs (coordinated by Dr. George Kaplan for the Section on Urology of the American Academy of Pediatrics*) may help determine the best form of initial management for Stage I disease. It may be inguinal orchiectomy alone or in combination with chemotherapy or node dissection or both. It is difficult to take strong exception to Brosman's recommendation of orchiectomy alone and careful follow-up with AFP studies, chest x-rays, and so forth. Still, when one looks back at the substantial number of metastatic deaths in series such as that of Abell and Holtz,[1] diagnostic unilateral retroperitoneal node dissection and adjuvant chemotherapy do not seem terribly radical. The current trend of management is away from routine node dissection for Stage I disease. The reliability of serum AFP as an indicator of higher stage disease is high, but not absolute. Orchiectomy with surveillance, with or without adjuvant chemotherapy, is usually satisfactory but not infallible for recognition of relapse. Prognosis will still be linked to the good fortune of having orchiectomy prior to metastases. If any form of adjuvant therapy is rational for Stage I disease, it would be chemotherapy.

Whereas the best form of management may not be known for many years, we believe that all options, regardless of an individual physician's bias, should be considered so that treatment of this urologic tumor can be tailored to the individual needs of each patient and his family rather than tailoring the patient to an algorithm. We strongly believe that this tumor is best managed by a urologist with a team that can address all treatment modalities.

---

*Since 1980, the Registry has collected 226 PPTTs, of which over half are YSTs. Analysis of this data, as it accrues, should point the way to rational management of PPTTs. Details of any patient with a PPTT should be sent to Dr. George Kaplan, 7930 Frost Street, Suite 407, San Diego, CA 92123. Dr. Kaplan is a great resource, willingly providing not only the Registry data but also his own invaluable thoughts regarding the management of any specific PPTT to anyone.

Extragonadal Yolk Sac Tumors

Extragonadal yolk sac tumors probably arise from totipotential germ cells that migrate aberrantly and tend to occur in midline locations. Extragonadal YSTs may also constitute a malignant component of a teratoma or cyst, a phenomenon Huntington explains by noting that any element in a teratoma can become malignant and such transformation is more likely in embryoid than in adult tissue components.[52] O'Sullivan's comprehensive review of 46 patients with yolk sac tumors included 24 with extragonadal primary lesions.[98] Females predominated (17 of 24 patients), and the most likely tumor location was sacrococcygeal. Vagina, liver, nasopharynx, mediastinum, bladder, and brain were less likely sites. These lesions had a high metastatic rate of 50%, usually to the lungs, in addition to a local recurrence rate of 20%. Cure of metastatic disease was still possible with chemotherapy. Ages ranged from one day to five years, with a mean of 21 months.[98] As with gonadal YST, AFP is a useful tumor marker.[130] Of the small number of case reports, two are of particular urologic interest. Allyn's case was an 11-month-old girl with bloody vaginal spotting and a rectal mass. Five months after hysterectomy and vaginectomy, a positive obturator node was found. She underwent node dissection, chemotherapy (actinomycin D), and radiation therapy and was free of disease at seven years.[2] Taylor reported on a one-year-old boy with a sudden onset of gross, total, painless hematuria.[132] A YST was found on the lateral bladder wall and serum AFP was elevated at 6000 ng/ml. Partial cystectomy and pelvic node dissection with negative results was performed, and combination chemotherapy (vincristine, actinomycin D, cyclophosphamide, and doxorubicin) was administered. The patient was free of disease with negative results of serum AFP tests at 14 months.[132]

Prepubertal Testicular Teratoma

Testicular teratoma accounts for 10 to 15% of PPTTs and is benign, unlike the potentially malignant testicular teratoma of postpubertal males. In children, the mean age of diagnosis is 18 to 20 months. ReMine believed these lesions to be congenital and reported 33 cases younger than one year of age in the literature.[108] Three patients in his review had metastatic disease, but no pathologic descriptions were available. Occasional cases are seen in older boys, such as Mosli's report involving a pubertal 12-year-old.[86]

Microscopically, teratomas consist of multiple cysts of varying size, although one third are composed of a solitary cyst. Various recognizable body tissues such as epidermoid structures, cartilage, bone, muscle, ciliated epithelium, intestinal epithelium, and nervous tissue are found in teratomas, which are identical microscopically in prepubertal and older patients. Johnson's case from 1856 is one of the first recorded cases.[55] The older worldwide literature and the more recent British literature describe most germ cell testicular tumors as variants of teratomas. Probably because of this semantic confusion, Spitalny called teratoma the most common testicular tumor in infancy,[127] whereas Moran, in 1917, noted that British surgeons saw only five cases in 30 years.[85] Current usage, however, restricts the definition of teratoma to a testicular tumor with differentiation into recognizable fetal or adult tissues from all three germ cell layers. Fraley's careful definition of teratoma allowed him to conclude that prepubertal teratoma was benign, although the same lesion in adults was potentially malignant, as demonstrated by its ability to metastasize.[35] Carney found 58 children with teratoma at the Mayo Clinic between 1935 and 1965; all were 16 years of age or younger.[15] He insisted on the presence of all three germ layers in each tumor in order to identify a lesion as a teratoma. One of the patients had a malignant testicular teratoma in combination with an endodermal sinus tumor. Abell and Holtz described 11 teratomas in 10 patients with a mean age of 3.5 years.[1] The mean duration of symptoms was eight months, and in one patient the testicular mass had been present since birth. All of the patients were treated by orchiectomy alone. Marshall had seven patients with teratoma who were from 10 months to seven years of age, and all were treated successfully with orchiectomy (follow-ups were 1.5 to 34 years).[79] In the series of 35 Nigerian boys with testicular tumors there were four with teratomas.[59] Familial prepubertal testicular teratomas were reported in two cousins, ages five months and 17 months, by Shinohara, who noted that similar occurrences had been described in 33 families.[121]

Epidermoid cysts are monolayer expressions of teratomas. They are composed of keratohyaline material bearing no skin appendages. Price reviewed 69 cases (1.2%) of testicular epidermoid cyst from the Testicular Tumor Registry of 5845 testicular tumors and defined four diagnostic criteria:

1. The lesion is intratesticular.
2. The lumen contains keratinized debris.
3. The cyst is fibrous tissue with an inner lining of squamous epithelium.
4. There is no teratomatous or adnexal structure (hair or sebaceous glands) within the testicular parenchyma.[102]

In postpubertal males, epidermoid cysts associated with teratomatous elements or parenchymal scars are best treated as teratomas.[5] Barnhouse, in 1972, recommended complete orchiectomy, commenting,

"In view of the probable origin of these epidermoid cysts from the totipotential stem cell of teratomas, it seems risky to treat them as though they were benign. . . . The question at the time of surgery should not be: is this benign or malignant, but is this lesion neoplastic or inflammatory? The pathologist can answer this question, and only if the aetiology is inflammatory may the testis be left in place."[4]

With the improvement of ultrasound imaging, some authors have suggested that epidermoid cysts may be safely treated by simple enucleation with conservation of the testis if the diagnosis can be ensured preoperatively.[21]

Dermoid cysts are keratinous cysts that contain skin appendages and may also contain elements from a second germ cell layer such as bone or cartilage. Some authors have suggested that dermoid cysts are bilayer expressions of teratomas.[39]

Some teratomas and related lesions are extratesticular and still intrascrotal. Cowen described an epididymal teratoma in an 18-month-old infant.[24] Bloom reported a three-year-old boy with an infratesticular dermoid cyst.[8] Gupta saw a 20-year-old patient with a calculus-containing dermoid cyst of the scrotal raphe that had been noted as a posterior scrotal mass since birth.[47]

Adult Types of Testicular Tumors in Children

Seminomas

Seminomas in prepubertal boys are extremely rare. At one time Mostofi, Melicow, and Anderson commented that they had seen none.[87] Grabstald suggested that they did not occur before puberty,[45] and Giebink and Ruymann found only 11 recorded cases.[38] The case that Collins described as a variant of seminoma in an undescended testis of a nine-year-old boy was described by other reviewers as a germinoma or a gonadoblastoma.[22] A bona fide seminoma, however, in a nine-year-old boy responded to orchiectomy and radiation therapy.[139] McCullough described a case in a 10-year-old boy with positive nodes who was treated with node dissection, chemotherapy, and radiation.[82] Karamehmedovic reported a case in a 15-year-old.[63]

Houser found fewer than 10 pediatric seminomas in the literature and reported one other in a 12-year-old.[51] An eight-year-old boy developed seminoma in a testis after having undergone orchidopexy two years previously.[9] Grechi removed an undescended polyorchid testis from a nine-year-old boy that contained anaplastic seminoma, but the boy subsequently succumbed with metastatic disease.[46] Osborn found a seminoma in a 12-year-old boy who had previously undergone contralateral orchidopexy for an undescended testis.[97] The patient was treated with radiation therapy and remained well until five years later, when the previously operated testis enlarged and was found to contain a yolk sac tumor. Boatman's series of 18 boys under 16 years of age with testicular tumors includes a 14-year-old with seminoma.[9] A review of 35 testicular tumors in Nigerian children includes three seminomas.[59] Seminoma and other germ cell testicular tumors have been described in patients with Down's syndrome.[61]

Adult Embryonal Carcinoma

Since the work of Magner and Bryant in 1951, it has been clear that YST is a lesion distinct from embryonal carcinoma.[77] The previous literature presents contradiction in distinguishing these two terms, but subsequent publications have sometimes perpetuated the myth that embryonal carcinoma is a frequent form of infantile testicular tumor. It is likely that most cases so reported would be redescribed as YSTs if the tissue could be reexamined. In older boys, however, there is a chance that embryonal carcinomas could occur, and it is possible to find embryonal elements in an otherwise distinctive YST. Treatment of boys with adult types of testicular tumors is generally identical to treatment of an adult with the same lesion.

GONADAL STROMAL AND INTERSTITIAL CELL TUMORS

Even though Leydig and Sertoli cells are found in separate locations in the testicular parenchyma, they probably share a common embryologic precursor and seem to have related neoplastic forms in children. These so-called interstitial cell tumors are rare in adults but are somewhat more common in children, representing the most common prepubertal non–germ cell testicular tumor. These lesions may or may not be hormonally active. Various terms have been applied to these lesions, including androblastoma, arrhenoblastoma, interstitial cell tumors, granulosa stromal tumors, and gonadal stromal tumors, in addition to the more specific designations of Leydig cell or Sertoli cell tumor, which form the two main subgroups. Mostofi describes these as specialized gonadal stromal tumors.[89] They are found in patients of all ages, the youngest being a 1000-gm, 30-week fetus.[27]

Leydig cell (interstitial cell) tumors (LCT) tend to occur between ages six and 12 years in children and in the third to seventh decades in adults. The experience at Walter Reed demonstrated a prevalence in blacks, in contrast to the well-known infrequency of most other testicular tumors in black males.[28] Symptoms may antedate diagnosis by a number of years, and in Cook's review this interval was two years.[23] In some situations there initially may not be a discernible testicular mass and random testicular biopsy fails to detect the tumor.[37] In children the tumors may present with precocious puberty, gynecomastia, or both.[60] The virilizing or feminizing manifestation is a feature of each individual tumor, but the feminizing forms are more likely in postpubertal patients: of the 38 feminizing Leydig cell tumors discussed by Gabrilove, five occurred in prepubertal boys, one occurred in a 13-year-old, and the rest of the patients were between 19 and 68 years of age.[37] An androgen-producing Leydig cell tumor in a prepubertal male is usually manifested by precocious puberty (i.e., early development of the penis, beard, muscles, and accelerated linear growth). Unusually aggressive behavior may be the main clinical feature in some patients.[60] The combination of precocious puberty and unilateral testicular enlargement should raise the possibility of a Leydig cell tumor. In young boys a Leydig cell tumor may produce elevated serum androgen levels as well as elevated plasma and urinary levels of 17-ketosteroids. These hormonal patterns may be mistaken for those caused by congenital adrenal hyperplasia, but in the latter situation exogenous corticosteroids will suppress the 17-ketosteroids; this is not the case in patients with testicular tumors. Ectopic adrenal rests adjacent to a testis can also be confusing, but, when recognized, these do not require orchiectomy. Franco-Saenz studied biopsies from bilateral testicular tumors in a patient with congenital adrenal hyperplasia (CAH) to determine whether the tumors were LCTs or aberrant adrenal tissue.[36] He concluded that the testicular tumors in CAH develop from pluripotential testicular cells that, under ACTH stimulation and LH suppression, differentiate into ACTH-dependent cells that are morphologically like LCT but functionally like adrenal cells in their behavior. Nonpalpable LCTs have been detected by spermatic vein sampling showing elevated estrogens and estrogen response to human chorionic gonadotropin (hCG).[7] The typical Leydig cell tumor is generally small and on cut section is yellow to brown. These tumors may be quite pleomorphic with many mitotic figures; however, the biologic behavior is predictably benign. Malignancy is defined behaviorally by the presence of metastatic disease, and prepubertal LCTs are unlikely to metastasize.[58] There is often a microscopic resemblance to adrenal rests. Inguinal orchiectomy alone is generally curative, although Yuval described an apparently successful case managed by tumor enucleation alone, with no evidence of recurrence at three years.[146] Signs and symptoms of precocious puberty or gynecomastia may or may not regress.[23] Postoperative supervision is necessary because metastases have been observed as late as nine years after orchiectomy.[124]

Sertoli cell (gonadal stromal) tumors are among the rarest of testicular tumors in children or adults, although these are common canine tumors that frequently metastasize.[111] Sertoli cell tumors, as most of the other PPTTs we have discussed, usually present clinically as a painless testicular mass. They may occur in patients with testicular feminization.[140] White discussed nine newborns with gonadal stromal tumors, all of which were benign.[142] Gynecomastia is a presenting feature in only 15 to 26% of patients with this tumor, and these tend to be older prepubertal or postpubertal boys.[34] Gynecomastia was evident in 60% of patients with malignant Sertoli tumors.[142] Occasional patients have both penile enlargement and gynecomastia,[34] and Gonder reported one of the early cases that documented androgen and estrogen production in an infant with a gonadal stromal tumor.[42] Microscopically, the tumor consists of uniform cells with rare mitotic figures. A unique pathognomonic feature of the benign and neoplastic Sertoli cell is the Charcot-Böttcher crystalloid.[140] The behavior of this tumor in children is usually benign. Malignancy is defined by metastatic behavior rather than histologic appearance, although there is one well-documented case of a malignant Sertoli cell tumor in a child with positive retroperitoneal nodes.[101] Metastases are more common in adults, occurring in 30% of patients.[11] An interesting variant is the large cell calcifying Sertoli tumor, which is often bilateral or multifocal and which may be related to an underlying endocrine disorder.

Waxman's patient had adjacent seminiferous tubules containing only Sertoli cells that ranged from atypical ones to neoplastic Sertoli cells in situ.[140] Rosenzweig described a 16-year-old with hard, nontender, nodular testes that contained the large cell calcifying variant.[110] Sertoli cell adenomas have been described in patients with testicular feminization.[140] Gabrilove reviewed 35 boys with Sertoli cell tumors and found that some of these lesions contained some identifiable Leydig cells. These may take the form of hyperplastic clusters adjacent to areas of Sertoli cell tumor.[37] Inguinal orchiectomy is adequate initial therapy. Abnormal hormonal levels normalize, unless residual disease is present. Gynecomastia, however, may never completely regress, and reduction mammoplasty may be required.[140]

GONADOBLASTOMA

This rare hormone-secreting tumor of germ cells and sex cord derivatives was initially described by Scully in 1953 in two phenotypic females.[117] Since then this lesion has been characterized microscopically by the presence in a tumor of discrete aggregates of intimately mixed germ cells and smaller epithelial cells that resemble immature Sertoli and granulosa cells. Leydig or lutein-type cells are found in about two thirds of the patients, especially in those that are postpubertal. These tumors have been described as dysgenetic gonadomas and gonadocytomas, but Scully offers good reasons for the preferred terminology of gonadoblastoma and explains why Leydig cells are more of an age-dependent concomitant that may or may not be present.

Gonadoblastomas are most common in phenotypic females who may or may not be virilized but are likely to have a Y chromosome. Less than 18% of the gonadoblastomas in Scully's review of 74 cases occurred in phenotypic males, and these patients ranged in age from one to 22 years. The males are usually male pseudohermaphrodites, but they may also be patients with mixed gonadal dysgenesis. The gonad involved is most often unidentifiable but may be a streak gonad or a testis. In any case these tumors occur almost entirely in patients with an underlying gonadal abnormality. In a third of the patients the tumor is bilateral.[11] An additional and different tumor may be found in the gonadoblastoma-bearing gonad or in the contralateral gonad.[117]

Gonadoblastomas do not metastasize but may be associated with a malignant neoplasm within the same gonad or in the contralateral gonad. When there is significant hormonal secretion, it is usually androgenic. In some gonadoblastomas the germ cells are no longer confined to epithelial nests but have invaded stroma. Scully refers to these as gonadoblastomas with germinoma and suggests this is a malignant progression of a gonadoblastoma, which can also progress to any other germ cell testicular tumor.

Proper treatment for a simple gonadoblastoma is orchiectomy. However, when admixed with a malignant germ cell testicular tumor, treatment is dictated by the more invasive element. When a dysgenetic or streak gonad is identified earlier in life, it is generally best to remove it before gonadoblastoma has a chance to develop.

TESTICULAR LEUKEMIA AND LYMPHOMA

The testicle is the first site of extramedullary relapse in 8 to 36% of boys with leukemia.[109, 128] Testicular relapse is more likely if the white blood count is greater than 20,000 at the time of initial diagnosis, and relapse follows quickly at other sites if treatment is not instituted.[128]

The testis seems to offer sanctuary for leukemic cells during chemotherapy, and explanations for this include the blood-testis barrier, scrotal temperature differential (1.7 to 3.8°C cooler than the rest of the body[125]), and the possibility of immunologic privilege in the testis.[109]

The usual presentation of testicular relapse is painless swelling, although in many boys there may be no discernible increase in size. Careful genital examination, however, revealed irregular testicular contours, enlargement, and induration in Shepard's series, which suggested that truly occult leukemic infiltration is rare.[120] Relapse may occur when the bone marrow is in complete remission, and many protocols advocate testicular biopsy prior to discontinuing chemotherapy and repeated biopsies for surveillance.[109]

Standard open biopsy is performed bilaterally, although we have found aspiration biopsy helpful adjunctively. In one of our patients wedge biopsies did not demonstrate leukemic infiltration, but concurrent aspiration biopsy did. Noninvasive methods such as ultrasound have not yet been able to replace biopsy. The leukemic infiltration mainly involves interstitial spaces but may enter seminiferous tubules.

The usual treatment for testicular relapse is local irradiation with 1200 to 2000 rads and resumption of systemic chemotherapy, although relapses have occurred in irradiated gonads.[114] Kim, however, advocated systemic induction therapy for testicular relapse without gonadal irradiation.[64] Tiedemann found 13% of boys with acute lymphoblastic leukemia had their first relapse in the testes, and, in over half of these patients, the relapse was found unexpectedly on routine biopsy or late after systemic therapy had been stopped.[136] After local gonadal irradiation, intrathecal methotrexate, and two years of cyclic chemotherapy, the majority remain in complete remission, leading the authors to suggest that late isolated testicular relapse offers a better chance than late marrow relapse.

Lymphoma may also involve the testes. Burkitt's lymphoma, a common malignancy of children in Africa, accounted for half of the children's testicular tumors in Junaid's series, whereas this lesion is rarely mentioned in any of the other pediatric gonadal tumor series.[59]

RHABDOMYOSARCOMA

Childhood rhabdomyosarcoma is as prevalent a pediatric malignancy as Wilms' tumor or neuroblastoma.[38] Urogenital rhabdomyosarcomas, however, account for only 15% of all rhabdomyosarcomas and usually occur in the prostate, bladder, or vagina. The paratesticular location is uncommon, composing only 7% of patients in the Intergroup Rhabdomyosarcoma Study.[106] Nonetheless, rhabdomyosarcoma is the most common pediatric spermatic cord tumor.[96] Paratesticular rhabdomyosarcoma is more prevalent in children than in adults. Littmann found 74 cases in his literature survey in 1972.[71] Nearly two thirds of these patients were under 15 years of age, and the best survivals were in the boys under five years. Olney's review in 1979 encompassed 162 patients from one month to 80 years of age, and nearly half of the patients were prepubertal.[96] When an anatomic origin could be identified, it was found in the spermatic cord in 34%, paratesticular in 31%, in testis in 15%, in the tunics in 8%, in epididymis in 8%, and in scrotum in 4%. Burrington noted that paratesticular rhabdomyosarcomas do not seem to occur in undescended testes.[14] A bimodal age distribution was noted with peaks at four and 16 years of age. Right- and left-sided lesions were of equal prevalence except in the children younger than 10 years, in whom the left side was involved 2.5 times as often as the right.

Paratesticular rhabdomyosarcomas usually present as painless scrotal or inguinal masses. They may encroach upon or invade the testis, and sometimes they grow so rapidly that the site of origin is obscured by the time of diagnosis. Grossly, these lesions may be rubbery and nodular with great variability in size (Fig. 36–5). The four pathologic types described are pleomorphic, alveolar, embryonal, and botryoid—the last three being the juvenile forms. Mostofi has defined the cellular characteristics of rhabdomyosarcoma.[88] Cross-striations may help make the diagnosis, but their presence is not required.

Evaluation of a paratesticular rhabdomyosarcoma is similar to that of other PPTTs. There is no useful tumor marker, and diag-

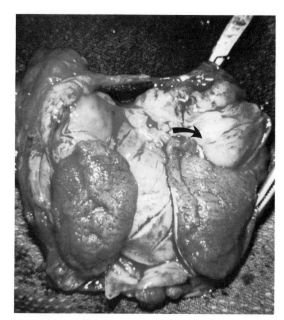

Figure 36–5. Gross appearance of a paratesticular rhabdomyosarcoma.

nosis is made by examination of the inguinal orchiectomy specimen. Scrotal exploration for this tumor produces a significant chance for local recurrence. Stage classification differs from that of testicular tumors, and the Intergroup Rhabdomyosarcoma Study Group system is generally employed: Group 1, localized and resected tumor; Group 2, grossly resected tumor with residual local microscopic disease or regional nodal tumor; Group 3, localized tumor not treated by initial resection; and Group 4, metastases present at diagnosis.[56]

Paratesticular rhabdomyosarcomas have a greater predilection for lymphatic dissemination than YSTs, and nodal involvement occurs in 40% of patients.[106] In the absence of an effective tumor marker, retroperitoneal lymph node dissection is an important diagnostic and therapeutic tool that also provides the opportunity to remove the remainder of the spermatic cord, which might still be a primary tumor site. We have generally favored node dissection as an initial step in management for most Group 1 or 2 paratesticular rhabdomyosarcomas. Burrington commented, "It is difficult to defend statements that aortic lymph node dissections are not indicated."[14] Some centers, however, prefer to withhold node dissection if results of a lymphangiogram are negative.[56] Recent clinical experiences reported by Olive[95] and Quesada[103] demonstrated favorable results without node dissection in Group 1 patients.

Chemotherapy has been refined by the Intergroup Study, and cyclic treatment with vincristine, actinomycin, and cyclophosphamide is usually given to Group 1 and 2 patients after, or instead of, lymphadenectomy.[106] Children with more extensive disease are best treated initially with chemotherapy to lessen the effects of the initial disease, and tumor resection or irradiation can follow.

Chances for survival seem to be increasing as more experience is gained with rhabdomyosarcoma, and recent reports illustrate this favorable trend. Burrington described eight patients in 1969, of which six were cured.[14] In the cure group, in addition to having orchiectomy, four patients underwent radiation therapy, two had node dissections, and one had chemotherapy. The two patients that died presented with metastatic disease and both were dead within a year of initial diagnosis. Tank, in 1972, reported on eight boys from three months to 16 years of age.[131] Four patients with Group 1 disease were cured by orchiectomy alone in three instances and orchiectomy and node dissection in another. Four other patients died of metastatic disease; three presented with extensive disease at the time of diagnosis and the fourth had positive results on retroperitoneal node dissection. Cromie's five patients were all alive at the time of his report in 1979; they underwent multimodality therapy.[26] That same year, in Olney's experience with seven patients (two deaths), the five retroperitoneal node dissections done as initial therapy all had negative results. Two of these patients with no diseased nodes subsequently developed disseminated disease.[96] Cheng described a technique to transpose the testis away from a field of intended scrotal irradiation in a boy with a paratesticular rhabdomyosarcoma. The lesion had been initially approached scrotally, and local recurrence followed.[19]

Occasional other intrascrotal sarcomas have been described in paratesticular locations, but these are extremely rare curiosities.[94, 113]

OTHER TESTICULAR TUMORS

Other testicular tumors in children are extremely uncommon. Tumors metastatic to the testis have been described occasionally. Haupt found two children among 127 patients with secondary testicular tumors, but the primary lesions were not noted.[48] Adrenal rest tumors are occasionally found, but these may be clinically evident only because of an underlying endocrinologic disorder such as congenital adrenal hyperplasia, and these disorders respond to steroids.[13] Townell described a juvenile xanthogranuloma of the testis in a seven-month-old.[137] Localized testicular infarction can mimic a mass.[57] Benign lesions of the tunica albuginea are seen in adults[138] but must be very rare in children, although hemangioma of the tunica albuginea was described in a 15-year-old.[119] Scrotal panniculitis, or fat necrosis, can also produce an indurated scrotal mass in children, although this lesion is usually located inferior to the testis.[30, 65, 93] Healed meconium peritonitis may present as an inguinal mass.[135] Paratesticular accessory spleen occurs in patients with splenogonadal fusion.[143] Adenomatoid tumor was noted in a five-month-old.[18]

Scrotal lymphangiomas and hemangiomas have been recognized in children.[44, 76] Myxoid neurofibroma has been reported in a young man.[72] Testicular or epididymal tuberculosis or sarcoidosis is not uncommon in young men,[118] although we have not seen these in the prepubertal ages. These various testicular and adnexal lesions are so unusual that principles of management of the more common intrascrotal neoplasms should generally apply.

References

1. Abell MR, Holtz F: Testicular neoplasms in infants and children. I. Tumors of germ cell origin. Cancer 16:965–981, 1963.
2. Allyn DL, Silverberg SG, Salzberg AM: Endodermal sinus tumor of vagina. Report of a case with 7-year survival and literature review of so-called "mesonephromas." Cancer 27:1231–1238, 1971.
3. Archson E, Cromie W: Yolk sac tumor: chemotherapy. Dial Pediatr Urol 5:4, 1982.
4. Barnhouse DH: Epidermoid cyst of the testicle. Br J Urol 44:364–367, 1972.
5. Bates RJ, Perrone TL, Althausen A: Simple epidermoid cysts of testis. Urology 17:560–562, 1981.
6. Belt E: Tumors of testicle. Am J Surg 38:201–219, 1937.
7. Bercovici JP, Nahoul K, Tater D, et al: Hormonal profile of Leydig cell tumors with gynecomastia. J Clin Endocrinol Metab 59:625–630, 1984.
8. Bloom DA, Dipietro MA, Gikas PW, McGuire EJ: Extratesticular dermoid cyst and fibrous dysplasia of the epididymis. J Urol (in press).
9. Boatman DL, Culp DA, Wilson VB: Testicular neoplasms in children. J Urol 109:315–317, 1973.
10. Brodeur GM, Howarth CB, Pratt CB, et al: Malignant germ cell tumors in 57 children and adolescents. Cancer 48:1890–1898, 1981.

11. Brosman SA: Male genital tract. In PP Kelalis, LR King, AB Belman (eds), Clinical Pediatric Urology, 2nd ed. Philadelphia, WB Saunders, 1985.
12. Brosman SA: Testicular tumors in prepubertal children. Urology 13:581–588, 1979.
13. Burke EF, Gilbert E, Uehling DT: Adrenal rest tumors of the testes. J Urol 109:649–652, 1973.
14. Burrington JD: Rhabdomyosarcoma of the paratesticular tissues in children. Report of eight cases. J Pediatr Surg 4:503–510, 1969.
15. Carney JA, Thompson DP, Johnson CL, Lynn HB: Teratomas in children: clinical and pathologic aspects. J Pediatr Surg 7:271–282, 1972.
16. Carroll WL, Kempson RL, Govan DE, et al: Conservative management of testicular endodermal sinus tumor in childhood. J Urol 133:1011–1014, 1985.
17. Chaffey WC: Early sarcoma of testis. Trans Pathol Soc London 36:302, 1885.
18. Chahla Y: Benign genital mesothelioma. Eur Urol 11:285–287, 1985.
19. Cheng BS, King LR, Kinney TR: Testicle transposition in children who undergo low-pelvic or scrotal irradiation. Urology 24:476–478, 1984.
20. Clark HJ: Malignant disease of the testicle in an infant. Lancet 2:145, 1901.
21. Cohen EL, Mandel E, Goodman JD, et al: Epidermoid cyst of testicle. Ultrasonographic characteristics. Urology 24:79–81, 1984.
22. Collins JD, Schoenenberger AP: An unusual germinal tumor of the testis in a nine-year-old boy: a variant of a seminoma. J Urol 87:710–714, 1962.
23. Cook CD, Gross RE, Landing BH, Zygmuntowicz AS: Interstitial cell tumor of the testis. Study of a 5-year-old boy with pseudoprecocious puberty. J Clin Endocrinol 12:725–734, 1952.
24. Cowen R: Teratoma of the epididymis: a mature adult type inclusion tumor of the epididymis in an 18-month-old child. J Urol 79:1001–1002, 1958.
25. Cromie W, Kaplan G, Kelalis P, et al: Prepubertal gonadal stromal tumors: a report for the Testicular Tumor Registry. American Academy of Pediatrics, Section on Urology, 54th Annual Meeting, San Antonio, Texas, October 20, 1985.
26. Cromie WJ, Raney RB Jr, Duckett JW: Paratesticular rhabdomyosarcoma in children. J Urol 122:80–82, 1979.
27. Crump WD: Juvenile granulosa cell (sex cord–stromal) tumor of fetal testis. J Urol 129:1057–1058, 1983.
28. Daniels JL Jr, Stutzman RE, McLeod DG: A comparison of testicular tumors in black and white patients. J Urol 125:341–342, 1981.
29. Donohue J: Personal communication.
30. Donohue R, Utler WL: Idiopathic fat necrosis in the scrotum. Br J Urol 47:331–333, 1975.
31. Doyle GB: Embryonal carcinoma of testis in infant. Br J Urol 27:287–291, 1955.
32. Drago JR, Nelson RP, Palmer JM: Childhood embryonal carcinoma of testes. Urology 12:499–503, 1978.
33. Exelby PR: Testicular cancer in children. Cancer 45(7 suppl):1803–1809, 1980.
34. Fligiel Z, Kaneko M, Leiter E: Bilateral Sertoli cell tumor of testes with feminizing and masculinizing activity occurring in a child. Cancer 38:1853–1858, 1976.
35. Fraley EE, Ketcham AS: Teratoma of testis in an infant. J Urol 100:659–660, 1968.
36. Franco-Saenz R, Antonipillai I, Tan SY, et al: Cortisol production by testicular tumors in a patient with congenital adrenal hyperplasia (21-hydroxylase deficiency). J Clin Endocrinol Metab 53:85–90, 1981.
37. Gabrilove JL, Nicolis GL, Mitty HA, Sohval AR: Feminizing interstitial cell tumor of the testis: personal observations and a review of the literature. Cancer 35:1185–1202, 1975.
38. Giebink GS, Ruymann FB: Testicular tumors in childhood. Review and report of three cases. Am J Dis Child 127:433–438, 1974.
39. Gilbaugh JH Jr, Kelalis PP, Dockerty MB: Epidermoid cysts of the testis. J Urol 97:876–879, 1967.
40. Gitlin D, Perricelli A, Gitlin GM: Synthesis of alpha-fetoprotein by liver, yolk sac, and gastrointestinal tract of the human conceptus. Cancer Res 32:979–982, 1972.
41. Goldberg JD, Deitch AD, Schevchuck M, et al: Comparison of histologic and flow cytometric evaluation of cyclophosphamide induced testicular damage. Urology 24:472, 1984.
42. Gonder MJ, Fadell EJ: Gonadal stromal tumor in an infant. J Urol 84:357–359, 1960.
43. Gonzalez-Crussi F, Roth LM: The human yolk sac and yolk sac carcinoma. Hum Pathol 7:675–691, 1976.
44. Gotoh M, Tsai S, Sugiyama T, et al: Giant scrotal hemangioma with azoospermia. Urology 22:637–639, 1983.
45. Grabstald H: Testis tumors. AUA/Roche History of Urology, Nutley, NJ, 1976.
46. Grechi G, Zampi GC, Selli C, et al: Polyorchidism and seminoma in a child. J Urol 123:291–292, 1980.
47. Gupta SK, Gupta S, Khanna S: Dermoid cyst of scrotal raphe containing calculi. Br J Urol 46:348, 1974.
48. Haupt HM, Mann RB, Trump DL, Abeloff MD: Metastatic carcinoma involving the testis. Clinical and pathologic distinction from primary testicular neoplasms. Cancer 54:709, 1984.
49. Homsy Y, Arrojo-Vila F, Khoriaty N, Demers J: Yolk sac tumor of the testicle: is retroperitoneal lymph node dissection necessary? J Urol 132:532–536, 1984.
50. Hopkins TB, Jaffe N, Colodny A, et al: The management of testicular tumors in children. J Urol 120:96–102, 1978.
51. Houser R, Izant RJ Jr, Persky L: Testicular tumors in children. Am J Surg 110:876–892, 1965.
52. Huntington RW Jr, Bullock WK: Yolk sac tumors of extragonadal origin. Cancer 25:1368–1376, 1970.
53. Huntington RW Jr, Morganstern NL, Sargent JA, et al: Germinal tumors exhibiting the endodermal sinus pattern of Teilum in young children. Cancer 16:34–47, 1963.
54. Ise T, Ohtsuki H, Matsumoto K, et al: Management of malignant testicular tumors in children. Cancer 37:1539–1545, 1976.
55. Johnson AA: Cystic disease of the testis occurring in an infant and probably congenital. Trans Pathol Soc London 7:241–246, 1856.
56. Johnson DE, McHugh TA, Jaffe N: Paratesticular rhabdomyosarcoma in childhood. J Urol 128:1275–1276, 1982.
57. Johnston JH: Localized infarction of the testis. Br J Urol 32:97–99, 1960.

58. Johnstone G: Prepubertal gynaecomastia in association with an interstitial-cell tumour of the testis. Br J Urol 39:211–220, 1967.

59. Junaid TA: Testicular cancer in children and adolescents in Ibadan, Nigeria. Urology 18:510–513, 1981.

60. Jungck EC, Thrash AM, Ohlmacher AP, et al: Sexual precocity due to interstitial cell tumor of the testis: report of 2 cases. J Clin Endocrinol 17:291, 1957.

61. Kamidono S, Takada K, Ishigami J, et al: Giant seminoma of undescended testis in Down syndrome. Urology 25:637, 1985.

62. Kaplan WE, Firlit CF: Treatment of testicular yolk sac carcinoma in the young child. J Urol 126:663–664, 1981.

63. Karamehmedovic O, Woodtli W, Plüss HJ: Testicular tumors in childhood. J Pediatr Surg 10:109–114, 1975.

64. Kim TH, Hargreaves HK, Brynes RK, et al: Pretreatment testicular biopsy in childhood acute lymphocytic leukaemia. Lancet 2:657–658, 1981.

65. Koster LH, Antoon SJ: Fat necrosis in the scrotum. J Urol 123:599–600, 1980.

66. Kramer SA: Embryonal cell carcinoma in children. Soc Pediatr Urol Newsletter, 1981.

67. Kramer SA: Pediatric urologic oncology. Urol Clin North Am 12:31, 1985.

68. Kramer SA, Wold LE, Gilchrist GS, et al: Yolk sac carcinoma: an immunohistochemical and clinicopathologic review. J Urol 131:315–318, 1984.

69. Lewis EL: Tumors of the testis in infants. US Armed Forces Med J 8:431, 1957.

70. Li FP, Fraumeni JF Jr: Testicular cancers in children: epidemiologic characteristics. Natl Cancer Inst Bull 48:1575–1581, 1972.

71. Littmann R, Tessler AN, Valensi Q: Paratesticular rhabdomyosarcoma: a case presentation and review of the literature. J Urol 108:290–292, 1972.

72. Livolsi VA, Schiff M: Myxoid neurofibroma of the testis. J Urol 118:341–342, 1977.

73. Logothetis CJ, Samuels ML, Trindade A, et al: The prognostic significance of endodermal sinus tumor histology among patients treated for stage III nonseminomatous germ cell tumors of the testes. Cancer 53:122–128, 1984.

74. Lynch JH, Maxted WC: Use of ephedrine in postlymphadenectomy ejaculatory failure: a case report. J Urol 129:379, 1983.

75. Mackinnon AE, Cohen SJ: Archenteronoma (yolk sac tumors). J Pediatr Surg 13:21–23, 1978.

76. MacMillan RW, MacDonald BR, Alpern HD: Scrotal lymphangioma. Urology 23:79–80, 1984.

77. Magner D, Bryant AJS: Adenocarcinoma of testis occurring in infants: report of 2 cases. Arch Pathol 52:82–89, 1951.

78. Magner D, Campbell JS, Wiglesworth FW: Testicular adenocarcinoma with clear cells, occurring in infancy. Cancer 9:165–175, 1956.

79. Marshall S, Lyon RP, Scott MP: A conservative approach to testicular tumors in children: 12 cases and their management. J Urol 129:350–351, 1983.

80. Martinez-Mora J, Cerquella VS, Padulles J, et al: Management of primary testicular tumors in children. J Pediatr Surg 15:283–286, 1980.

81. Matsumoto K, Nakauchi K, Fujita K: Radiation therapy for the embryonal carcinoma of testis in childhood. J Urol 104:778–780, 1970.

82. McCullough DL, Carlton CE, Seybold HM: Testicular tumors in infants and children: report of 5 cases and evaluation of different modes of therapy. J Urol 105:140–148, 1971.

83. Minghetti PP, Harper ME, Alpert E, Dugaiczyk A: Chromosomal structure and localization of the human alpha-fetoprotein gene. Ann NY Acad Sci 417:1–12, 1983.

84. Mizejewski GJ, Bellisario R, Carter TP: Birth weight and alpha-fetoprotein in the newborn [letter]. Pediatrics 73:736–737, 1984.

85. Moran HM: Notes on a case of embryoma testis. Med J Austral 2:5, 1917.

86. Mosli HA, Carpenter B, Schillinger JF: Teratoma of the testis in a pubertal child. J Urol 133:105–106, 1985.

87. Mostofi FK: Infantile testicular tumors. Bull NY Acad Med 28:684, 1952.

88. Mostofi FK, Price EB Jr: Tumors of the male genital system. Atlas of Tumor Pathology, Second series, Fascicle 8, Washington, DC, Armed Forces Institute of Pathology, 1973.

89. Mostofi FK, Theiss EA, Ashley DJB: Tumors of specialized gonadal stroma in human male patients: androblastoma, Sertoli cell tumor, granulosa-theca cell tumor of the testis, and gonadal stromal tumor. Cancer 12:944–957, 1959.

90. Muir CS, Nectoux J: Epidemiology of cancer of the testis and penis. NCI Monogr 53:157–164, 1979.

91. Narayana AS, Loening S, Weimar G, Culp DA: Serum markers in testicular tumors. J Urol 121:51–53, 1979.

92. Nelson RP: Malignant testicular tumors in children. Urology 10:290, 1977.

93. Nemoy NJ, Rosin S, Kaplan L: Scrotal panniculitis in the prepubertal male patient. J Urol 118:492–493, 1977.

94. O'Brien MG: Primary sarcoma of epididymis: case report. J Urol 47:311–319, 1942.

95. Olive D, Flamant F, Zucker JM, et al: Paraaortic lymphadenectomy is not necessary in the treatment of localized paratesticular rhabdomyosarcoma. Cancer 54:1283–1287, 1984.

96. Olney LE, Narayana A, Loening S, Culp DA: Intrascrotal rhabdomyosarcoma. Urology 14:113–116, 1979.

97. Osborn DE, Jeffery PJ: Testicular tumor in children: report of 4 cases. Urology 7:433–435, 1976.

98. O'Sullivan P, Daneman A, Chan HS, et al: Extragonadal endodermal sinus tumors in children: a review of 24 cases. Pediatr Radiol 13:249–257, 1983.

99. Parker RW: Congenital adeno-sarcoma of testis. Trans Pathol Soc London 36:299, 1885.

100. Perry C, Servadio C: Seminoma in childhood. J Urol 124:932–933, 1980.

101. Pierce GB, Bullock WK, Huntington RW Jr: Yolk sac tumors of the testis. Cancer 25:644–658, 1970.

102. Price EB Jr: Epidermoid cysts of the testis: a clinical and pathologic analysis of 69 cases from the testicular tumor registry. J Urol 102:708–713, 1969.

103. Quesada EM, Diez B, Silva M, Sackmann MF: Paratesticular rhabdomyosarcoma in children. American Academy of Pediatrics, Section on Urology, 54th Annual Meeting, San Antonio, Texas, October 20, 1985.

104. Quintana J, Beresi V, Latorre JJ, et al: Infantile embryonal carcinoma of testis. J Urol 128:785–787, 1982.

105. Rabinovitch HH: Simple innocuous treatment of massive cyclophosphamide hemorrhagic cystitis. Urology 13:610–612, 1979.

106. Raney RB Jr, Hays DM, Lawrence W Jr, et al: Paratesticular rhabdomyosarcoma in childhood. Cancer 42:729–736, 1978.

107. Ravich L, Lerman PH, Drabkin JW, Noya J: Embryonal carcinoma of testicle in childhood: review of literature and presentation of 2 cases. J Urol 96:501–507, 1966.

108. ReMine WH, Woolner LB, Judd ES, Hopkins DM: Testicular teratoma in infancy: report of a case with a 10-year follow-up. Proc Mayo Clinic 36:661–664, 1961.

109. Rosenkrantz JG, Wong KY, Ballard ET, et al: Leukemic infiltration of the testis during long-term remission. J Pediatr Surg 13:753–756, 1978.

110. Rosenzweig JL, Lawrence DA, Vogel DL, et al: Adrenocorticotropin-independent hypercortisolemia and testicular tumors in a patient with a pituitary tumor and gigantism. J Clin Endocrinol Metab 55:421–427, 1982.

111. Rosvoll RV, Woodard JR: Malignant Sertoli cell tumor of the testis. Cancer 22:8–13, 1968.

112. Roth LM, Panganiban WG: Gonadal and extragonadal yolk sac carcinomas: a clinicopathologic study of 14 cases. Cancer 37:812–820, 1976.

113. Rusche C: Twelve cases of testicular tumors occurring during infancy and childhood. J Pediatr 40:192–199, 1952.

114. Saiontz HI, Gilchrist GS, Smithson WA, et al: Testicular relapse in childhood leukemia. Mayo Clinic Proc 53:212–216, 1978.

115. Sakashita S, Koyanagi T, Tsuji I, et al: Congenital anomalies in children with testicular germ cell tumor. J Urol 124:889–891, 1980.

116. Scobie WG: Orchioblastoma. A report of six cases. Br J Urol 42:332–335, 1970.

117. Scully RE: Gonadoblastoma. A review of 74 cases. Cancer 25:1340–1356, 1970.

118. Seaworth JF: Aggressive diagnostic approach indicated in testicular sarcoidosis. Urology 21:396, 1983.

119. Shental J, Fischelovitz J, Sudarsky M, Rizescu J: Hemangioma of the tunica albuginea testis. Eur Urol 8:370–371, 1982.

120. Shepard BR, Hensle TW, Marboe CC: Testicular biopsy and occult tumor in acute lymphocytic leukemia. Urology 22:36–38, 1983.

121. Shinohara M, Komatsu H, Kawamura T, Yokoyama M: Familial testicular teratoma in 2 children: familial report and review of the literature. J Urol 123:552–555, 1980.

122. Shirai T, Itoh T, Yoshiki T, et al: Immunofluorescent demonstration of alpha-fetoprotein and other plasma proteins in yolk sac tumor. Cancer 38:1661–1667, 1976.

123. Silcock AQ: Congenital sarcoma of the testis. Trans Pathol Soc London 36:301, 1885.

124. Silverberg SG, Thompson JW, Higashi G, Basin AM: Malignant interstitial cell tumor of the testis: case report and review. J Urol 96:356–363, 1966.

125. Smith SD, Trueworthy RC, Klopovich PM, et al: Management of children with isolated testicular leukemia. Cancer 54:2854–2858, 1984.

126. Snyder HM, D'Angio GJ, Evans AE, Raney RB Jr: Pediatric oncology. In PC Walsh, RF Gittes, AD Perlmutter, TA Stamey (eds), Campbell's Urology, 5th ed. Philadelphia, WB Saunders, 1985.

127. Spitalny A, Bronstein B: Teratoma of the testis in an infant: case report. J Urol 85:63–64, 1961.

128. Stoffel TJ, Nesbit ME, Levitt SH: Extramedullary involvement of the testes in childhood leukemia. Cancer 35:1203–1211, 1975.

129. Talerman A: The incidence of yolk sac tumor (endodermal sinus tumor) elements in germ cell tumors of the testis in adults. Cancer 36:211–215, 1975.

130. Talerman A, Haije WG, Baggerman L: Serum alphafetoprotein (AFP) in patients with germ cell tumors of the gonads and extragonadal sites: correlation between endodermal sinus (yolk sac) tumor and raised serum AFP. Cancer 46:380–385, 1980.

131. Tank ES, Fellmann SL, Wheeler ES, et al: Treatment of urogenital tract rhabdomyosarcoma in infants and children. J Urol 107:324–328, 1972.

132. Taylor G, Jordan M, Churchill B, Mancer K: Yolk sac tumor of the bladder. J Urol 129:591–594, 1983.

133. Teilum G: Endodermal sinus tumors of the ovary and testis. Comparative morphogenesis of the so-called mesonephroma ovarii (Schiller) and extraembryonic (yolk-sac allantoic) structures of the rat's placenta. Cancer 21:1092–1105, 1959.

134. Teoh TB, Steward JK, Willis RA: The distinctive adenocarcinoma of the infant's testis: an account of 15 cases. J Pathol Bacteriol 80:147–156, 1960.

135. Thompson RB, Rosen DI, Gross DM: Healed meconium peritonitis presenting as an inguinal mass. J Urol 110:364–365, 1973.

136. Tiedemann J, Chessells JM, Sandland RM: Isolated testicular relapse in boys with acute lymphoblastic leukaemia: treatment and outcome. Br Med J 285:1614–1616, 1982.

137. Townell NH, Gledhill A, Robinson T, Hopewell P: Juvenile xanthogranuloma of the testis. J Urol 133:1054–1055, 1985.

138. Turner WR Jr, Derrick FC, Sanders P III, Rous SN: Benign lesions of the tunica albuginea. J Urol 117:602–603, 1977.

139. Viprakasit D, Navarro C, Guarin UK, Garnes HA: Seminoma in children. Urology 9:568–570, 1977.

140. Waxman M, Damjanov I, Khapra A, Landau SJ: Large cell calcifying Sertoli tumor of the testis: light microscopic and ultrastructural study. Cancer 54:1574–1581, 1984.

141. Weissbach L, Altwein JE, Stiens R: Germinal testicular tumors in childhood. Report of observations and literature review. Eur Urol 10:73–85, 1984.

142. White JM, McCarthy MP: Testicular gonadal stromal tumors in newborns. Urology 20:121–124, 1982.

143. Wick MR, Rife CC: Paratesticular accessory spleen. Mayo Clin Proc 56:455–456, 1981.

144. Wobbes T, Oldhoff J, Koops H, de Vries JA: The treatment of infantile embryonal carcinoma (yolk-sac tumour) of the testis in children. Z Kinderchir 33:349–354, 1981.

145. Young PG, Mount BM, Foote FW Jr, Whitmore WF Jr: Embryonal adenocarcinoma in the prepubertal testis. A clinicopathologic study of 18 cases. Cancer 26:1065–1075, 1970.

146. Yuval E, Eidelman A, Beer SI, Vure E: Local excision of a virilising Leydig-cell tumour of the testis. Br J Urol 46:237–240, 1974.

E. DAVID CRAWFORD, M.D.
CRAIG A. DAWKINS, M.D.

CHAPTER *37*   *Cancer of the Penis*

"He that is wounded in the stones or has his private member cut off shall not enter into the congregation of the Lord."

DEUTERONOMY 23:1

HISTORICAL PERSPECTIVE

One of the earliest references to the management of penile cancer dates to the first century AD, when Celsus reported the amputation and subsequent cautery of the penile stump.[46] The disease was relatively common and was mentioned in writings by the Egyptians, Hebrews, Persians, and Indians.[34] In 1761 the famed anatomist Morgagni, who was present at a partial penectomy performed by Valsalva, reviewed the procedure in amusing detail.[44] The first detailed description of an operation for radical cure of carcinoma of the penis is credited to Thiersch in 1875.[35] Sir William MacCormack reported on five cases in 1886, whereby he performed a total penectomy, dividing the scrotum with bilateral inguinal incisions similar to the procedure of Thiersch.[26] In 1898, Curtis[12] advised removing the lymph nodes from the groin en bloc and the penis being amputated at the pubic symphysis. In 1912, Gibson[19] advocated the en bloc dissection of the penis and bilateral inguinal nodes and removal of the corpora. The corpus spongiosum was transected at the pubic symphysis and brought out the anterior wall of the scrotum, allowing the patient control of his stream through scrotal manipulation. By 1924, Barringer and Dean[7] recommended only partial amputation of the penis 1.5 cm proximal to the lesion followed by radiation therapy to the groin. In 1931, Young[64] reported his results with partial penectomy and unilateral groin dissection for management of squamous cell carcinoma of the penis, a technique he initiated in 1907. This operation differed from those previously described in that, along with the glands of the inguinal region, femoral nodes were additionally removed en bloc with the primary penile tumor.

The role of lymph node dissection in penile cancer was advanced with Daseler's[13] anatomical description in 1948 of the lymph nodes in the inguinal region. Five years later, Baronofsky[5] described the ilioinguinal node dissection, including the transposition of the proximal sartorius muscles for coverage of the femoral vessels.

Cabanas,[10] in 1977, described a "sentinel node" in the inguinal node chain that was the first involved with metastatic disease. This node was sampled and, if results were negative, then a complete node dissection could be avoided. The reliability of sentinel node biopsy, however, has not been supported by others.[48, 50] Currently the primary penile lesion may be managed by local excision, chemosurgery,[55] partial amputation, total penectomy, or laser therapy. For metastatic disease the techniques for lymph node dissection are consistently being improved to minimize morbidity.[11]

EPIDEMIOLOGY

Carcinoma of the penis accounts for 0.3 to 1.0% of cancer in the male population in the United States.[4, 36, 49, 59] In the hot, humid regions of South America, Africa, and the Far East, squamous cell carcinoma may compose 10 to 20% of malignant tumors in males.[36, 49] Indeed, unusually high incidences are reported in tropical areas such as Puerto Rico, Mexico, Paraguay, Venezuela, Vietnam, Ceylon, Thailand, China, Uganda, and parts of India.[25, 49, 61] Migrants into an area with a high incidence of squamous cell carcinoma of the penis tend to assume the incidence of that area.[49]

Race seems not to be a factor in the predisposition to penile cancer, but hygiene and retained phimotic foreskin are implicated. Schrek and Lenowitz[57] compared the frequency of squamous cell carcinoma of the penis in blacks and whites with that for controls and noted no increased incidence of tumor in blacks. It is well known that squamous cell carcinoma of the penis is extremely rare among Jews, who ritualistically circumcise in the neonatal period.[4, 14, 25, 34, 35, 37, 49, 50, 57] The disease has been infrequently reported in Jews who have been circumcised, but these have been unusual situations of chronic irritation or retained foreskin from inadequate circumcision.[50] Consequently, there is a low incidence of penile cancer in Israel, with only one case reported in 1969, less than 0.1 case per 100,000 males.[49] The incidence of nongenital epidermoid cancers in Jewish males parallels that of other populations, further supporting the prophylactic role of circumcision.[14]

This disease is seldom found in any male circumcised in infancy.[25, 30] The most convincing evidence demonstrating the effectiveness of circumcision in preventing squamous cell carcinoma of the penis comes from areas where two cultures live in proximity and differ mainly in the practice of circumcision. For example, the Gisu tribe in Uganda, which practices infant circumcision, has a markedly lower incidence of penile cancer than the general Ugandan male population, which does not practice circumcision.[15] In addition, the difference in incidence of penile cancer among the Mohammedans and Hindus in India supports the efficacy of the Mohammedan ritual of infant circumcision.[14, 46]

Cancer of the penis occurs most commonly in the sixth decade, with an age range from 20 to 90.[4, 14, 49] It has been reported in children[31] but rarely occurs in males under 40 years of age in the United States. Hoppmann and Fraley[25] combined several large series and quote a mean age of 58 years at presentation.

Although most epidermoid tumors arise in exposed parts of the body, this tumor is unique in its closed-space origin.[58] The presence of phimosis or paraphimosis is the one factor that is most consistently implicated with penile cancer, suggesting the retention or production of a carcinogen under the foreskin. In addition, it is known that circumcision performed early in life is protective against carcinoma of the penis, whereas circumcision performed in adult life has no prophylactic effects.[57] This implies the action of a carcinogen in a closed space. Prolonged irritation and chronic inflammation are thought by most investigators to stimulate epithelial tumor growth.[44]

In the normal uncircumcised male, smegma, or the admixture of desquamated cells and *Mycobacterium smegmatis*, begins to form during the first days of life. It forms from surface epithelial cells and under normal conditions is the only material in the preputial cavity, suggesting its possible role as a carcinogen.[52] The same surface is accessible to daily retraction and washing. It has been suggested that *Mycobacterium smegmatis* may convert the smegma sterols into carcinogenic sterols.[60]

PATHOLOGY

Generally, cancer of the penis presents as a papillary or ulcerative lesion under the prepuce on the glans. The majority of lesions are well-differentiated squamous cell carcinomas. However, the histologic grade of the tumor seems to influence the propensity of the primary tumor to metastasize. Neither the age of the patient nor the duration of symptoms affect the metastatic behavior of the tumor.[61]

CLINICAL PRESENTATION

Cancer of the penis begins as a small papillary or chronic ulcerative lesion with symptoms largely dependent on the degree

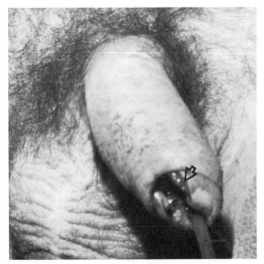

Figure 37–1. Squamous cell carcinoma of glans penis (arrow) in 42-year-old male.

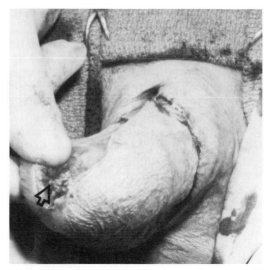

Figure 37–3. Squamous cell carcinoma in patient with epispadias (arrow)

of phimosis (Figs. 37–1 to 37–3). Usually there is some itching and burning under the prepuce and an occasional foul discharge. A paraphimosis may develop in an otherwise normal retractile foreskin. Signs and symptoms may be ignored for several months, the results of a form of denial or fear of venereal disease regardless of exposure.

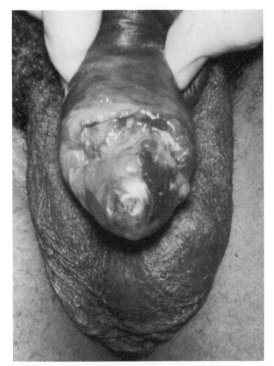

Figure 37–2. Extensive squamous cell carcinoma of glans penis and foreskin.

DIFFERENTIAL DIAGNOSIS

In a number of large series, squamous cell carcinoma of the penis composed more than 95% of penile malignancies. Other cancerous lesions included basal cell carcinomas, melanomas, mesenchymal tumors including fibrosarcoma and Kaposi's sarcoma, and metastatic tumors to the penis.[25] There are several diseases that may closely resemble cancer of the penis. These include balanitis, the chancre of syphilis, the ulcerative chancre of granuloma inguinale, herpes ulcers, tuberculosis, and papilloma of the penis. In addition, tumor-like premalignant lesions that include leukoplakia, balanitis xerotica obliterans, erythroplasia of Queyrat, bowenoid lesions, Buschke-Löwenstein tumors, and Paget's disease can mimic squamous cell carcinoma.

Precancerous Dermatologic Lesions

Leukoplakia of the glans penis is a rare condition, more commonly occurring in diabetics. It appears as one or more scaly patches generally originating at the meatal area with occasional meatal stenosis. Pathologically, it is characterized by acanthosis, hyperkeratosis, and parakeratosis.[8, 43] The differential diagnoses include balanitis xerotica obliterans, lichen planus, lichen simplex chronicus, and candidiasis.[43] Local hygiene and excisional biopsy with close follow-up usually are required for treatment.

Balanitis xerotica obliterans presents with white, atrophic, slightly edematous plaques resulting in phimotic adhesions between the prepuce and glans. Meatal stenosis may appear as a complication. The disease can resemble carcinoma in situ. Although it occurs generally in elderly diabetics, the disease has been reported in pediatric patients.[41] Treatment consists of circumcision and topical steroid therapy. Squamous cell carcinoma has been reported in very rare instances in association with balanitis xerotica obliterans.[43]

Bowen's disease is squamous cell carcinoma in situ that may involve the shaft of the penis as well as the hairy skin of the inguinal and suprapubic area. Clinically, the lesion is a solitary, dull-red plaque with areas of crusting and oozing. Approximately 25% of patients who have this disease will have a concomitant visceral malignancy.[45] Treatment is predicated by the size of the lesion and the area involved. Topical 5-fluorouracil (5-FU) is effective for lesions on the shaft or glans. However, if hair-bearing areas are involved, the epithelium of the follicles frequently contains in situ cancer requiring surgical excision.[20, 63]

Erythroplasia of Queyrat is an epidermoid carcinoma in situ that occurs primarily on the glans or coronal sulcus. Clinically, it appears as a reddened, elevated, or ulcerated lesion. Mikhail[43] reported that five of 15 patients presenting with erythroplasia of Queyrat had invasive squamous cell carcinoma at diagnosis. Erythroplasia of Queyrat is not associated with internal malignancies. Treatment consists of topical 5% 5-FU cream applied twice a day for 3 to 4 weeks.[20] With this treatment, inflammation usually resolves over a period of weeks to months. After application of the cream, it is advisable to have the patient wear a condom over his penis so that intense dermatitis of the scrotum or inguinal region does not occur. Circumcision is the treatment of choice when Queyrat's erythroplasia is limited to the prepuce.

Extramammary *Paget's disease* is a rare intraepithelial apocrine carcinoma. The most common sites are the scrotum, inguinal folds, and perianal region.[43] Extramammary Paget's disease should be treated by surgical excision. However, recurrences are common because of the multicentricity of the process. The lesion has a propensity to metastasize, necessitating frequent assessment of regional nodes. Radiotherapy has been recommended as palliative treatment.[43]

Giant condyloma acuminatum (Buschke-Löwenstein's tumor) is believed to be caused by a papovavirus,[43] yet the virus has not been clearly demonstrated in this lesion, leading some to postulate that it is a low-grade malignancy with slow, locally aggressive growth.[32] It presents as a cauliflower-like lesion arising from the glans and foreskin. Deep biopsies are indicated because of the inward growth of the tumor. Mostofi and Price[45] reserve the term "giant condyloma" for well-differentiated papillary squamous cell tumors with no true invasion and no capacity to metastasize. Giant condylomas with invasion are classified as verrucous carcinomas. Partial or total penectomy is recommended in the majority of the cases.

Soft Tissue Tumors of the Penis

Penile soft tissue tumors are uncommon lesions. Approximately one half of the tumors are benign and may include angiomatous, neurogenous, myogenous, fibrous, and lymphoreticular tumors.[39] Table 37–1 classifies soft tissue penile tumors by location and malignancy. Most soft tissue tumors occur on the shaft and are malignant. Macaluso and associates[39] have reported a rare case of a glomus tumor of the penis, which was cured by simple surgical excision.

Nonpenile Primary Tumors with Penile Metastasis

Cancers metastatic to the penis are rare and usually represent a late manifestation of advanced carcinomatosis. Paquin and Roland[47] have emphasized the dismal prognosis, in that 61 of 64 patients with this metastatic site were dead within "a few weeks to a few months."

The most common neoplasms accounting for metastatic disease to the penis are from

Table 37–1. PENILE SOFT TISSUE TUMORS*

Location (%)	Percentage Malignant
Penile shaft (46.7)	66.7
Glans penis (35.6)	31.3
Prepuce (13.3)	33.3
Frenulum (2.2)	0.0
Ischiocavernosus muscle (2.2)	100.0
Total = 100%	

*From Macaluso JN Jr, et al: Glomus tumor of glans penis. Urology 25:409–410, 1985.

the genitourinary organs, followed by the gastrointestinal tract and respiratory system.[51] Table 37–2 summarizes a series of 219 primary malignancies associated with penile metastases. The predominant cell type is carcinoma, occurring in 202 of 219 cases. Sarcoma, lymphoma, and tumors of unknown histologic type comprise the remainder. Metastases to the penis from nonpenile primary malignancies are diagnosed synchronously in approximately 20% of presentations, whereas 50% are manifested within two years from the time of initial diagnosis. Obstructive uropathy leading to urinary retention is a common presenting symptom. A palpable mass, swelling, nodule, or skin change frequently occurs. Priapism as an initial presenting feature or subsequent development occurs in 40% of patients.[51]

The rarity of case reports of metastases to the penis is perplexing in view of the rich vascular network to this organ. Three routes of metastases have been postulated: direct extension of bladder, prostatic, or rectal tumors via the ischiorectal fossa to the superficial perineal space and then to the corpus; retrograde venous flow secondary to obstruction or compromise of more proximal venous channels; and arterial dissemination from distant sites.[1, 62]

Treatment of penile metastases depends upon the histologic features of the primary tumor and may include chemotherapy, local radiation therapy, hormonal therapy, nerve root block, arterial chemotherapy, and corporal shunting for resolution of pain and priapism.[51] Radical amputation is rarely indicated and is reserved for patients with uncontrollable local symptoms or those with the penile lesion as a solitary metastatic site. Obstructive uropathy is managed with simple urethral catheter drainage, perineal urethrostomy, suprapubic cystostomy, or percutaneous nephrostomy. Survival of patients with penile metastases from genitourinary primaries is six weeks if untreated and 47 weeks with appropriate treatment.[54] Generally, the prognosis for all lesions is poor, and most patients die within a year.

STAGING OF PRIMARY PENILE CANCER

Following the initial assessment of the penile lesion, the inguinal regions are examined and clinically assessed. The penile

lesion is biopsied or excised and the pathologic diagnosis made. At this time the patient is clinically staged. The most common staging system employed in this country is the Jackson Staging System,[28] which is as follows:

Stage		Tumor Presentation
Stage I	(A)	Tumor confined to glans or prepuce or both
Stage II	(B)	Tumor involving the penile shaft
Stage III	(C)	Operable inguinal node metastasis
Stage IV	(D)	Tumor extending beyond the penile shaft; inoperable inguinal or distant metastases

In 1967 the International Union Against Cancer (UICC) proposed the TNM Classification System. The proposed system for penile tumors is as follows:[3]

TMN Classification of Penile Carcinoma

T = *Primary Tumor*	
TIS	Preinvasive carcinoma (carcinoma in situ)
T0	No evidence of primary tumor
T1	Tumor 2 cm or less in its largest dimension, strictly superficial or exophytic
T2	Tumor more than 2 cm but not more than 5 cm in its largest dimension, with minimal infiltration
T3	Tumor more than 5 cm in its largest dimension, or tumor of any size with deep infiltration, including the urethra
T4	Tumor infiltrating neighboring structures
N = *Regional Lymph Nodes*	
	The clinician may record whether palpable nodes are considered to contain growth
N0	No palpable nodes
N1	Movable unilateral nodes
	N1$_a$ Nodes not considered to contain growth
	N1$_b$ Nodes considered to contain growth
N2	Movable bilateral nodes
	N2$_a$ Nodes not considered to contain growth
	N2$_b$ Nodes considered to contain growth
N3	Fixed nodes
M = *Distant Metastases*	
M0	No evidence of distant metastases
M1	Distant metastases present

SURGICAL TREATMENT OF PRIMARY TUMOR

Carcinoma of the penis limited to the prepuce can be treated with circumcision alone. The survival rates do not appreciably differ from those of patients treated by a partial penectomy. Tumors 2 to 5 cm in diameter located on the distal third of the penile shaft should be treated with partial penectomy. However, more proximal lesions will require a total penectomy because an inadequate stump length remaining after a

Table 37–2. PRIMARY MALIGNANCIES
ASSOCIATED WITH SECONDARY CANCERS
OF THE PENIS IN 219 PATIENTS*

Site of Primary Malignancy	Number of Patients
Genitourinary Tract	
Bladder	65
Prostate	65
Kidney	23
Testis	10
Ureter	1
Gastrointestinal Tract	
Rectum/sigmoid	34
Colon	1
Anus	1
Liver	1
Pancreas	1
Respiratory Tract	
Lungs	8
Nasopharynx	1
Other	
Lymphosarcoma/reticulum cell sarcoma	4
Bone	2
Burkitt's lymphoma	1
Skin (malignant melanoma)	1

*From Powell BL, et al: Secondary malignancies of
the penis and epididymis: a case report and review of
the literature. J Clin Oncol 3:110–116, 1985.

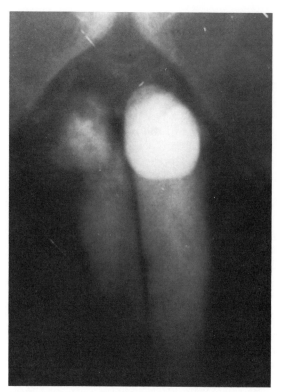

Figure 37–4. Corpus cavernosogram in patient with
deeply invasive penile cancer.

partial excision results in perineal soiling
and spraying. Local recurrence rates for T1
and T2 tumors are less than 2% when treated
with a partial penectomy. Since deeply infiltrating (T3 and T4) tumors, regardless of
their location, require total penectomy, a
corpus cavernosogram is useful to distinguish T2 from T3 tumors. Comparing results
for this technique with those for clinical
staging by physical examination, Raghavaiah[53] reported that 22% of Stage I
(approximated by T1 and T2) tumors were
clinically understaged. The corpus cavernosogram showed filling defects even if there
was minimal tumor infiltration into the cav-
ernous tissue. Because of the propensity for
Stage II tumors [T3] to metastasize to lymph
nodes, recognition of corporal infiltration is
important. A corpus cavernosogram is also
helpful for planning the margins of surgical
resection. The procedure can be performed
on an out-patient basis. The base of the penis
is infiltrated with a 1% lidocaine solution.
The anesthetized organ is then placed on
stretch and one corpus infiltrated with 20
ml of a 65% diatrizoate solution via a fine
needle. Infiltration of only one side is necessary because of vascular cross communication. Figure 37–4 shows a corpus cavernosogram from a patient with an infiltrating

penile cancer and extensive infiltration of
the corpora.

Partial Penectomy

Appropriate antibiotic therapy is instituted prior to local surgical resection. This
is designed to sterilize the urine and treat
pathogens as identified by culture of the
lesion. Sodium biphosphate–sodium phosphate (Fleet's) enemas the evening prior to
the operation will decrease postoperative
contamination of the wound and dressing.
The distal penis containing the tumor is
covered by a sterile glove finger after the
area is prepped and draped. A tourniquet is
placed at the penile base. An encircling
incision is made on the penile shaft approximately 2 cm proximal to the primary lesion
(Fig. 37–5A). The subcutaneous veins are
either cauterized or suture-ligated, and the
dorsal veins and arteries are ligated and
divided with 4-0 chromic sutures. The corpora bodies are divided 1 cm proximal to
the line of the skin incision on the ventral
aspect. The profunda arteries in each corpus
are individually ligated. The urethra is dis-

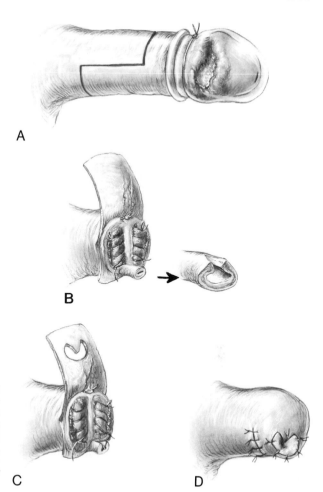

A

B

Figure 37–5. A, Solid line shows proposed skin incision; condom covers the lesion. B, The amputation has been performed. The corpora cavernosa have been sutured, and a 2-cm cuff of urethra has been left extending. C, Cutaneous flap is fashioned to fit over spatulated end of urethral stump. D, Mucocutaneous junction and dorsal-ventral junction are sutured. New orifice has been tailored for urethral exit.

C   D

sected free from the corpus spongiosum, extending the division 1 cm distal to the transected corpora. Horizontal 2-0 chromic mattress sutures are placed through the tunica albuginea, Buck's fascia, and the intercavernous septum between the corpora bodies (Fig. 37–5B). The tourniquet is released to expose any bleeding points. The dorsal skin flap is swung inferiorly over the penile stump, and the urethra is brought through a 1-cm spatulated opening in the flap (Fig. 37–5B). The cutaneous flap is then fashioned to accommodate urethral flattening. A mucocutaneous junction is established with the use of 4-0 chromic sutures, and the ventral dorsal junction is closed with 2-0 chromic sutures (Fig. 37–5C and D). A No. 18 to 20 French catheter is left indwelling for five to seven days.

Radical Penectomy

Preoperative antibiotic therapy and enemas are instituted similar to the program for partial penectomy. A vertical elliptical incision is made over the base of the penis. In patients having extensive lesions involving the base, the incision is carried at least 2 cm away from the carcinoma. The incision is extended over the anterior surface of the scrotum in the midline through the skin and dartos fascia (Fig. 37–6A). Blunt dissection is employed to separate the tunica of the testicles in such a manner to expose the corporal bodies (Fig. 37–6B).

With both blunt and sharp dissection, the corporal bodies are dissected proximally by dividing the suspensory and fundiform ligaments as well as the dorsal vessels. Buck's fascia is divided at its ventral aspect over the urethra, exposing the corpus spongiosum (Fig. 37–7). The urethra is dissected both proximally and distally and divided. Ventral traction on the proximal end will assist in the dissection. The paired corpora cavernosa are divided sharply and suture ligated with 2-0 chromic catgut sutures. With extensive carcinoma infiltrating the corpora, these

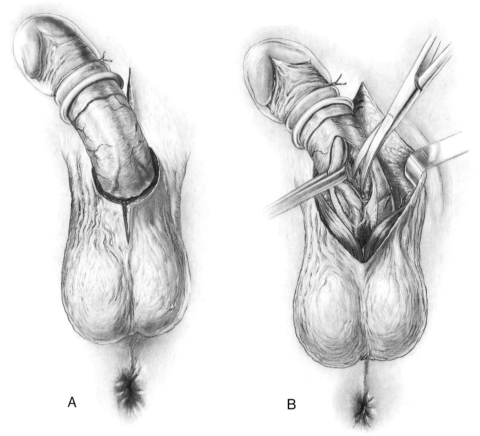

Figure 37–6. A, Circumferential incision around base of penis with extensions at 12 o'clock and 6 o'clock positions. B, Mobilization of the urethra through incision in Buck's fascia.

structures are dissected proximal from the ischiopubic rami. A No. 18 French catheter is inserted through the urethra to facilitate palpation in the perineum (Fig. 37–7). At this point, a 1-cm ellipse of skin is removed from the region of the central tendon of the perineum over the urethra, and a subcutaneous tunnel is created bluntly (Fig. 37–8). The urethra is transposed, taking care not to create any acute angle of exit (Figs. 37–9 and 37–10). The urethra is spatulated and approximated to the skin with 4-0 chromic catgut sutures (Fig. 37–11). The primary incision is closed in a horizontal fashion, resulting in some elevation of the scrotum (Fig. 37–12). This serves to elevate it above the perineal urethrostomy to facilitate urination. A Penrose drain is placed "through and through" the inferior corners of the incision and removed in two to four days. A urethral catheter is left indwelling for approximately five days.

Management of Regional Lymph Nodes

Regional lymph node metastases, in the absence of documentation of distant metastases from penile cancer, represent a clear indication for ilioinguinal lymphadenectomy, as patients will succumb to their disease if treated by penectomy alone (Fig. 37–13A and B). Prophylactic ilioinguinal lymph node dissection without biopsy-confirmed evidence of metastases remains controversial.[1] One third of patients with penile cancer will harbor metastatic nodal disease at the time of presentation.[22] Penile cancers are frequently infected, and palpable inguinal adenopathy is common. Approximately 50% of these enlarged lymph nodes are secondary to infection rather than metastatic involvement. Twenty per cent of patients with penile cancer without synchronous evidence of nodal involvement will

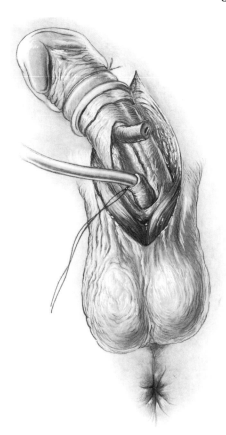

Figure 37–7. The urethra has been transected, and a No. 15 French catheter is placed proximally to aid in location of the urethra in the perineum.

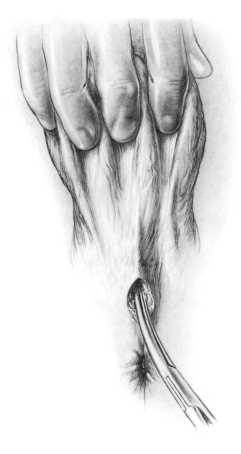

Figure 37–8. A 1-cm elliptical incision is made and a tunnel created to the base of the penis.

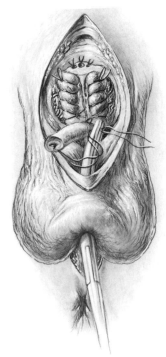

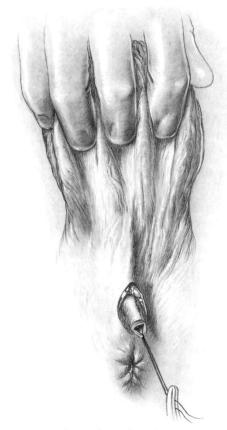

Figure 37–9. The suture used to provide traction to assist urethral dissection is grasped with a Kelly clamp, after a subcutaneous tunnel has been created bluntly in preparation for transposition of the urethra to the perineum.

Figure 37–10. The urethra is brought to the midline of the perineum through the elliptical opening.

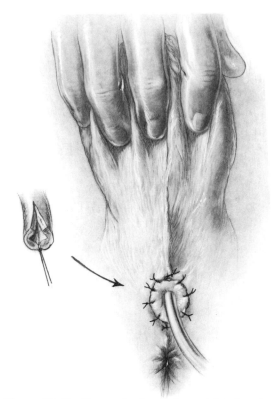

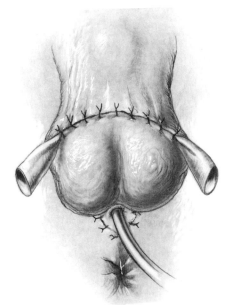

Figure 37–11. The urethral end is spatulated and sutured to the skin edges of the elliptical opening in the perineum.

Figure 37–12. The original amputation incision is closed horizontally, raising the scrotum slightly.

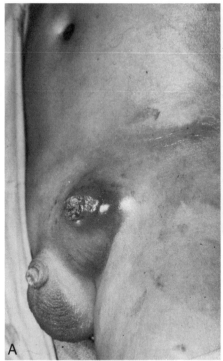
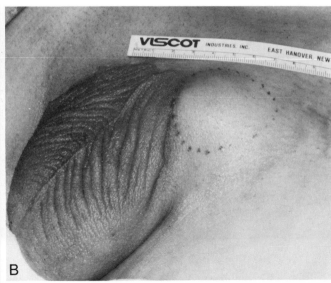

Figure 37–13. A, Advanced inguinal lymph node metastases. B, Inguinal node metastases developing six months after radical penectomy.

develop metastases metachronously. Because the removal of the ilioinguinal lymph nodes is associated with substantial morbidity, proper patient selection for this surgical procedure is imperative.

Cabanas[10] has championed the sentinel lymph node biopsy as a means of identifying patients for lymph node dissection. Anatomically, the sentinel nodes are encountered bilaterally at the epigastric-saphenous junction and represent the first echelon of tumor metastases. In Cabanas's series, the five-year survival of patients with negative results from sentinel lymph node biopsy approaches 90%, implying that 10% are understaged with sentinel node biopsies. It would appear that if both sentinel nodes are free of tumor, then no further surgical therapy is indicated after removal of the primary. However, if either or both sentinel lymph nodes contain tumor, then a unilateral or bilateral ilioinguinal node dissection should be performed. Clinical evaluation by palpation results in understaging in only 20% of cases, which does not differ significantly from Cabanas's 10% failure rate. Recently, Perinetti[48] has reported a patient who developed unresectable lymph node metastases after a bilateral negative finding on sentinel lymph node biopsy. Daseler[13] has described seven

lymph nodes located in the area designated by Cabanas. This may be an explanation for Perinetti's reported failure.

Luciani and co-workers[38] from Italy have reported favorable results from percutaneous regional node aspiration cytologic testing for staging of the regional lymph nodes. Penile and pedal lymphography opacifies all lymph nodes anatomically involved by carcinoma of the penis, making fine-needle aspiration of these nodes possible. By using fluoroscopic guidance, a modified Chiba needle attached to a 20-ml syringe is directed to the superficial inguinal, sentinel, and deep inguinal lymph nodes. Aspirations were subjected to cytopathologic review. Based upon the cytologic and lymphographic results, the patients were judged to be either positive or negative for metastatic disease. Patients with pathologically confirmed nodal involvement received either ilioinguinal lymphadenectomy or irradiation therapy. Lymphography alone is an inaccurate method for detecting lymphatic spread of urologic malignancies, and we believe that all opacified nodes should be aspirated regardless of lymphography findings.[38] Several aspirations should be performed in different parts of the node. Repeat fine-needle aspiration can be performed up to nine months later, since the

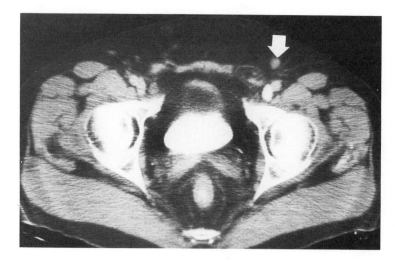

Figure 37–14. *CT scan demonstrating inguinal lymph node metastases (arrow).*

contrast will remain in the nodes. This later aspiration may allow detection of delayed nodal metastases.

Johnson and Lo,[29] from MD Anderson Hospital, retrospectively reviewed the records of 22 patients with squamous cell carcinoma of the penis undergoing ilioinguinal lymph node dissection at their institution. Fourteen patients underwent ilioinguinal dissection for clinically suspicious nodes at the time the primary tumor was diagnosed, and their five-year survival rate was 57%. Eight patients who appeared clinically free of lymphatic metastases at the time of diagnosis subsequently developed palpable nodes and underwent therapeutic lymph node dissection. Their five-year survival rate was 13%. In this study, survival appeared to correlate with the number of inguinal lymph nodes found to harbor metastatic cancer. Only one patient with more than two positive lymph nodes survived longer than five years. Six of the eight patients who underwent late therapeutic dissection had more than two positive nodes, with the median number being four. Only one patient in this group survived, and he had a solitary metastatic node. They conclude that a policy of wait and watch in patients with clinically negative nodes at the time of diagnosis does not appear justified.

Nevertheless, there remains no proof that prophylactic superficial and deep groin dissection yields a higher percentage of survival than therapeutic node dissection. In support of Raghavaiah's results,[53] it appears that a cavernosogram is a valuable procedure to assess the primary tumor accurately and

plan the level of resection during penectomy. It is our opinion that lesions of the corpora require an ilioinguinal lymphadenectomy and that this radiologic evaluation is useful in establishing its presence. CT scans are helpful in evaluation of the pelvic and inguinal lymph node regions (Fig. 37–14).

At the present time, we recommend bilateral ilioinguinal lymphadenectomy for penile cancer in the presence of one or more of the following conditions:

1. Lymphadenopathy persisting more than four weeks after penectomy and adequate antimicrobial treatment
2. Pathologic confirmation of nodal metastases
3. Subsequent development of adenopathy in the patient with a history of penile cancer, in the absence of any other inflammatory or infective process
4. Extensive lesions at the base of the penis at presentation
5. Any lesion involving the corpora cavernosa

RADIATION THERAPY

Grabstald and associates[21] have reported a select group of 10 patients with infiltrating penile cancer who were treated with irradiation therapy. Six- to ten-year follow-up revealed that only one patient failed therapy, with the development of a new primary eight years after his initial treatment. Long-term complications from irradiation included telangiectasia in all 10 patients and urethral stricture in four patients. The obvious advantage of radiotherapy is that the penis is spared. However, factors such as size and grade of the tumor are key variables in determining the appropriate primary modality of therapy. Krieg and Luk[33] retrospectively evaluated the management of 29 patients with penile cancer. In 17 patients who had surgical treatment, 15 of 17 (88%) had good local control, whereas nine of 12 (75%) who received radiation therapy as the primary modality of treatment achieved local control. Two of the patients who received radiotherapy as the primary treatment subsequently relapsed and required surgical resection. Doses of irradiation employed varied from 5000 to 7000 rads. The conclusion from this series suggests that irradiation therapy is the treatment of choice for early stage lesions and that surgery should be reserved for those patients refractory to radiotherapy. However, we believe that patients with tumors greater than 3 cm in size, or invasion of deeper structures, including the corpora cavernosa, are not candidates for radiotherapy as the primary treatment modality.

In Gursel's series[23] of 15 patients with regional node metastases treated with radiotherapy as a primary treatment, only two survived for five years. However, irradiation therapy does offer palliation for patients who, either because of advanced disease or pre-existing medical conditions, are not candidates for curative surgical procedures.

CHEMOTHERAPY

The initial enthusiasm for chemotherapy as an effective treatment modality for penile cancer emanated from the reports of Ichikawa.[27] This enthusiasm has tempered with time. Because of the rarity of the disease, large multicenter clinical trials evaluating single or combination chemotherapy, or both, are lacking. The oncology literature contains anecdotal case reports of long-term, complete responses with chemotherapeutic agents. Unfortunately, few controlled clinical trials accrue more than 15 patients, and results fail to substantiate the responsiveness of this disease to chemotherapy.

Bleomycin was reported by Ichikawa[27] to be an extremely effective chemotherapeutic agent in penile cancer. The drug used as a single agent was reported to result in a 50% response rate in 24 patients. In a large series of 188 patients, Ichikawa reported objective responses in all patients treated with bleomycin and surgery, with or without radiation therapy. Blum,[9] reviewing the world literature on treatment of penile cancer with bleomycin, has reported response rates between 29 and 100% (Table 37–3). Matveev and Gotsadze[40] administered the drug alone or in combination with other chemotherapeutic agents, with or without radiation therapy, in 25 patients. Complete response status was achieved in four of four (100%) clinical Stage I tumors, six of 10 (60%) Stage II tumors, and one of four (25%) Stage III tumors. Based upon this and other studies, bleomycin may be capable of curing a subset of patients with localized Stage I and II cancer but lacks sufficient activity in metastatic disease to recommend its continued use as the "gold standard."

Cisplatin is an effective chemotherapeutic agent producing durable complete response in a number of tumors. Merrin,[42] using a dose of 50 mg/m^2 weekly for six weeks, reported responses in two of three evaluated patients with metastatic penile cancer. Recently, the Southwest Oncology Group[16] has completed a Phase II trial of cisplatin in Stage III and IV penile cancer in patients

Table 37–3. EFFECT OF BLEOMYCIN ON SQUAMOUS CELL CARCINOMA OF THE PENIS*

| Source | Number of Patients Entered | Number of Patients Evaluated | Response | | | Response Rate (%) |
			Complete	50%	25 to 50%	
United States	9	7	0	0	2	29
European Organization for Research on Treatment of Cancer	2	1	1	0	0	100
Japan	58	53	8	27	8	81
Scandinavia	—	6	1	1	1	50
Total		67	10	28	11	73

*From Blum RH, et al: A clinical review of bleomycin—a new antineoplastic agent. Cancer 31:903–914, 1973.

refractory to surgery, irradiation therapy, or both. The agent was chosen because of its reported activity in other squamous cell tumors. Of 13 evaluated patients, three had a partial response. Fewer than 50 patients have been prospectively treated with chemotherapeutic drugs in Phase I, II, and III trials.[2] The antifolate agent methotrexate appears to induce responses in metastatic epidermoid carcinoma of the penis. In Ahmed's report of 13 patients treated with methotrexate, one complete and seven partial responses of more than five months' duration were achieved.[17] Five of the 13 patients had been previously treated with bleomycin or cisplatin. Of eight patients with no prior therapy, five responded as well as three who failed cisplatin. There were no responses seen in patients failing bleomycin chemotherapy. In this series methotrexate appeared superior to either bleomycin or cisplatin. Garnick and associates[18] have reported a complete remission in a patient with advanced penile cancer treated with high-dose methotrexate. This lasted nine months, at which time the patient died of a noncancerous cause and at autopsy was found to harbor only two foci of well-differentiated squamous cell cancer.[17]

We have employed intra-arterial cisplatin in one patient with advanced localized penile cancer unresponsive to radiation therapy. The patient failed to respond to the intra-arterial cisplatin. However, he received only one course, declining subsequent therapy.

The results of chemotherapeutic management of disseminated penile cancer remain dismal. Organized multicentered clinical trials are indicated to evaluate investigational agents as well as new regimens and dosages of combination agents.

YAG LASER TREATMENT OF PENILE CARCINOMA

A variety of lesions of external genitalia treated with the Neodymium-YAG laser may demonstrate cosmetically superior results, compared with those for traditional surgical or radiotherapeutic management.[24] Carcinoma in situ may be effectively managed with YAG laser therapy.

Rothenberger and associates[56] reported 16 patients with localized squamous carcinoma of the penis treated with the YAG laser. One of the 16 patients has developed a local recurrence in the brief follow-up period. We believe that this treatment offers an exciting alternative to standard therapy for early stage lesions. However, carefully controlled clinical trials are necessary to substantiate the therapeutic as well as cosmetic benefits.

References

1. Abeshouse BS, Abeshouse GA: Metastatic tumors of the penis: a review of the literature and a report of two cases. J Urol 86:99–112, 1961.
2. Ahmed T, Sklaroff R, Yagoda A: Sequential trials of methotrexate, cisplatin and bleomycin for penile cancer. J Urol 132:465–468, 1984.
3. American Joint Committee for Cancer Staging and End Results Recording: Staging of cancer at genitourinary sites. In Manual for Staging of Cancer. Chicago, American Joint Committee, 1977.
4. Barney JD: Epithelioma of the penis. An analysis of one hundred cases. Ann Surg 46:890–914, 1907.
5. Baronofsky IA: Technique of inguinal node dissection. Surgery 33:886, 1953.
6. Barringer BS: Inguinal gland metastases in carcinoma of the penis. JAMA 106:21–24, 1936.
7. Barringer BS, Dean AL Jr: Epithelioma of the penis. J Urol 11:497–514, 1924.
8. Bergreen PW: Penile and urethral carcinoma: an overview. In ED Crawford, TA Borden (eds), Genitourinary Cancer Surgery. Philadelphia, Lea & Febiger, 1982, pp 303–309.
9. Blum RH, Carter SK, Agre K: A clinical review of bleomycin—a new antineoplastic agent. Cancer 31:903–914, 1973.
10. Cabanas RM: An approach for the treatment of penile carcinoma. Cancer 39:456–466, 1977.
11. Crawford ED: Radical ilioinguinal lymphadenectomy. Urol Clin North Am 11:543–552, 1984.
12. Curtis BF: American Textbook of Diseases of the Skin. Philadelphia, WB Saunders, 1898, p 76.
13. Daseler EH, Anson BJ, Reimann AF: Radical excision of the inguinal and iliac lymph glands. Surg Gynec Obstet 87:679–694, 1948.
14. Dean AL Jr: Epithelioma of the penis. J Urol 33:252–283, 1935.
15. Dodge OG, Linsell CA: Carcinoma of the penis in Uganda and Kenya Africans. Cancer 16:1255–1263, 1963.
16. Gagliano R, Crawford ED: Cis-platinum in advanced squamous cell penile carcinoma: a Southwest Oncology Group Study. Proc ASCO 4:96, 1985.
17. Garnick MB: Personal communication.
18. Garnick MB, Skarin AT, Steele GD Jr: Metastatic carcinoma of the penis: complete remission after high dose methotrexate chemotherapy. J Urol 122:265–266, 1979.
19. Gibson CL: Cancer of the penis. Ann Surg 56:471, 1912.
20. Goette DK, Carson TE: Erythroplasia of Queyrat: treatment with topical 5-fluorouracil. Cancer 38:1498–1502, 1976.
21. Grabstald H: Cancer of the penis. Urology 18:15, 1979.
22. Grabstald H: Controversies concerning lymph node

dissection for cancer of the penis. Urol Clin North Am 7:793–799, 1980.

23. Gursel EO, Georgountzos C, Uson AC, et al: Penile cancer: clinicopathologic study of 64 cases. Urology 1:569–578, 1973.

24. Hofstetter A, Frank F: The Neodymium-YAG Laser in Urology. Basel, Switzerland, Hoffman-LaRoche, 1980, p 9.

25. Hoppmann HJ, Fraley EE: Squamous cell carcinoma of the penis. J Urol 120:393–398, 1978.

26. Hovnanian AP: The evolution and present status of pelvi-inguinal lymphatic excision. Surg Gynec Obstet 124:851–865, 1967.

27. Ichikawa T: Chemotherapy of penis carcinoma. Recent Results Cancer Res 60:140–156, 1977.

28. Jackson SM: The treatment of carcinoma of the penis. Br J Surg 53:33–35, 1966.

29. Johnson DE, Lo RK: Management of regional lymph nodes in penile carcinoma: five-year results following therapeutic groin dissections. Urology 24:308–311, 1984.

30. Kaufman JJ, Sternberg TH: Carcinoma of the penis in a circumcised man. J Urol 90:449–450, 1963.

31. Kini MG: Cancer of the penis in a child, aged 2 years. Indian Med Gazette 79:66–68, 1944.

32. Kraus FT, Perezmesa C: Verrucous carcinoma, clinical and pathologic study of 105 cases involving oral cavity, larynx and genitalia. Cancer 19:26–38, 1966.

33. Kreig RM, Luk KH: Carcinoma of the penis. Review of cases treated by surgery and radiation therapy 1960–1977. Urology 18:149–154, 1981.

34. Lenowitz H, Graham AP: Carcinoma of the penis. J Urol 56:458–484, 1946.

35. Lewis LG: Young's radical operation for the cure of cancer of the penis. A report of 34 cases. J Urol 26:295–316, 1931.

36. Lichtenauer P, Scheer H, Louton T: On the classification of penis carcinoma and its 10 year survival. Recent Results Cancer Res 60:110–119, 1977.

37. Licklider S: Jewish penile carcinoma. J Urol 86:98, 1961.

38. Luciani L, Piscioli F, Scappini P, Pusiol T: Value and role of percutaneous regional node aspiration cytology in the management of penile carcinoma. Eur Urol 10:294–302, 1984.

39. Macaluso JN Jr, Sullivan JW, Tomberlin S: Glomus tumor of glans penis. Urology 25:409–410, 1985.

40. Matveev BP, Gotsadze DT: Khimioterapiia raka polcvogo chiena. (Chemotherapy of penile carcinoma). Urol Nefrol (Mosk) 4:39–42, 1981 (English abstract).

41. McKay DL Jr, Fuque F, Weinberg AG: Balanitis xerotica obliterans in children. J Urol 114:773–775, 1975.

42. Merrin CE: Treatment of genitourinary tumors with cis-dichlorodiammineplatinum (II): Experience in 250 patients. Cancer Treat Rep 63:1579–1584, 1979.

43. Mikhail GR: Cancers, precancers, and pseudocancer on the male genitalia: a review of clinical appearances, histopathology, and management. J Dermatol Surg Oncol 6:1027–1035, 1980.

44. Morgagni GB: The Seats and Causes of Disease, Book IV, Letter L, Article 50, 1761.

45. Mostofi FK, Price EB: Tumors of the Male Genital System. Washington DC, Armed Forces Institute of Pathology, 1973, p 205, 283.

46. Murphy LJT: The History of Urology. Springfield, IL, Charles C Thomas, 1972, p 486–487.

47. Paquin AJ Jr, Roland SI: Secondary carcinoma of the penis: a review of the literature and a report of nine new cases. Cancer 9:626–632, 1956.

48. Perinetti E, Crane DB, Catalona WJ: Unreliability of sentinel lymph node biopsy for staging penile carcinoma. J Urol 124:734–735, 1980.

49. Persky L: Epidemiology of cancer of the penis. Recent results. Cancer Res 60:97–109, 1977.

50. Persky L: Commentary: Problems and management of squamous cell carcinoma of the penis. In ED Whitehead, E Leiter (eds), Current Operative Urology, 2nd ed. Philadelphia, Harper & Row, 1984, pp 1180–1183.

51. Powell BL, Craig JB, Muss HB: Secondary malignancies of the penis and epididymis: a case report and review of the literature. J Clin Oncol 3:110–116, 1985.

52. Pratt-Thomas HR, Heins HC, Lathame E, et al: The carcinogenic effect of human smegma: an experimental study. Preliminary report. Cancer 9:671–680, 1956.

53. Raghavaiah NV: Corpus cavernosogram in the evaluation of carcinoma of the penis. J Urol 120:423–424, 1978.

54. Robey EL, Schellhammer PF: Four cases of metastases to the penis and a review of the literature. J Urol 132:992–994, 1984.

55. Rosenberg SK: Carbon dioxide laser treatment of external genital lesions. Urology 24:555, 1985.

56. Rothenberger K, Hofstetter A, Frank F, et al: The Neodymium-YAG laser in the treatment of penis carcinoma. Proc 4th Cong Int Soc Laser Surg, Tokyo, 1981.

57. Schrek R, Lenowitz H: Etiologic facts in carcinoma of the penis. Cancer Res 7:180–187, 1947.

58. Shabad AL: Some aspects of etiology and prevention of penile cancer. J Urol 92:696–702, 1964.

59. Skinner DG, Leadbetter WF, Kelly SB: The surgical management of squamous cell carcinoma of the penis. J Urol 107:273–277, 1972.

60. Sobel H, Plaut A: The assimilation of cholesterol by Mycobacterium smegmatis. J Bacteriol 57:377–382, 1949.

61. Staubitz WJ, Lent MH, Oberkircher OJ: Carcinoma of the penis. Cancer 8:371–378, 1955.

62. Stein JJ, Hantsch FK: Adenocarcinoma of the rectum with unusual sites of metastases. Report of two cases. JAMA 108:1776–1779, 1937.

63. Tolia BM, Castro VL, Mouded IM, Newman HR: Bowen's disease of the shaft of the penis: successful treatment with 5-fluorouracil. Urology 7:617–619, 1976.

64. Young HH: A radical operation for the cure of cancer of the penis. J Urol 26:285–294, 1931.

MALCOLM S. MITCHELL, M.D.

Immunology and Immunotherapy of Genitourinary Cancers

An understanding of the attempts of a tumor-bearing individual, the "host," to deal with a tumor is fundamental to any therapeutic approach to that tumor. Even if immunotherapy is not specifically entertained as a possibility, it is still important to be aware of the ways in which standard modalities affect the ability of the patient to react against the tumor. This in itself would justify the study of tumor immunology, but beyond that there is increasing evidence that appropriately designed modifications of the immune response can be useful as treatment for several types of cancer.

Genitourinary tract cancers are no exception to these general remarks. Before embarking on a specific discussion of some of the most interesting findings concerning the immunotherapy of these neoplasms, it might be helpful to present some general principles of tumor immunology and to outline the categories of immunotherapy that might be applied to the treatment of any tumor. This will provide a framework for the more specific discussion to follow. These topics have been addressed in two recent reviews,[63, 86] to which the interested reader is referred for a more complete treatment of the subject.

PRINCIPLES OF TUMOR IMMUNOLOGY

Tumor Antigens

Fundamental to this entire discussion is the concept that tumors are antigenic in the host. Recent data indicate that the tumor cells in fact have differences from normal cells that can be detected by immunity, i.e., that they have tumor-associated antigens (TAAs). The weak ability of "spontaneous" tumors, those that arise without purposeful induction by chemicals or viruses, to elicit an immune response has been the single factor most responsible for confusion. Now that antitumor monoclonal antibodies have been successfully generated experimentally, there is substantial agreement that TAAs exist in man.

Since the discovery of blood group antigens by Landsteiner in 1900, antigens that were specific for the surface of tumor have been actively sought, mainly through transplantation experiments. It was only with the development of inbred strains of mice that these experiments could be properly performed. Before then, the outcome of transplantation had been influenced by histocompatibility antigens on the tumor far more than by its TAAs and had given erroneous conclusions about the strength of the TAAs. Carcinogen-induced tumors were the subject of the first conclusive investigations for the existence of tumor antigens in the 1950s. Prehn and Main[82] demonstrated that mice with methylcholanthrene-induced sarcomas could be made specifically resistant to rechallenge with their sarcoma by allowing the tumor to grow briefly and then amputating it. Thus, a true immunity to the tumor developed in an autologous host. A large number of chemically and virally induced tumors have been studied in rodents since then, always with the finding that TAAs are present on the tumor cells.

It is important to distinguish TAAs from tumor-*specific* antigens (TSAs), since the former term implies only that the tumor has antigens that are preferentially expressed on it but are not necessarily unique. Thus differentiation antigens and embryonic (fetal) antigens are tumor-associated but not unique in the ontogeny of the host. Nevertheless, these TAAs may be very useful in detecting the tumor amidst normal tissues or detecting tumor antigens shed into the circulation, as long as there are no antigenically similar normal cells or circulating substances that might be confused with them. We should stress that TSAs have not yet been conclusively demonstrated either in animals or in human beings. TAAs appear to be relatively weak immunogens (i.e., do not generate a strong immune response in the autologous host) and therefore may be difficult to demonstrate using the patient's own serum or lymphoid cells as the reactants. Ethical constraints and genetic heterogeneity prevent transplantation of the tumors among human beings to look for the antigens, and even the alternative of injecting animals with human tissues to obtain antisera may be precluded by the possible limitations of the animal's genetic repertoire, which could prevent it from recognizing the human neoantigens as immunogens. There are so many strong antigens that an animal's lymphoid cells recognize on human cells, such as histocompatibility antigens, that the weaker tumor antigens might be "hidden" by their proximity to the stronger ones.

Monoclonal antibodies will almost certainly be the means by which the existence and nature of human TSAs will be demonstrated conclusively. Monoclonal antibodies are prepared by fusing lymphoid cells from immunized mice or cancer patients with myeloma cell lines, usually from mice. The reactivity of monoclonal antibodies of any derivation is to a single antigenic determinant (epitope), affording an exquisitely sensitive and specific way to detect differences between tumor and normal cells. Even if TSAs do not exist, the current approach of using surface antigens of tumor cells for the diagnosis and treatment of malignant disease will not be invalidated. As long as the antigens in question are sufficiently restricted to malignant cells, their usefulness as targets should be very similar to that of true TSAs for applications such as detection of tumor cells in metastatic sites.

Carcinogen-induced tumor antigens in rodents appear to be unique to the tumor on which they are present. They are even different from other tumors induced by the same carcinogen in other inbred littermates. In direct contrast, virus-induced tumor antigens are characteristic of the inducing virus.[49] Specifically, methylcholanthrene-induced tumor in one DBA/2 mouse is different from a methylcholanthrene-induced tumor in another DBA/2 mouse, whereas a polyoma virus–induced tumor in a C57BL/6 mouse, or even a *rat* for that matter, has antigens that indicate that polyoma virus was the inducing agent. This major difference has made it difficult to develop a unitary theory of the cause of cancer. If, as some suggest, carcinogens simply release latent tumor viruses in the cell, why are not more common antigens found? The discrepancy may not be as great as first thought, however, since fetal antigens common to several rat colonic tumors have been described. More fundamentally, perhaps, monoclonal antibodies have recently detected a 70,000-dalton retrovirus envelope protein present consistently in a series of chemically induced mouse tumors.[53] If these findings are confirmed, it would indicate that each host may simply modify somewhat the viral structure proteins represented on the tumor cell surface, leading to the apparent uniqueness of carcinogen-induced antigens on each tumor.

The Immune Response To Tumor Antigens

There have been many clinical anecdotes that suggest that antitumor immunity exists in man and, in fact, influences the course of malignant disease. The possible involvement of tumor immunity has been manifested in such things as:

1. Spontaneous regression of tumors (rare)
2. Prolonged survival or cure of patients after complete removal of malignant lesions
3. Sudden appearance of metastases many years after successful therapy, with the tumor having ostensibly been "dormant" until then
4. Regression of metastases after removal of

the primary lesion (rare). The behavior of renal cell carcinoma fits many of these categories.

Much firmer evidence has been obtained recently, documenting that patients as well as animals can mount an antibody or cell-mediated immune response against tumor cells. Reactivity to autologous tumors of lymphoid cells and antibodies is most compelling here and has been demonstrated in sarcomas, melanoma, ovarian carcinomas, and lung cancer. The controversy about specificity of these reactions, particularly those mediated by lymphocytes and monocytes in the patient's blood, is rapidly being resolved by improved techniques of testing.

There are two principal components to immunity to tumors, as to any antigenic materials: antibodies (humoral immunity) and cell-mediated immunity. The latter appears to be more universally important in the rejection of tumors, although cells may well require the cooperative participation of antibodies to achieve their maximal effectiveness.

Thymus-derived small lymphocytes (T-cells) and macrophages are perhaps most important types of cell, with "natural killer" (NK) cells, antibody-dependent killer (K) cells, and perhaps polymorphonuclear leukocytes also involved. T-cells can lyse tumor cells to which they have been sensitized in four to 18 hours in vitro, but it is likely that their major role in vivo is to recruit other effector cells, particularly macrophages, through the production of "lymphokines," soluble mediators that attract and activate cells. A recently discussed subgroup of T-cells, lymphokine-activated killer (LAK) cells, can selectively kill tumor cells and not normal cells after they are activated in vitro by interleukin 2 and can presumably perform a similar function in vivo as well. However, the predominant cell at the site of active experimental tumor rejection is the macrophage, which, when activated by various means, can kill tumor cells nonspecifically. Macrophages are not only effector cells but can also make soluble mediators, "monokines," that affect the function of T-cells. Further, macrophages process and present antigens to T-cells during antibody production and have been increasingly recognized as critical cells in any immune response. NK cells, currently thought to be a variety of lymphocyte, lyse selected tumor targets in vitro and may be important in surveillance against the emergence of tumor cells, which we will shortly discuss. K-cells require antibody-coated tumor cells in order to be effective in antibody-dependent cell-mediated cytotoxicity (ADCC). They may be important in the rejection of dispersed tumors such as leukemia and ovarian cancer, and perhaps solid tumors such as bladder cancer.

Cell-mediated immunity and antibody synthesis are regulated by helper and suppressor cells, which are both subpopulations of T-cells and macrophages. T-cells and macrophages are thus not simply effector cells that kill tumor cells, they also interact considerably with each other and regulate each other's activity. Both suppressor and activator substances have been identified from each type of cell.

Antibody synthesis in response to tumor cells occurs in animals and in patients. Cytotoxic antibodies, which kill tumor cells in the presence of complement, may not be as important in vivo as cytophilic antibodies, which arm macrophages and other cells that have receptors for the Fc portion of antibody. Cytophilic antibodies enable immunologically neutral macrophages to specifically seek out and destroy tumor cells. Together with nonspecific activators of macrophages, such as lymphokines or bacille Calmette-Guérin (BCG), the cytophilic (arming) antibodies help to create a very potent, directed antitumor cellular response.

The titration of serologic responses to cancer in patients will be greatly facilitated by the availability of monoclonal antibodies as reference reagents, to be used in competitive binding assays, for example. Serologic detection of tumor antigens by Old and collaborators with sera from patients with several types of tumors has already strongly reaffirmed the existence of tumor immunity in humans.[74] This group of investigators has defined three classes of antigens based upon this serologic analysis. Class 1 antigens are those found uniquely on a patient's own tumor and not on any other, even within the same histologic class. Class 2 antigens are found on all tumors of a certain histologic class, and on a few other, related tumors. Class 3 antigens are found on a wide variety of tumor cells and normal cells. The last group may be differentiation antigens or in some cases may simply be artifacts due to adsorption of components of the medium in which the tumor cells are grown.

Immunologic Surveillance

If tumor cells are antigenic, why are they not detected when they are present in small numbers and rejected before they can become frank malignancy? This question has not yet been completely answered, but the existence of a tumor should not be taken as sufficient reason to reject the existence and importance of tumor immunity. To the contrary, it may well be that only when immunity is defective do we develop a tumor at all. The immunosurveillance theory, first postulated by Thomas and popularized by Burnet,[14] states in its simplest form that tumor cells arise frequently in every individual by somatic mutations but are recognized as foreign and destroyed by immunologic mechanisms before a frank tumor develops. This surveillance was postulated to be T-cell–mediated and directed against TSAs. Cellular immunity in animals, it was theorized, developed phylogenetically mainly to prevent the emergence of cancer.

The presence of an antitumor response in patients with an established tumor is unquestionable, but it is logistically impossible to prove whether there is antitumor immunity at the time the tumor first develops from a single cell. Thus, the evidence for immunologic surveillance against cancer necessarily comes mainly from examples in which its predictions seem to have been borne out clinically. Patients with immunodeficiency disorders, such as those with T-cell deprivation, would be expected to have a greater than normal frequency of cancers. In fact, patients with ataxia telangiectasia variable immunodeficiency, or Wiskott-Aldrich syndrome, have at least a 200-fold excess risk of cancer over age- and sex-matched controls. Most of these cancers are lymphomas or Hodgkin's disease and are particularly aggressive forms of these diseases. Similarly, in patients with renal transplants, who are given long-term immunosuppressive therapy, there is at least a 300-fold increased incidence of malignancies, not only of lymphomas but also epithelial neoplasms of many kinds. This lends credence to the assertion that surveillance in general has broken down, rather than that the lymphoid system is the target for malignant degeneration. Virally induced tumors are increased in animals experimentally given antilymphocyte serum chronically or subjected to thymectomy. Finally, homosexual men with

acquired immunodeficiency syndrome (AIDS), whose total lymphocyte count, (and particularly number of T-cells) is decreased, have a high incidence of Kaposi's sarcoma, Burkitt's lymphoma, carcinoma of the tongue, and cloacogenic carcinoma of the rectum.[54]

It is not necessary to postulate a complete loss of the ability to respond immunologically to explain a loss of surveillance. It is likely that the immunodeficiency is usually highly selective for the cancer cell or its etiologic agent, and of short duration. The extreme examples of profound immunodeficiency states are simply more dramatic evidence. Moreover, the surveillance may well be performed by non-T-cells, such as macrophages or NK cells, and the target of surveillance may be the etiologic agent rather than the cancer cell itself. Fundamentally, however, the immunosurveillance theory is still a useful hypothesis with which to assess observations on the occurrence of cancer under various circumstances.

The Escape of Established Tumors From Immunologic Rejection

Regardless of whether immunity plays a role in preventing the occurrence of a tumor, once a frank tumor is established there is little doubt that the host can mount an immune response against it. The response may, however, be relatively deficient, failing to reject the cancer. It seems that the mechanisms originally intended to regulate immune responses in general are exaggerated by the presence of the tumor, which thus fosters its own growth. Tumors shed antigens into the circulation, which by themselves or in the presence of admixed host antibody, can induce suppressor T-cells.[31, 61, 64] The serum "blocking factors" described in humans[32] are undoubtedly the counterpart of these, and of the serum factors that caused enhancement of tumor growth in experimental animals in the 1950s.[42] Tumor cells, which are only weakly immunogenic in most cases, further lose antigenic strength through prolonged residency in the host and immunoselection, which is called "antigenic modulation." The role of macrophage suppressor cells in perpetuation of a cancer is uncertain. It is perhaps more closely related to other, cancer-associated phenomena, such as skin test anergy and depressed ability to

respond to microorganisms found in Hodgkin's disease.

Immunotherapy

There are at least four categories of immunotherapy that one can use to classify
most existing forms of such treatment. However, it should be noted that the field has
recently been expanded to include strategies
that affect the growth and behavior of the
tumor itself. The reader should be aware
that the term "immunotherapy" is rapidly
being replaced and subsumed under the
broader heading of "biological response
modification," or "biomodulation" as we
abbreviate it.[62]

The principal types of immunotherapy are
listed in Table 38–1. Active immunotherapy
attempts to stimulate the tumor-bearing host
to respond more vigorously against the tumor, either through augmentation of specific
(T) cells or nonspecific (macrophage, NK, or
K) cells. Adoptive immunotherapy transfers
immunologically active histocompatible
lymphoid cells or subcellular immunologic
"information," such as "immune" RNA, that
will be accepted by the host largely in place
of a defective intrinsic immunity. Restorative immunotherapy attempts to boost the
immune response of a host to normal levels,
before attempts are made to augment it above
those levels. Passive immunotherapy attempts by transfer of antibodies to supplement the host's existing antibody response,

particularly to attack dispersed tumors in
circulation or ascites that are most easily
accessible to direct coating by antibodies.

Most of the agents used during the 1970s
were nonspecific stimulants of active immunity, such as BCG and *Corynebacterium
parvum*. These agents are best used in humans together with specific immunization
procedures, such as with killed tumor cells
or antigenic extracts, rather than by themselves, since they are principally stimulants
of macrophages and can affect immunity
longer and more specifically when used as
true adjuvants. Adoptive immunotherapy
with transferred T lymphocytes has been
particularly very effective for treatment of
rodent leukemias and lymphomas.[26] With
our present ability to immunize and clone
T-cells in vitro and then expand the number
of highly specific cytolytic and helper T-
cells for adoptive transfer, the capacity to
attack tumors by this means is now greater
than ever. Bone marrow transplantation,
with its consequent transfer of immunocom-
petent cells and their precursors, is also a
form of adoptive immunotherapy besides its
obvious function in replacing hematopoietic
stem cells.

The use of "immune" RNA, which is more
correctly a phenol extract of cellular RNA
rather than the messenger RNA relating to
the specific immune response, has been attempted as a means of adoptive immunotherapy of subcellular information. In genitourinary tract cancers this form of therapy
has been given with variable success, as we
will note in detail below.

Restorative immunotherapy refers to the
repletion of competent effector cells by the
administration of thymic hormones or agents
such as levamisole that have a similar effect.
These materials stimulate precursors to differentiate into mature T-cells. Antagonism
of suppressor T-cells by the administration
of low doses of cyclophosphamide or antagonism of suppressor macrophages by the
administration of inhibitors of prostaglandins (by which suppressor macrophages produce their effect) are other forms of restorative immunotherapy.

Passive immunotherapy was the form that
seemed in the past to have the least likelihood of significant utility, since it is by
definition a short-lived therapy. Antibodies
transferred in the form of antisera have been
of some use in treating rodent leukemias,
primarily by "arming" effector cells, but

Table 38–1. TYPES OF IMMUNOTHERAPY

1. **Active:** Stimulation of the host's intrinsic antitumor immunity.
   a. Nonspecific: Use of microbial or chemical immunomodulators (adjuvants). Activates macrophages, NK cells and other nonspecific effectors, and T-cells secondarily through macrophages.
   b. Specific: Use of antigenic tumor cells or extracted tumor antigens, often altered by added chemical groups or treatment with enzymes. Activates specific effector cells such as T-cells and "armed" macrophages.
2. **Adoptive:** Transfer of immunologic cells or informational molecules.
3. **Restorative:** Repletion of deficient immunologic subpopulations (principally T-cells) or inhibition of suppressor influences (T-cells or macrophages).
4. **Passive:** Transfer of antibodies or short-lived anti-tumor "factors".

raising the antisera posed a significant problem, as did the issue of transfusing large amounts of foreign proteins (albumin and globulin) into patients. The advent of monoclonal antibodies, with their great inherent specificity and potency, has made it possible to give relatively small amounts of protein from foreign species (usually a mouse), reducing the risk of anaphylactic reactions. Furthermore, human monoclonal antibodies are now being developed, and this should further improve the situation.

Interferon, a group of three types of antiviral and antitumor substances from human cells, now manufactured in pure form by recombinant DNA technology, does not easily fit into just one of the categories of immunotherapy outlined above. This illustrates in fact why the broader term of biomodulation is preferable. Interferon stimulates several types of cell (particularly macrophages and NK cells), directly inhibits tumor cell growth, and has antiviral activity, and one subclass of interferon (interferon-gamma) is a true lymphokine. This potent material will almost certainly be of use in treating several types of cancer, including renal cell carcinoma, judging from recent phase II trials. Similarly, retinoids and vitamin A derivatives, of which 13-cis-retinoic acid is perhaps the best known, are both maturational agents and antitumor agents to some extent and may be helpful in preventing dysplastic conditions from becoming frankly cancerous: a situation frequently noted in various squamous and transitional carcinomas.

IMMUNOLOGY OF GENITOURINARY CANCERS

Tumor Antigens

There is ample evidence that there are tumor-associated antigens in genitourinary tract cancers of all varieties. Much of the better evidence comes from recent work with monoclonal antibodies. It should be noted, however, that none of the antigens thus far identified is tumor-specific; instead, all are found on one of several other tumors and on normal tissues.

Prostatic Cancer

Prostatic acid phosphatase is a well-known tumor marker for prostatic cancer[13, 27] and can be considered a tumor-associated antigen, even though it is found in the cytoplasm rather than on the surface of the cell. In this respect it is very similar to α-fetoprotein as a TAA in testicular cancers. Another such marker is creatine kinase BB, found in the brain; levels of this substance are elevated in the serum of prostatic carcinoma patients.[91]

An antigen claimed to be specific for the human prostate, though not specific for prostatic cancer, was identified by a rabbit antiserum made against human prostatic tissue. In the late 1970s, Chu and co-workers[17] described this interesting antigen, which they have called "prostate-specific antigen" (PA), possibly related to the prostate antigens found in normal prostate but to a far lesser extent in malignant prostate by Ablin and associates.[3] PA is found in both normal and malignant prostatic tissue, including primary and metastatic tumors. It appears to be a glycoprotein of approximately 34,000 daltons (34Kd) molecular weight, with distinct proteinase activity.[7] Radioimmunoassay and other sensitive methods have made it possible to detect the antigen more successfully than was originally possible, such that 371 of 442 patients with prostatic cancer and 13 of 19 with benign prostatic hyperplasia had levels elevated above that found in normal males.[51] In a recently reported study of 602 serum samples from the National Prostatic Cancer Project,[45] the presence of PA in the serum was a useful marker for recurrence of the disease in patients with Stage B_2 to D_1 disease. Moreover, the authors contended that an elevation of PA portended recurrence in 92% of the patients, with a lead time of 12 months before clinical detection. However, many factors could have influenced this assessment. For example, the frequency of collection of the sera versus the frequency of clinical examinations (every six weeks for the latter), and the intensity of the clinical assessment both strongly influence the relative effectiveness of the two evaluations. However, the times at which sera were collected and the specific clinical studies that were performed were both omitted from the report. Nevertheless, PA seems to be a useful antigenic marker for the disease in the serum and on prostatic tissue itself. In fact, a study by Allhoff and associates[5] found that primary and metastatic prostate tumors whose histologic diagnosis was uncertain could readily be identified through immunoperoxidase staining of the tissues with antibodies to prostatic acid phosphatase and to PA. Nine of 12 primary tumors thought to be prostatic were stained with antibodies to both substances, and two more stained only with antibody to PA. Six of 12 metastatic lesions had both antigens, and an additional one manifested PA only.

Antibodies to PA have also been detected in the sera of patients with prostatic cancer,[16] usually in patients with advanced disease. Some of the antibody appeared to be complexed with PA, identified on high-performance liquid chromatography at a molecular weight of more than 240 Kd, rather than at 150 Kd, where IgG would be expected. It is found to be characteristic of both primary and metastatic prostatic malignancy.[68] The same group of investigators also reported that the sera of 8% of 219 prostatic cancer patients contained a prostate antigen, a glycoprotein of approximately 34 to 36 Kd molecular weight.[76] Radioimmunoassay and other sensitive methods are now available to detect the antigen more readily, such that 371 of 442 prostate cancer patients and 13 of 19 prostatic hypertrophy patients had elevated levels (i.e., above the normal levels found in males).[51]

Monoclonal antibodies have now been developed to prostatic antigens, most of which identify normal prostatic tissue-specific antigens rather than tumor-associated antigens. Benign prostatic hypertrophy (BPH) is usually stained even when normal prostate tissue is not.[56, 75, 85] There are monoclonal antibodies, one set from mice[105] and another derived from human beings,[43] that appear to distinguish between benign prostatic hypertrophy and carcinoma. The antigens, called 83.21 and 6.2 by Wright and associates,[105] were found in 70 to 80% of 19 primary prostatic cancers, as well as in the majority of bladder cancers, but not in nine specimens of BPH or in normal tissues. The human monoclonal antibodies we have derived from patients with melanoma[43] have cross-reacted strongly with colon and prostatic carcinomas but have failed to react with BPH. Although none of the monoclonal antibodies is entirely tumor-specific, since they react with a number of other types of cancer, those antibodies that react with prostatic cancer rather than normal tissues, such as 83.21, 6.2, and our human monoclonal anti-melanoma antibodies, may ultimately prove

very useful for detecting and monitoring the course of the tumor.

Monoclonal antibodies have detected both a 94-Kd TAA, a glycoprotein, and HLA-Ia-like antigens on prostatic carcinoma cell lines.[73] The Ia-like molecules, which are products of the genes controlling the immune response, resemble those found on B lymphoid cell lines. Ia-like antigens (also called "DR" in humans) are also found in other tumors, such as melanomas. Significantly, both the glycoprotein antigen and the Ia-like antigens could serve as targets for the monoclonal antibodies in ADCC in vitro.[73] A monoclonal antibody called Anti-Pro 3 recognizes an antigen in human prostatic carcinoma that was also present in extracts of human normal and malignant nonprostatic tissues, and in normal prostatic tissue. However, there was a greater quantity of the antigen in malignant prostatic tissue. The antigen had an apparent molecular weight of 175 Kd, with a subunit of approximately 54 Kd.[102] Since serum from patients had antibodies that competed with the monoclonal antibody for the 54-Kd protein antigen, it seemed that this "p54" antigen might be a significant in vivo target for immunity in human prostatic cancer. This antigen is clearly a Class 3 antigen, as defined above, but might be of clinical importance nonetheless.

Bladder Cancer

ABO(H) Antigens and Invasiveness. An important antigenic change on the surface of TCC cells of prognostic significance is the decrease in expression of blood group antigens associated with a change of normal urothelial cells to neoplastic ones. Well-differentiated noninvasive TCC cells generally retain the ABO(H) antigens of normal urothelium, whereas less well differentiated tumors lose these antigens. Even among histologically well-differentiated TCC, those with a poor ABO(H) antigenic content have a strong tendency to become invasive later.[18, 55, 72, 103] It is somewhat paradoxical that one of the changes most related to the tumorous nature of bladder cancer cells might be the deletion of a normal set of antigens rather than the appearance of a new TSA specifically characterizing the tumor.

We should note, however, that several attempts to confirm these data on the usefulness of ABO(H) antigens as markers for invasive bladder carcinoma have led to equivocal results. Three carefully done studies, albeit with immunoperoxidase and immunofluorescence measurement of the presence of the antigens rather than the specific red cell adherence assay, found essentially no correlation between the blood group antigens and the grade of the tumor in the bladder.[24, 69, 100] However, a study of intravesical doxorubicin for bladder cancer noted a loss of ABO(H) antigens by specific red cell adherence, which correlated with ultrastructural changes in the membrane of the tumor cells.[40] The 12 patients who achieved a remission after topical chemotherapy had a return of blood group isoantigens that antedated the ultrastructural changes to normalcy. Studies that have utilized the original technique of specific red cell adherence to examine tumors of the upper urothelium, renal pelvis, and ureter have varied from confirming[23] to disputing[47] the validity of the original observations. A similar discrepancy occurred in two studies on prostatic cancer, one of which noted a strong correlation of ABO(H) antigen loss and invasiveness[101] and another that found no such correlation.[23] In bladder cancer after schistosomiasis, no loss of blood group substances was found, but there the majority of the tumors were squamous cell carcinomas. It is noteworthy that the few transitional cell carcinomas that were found were largely devoid of blood group substances, as would have been predicted.[21]

Methodologic problems have undoubtedly accounted in part for the discrepancies among the studies. Among these are the difficulties caused by the weak antigenicity of the O(H) antigen, present in 45% of the population, emphasized by Javadpour,[41] and the inadvertent removal of the blood group antigens during routine fixation of tissue specimens.[96] Thorpe and co-workers[96] have suggested that only frozen, unfixed tissue sections be used, to avoid extraction of the glycolipid antigens that occurs with formalin fixation. A significant improvement in technology should involve the use of immunoperoxidase techniques on tissues, preferably with highly specific monoclonal antibodies to blood group–specific antigens. In fact, in one such study[22] it was noted that 50% of the patients whose tumors had absent blood group substances had an invasive re-

currence, whereas only 13% of the blood group–positive population had invasive disease.

At the moment, it seems likely that the original observations on the inverse relationship between the presence of blood group antigens on the tumor and its invasiveness will prove correct for transitional cell carcinoma of the bladder, but data are too scanty and conflicting even to suggest that a similar relationship will be obtained in other types of urothelial cancer.

Cell Surface Glycoproteins Associated With Bladder Cancer. A newer line of investigation of bladder cancer that promises to be useful in many types of cancer involves the determination of the sugars present on the cell membrane, as detected by binding or microprecipitation with plant lectins. These sugars are an integral part of the tumor-associated glycoproteins, one of which could conceivably prove to be a TSA. Paulie and colleagues[77] have identified a 115-Kd glycopeptide that was precipitated by the lectin leukoagglutinin (La). This glycopeptide was present on transitional cell bladder carcinoma cells but not on normal urothelial cells or a squamous bladder carcinoma line. Similarly, with renal cell carcinoma, increased binding of several lectins, but not all, was noted with frozen sections and cell suspensions of renal cell carcinoma compared with preparations from normal kidney.[84] An analogous binding of lectins, though with less specificity for cancer versus hyperplasia, was also noted recently with prostatic carcinoma.[30]

Several investigators have reported monoclonal antibodies to bladder cancer cells that identify protein antigens. One recent example is a mouse antibody called 3G2-C6, which has identified one half to three quarters of the limited number of fresh and cultured bladder cancer cell preparations against which it has been tested, and has reacted with kidney and other urothelial tumor cells. It does not react against normal urothelial cells in culture, nor with most other types of tumor, and it identifies a 90-Kd cell surface protein.[106] Perlmann and colleagues[50, 78] have reported six monoclonal antibodies, several of which are reactive with malignant but not normal urothelium, including transitional cell carcinomas of the bladder and to some degree prostatic carcinomas. The antibodies were not tested against a broad range of other tumors, but they did not react against normal hematopoietic cells or normal urothelium. Several different antigenic targets were found with the six antibodies, but the clinical usefulness of any or all of these antigens remains to be seen.

In bladder cancer, much of the investigation into reactions to the presence of tumor antigens has involved the use of cell-mediated immunity, in particular ADCC. For example, with rabbit polyclonal antibodies to T24, a cell line derived from a transitional cell carcinoma (TCC) of the human bladder, Schneider and colleagues[88] found evidence of reactivity to antigens found on normal and cancerous urothelium. In further experiments, the same group found that a 110-Kd polypeptide was confined to the membrane of the urothelium cells, both normal and malignant (Class 3), but was absent from the colon carcinoma and malignant melanoma cells used as controls.[89]

Rat monoclonal antibodies to mouse bladder carcinoma were produced by the Hellstrom group and were then tested against a variety of target tumor lines. An antibody was produced that reacted against cell membranes from five of seven human TCCs but not to membranes from normal tissues. The antigen detected was a 140-Kd protein on the surface of the TCC. Another antigen found on TCC, normal liver, and several other normal and neoplastic tissues was detected by a second monoclonal antibody, but its nature has not yet been defined.[33]

Kidney Cancer

Kidney cancer has also been investigated for tumor-associated antigens. Monoclonal antibodies made in a mouse against human renal carcinoma cell lines by Ueda and colleagues[99] detected nine cell-surface antigenic systems. Three of them were related to histocompatibility (HLA) antigens and A and B blood group antigens, which interestingly are also found on these cells. The other six systems detected other antigens, but none of the antigens proved to be specific for renal carcinoma. They were more likely broadly expressed differentiation antigens found on other tumor cell lines and on normal cells, such as fibroblasts. The ABO(H) antigen expression detected here was used as the basis of an attempt to prog-

nosticate the outcome of tumors.[87] Thirty-nine of 42 patients had ABO(H) antigens on the renal tumor. These results are of course in strong contradistinction to those with TCCs that we have just noted. Despite the paucity of evidence for TAAs in renal cancer, there is strong circumstantial evidence for them, since such phenomena as the occasional spontaneous regression and disappearance of metastatic pulmonary nodules after removal of the primary tumor, and the very encouraging results with immunotherapy all suggest that the immune response plays a role in this tumor. Bander and colleagues[8] have described a series of mouse monoclonal antibodies that may represent the early stage of generation of a panel of antibodies for the typing of renal cell tumors. An antigen called gp 120nr, a differentiation antigen of proximal tubules, defines a large subset of the tumors, which also express at least two of the other proximal tubule differentiation antigens. Data thus far suggest that those tumors derived from parts of the nephron other than the proximal tubule, defined by their lack of reactivity to these monoclonal antibodies, tend to disseminate earlier than those expressing the antigens defined by these antibodies.

Testicular Cancer

Testicular cancers have received fairly little attention as far as investigation of their TAAs is concerned. Alpha-fetoprotein (AFP) is a fairly sensitive, though not entirely specific, marker for the presence and extent of the tumor, and it is used in much the same way as carcinoembryonic antigen (CEA) for colon carcinoma or prostatic acid phosphatase for prostatic carcinoma, to monitor the course of the disease rather than to screen for it. AFP can be used to localize testicular cancer in metastatic sites in the body, as Goldenberg and associates have nicely shown.[25] After radiolabeling with ^{131}I, goat anti-AFP IgG antibodies were injected into 12 patients with various neoplasms. After computer subtraction of background radioactivity, all tumor sites known to be present were visualized in the four patients who had either hepatocellular or germ cell carcinoma. The other eight patients, with other tumors, had radioactivity at five of 19 tumor sites, although the accumulation was less than in the patients with cancers known to make

AFP. Even circulating AFP levels of as much as 15 μg/ml did not prevent the antibodies from reaching metastatic sites in the tissues. Kim and associates[46] in an update of this work, indicated that all sites involved by five AFP-producing tumors could be demonstrated with the specific radiolabeled IgG, whereas normal goat IgG did not achieve similar results in one of the patients. The results with goat antibodies are of importance in paving the way for the use of highly specific monoclonal antibodies for the same purpose, for which they seem ideally suited.

It is worth noting, too, that HLA antigens and β2-microglobulin are expressed on testicular cancer cell lines in humans.[6] All of the cells examined had low levels of HLA-A, B, and C antigens and β2-microglobulin, but there were no discrete subpopulations positive or negative for these antigens. Mice, in contrast, did not express histocompatibility antigens on the surface of their testicular cancer cells.

Antibody-Mediated Immunity

ADCC reactions have been used to detect circulating antibodies in bladder cancer.[88, 89, 97] An antibody-mediated immune response of patients with bladder cancer to a panel of target cells was detected by ADCC.[97] Reactivity to bladder cancer cell lines was generally stronger than for the colon carcinoma cells used as control targets. Moreover, the reactivity to the same target cells was stronger than that of healthy normal donors. Whether the antigens reacted against by autologous antibodies were similar to those detected by the rabbit antibodies from the same laboratory was not determined by the investigators.[89] Circulating immune complexes have also been detected in 15% of the bladder cancer patients, suggesting an antibody response to tumor antigens in the circulation.[79] Both antibodies and cell-mediated cytotoxicity have been demonstrated concomitantly to transitional cell carcinoma of the bladder by Hansson and associates.[29] They found a strong statistical correlation between the presence of both types of immune response in a given patient, and they suggested that antibody-directed cytotoxicity was at the root of all specific cell-mediated reactions. It is at least certain that strong *specific* immunity (as opposed to the type exemplified by "natural" killing), both humoral and cellular, is elicited by the bladder cancer in many patients.

Antibodies to testicular carcinoma have been detected in 15 of 23 sera examined, with human and mouse sperm and a mouse teratocarcinoma cell line as the target cells. Six of the 15 positive sera reacted against both sperm and tumor cells.[95]

Leukocyte adherence-inhibition (LAI), a test that measures the ability of tumor antigens to prevent adherence of macrophages armed with cytophilic antibodies, has been used in a variety of cancers to demonstrate a patient's immune response to the tumor. In prostatic carcinoma in particular, Ablin and co-workers have found evidence for an antibody-directed cell-mediated immune response by this means.[1, 2] These investigators have also stressed that suppressor mechanisms in prostatic cancer include immunosuppressive substances found in seminal plasma that are active against the arming of peripheral blood mononuclear cells in the LAI test. These substances may play a role not only in the suppression of an ongoing immune response but perhaps in the pathogenesis of the disease, since normal human seminal plasma also contains such inhibitors.[1, 2, 10]

Miller and colleagues[60] noted the development of antibodies to autologous tumor cell lines in the majority of patients undergoing specific active immunization with irradiated autologous renal carcinoma cells, given together with *Corynebacterium parvum*. The autologous immunization induced IgG antibodies specifically reactive against autologous renal carcinoma cells in 50 of 70 serum samples from 11 patients, with an increase in antibody titer during the period of immunization in three of five patients studied serially. In a companion study, Huben and associates[38] found lymphocyte-mediated cytotoxicity against autologous tumor cells in these patients that did not correlate with the level of NK activity. The degree of reactivity against autologous cells was significantly higher than against allogeneic renal cells, although the levels of both were substantial (76% lysis versus 56%) at a 100:1 ratio of effectors to target cells.

Cytotoxic antibodies against a cultured renal cell carcinoma cell line were studied by Japanese investigators.[39] These workers found antibodies in eight of 18 patients who were about to undergo nephrectomy, partic-

ularly in those patients with a low pathologic grade of tumor.

Cell-Mediated Immunity

Specific T-cell–mediated cytotoxicity to
tumor cells has been studied in very few
human cancers and in none of the genitourinary cancers, to our knowledge. Specific
techniques for obtaining purified T-cells
from human peripheral blood, such as by
fluorescence-activated cell sorting (FACS),
may now make it possible to study only T-
cell activities, especially after the T-cells are
cloned in vitro. It is very likely that, as in
animal tumors, specific T-cell–mediated
reactivity of patients against their own tumor
will be demonstrable in humans. As a start,
macrophage mobility has been used as a
measurement of the release of specific lymphokines from T-cells in renal cell carcinoma.[58] These workers found that 16 of 21
patients were sensitized to antigens contained in an extract of an allogeneic kidney
tumor. Four of 19 were sensitized to fetal
kidney antigens, four of 21 to normal kidney
antigens, and three of 19 to urinary bladder
carcinoma extracts.

Suppressor Cells

Suppressor cells have been found in patients with bladder and prostatic carcinoma
by at least two investigative groups.[35, 93] Macrophage suppressor cells were found in 15
of 23 patients with bladder or prostatic cancer whose lymphocytes responded poorly in
vitro to nonspecific mitogens such as phytohemagglutinin and concanavalin A. These
patients generally had advanced disease.
Such suppressor macrophages may explain
the reduced skin test reactivity found in
patients with advanced urologic cancer.[35]
Spina and associates[93] confirmed these findings in bladder cancer, in that patients with
advanced disease had a decreased ability to
generate a cytotoxic response against allogeneic lymphoid cells in vitro, which was
improved after the patient's adherent cells
(predominantly macrophages) were removed
from the culture. Removal of the tumor in
patients with superficial disease restored
their in vitro response to normal without the
need for other maneuvers in vitro. In contrast, patients with invasive disease had only
minimal improvement of their ability to gen-

erate a cytotoxic response in vitro after surgery.

The mixed lymphocyte reaction (MLR),
the proliferative response of lymphocytes to
normal lymphocytes, was diminished in patients with bladder papillomas who later
developed a frank malignancy.[36] Usually
only 10% of such patients have lesions that
progress to malignancy. Twelve of 27 patients with papillomas were found to have a
depressed MLR. Strikingly, 10 of these 12
developed bladder cancer within five years.
Of the 15 patients with a normal MLR, only
three of 15 developed cancer during that
time. Survival of patients with a normal
MLR was 80% at five years versus 17% for
those with a depressed MLR. This sort of
gross immunological deficit in reactivity is
not usually found in patients with premalignant lesions, but where it does exist, strong
correlations like those described here can
emerge.

Suppressor T-cells specific for the tumor
have not been demonstrated routinely in any
urologic cancer, but Akiyama and colleagues
found that re-exposure of lymphocytes from
a renal or bladder cancer patient to the
patient's own tumor elicited suppressor T-
cells in vitro that were capable of nonspecifically suppressing mixed lymphocyte
reactions.[4] These cells were rarely demonstrable before restimulation in vitro. Immune
complexes, presumably the "blocking factors" previously described in genitourinary
cancer by the Hellstroms,[32] have been demonstrable in approximately 15% of patients
with TCC of the bladder,[79] and perhaps in
prostatic cancer, too.[15] It is probable that
persistent study will also reveal the existence of tumor-specific suppressor T-cells
elicited by the complexes.

Even though it is difficult to do immunologic testing for specific tumor-associated
immunity in any cancer patient, this sort of
activity should be the focus of our energies,
not nonspecific immunologic profiles. All
the latter can tell us is the burden of tumor
cells in the body, and by a far less direct
means than clinical examination, radiography, and blood values. It is highly doubtful
whether the prognosis or even the likelihood
of response to immunotherapy can be predicted by skin test reactivity to microbial
antigens such as tuberculin or Candida. Our
reexamination of data that were originally
interpreted as being prognostic for outcome

has revealed that patients with good or poor reactivity to such antigens have an equal response to therapy.[9]

IMMUNOTHERAPY OF GENITOURINARY CANCERS

Bladder Cancer

Bacille Calmette-Guérin (BCG)

The most interesting advance in the field of immunotherapy for bladder cancer has been the use of BCG instillations for the treatment of superficial bladder carcinomas. Several groups have reported success with this therapy. In the original study by Morales and associates[66] 16 patients who had had 53 tumors before BCG during 162 patient-months received this treatment. After six instillations of BCG (from Institut Armand Frappier, Montreal), there were only seven recurrences in 222 patient-months. In a later report, 14 of 26 patients (54%) remained tumor-free for the duration of follow-up, which was nine to 56 months after treatment. There was a highly significant (p <0.00001) decrease in the frequency of recurrence of the tumors.[67]

Morales has now treated 93 patients with intravesical BCG. Seventy per cent of the patients remained disease-free at 24 months, but recurrences were noted between 24 and 36 months after the beginning of therapy with no further decline. Side effects were self-limited and ended within a short time after treatment was discontinued. Only 20% had symptoms warranting discontinuation of treatment or antituberculous medication. No permanent structural or functional alterations in the bladder occurred in any patient.[65] Brosman[12] and Pinsky and associates[80] have confirmed these findings in independent trials. In Brosman's study there were no recurrences in the BCG group of 39 patients, versus nine recurrences of 22 in the other group given instillations of the alkylating agent thio-tepa. Six of 12 patients with visible tumors had a complete response after 18 instillations and in two this effect was seen after 24 weeks. Two further patients were free of tumor after only six weeks of BCG instillations. Five of the seven patients with carcinoma in situ had a complete response after 18 weeks, with no cellular atypia cytologically.

Pinsky and associates[80] randomly gave 51 patients either fulguration or BCG treatment (six weekly instillations plus cutaneous inoculation of BCG). The number of recurrences in the BCG group was reduced and the time to recurrence was prolonged. Only in the BCG group was the incidence of positive cytologic results decreased. The same group has recently updated their data in a randomized trial, in which 43 patients were assigned either to transurethral resection alone or transurethral resection followed by therapy with the Pasteur strain of BCG, given intravesically and intradermally weekly for six weeks. The number of tumors per patient-month was reduced from 3.6 to 0.7, and the median time to relapse was increased from nine to 36 months in the BCG group. Moreover, symptomatic flat carcinomas in situ were also beneficially affected by the BCG regimen in an extension of the study. Nineteen of the 24 patients with carcinomas in situ responded completely, with a median followup of 24 months.[37]

Urine cytologic findings returned to normal in 22 of 33 BCG-treated patients in the randomized study group, versus only three of 34 with transurethral resection alone.[37] Flow cytometric monitoring of the bladder washings from these patients also has been performed.[104] In patients who originally had more than 15% hyperdiploid cells in their bladder washings or in those with a hyperdiploid stemline, intravesical BCG led to reversion of the cells to a normal phenotype. Thirteen patients with more than 15% hyperdiploid cells before therapy had less than 15% afterward, and 11 had complete response by all criteria. Two were treatment failures. Four of 17 continued to have more than 15% hyperdiploid cells, three of whom were treatment failures, with the fourth considered to have a flow-cytometry false-positive result. Similarly, 10 of the 12 patients who had a hyperdiploid stemline lost that line after therapy. Seven of these 10 had complete remission and another two were clinically without evidence of disease.

Lamm and associates have reported on 55 randomized and 30 high-risk nonrandomized patients treated since 1978 with intravesical BCG, usually with additional cutaneous BCG immunization.[52] Recurrences have been fewer (six of 29 versus 14 of 26) in the BCG group relative to controls, and those whose skin test results converted appeared to be best protected. High-risk patients have thus far shown a considerable reduction or prevention of recurrences. A temporary ureteral obstruction due to BCG cystitis was the only major toxicity observed.[52] With the availability of purified components of BCG, such as muramyl dipeptide (MDP) and "P3," the principal lipid component of BCG, it may now be possible to obtain these results without the severe systemic toxicity of whole, viable BCG organisms. Marked bladder irritability, which frequently accompanies BCG instillation, may be somewhat more difficult to circumvent, however.

Interleukin-2

Another interesting approach along the same lines has involved intralesional injection of bladder carcinoma with interleukin 2 (IL-2), the lymphokine secreted by helper T-cells that causes proliferation and maturation of other T-cells, especially cytolytic ones. A preliminary report[81] suggests that repeated injections of xenogeneic IL-2 of high biologic activity over a period of one to eight weeks caused complete or partial regression in five of six patients, with massive necrosis in the sixth noted at the time of cystectomy. This is undoubtedly similar to the striking local (inflammatory) results obtained with intralesional BCG in the past in melanoma and other cutaneous diseases. Whether the results will be translated into a prolonged disease-free interval for these patients, as with *intravesical* BCG, or will mimic the less satisfactory course of the *intralesional* BCG patients remains to be seen.

Retinoic Acid

A study was planned by the National Bladder Cancer Cooperative Group A to include 80 patients with recurrent superficial TCC, 70% of whom were expected to develop further recurrences. These patients received 13-*cis*-retinoic acid for six months, followed by 24 months of observation. Rates of recurrence were then compared with those of historic controls. Unfortunately, the study was terminated early because, of the first 17 patients to complete six months of therapy with the retinoid, only two were free of disease at the end of the study period. This

represented a recurrence rate of 88%. Seven further patients were withdrawn from the study because of unacceptable toxicity. There was even an apparent acceleration of disease with extravesicle involvement. Thus, after the tumor has developed, retinoids may be ineffective, and it is very likely that this group of patients had many subclinical but nevertheless established tumors. Treatment of individuals with dysplasia in order to prevent their development of TCC might have been a better setting for the use of retinoic acid.[11]

Kidney Cancer

Specific Active Immunotherapy

Two impressive early studies with tumor vaccines are noteworthy. McCune and associates[57] found that autologous irradiated renal carcinoma cells mixed with *C. parvum*, administered weekly to 14 patients with metastatic renal cell carcinoma, led to regression of metastatic disease in four (28%). A fifth patient had stable disease for more than 27 months. There was a considerable variation in the response of different sites of metastatic disease and even among lesions (particularly pulmonary) in the same organ. Patients who responded best were those in the best physical condition, which generally is true also as a predictor of response to chemotherapy. These were presumably the individuals whose immunity was least impaired, although specific measurements of antitumor immunity were not made in this study.

Neidhart and co-workers[71] performed a similar trial in 24 patients, except that instead of killed tumor cells they used an extract of the tumor aggregated with ethylchlorformiate mixed with tuberculin or with phytohemagglutinin as nonspecific adjuvants. BCG inoculations were also given to sensitize the patients to tuberculin. The patient's own tumor was used in 30 patients until the extract was exhausted; allogeneic renal cell carcinoma was used thereafter. The other six patients had only autologous tumor extracts. Two patients (7%) had a complete remission of pulmonary metastases, lasting more than 30 weeks, and two other patients had a partial remission or mixed response lasting 22 weeks. Eleven more patients (37%) were stabilized for a mean of more than 26 months, whereas the remaining 15 (50%) had progressive disease. It is of interest that the best responses, the two complete remissions, occurred in patients after they were switched to allogeneic vaccine from autologous extracts. Bone metastases as well as pulmonary lesions disappeared or regressed after treatment. One of the patients with disease judged "stable" had no measurable disease at entry, but it had not recurred in five years. These results were very similar to those previously reported by Tykka and associates,[98] who used only autologous aggregated extracts. Patients with the smallest tumor cell burden did the best in both of these studies with aggregated tumor extracts.

Neidhart and associates[70] recently have begun an attempt to confirm their results in a randomized trial. One of 27 evaluated patients receiving the vaccine has had a complete remission and one has had a partial response. None of the 31 patients randomly chosen to receive medroxyprogesterone acetate (Provera) has improved. After cross-over to vaccine, two patients formerly on Provera had partial responses. Although the duration of this randomized study has been very short, the results are still suggestive of efficacy for the vaccine.

Adoptive Immunotherapy With "Immune" RNA

The results of treatment with "immune" RNA have been more variable. This material was extracted from the lymphocytes of sheep after immunization of the animal with the patient's own renal carcinoma obtained at the time of nephrectomy. None of the studies has been randomized and only one has involved even a moderately large number of patients. Whereas Skinner[92] found only one response in 12 patients, with stabilization in two others for two years, in another study three of six patients treated with autologous lymphocytes previously incubated with "immune" RNA in vitro had a measurable response.[94] The pulmonary lesions of two other patients stabilized. In this study, an attempt was made to measure reactivity of the patient's peripheral blood mononuclear cells, which showed progressive increase in their ability to kill allogeneic renal carcinoma cells in vitro. deKernion and Ramming found that the median survival among

25 patients treated with "immune" RNA intradermally was improved, compared with that of 85 retrospective controls, if their metastases were limited to the lungs.[19] Those with disease at other sites, specifically bones, or with multiple sites involved, had no such increase in survival. The increases in delayed hypersensitivity reactions and mononuclear cell–mediated cytotoxicity to renal carcinoma cells were related to changes in the tumor burden and not to the RNA administered, in direct contrast to the findings of Steele and associates.[94] The use of "immune" RNA has largely been restricted to this disorder, perhaps because the amount of tumor material required to immunize a large animal is found only in this and a few other solid tumors. Whether "immune" RNA will prove to be active objectively in large-scale trials remains to be seen.

Alpha-Interferon

Interferon (IFN), particularly pure α-IFN obtained by recombinant DNA technology, is proving to be effective in the treatment of renal cell carcinoma, not only as an immunotherapeutic agent but also as a cytostatic agent directly affecting tumor cells. Nevertheless, this represents a rare instance in which even putative immunotherapy appears to be superior to chemotherapy as the principal treatment for metastatic disease, because there really is no effective chemical (or hormonal) therapy for renal cell carcinoma. Objective complete and partial responses have been noted with both extracted (partially purified) human leukocyte α-IFN[20, 48, 83] and more recently with pure recombinant α-IFN.[44] A substantial number of patients have also had minimal response (less than the 50% regression required for a partial response) and stabilization of previously advancing disease during the treatment. The proportion of patients who respond to the treatment with either the partially purified leukocyte α-IFN or the pure recombinant material is probably no greater than 20%, judging from several independent studies, including our own. Subcutaneous and lung metastases have been most affected by IFN, with other sites remaining relatively resistant. Objective response usually has required several months to achieve during what was previously considered the "maintenance" period, so that a prolonged, continued treatment of patients who have minimal responses or stable disease in the first few weeks of treatment is mandatory. Toxicity has been moderate to severe, with severe malaise the main symptom. Alpha-IFN appears to be effective at either "low" doses of 1 to 3 million IU per day, "intermediate" doses of 10 million IU per day or "high" doses of 30 to 50 million IU. It is interesting that α-IFN is immunosuppressive at doses higher than approximately 3 million IU per day,[34] meaning that its effects on the tumor at the high dose level is through its cytostatic effects rather than through any biomodulatory influences on the host.

Clinical trials of recombinant β- and γ-IFN in renal cell carcinoma are now in progress.

Restorative Immunotherapy: Thymosin

Thymosin factor 5 has also shown promise in a preliminary trial of 21 patients. Schulof and associates[90] have noted three partial responses and two stable disease patterns of 20 evaluated patients. Lung metastases were the dominant disease in the responding patients, similar to the responsive site in other immunotherapy trials.

Prostatic Cancer

Thirty-three patients were randomly chosen to receive BCG intradermally every four weeks, with or without "standard" therapy for prostatic cancer.[28] In this study, the standard treatment consisted of administration of estrogens, with or without orchiectomy, or simple observation. A 42-week survival was noted in the group receiving BCG, versus 29 weeks in those that did not. Direct intratumoral injection of BCG was performed by Merrin and associates,[59] with success in causing regression of disease in three of seven tuberculin-positive patients. There was no attempt to modify systemic disseminated tumor by these workers. Except for these studies, there has been little or no approach to prostatic cancer through immunotherapy, but this is likely to occur as more data on the fundamental immunology of this tumor are accrued.

Testicular Cancer

The dramatic success in the chemotherapeutic approach to disseminated testicular cancer has understandably made the development of immunotherapy a low-priority issue. However, the same approach that Goldenberg and others have taken to the localization of these tumors in their metastatic sites could be used to kill the tumors, if the radiolabel attached to antibodies emits alpha particles or carries a toxic moiety to the metastatic sites. These could well be future approaches to those who are not cured by intensive chemotherapy.

SUMMARY AND CONCLUSIONS

Although the field of genitourinary cancer immunology is just now undergoing considerable development, it is already clear that these tumors are governed by the same immunologic conditions as tumors in other parts of the body. Fundamental observations remain to be made about the nature of the antigens in these tumors, and the variety of immunologic techniques used to identify the host's response to autologous tumors should and will certainly be applied to them as well. Finally, the already dramatic results of some forms of immunotherapy in treating even disseminated disease make it imperative to explore this avenue extensively in the near future. Although surgery, radiation therapy, and often chemotherapy are useful in the standard treatment of genitourinary cancers, the broad approach to the tumor known as biomodulation, which includes immunotherapy, may well have a significant impact very shortly.

References

1. Ablin RJ, Bhatti RA, Bush IM, Guinan PD: Immunosuppression of cell- and serum-mediated tumour-associated immunity in prostatic cancer by human seminal plasma. Eur J Cancer 15:775–780, 1980.
2. Ablin RJ, Bhatti RA, Bush IM, Guinan PD: Suppression of tumor-associated immunity by human seminal plasma and its possible role in the natural history of prostatic cancer. Eur Urol 6:225–228, 1980.
3. Ablin RJ, Bronson P, Soanes WA, Witebsky E: Tissue- and species-specific antigens of normal human prostatic tissue. J Immunol 104:1329–1339, 1970.
4. Akiyama M, Bean MA, Sadamoto K, et al: Suppression of the responsiveness of lymphocytes from cancer patients triggered by co-culture with autologous tumor-derived cells. J Immunol 131:3085–3090, 1983.

5. Allhoff EP, Proppe KH, Chapman CM, et al: Evaluation of prostate specific acid phosphatase and prostate specific antigen in identification of prostatic cancer. J Urol 129:315–318, 1983.

6. Andrews PW, Bronson DL, Wiles MV, Goodfellow PN: The expression of MHC antigens by human teratocarcinoma derived cell lines. Tissue Antigens 17:493–500, 1981.

7. Ban Y, Wang MC, Chu TM: Biological nature of the human prostate-specific antigen. Fed Proc 42:406, 1983.

8. Bander N, Cordon-Cardo C, Finstad C, et al: Immunopathology of renal cancer: identification of antigenically and clinically distinct subtypes with monoclonal antibodies. Proc Am Assoc Cancer Res 25:253, 1984.

9. Bennett JA, Mitchell MS: Principles of tumor immunology. In SK Carter, E Glatstein, RB Livingston (eds), Principles of Cancer Treatment. New York, McGraw Hill, 1981, pp 162–169.

10. Bhatti RA, Ablin RJ, Zamora S, et al: Suppression of cytophilic antibody ("arming" factor) in the sera of patients with prostatic cancer by human seminal plasma. Experientia 36:349–350, 1980.

11. Biological Response Modifiers: Subcommittee report. National Cancer Institute Monogr #63, NIH Publication No. 83-2606, Bethesda, MD, 1983.

12. Brosman SA: Experience with bacillus Calmette-Guérin in patients with superficial bladder carcinoma. J Urol 128:27–30, 1982.

13. Bruce AW, Mahan DE: The role of prostatic acid phosphatase in the investigation and treatment of adenocarcinoma of the prostate. Ann NY Acad Sci 390:110–121, 1982.

14. Burnet FM: The concept of immunological surveillance. Prog Exp Tumor Res 13:1–27, 1970.

15. Catalona WJ: Immunobiology of carcinoma of the prostate. Invest Urol 17:373–377, 1980.

16. Chu TM, Kuriyama M, Johnson E, et al: Circulating antibody to prostate antigen in patients with prostatic cancer. Ann NY Acad Sci 417:383–389, 1983.

17. Chu TM, Wang MC, Lee CL, et al: Enzyme markers for prostatic cancer. Cancer Detect Prev 2:693–706, 1979.

18. DeCenzo JM, Howard P, Irish CE: Antigenic deletion and prognosis of patients with Stage A transitional cell bladder carcinoma. J Urol 114:875–878, 1975.

19. deKernion JB, Ramming KP: The therapy of renal adenocarcinoma with immune RNA. Invest Urol 17:378–381, 1980.

20. deKernion JB, Sarna G, Figlin R, et al: The treatment of renal cell carcinoma with human leukocyte alpha-interferon. J Urol 130:1063–1066, 1983.

21. El Adl MM, Yamase HT, Nieh PT, et al: ABH cell surface isoantigens in invasive bladder carcinoma associated with schistosomiasis. J Urol 131:249–251, 1984.

22. Finan PJ, Anderson JR, Doyle PT, et al: The prediction of invasive potential in superficial transitional cell carcinoma of the bladder. Br J Urol 54:720–725, 1982.

23. Ghazizadeh M, Numata A, Kagawa S, et al: Prognostic validity of the specific red cell adherence test in upper urothelial tumours. Br J Urol 55:473–476, 1983.

24. Giraldo AA, Ruby SG, Humes JJ: Blood group antigens in urothelium in transitional cell carcinoma. Ann Clin Lab Sci 13:307–314, 1983.

25. Goldenberg DM, Kim EE, Deland F, et al: Clinical studies on the radioimmunodetection of tumors containing alpha-fetoprotein. Cancer 45:2500–2505, 1980.

26. Greenberg PD, Cheever MA, Fefer A: Prerequisite for successful adaptive immunotherapy: nature of effector cells and role of H-2 restriction. In A Fefer, AL Goldstein (eds), The Potential Role of T Cells in Cancer Therapy. New York, Raven Press, 1982, pp 31–50.

27. Griffiths J: The appropriate uses of prostatic acid phosphatase determination in the diagnosis of adenocarcinoma of the prostate. Ann NY Acad Sci 390:100–103, 1982.

28. Guinan PD, John T, Baumgartner G, et al: Adjuvant immunotherapy (BCG) in Stage D prostate cancer. Am J Clin Oncol 5:65–68, 1982.

29. Hansson T, Paulie S, Larsson A, et al: Humoral and cellular immune reactions against tumor cells in patients with urinary bladder carcinoma. Correlation between direct and antibody-dependent cell-mediated cytotoxicity. Cancer Immunol Immunother 16:23–29, 1983.

30. Heaney J, Orgad U, Alroy J, et al: Comparative studies of cell surface sugars in neoplastic metaplastic and atrophic prostatic epithelium (abstr). American Urological Association 78th Annual Meeting, Las Vegas, NV, April 17–21, 1983.

31. Hellström KE, Hellström I: Evidence that tumor antigens enhance tumor growth in vivo by interacting with a radiosensitive (suppressor?) cell population. Proc Natl Acad Sci USA 75:436–440, 1978.

32. Hellström KE, Hellström I: Lymphocyte-mediated cytotoxicity and blocking serum activity to tumor antigens. Adv Immunol 18:209–277, 1974.

33. Hellström I, Rollins N, Settle S, et al: Monoclonal antibodies to two mouse bladder carcinoma antigens. Int J Cancer 29:175–180, 1982.

34. Hengst JC, Kempf RA, Kan-Mitchell J, et al: Immunological effects of recombinant interferon-alpha 2 in cancer patients. J Biol Response Mod 2:516–527, 1983.

35. Herr HW: Suppressor cells in immunodepressed bladder and prostate cancer patients. J Urol 123:635–639, 1980.

36. Herr HW: Association of depressed mixed lymphocyte reactivity with the development of bladder carcinoma in patients with papillomas. Cancer 51:344–347, 1983.

37. Herr HW, Pinsky CM, Whitmore WF, et al: Intravesical bacillus Calmette-Guérin (BCG) therapy of superficial bladder tumors (abstr). American Urologic Association 78th Annual Meeting, Las Vegas, NV. April 17–21, 1983.

38. Huben RP, Connelly RW, Goldrosen MH, et al: Cell-mediated cytotoxicity in patients undergoing active specific immunotherapy (abstr). American Urologic Association 78th Annual Meeting, Las Vegas, NV, April 17–21, 1983.

39. Ishibashi M, Matsuda M, Osafune M, et al: Circulating cytotoxic anti-RCC antibody responses in renal cell carcinoma patients. Hinyokika Kiyo 29:121–129, 1983.

40. Jakse G, Hofstadter F: Mechanisms of action of intravesical treatment. Effect on the ABH surface antigens of urothelial cells. Cancer Chemother Pharmacol 11(Suppl):574–578, 1983.

41. Javadpour N, Vafrier J, Worsham GF, O'Connel K: Peroxidase antiperoxidase versus specific red cell adherence in detection of O(H) antigen in bladder

cancer: a blind study. J Surg Oncol 27:112–115, 1984.

42. Kaliss N: Immunological enhancement of tumor homografts in mice: a review. Cancer Res 18:992–1003, 1958.

43. Kan-Mitchell J, Imam A, Kempf RA, et al: Human monoclonal antibodies directed against melanoma tumor-associated antigens. Cancer Res 46:2490–2496, 1986.

44. Kempf RA, Grunberg SM, Daniels JR, et al: Recombinant interferon alpha-2 (Intron A) in a phase II study of renal carcinoma. J Biol Response Mod 5:27–35, 1986.

45. Killian CS, Yang N, Emrich LJ, et al: Prognostic importance of prostate-specific antigen for monitoring patients with stages B_2 to D_1 prostate cancer. Cancer Res 45:886–891, 1985.

46. Kim EE, DeLand FH, Nelson MO, et al: Radioimmunodetection of cancer with radiolabeled antibodies to alpha-fetoprotein. Cancer Res 40:3008–3012, 1980.

47. King CT, Clark TD, Lovett J, et al: A comparison of clinical course with blood group antigen testing by specific red cell adherence and immunoperoxidase in ureteral and renal pelvic tumors. J Urol 130:871–873, 1983.

48. Kirkwood JM, Harris JE, Vera R, et al: A randomized study of low and high doses of leukocyte alpha-interferon in metastatic renal cell carcinoma: The American Cancer Society Collaborative Trial. Cancer Res 45:863–871, 1985.

49. Klein G: Tumor-specific transplantation antigens: GHA Clowes Memorial Lecture. Cancer Res 28:625–635, 1968.

50. Koho H, Paulie S, Ben-Aissa H, et al: Monoclonal antibodies to antigens associated with transitional cell carcinoma of the human urinary bladder. I. Determination of the selectivity of six antibodies by cell Elisa and immunofluorescence. Cancer Immunol Immunother 17:165–172, 1984.

51. Kuriyama M, Wang MC, Papsidero LD, et al: Quantitation of prostate-specific antigen in serum by a sensitive enzyme immunoassay. Cancer Res 40:4658–4662, 1980.

52. Lamm DL, Stogdill VD, Radwin HM: The current status of BCG in the treatment of human bladder cancer (abstr). American Urologic Association 78th Annual Meeting, Las Vegas, NV, April 17–21, 1983.

53. Lennox ES, Lowe AD, Cohn J, Evan G: Specific antigens on methylcholanthrene-induced tumors of mice. Transplant Proc 13:1759–1761, 1981.

54. Levine AS: The epidemic of acquired immune dysfunction in homosexual men and its sequelae—opportunistic infections, Kaposi's sarcoma, and other malignancies: an update and interpretation. Cancer Treat Rep 66:1391–1395, 1982.

55. Limas C, Lange P: Altered reactivity for A,B,H antigens in transitional cell carcinomas of the urinary bladder. A study of the mechanisms involved. Cancer 46:1366–1373, 1980.

56. Lowe DH, Handley HH, Schmidt J, et al: A human monoclonal antibody reactive with human prostate. J Urol 132:780–785, 1984.

57. McCune CS, Schapira DV, Henshaw EC: Specific immunotherapy of advanced renal carcinoma: evidence for the polyclonality of metastases. Cancer 47:1984–1987, 1981.

58. Malkovsky M, Bubeník J, Jakoubková J, et al: The macrophage electrophoretic mobility assay in patients with renal cell carcinoma. Neoplasma 28:245–251, 1981.

59. Merrin C, Han T, Klein E, et al: Immunotherapy of prostatic carcinoma with bacillus Calmette-Guérin. Cancer Chemother Rep 59:157–163, 1975.

60. Miller GA, Pontes JE, Huben R, et al: Characterization of the serological response of renal cell carcinoma (RCC) patients receiving specific active immunotherapy by the mixed hemadsorption assay (MHA) (abstr). American Urologic Association 78th Annual Meeting, Las Vegas, NV, April 17–21, 1983.

61. Mitchell MS: Role of "suppressor" T lymphocytes in antibody-induced inhibition of cytophilic antibody receptors. Ann NY Acad Sci 276:229–242, 1976.

62. Mitchell MS: Biomodulation: a classification and overview. In AE Reif, MS Mitchell (eds), Immunity to Cancer. Orlando, FL, Adademic Press, 1985, pp 401–411.

63. Mitchell MS, Bertram JH: Tumor immunology and biomodulation. In P Calabresi, PS Schein, SA Rosenberg (eds), Medical Oncology. New York, Macmillan, 1985, pp 363–391.

64. Mitchell MS, Rao VS: Interaction of immune complexes and suppressor T cells in the inhibition of cytophilic antibody receptors on macrophages. In RG Crispen (ed). Neoplasm Immunity: Experimental and Clinical. New York, Elsevier, 1980, pp 61–83.

65. Morales A: Long-term results and complications of intracavitary bacillus Calmette-Guérin therapy for bladder cancer. J Urol 132:457–459, 1984.

66. Morales A, Eidinger D, Bruce AW: Adjuvant BCG immunotherapy for recurrent superficial bladder cancer. In WD Terry, D Windhorst (eds), Immunotherapy of Cancer: Present Status of Trials in Man. New York, Raven Press, 1978, pp 225–231.

67. Morales A, Ersil A: Adjuvant BCG immunotherapy in the prophylaxis and treatment of noninvasive bladder cancer. In WD Terry, SA Rosenberg (eds), Immunotherapy of Human Cancer. New York, Elsevier, 1982, pp 301–306.

68. Nadji M, Tabei SZ, Castro A, et al: Prostatic-specific antigen: an immunohistologic marker for prostatic neoplasms. Cancer 48:1229–1232, 1981.

69. Nakatsu H, Kobayashi I, Onishi Y, et al: ABO(H) blood group antigens and carcinoembryonic antigens as indicators of malignant potential in patients with transitional cell carcinoma of the bladder. J Urol 131:252–257, 1984.

70. Neidhart JA, Gagen M, Young D, Wise HA: A randomized study of polymerized tumor antigen admixed with adjuvant (PTA) for therapy of renal cancer (abstr). Proc Am Soc Clin Oncol 2:C-189, 1983.

71. Neidhart JA, Murphy SG, Hennick LA, Wise HA: Active specific immunotherapy of Stage IV renal carcinoma with aggregated tumor antigen adjuvant. Cancer 46:1128–1134, 1980.

72. Newman AJ Jr, Carlton CE Jr, Johnson S: Cell surface A,B, or O(H) blood group antigens as an indicator of malignant potential in Stage A bladder carcinoma. J Urol 124:27–29, 1980.

73. Ng AK, Pellegrino MA, Imai K, Ferrone S: HLA-A,B antigens, la-like antigens, and tumor-associated antigens on prostate carcinoma cell lines: serologic and immunochemical analysis with

monoclonal antibodies. J Immunol 127:443–447, 1981.

74. Old LJ: Cancer immunology: the search for specificity. GHA Clowes Memorial Lecture. Cancer Res 41:361–375, 1981.

75. Papsidero LD, Croghan GA, Wang MC, et al: Monoclonal antibody (F5) to human prostate antigen. Hybridoma 2:139–147, 1983.

76. Papsidero LD, Wang MC, Valenzuela LA, et al: A prostate antigen in sera of prostatic cancer patients. Cancer Res 40:2428–2432, 1980.

77. Paulie S, Hansson Y, Lundblad ML, Perlmann P: Lectins as probes for identification of tumor-associated antigens on urothelial and colonic carcinoma cell lines. Int J Cancer 31:297–303, 1983.

78. Paulie S, Koho H, Ben-Aissa H, et al: Monoclonal antibodies to antigens associated with transitional cell carcinoma of the human urinary bladder. II. Identification of the cellular target structures by immunoprecipitation and SDS-Page analysis. Cancer Immunol Immunother 17:173–179, 1984.

79. Pesce AJ, Phillips TM, Ooi BS, et al: Immune complexes in transitional cell carcinoma. J Urol 123:486–488, 1980.

80. Pinsky CM, Camacho FJ, Kerr D, et al: Treatment of superficial bladder cancer with intravesical BCG. In WD Terry, SA Rosenberg (eds), Immunotherapy of Human Cancer. New York, Elsevier, 1982, pp 309–314.

81. Pizza G, Severine G, Menniti D, et al: Tumour regression after intralesional injection of interleukin 2 (IL-2) in bladder cancer: preliminary report. Int J Cancer 34:359–367, 1984.

82. Prehn RT, Main JM: Immunity to methylcholanthrene-induced sarcomas. JNCI 18:769–778, 1957.

83. Quesada JR, Swanson DA, Trindade A, Gutterman JU: Renal cell carcinoma: antitumor effects of leukocyte interferon. Cancer Res 43:940–947, 1983.

84. Raedler A, Boehle A, Otto U, Raedler E: Differences of glycoconjugates exposed on hypernephroma and normal kidney cells. J Urol 128:1109–1113, 1982.

85. Raynor RH, Hazra TA, Moncure CW, Mohanakumar T: Characterization of a monoclonal antibody, KR-P8, that detects a new prostate-specific marker. JNCI 73:617–625, 1984.

86. Reif AE, Mitchell MS (eds): Immunity to Cancer. Orlando, FL, Academic Press, 1985.

87. Sarosdy MF, Lamm DL: Application of the mixed cell agglutination test for cell surface antigens to renal cell carcinoma. J Urol 128:693–696, 1982.

88. Schneider MU, Troye M, Paulie S, Perlmann P: Membrane-associated antigens on tumor cells from transitional-cell carcinoma of the human urinary bladder. I. Immunological characterization by xenogeneic antisera. Int J Cancer 26:185–192, 1980.

89. Schneider MU, Paulie S, Troye M, Perlmann P: Plasma membrane-associated antigens on tumor cells derived from transitional-cell carcinoma of the human urinary bladder. II. Identification at the molecular level of plasma membrane–associated antigens. Int J Cancer 26:193–202, 1980.

90. Schulof RS, Lloyd MJ, Ueno WM, et al: Phase II trial of thymosin fraction 5 in advanced renal cancer. J Biol Response Mod 3:151–159, 1984.

91. Silverman LM, Chapman JF, Jones ME, et al: Creatinine kinase BB and other markers of prostatic carcinoma. Prostate 2:109–119, 1981.

92. Skinner DG, deKernion JB, Brower PA, et al: Advanced renal cell carcinoma: treatment with xenogeneic immune ribonucleic acid and appropriate surgical resection. J Urol 115:246–250, 1976.

93. Spina CA, Dorey F, Vescera C, et al: Depression of the generation of cell-mediated cytotoxicity by macrophage-like suppressor cells in bladder carcinoma patients. Cancer Res 41:4324–4330, 1981.

94. Steele G Jr, Wang BS, Richie JP, et al: Results of xenogeneic I-RNA therapy in patients with metastatic renal cell carcinoma. Cancer 47:1286–1288, 1982.

95. Teodorczyk-Injayan J, Jewett MA, Burke CA, Ostrand-Rosenberg S: Detection of the circulating antibodies to teratocarcinoma defined antigens in patients with testicular tumours. Clin Exp Immunol 40:438–444, 1980.

96. Thorpe SJ, Abel P, Slavin G, Feizi T: Blood group antigens in the normal and neoplastic bladder epithelium. J Clin Pathol 36:873–882, 1983.

97. Troye M, Hansson Y, Paulie S, et al: Lymphocyte-mediated lysis of tumor cells in vitro (ADCC), induced by serum antibodies from patients with urinary bladder carcinoma or from controls. Int J Cancer 25:45–51, 1980.

98. Tykkä H, Hjelt L, Oravisto KJ, et al: Disappearance of lung metastases during immunotherapy in five patients suffering from renal carcinoma. Scand J Respir Dis [Suppl] 89:123–134, 1974.

99. Ueda R, Ogata S, Morrissey DM, et al: Cell surface antigens of human renal cancer defined by mouse monoclonal antibodies: identification of tissue-specific kidney glycoproteins. Proc Natl Acad Sci USA 78:5122–5126, 1981.

100. Vallancien G, Rouger PH, LeClerc JP, Kuss R: Immunofluorescence study of the distribution of A, B, and H cell surface antigens in bladder tumors. J Urol 130:67–70, 1983.

101. Walker PD, Karnik S, deKernion JB, Pramberg JC: Cell surface blood group antigens in prostatic carcinoma. Am J Clin Pathol 81:503–506, 1984.

102. Ware JL, Paulson DF, Parks SF, Webb KS: Production of monoclonal antibody alpha Pro 3 recognizing a human prostatic carcinoma antigen. Cancer Res 42:1215–1222, 1982.

103. Wiley EL, Mendelsohn G, Droller MJ, Eggleston JC: Immunoperoxidase detection of carcinoembryonic antigen and blood group substances in papillary transitional cell carcinoma of the bladder. J Urol 128:276–280, 1982.

104. Wolf RM, Coice LS, Melamed MR, et al: Flow cytometric monitoring of adjuvant intravesical BCG therapy of superficial bladder cancer. Proc Am Soc Clin Oncol 2:C-548, 1983.

105. Wright GL, Starling JJ, Beckett ML, et al: Immunoperoxidase staining of prostate adenocarcinoma tissue sections with monoclonal antibodies to prostate tumor-associated antigens. Fed Proc 42:399, 1983.

106. Young DA, Prout GR, Lin CW: Production and characterization of a mouse monoclonal antibody to a human bladder tumor cell surface antigen. Proc Am Assoc for Cancer Res 25:255, 1984.

TERRY W. HENSLE, M.D.
JEFFREY ASKANAZI, M.D.

Nutritional Support of The Urologic Patient

There have been in the past, and continue to be, a number of misconceptions with regard to nutrition and cancer. Miraculous cures of different tumors on a nutritional basis are regrettably rare but remain a very salable item for the lay press. The Food and Drug Administration adds to this sensationalism with various bans and injunctions against certain dietary items on the basis of their oncogenic effect. It is well recognized that there are a number of disease states, including arteriosclerosis, hypertension, diabetes, and degenerative diseases, that have a clearly definable interaction with nutrition. There are also a number of tumors that are clearly nutritionally related. As far as bladder cancer is concerned, however, the data to support or refute a nutritional role in its development or resolution are nonexistent. Saccharin when administered in concentrations of greater than 5% of the normal rat diet for two generations, has been shown to cause bladder cancer in rats in a number of studies.[12] Epidemiologic studies in humans, however, have shown that saccharin does not pose a major cancer risk.[2] Cyclamate itself has not been demonstrated to be carcinogenic; however, it does give rise to a metabolite, cyclohexylamine, which can cause testicular atrophy in rats.[13] Zylytol, a newer compound introduced as a sweetener, has been reported in unpublished material to give rise to bladder cancer in mice and adrenal tumors in rats when given in very high concentrations in single-generation studies. Even though specifics of drug action and impurity data have not been worked out, it would appear that this compound is not a major cause of human bladder cancer.

What is clear, however, is the fact that protein-calorie malnutrition is the single most common secondary diagnosis that we find in patients with major urologic cancers, especially bladder cancer. The malnutrition probably has little to do with the pathophysiology of the tumor and is more realistically related to the patient's altered oral intake of nutrients. When first seen, many bladder cancer patients have already begun to lose weight because of the tumor itself, anxiety over their symptoms, or diminished oral intake secondary to the pain of their tumors. Not infrequently, at some point during the course of their treatment, malnutrition will become a problem. Treatment modalities such as chemotherapy, radiotherapy, immunotherapy, and surgery generally result in tissue injury and the consequent need for tissue repair. In this setting, then, nutrition becomes a realistic problem for the physician dealing with the bladder cancer patient.

CANCER CACHEXIA

Cachexia in the cancer patient is not a new concept—it has been recognized for centuries. The etiology of this cachexia is not straightforward, however, and would

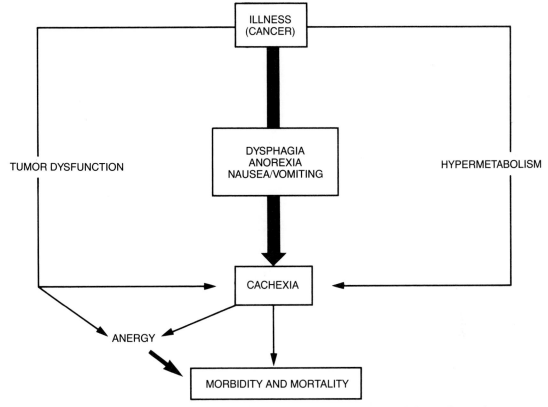

Figure 39–1. The etiology of cancer cachexia and its relationship to morbidity and mortality.

now appear to be, at least in part, multifactorial (Fig. 39–1).

Tumor Dysfunction

There is some evidence to suggest that growing tumors preferentially consume glucose in their glycolytic cycles and act as energy traps.[15] Furthermore, the amount of energy produced by the anaerobic cycle of tumor metabolism is very low (8 moles of ATP per mole of glucose metabolized), as compared with the energy produced by normal host metabolism via the Krebs cycle (36 moles of ATP per mole of glucose metabolized). Amino acid metabolism in tumors is also abnormal in that, once incorporated into most cancer cells, amino acids are no longer available for recycling into the protein pool of the host. Therefore, although gluconeogenesis takes place within cancer cells, the nitrogen released by this process is only available for the production of tumor protein.

Hypermetabolism

Although basal energy expenditure (BEE) is not elevated in most bladder cancer patients, there has been some suggestion that weight loss is correlated with high Cori cycle activity.[17] This increase in energy expenditure, however, is but a small fraction of the total energy expenditure of the host and is therefore of little significance.

Dysphagia, Anorexia, Nausea, and Vomiting

Obviously, this is the area of primary importance in the etiology of cancer cachexia. There is not only a relative but an absolute dysphagia in patients with cancers of all kinds.[21] It has been proposed that peptides, oligonucleotides, and other small metabolites produced by the cancer are responsible for the genesis of this anorexia. They produce the anorexia through a peripheral effect on neuroendocrine cells and neuroreceptors, as well as through a direct effect on the hypothalamus and other central nervous system responder cells.[30] The capacity for cancer patients to increase intake on the basis of nutritional need seems to be impaired, and most evidence now points to the lack of nutrient intake as the primary origin of cancer cachexia.

Tumors in general require energy substrate in order to grow. If host intake meets tumor demands as well as the normal metabolic demands of the host, then weight is maintained. As the tumor increases in size and bulk, however, nutritive demands become greater, and host intake usually becomes less. The result may be extreme weight loss and severe malnutrition.

NUTRITIONAL ASSESSMENT

Once we accept the concept of protein-calorie malnutrition in the cancer patient, we can then identify a definite interplay between nutritional status and disease. Altered host metabolism is associated with cancer in general, and the side effects of oncologic therapy simply compound the problem of impending protein-calorie malnutrition. In turn, this malnutrition can produce a vicious circle by interfering with response to oncologic therapy and enhancing morbidity. It therefore becomes essential for the clinician to establish accurately the nature and extent of the individual patient's nutritional needs in order to formulate a reasonable plan of nutritional support.

Nutritional assessment should be an integral part of the evaluation of all hospitalized cancer patients, particularly those scheduled for some form of antineoplastic therapy.[6] It has been clearly shown that such surveillance can minimize the risk of elective or semielective surgical procedures and should become a part of routine preoperative evaluation.[14] Nutritional assessment should consist basically of the measurement of body protein stores, fat stores, and metabolic rate. The specific method for each of these has been well described.

Skeletal Muscle Protein

A simple and accurate method of assessing the skeletal muscle compartment is to measure the mid-arm muscle circumference and compare this value with known standards for age and sex (Fig. 39–2). Estimation of creatinine height index (CHI) also indicates the quantity of muscle stores and is a sensitive measure of protein depletion in cachectic and marasmic states.[4] In obese or edematous patients, height/weight index may not provide an accurate estimate of the nutritional status and, therefore, has limited application in nutritional assessment.

Visceral Protein

In stress conditions, loss of secretory or visceral protein occurs rapidly. Estimation of serum albumin and transfer in iron-binding protein levels indicate the extent of depletion of this vital tissue compartment. The cellular immune system also reflects important visceral function. Measurements of the total lymphocyte count, together with delayed cutaneous hypersensitivity reaction to recall skin test antigens (SK-SD, mumps, Candida), are particularly useful indicators of the visceral protein compartment.[4]

Fat Stores

The major energy store in the body is fat, and fat mass can be measured adequately by triceps skinfold (Fig. 39–2).[6] This is not as accurate as weighing patients under water; however, it is usually more readily accepted by the patients and much easier to carry out. Given the fact that each pound of fat contains 3500 cal, only a severe loss (<60% of standard) represents significant depletion of stored energy.

Extent of Hypermetabolism

It is interesting to note in the patient undergoing radical cystectomy that the degree of hypermetabolism, as measured by urinary nitrogen loss, places the patient in a category of metabolic injury that is the same as for patients with multiple long bone fractures and just below the category for patients with severe sepsis and major body burns.[16] Unless nutritional support is provided, this can lead to extensive cumulative protein loss (Fig. 39–3). The relationship between urea nitrogen excretion and metabolic rate is a result of the obligatory oxidation of body cell mass that occurs with stress or starvation. Thus, energy expenditure and extent of

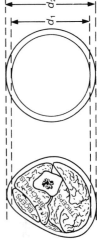

MEASUREMENT OF TRICEPS SKINFOLD WITH HARPENDEN CALIPERS

ASSESSING MIDPOINT OF UPPER ARM (HALFWAY BETWEEN THE ACROMIAL PROCESS OF THE SCAPULA AND THE OLECRANON PROCESS OF THE ULNA)

MEASUREMENT OF MIDDLE UPPER ARM CIRCUMFERENCE

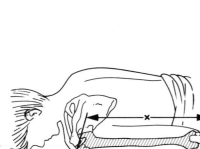

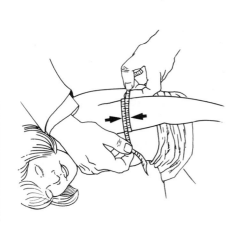

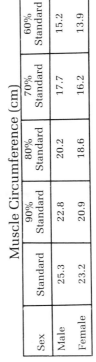

CALCULATION OF MIDDLE UPPER ARM MUSCLE CIRCUMFERENCE

MUSCLE CIRCUMFERENCE, ADULTS, SEXES SEPARATE

Muscle Circumference (cm)

Sex	Standard	90% Standard	80% Standard	70% Standard	60% Standard
Male	25.3	22.8	20.2	17.7	15.2
Female	23.2	20.9	18.6	16.2	13.9

ARM CIRCUMFERENCE, ADULTS, SEXES SEPARATE

Arm Circumference (cm)

Sex	Standard	90% Standard	80% Standard	70% Standard	60% Standard
Male	29.3	26.3	23.4	20.5	17.6
Female	28.5	25.7	22.8	20.0	17.1

TRICEPS SKINFOLD, ADULTS, SEXES SEPARATE

Triceps Skinfold (mm)

Sex	Standard	90% Standard	80% Standard	70% Standard	60% Standard
Male	12.5	11.3	10.0	8.8	7.5
Female	16.5	14.9	13.2	11.6	9.9

Figure 39-2. Method of assessing muscle compartment.

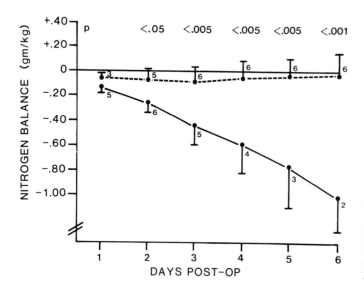

Figure 39–3. Cumulative nitrogen balance in patients receiving postoperative total parenteral nutrition (TPN, dashed line) or 5% dextrose in water (D5W, solid line). Note the marked difference after one week and the significant loss of nitrogen in the group receiving D5W.

hypermetabolism (percentage above normal) can be predicted from simple clinical determination of urea nitrogen in a 24-hour urine collection.

MODES OF THERAPY*

Various techniques are available to the clinician treating a malnourished patient, and several points must be considered in formulating a nutritional support plan. These include the type and extent of malnutrition, the extent of hypermetabolism, the presence or absence of sepsis, the protein and calorie requirements of the patient, the goal of nutritional therapy, the status of gastrointestinal function, the appetite of the patient, the route of delivery, and the presence of specific organ dysfunctions such as renal failure that necessitate restrictions in the volume or the nutrients delivered.

Enteral Hyperalimentation

The enteral route is preferred for nutritional support of all patients in whom the gastrointestinal tract is functional. We now have many commercially prepared liquid diets and formulas for adult and pediatric

*This section on modes of therapy is reproduced from Hensle TW: Nutritional support of the urologic patient. Urol Clin North Am 10:109–118, 1983, with permission.

use that provide aproximately 1 kcal/ml in their recommended concentrations. The particular carbohydrate, fat, and protein contents of these diets differ widely, and often it is necessary to have several preparations available to meet particular needs. Recent advances in the use of feeding modules, such as pure carbohydrate, fat, or protein, may eventually allow the physician more flexibility to meet particular needs without necessitating a large inventory of commercial formulations.

Generally, defined-formula diets are categorized as clear liquid, minimum residue, or lactose-free formulas. Their protein content ranges from 8 to 16% of total calories, and they contain 50 to 90% of their total calories as carbohydrate. They are hyperosmolar (450 to 800 mOsm) and should be started in dilute form by slow continuous drip. If given orally, they should be taken in sips throughout the day to minimize the effects of the hyperosmolarity. Obviously, patients who have glucose intolerance or sensitivity to hyperosmolar loads require especially close monitoring. When these formulas are given in the volumes needed to meet caloric requirements, the Recommended Dietary Allowances (RDAs) for vitamins and minerals are met or exceeded. Therefore, these formulas are nutritionally complete and provide approximately 1 calorie/ml. They require little digestion. Some may be given either orally or by tube, but formulas containing hydrolyzed protein or crystalline amino acids should be given only by tube because of their objectionable taste.

Meal-replacement formulas are low in residue, with approximately 30% of their calories as fat and 12 to 16% as protein. They have various amounts of lactose, and some are milk-based; others are lactose-free. The vitamin and mineral contents also differ, but in calorically adequate volumes all meet or exceed the RDAs for these nutrients. The nutrient sources are more complex than are those in the defined-formula diets, and thus intact digestive and absorptive capacity is required. Meal replacements are nutritionally complete in calorically adequate volumes, provide 1 calorie/ml, and may be given orally or by tube. Added flavorings help make some of the formulas more palatable. The formulas have osmolalities of 300 to 450 mOsm, and patients often tolerate them better if they are given at half-strength the first day.

As the name indicates, supplements are designed to be used in conjunction with food or a dietary formula to increase the intake of one or more nutrients. Some, for example, are concentrated sources of a single nutrient, such as protein, fat, or carbohydrate. They are not nutritionally complete formulations and should not be used as the sole source of nutrients. Their vitamin and mineral contents differ, as do their amounts of residue. When they are combined with oral or formula diets, the resulting changes in caloric amounts and distribution and changes in osmolality should be remembered.

The nausea, vomiting, and diarrhea that limited the acceptability and use of enteral preparations in the past may largely be obviated by the use of the more sophisticated methods of enteral feeding. Most of the commercial products must be given by continuous drip infusion or pump, and increasing the concentration and rate in small steps largely prevents gastrointestinal intolerance

(Table 39–1). Also, the hardware has been improved by the introduction of small Silastic mercury-tipped feeding tubes that have a high degree of patient acceptance.

The recent advent of needle catheter jejunostomy and postoperative jejunal feeding has added another very effective method of delivery of enteral hyperalimentation to our armamentarium. The indications, surgical technique, and complications of this procedure have been well described,[7] and it appears to be applicable to many urologic patients especially those who face postoperative irradiation or chemotherapy. Jejunal feedings in the early postoperative period help to maintain a positive nitrogen balance, prevent significant weight loss, and maintain the fluid and electrolyte balance, which facilitate early discontinuation of intravenous therapy. We have found the method to be safe, and it has often eliminated the need for total parenteral nutrition.

Despite the success of enteral hyperalimentation in the support of many cancer patients, patients with chronic renal failure, and some geriatric patients, unfortunately, the delivery of adequate nutrients via the enteral route is not always rapid and efficient enough to restore the severely depleted patient. Furthermore, malnutrition itself can cause changes in the gastrointestinal tract, such as reduction in the height of the mucosal brush border and changes in the morphology of the columnar cells to more cuboidal forms, that lead to malabsorption. Also, gastrointestinal motility is markedly reduced, which can lead to overgrowth of anaerobic bacteria and impairment of absorption of carbohydrate, fat, and protein. These changes are all reversible if nutrition improves, but this often is a slow process. A more aggressive approach to nutritional restoration is often warranted in the depleted patient, because of either time constraints or the extent of malnutrition.

Table 39–1. DILUTION SCHEDULE FOR TUBE FEEDING OF ELEMENTAL DIETS

Day	Volume Added to One Packet	Calories/ml	Rate ml/hr	ml/day	Calories/Day
1	600	0.5	50	1200	600
2	450	0.75	50	1200	900
3	450	0.75	75	1800	1200
4	300	1.0	75	1800	1800
5	300	1.0	100	2400	2400

Central Intravenous Hyperalimentation

The development of intravenous hyperalimentation by Dudrick and associates in 1968[10] has proved to be one of the most significant recent advances in the care of critically ill patients. The delivery of 25% dextrose and 4.25% amino acids mixed with vitamins and micronutrients delivered into the central venous system has been widely accepted.

Standard intravenous hyperalimentation solutions for use in nutritionally depleted geriatric and cancer patients contain approximately 1000 calories and 6 gm of nitrogen per liter and exert 2000 mOsm of pressure at the point of delivery. Because of this hypertonicity, these solutions must be delivered into the central venous system at a carefully controlled rate. The techniques of insertion and maintenance of catheters have been well described.[19]

In the patient with renal failure, hyperalimentation is especially complicated and must be done within strict guidelines. For instance, fluid tolerance must be determined beforehand, particularly during periods of oliguria. Insensible water losses will usually permit infusion of 700 to 800 ml of renal failure hyperalimentation solution per day. Losses via nasogastric tube, fistulae, and the stool will, of course, increase the tolerance for fluid intake. Once the urine output is satisfactory, the rigid volume restrictions can be liberalized, and 1500 and 2000 ml of renal failure hyperalimentation solution can be administered per day, with an optimum calorie-to-protein ratio of between 300:1 and 450:1.

Because of the high caloric density of the solutions used for intravenous hyperalimentation, it is often necessary to include large amounts of regular insulin to maintain the blood sugar in the range of 125 to 150 mg/dl. Insulin is important in promoting the uptake of glucose to meet the energy demands of cells; it also has a marked effect on the uptake of amino acids by muscles and on reducing the breakdown of protein. High circulating insulin levels also promote the uptake of potassium, phosphate, and magnesium by the regenerating cell mass.

When dealing with the patient in acute renal failure it is important not to substitute the administration of renal failure hyperalimentation solution for dialysis, because, al-though the two therapies may potentiate each other, neither can be substituted for the other. Administration of the solution tends to increase the intravascular volume and the blood flow. Dialysis removes products created by the breakdown of tissue and can inhibit the anabolism of protein and also permits the intake of more protein and calories through its capacity to control fluid, electrolyte, and serum urea nitrogen concentrations. The combination of the administration of renal failure hyperalimentation solution and dialysis thus leads to an optimal positive nitrogen balance and maximum protein synthesis. The early and vigorous use of hypertonic dextrose, together with provision of protein with high biologic value, represents a valuable ancillary treatment of acute renal failure.

Complications. The complications of intravenous hyperalimentation can be divided into three groups: technical, septic, and metabolic.

Technical complications are associated primarily with the placement of the central venous catheter and include pneumothorax, hydrothorax, brachial plexus injury, subclavian artery injury, venous thrombosis, and air embolism. *The frequency of technical complications is directly related to the extent of experience of the person inserting the catheter.*

Septic complications of intravenous hyperalimentation are attributable either to the catheter or to the solution itself. Although sepsis rates of 10 to 30% were common in the past, most medical centers that utilize hyperalimentation teams and a controlled approach to the manufacture and delivery of solutions consistently report sepsis rates of only 2 to 3%.[25] Routine procedures have been outlined for the evaluation and treatment of septic episodes in the patient receiving intravenous hyperalimentation.

Numerous metabolic complications can be associated with intravenous hyperalimentation. The most common are alterations in the metabolism of glucose that result in various degrees of hyperglycemia or hypoglycemia. The most dangerous result is hyperosmolar nonketotic coma, which is caused by unchecked hyperglycemia, glucosuria, and massive osmotic diuresis. The resultant cerebral dehydration often leads to coma and sometimes to death. Although this problem was once prominent, it has become far less common because of strict monitoring of the delivery of the intravenous hyperalimentation and close supervision of the metabolic status of the patient.

Other metabolic problems, such as hyperphosphatemia, hypercalcemia, hypocalcemia, and hypomagnesemia, tend to reflect simply the amount of these substances delivered and are not life-threatening. These conditions are easily reversible.

Deficiencies in essential fatty acids and trace metals have been associated with long-term use of intravenous hyperalimentation. Although these conditions can be worrisome and difficult to diagnose, they are easily remedied. In the case of a deficiency of essential fatty acids, incorporation of a commercial fat source as part of the daily calorie supply will more than remedy the problem. Similarly, the routine addition of solutions of trace metals to standard preparations used for intravenous hyperalimentation will eliminate deficiencies.

Another metabolic abnormality linked to long-term administration of intravenous hyperalimentation is an alteration in liver enzymes, which is caused largely by the delivery of calories in excess of the patient's needs. Such excess calories probably stimulate increased release of insulin and lead to hepatic lipogenesis and enzyme derangements. Various regimens of cyclic hyperalimentation have been proposed as one method of dealing with the problem of hepatic lipogenesis;[20] however, simple readjustment of the calorie-to-nitrogen ratio of the solution often will eliminate the problem or at least minimize it.

Peripheral Intravenous Hyperalimentation

The provision via peripheral veins of adequate calories and protein to support or rebuild the body's cell mass must involve the use of lipid as the principal calorie source, and this use of fat preparations is controversial in the United States. The introduction of fat as a calorie source in the 1950s was marred by the occurrence of severe febrile reactions, jaundice, and defects of coagulation. However, these reactions were specifically attributable to the type of fat used, which was cottonseed-oil emulsion, as found in Lipomul. The present fat source, soybean oil emulsified with egg phospholipid, as found in Intralipid from Cutter Laboratories and Liposyn from Abbott, has none of the untoward effects seen with the earlier substance.

More recently, there has been some controversy about the use of fat as a calorie source in the severely hypermetabolic patient. In burn patients, for example, fat may not be as appropriate as carbohydrate. There is recent evidence, however, to suggest that fat is a very important calorie source of patients with compromised pulmonary function. The advent of safe lipid preparations and the development of a domestic source should help with both the availability and price of fat preparations.

The peripheral system of total parenteral nutrition (TPN) involves administration of 3% amino acids, 5 to 7.5% dextrose, and 10% lipid, a solution that provides approximately 40% of its calories as carbohydrate and the rest as lipid. The advantages of using peripheral intravenous hyperalimentation are obvious: there are far fewer technical and septic complications in comparison with central intravenous hyperalimentation, and the time involved in running the system is much less. However, peripheral intravenous hyperalimentation requires the administration of larger volumes of fluid to deliver the same number of calories as intravenous hyperalimentation, and in patients who are critically ill or elderly, this may be a limiting factor. With the current price of fat preparations, there is little difference in the cost of peripheral intravenous hyperalimentation and central intravenous hyperalimentation.

Preoperative Nutritional Support

A low serum albumin level (<3.5 g/dl), depressed total lymphocyte count (<1500/mm^3), and negative reactivity to skin test antigens along with a history of recent weight loss are all indicators of nutritional depletion. By using the simple techniques outlined, adequate estimates can be made of the risk of morbidity associated with malnutrition. Given the fact that these tests are simple, quick, and easily obtainable at minimal cost, they should become a standard part of the evaluation of the patient with urologic cancer.

We believe that once moderate or severe nutritional deficits have been identified, nutritional support is mandatory prior to any form of antineoplastic therapy. It has been standard dogma that a period of at least two

Table 39–2. EFFECTS OF NUTRITION
AND BODY COMPOSITION ON
EXTRACELLULAR WATER*

Condition	Total Amount of Water (%)		
	Observed	*Predicted*	*Difference*
Injury	55	48	+7
Malnutrition	59	48	+11

*Expansion of the extracellular fluid compartment area seen both in injury and in malnourished surgical patients.

to three weeks is necessary for an objective response to nutritional therapy. However, the impact of perioperative nutritional support on mortality and morbidity is unclear,[9, 18] and the optimal duration of nutritional support and criteria for the use of perioperative TPN remain undefined.[22, 23] The cost and morbidity associated with TPN itself require that the minimum period of preoperative nutritional support be utilized. Extended periods of nutritional support that improve laboratory values but do not affect overall morbidity are contraindicated.

We have tried to look at the question of whether the application of parenteral nutrition preoperatively will reduce mortality and morbidity. We have shown that an expanded extracellular fluid compartment occurs in both injury and in malnourished surgical patients (Table 39–2). This process is due in part to malnutrition and in part to the patient's disease. We believe that this alteration in body composition is the primary factor in the increased morbidity and mortality seen in the malnourished patient and that it is associated with low serum albumin levels due to a dilutional effect.[27]

Table 39–3. CHANGES IN BODY WEIGHT AND
SERUM ALBUMIN DURING TPN*

	Pre-TPN	Preoperative	Statistical Significance
	Weight (LBS)		
Group I	127	124	0.001
Group II	119	121	0.025
	Albumin (gm %)		
Group I	3.28	3.46	0.001
Group II	3.14	3.00	0.01

*Group I represents those patients who contract the ECF, lose weight, and increase serum albumin levels during one week of preoperative TPN. Group II represents those patients who expand the ECF, gain weight, and lower serum albumin levels in response to one week of preoperative TPN.

The uncomplicated patient with an expanded extracellular fluid space (ECF, which characteristically develops during progressive malnutrition) contracts the ECF in response to nutritional support (Table 39–3, Group I). This is evidenced by a loss of weight and a rise in serum albumin during the first weeks of nutritional support.[27] This diuresis is not only an indication of a normalization in body composition but has been associated with improvement in immune function.[11, 26] Patients who undergo this early diuresis have been shown to have a very low postoperative morbidity and mortality, with a complication rate of 4.3%, whereas patients who fail to show diuresis during a week of preoperative TPN (Table 39–3, Group II) derive virtually no benefit from this nutritional support with regard to postoperative complications.[28] This means that these patients do not experience a normalization of body composition or an improvement in immune function. This is reflected in their postoperative complication rate of 45%, which is similar to that of malnourished patients receiving no preoperative support, who have been shown to have postoperative complication rates of 40 to 80%.[8, 24]

We have further examined, with regard to the efficacy of prolonged preoperative nutritional support, this subset of malnourished patients who do not initially achieve their normal body composition. Prior to the administration of TPN, the standard nutritional measurements are not adequate to distinguish those patients who will respond to one week of TPN from those patients who will not. In another group of operative candidates, those who did not respond initially with normalization of body composition (i.e., those who showed weight loss and a rise in serum albumin) were then treated with an extended period of preoperative TPN. After three to six weeks of nutritional support, normalization of body composition was achieved (Table 39–4) and the postoperative complication rate in these patients was only 12.5% (Table 39–5). This is markedly reduced from the complication rate of 45% in the group of patients who had a similar initial response pattern but were operated on after only one week of preoperative TPN.

Clearly, a reduction in postoperative morbidity can be achieved in the malnourished patient with preoperative nutritional sup-

Table 39–4. CHANGES IN NUTRITIONAL STATUS DURING PREOPERATIVE TPN*

	Group I†	Group IIA†	Group IIB
Number of patients	23	20	16
Body weight (lb)	126.3 ± 5.2	118.2 ± 6.4	117.6 ± 5.2
Pre/post one week TPN	123.2 ± 5.2*	120.1 ± 6.4§	119.8 ± 5.4‡
			(121.9 ± 5.8)‖
Serum albumin (gm %)	3.19 ± 0.10	3.14 ± 0.12	3.11 ± 0.6
Pre/post one week TPN	3.44 ± 0.11‡	3.00 ± 0.13§	2.90 ± 0.16§
			(3.27 ± 0.10)‖**
Days of preoperative TPN	7.3 ± 0.8	6.8 ± 0.8	33.4 ± 3.2
Time in operating room (hr)	3.6 ± 0.4	4.4 ± 0.7	3.0 ± 0.4

*Group I represents those patients who respond to one week of preoperative TPN. Group IIA represents those patients who did not respond to one week of preoperative TPN. Group IIB represents those patients who did not respond initially but were treated with TPN until a response was seen.

†Sixteen patients in each group were previously reported upon (Starker PM, et al.: Ann Surg 198:720–724, 1983).

‡$p < 0.001$ (comparing pre-TPN values with those obtained ofter one week of TPN).

§$p < 0.01$ (comparing pre-TPN values with those obtained after one week of TPN).

‖Numbers in parentheses represent the values prior to operation but following the entire period of nutritional support.

**$p < 0.01$ (comparing values after one week of TPN with those obtained after three to six weeks of TPN).

port. These patients develop nutrition-related complications in part because of abnormalities in body composition and immune function. Such abnormalities must be at least partially reversed before these patients are subjected to operation if a decrease in postoperative complications is to be achieved. Therefore, the duration of preoperative support must be individualized. Some patients require as little as one week of preoperative TPN in order to improve their postoperative course, whereas others benefit only after a prolonged course of preoperative support.

Changes in body weight and serum albumin levels during the period of preoperative nutritional support provide an important determinant for the timing of operations. This represents a normalization of body fluid compartments. Patients who lose weight and show a rise in serum albumin levels during one week of preoperative TPN are at a reduced risk for postoperative complications. In our experience, a rise in albumin levels of 0.5 gm/dl should be observed before an elective operation is considered. This will often be accompanied by a decrease of two to three pounds in body weight during the first weeks, indicating a contraction of the extracellular fluid compartment. A weight gain, with no change or a decrease in already depressed serum albumin levels during the first week of preoperative TPN, is an indication that the abnormalities in body composition and immune function characteristic of malnutrition persist. In prolonged preoperative TPN, the weight gain presumably reflects an increase in body cell mass with a relative decrease in ECF, accompanied by a rise in serum albumin levels. Patients who respond to early nutritional support with decreased serum albumin levels and increased weight remain at high risk for postoperative complications and should be

Table 39–5. POSTOPERATIVE COMPLICATIONS*

Complications	Group I	Group IIA	Group IIB
Mechanical			
Prolonged ventilatory support	0	4	0
Fistula	0	0	1
Wound dehiscence	0	1	0
Anastomotic leak	0	1	0
Total mechanical complications	0	6	1
Infections			
Sepsis	0	2	0
Pneumonia	1	3	0
Wound infection	0	3	1
Abscess	0	1	0
Total infectious complications	1	9	1
Death (nutritionally related)	0	2	0
Total complications	1	17	2
Total number of patients developing complications	1†	9	2‡
Percentage of patients developing complications	4.3	45	12.5

*Groups are the same as those in Table 39–4.

†$p < 0.01$ (Group I/Group IIA).

‡$p < 0.05$ (Group IIB/Group IIA).

considered candidates for prolonged preoperative nutritional support.

POSTOPERATIVE NUTRITIONAL SUPPORT

As we have shown, preoperative TPN in patients with malnutrition, particularly when this is associated with a low level of albumin, can be a useful therapeutic intervention. Mullen and associates have demonstrated a reduction in major complications with preoperative parenteral nutrition in patients with gastrointestinal carcinoma.[23] These investigators used the prognostic nutritional index (PNI) to identify malnourished patients at risk for postoperative complications and demonstrated a reduction in operative mortality and morbidity with preoperative nutritional support. We have demonstrated that one week of preoperative nutritional support resulted in a reduction in complication rates when a rise in serum albumin occurred. In patients who did not show a clear rise in albumin levels after one week of nutritional support, a three to five

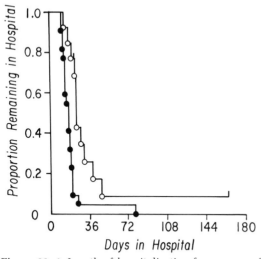

Figure 39–4. Length of hospitalization for a group of well-nourished patients undergoing radical cystectomy for bladder cancer. Solid circles represent those patients who received total parenteral nutrition (TPN) after the procedure (22 patients, 0 died), and the open circles denote patients who received postoperative 5% dextrose in water (D5W, 13 patients, 2 died). A tick mark indicates the last follow-up. The data demonstrate a markedly shorter length of hospital stay for patients receiving postoperative TPN (median stay, 17 days) than for those given D5W (median stay, 24 days).

week period of TPN was necessary to reduce complication rates.[29]

The efficacy of parenteral nutrition in the postoperative period is less well established. This is particularly true in previously well-nourished patients undergoing elective surgery in whom a return to oral intake is expected within five to seven days. Abel and associates[1] studied the effect of immediate postoperative parenteral hyperalimentation and found no improvement of the course of malnourished patients undergoing cardiac surgery. However, the nutritional regimen that they used supplied a daily caloric intake of only 1000 to 1400 kcal/day. Holter and Fischer[18] demonstrated that a combined pre- (three-day) and postoperative (10-day) period of nutritional support reduced complication rates in malnourished patients with gastrointestinal carcinoma and weight loss.

Recently, however, we have shown that immediate postoperative parenteral nutrition reduced hospitalization time in a group of bladder cancer patients undergoing radical cystectomy and diversion.[3] This occurred in patients with no significant degree of preoperative malnutrition. There was a markedly shorter length of hospitalization for patients receiving TPN in the postoperative period (median stay, 17 days) as compared with the stay for those receiving 5% dextrose (median stay, 24 days) (Fig. 39–4). This difference was found to be highly significant ($p < 0.002$). It should be noted that this investigation was randomized but not double-blind, and it was a retrospective review of data not analyzed during the actual performance of a study aimed at instituting immediate postoperative parenteral nutrition and examining the metabolic effects of nutrients in the stress state. We did not originally intend to examine duration of hospitalization. Furthermore, after the period of randomized nutritional therapy and metabolic measurements, the patients were transferred out of the Surgical Metabolism Unit to routine ward care; we did not follow the course of the patients beyond this point. The data presented here were obtained by retrospective review of hospital charts. So far as we could determine, the reduction in hospitalization time in the group that received early aggressive nutritional therapy was not due to individual, clearly identifiable factors (e.g., improved wound healing). Rather, it seemed that the group receiving dextrose had a longer convalescence and a decreased rate of return to normal activity. Further studies are necessary to document the application of this finding to patients undergoing other major surgical procedures. The cost saving achieved by shorter hospitalization following elective surgery warrants that the effect of nutrient support following injury be seriously examined, particularly as the age of the population increases. However, it seems advisable that the routine use of 5% dextrose solution for postoperative nutrition should be re-evaluated.

THE TERMINAL PATIENT

Occasionally, TPN has been started only to find that the patient has a metastatic malignant process for which there is no remaining treatment. In such a situation, we attempt to nourish the patient by enteral means and discontinue TPN. Forced enteral nutritional replenishment of terminal cancer patients as well as the administration of TPN have been reported to improve the quality of remaining life. Despite this we continue to recommend that TPN not be used for patients who have received all possible modalities of oncologic therapy and are dying of the combined effects of malnutrition and progressive cancer growth. The nutritional states of these patients should be maintained as adequately as possible, utilizing all available enteral diets, but with the current state of the art, TPN is not often indicated. Terminal patients may feel somewhat better during TPN infusion, but this effect ceases immediately upon discontinuing TPN. Prolongation of pain for the patient and anguish for the family do not seem justified as indications for the use of TPN in terminal cancer patients.

References

1. Abel RM, Fischer JE, Buckley MJ, et al: Malnutrition in cardiac surgical patients. Results of a prospective, randomized evaluation of early postoperative parenteral nutrition. Arch Surg 111:45–50, 1976.
2. Armstrong B, Doll R: Bladder cancer mortality in diabetics in relation to saccharin consumption and smoking habits. Br J Prev Soc Med 29:73–81, 1975.
3. Askanazi J, Hensle TW, Starker PM, et al: Effect of immediate postoperative nutritional support on length of hospitalization. Ann Surg 23:236–239, 1986.
4. Bistrian BR, Blackburn GL, Sherman M, et al: Therapeutic index of nutritional depletion in hospitalized patients. Surg Gynecol Obstet 141:512–516, 1975.
5. Blackburn GL: Nitrogen conservation using fat as a nonprotein calorie source. In Proceedings AMA Symposium on Fat Emulsion in Parenteral Nutrition. Chicago, 1975.
6. Blackburn GL, Bistrian BR, Maini BS, et al: Nutritional and metabolic assessment of the hospitalized patient. JPEN 1:11–22, 1977.
7. Bongiorno FP: The needle catheter jejunostomy: present indications, future use. Surg Rounds 5:52, 1982.
8. Buzby GP, Mullen JL, Matthews DC, et al: Prognostic nutritional index in gastrointestinal surgery. Am J Surg 139:160–167, 1980.
9. Copeland EM III, Daly JM, Ota OM, Dudrick SJ: Nutrition, cancer, and intravenous hyperalimentation. Cancer 43(Suppl 5):2108–2116, 1979.
10. Dudrick SJ, Wilmore DW, Vars HM, et al: Long-term parenteral nutrition with growth development and positive nitrogen balance. Surgery 64:135, 1968.
11. Forse RA, Christou N, Meakins JL, et al: Reliability of skin testing as a measure of nutritional state. Arch Surg 116:1284–1288, 1981.
12. Friedman L, Richardson HL, Richardson ME, et al: Toxic response of rats to cyclamates in chow and semisynthetic diets. JNCI 49:751–764, 1972.
13. Gaunt IF, Sharratt M, Grasso P, et al: Short-term toxicity of cyclohexylamine hydrochloride in the rat. Food Cosmet Toxicol 12:609–624, 1974.
14. Gibbons GW, Blackburn GL, Harken DE, et al: Pre- and postoperative hyperalimentation in the treatment of cardiac cachexia. J Surg Res 20:439–444, 1976.
15. Gold J: Proposed treatment of cancer by inhibition of gluconeogenesis. Oncology 22:185–207, 1968.
16. Hensle TW, et al: Metabolic changes associated with radical cystectomy. J Urol 134:1032–1036, 1985.
17. Holroyde CP, Gabuzda TG, Putnam RC, et al: Altered glucose metabolism in metastatic carcinoma. Cancer Res 35:3710–3714, 1975.
18. Holter AR, Fischer JE: The effects of perioperative hyperalimentation on complications in patients with carcinoma and weight loss. J Surg Res 23:31–34, 1977.
19. Kaminski MV, Burke WA, Blackburn GL: Intravenous hyperalimentation. In Modern Hospital Practice. USV Laboratory Monograph, Tuckahoe, New York, USV Pharmaceutical Corp., 1977.
20. Maini B, Blackburn GL, Bistrian BR, et al: Cyclic hyperalimentation: an optimal technique for preservation of visceral protein. J Surg Res 20:515, 1976.
21. Mider G: Some aspects of nitrogen and energy metabolism in cancerous subjects: a review. Cancer Res 11:821–829, 1951.
22. Mullen JL: Consequences of malnutrition in the surgical patient. Surg Clin North Am 61:465–487, 1981.
23. Mullen JL, Buzby GP, Matthews DC, et al: Reduction of operative morbidity and mortality by combined preoperative and postoperative nutritional support. Ann Surg 192:604–613, 1980.
24. Mullen JL, Buzby GP, Waldman MT, et al: Predic-

tion of operative morbidity and mortality by pre-operative nutritional assessment. Surg Forum 30:80–82, 1979.

25. Ryan JA Jr, Abel RM, Abbott WM, et al: Catheter complications in total parenteral nutrition: a prospective study of 200 consecutive patients. N Engl J Med 290:757, 1974.

26. Spanier AH, Pietsch JB, Meakins JL, et al: The relationship between immune competence and nutrition. Surg Forum 27:332–336, 1976.

27 Starker PM, Gump FE, Askanazi J, et al: Serum albumin levels as an index of nutritional support. Surgery 91:194–199, 1982.

28. Starker PM, Lasala PA, Askanazi J, et al: The response to TPN. A form of nutritional assessment. Ann Surg 198:720–724, 1983.

29. Starker PM, LaSala A, Askanazi J, et al: The influence of preoperative TPN on mortality and morbidity. Ann Surg 162:569–574, 1986.

30. Theologides A: Anorexia producing intermediary metabolites. Am J Clin Nutr 29:552–558, 1976.

JOHN F. VILJOEN, M.D.
DURAIYAH THANGATHURAI, M.D.

CHAPTER 40 ⚫

Anesthetic Management in Radical Surgery for Urologic Malignancies

The combined use of aggressive surgical techniques and new chemotherapeutic agents has greatly improved the prognosis of patients with urologic malignances. The operations are complicated and are often performed on patients in poor physical condition. It is essential for the anesthesiologist to understand each step of the surgical procedure so that the appropriate pharmacologic and physiologic adjustment can be made.

PREOPERATIVE ASSESSMENT

Preoperative evaluation should include consideration of the patient's age, physical and emotional state, coexisting disease (with particular emphasis on the cardiovascular and respiratory systems) and drug therapy.

Age. Patients with cancer of the bladder and prostate tend to be from 60 to 85 years of age. Increased morbidity and mortality associated with anesthesia and surgery are found in this age group.

Physical Status. The patient's general physical condition is often compromised by the malignancy and the side effects of chemotherapy. These can result in poor nutrition, weight loss, anemia, and hypoalbuminemia, all of which adversely affect the patient's tolerance to anesthetic agents.

Psychological State. Patients with uro-logic malignancies present two extremes of the emotional spectrum. They may experience either a high level of anxiety due to the fear of dying, which is compounded by apprehension in the face of a major surgical procedure, or they may eagerly anticipate the surgery as their only hope of survival.

Coexistent Cardiovascular Disease. Patients with bladder or prostatic carcinoma are older and often have a history of smoking. A thorough cardiovascular work-up is essential. Atherosclerosis is common, and this condition predisposes to hypertension and ischemic heart disease. These patients often have a history of angina, myocardial infarction, arrhythmias, or episodes of congestive cardiac failure. Although decisions pertaining to preoperative drug therapy and cardiovascular monitoring are the responsibility of the anesthesiologist, a cardiologist's assistance is valuable in interpreting echocardiogram findings, or electrocardiographic responses to stress testing.

Preoperative placement of a Swan-Ganz catheter will facilitate intra- and postoperative management in the patient with a history of severe ischemic heart disease, prior myocardial infarction, cardiac failure, or labile hypertension. Hypertension is particularly common, and efforts should be made to avoid the wide swings of pressure to which these patients are susceptible. Vasodilators and β-blockers should be immedi-

595

ately available to achieve rapid control of any such exacerbations.

A history of stroke or symptoms related to cerebrovascular insufficiency must be viewed seriously, as even well-controlled hypertension may precipitate a cerebrovascular accident. It is unwise to initiate treatment with drugs such as dipyridamole or aspirin, which may cause platelet dysfunction and aggravate intraoperative bleeding.

Respiratory Disease. The incidence of chronic obstructive pulmonary disease (COPD) increases with age. Because of this reduced pulmonary reserve and the fact that many patients with urologic malignancies have a history of excessive smoking, simple pulmonary function tests, such as forced expiratory volume (FEV-1) and blood gas analysis, are performed routinely. This information is particularly helpful in guiding postoperative oxygen therapy. It is futile to attempt to elevate the arterial oxygen tension in a patient whose levels have been low for many years!

In patients with small airway obstruction, response to bronchodilator therapy should be evaluated. An increase of 15% or more in FEV-1 is regarded as encouraging. The following formula is used to quantitate the response:

$$\frac{\text{Post-BD FEV-1} - \text{Pre-BD FEV-1} \times 100}{\text{Pre-BD FEV-1}}$$

Patients treated with bleomycin may develop pulmonary fibrosis with consequent reduction in lung reserve. Measurement of forced vital capacity (FVC) and blood gas analysis should be performed. Testicular and renal cell carcinomas metastasize early to the lungs, so x-rays, tomograms, and CT scans should be carefully examined.

Patients with renal cell malignancies are prone to develop pulmonary embolism, and if this complication is suspected, angiography is important.

Liver and Renal Dysfunction. Although it is unusual for liver function to be affected by metastases, fatty infiltration of the liver may be seen in patients with poor nutritional status who have received chemotherapy. Renal cell carcinoma can extend into the hepatic vein, and venography should be performed to exclude this complication. The presence of ascites does not necessarily indicate a severe liver disorder as it can be an early development when the inferior vena

cava is obstructed. In this situation there is minimal alteration in liver function.

If the malignant growth obstructs urine flow, renal function will be compromised. In all patients with renal cell carcinoma, it is important that the function of the contralateral kidney be assessed. Chemotherapeutic drugs such as cyclophosphamide and cisplatin can cause renal dysfunction. Levels of blood urea nitrogen and creatinine and clearance tests will unmask subclinical involvement; these are performed whenever patients have been treated with these drugs.

Hematologic and Immunologic Functions. Cytotoxic drugs can cause bone marrow suppression, resulting in neutropenia, anemia, and thrombocytopenia. Patients with platelet counts less than 75,000 are at risk from hemorrhage both intra- and postoperatively. Neutropenia will increase susceptibility to bacterial infections.

Nitrous oxide should be avoided whenever cytotoxic drugs have been used. Cancer patients tend to have depressed immune function (both cellular and humoral). All general anesthetic agents compound this effect. Combining "light" general anesthesia with an epidural block will reduce the overall requirement for anesthetic drugs.

Drug Therapy. It has been reported that bleomycin therapy is associated with an increased incidence of postoperative pulmonary problems (manifesting as ARDS). High inspired oxygen concentrations and crystalloid therapy are believed to be contributory factors. Doxorubicin therapy may cause cardiac toxicity, and cisplatin can compromise renal function. Beta-blockers, antihypertensives, and antiarrhythmic agents should be continued up to and including the day of surgery.

MANAGEMENT OF SOME SPECIFIC DISEASE ENTITIES

Renal Cell Carcinoma

Renal cell carcinoma is manifested in various ways, and the surgical approach is modified accordingly. When the malignancy is confined to the kidney, a standard anesthetic technique can be used. When the tumor invades or obstructs the inferior vena cava, the problem becomes far more complicated. If the tumor extends into the right atrium, all the anesthetic techniques associated with cardiac surgery must be considered.

Renal cell carcinoma extending through the inferior vena cava into the right atrium demands immediate surgical intervention, as the tumor can suddenly obstruct the tricuspid valve or embolize to the pulmonary artery. If the atrial thrombus occupies more than 40% of the atrium, cardiopulmonary bypass is advisable. Of importance are the following:

1. Right heart catheterization is potentially hazardous, since there is a danger that part of the tumor can be dislodged and embolize to the pulmonary artery. An echocardiogram is therefore recommended for assessing both the size of the tumor and the mobility of the tricuspid valve. If there is a pulmonary embolus, one may see a dilated right ventricle. A ventilation/perfusion scan of the lungs is used in detecting pulmonary emboli, and although pulmonary angiography is more accurate, it should probably not be performed in patients who have renal cell cancer with intracardiac extension.

2. Because of the obstruction of the inferior vena cava and atrial flow, central venous pressures are high and do not accurately reflect volume status or cardiac function. Nevertheless, we recommend utilizing a CVP catheter inserted via the left internal or external jugular vein. If the latter approach is used, a J-wire will facilitate passage of the catheter, the tip of which should not be advanced farther than the superior vena cava. The use of a Swan-Ganz catheter is hazardous because of the presence of tumor in the right atrium.

3. Hypotension may occur at the time of induction because of inflow obstruction, even though the total blood volume remains adequate.

4. Excessive blood loss should be anticipated. The dilated veins of the abdominal wall, which act as collaterals, are a common source of bleeding. Retroperitoneal dissection exposes large areas of the capillary bed, leading to excessive loss of blood, plasma, and lymphatic fluid. Heparinization (in patients in whom cardiopulmonary bypass is used) interferes with hemostasis and compounds any bleeding problems. Extracorporeal circulation may contribute to abnormal coagulation, particularly when prolonged.

It is difficult to estimate actual blood loss because hemodynamic measurements are distorted by venous obstruction. Replacement volume should include whole blood, fresh frozen plasma, and platelets. As a temporary measure, vasopressors (for example, phenylephrine) can be useful in maintaining adequate perfusion pressures. Cardioplegia is not necessary, since the aorta is not cross-clamped.

5. Renal function must be preserved both during episodes of unexpected hypotension and when the renal artery is clamped. Total ischemic time of the functional kidney should not exceed 30 minutes. The margin of safety can be increased by mild hypothermia, ventilation with 100% oxygen, adequate perfusion pressures, and use of mannitol before the major vessels are clamped.

6. The liver can be affected by extension of thrombus into the hepatic vein, giving rise to symptoms and signs of a Budd-Chiari syndrome. Venography should be performed to exclude hepatic vein involvement. Perioperative monitoring of hepatic function is of great importance, as hepatic circulation may be compromised during surgery.

7. The volume of the epidural space is reduced in patients with inferior vena caval obstruction. Epidural veins are dilated and act as collaterals of venous drainage, accounting for the increased incidence of inadvertent intravenous injection or an unexpectedly high level of block.

8. Despite having normal blood volumes, these patients behave as if they were hypovolemic. A smooth anesthetic induction with minimal fluctuations in hemodynamics is important because compensatory mechanisms are less effective. Hydration with a mixture of colloids (such as 5% albumin) and crystalloid (lactated Ringer's) in a ratio of 1:2 will not only reduce the incidence of hypotension at the time of induction but will maintain adequate perfusion of the liver and functional kidney. The tumor functions as a "safety valve," reducing venous return, so left ventricular failure is uncommon.

9. There is a high risk of pulmonary embolism during mobilization of the tumor. End tidal carbon dioxide monitoring can give an early warning of pulmonary emboli and is routinely employed.

10. If extracorporeal circulation is utilized, aortic and venous cannulae are inserted through a right thoracoabdominal incision. This approach is different from the more commonly used median sternotomy. Venous return to the pump is compromised if the inferior vena cava is obstructed be-

cause venous return from the lower extremities is restricted.

Patients with Testicular Cancer Treated with Bleomycin

Patients treated with bleomycin who undergo radical cancer surgery present a number of problems:

1. There is an increased risk of postoperative pulmonary complications, particularly adult respiratory distress syndrome (ARDS). Contributing factors are thought to include sensitivity to high inspired oxygen concentrations and overaggressive intraoperative fluid replacement. Some recent evidence disputes that ARDS is caused by hyperoxia, but the data are sufficiently compelling to respect this possibility. The use of ear oximetry for continuous monitoring of oxygen saturation helps to avoid unnecessarily high inspired oxygen concentrations. The modified flank position used during surgery is associated with a reduction of functional residual capacity (FRC) and predisposition to microatelectasis. Prophylactic positive end-expiratory pressure will not only increase FRC and prevent atelectasis but also protect against pulmonary congestion due to excessive fluid therapy. Preoperative pulmonary function studies are important, as lung function may be compromised by pulmonary fibrosis associated with bleomycin therapy. Forced vital capacity (FVC) is a reliable index of the extent of fibrosis. Diffusion tests are unreliable and misleading.

It is also thought that an intolerance to excessive intravenous fluid may cause postoperative pulmonary complications. The use of colloid versus crystalloid in the perioperative period is controversial. We have used colloid and crystalloid in a 1:2 ratio without any apparent deleterious effects.

Postoperative pain associated with a thoracoabdominal incision and chest tubes can be severe, interfering with breathing and causing splinting of the diaphragm. The resultant hypoventilation and atelectasis increase the need for a high fractional concentration of oxygen (F_{IO_2}), which we believe should be avoided. Pain should therefore be managed by the judicious use of epidural bupivacaine or narcotics, or both. This regimen will provide pain relief without causing respiratory depression, and we have found a 20 to 40% improvement in lung function as measured by incentive spirometry.

2. There is a risk of bone marrow suppression, increasing the likelihood of infection and septicemia. The use of nitrous oxide is to be avoided in patients who are neutropenic from previous chemotherapy, as prolonged exposure will reduce neutrophil production. Oxygen-enriched air is a satisfactory alternative.

3. Thrombocytopenia leads to increased intra- and postoperative blood loss, particularly during retroperitoneal dissection. Epidural analgesia will not only reduce the need for anesthetic agents but will also produce hypotension, thereby minimizing blood loss. With induced hypotension (i.e., pressures ± 30% below the preoperative level), blood loss is usually less than 700 ml; by comparison, normotensive patients can lose up to 2500 ml. Avoidance of multiple transfusions will also help to reduce postoperative pulmonary complications, hepatitis, and the potential for AIDS.

Since the mechanism of bleomycin-related ARDS remains unclear, we recommend the following: (1) Avoidance of high inspired oxygen concentrations (less than 30%). Ear oximetry or transcutaneous oxygen monitoring are used to ensure adequate oxygenation with the lowest F_{IO_2}. (2) Conservative use of intravenous fluids. Multiple transfusions are avoided because they may be associated with pulmonary insufficiency. (3) Prophylactic use of positive end-expiratory pressure (PEEP of 10 cm water), to reduce lung complications such as atelectasis and pulmonary congestion. (4) Aggressive postoperative pain relief combined with early ambulation. (5) In neutropenic patients, scrupulous attention should be paid to aseptic technique. Drugs associated with neutropenia, such as nitrous oxide, are avoided.

Patients Undergoing Radical Cystectomy and Creation of a Kock Pouch

Patients undergoing radical cystectomy and creation of a continent ileal pouch (Kock) belong to an older age group and are often in a debilitated condition. Anesthetic problems associated with this procedure are: (1) Significant blood loss during the cystectomy and lymph node dissection. (2) Adverse hemodynamic consequences of the hyperextended position. This is aggravated by manipulations in the pelvis, during which procedure the iliac veins are compressed.

This causes a reduction in venous return with a resultant fall in cardiac output and blood pressure. (3) Difficulty in measuring urine output after the ureters have been separated from the bladder. This maneuver is carried out early in the procedure. (4) Maintenance of normal intestinal tone during the creation of the pouch. Hypertonicity of the ileum can lead to technical difficulties.

Intraoperative management can be conveniently divided into two phases; the cystectomy and lymph node dissection, and the creation of the pouch. As has been pointed out, the first phase is often accompanied by significant blood loss, and a technique of deliberate hypotension will reduce the need for blood replacement.

Of note is the increasing awareness of patients and their families of acquired immunodeficiency syndrome (AIDS) and post-transfusion hepatitis. As a result, the anesthesiologist is frequently requested to avoid or minimize administration of blood products. The technique of epidural analgesia combined with light general anesthesia and controlled ventilation has been developed to achieve this goal.

It should be remembered that many of these patients have cerebral arteriosclerosis, and excessive lowering of blood pressure can cause a catastrophic reduction in cerebral perfusion with resultant neurologic deficits. A general guideline is a 30% reduction of the preoperative blood pressure level. An intra-arterial catheter and central venous cannula should be inserted in all these patients, and the use of a pulmonary artery catheter should be considered if severe or unstable cardiovascular disease is present.

Excessive hyperventilation should be avoided, as a combination of hypotension and cerebral vasoconstriction resulting from hypocapnea can cause significant reductions in cerebral blood flow. Use of an end-tidal carbon dioxide analyzer is strongly recommended to monitor ventilation and to adjust end tidal carbon dioxide levels between 35 and 40 mm Hg. Moderate hemodilution is desirable, as a reduction in viscosity will enhance tissue perfusion when low pressures occur. A hematocrit of 35% will achieve this goal without deleteriously affecting oxygen-carrying capacity. The patient is ventilated with 100% oxygen during the period of hypotension and a thiopental infusion of 10 mg/kg/hr is also given, since

it is believed that some degree of cerebral protection will be conferred. Mild hypothermia may also have a protective effect on organ function.

Maintenance of adequate blood volume is essential to avoid uncontrollable hypotension while the cystectomy is performed. A combination of colloid and crystalloid in a ratio of 1:2 will compensate for "third spacing" and maximize hemodynamic stability.

Once the cystectomy and lymph node dissection have been completed, there is no need for continuing the hypotensive technique; indeed, it is highly undesirable from several points of view. First, the persistence of epidural blockade at this stage will lead to unopposed parasympathetic activity. This causes a constricted and hyperactive ileum, which poses considerable technical problems for the surgeon. Every effort should be made to ensure that the effects of the epidural block have dissipated by the time the creation of the Kock pouch has begun. To this end, we advise initially activating the epidural catheter with 1.5% lidocaine. If the intestinal tone has not returned, scopolamine (or atropine) can be administered and will achieve the desired effect in most patients.

Secondly, multiple anastomoses are utilized in the creation of the ileal reservoir and it is important that splanchnic blood flow be adequate. If visceral perfusion is compromised, there is a likelihood of postoperative anastomotic leakage.

We believe that attention to all the details outlined above will not only enhance the likelihood of a successful surgical outcome but will reduce morbidity and mortality in this group of patients.

References

1. Ahlering TE, Henderson JB, Skinner DG: Controlled hypotensive anesthesia to reduce blood loss in radical cystectomy for bladder cancer. J Urol 129:953–954, 1983.
2. Aitkenhead AR, Wishart HY, Brown DA: High spinal nerve block for large bowel anastomosis. A retrospective study. Br J Anaesth 50:177–183, 1978.
3. Arkless R: Renal carcinoma: how it metastasizes. Radiology 84:496–501, 1965.
4. Bokey L, Fazio VW: The mesenteric sling technique: new method of constructing an intestinal nipple valve for the continent ileostomy. Cleve Clin Q 45:231–236, 1978.
5. Chung F: Cancer, chemotherapy and anaesthesia. Can Anaesth Soc J 29:364–371, 1982.
6. Einhorn LH, Donohue JP: Improved chemotherapy

in disseminated testicular cancer. J Urol 117:65–69, 1977.

7. Goldiner PL, Carlon GC, Cvitkovic E, et al: Factors influencing postoperative morbidity and mortality in patients treated with bleomycin. Br Med J 1:1664–1667, 1978.

8. Krane RJ, White RD, Davis Z, et al: Removal of renal cell carcinoma extending into the right atrium using cardiopulmonary bypass, profound hypothermia and circulatory arrest. J Urol 131:945–947, 1984.

9. Lewis BM, Izbicki R: Routine pulmonary function tests during bleomycin therapy. Tests may be ineffective and potentially misleading. JAMA 243:347–351, 1980.

10. Milne B, Cervenko FW, Morales A, Salerno TA: Massive intraoperative pulmonary tumor embolus from renal cell carcinoma. Anesthesiology 54:253–255, 1981.

11. Neely J, Catchpole B: Ileus: the restoration of alimentary-tract motility by pharmacological means. Br J Surg 58:21–28, 1971.

12. Ney C: Thrombosis of inferior vena cava associated with malignant renal tumors. J Urol 55:583–590, 1946.

13. Novick AC, Cosgrove DM: Surgical approach for removal of renal cell carcinoma exending into the vena cava and the right atrium. J Urol 123:947–950, 1980.

14. Nygaard K, Smith-Erichsen N, Hatlevoll R, Refsum SB: Pulmonary complications after bleomycin, irradiation and surgery for esophageal cancer. Cancer 41:17–22, 1978.

15. Pawlik W, Mailman D, Shanbour LL, et al: Dopamine effects on the intestinal circulation. Am Heart J 91:325–331, 1976.

16. Prager RL, Dean R, Turner B: Surgical approach to intracardiac renal cell carcinoma. Ann Thorac Surg 33:74–77, 1982.

17. Rennie JA, Christofides ND, Mitchenere P, et al: Neural and humoral factors in postoperative ileus. Br J Surg 67:694–698, 1980.

18. Selvin BL: Cancer chemotherapy: implications for the anesthesiologist. Anesth Analg (Cleve) 60:425–434, 1981.

19. Skinner DG, Pfister RF, Colvin R: Extension of renal cell carcinoma into the vena cava: the rationale for aggressive surgical management. J Urol 107:711–716, 1972.

20. Skinner DG, Scardino PT, Daniels JR: Testicular cancer. Annu Rev Med 32:543–557, 1981.

21. Stirt JA, Korn EL, Reynolds RC: Sodium nitroprusside-induced hypotension in radical thoraco-abdominal dissection of retroperitoneal lymph nodes. Br J Anaesth 52:1045–1048, 1980.

22. Svane S: Tumor thrombus of the inferior vena cava resulting from renal carcinoma. A report on 12 autopsied cases. Scand J Urol Nephrol 3:245–256, 1969.

23. Utley JR, Mobin-Uddin K, Segnitz RH, et al: Acute obstruction of tricuspid valve by Wilms' tumor. J Thorac Cardiovasc Surg 66:626–628, 1973.

DURAIYAH THANGATHURAI, M.D.
MAGED S. MIKHAIL, M.D.

Intensive Care of the Postoperative Urologic Patient

CHAPTER 41

Patients undergoing radical surgery for urologic malignancies commonly require intensive care postoperatively. The need for such care arises from the extensive nature of the operative procedure and the physical state of the patient. Pre-existing systemic illnesses, chemotherapy, advanced age, and even the malignancy itself place such patients at high risk for developing postoperative complications.[7, 36]

Ideal intensive care starts in the preoperative period and continues intra- and postoperatively. The purpose of intensive care is the prevention, early detection, and aggressive treatment of postoperative complications.

PREOPERATIVE INTENSIVE CARE

The intensive care specialist should plan and coordinate the patient's management with the surgeon and the anesthesiologist. Prevention is the most effective treatment for postoperative complications. Pulmonary as well as cardiac complications have been reduced or prevented in high-risk patients who are identified preoperatively.[13, 37, 42] A more detailed discussion of preoperative evaluation and management of high-risk patients is found in Chapter 40.

Preoperative involvement allows for more accurate assessment of the patient's baseline values. For example, only preoperative placement of a Swan-Ganz catheter yields true baseline data. When introduced intra- or postoperatively, data represent hemodynamic changes associated with fasting, anesthesia, surgical stimulation, and blood loss and thus may be misleading. Moreover, preoperative measurements allow for more rational decisions about perioperative hydration and vasodilator or inotropic therapy.

INTRAOPERATIVE CARE

Although discussed in the chapter on anesthetic management, the role of the intensive care specialist must be emphasized in complex operations, particularly those concerning renal cell carcinoma involving the vena cava and atrium. In such cases, maintaining adequate perfusion of vital organs (brain, heart, kidneys, and liver) is critical during hypotensive episodes.

POSTOPERATIVE CARE

The goals of postoperative management are pain relief, respiratory care, careful monitoring, and the early detection and aggressive treatment of complications.

601

Pain Relief

Following major thoracoabdominal and upper abdominal procedures, the normal respiratory pattern is altered markedly. Lung volume, particularly functional residual capacity (FRC), decreases owing to the effects of pain, surgery, and anesthesia.[23, 30] The net result is predisposition to atelectasis and hypoxia. Adequate pain relief can reverse these effects.[5, 34] Intense pain is also often associated with agitation, tachycardia, and hypertension, all of which increase myocardial oxygen demand and may also enhance the likelihood of postoperative bleeding. Good analgesia blunts these effects.

The recent use of epidural narcotics has had a major impact on management of pain in the ICU. Multiple studies have documented the superiority of the lumbar epidural route over the parenteral route for narcotics.[5, 11, 29] Epidural morphine provides more effective, longer-lasting pain relief with greater preservation of respiratory function and minimal hemodynamic effect. High lumbar or thoracic epidural injections may be more effective in patients with thoracoabdominal incisions. If pain persists, intercostal or paravertebral blocks can also be tried. The use of epidural bupivacaine (0.25 to 0.5%) intermittently or as a continuous infusion is also extremely effective but is not associated with the respiratory depression seen with opioids. Additional benefits include enhancement of gut motility and blunting of stress response with stable hemodynamics.

Parenteral narcotics are most effective when titrated intravenously to the desired effect. Morphine and meperidine remain the most useful. Newer agents such as butorphanol, nalbuphine, and buprenorphine are also useful, but because of their mixed antagonist activity, they may precipitate withdrawal in the morphine-dependent patient.

Respiratory Care

Nonventilated Patients

Hypoxemia due to ventilation and perfusion mismatching is common following upper abdominal and thoracic incisions.[19, 30] Many patients require supplemental oxygen via facemask or nasal cannula. The fractional inspired oxygen concentration (FI_{O2}) should be monitored carefully, however, in patients with testicular cancer who have received bleomycin. The lowest inspired concentration associated with adequate oxygen saturation should be used, as postoperative respiratory failure has been associated with high oxygen tensions in these patients.[15, 21] Careful controlled oxygen therapy is also necessary in patients known to retain carbon dioxide.

The sequence of hypoventilation, atelectasis, and pneumonia is common postoperatively. Aggressive pulmonary physiotherapy (particularly incentive spirometry) effectively reduces the incidence of these complications[3] and should be used in all patients. We have found doxapram, 0.5 to 1.0 mg/minute infusion, to be useful in oversedated or uncooperative patients. Doxapram increases tidal volume as well as respiratory rate.

Patients on a Ventilator

Management of patients on ventilators should be directed at aggressive supportive care with the goal of early extubation to avoid respirator-related complications such as barotrauma, nosocomial pneumonia, and malnutrition.

Ventilation is best accomplished with 12 to 15 ml/kg tidal volumes with the rate adjusted to maintain eucapnia. Large tidal volumes help maintain normal lung volumes and eliminate the need for sighs. "Physiologic" PEEP (5 cm water) may also help maintain normal FRC. PEEP should be used to reduce FI_{O2} to nontoxic levels (<0.5). Although controversial, aggressive use of PEEP may prevent the onset or reduce the severity of the adult respiratory distress syndrome (ARDS).[33, 41] Higher levels of PEEP may be associated with a reduction in cardiac output,[39] urine output,[18] fluid retention, and an increased risk of pulmonary barotrauma. The major mechanisms in reduction of cardiac output are decreased venous return and a decrease in left ventricular diastolic volume.[8, 25, 27] Increasing intravenous fluids and use of intermittent mandatory ventilation (IMV)[12] are helpful in maintaining cardiac output. With higher levels of PEEP (10 to 15 cm water) a Swan-Ganz catheter is useful in fluid management. Agitation in some patients may necessitate the use of narcotics or, less commonly, muscle relaxants.

Weaning should be attempted only upon improvement in clinical condition, blood gas levels, and radiographic appearance. Diuretic therapy may be beneficial as PEEP is decreased. Early nutritional support increases the likelihood of successful weaning.[20, 31] Persistent carbon dioxide retention may be caused by narcotics, metabolic alkalosis, sepsis, or excessive glucose loads.[2] Other contributing factors may include cardiac decompensation, uncontrolled sepsis, and abdominal distention. High-frequency jet ventilation can be useful, particularly in patients with bronchopleural fistulae,[14] and possibly in those with bronchorrhea. Antacids and histamine Type II receptor blockers (cimetidine or ranitidine) decrease the high incidence of upper gastrointestinal bleeding in patients with respiratory failure.[26]

Hemodynamic Monitoring

The radical nature of most of the surgical procedures for malignancy gives rise to many potential bleeding sites. Bleeding can occur postoperatively despite meticulous hemostasis. Although use of hypotensive anesthetic techniques reduces intraoperative blood loss,[1] failure to elevate the blood pressure to normal levels at the end of the surgical procedure so that the surgeon can ensure adequate hemostasis may result in postoperative bleeding.

Monitoring for postoperative bleeding involves measurement of vital signs, serial hematocrit, output from drains, abdominal girth, and urine output. Each measurement, however, has its limitations and is often affected by other factors. Blood pressure changes are very late signs of bleeding, and the expected increase in heart rate is often blunted by the residual effects of anesthesia, drug therapy, or even age. Serial hematocrits are useful when obvious changes occur, but changes are often difficult to interpret because of compartmental fluid shifts. Occult bleeding often occurs even when surgical drains are properly placed and in the absence of increase in abdominal girth. Such bleeding is usually in the retroperitoneal space. We have found that the most sensitive monitor of bleeding is the measurement of urine output, particularly in the presence of other evidence of bleeding. The diagnosis of postoperative bleeding is ultimately based on overall clinical assessment of the patient by utilizing all the above measurements.

Retroperitoneal hemorrhage is a complication that may occasionally occur, owing to bleeding from venous plexuses. The clots that form often cause tamponade, however, and result in cessation of bleeding. Therefore, early re-exploration is usually unnecessary and may lead to further complications. All that is required is replacement of the blood lost in the retroperitoneal space. Rapid blood loss and acute respiratory and cardiac embarrassment are the only indications for re-exploration.

Even healthy patients undergoing radical surgery experience major hemodynamic changes because of the residual effects of anesthesia combined with rapid fluid shifts ("third spacing"). The need for fluid resuscitation and transfusion does not stop at the end of surgery and often continues for the following six to 12 hours, even in the absence of major bleeding. Although the controversy of colloid versus crystalloid fluid therapy continues,[35, 40] we have observed that a 1:2 ratio of colloids to crystalloids provides the best hemodynamic stability in the first 24 hours. The ratio can be increased to 1:1 for patients with low albumin levels and for those with prior bleomycin therapy.[15] Central venous pressure and urine output are invaluable monitors in assessing adequacy of fluid therapy. In patients with reduced urine output, early therapy with mannitol is helpful. Infusion of mannitol can lead to cardiac decompensation, however, and patients with borderline cardiac function should be carefully observed.

Electrocardiographic Monitoring

Cardiac arrhythmias are common postoperatively, particularly in elderly patients. Arrhythmias are usually secondary to underlying medical problems, metabolic abnormalities, or drug therapy.[16] Bradyarrhythmias or sinus bradycardia, which are common with the use of epidural bupivacaine and hypothermia, are well tolerated and only occasionally require the use of atropine and ephedrine. Tachycardia is often associated with pain, hypovolemia, anemia, or hypoxia, and treatment should be directed at these factors. The commonest types of tachyarrhythmias are atrial fibrillation and paroxysmal, supraventricular tachycardias, which usually respond to calcium channel blockers and digitalis. Ventricular ectopy is not uncommon in the postoperative period and, if it is a frequent or complex finding, particularly in the presence of underlying heart disease, treatment with lidocaine or procainamide infusions is indicated.[32]

Intravenous nitroglycerin should be started in elderly patients with ischemic heart disease and in those who show evidence of ischemia. Often ST segment abnormalities in the EKG are associated with digitalis, hypokalemia, local anesthetics, and hypothermia. Therefore, ST abnormalities should be interpreted very carefully. Patients receiving β-blockers or calcium channel blocker therapy for angina or hypertension should be continued on these drugs in the postoperative period.[17]

Hematologic Abnormalities

Anemia, thrombocytopenia, and neutropenia are common in patients who have received chemotherapy. The additional stress of surgery and the ensuing blood loss impose additional demands on the bone marrow, accentuating or unmasking these deficiencies. Platelet transfusions should be given when the count falls below 75,000 in the early postoperative period.[24]

Patients who develop platelet antibodies require single donor platelets. In addition to replacement of red cells and platelets following massive blood loss, clotting factors should be given based on coagulation studies. Neutropenic patients are prone to nosocomial infections and septicemia. A rapid fall in neutrophils may be an early sign of the adult respiratory distress syndrome.[4]

Electrolyte Abnormalities

Electrolyte abnormalities are very common in postoperative urologic patients. Deficiencies are more common than excesses and often require aggressive replacement. Excess electrolytes are usually due to increased intake along with renal impairment.

Hypokalemia is the most common abnormality encountered postoperatively. Preoperative deficiency, diuresis, nasogastric suctioning, and metabolic alkalosis are often contributing factors. Hypokalemia predisposes to both ventricular and supraventricular arrhythmias. Potentiation of muscular weakness and paralytic ileus may contribute to ventilatory impairment. Hypomagnesemia often accompanies hypokalemia, owing to abnormal renal and gastrointestinal losses.

Clinical signs include neurologic and cardiac irritability and ileus.

Hypocalcemia is common in critically ill patients.[10] Ionized calcium concentration is affected by serum proteins and pH but is more reliable than total serum measurements. Hypocalcemia occurs after massive transfusion with citrated blood products in patients with decreased citrate clearance (renal or hepatic disease and hypothermia) and can cause cardiovascular compromise.[38] Other causes of hypocalcemia include severe hyperphosphatemia, pancreatitis, parathyroid hypofunction, and vitamin D deficiency. Manifestations include neurologic and muscular irritability, cardiac failure, and arrhythmias.

Hypophosphatemia in the intensive care unit can occur during prolonged parenteral nutrition and may be associated with weakness, neurologic impairment, and hemolysis.

Sepsis

Many patients admitted postoperatively to the intensive care unit have an acquired immunodeficiency due to their malignancy, malnutrition, and prior chemotherapy.[9] Both cellular and humoral defects are often present. The stress of surgery, antibiotic administration, alteration of the normal bacterial flora, and breaches of cutaneous barriers and respiratory, gastrointestinal, and genitourinary tracts further predispose the patient to infectious complications.[6, 22] The presence of cutaneous anergy is common and markedly increases the risk of sepsis.

Gram-negative bacteria are responsible for most episodes of sepsis. Postoperative urologic patients, however, are also susceptible to gram-positive bacteria and fungi, particularly Candida. Multiple preventive measures can decrease the incidence of sepsis. All invasive catheters should be placed under aseptic conditions and should be removed as soon as they are no longer necessary. Lastly, prophylactic antibiotics should be narrow-spectrum agents and should be given only for a limited course.

Sepsis in critically ill patients tends to be overwhelming, consequently a clinical diagnosis must be made rapidly and, following appropriate cultures and gram stains, broad-spectrum antibiotic coverage including an aminoglycoside should be started. Surgical débridement and drainage, if appropriate, should be undertaken. Aggressive nutritional support can improve immune function and may enhance the likelihood of a favorable outcome.

CONCLUSION

Advances in both surgical and anesthetic techniques now allow an increasing number of patients with urologic malignancies, previously considered inoperable or at prohibitively high risk, to undergo major surgical procedures. Pre-existing systemic illness, advanced age, and the radical nature of many procedures place these patients at high risk for developing complications. The care of such patients is challenging and requires careful coordination of pre-, intra- and postoperative care to optimize chances for successful outcome.

Ideally, intensive care should start before surgery in high-risk patients, when an accurate baseline can be established and preventive interventions instituted. Involvement of the intensive care specialist in intraoperative care may also be desirable, particularly in patients with renal cell carcinoma involving the vena cava and atrium.

Postoperative intensive care is directed at thorough pain relief, with rational respiratory care and careful monitoring, allowing for the early detection of complications and appropriate treatment. Recently, use of epidural narcotics has provided more effective, longer-lasting pain relief with greater preservation of respiratory function and minimal hemodynamic side effects. Aggressive pulmonary physiotherapy effectively reduces the incidence of postoperative respiratory complications. Early detection of postoperative bleeding, dysrhythmias, myocardial ischemic changes, and hematologic and metabolic abnormalities also reduces the morbidity associated with these complications. Sepsis in critically ill postoperative patients, who are often immunocompromised, requires early recognition and prompt treatment with appropriate antibiotics.

References

1. Ahlering TE, Henderson JB, Skinner DG: Controlled hypotensive anesthesia to reduce blood loss in radical cystectomy for bladder cancer. J Urol 129:953–954, 1983.
2. Askanazi J, Rosenbaum SH, Hyman AT, et al: Respiratory changes induced by the large glucose loads of total parenteral nutrition. JAMA 243:1444–1447, 1980.
3. Bartlett RH, Gazzaniga AB, Geraghty TR: Respiratory maneuvers to prevent postoperative pulmonary complications. JAMA 224:1017–1021, 1973.
4. Brigham KL: Mechanisms of lung injury. Clin Chest Med 3:9–24, 1982.
5. Bromage PR, Camporesi E, Chestnut D: Epidural narcotics for postoperative analgesia. Anesth Analg 59:473–480, 1980.
6. Brun Biusson C, Meakins JL: Host defense mechanisms in acutely ill patients. In IMcA Ledingham, CD Manning (eds), Recent Advances in Critical Care Medicine. Edinburgh, Churchill Livingstone, 1983, pp 97–127.
7. Burnett W, McCaffrey J: Surgical procedures in the elderly. Surg Gynecol Obstet 134:221–226, 1972.
8. Calvin JE, Driedger AA, Sibbald WJ: Positive end-expiratory pressure (PEEP) does not depress left ventricular function in patients with pulmonary edema. Am Rev Respir Dis 124:121–128, 1981.
9. Chandra RK: Rosette-forming T lymphocytes and cell-mediated immunity in malnutrition. Br Med J 3:608–609, 1974.
10. Chernow B, Zaloga G, McFadden E, et al: Hypocalcemia in critically ill patients. Crit Care Med 10:848–851, 1982.
11. Cousins MJ, Mather LE: Intrathecal and epidural administration of opioids. Anesthesiology 61:276–310, 1984.
12. Downs JB, Douglas ME, Sanfelippo PM, et al: Ventilatory pattern, intrapleural pressure, and cardiac output. Anesth Analg 56:88–96, 1977.
13. Dripps RD, Deming MV: Postoperative atelectasis and pneumonia: diagnosis, etiology and management based upon 1,240 cases of upper abdominal surgery. Ann Surg 124:94–110, 1946.
14. Froese AB: High frequency ventilation: a critical assessment. In WC Shoemaker (ed): Critical Care State of the Art. Fullerton, CA, Soc Crit Care Med, Vol 5, 1984.
15. Goldiner PL, Carlon GC, Cvitkovic E, et al: Factors influencing postoperative morbidity and mortality in patients treated with bleomycin. Br Med J 1:1664–1667, 1978.
16. Goldman L: Supraventricular tachyarrhythmias in hospitalized adults after surgery. Clinical correlates in patients over 40 years of age after major noncardiac surgery. Chest 73:450–454, 1978.
17. Goldman L: Noncardiac surgery in patients receiving propranolol. Case reports and recommended approach. Arch Intern Med 141:193–196, 1981.
18. Järnberg PO, de Villota ED, Eklund J, et al: Effects of positive end-expiratory pressure on renal function. Acta Anaesthesiol Scand 22:508–514, 1978.
19. Latimer RG, Dickman M, Day WC, et al: Ventilatory patterns and pulmonary complications after upper abdominal surgery determined by preoperative and postoperative computerized spirometry and blood gas analysis. Am J Surg 122:622–632, 1971.
20. Lopes J, Russell DM, Whitwell J, Jeejeebhoy KN: Skeletal muscle function in malnutrition. Am J Clin Nutr 36:602–610, 1982.
21. Luna MA, Bedrossian CW, Lichtiger B, et al: Interstitial pneumonitis associated with bleomycin therapy. Am J Clin Pathol 58:501–510, 1972.
22. Meakins JL, Christou NV, Shizgal HM, MacLean LD: Therapeutic approaches to anergy in surgical patients. Surgery and levamisole. Ann Surg 190:286–296, 1979.

23. Meyers JR, Lembeck L, O'Kane H, et al: Changes in functional residual capacity of the lung after operation. Arch Surg 110:576–583, 1975.
24. Miller RD: Complications of massive blood transfusions. Anesthesiology 39:82–93, 1973.
25. Prewitt RM, Oppenheimer L, Sutherland JB, Wood LD: Effect of positive end-expiratory pressure on left ventricular mechanics in patients with hypoxemic respiratory failure. Anesthesiology 55:409–415, 1981.
26. Priebe HJ, Skillman JJ, Bushnell LS, et al: Antacid versus cimetidine in preventing acute gastrointestinal bleeding. A randomized trial in 75 critically ill patients. N Engl J Med 302:426–430, 1980.
27. Qvist J, Pontoppidan H, Wilson RS, et al: Hemodynamic responses to mechanical ventilation with PEEP: the effect of hypervolemia. Anesthesiology 42:45–55, 1975.
28. Rao TL, Jacobs KH, El-Etr AA: Reinfarction following anesthesia in patients with myocardial infarction. Anesthesiology 59:499–505, 1983.
29. Rawal N, Sjöstrand U, Dahlström B: Postoperative pain relief by epidural morphine. Anesth Analg 60:726–731, 1981.
30. Rehder K, Sessler AD, Marsh HM: General anesthesia and the lung. Am Rev Respir Dis 112:541–563, 1975.
31. Roulet M, Detsky AS, Marliss EB: A controlled trial of the effect of parenteral nutritional support on patients with respiratory failure and sepsis. Clin Nutrition, 1983.
32. Ruberman W, Weinblatt E, Goldberg JD, et al: Ventricular premature beats and mortality after myocardial infarction. N Engl J Med 297:750–757, 1977.
33. Schmidt GB, O'Neill WW, Kotb K, et al: Continuous positive airway pressure in the prophylaxis of the adult respiratory distress syndrome (ARDS). Surg Gynecol Obstet 143:613–618, 1976.
34. Shulman M, Sandler AN, Bradley JW, et al: Postthoracotomy pain and pulmonary function following epidural and systemic morphine. Anesthesiology 61:569–575, 1984.
35. Skillman JJ, Restal DS, Salzman EW: Randomized trial of albumin vs electrolyte solutions during abdominal aortic operations. Surgery 78:291–303, 1975.
36. Stahlgren LH: An analysis of factors which influence mortality following extensive abdominal operations upon geriatric patients. Surg Gynecol Obstet 113:283–292, 1961.
37. Stein M, Cassara EL: Preoperative pulmonary evaluation and therapy for surgery patients. JAMA 211:787–790, 1970.
38. Stulz PM, Scheidegger D, Drop LJ, et al: Ventricular pump performance during hypocalcemia: clinical and experimental studies. J Thorac Cardiovasc Surg 78:185–194, 1979.
39. Suter PM, Fairley B, Isenberg MD: Optimum end-expiratory airway pressure in patients with acute pulmonary failure. N Engl J Med 292:284–289, 1975.
40. Virgilio RW, Rice CL, Smith DE, et al: Crystalloid vs. colloid resuscitation: is one better? A randomized clinical study. Surgery 85:129–139, 1979.
41. Weigelt JA, Mitchell RA, Snyder WH 3d: Early positive end-expiratory pressure in the adult respiratory distress syndrome. Arch Surg 114:497–501, 1979.
42. Williams CD, Brenowitz JB: "Prohibitive" lung function and major surgical procedures. Am J Surg 132:763–766, 1976.

DONALD G. SKINNER, M.D.
GARY LIESKOVSKY, M.D.

CHAPTER 42

Technique of Radical Cystectomy

Radical cystectomy implies the en bloc removal of the anterior pelvic organs: the prostate, seminal vesicles, and bladder with its visceral peritoneum and perivesicle fat in males, and the urethra, bladder, cervix, vaginal cuff, uterus, ovaries, and anterior pelvic peritoneum in females. A pelvic iliac lymph node dissection of varying extent is usually included but should be denoted together with the term radical cystectomy to clarify whether or not a meticulous dissection was performed. Particularly in females, the operation is sometimes called an anterior exenteration with bilateral pelvic iliac lymph node dissection. This is the optimal ablative surgical procedure for the treatment of invasive carcinoma of the bladder in the properly selected patient who is an appropriate surgical risk. Many urologic oncologists use planned, preoperative radiation therapy before radical cystectomy, and results indicate that doses up to 5000 rads have little impact on the operation in terms of morbidity or the ability to perform the operation successfully as described. Our own experience reveals an insignificant increase in the occurrence of superficial wound infection and postoperative partial small bowel obstruction among irradiated as compared with nonirradiated patients. Prior radiation therapy in excess of 6000 rads, however, is associated with increased operative morbidity and mortality. Usually it is not feasible or safe to perform a pelvic node dissection in such cases because of the dense desmoplasia resulting from accumulated radiation doses of this magnitude.

PREOPERATIVE PREPARATION

In general, patients are admitted two days prior to surgery or by 0900 hours the day before surgery. They remain on a regular diet through breakfast the morning before surgery and thereafter receive only clear liquids by mouth until midnight before the day of surgery. At 0900 hours the day before surgery, 120 ml of Neoloid, a palatable emulsion of castor oil, is given by mouth. Patients then receive 1 gm of neomycin orally at 1000, 1100, 1200, 1300, 1600, 2000, and 2400 hours and 1 gm of erythromycin base orally at 1200, 1600, 2000, and 2400 hours. This program of bowel preparation, adapted and modified from that originally described by Nichols and associates,[4] is short and exceedingly effective in cleansing and decompressing the small and large bowel, prevents dehydration associated with prolonged catharsis, obviates the use of enemas, and maintains good nutritional support.

Patients over the age of 50 years are routinely digitalized prophylactically prior to surgery unless there is a specific contraindication. Digoxin, 0.5 mg, is given orally the afternoon of admission, followed by 0.25 mg that evening and 0.125 mg orally the day before surgery. If the patient is admitted 24

607

hours before surgery, 0.5 mg is given on admission, 0.25 mg the afternoon before surgery, and 0.125 mg that evening. No digoxin is given the morning of surgery. Evidence suggests that prophylactic preoperative digitalization may reduce the incidence of intraoperative or postoperative arrhythmias as well as minimize the development of congestive heart failure in elderly patients undergoing an operation of the magnitude of cystectomy.[5] This dosage schedule has resulted in no toxicity in more than 300 consecutive patients.

Preoperative hydration with intravenous Ringer's lactate or 5% dextrose with 0.5 normal saline at a rate of 125 ml/hour is initiated the evening before surgery. One of the most important preparations for surgery is determining the ileal stoma site. This is accomplished jointly by the surgeon and the enterostomal therapist by examining the patient in supine, sitting, and standing positions. Optimal stomal placement is essential to postoperative management, patient acceptance of the procedure, and the ability to care for the ileostomy effectively. In patients opting for the continent internal ileal reservoir (Kock pouch), the position for the ileostomy location may be lower (well caudal to the belt or underwear line), and close to the pubis for concealment, since these patients do not wear an external appliance and skin folds or creases are unimportant. However, if cosmetic concealment is of little concern to the patient, placement higher on the abdominal wall, in a position similar to one selected for a standard ileostomy, may facilitate intermittent catheterization.

Anesthesia selection can further facilitate the performance of the operation and postoperative comfort for the patient. Preoperative placement of an epidural catheter allows intraoperative use of lidocaine, which reduces the need for depolarizing muscle relaxants, facilitates controlled hypotensive anesthesia, and in turn reduces blood loss and the need for blood replacement.[1] The indwelling epidural catheter can also be used during the first 24 to 48 hours postoperatively for pain management by administration of intermittent epidural morphine.

OPERATIVE TECHNIQUE

The patient is positioned in the hyperextended supine position (Fig. 42–1). A catheter is routinely placed in the bladder and is drained. Thirty to 60 ml of 10% formalin solution can be infused into the bladder under gravity if there is no known vesicoureteral reflux. This was routine in our practice until 1980, when we stopped using formalin in order to grow in vitro the removed tumors in an effort to search for effective cytotoxic drugs as well as collaborate with basic science investigations. We have observed no change in the incidence of pelvic recurrence since stopping formalin instillation. Nonetheless, the use of formalin seems to offer theoretical advantage, as it may lessen the risk of pelvic tumor recurrence should the bladder inadvertently be entered during surgery, and we have recognized no postoperative complication from its use. The catheter is clamped for 10 minutes and then drained. Gravity drainage is then maintained.

The operation commences with a long midline incision. The vertical incision is directed laterally to the paramedian position at the level of the stoma site to ensure that the incision is as far from the stoma as possible. The anterior rectus fascia is incised, the rectus muscle retracted laterally, and the posterior rectus fascia and peritoneum entered in the superior aspect of the incision. As the peritoneum and posterior fascia are incised inferiorly, care is taken to identify the urachal remnant, which should be circumscribed so that it can be removed en bloc with the bladder. This maneuver avoids potential early entry into a high-rising bladder. Similarly, if the patient has had a previous segmental resection or cystotomy through a vertical incision, that in-

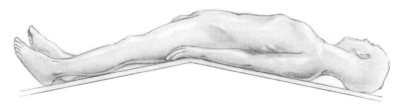

Figure 42–1. *Proper position of the patient for cystectomy. Note that the table is hyperextended; this opens up the pelvis and facilitates exposure.*

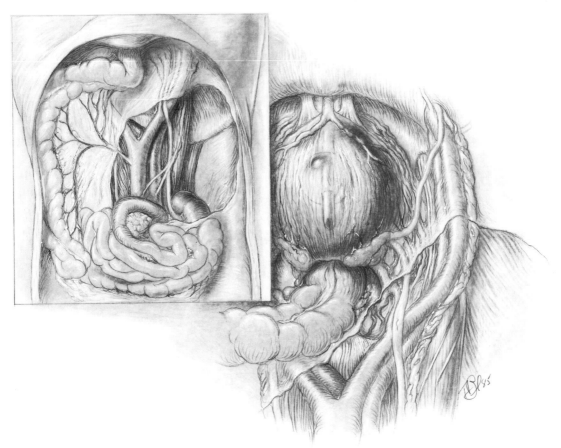

Figure 42–2. *Diagrammatic view of the pelvis from overhead, after the ascending colon and peritoneal attachment to the small bowel mesentery have been mobilized up to the level of the duodenum (inset). This mobilization is important to allow the bowel to be packed in the epigastrium and to provide exposure to the area of the aortic bifurcation for initiation of the node dissection.*

cisional tract should be circumscribed, full-thickness, to be removed en bloc with the bladder.

Once the peritoneum has been opened, careful intra-abdominal exploration is undertaken to determine the extent of disease, to search for possible intrahepatic metastatic disease, and to detect any concomitant unrelated pathologic processes. All intra-abdominal adhesions should be incised and freed at this time.

A right-angle Richardson retractor is utilized to elevate the right abdominal wall, and the ascending colon and peritoneal attachments to the small bowel mesentery directed toward the ligament of Treitz are then mobilized (Fig. 42–2). Conceptually, the ascending colon and peritoneal attachments to the small bowel mesentery are triangular, with the ileal cecal region at the apex of this triangle. The retroperitoneal transverse por-

tion of the duodenum is at the base, the medial portion of the descending left colonic mesentery at the left border of the triangle, and the peritoneal attachment to the ascending colon (avascular line of Toldt) at the right side of the triangle. This mobilization is an important part of setting up the operative field to perform a cystectomy and is necessary to allow proper subsequent packing of the intra-abdominal contents.

The left colon and sigmoid mesentery are then widely mobilized by incising the avascular line of Toldt along the left gutter. This dissection extends up to the lower pole of the left kidney, and the sigmoid mesentery is mobilized off the sacral promontory and distal aorta up to the origin of the inferior mesenteric artery. In this way, the base of the sigmoid mesentery is freed from the sacral promontory, with numerous adherent bands divided so that the left ureter can

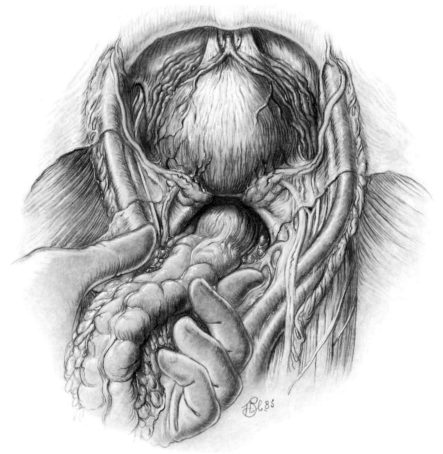

Figure 42–3. *Diagrammatic view of the pelvis after the ascending colon and small bowel have been packed in the epigastrium. Note that the sigmoid mesentery is being mobilized off the sacral promontory and distal aorta. This will facilitate the node dissection and allow the left ureter to pass under the sigmoid mesentery without angulation.*

eventually be brought under the mesentery without angulation or tension.

A self-retaining retractor is then positioned. The authors prefer to use a Finochietto retractor. The right colon and small bowel are then packed in the epigastrium, utilizing three moist lap pads and a moist towel rolled to the width of the abdomen. No attempt is made to pack the descending colon, which should be left as mobile as possible. Successful packing is an art that greatly facilitates the operation. In general, the surgeon's left hand should be used to position the small bowel where desired. Opened, moist lap pads then can be swept along the palm of the left hand, using the right hand to tuck them under the viscera. It is best to first pack each gutter and then the remaining small bowel with the third lap pad. The rolled moist towel can then be positioned to complete the packing as it lies

horizontally above the level of the aortic bifurcation. Occasionally, a large Deaver retractor on the rolled towel facilitates the cephalad exposure, but usually the region above the aortic bifurcation is readily visible without retraction (Fig. 42–3).

At this point, both ureters are dissected in the deep pelvis to several centimeters beyond the point where they cross the common iliac arteries. Two large right-angle hemoclips are then placed on the distal mobilized ureter, 1.5 to 2.0 cm apart, and the ureter is divided just proximal to the distal hemoclip. A small portion of the proximal ureter is then excised and sent to the pathology laboratory for frozen section. The proximal ureter is further mobilized cephalad and safely tucked beneath the rolled towel packing. Usually, a medial vessel requires clipping and division to allow adequate mobilization. It is advisable to maintain the ureteral attachment with the spermatic cord in the male, and the infundibulopelvic ligament in the female, since the gonadal artery provides important collateral blood supply to the ureter, improving the viability of the subsequent ureteroileal anastomosis. This is particularly important in irradiated patients or those with undilated ureters. Placement of a hemoclip on the distal ureter at the time it is divided allows the ureter to dilate hydrostatically while the cystectomy is being performed, facilitating the ureterointestinal anastomosis.

The proximal extent of the lymph node dissection is then initiated 1 to 2 cm above the aortic bifurcation. All fibroareolar and lymphatic tissue is dissected off the distal aorta and vena cava, extending laterally to the genitofemoral nerve, which represents the lateral limits of the dissection. Large or medium hemoclips are placed on the proximal limits of dissection to reduce lymphatic leak. The distal fibroareolar lymphatic tissue is not clipped unless a vessel is identified, since this tissue will be removed. In the female, the infundibulopelvic ligament, including the ovarian vein, is ligated and divided at the pelvic brim.

All tissue is swept off the distal aorta, vena cava, and the common iliac vessels, and over the sacral promontory into the deep pelvis. The common iliac arteries are mobilized. Care must be taken to secure small arterial and venous branches running on the sacral promontory. This is one area where cautery can be very helpful as hemoclips are often dislodged and, if these vessels are not well controlled, annoying bleeding can result.

Once the proximal portion of the dissection is complete, a finger is passed under the pelvic peritoneum and over the external iliac artery and vein to the femoral canal. The opposite hand may be used to strip the peritoneum from the undersurface of the fascia transversalis in order to connect with the dissection from above. This elevates the peritoneum and defines the limits of lateral peritoneum to be excised. The peritoneum is then incised medial to the spermatic vessels in males and lateral to the ovarian vein in females, with the vas deferens in the male and the round ligament in the female clipped and divided. These are the only structures of consequence encountered in this divided tissue.

A large right-angle rake retractor (also called an Israel retractor) is then used to elevate the lower abdominal wall. Tension on this retractor should be directed to the ceiling, not caudally, and the distal round ligament in the female and spermatic cord in the male should be retracted in order to provide maximal visualization of the area around the femoral canal.

Medium hemoclips are meticulously placed on the fibroareolar and lymphatic tissue at the distal limits of dissection on the external iliac artery and vein to prevent leakage of lymph. The circumflex iliac vein represents the distal limits of dissection along the artery, the genitofemoral nerve the lateral limits, and Cooper's ligament the medial distal boundary of dissection. The lymph node of Cloquet, or Rosenmüller, represents the distal limit of lymphatic dissection medial to the external iliac artery at the femoral canal. Lymphatics draining into this node should be clipped. Then the external iliac artery and vein are circumferentially dissected. The surgeon should look for an accessory obturator vein draining into the back wall of the external iliac vein at this level, present in approximately 40% of patients. This vessel is ligated and divided.

Once the distal limits of dissection have been defined and completed, the proximal portions of the external iliac artery and vein are skeletonized. Usually a small muscular arterial and venous branch is found along the proximal portion of the external iliac vessels, but other major vascular branches usually are not encountered. The fibroareolar tissue overlying the psoas muscle can then be incised medial to the genitofemoral nerve. On the left side, branches of the genitofemoral nerve often pursue a more medial course and may be intimately related to the vessels, in which case they are excised.

At this point, the external iliac vessels are retracted medially and gauze x-ray sponge is used to dissect bluntly all fibroareolar and lymphatic tissue off the lateral wall of the pelvis, pushing the tissue with one or two sponges into the obturator fossa (Fig. 42–4). The vessels are retracted laterally and with traction by using the left hand; all lymphatic and fibroareolar tissue can thus be swept bluntly out of the obturator fossa. Great care should be taken to identify and protect the obturator nerve; the hypogastric vein should not be torn. The nerve is carefully dissected free and retracted laterally so that the index

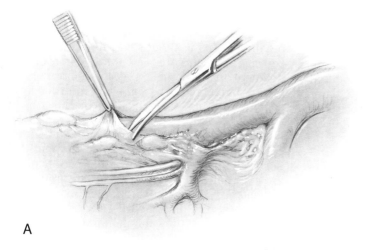

A

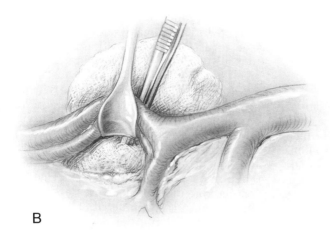

B

Figure 42–4. Diagrammatic view of the technique of skeletonization of the external iliac artery and vein. A gauze sponge is used to dissect out the obturator fossa, sweeping all fibroareolar and lymphatic tissue, en bloc, toward the bladder.

Illustration continued on opposite page

finger of the left hand can be placed medial to it, parallel to the endopelvic fascia. The second finger is passed along the endopelvic fascia medial to this region, isolating the obturator vessels between the two fingers, medial to the obturator nerve. These vessels should be ligated and divided, allowing the obturator group of nodes to be stripped medially with the specimen. Once the obturator fossa has been dissected free, the lateral pedicle is developed.

Perhaps the most important point in the safe performance of a radical cystectomy is the next step. Counter-traction is used with the left hand, and the left index finger gently moves medial to the hypogastric artery in the deep pelvis, parallel to the sweep of the sacrum, extending all the way to the endo-

pelvic fascia. This helps define two pedicles, one extending from the anterior pelvic organs to the hypogastric vessels, and the other posteriorly to the rectum. Again, with the left index finger behind the lateral pedicle for counter-traction, the hypogastric artery is further skeletonized (Fig. 42–5). The first branch off the posterior portion of the hypogastric artery, the posterior superior gluteal artery, should be identified and protected if possible. A right-angle clamp then should be passed carefully behind the hypogastric artery, distal to the posterior superior gluteal artery. The hypogastric artery is ligated at this level. Occasionally, because of the extent of disease or anatomic variation, it will be necessary to ligate the hypogastric artery proximal to its first posterior

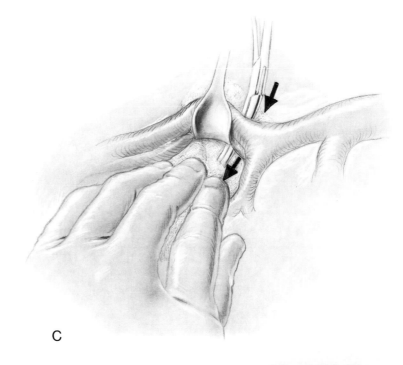

Figure 42–4 Continued

C

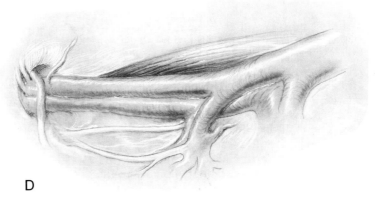

D

muscular branch. Some patients in whom this is done will complain of buttock claudication with exercise following surgery, but this sequela can be avoided by preserving the posterior superior gluteal artery whenever possible.

The lateral pedicle is then divided between large hemoclips all the way to the endopelvic fascia or as far as is technically feasible (Fig. 42–5). Blunt dissection with the index finger will allow development of this plane and protection of the rectum. Large, right-angle hemoclip appliers are ideally suited for proper placement of clips, and it is important to position the dual set of clips as far apart as possible so that at least 0.5 to 1 cm of tissue projects beyond each clip as the pedicle is divided. This prevents the clips from being dislodged and allowing subsequent troublesome bleeding.

Once the lateral pedicle has been divided, attention is directed toward the posterior pedicle. A large clamp can be placed on the urachal peritoneal remnant in the male, or a double-hook thyroid tenaculum placed on the body of the uterus in the female, to give anterior traction for visualization of the cul-de-sac, or pouch of Douglas. The peritoneum lateral to the rectum is then incised, with extension of incision anteriorly into the cul-de-sac to join the incision from the opposite side. One should remember that the anterior and posterior peritoneal reflections meet in the cul-de-sac to form Denonvilliers' fascia, which extends caudally to the urogenital diaphragm. This is an extremely important

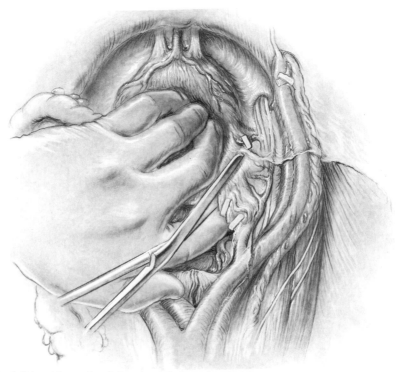

Figure 42–5. *The left hand is used to define the right lateral pedicle, extending from the bladder to the hypogastric artery. To develop this plane, the index finger is inserted just behind the hypogastric artery. This thin vascular pedicle can then be clipped and divided all the way to the endopelvic fascia. Traction with the left hand defines the pedicle, allows direct visualization, and protects the rectum from injury.*

anatomic boundary in the male, lying between the posterior surface of the prostate and seminal vesicles and the anterior surface of the rectum (Fig. 42–6). The peritoneal incision in the cul-de-sac should be made immediately on the rectal side rather than the bladder side so that the plane behind the posterior leaf of Denonvilliers' fascia and the anterior rectal wall is developed (Fig. 42–7). This allows entry into Denonvillier's space. In this plane, the rectum can be easily swept off the bladder, the seminal vesicles, and prostate in the male, and off the posterior vaginal wall in the female. If the peritoneal incision in the cul-de-sac is made anteriorly, entry between the two planes of Denonvilliers' fascia or anterior to that fascial plane may occur, making dissection of the rectum difficult and increasing the risk of incidental rectal injury. Occasionally, carcinoma may obliterate this plane or prior high-dose radiation therapy may cause severe fibrosis, complicating the dissection. In such instances, when patients have received a high prior cumulative dose of radiation (greater than 6000 rads), dissection of this plane may be facilitated by an initial peri-

neal dissection.[3] To finish the dissection of this plane, a posterior motion of the hand should be used to free the rectum from Denonvilliers' fascia and to develop the posterior pedicles (Fig. 42–8). This motion thins and develops the posterior pedicle, facilitates use of hemoclips, and protects the rectum from inadvertent injury during division of the posterior pedicles. Once the posterior pedicles have been defined, they are clipped and divided all the way to the endopelvic fascia (in the male), which is also incised on the ipsilateral side of the prostate and cleaned off the posterior and side walls of the prostate (Fig. 42–8).

In the female the posterior pedicles, including the cardinal ligaments, are clipped and divided for approximately 4 to 5 cm beyond the cervix. At this point the posterior vaginal wall is opened and the vagina circumscribed anteriorly. The anterior vaginal wall is dissected off the posterior wall of the bladder down to the region of the urethra. This maneuver further defines the two distal posterior pedicles extending from the bladder to the lateral vagina on either side. These are further clipped and divided distally,

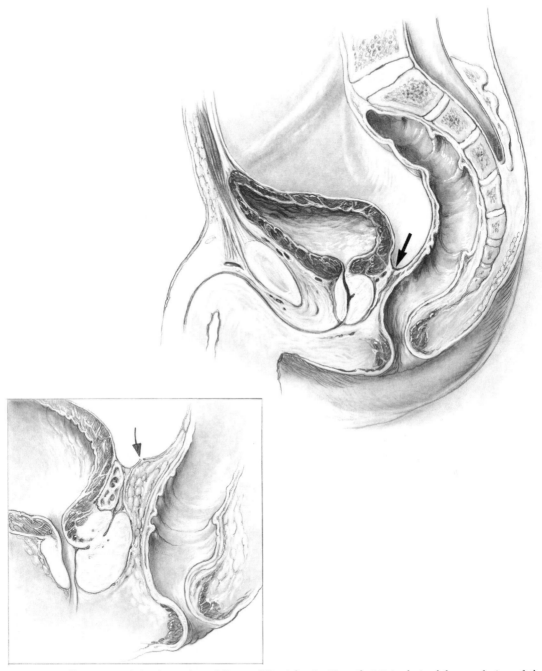

Figure 42–6. *Illustration of the formation of Denonvilliers' fascia. Note that it is derived from a fusion of the anterior and posterior peritoneal reflections, and that Denonvilliers' space lies behind the fascia. Therefore, to successfully enter this space so as to facilitate mobilization of the anterior rectal wall off Denonvilliers' fascia, the incision in the cul-de-sac should be close to the peritoneal fusion at the anterior rectal wall and not close to the bladder (arrow). See inset for detail.*

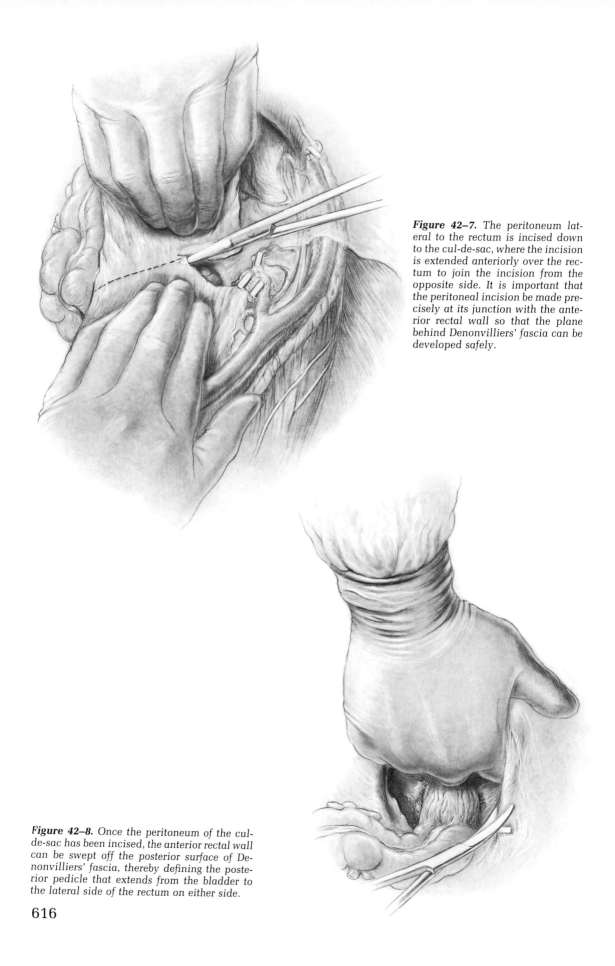

Figure 42–7. The peritoneum lateral to the rectum is incised down to the cul-de-sac, where the incision is extended anteriorly over the rectum to join the incision from the opposite side. It is important that the peritoneal incision be made precisely at its junction with the anterior rectal wall so that the plane behind Denonvilliers' fascia can be developed safely.

Figure 42–8. Once the peritoneum of the cul-de-sac has been incised, the anterior rectal wall can be swept off the posterior surface of Denonvilliers' fascia, thereby defining the posterior pedicle that extends from the bladder to the lateral side of the rectum on either side.

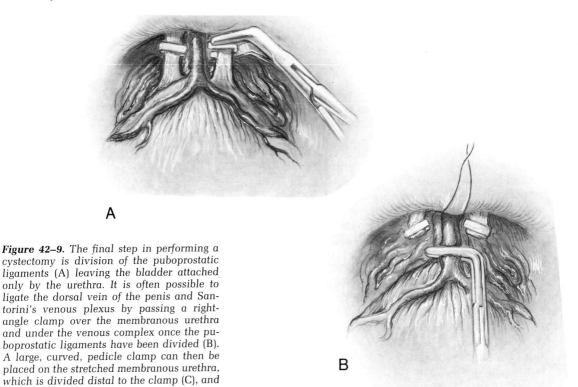

A

Figure 42–9. The final step in performing a cystectomy is division of the puboprostatic ligaments (A) leaving the bladder attached only by the urethra. It is often possible to ligate the dorsal vein of the penis and Santorini's venous plexus by passing a right-angle clamp over the membranous urethra and under the venous complex once the puboprostatic ligaments have been divided (B). A large, curved, pedicle clamp can then be placed on the stretched membranous urethra, which is divided distal to the clamp (C), and the specimen can then be removed.

B

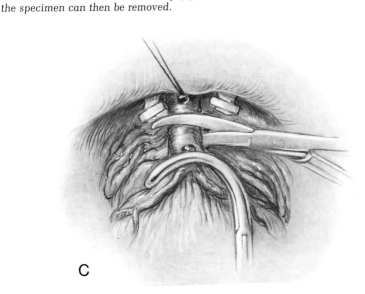

C

freeing the bladder from its posterior attachments except for the urethra. In some patients with large, deeply penetrating posterior tumors, it may be advantageous to remove the anterior vaginal wall completely, in which case the lateral vaginal wall is incised to the urethral meatus.

A similar dissection is then performed on the opposite side. As the authors are right-handed, it is customary for the surgeon to move to the opposite side of the table to initiate the dissection on the left side. Once the lateral and posterior pedicles have been delineated, the surgeon usually returns to the ipsilateral side of the operating table, which facilitates clipping and division of the pedicles.

With completion of the posterior and lateral portion of the operation, attention is directed anteriorly for the first time. Fibroareolar connections between the anterior bladder wall and proximal prostate are divided from the undersurface of the pubis. In patients who have had a prior segmental resection or open prostatectomy, this plane may be difficult to develop. In such situations, the procedure may be facilitated by incising the periosteum of the pubis with the cautery. A periosteal elevator then can be used to develop this subperiosteal plane down to the region of the urethra.

The puboprostatic ligaments are then stretched and separated in the midline, immediately adjacent to the undersurface of the pubis. These ligaments are clipped close to the pubis and divided with angled scissors vertical to the membranous urethra. Once the puboprostatic ligaments have been divided, the prostate is mobilized and the membranous urethra is stretched well above the urogenital diaphragm. It is often possible to pass a right-angled clamp under the dorsal vein of the penis and Santorini's plexus just anterior to the urethra and to ligate this venous plexus as described by Walsh in Chapter 53. Next, a large, curved pedicle clamp is placed on the urethra just beyond the apex of the prostate (Fig. 42–9). This clamp must be placed carefully to avoid rectal injury and to ensure that the end of the clamp extends beyond the urethra, preventing the spilling of intravesical contents once the urethra is divided. The index finger of the left hand is then placed beyond the clamp and the urethra divided with the catheter distal to the clamp. Placement of the finger prevents injury to the rectum during division of the urethra. The entire specimen is then removed en bloc with the pelvic nodes and lymphatics.

Once the urethropubic ligaments have been divided in the female, a large, curved Kocher clamp is placed on the urethra, and the anterior vaginal wall is opened distally and circumferentially incised around the urethral meatus. The vaginal cuff is closed with interrupted size 0 Dexon or chromic sutures. Preservation of the anterior vaginal wall, when feasible, retains a functional vagina. When the anterior vaginal wall is removed because of the local extent of the primary tumor, closure results in a small, largely obliterated vagina. It is important to suspend the closed vagina to Cooper's ligament on each side in order to prevent vaginal prolapse or the development of an enterocele.

In both males and females, a figure-of-eight suture with size 0 chromic or Dexon suture material is placed through the levators anteriorly, immediately adjacent to the pubis. This effectively controls venous bleeding from the region of the dorsal vein of the penis and the large venous plexus found in this region. When inspection of the side walls of the pelvis confirms that all bleeding is controlled, a dry lap pad is placed in the deep pelvis.

In more than 300 consecutive patients, major bleeding from the region of the dorsal vein has not been a factor, and the use of a Foley catheter inserted through the urethra or penis has been unnecessary to control bleeding. In fact, that maneuver may contribute to a greater incidence of pelvic abscess. If the pelvis continues to ooze, a large Hemovac tube has been used and left on suction for 24 to 48 hours. In most cases, the pelvis is not drained by any means unless a Kock pouch is used for urinary diversion.

Following cystectomy as described in this chapter, nearly all male patients will be impotent, although many will retain penile and perineal feelings of excitement and achieve psychogenic climax. However, they cannot develop an erection. This problem should be discussed at length before surgery. In selected patients, placement of a semirigid or a Scott inflatable prosthesis proves effective in restoring potency and is an important consideration psychologically. In those patients opting for the Scott prosthesis, the reservoir and pump components are placed at the time of cystectomy. At a later date, the inflatable cylinders are inserted and the apparatus connected. Implanting the reservoir and pump at the time of cystectomy reduces much of the discomfort usually associated with placement of the Scott prosthesis and, in our hands, has not been accompanied with increased morbidity. A detailed discussion of this, with surgical technique, will be found in Chapter 47. Walsh[11] has suggested utilization of his technique for radical retropubic prostatectomy when performing cystectomy in order to preserve potency. Although potency has been achieved in more than 50% of such patients, the impact of this modification in terms of compromising the cancer operation or increasing blood loss at the time of cystectomy remains unknown. Pelvic recurrence following prostatectomy for cancer of the prostate seems less of a problem than that following cystectomy. In the latter, nearly all patients are dead within two years, since there is no effective therapeutic alternative (e.g., hormone therapy). Furthermore, as discussed in Chapter 14, clinical staging techniques carry at least a 50% error in understaging bladder cancer, and cure seems dependent on the effectiveness of the surgical procedure. Perhaps the Walsh modification will prove effective in the future, but not until the true incidence of pelvic recurrence and long-term survival figures are reported.

In patients with normal cardiogram results, use of controlled hypotensive anesthesia during performance of the cystectomy substantially reduces blood loss and the need for blood replacement. We have reviewed our experience, comparing similarly staged patients who have undergone our standard surgical technique. The mean blood loss among 16 patients undergoing surgery with controlled hypotensive anesthesia was 821 ± 78 ml compared with 1740 ± 134 ml for a similar group undergoing the operation under standard anesthesia. Similarly, the group having hypotensive anesthesia required less blood replacement during their hospital stay than those operated under routine anesthesia (700 ml to 1600 ml, respectively).[1] Further, analysis of the number of patients who required blood revealed that 90% of the normotensive patients received blood, compared with 69% of those in the hypotensive group.[1]

MANAGEMENT OF THE URETHRA

In the female, urethrectomy is routinely performed with cystectomy. In males, en bloc urethrectomy is performed according to guidelines discussed in detail in Chapter 43. In general, simultaneous urethrectomy is performed only when overt tumor is seen in the membranous urethra or known to involve the prostatic urethra, and in selected patients in whom multifocal carcinoma in situ is known to exist. In these circumstances, the patient is positioned initially in the hyperextended frog-leg position, with the perineum prepped and draped into the operative field. An associate initiates the urethrectomy at the same time the cystectomy is started above. This two-team approach eliminates the added time associated with cystourethrectomy performed by one surgeon,

and in our hands, the urethrectomy portion of the procedure is completed at about the same time the bladder is ready to be removed and the entire specimen can be delivered en bloc with the pelvic lymph nodes.

When this two-team approach is not utilized, the operation is started perineally, with the patient placed in the exaggerated lithotomy position and the perineum parallel to the floor. This position is similar to that used to perform perineal prostatectomy. The entire urethra within the corpus spongiosum is mobilized out to the glans by inverting the penis according to the method of Whitmore.[12] However, the distal urethra is not divided, so that a catheter may be maintained within the bladder. In the occasional case when inoperable disease is unexpectedly encountered at the time of abdominal exploration, it is not necessary to divert the urine or remove the bladder because the urethra has not been divided.

In most cases, the pathologic findings of the cystectomy specimen determine the candidates for secondary urethrectomy. The histologic findings of carcinoma in situ, or overt transitional cell carcinoma in the prostatic urethra, are indications for a secondary urethrectomy. In patients with multifocal disease or carcinoma in situ that is remote from the primary tumor, secondary urethrectomy is performed only when saline urethral washings performed four months following cystectomy reveal cells positive for malignancy.

A complete discussion on indications for urethrectomy and its surgical technique is addressed in Chapter 43.

COMMENTARY

Between 1971 and 1982, 202 patients were explored with the intention of performing a single-stage radical cystectomy along with en bloc dissection of the pelvic iliac lymph nodes and urinary diversion for cure of primary urothelial carcinoma of the bladder. Five patients (2.5%) were found to have unresectable disease, usually attributable to the unexpected findings of extensive involvement above the aortic bifurcation. Urinary diversion and a total cystectomy was performed in these patients unless the ureters were involved or encased by tumor. We believe this provides reasonable palliation in terms of local control, reduced bleeding

Table 42–1. BLADDER CANCER MORBIDITY RATES

Complications	1600 rads + Cystectomy		Cystectomy Only	
	Number of Patients (out of 100)	Average Postoperative Stay (days)	Number of Patients (out of 97)	Average Postoperative Stay (days)
None	82	12.0	83	11.2
Wound infection/dehiscence	6	25.5	1	14
Prolonged ileus/partial small bowel obstruction	7	29.1	4	28.2
Sepsis ± urine leak	1	OP mort.	2	OP mort.
Loop infarction—reoperated			1	22
Vascular—clot to toe			1	11
Occlusion—femoral-femoral bypass			1	12
Rectal fistula	1	31		
Pyelonephritis/colic	1	32		
Cardiac arrhythmia			1	18
Thrombophlebitis/pulmonary embolism	0		0	
Ureteroileal obstruction (N tube)	1	28		
Acute cholecystitis	1	28		
Brachial palsy (temporary)			1	9
Stoma—relocation			1	21
Entero-loop fistula			1	50
Any complication	18	27.7	14	22.3

from the retained bladder, and relief of urgency and strangury without significantly increasing the operative morbidity.

During this period, 197 patients underwent the operation with the intent of cure. The postoperative mortality, defined as death for any reason before discharge from the hospital, or death within 30 days as a result of the operation regardless of location, was 1.5% (three of 197 patients). Most of the patients treated from 1971 to 1978 were part of a protocol utilizing high-dose, short-course, preoperative radiation therapy and single-stage radical cystectomy for the management of invasive bladder carcinoma.[10] Data from that study in terms of morbidity and efficacy have been reported elsewhere and are discussed in detail in Chapter 16.[7, 10] Since 1978, preoperative radiation has been used rarely. Early postoperative complications that prolonged hospitalization occurred in 32 of the 197 patients (16%).[9] Table 42–1 lists the complications and their impact on hospitalization. It should be empha-

Table 42–2. BLADDER CANCER STUDY OF 197 PATIENTS

	Pathologic Stage												
				TNM							Marshall-Jewett			
	P0	P1/PIS	P2	P3a	P3b	P4	N+	0	A	B₁	B₂	C	D
1600 rads + Cystectomy	16	34	17	7	18	8	29	26	22	10	4	5	33
Number of patients with positive nodes		3	7	3	12	4							
Cystectomy only	2	33	19	7	26	10	21	11	21	17	6	15	27
Number of patients with postive nodes		2	2	1	12	4							
Total	18	67	36	14	44	18	50	37	43	27	10	20	60
Number of patients with positive nodes		5	9	4	24	8							
Percentage of patients with positive nodes, per stage		7	25	28	55	44	25						

sized that 165 patients suffered no complication, and their average hospitalization was only 11.5 days.

Since 1971, it has been our policy to give anticoagulants to patients prophylactically, utilizing parenteral crystalline warfarin sodium (Coumadin) postoperatively. Ten mg of Coumadin are given intramuscularly in the recovery room, usually followed by 5 mg the following day unless the patient's prothrombin time exceeds 24 seconds; anticoagulation should be reversed with phytonadione (AquaMEPHYTON) as the complications of excessive anticoagulation exceed its possible benefits. Utilization of this protocol has virtually eliminated pulmonary embolism in this group of high-risk patients.[7]

Further analysis of the patient undergoing radical cystectomy for management of invasive bladder carcinoma reveals important implications in terms of node involvement according to the extent of primary disease. Table 42–2 reveals the incidence of positive nodes according to pathologic (P) stage. Although the incidence of positive postoperative nodes becomes greater with increasing depth of penetration of the primary tumor, 7% of patients with pathologically superficial tumor and 25% of patients with superficial muscle invasion already have metastases to the pelvic nodes.[6, 9] This implies the need to treat the pelvic nodes whenever cystectomy seems indicated for carcinoma. Five-year survival curves indicate that more than 35% of patients with positive nodes can be cured by pelvic node dissection.[6, 9, 10] Perhaps standard fractionation radiation therapy (4000 to 5000 rads) can sterilize pelvic nodal metastatic disease, but it is unlikely that 1600 to 2000 rads can control metastatic disease in these patients. Therefore, whenever cystectomy is indicated for the treatment of transitional cell carcinoma of the bladder, the incidence of nodal metastatic disease implies the need to treat that area effectively. A pelvic node dissection can cure some patients with minimal metastatic disease and identifies those at high risk for the development of disseminated disease. In these cases, the early use of systemic adjuvant chemotherapy may improve survival, although this is as yet unproved.[8]

CONCLUSION

In summary, a single-stage radical cystectomy with bilateral pelvic iliac lymph node dissection and urinary diversion can be performed with an acceptably low rate of operative mortality and morbidity. Attention to preoperative preparation, operative technique, and postoperative details make a real difference in mortality and morbidity. The operation remains the optimal procedure for the management of multifocal or invasive bladder cancer.

References

1. Ahlering TE, Henderson JB, Skinner DG: Controlled hypotensive anesthesia to reduce blood loss in radical cystectomy for bladder cancer. J Urol 129:953–954, 1983.
2. Burman SO: The prophylactic use of digitalis before thoracotomy. Ann Thorac Surg 14:359, 1972.
3. Crawford ED, Skinner DG: Salvage cystectomy after irradiation failure. J Urol 123:32, 1980.
4. Nichols RL, Broido P, Condon RE, et al: Effect of preoperative neomycin-erythromycin intestinal preparation on the incidence of infectious complications following colon surgery. Ann Surg 178:453, 1973.
5. Pinaud MLJ, Blanloeil YAG, Souron RJ: Preoperative prophylactic digitalization of patients with coronary artery disease—a randomized echocardiographic and hemodynamic study. Anesth Analg 62:865–869, 1983.
6. Skinner DG: Management of invasive bladder cancer: a meticulous pelvic node dissection can make a difference. J Urol 128:34–36, 1982.
7. Skinner DG, Crawford ED, Kaufman JJ: Complications of radical cystectomy for carcinoma of the bladder. J Urol 123:640–642, 1980.
8. Skinner DG, Daniels JR, Lieskovsky G: Current status of adjuvant chemotherapy after radical cystectomy for deeply invasive bladder cancer. Urology 24:46–52, 1984.
9. Skinner DG, Lieskovsky G: Contemporary cystectomy with pelvic node dissection compared to preoperative radiation therapy plus cystectomy in management of invasive bladder cancer. J Urol 131:1069, 1984.
10. Skinner DG, Tift JP, Kaufman JJ: High dose, short course preoperative radiation therapy and immediate single stage radical cystectomy with pelvic node dissection in the management of bladder cancer. J Urol 127:671, 1982.
11. Walsh PC, Lepor H, Eggleston JC: Radical prostatectomy with preservation of sexual function: anatomical and pathological consideration. Prostate 4:473–485, 1983.
12. Whitmore WF Jr, Mount BM: A technique of urethrectomy in the male. Surg Gynecol Obstet 131:303, 1970.

THOMAS E. AHLERING, M.D.
GARY LIESKOVSKY, M.D.

Surgical Treatment of Urethral Cancer in the Male Patient

CHAPTER 43

Carcinoma of the urethra may arise primarily in the urethra or more commonly in association with transitional cell cancer of the lower urinary tract. The first section of this chapter will discuss the management of primary carcinoma of the urethra and will include tumors of Cowper's and Littre's glands. The second section will outline our management of the urethra in patients with transitional cell carcinoma of the bladder.

PRIMARY CARCINOMA OF THE URETHRA

History

The first reported case of primary urethral carcinoma was described by Thiaudierre in 1834.[30] Kirwin in 1932 questioned the validity of that case because it was a small lesion in a young man who was cured by local excision and cautery.[14] Hutchinson reported the first apparently verified case of primary urethral cancer in 1861 in London, but Wasserman is credited for the first significant paper, on a series of 20 men, in 1895.[32] More than four decades later, Kreutzmann and Colloff[18] divided primary urethral carcinoma according to the urethral segment from which the tumor arose: (1) anterior portion (penile urethra) and (2) the posterior portion (bulbomembranous and prostatic urethra).

They reported that 35 of 65 patients with anteriorly placed lesions recovered after partial penile amputations, whereas only 10 of 77 recovered after treatment for posteriorly located tumors. These posterior lesions were generally treated by radical excision, including emasculation and perineal urethrostomy. In the same year, Hugh Hampton Young demonstrated that small posterior urethral lesions could be radically excised while the penis and testicles were spared.[32] In the 1950s treatment of larger lesions of the posterior urethra was altered to allow preservation of the scrotum, testes, and, if feasible, the penis, along with ureterocolonic supravesical diversion.[12, 20, 31] Little has changed since the 1950s except for better urinary diversion and the adoption of a staging system by Ray and Whitmore in 1977.[23] To date, fewer than 600 cases of primary urethral carcinoma have been reported.[10]

Anatomy

The urethra, with an average length of 21 cm, can be divided into three regions: the prostatic, the bulbomembranous, and the penile. The prostatic portion is lined with transitional epithelium, the bulbomembranous and penile portions with pseudostratified or stratified columnar epithelium, and the meatus with squamous epithelium. The urethra consists of a mucosal lining, submucosa, and, from the bulbous portion to

622

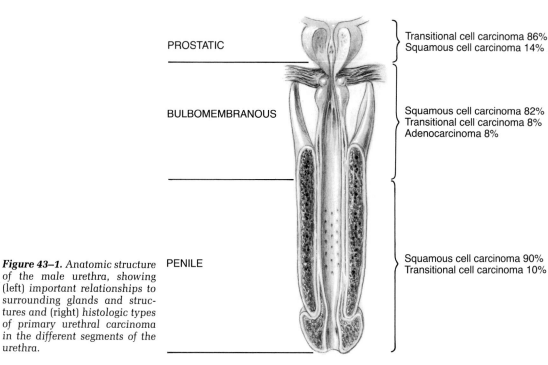

PROSTATIC — Transitional cell carcinoma 86%
Squamous cell carcinoma 14%

BULBOMEMBRANOUS — Squamous cell carcinoma 82%
Transitional cell carcinoma 8%
Adenocarcinoma 8%

PENILE — Squamous cell carcinoma 90%
Transitional cell carcinoma 10%

Figure 43–1. *Anatomic structure of the male urethra, showing* (left) *important relationships to surrounding glands and structures and* (right) *histologic types of primary urethral carcinoma in the different segments of the urethra.*

the meatus, a surrounding corpus spongiosum. Through most of its course the urethra is in apposition with the ventrally placed paired corpora cavernosa, and all three are surrounded by Buck's fascia. Cowper's glands are paired and lie within the urogenital diaphragm and drain into the bulbous urethra. The glands of Littre are small lubricating glands located in the bulbous urethra (Fig. 43–1).

The major blood supply to the penis and urethra is from the internal pudendal artery; however, sufficient collateral supply from the surrounding skin is usually present to allow vitality even if both pudendal arteries are ligated.[12] Lymphatic drainage of lesions in the anterior or penile urethra confined within Buck's fascia drain to the deep inguinal and external iliac nodes. Lesions penetrating Buck's fascia drain to the superficial inguinal nodes. Lesions of the posterior urethra drain to (1) the deep inguinal nodes along the dorsal vein, (2) the obturator and iliac nodes along the pudendal vessels, and (3) posterior to the presacral nodes.

Histopathology

The histologic type of carcinoma varies with the urethral segment from which it arises (Fig. 43–1). The prostatic portion accounts for 9% of primary urethral carcinomas; the bulbomembranous, 55%; and the penile portion, 36%.[29] In addition to development of squamous and transitional cell carcinoma within the bulbomembranous portion, adenocarcinomas, which may arise from glandular metaplasia or from Cowper's gland or the glands of Littre, may also appear. Frequently, the origin of these tumors cannot be exactly localized. Nevertheless, they present and are managed in the same manner as all other posterior urethral carcinomas. Some of these adenocarcinomas may have striking similarities histologically to colonic adenocarcinoma, as reported by Scott in 1952[26] and others since.[4, 19]

Etiology

The association of urethral stricture disease to primary carcinoma of the urethra was suggested as early as 1895 by Wasserman.[32] About 50% of all urethral tumors are associated with urethral stricture[11] and its attendant inflammation. Chronic inflammation may induce squamous metaplasia followed by malignant transformation similar to squamous cell cancer of the lung. Venereal disease seems to be related through subsequent stricture disease. Gonorrhea as a direct cause seems unlikely because, as stated by Kretschmer in 1923,[17] "gonococcal infection of the male urethra is common and carcinoma rare, the gonococcus plays little if any etiologic role in the production of this disease." Trauma to the urethra and recurrent dilations have also been cited.[32]

Symptoms

The average age for primary urethral carcinoma is 60 years, with a range of 13 to 90 years. The nature of this lesion would lead one to expect patients to present with urinary obstructive symptoms (occurring in approximately 50% of cases) similar to urethral stricture disease. The lack of specificity of these symptoms usually results in delayed diagnosis, and the association of a urethral mass (40 to 60%) with these symptoms should alert one to carcinoma. Other symptoms may include hematuria, blood per meatus, and hemospermia. Urethral carcinoma has been found in conjunction with periurethral abscesses and urethrocutaneous fistulae.[10, 11]

Diagnosis

The most difficult problem with primary urethral carcinoma is the initial suspicion for the disease. Evaluation begins with palpation of the urethra and retrograde urethrography. Figure 43–2 demonstrates radio-

Table 43–1. STAGING SYSTEM FOR CARCINOMA OF THE URETHRA*

Stage	Characteristic
Stage 0	Confined to the mucosa (in situ)
Stage A	Into but not beyond the lamina propria
Stage B	Into but not beyond the substance of the corpus spongiosum (or into but not beyond the prostate)
Stage C	Direct extension into tissues beyond the corpus spongiosum, e.g., the corpora cavernosa, muscle, fat, fascia, skin, direct skeletal involvement (or beyond the prostatic capsule)
Stage D_1	Regional metastasis including inguinal or pelvic lymph nodes
Stage D_2	Distant metastasis

*From Ray B, et al: Experience with primary carcinoma of the male urethra. J Urol 117:591–594, 1977.

graphically a small lesion in a patient with primary carcinoma in the proximal third of the urethra. If a mass is palpated in a patient with stricture disease, one should include, in addition to more common problems such as periurethral fibrosis, periurethral abscess, or urethrocutaneous fistula, the possibility of urethral carcinoma. Definitive diagnosis is established by cystoscopic or percutaneous biopsy. In difficult mass lesions associated with periurethral abscesses or fistulae, urine cytologic studies may establish the presence of tumor,[13] but open biopsy is often necessary.

The natural history of primary urethral carcinoma is characterized by extensive local disease with metastasis to regional nodes. Even though these tumors frequently invade the vascular corporal bodies of the penis, widespread metastases are typically found late in the course of the disease. Thorough evaluation under anesthesia should include panendoscopy, bimanual examination, and rectoperineal examination of the perineum to assess involvement of the prostate, urogenital diaphragm, and the corporal bodies of the penis. Palpable inguinal lymphadenopathy is highly indicative of metastatic nodal disease and usually is secondary to tumors of the penile portion of the urethra. This is in distinction to squamous cell cancer of the penis, in which lymphadenopathy is often secondary to infection.

Assessment for metastasis should include chest x-ray, intravenous urogram, liver function tests, bone scan, and CT scan of the abdomen and pelvis. The most widely accepted staging system is that proposed by Ray and associates in 1977 (Table 43–1).[23]

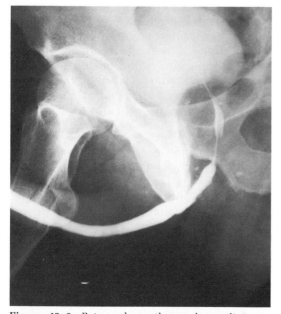

Figure 43–2. Retrograde urethrography outlining a mass in the proximal urethra that proved to be invasive.

TREATMENT OF ANTERIOR URETHRAL TUMORS

Surgical management of anterior tumors is directed at complete resection with adequate margins. Generally, partial amputation of the penis, including 2 cm of tissue free of disease proximal to the lesion, has resulted in a very low recurrence rate.[10, 11, 23] The limit of partial penectomy is a shaft long enough to allow the patient to direct his urinary stream. If there is insufficient length after resection of the tumor, then the patient usually requires total penectomy and a permanent perineal urethrostomy. Recurrence rates are higher after total penectomy than for partial amputation because of the extensiveness of the lesions.[11, 23] Prophylactic inguinal lymph node dissection has not demonstrated a significant survival advantage but, for palpable inguinal nodes, lymphadenectomy can control regional disease.[2, 10, 11, 23]

Radiation and chemotherapy have had limited use in the management of these tumors and should be used only as an adjunct to surgery. These tumors are not sensitive to hormonal manipulation and thus estrogens or orchiectomy should be avoided.

Durable survival rates for anterior urethral tumors treated surgically have generally been 50 to 60%,[2, 10, 11, 23] whereas untreated patients have generally fared very poorly.[11]

TREATMENT OF POSTERIOR URETHRAL TUMORS

In Kaplan's review of 46 patients who received no treatment or palliative treatment only, 44 were known to have died, with a median survival of three months and a range of one week to 15 months.[11] The disease is characterized by local extension rather than early dissemination, and Ray[23] reported that 12 of 14 patients presented with Stage C or D disease. Patients treated with radiation have high recurrence rates, and there are only rare instances of long-term survivors.[12] Since Marshall's report[20] in 1957 that four of five patients treated with radical excision survived five years or more without evidence of disease, management has been directed at surgical extirpation. Most authors agree that disease in Stage C or D is best controlled by en bloc radical excision of the urethra and mass, resection of the urogenital diaphragm, cystoprostatectomy, and bilateral pelvic and iliac lymph node dissection. The testis, distal corpora cavernosa, and penis are not involved and should be spared if possible. To improve surgical margins, some authors have advocated en bloc pubectomy or resection of the inferior pubic rami.[5, 15, 27] Urinary diversion usually is carried out by using an ileal loop. As with anterior tumors, inguinal node dissection is withheld unless there is palpable inguinal lymphadenopathy. Historically, the five-year survival rates of 10 to 20% have been dismal.[29] In a review of published series since 1981, fifteen patients were treated for cure using radical extirpation with or without preoperative radiation therapy (Table 43–2).[2, 5, 10, 15] Four patients died of progressive disease, and two patients died (at 101 and 39 months, respectively) without evidence of disease. Nine patients (60%) are alive without evidence of disease (range, 7 to 82 months), with a median follow-up of 40 months.

Table 43–2. SUMMARY OF SURVIVAL STATUS FOR PATIENTS WITH PRIMARY URETHRAL CARCINOMA TREATED WITH RADICAL SURGERY, REPORTED SINCE 1981

First Author	Reference	Dead of Disease (range, in months)	Survival Status (range, in months) Alive, No Evidence of Disease	Dead, No Evidence of Disease
Klein	15	1–13*	1–82†	1–101
		1–9*	1–9†	1–39
			1–9†	
Bracken	5		1–18	
			1–48	
			1–60	
Anderson	2	1–8	1–7	
			1–9	
Hopkins	10	1–30‡	1–122	
Total, mean follow-up		4–15	9–40	2–70

*Received 6000 rads preoperative radiation
†Received 2000 rads preoperative radiation.
‡Received 3000 rads postoperative radiation.

Stage A or B disease may be successfully treated with local resection and urethral anastomosis.[2, 19, 23, 32] A combination of trans-urethral resection and topical chemotherapy has recently been espoused, but follow-up has been too short to recommend this form of management.[10, 16] However, we feel that the aggressive nature of posterior urethral carcinoma, inherent inaccuracy of staging small lesions, and the lethal consequences of inadequate treatment of Stage A or B disease suggest urethrocystoprostatectomy as the optimal treatment of choice.

Preoperative radiation as an adjunct may be helpful and has been advocated by the group at Memorial Sloan-Kettering Cancer Center.[15] Chemotherapy has not yet been shown to be beneficial, but trials similar to those currently in use to study bladder cancer are likely to reveal the area of greatest improvement in the management of this disease.

URETHRAL CARCINOMA FOLLOWING BLADDER CANCER

History

In 1945 Melicow[21] reported that transitional cell cancer of the renal pelvis may be associated with tumors in the ureter, bladder, and urethra. Three cases documenting recurrence of carcinoma in the urethra in patients who had their bladders removed were reported in 1948.[6] Melicow and Hollowell later pointed out that urothelium can be multicentrically involved with carcinoma in situ (CIS) and that these sites may be responsible for temporally separated recurrences.[22] Ashworth,[3] in 1956, was the first to statistically associate urethral recurrence after treatment for bladder cancer. He reviewed 1307 patients with bladder tumors and found that 54 subsequently developed urethral papillomas (4.1%). Cordonnier and Spjut[6] similarly reported 4.02% urethral tumor occurrence after cystectomy in 174 patients in 1962. Gowing,[8] in 1960, drew attention to the relatively high incidence of urethral CIS in patients with bladder cancer. His autopsy study of 33 men who died of bladder cancer showed 18% to have urethral CIS. In an expanded series of 101 men who died of bladder cancer, Hendry, Gowing, and Wallace[9] confirmed their initial finding that

19% had urethral CIS. Because the urethra may recur with overt tumor or CIS, large series since 1970 put the incidence of subsequent urethral involvement between 8 and 12%.[1, 7, 24]

Indications for Urethrectomy

Some urologists have advocated prophylactic urethrectomy in all patients undergoing radical cystectomy.[1,7] It is evident that patients with overt anterior urethral tumor or tumor extending into the prostatic urethra should undergo simultaneous total urethrectomy in continuity with the radical cystectomy. It is our opinion that patients at low risk for urethral recurrence may be safely managed without routine prophylactic urethrectomy.[9]

All male patients who have cystectomy need careful examination of the pathologic slides for: (1) invasion of the prostate (P4), (2) carcinoma in situ of the prostatic urethra, and (3) carcinoma in situ of the bladder. If there is invasion of the prostate or carcinoma in situ of the prostatic urethra, the patient is scheduled for prophylactic total urethrectomy including excision of the fossa navicularis.[25] The rest of our patients and especially those with multifocal CIS of the bladder need urethral cytologic examinations every 6 to 12 months indefinitely. If the urethral cytologic results become positive, then total urethrectomy is performed.

Symptomatic development of a urethral tumor is most commonly heralded by blood per meatus. The average interval between cystectomy and development of recurrence among our patients was 42 months (range, 12 to 106 months).[1] Less frequently, a patient may present with a mass along the urethra or with pruritus of the glans. If a patient develops blood per meatus, we proceed to total urethrectomy; otherwise, if there is doubt about the origin of the symptom, we recommend urethral cytologic examination and occasionally urethroscopy and biopsy.

Urethral cytologic specimens are obtained by inserting a small red Robinson catheter in the urethra, lavaging about 20 ml of normal saline back and forth, and collecting the wash.

Anatomy

The important anatomic features of the urethra with regard to transitional cell cancer following bladder cancer focus around the corpus spongiosum. Lesions confined to the submucosa should be cured after total urethrectomy, whereas lesions that infiltrate the corpus spongiosum are at risk for lymphatic or hematogenous dissemination. The lymphatic drainage of the corpus spongiosum is normally to the deep inguinal and external iliac nodes; however, after interruption of these channels with prior pelvic lymph node dissection, the primary nodes become the superficial inguinal nodes.

Preoperative Care

Preoperative care of patients undergoing radical cystectomy alone or combined with en bloc cystourethrectomy is described in Chapter 42. In patients undergoing delayed urethrectomy, no specific preparation is required. The exception is for insertion of a penile prosthesis; an aminoglycoside is administered parenterally to such a patient the evening before surgery.

SURGICAL TECHNIQUE OF EN BLOC CYSTECTOMY AND URETHRECTOMY

Since radical cystectomy in a woman includes removal of the entire urethra, the following discussion of en bloc cystourethrectomy applies only to men.

After the patient has been prepped and draped in the frog-leg position (Fig. 43–3), a Foley catheter is inserted, the bladder drained, and the catheter clamped. At the same time that one team starts on the abdominal portion of the procedure, a midline perineal skin incision is made in the area of the bulbous urethra for a distance of about 6 cm and is carried through the subcutaneous fascia onto the bulbocavernosus muscle (Fig. 43–4A). This muscle is divided in the midline, exposing the palpable bulbous urethra. Incision of Buck's fascia on either side of the bulbous urethra permits separation of the urethra from the corpora cavernosa (Fig. 43–4B). An umbilical tape can then be passed around the urethra for traction to facilitate dissection (Fig. 43–5). Continued sharp dissection of Buck's fascia allows the corpus spongiosum to be separated from both corpora cavernosa, proximally to the membranous urethra and distally to the glandular urethra. Invagination of the glans further assists in sharply dissecting the urethra from attachments within the glans (Fig. 43–6). Throughout the dissection, meticulous hemostasis is maintained by diathermy. Then the meatus is circumcised and the urethra is dissected free from its intraglandular investments (Fig. 43–7). The distal

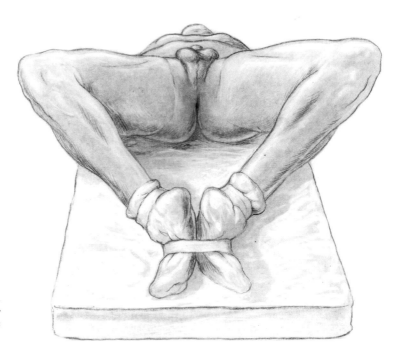

Figure 43–3. Frog-leg position allows simultaneous exposure for perineal and abdominal incisions for en bloc cystourethrectomy.

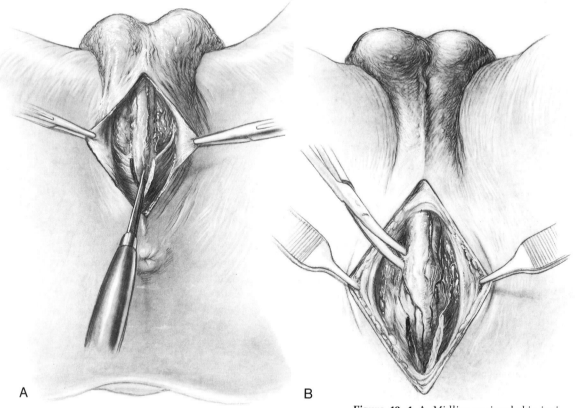

A

B

Figure 43–4. A, Midline perineal skin incision is created at the level of the bulbous urethra. B, The bulbocavernosus muscle is divided in the midline, and the plane between the corpus spongiosum and corpora cavernosa is developed.

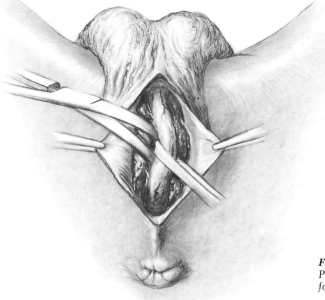

Figure 43–5. An umbilical tape or small Penrose drain passed around the urethra for traction facilitates urethral dissection.

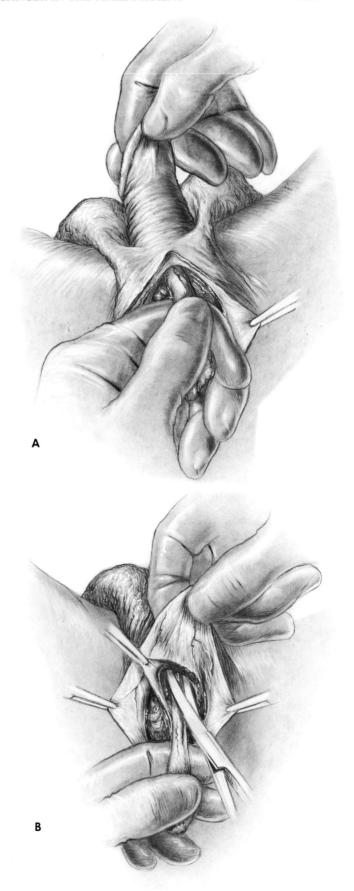

Figure 43–6. *A, The glans is invaginated.*
B, The glans is invaginated to allow distal
dissection of the urethra under direct vision.

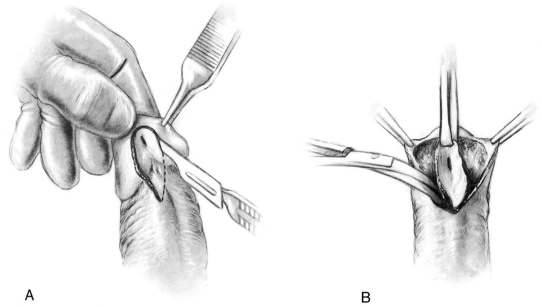

A   B

Figure 43–7. A, *The meatus is sharply circumcised.* B, *The glandular urethra is dissected from its investments.*

urethra is freed and then clamped (to prevent spillage) and delivered into the perineal wound. The membranous urethra can be dissected from the urogenital diaphragm and removed en bloc with the prostate and bladder (Fig. 43–8).

The glans is then closed with interrupted mattress sutures of 3-0 Dexon. A small Penrose drain is placed to the level of the glans, exiting from the perineal incision site (Fig.

43–9); it is removed on the following day. The perineal incision is loosely approximated, and the bulbocavernosus muscle and subcutaneous fascia are closed with interrupted 3-0 Dexon sutures. After both the abdominal and perineal wounds are closed, the abdominal incision is appropriately dressed; a loose gauze dressing, held in place by a T binder, is applied to the perineal incision. The penis should be loosely se-

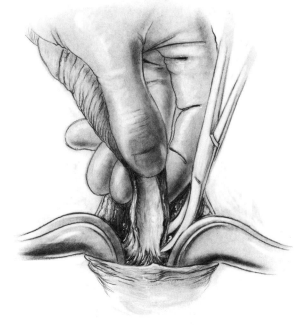

Figure 43–8. *The membranous urethra is dissected free of the urogenital diaphragm in preparation for en bloc removal of the bladder and urethra.*

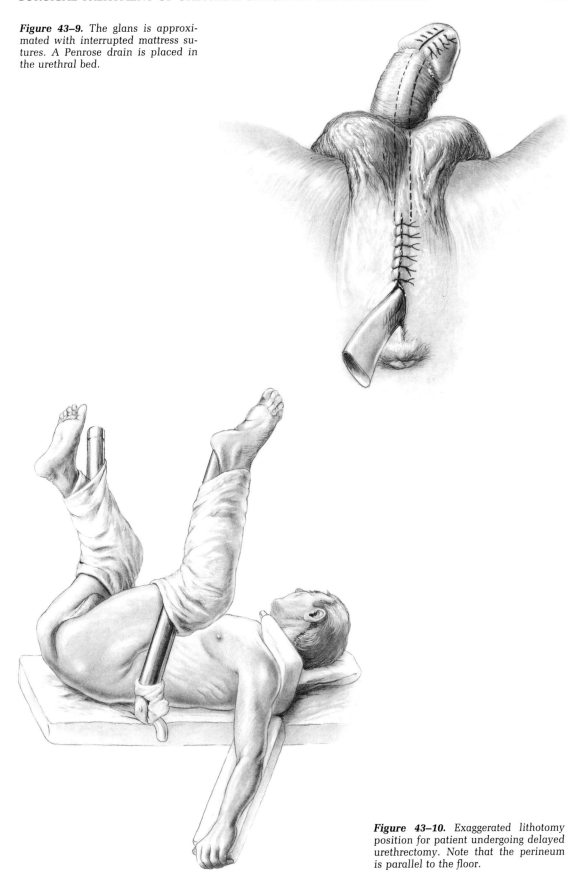

Figure 43–9. The glans is approximated with interrupted mattress sutures. A Penrose drain is placed in the urethral bed.

Figure 43–10. Exaggerated lithotomy position for patient undergoing delayed urethrectomy. Note that the perineum is parallel to the floor.

cured to the abdomen to facilitate venous return and decrease penile edema, which follows when the penis is allowed to hang in the dependent position. Circumferential penile dressings are not recommended, since they tend to impede the vascular supply to the penis.

DELAYED URETHRECTOMY

In patients undergoing delayed urethrectomy for urethral recurrence, a similar approach is used, albeit with some minor modifications. The patient is positioned in the exaggerated lithotomy position and the external genitalia are suitably prepared (Fig. 43–10). The bulbous urethra is dissected free and the severed membranous urethra identified. This is facilitated by inserting a catheter into the apex of the retained urethra, allowing accurate dissection of the urethra off the urogenital diaphragm and preventing inadvertent opening of the urethra. After the bulbous and pendulous portions of the urethra have been completely freed from the corpora cavernosa, a Penrose drain is applied as a tourniquet to the base of the penis for hemostasis in preparation for dissecting the fossa navicularis, as previously described. The entire urethra is then removed.

POSTOPERATIVE CARE AND COMPLICATIONS

In patients undergoing either en bloc cystourethrectomy or delayed urethrectomy, the site previously occupied by the urethra is the only area requiring drainage. This is accomplished by inserting a one-half–inch Penrose drain to the level of the glans penis, exiting from the perineal incision. Unless drainage is excessive, the drain is removed on the following day.

It has been our policy to give anticoagulants prophylactically to all patients undergoing radical cystectomy or cystourethrectomy by using oral warfarin (Coumadin). Ten mg are given down the nasogastric tube in the recovery room, and a subsequent individualized daily dose sufficient to maintain the prothrombin time between one and a half to two times control is administered until the patient is ambulatory. Patients undergoing delayed urethrectomy

are not given prophylactic anticoagulants, but early ambulation is encouraged.

In our experience, complications resulting from urethrectomy have been minimal with one major exception. A 70-year-old black man who had undergone total urethrectomy developed delayed hemorrhage from the glans the evening of surgery. The bleeding was controlled by packing the area; however, the patient subsequently developed extensive necrosis of the glans and distal shaft of the penis, necessitating total penectomy. Based on this experience, we recommend that any significant postoperative bleeding following urethrectomy should be managed by immediate surgical exploration, and that the source of bleeding be identified and ligated by suture.

References

1. Ahlering TE, Lieskovsky G, Skinner DG: Indications for urethrectomy in men undergoing single stage radical cystectomy for bladder cancer. J Urol 131:657–659, 1984.
2. Anderson KA, McAninch JW: Primary squamous cell carcinoma of anterior male urethra. Urology 23:134–140, 1984.
3. Ashworth A: Papillomatosis of the urethra. Br J Urol 28:3–13, 1956.
4. Bourque JL, Charghi A, Gauthier GE, et al: Primary carcinoma of Cowper's gland. J Urol 103:758–761, 1970.
5. Bracken RB: Exenterative surgery for posterior urethral cancer. Urology 19:248–251, 1982.
6. Cordonnier JJ, Spjut HJ: Urethral occurrence of bladder carcinoma following cystectomy. J Urol 87:398–403, 1962.
7. Faysal MH: Urethrectomy in men with transitional cell carcinoma of the bladder. Urology 16:23–26, 1980.
8. Gowing NF: Urethral carcinoma associated with cancer of the bladder. Br J Urol 32:428–439, 1960.
9. Hendry WF, Gowing NF, Wallace DM: Surgical treatment of urethral tumours associated with bladder cancer. Proc R Soc Med 67:304–307, 1974.
10. Hopkins SC, Nag SK, Soloway MS: Primary carcinoma of male urethra. Urology 23:128–133, 1984.
11. Kaplan GW, Bulkley GJ, Grayhack JT: Carcinoma of the male urethra. J Urol 98:365–371, 1967.
12. Kaufman JJ, Goodwin WE: Carcinoma of the male urethra: one stage surgical treatment by radical perineal excision and rectal transplantation of the divided trigone. Surg Gynec Obstet 97:627–632, 1953.
13. King LR: Carcinoma of the urethra in male patients. J Urol 91:555–559, 1964.
14. Kirwin TJ: Primary epithelioma of the urethra. J Urol 27:539–560, 1932.
15. Klein FA, Whitmore WF Jr, Herr HW, et al: Inferior pubic rami resection with en bloc radical excision for invasive proximal urethral carcinoma. Cancer 51:1238–1242, 1983.
16. Konnak JW: Conservative management of low grade

neoplasms of the male urethra: a preliminary report. J Urol 123:175–177, 1980.

17. Kretschmer HL: Primary carcinoma of the male urethra. Arch Surg 6:830–836, 1923.

18. Kreutzmann HAR, Colloff B: Primary carcinoma of the male urethra. Arch Surg 39:513–529, 1939.

19. Lieber MM, Malek RS, Farrow GM, McMurtry J: Villous adenocarcinoma of the male urethra. J Urol 130:1191–1193, 1983.

20. Marshall VF: Radical excision of locally extensive carcinoma of the deep male urethra. J Urol 78:252–266, 1957.

21. Melicow MM: Tumors of the urinary drainage tract: Urothelial tumors. J Urol 54:186–193, 1945.

22. Melicow MM, Hollowell JW: Intra-urothelial cancer: carcinoma in situ, Bowen's disease of the urinary system: discussion of 30 cases. J Urol 68:763–772, 1952.

23. Ray B, Canto AR, Whitmore WF Jr: Experience with primary carcinoma of the male urethra. J Urol 117:591–594, 1977.

24. Schellhammer PF, Whitmore WF Jr: Transitional cell carcinoma of the urethra in men having cystectomy for bladder cancer. J Urol 115:56–60, 1976.

25. Schellhammer PF, Whitmore WF Jr: Urethral meatal carcinoma following cystourethrectomy for bladder carcinoma. J Urol 115:61–64, 1976.

26. Scott EV, Barelare B: Adenocarcinoma of the male urethra. J Urol 68:311–319, 1952.

27. Shuttleworth KE, Lloyd-Davies RW: Radical resection for tumours involving the posterior urethra. Br J Urol 41:739–743, 1969.

28. Stams UK, Gursel EO, Veenema RJ: Prophylactic urethrectomy in male patients with bladder cancer. J Urol 111:177–179, 1974.

29. Sullivan J, Grabstald H: Management of carcinoma of the urethra. In DG Skinner, JB deKernion (eds), Genitourinary Cancer. Philadelphia, WB Saunders, 1978, p 419.

30. Thiaudierre PD: Nouvelle espece de retrecissment de l'uretre; nouveau procede operatoire. Bull Gen de Therap 1834, p 210.

31. Uhle CAW, Holfelner ED: Treatment of carcinoma of the male urethra by radical surgical infrapubic removal: a case report. J Urol 68:302–310, 1952.

32. Young HH: A new radical operation for carcinoma of the bulbous urethra: new use for penis. Surg Gynec Obstet 68:77–86, 1939.

STUART D. BOYD, M.D.
GARY LIESKOVSKY, M.D.
DONALD G. SKINNER, M.D.

Cutaneous Urinary Diversion in the Cancer Patient

CHAPTER 44

In the early 1980s, the most readily accepted and frequently employed forms of supravesical urinary diversion were ureteroenterostomies that required wearing an external collecting appliance. The most popular of these cutaneous diversions utilized the ileum, the ileocecal segment, the jejunum, or the sigmoid colon as a transporting conduit. Each type of conduit had its own peculiar limitations, and no one diversion found universal acceptance.

Recently, various forms of continent urinary diversions have drawn attention away from the previously more established conduit diversions. There is a cosmetic as well as a functional appeal to the continent form. It is important to remember, however, that the cutaneous diversions have had more than 30 years of follow-up, along with a predictability and flexibility that continue to make them a good alternative to any of the more complicated continent forms. Urologic surgeons need to be familiar with several types of conduits in order to be able to respond to any of the variety of circumstances that may present at the time of diversion. It is the purpose of this chapter to describe the surgical technique, possible complications, and advantages of each of the major cutaneous conduit forms of ureterointestinal diversion.

ILEAL CONDUIT DIVERSION

Although Seiffert is credited with performing the first ureteroileal cutaneous urinary diversion in 1935, it was not until after Bricker's description of the procedure in 1950 that the technique achieved widespread acceptance to become the most common type of supravesical diversion.[3, 26] Over the years, the basic surgical technique has remained unchanged; however, there have been modifications in stomal construction (see Chapter 45) and ureteral implantation into the isolated ileal segment. Individual ureteral implantation into the proximal end of the ileal segment (Bricker technique) combined with anchoring the base of the conduit to the periosteum of the sacral promontory[14] has been previously described and extensively studied.[22] This technique has proved to be extremely reliable and virtually free of early technical failure.[24] Alternatively, Wallace and Barzilay have described methods of joining the two ureters together and implanting the conjoined unit into the side of the ileal segment or anastomosing it to the open end of the proximal conduit.[2, 31] In a comparison of these methods of ureteral implantation, Esho reported that in a group of nonirradiated patients, no significant difference was demonstrated between the Bricker

634

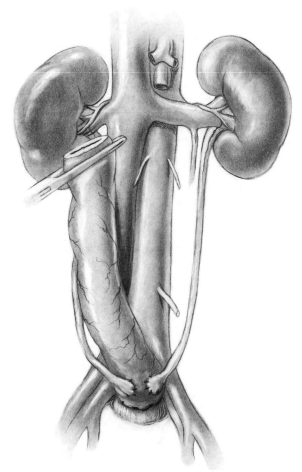

Figure 44–1. *Leadbetter's technique of ileal loop diversion. Ureters are anastomosed end to side near the base of the conduit, and the base is further sutured to the sacral promontory or the overlying fibrous tissue.*

versus the Wallace technique regarding deterioration of the upper urinary tracts.[5]

Our personal experience with more than 300 patients undergoing ureteroileal cutaneous diversion favors a modified Leadbetter ureteroileal anastomosis, joining the spatulated ureters end-to-side to the ileal segment near its base, and, when feasible, anchoring the base to the sacral promontory (Fig. 44–1). This technique combined with that for the Turnbull stoma is the basis of our approach.[29]

Patient Preparation

Generally, patients undergoing ureteroileal cutaneous diversion with or without a concomitant cystectomy are admitted the day prior to surgery. They are encouraged to be on a low-roughage diet at home before entering the hospital. Following breakfast on the admission day, the patients receive only a clear liquid diet. That morning an emulsified castor oil preparation (Neoloid, 120 ml) is administered; this provides an excellent mechanical component for cleansing the bowel. In addition, patients receive 1 gm of neomycin orally every hour for four doses, beginning at 1000 hours, and then 1 gm every four hours from 1600 hours until midnight. Erythromycin base, 1 gm, is added at 1200, 1600, 2000, and 2400 hours to more effectively inhibit the growth of anaerobic colonic bacteria, particularly *Bacteroides fragilis*. For patients in whom additional colonic surgery is planned, a neomycin retention enema (200 ml of a 1% solution) is given the night before, as well as the morning of surgery. This extremely effective yet short bowel preparation program is very well tolerated by the patients and prevents the dehydration phenomenon commonly associated with prolonged catharsis. Patients also receive additional preoperative hydration with intravenous Ringer's lactate or 5% dextrose and 0.5 normal saline at a rate of 125 ml per hour beginning the evening prior to surgery. When urinary diversion is combined with a radical cystectomy or anterior exenteration, preoperative preparation also includes prophylactic digitalization, especially in patients over the age of 50 years, in whom there is no specific contraindication.

Perhaps the most crucial point in preparing the patient for surgery is to identify accurately the most suitable position for the cutaneous stoma. This should be done with the assistance of an enterostomal therapist while examining the patient in the supine, sitting, and standing position. It is essential that the external appliance over the predetermined stoma site not impinge on adjacent bony structures such as the anterior-superior iliac spine or costal margin, or overlie abdominal scars, creases, or belt lines. In difficult patients, particularly the obese, it is helpful to have the patient wear the appliance for several days preoperatively to ensure proper stomal placement. An additional consideration in the obese patient is to position the stoma slightly higher than usual in order to allow easier visualization when changing the appliance. A preoperative scratch mark or tattoo with subcutaneous methylene blue will prevent removal of an erasable mark during the surgical preparation.

Operative Technique

A lower midline incision converted to an upper paramedian incision above the umbilicus is utilized to enter the peritoneal cavity. The ascending colon is mobilized from the right paracolic gutter. The peritoneal attachments between the terminal ileum and the sacral promontory are divided, thus mobilizing the ascending colon and terminal ileum up to the point at which the retroperitoneal portion of the duodenum crosses the midline. The descending and sigmoid colon are mobilized along the left paracolic gutter laterally, while medially the base of the sigmoid mesentery is freed distally from the sacral promontory and distal aorta up to the origin of the inferior mesenteric artery. This permits easy passage under the sigmoid mesentery of the left ureter without kinking or angulation that may subsequently result in necrosis or hydroureteronephrosis. After the bowel has been adequately mobilized, each ureter is identified and traced into the pelvis distal to the iliac vessels, where they are individually divided between ligatures or hemostatic clips. It is important to inform the anesthesiologist that the ureters have been divided, to prevent excessive administration of IV fluids based on diminished urine output. Ligating the proximal ends of the ureters allows them to hydrodilate, further facilitating the subsequent ureteroileal anastomosis.

It is important to avoid excessive proximal mobilization of the ureter from the spermatic cord or infundibulopelvic ligament, both of which provide additional collateral blood supply to the midureter. Frozen section of the proximal ends of each ureter is routinely performed in patients with bladder cancer to determine the presence or absence of significant urothelial changes prior to ureteral implantation into the ileal segment. It is our preference, in patients also undergoing a radical cystectomy and bilateral pelvic iliac lymph node dissection, to complete that portion of the surgery before proceeding with the urinary diversion in order to avoid inadvertent damage to the conduit from overzealous retraction during subsequent cystectomy. Others may prefer to complete the ureteroileal anastomosis after the proximal pelvic node dissection is completed. In this way the operative team is fresh and more careful attention can be directed to the critical details of the ureteroileal anastomosis.

Removal of the appendix is performed routinely, after which a suitable segment of distal ileum is identified and isolated, as illustrated in Figure 44–2. The avascular plane in the mesentery between the ileocolic artery and the terminal branches of the superior mesenteric artery, or alternatively the region between the right colic artery and the ileocolic artery, is easily identified, defining a broad vascular pedicle to the ileal segment to be isolated. Rarely is it necessary to use illumination to identify this vascular pedicle, which is readily palpable.

We prefer to divide the mesentery between the ileocolic artery and the terminal branches of the superior mesenteric artery, extending the incision into the base of the mesentery, which provides for a lengthy distal mesenteric division. The distal small bowel is then transected between well-positioned Welsh-Allyn bowel clamps, usually at a point approximately 15 cm from the ileocecal junction. Alternatively, the bowel can be divided by using an automatic stapling apparatus, depending on the surgeon's preference. After determining an appropriate length of small bowel required for the con-

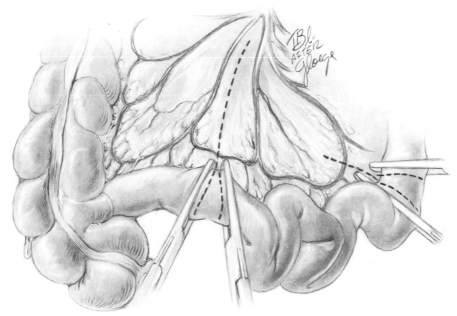

Figure 44–2. A suitable segment of ileum is selected for the conduit. Note that the distal mesenteric division should be lengthy and can usually utilize the avascular plane extending almost to the origin of the ileocolic artery. The proximal mesenteric division should be short in order to provide a broad vascular pedicle for the conduit.

duit, a short division of the proximal mesentery is made, providing a broad vascular pedicle to the segment (Fig. 44–3). The bowel at this point is once again divided by using a stapling device or between Welsh-Allyn bowel clamps. When the latter are used, the proximal end of the isolated intestinal segment is then closed with standard 3-0 chromic Parker-Kerr suture in two layers and reinforced by an additional interrupted

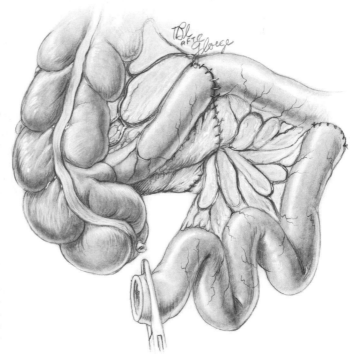

Figure 44–3. A lengthy distal mesenteric division provides maximal mobility and length so that the conduit can reach the skin without tension. The bowel anastomosis can be performed either with sutures or staples, depending on the surgeon's preference. It is also important to close the mesenteric trap above the conduit.

seromuscular layer of 4-0 silk. The stapled closure may be oversewn with a running suture of 3-0 polyglycolic acid (PGA).

When technically feasible, the base of the conduit is anchored either to the periosteum overlying the sacral promontory or to retroperitoneal fibroareolar tissue in the region of the aortic bifurcation. Traction on the ileal loop during construction of the stoma must be avoided to prevent avulsion of the anchored proximal end, which may result in urinary leakage from the base of the conduit. An end-to-side ureteroileal anastomosis is then performed approximately 2 to 3 cm above the closed end of the loop (Fig. 44–4).

After the appropriate length of ureter required to perform a tension-free anastomosis is determined, the ureter is partially transected from lateral to medial in an oblique fashion. One must first make certain that the ureter has not been twisted and that the left ureter passes under the base of the sigmoid mesentery without angulation or tension. A 4-0 PGA suture is placed at the lateral tip of the proximal ureter and used as a stay suture to avoid trauma to the ureter by forceps. Transection of the remaining ureter is completed and a small hemoclip is placed on the periadventitial blood vessel along the medial side of the ureter above a point destined to be the ureteral apex.

Fine atraumatic forceps are placed into the ureter, spread, and the ureter incised and spatulated medially. An apical suture of 4-0 PGA is placed, after which a small full-thickness ellipse of conduit is removed. The previously placed apical suture is then accurately positioned through the small ileal opening and tied (Fig. 44–4). A meticulous mucosa-to-mucosa anastomosis of interrupted 4-0 PGA suture is performed, proceeding from the proximal apical suture along the spatulation toward the stay suture. The last three or four distal sutures are placed prior to tying the knots to ensure accurate suture placement and ureteral patency.

An important feature of the ureteroileal anastomosis is placement of the suture in the ileum. This suture should include a

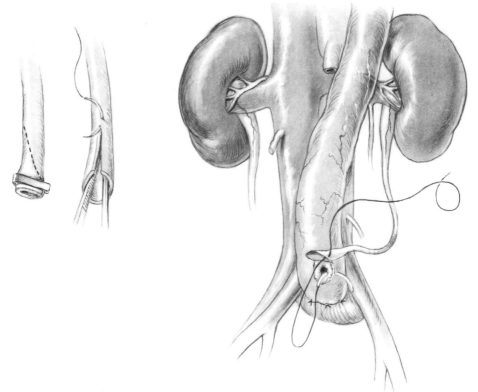

Figure 44–4. The ureteral anastomosis is performed after first obliquely transecting the ureter in a lateral to medial direction and then spatulating the ureter as necessary to provide a generous anastomosis. The anastomosis with interrupted 4-0 polyglycolic acid (PGA) suture (end to side) proceeds after a small full thickness ellipse of conduit has been removed. The first suture is placed at the apex of the ureteral spatulation and then into the lateral edge of the ileal mucosa, including a large bite of muscularis and serosa. Important are a tension-free anastomosis and minimal mechanical manipulation of the ureter with forceps.

small edge of the mucosa but should incorporate a larger bite of the muscularis and serosa. This tends to telescope the anastomosis into the ileum, taking tension off the mucosal portion of the anastomosis. Stents are not routinely employed, and the use of drains is left to the discretion of the responsible surgeon. No attempt is made to ensure that the ureteroileal anastomosis is retroperitoneal, and we have yet to see any problems related to this. There is always a small trap between the sigmoid mesentery, the base of the small bowel mesentery, and the base of the ileal loop that should be closed carefully with several interrupted 4-0 silk sutures to prevent late small bowel herniation and obstruction.

Our experience has shown that the loop stoma, as described by Turnbull, is the most versatile and complication-free.[29] The technique for this stoma is well documented in Chapter 45. Regardless of the type of stoma chosen, several key points should be emphasized about stoma construction: (1) all layers of the abdominal wall should be aligned with heavy clamps in order to ensure a straight exit for the urine; (2) when incising and splitting the rectus, special care must be taken not to injure the epigastric vessels; (3) the bowel should be well secured to the rectus fascia with at least four to six interrupted sutures; and (4) if internal stents are not used, the stoma and conduit should be stented for five to seven days with a No. 16 French fenestrated Robinson catheter to prevent obstruction of urine outflow from early postoperative edema or mucus retention.

A gastrostomy tube is often placed in older patients undergoing a simultaneous cystectomy, in whom prolonged ileus is expected. The abdominal wall is closed in layers and retention sutures are used if any problem of delayed healing is anticipated.

A final note should be made about the irradiated patient. Ileum that has been trapped in the pelvis and then has received more than 6000 rads should be inspected closely for viability. Pale color and a thickened serosa indicate significant radiation damage, and this portion of bowel should be avoided at all costs. Judgment needs to be exercised in selecting the proper segment of bowel. More proximal ileum, jejunum, or colon may be preferable. The urologic surgeon must be prepared to make this selection at the time of surgery and proceed with other options as circumstances dictate.

JEJUNAL CUTANEOUS DIVERSION

The surgical principles and technique of substituting jejunum for ileum as a urinary conduit varies minimally and has been advocated particularly in patients in whom severe radiation damage to the ileum is noted.[7, 12, 20] Originally it was hypothesized that the jejunal conduit might be superior to ileum for urinary diversion since preliminary experiments by Rangel and Jankengt suggested that jejunal segments absorbed less than their ileal counterparts.[11, 24] Clinical experience has not substantiated these earlier experimental claims. In fact, follow-up in jejunal conduit patients has revealed an unusual syndrome of electrolyte disturbances characterized by azotemia, acidosis, hyponatremia, hypovolemia, and hyperkalemia. This jejunal conduit syndrome develops in 25 to 40% of patients, and it is most serious in patients with a creatinine clearance of less than 55 ml/minute and with excessively long conduits.[7, 12] Studies have indicated that the major electrolyte abnormality is one of salt loss, which leads to a further electrolyte disturbance by stimulation of the renin-aldosterone system. Potassium absorption from the conduit and shifts of potassium from intracellular to extracellular spaces secondary to metabolic acidosis can cause an alarming level of hyperkalemia. Supplemental salt intake is required in all patients with this syndrome, in order to provide equilibrium between the amount of salt ingested and that excreted from the conduit.

Current evidence suggests that jejunal conduits are poor alternatives to the standard ileal loop diversion or colon conduits except for the rare patient for whom no other alternative exists. In these cases, the risk of jejunal conduit syndrome can be minimized by selecting patients with normal baseline renal function, constructing the shortest conduit possible, and prophylactically supplying oral electrolytes as needed.

SIGMOID CONDUIT DIVERSION

The concept of utilizing an isolated segment of sigmoid conduit for urinary diversion dates back to 1894, when Mauclaire implanted the ureters of a dog into the intact rectosigmoid previously excluded from the fecal stream by a proximal sigmoid colostomy.[17] Kronig subsequently used this method in 1906 in performing a two-stage procedure for a sarcoma of the uterus.[13] The first stage included exclusion of the rectosigmoid segment and a proximal colostomy, followed subsequently by an anterior exenteration and implantation of the ureters into the defunctionalized rectosigmoid segment. Later, Verhoogen (1908) and Lengemann (1911) isolated either an ileocecal segment or the entire asending colon and anastomosed the ureters to the cecal end while performing an ileal transverse appendicocutaneous transplant.[15, 30] Bricker also utilized an isolated sigmoid segment some 10 years before he made popular the ureteroileal cutaneous form of diversion. None of these approaches achieved widespread acceptance in their day.

Currently, Mogg is given credit for reintroducing ureterocolocutaneous diversion following his report in 1967 on 65 patients who underwent a sigmoid conduit diversion for the treatment of urinary incontinence.[19] He claimed good overall results without operative mortality. Although Mogg used a nipple technique described by Mathisen to prevent ureteral reflux, equally effective antirefluxing procedures using the Leadbetter combined approach or Goodwin's transcolonic technique have been well described with considerable clinical study.[8, 14, 16] We prefer a technique similar to that described by Leadbetter. The type of ureteral implantation used should be dependent on both the surgeon's familiarity with the procedure and intraoperative conditions that may favor one technique over the other. The major advantage of using colon rather than a small bowel segment for urinary diversion obviously is the fact that the thicker colonic musculature allows creation of antirefluxing submucosal tunnels. In addition, the colon provides for a larger and more trouble-free cutaneous stoma.

Preparation

Preparation of the colon is identical to that previously described for ileal conduit urinary diversion, with the addition of a neomycin retention enema (200 ml of a 1% solution) administered the night before surgery and the morning of the operation.

Indications for the use of a sigmoid conduit include: (1) patients, particularly children, with neurogenic bladder dysfunction requiring cutaneous diversion in which reflux should be prevented; (2) patients undergoing total pelvic exenteration that would require creation of a colostomy and thus obviate the need for an additional bowel anastomosis; and (3) patients requiring temporary cutaneous diversion while a major bladder disorder is corrected. In patients undergoing either radical cystectomy or anterior exenteration, the potential impairment of blood supply from the inferior and middle hemorrhoidal arteries to the distal rectosigmoid due to division of the hypogastric artery precludes using the sigmoid as a cutaneous conduit, in our opinion. If colocutaneous diversion is desirable in such patients, we recommend using the transverse colon instead. The best results with this form of diversion are achieved in patients with ureters of normal caliber. In selected patients, however, Hendren has demonstrated that even dilated ureters can be tapered and implanted according to the Leadbetter combined technique with equally good results.[9] Selection of the stoma site, usually in the left lower quadrant, is based on similar criteria to those applied for any stoma requiring an external appliance. It is important preoperatively to exclude patients with significant disorders of the bowel, such as diverticulitis. Barium enema studies and coloendoscopy, especially in patients with a suspicious medical history, should be performed routinely.

Operative Technique

A right paramedian or midline incision is used to enter the peritoneal cavity. The descending and sigmoid colon are extensively mobilized by incising the peritoneal reflection laterally along the line of Toldt. It is imperative that the base of the sigmoid mesentery be freed from the sacral promontory and, cephalad, to the origin of the inferior mesenteric artery. Mobilization of the splenic flexure is rarely required because of redundancy of the sigmoid colon.

An appropriate length of sigmoid colon, usually 15 to 20 cm, is selected and should be longer than anticipated because of the tendency of the bowel to contract once it is divided. A key to selection of this segment is a thorough understanding of the vascular supply to the descending and sigmoid colon. The inferior mesenteric artery gives rise to several sigmoid branches (left colic and superior rectal arteries). These anastomose with the middle rectal artery, which originates from the hypogastric artery (Fig. 44–5). This abundant anastomotic plexus ensures an adequate blood supply to the distal colonic segment.

Maximum mobility is provided by division of a lengthy distal segment of mesentery all the way to the sacrum. This results in division of the superior rectal artery and ensures an excellent blood supply to the isolated segment of colon from the proximal division of the inferior mesenteric artery. The proximal division in the mesentery should be very short, in order to preserve blood supply to the isolated segment of colon. Then the colonic conduit is usually placed laterally and the continuity of the bowel reestablished with a meticulous end-to-end sigmoid bowel anastomosis with interrupted 4-0 silk sutures in two layers (Fig. 44–6). Proximally, the sigmoid conduit is closed with a two-layer Parker-Kerr suture of 3-0 chromic and an additional layer of interrupted 4-0 silk inverting the sutures.

Two 4-0 silk holding sutures are positioned in each tenia approximately 4 cm apart to prepare for the ureteral anastomoses (Fig. 44–7A). The incisions in the teniae for the submucosal tunnels should be staggered, with the right side beginning just distal to the closed end of the conduit and the left side 3 cm or more distally. Developing the submucosal tunnels is further facilitated by injecting several milliliters of a 1:100,000 solution of adrenaline in saline just beneath the muscularis. This also diminishes bleeding and allows for a clear surgical field. A long incision, 3 to 4 cm in length, is made in the teniae and carried through the circular muscle fibers of the colon until the outer mucosa of the bowel is visualized. With traction on the previously placed holding sutures, blunt and sharp dissection with fine scissors or a No. 15 blade allows the submucosal plane to be easily developed. Once the proper plane has been reached, further blunt dissection can be performed using a Kitner dissector. It is important to direct the dissection of each tunnel toward the mesenteric side to prevent devascularization of the area between the two teniae. This technique is not unlike that described by Leadbetter for ureteral implantation in patients undergoing ureterosigmoidostomy, and it has been demonstrated in a film by Skinner and Richie, available from the American

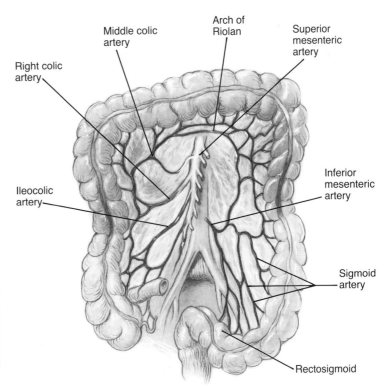

Figure 44–5. The vascular supply of the colon. The sigmoid is supplied by an abundant anastomotic plexus of arteries arising from the inferior mesenteric artery and its sigmoid and superior rectal branches and from the inferior and middle rectal arteries.

Middle colic artery

Arch of Riolan

Superior mesenteric artery

Right colic artery

Ileocolic artery

Inferior mesenteric artery

Sigmoid artery

Rectosigmoid

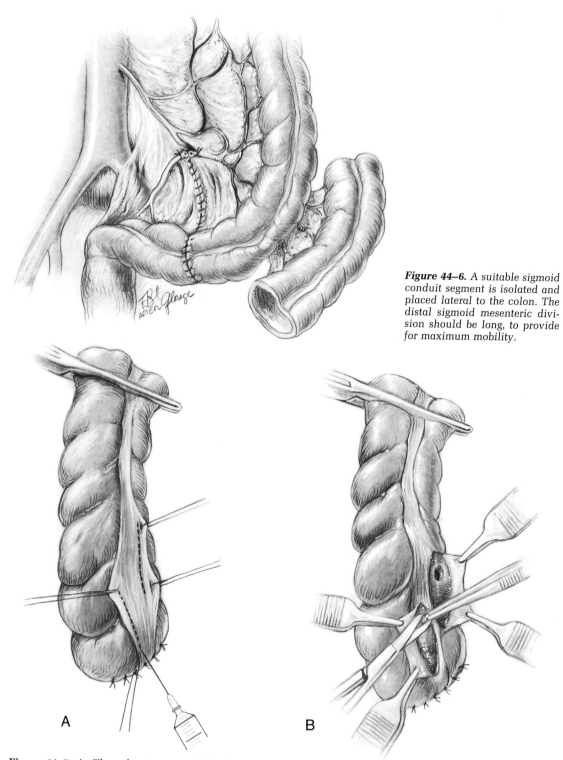

Figure 44–6. A suitable sigmoid conduit segment is isolated and placed lateral to the colon. The distal sigmoid mesenteric division should be long, to provide for maximum mobility.

A

B

Figure 44–7. A, The colon is prepared for the creation of antirefluxing submucosal tunnels. Marking sutures, approximately 4 cm apart, are placed in each tenia. The incisions in the two teniae are staggered by at least 3 cm, and the submuscularis is infiltrated with a solution of 1:100,000 adrenaline in saline to further facilitate dissection. B, The antirefluxing tunnels are created by incising the teniae down to the submucosa between the stay sutures. The muscularis is dissected off laterally by means of blunt and sharp dissection with fine scissors. Do not dissect between the two tunnels. A small ellipse of bowel mucosa is excised just proximal to the distal extent of the tunnels.

College of Surgeons Film Library and the Eaton Medical Film Library.

The submucosal tunnels should be at least 4 cm in length and capacious enough to allow the ureter to lie comfortably within the trough and be adequately covered by the seromuscular layer. If during development of either tunnel the mucosa is inadvertently entered, the opening should be closed with fine interrupted PGA sutures. Once the tunnels are completed, the base of the conduit is secured to the psoas muscle with 4-0 silk suture. The right ureter is passed beneath the sigmoid mesentery without being twisted or angulated. A stay suture in the ureter, similar to that described previously for ureteral implantation into an ileal conduit, minimizes trauma resulting from excessive handling of the ureter. The ureter is spatulated and a small ellipse of bowel mucosa is removed immediately proximal to the distal extent of the tunnel in the right tenia (Fig. 44–7B). A meticulous mucosa-to-mucosa anastomosis between the ureter and bowel is completed using interrupted 4-0 PGA sutures (Fig. 44–8A). The muscularis of the tenia is then reapproximated over the underlying ureter with interrupted 4-0 silk sutures; the surgeon should make certain that the hiatus at the proximal extent of the tunnel is not too tight. A right-angled clamp should easily pass alongside the ureter at

this point (Fig. 44–8B). If this junction appears too tight, the first sutures should be removed and replaced if necessary, otherwise obstruction to urine flow may occur. A similar procedure is performed for the left ureter.

Hendren preferred to position the conduit medial to the reconstituted colocolostomy, anchoring it to the sacral promontory and bringing the distal end out on the right side. It is our opinion that only when a total pelvic exenteration is performed should the stoma of the conduit be positioned on the right side, inasmuch as a permanent sigmoid colostomy is best performed on the left. In all other circumstances the most natural position for the cutaneous stoma is on the left side, decreasing the possibility of small bowel obstruction and excluding from the peritoneal cavity the ureteral colonic anastomosis by virtue of the sigmoid colonic mesentery.

Creation of the Stoma

A circular plug of skin, 2 to 3 cm in diameter, is removed from a predetermined site in the left lower quadrant. It is important that the opening in the skin not be too large, since colonic stomas have a tendency to become larger than their ileal counterparts. A long incision is made in the anterior rectus

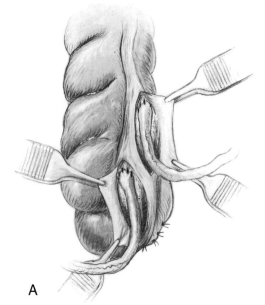

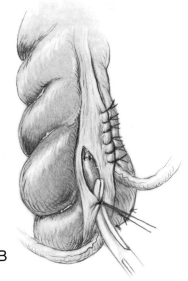

A   B

Figure 44–8. A, The ureterocolonic anastomoses are accomplished with interrupted 4-0 PGA sutures after the ureters are made to lie in the submucosal tunnels. B, The antirefluxing tunnels are completed by reapproximating the muscularis of the tenia over the underlying ureter. A right-angled clamp should easily pass alongside the ureter at its entrance to the tunnel, ensuring that the closure is not too tight.

fascia, the rectus muscle split, and the posterior fascia and peritoneum incised to enter the abdominal cavity. After it is determined that the opening is adequate in size (usually two fingers in breadth), the distal end of the conduit is brought through this opening and the seromuscular layer secured to the anterior rectus fascia in four quadrants with interrupted 2-0 chromic suture. A short everting nipple stoma is created by using interrupted 3-0 PGA sutures, which join the edge of the skin to the serosa of the colon at the level of the skin and then through the full thickness of the everting edge of the distal bowel. Myotomies or loop stomas are unnecessary because long-term complications of colonic stomas are very rare.

ILEOCECAL CUTANEOUS DIVERSION

The concept of utilizing the ileocecal segment for urinary diversion dates back to 1950, when both Gilchrist and Bricker described a technique of ureterocecocutaneous ileostomy for continent urinary diversion.[3, 6] Prevention of reflux was accomplished by a Leadbetter-type ureterocecal anastomosis, and continence was provided by antiperistalsis of the terminal ileum, the action of the ileocecal valve, and a tight cutaneous stoma. Sullivan in 1973 reported a followup of 40 patients undergoing the Gilchrist procedure.[27] Total continence was achieved in 37 of 40 patients (94%), and only three patients (7%) developed evidence of ureteral reflux or ileocecal calculi. Significant electrolyte disturbances did not occur. Similar successes, unfortunately, have not been duplicated. Bricker became discouraged that the ileocecal valve usually failed to provide acceptable continence, and abandoned the procedure in favor of the more dependable ileal conduit (Bricker procedure). Still others continued to modify the original principles of the Gilchrist procedure for construction of a continent ileocecal urinary reservoir, but with variable success. Incompetence of the nipple valve mechanism continues to be the major hurdle for success of these surgical procedures.

In contrast to the previous authors who focused attention on the ileocecal segment as a urinary reservoir for collection of urine, Zinman and Libertino utilized the ileocecal segment as a conduit for patients requiring urinary diversion.[32] This attractive method has certain appeal over conventional ileal conduits, since it combines the advantage of a colonic stoma that seldom develops stenosis with the antireflux mechanism provided by enhancing the competency of the ileocecal valve.

Operative Technique

Preoperatively, these patients are prepared identically to those described earlier in this chapter who are undergoing ileal conduit diversion. At surgery, after the abdomen is entered, the ascending colon is dissected from the right gutter and the peritoneal attachments between the terminal ileum and the sacral promontory are divided. This enables mobilization of the ascending colon and terminal ileum up to the duodenum where it is seen crossing the midline. The ileocolic artery lateral to the avascular plane is identified and the region of the mesentery between this vessel and the right colic artery is noted (Fig. 44–9). The length and mobility of the segment required depends on an adequate incision in the mesentery between these vessels. A long ascending colonic portion is not essential when this segment is used as a conduit, in contrast to that required for augmentation cecocystoplasty. A standard end-to-end ileal-ascending colonic bowel anastomosis is performed above the isolated segment by using either an interrupted 4-0 silk suture closure in two layers or a stapled bowel anastomosis. The competency of the ileocecal valve sufficient to prevent reflux can be enhanced by circumferential plication and intussusception of the terminal ileum into the cecum (Fig. 44–10). The intussusception can be further improved by first dividing the mesentery of that portion of ileum to be intussuscepted usually for a distance of 7 to 8 cm, a technique popularized by Hendren.

Zinman and Libertino prefer a Wallace conjoint ureteroureterostomy joined to the proximal ileal lumen, using interrupted 4-0 chromic sutures. We continue to prefer a Bricker type mucosa-to-mucosa ureteroileal anastomosis of interrupted 4-0 PGA suture. The proximal end of the ileum is closed with a running inverting Parker-Kerr suture of 3-0 chromic in two layers, whereas a third layer of interrupted 4-0 silk inverting serosal suture is used for reinforcement. The stoma is created by utilizing the already described colonic technique.

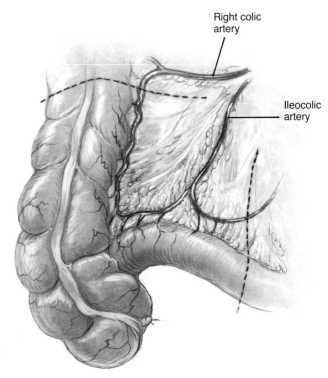

Figure 44–9. The ileocecal segment is selected. Adequate incisions in the mesentery ensure mobility.

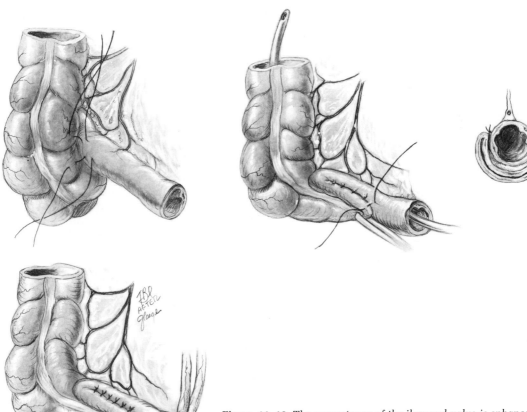

Figure 44–10. The competency of the ileocecal valve is enhanced by intussusception and plication. The intussusception may be facilitated by division of the mesentery of that portion of ileum to be intussuscepted, for a distance of up to 8 cm.

In 1975, Zinman and Libertino reported their initial experience of 15 patients undergoing an ileocecal conduit diversion and more recently reported their total clinical experience in 62 patients undergoing surgery between 1969 and 1978. This included 15 patients who had ileocecal conduit conversion from a previously troublesome ileal conduit. Six patients subsequently were undiverted to a cecocystoplasty one to two years later. The results have been uniformly good. Cecograms in 38 patients revealed a competent ileocecal valve in all but two patients.

Application of this form of diversion appears to be ideally suited for patients with dilated upper tracts, and particularly in those for whom a secondary lower urinary tract reconstruction may be possible. Sigmoid conduits would be an alternative to the ileocecal segment for cutaneous diversion of normal upper collecting systems.

COMMENTS

The ileal conduit remains the cornerstone of cutaneous diversions. It has been the most widely employed form of diversion since 1950, and it is well tested and reproducible. Long-term studies of the ileal conduit, however, reveal it not to be the panacea that urologists had hoped it would be. Significant late complications continue to be noted as experience mounts.

All ureterointestinal diversions have built-in early problems occurring in the first month after surgery. For the ileal conduit these include wound infections, enteric fistulas, urine leaks, ureteral obstruction, bowel obstruction, pelvic abscesses, and loop necrosis. The early complication rate for ileal conduits has been found to be at least 15 to 20%, but fortunately many of these problems can be handled by appropriately placed tubes and drains.[28] Anuria in the immediate postoperative period requires the most systematic evaluation. We recommend placement of a No. 16 French fenestrated Robinson catheter through the stoma to the base of the loop at the time of surgery to make certain that obstruction at the abdominal wall is not the problem. Since this catheter can also become plugged with mucus, the catheter should be irrigated as needed. Hypovolemia can be monitored with a central venous line and additional fluid administered as indicated. The need for reexploration in cases of undrained urine leaks and with conduit infarction, however, must be promptly recognized. Once a downhill course is begun, these cases carry a significant mortality rate.

The increasing rate of late complications is more distressing. These will include stomal stenosis, peristomal hernias, chronic pyelonephritis, ureteroileal obstruction, intestinal obstruction, calculi, and problems with hyperchloremic acidosis. Many of these problems appear to be particularly exacerbated in children. Stomal stenosis, which most often appeared with flush stomas, is noted in approximately 5% of adults but in up to 33% of children.[22, 28] Furthermore, in children followed for more than 10 years, there has been noted up to a 41% renal deterioration rate.[18] This deterioration is secondary to ureteroileal obstruction, reflux, or urinary infection. Renal calculi appear in approximately 4% of all cases.[28]

Hyperchloremic acidosis is noted in patients who already have impaired renal function and who often have an excessively long conduit. This usually can be controlled by taking an alkalizing solution (Polycitra), but shortening the loop may be necessary. Intestinal obstruction is often unpredictable and may occur at any time. The use of mechanical stapling devices to perform the bowel anastomoses takes less time than hand-sewn anastomoses but does not seem to affect significantly the postoperative recovery or long-term complications.[21]

The early and late complications for the jejunal conduit will be similar to those for the ileal conduit. The only unique problem is the jejunal syndrome, which results primarily from the greater absorptive and secretory capacity of the jejunal mucosa, compared with that for other intestinal segments. There is a loss of sodium and chloride into the urine, with reabsorption of potassium and urea. The resulting hyponatremia, hypochloremia, hyperkalemia, azotemia, and acidosis can be debilitating and needs to be treated with supplemental salt and sodium bicarbonate.

The key to colon and ileocecal conduits is the prevention of reflux. When this is accomplished, the preservation or restoration of the upper tracts can be remarkable. Elder reported a long-term review of patients undergoing sigmoid conduit diversion with a mean follow-up of 13 years (range, nine to

20 years).[4] In this study, 75% of the kidneys protected from reflux remained normal, whereas only 21% of refluxing units remained normal despite the use of the sigmoid conduit. The prevention of reflux, however, is not always easily achieved. Two long-term studies of colon conduits showed refluxing rates of 12 to 48%.[1, 10] The excellent results that Zinman and Libertino had in stabilizing the ileocecal valve (95%) have not always been as readily reproduced by others. For colon conduits, the integrity of the antireflux mechanism is dependent on ureters of normal caliber. The action of the ileocecal valve is independent of the condition of the ureters, and prevention of reflux depends only on the competency of the valve itself.

As we become more aware of the long-term results, the indications for the various types of conduit diversions are becoming more specific. The ileal conduit appears most effective in the older patient and in those adults requiring a cystectomy who are not otherwise going to have a continent form of diversion. Diversions for benign disease, especially in children, are probably best performed via one of the nonrefluxing versions, cutaneous or continent. The sigmoid conduit is most useful in patients with ureters of normal caliber, whereas the ileocecal segment is particularly appealing in those patients with dilated ureters. The use of jejunal conduits should be limited to that small subset of patients in whom none of the other bowel options are available because of concurrent disease or previous irradiation or surgery.

References

1. Altwrein JE, Jonas U, Hohenfellner R: Long-term followup of children with colon conduit urinary diversion and ureterosigmoidostomy. J Urol 118:832–836, 1977.
2. Barzilay BI, Goodwin WE: Clinical application of an experimental study of uretero-ileal anastomosis. J Urol 99:35–41, 1968.
3. Bricker EM: Symposium on clinical surgery: bladder substitution after pelvic evisceration. Surg Clin North Am 30:1511–1521, 1950.
4. Elder DD, Moisey CU, Rees RW: A long-term follow-up of the colonic conduit operation in children. Br J Urol 51:462–465, 1979.
5. Esho JO, Vitko RJ, Ireland GW, Cass AS: Comparison of Bricker and Wallace methods of ureteroileal anastomosis in urinary diversions. J Urol 111:600–602, 1974.
6. Gilchrist RK, Merricks JW, Hamlin HH, Rieger IT: Construction of substitute bladder and urethra. Surg Gynecol Obstet 90:752–760, 1950.
7. Golimbu M, Morales P: Jejunal conduits: technique and complications. J Urol 113:787–795, 1975.
8. Goodwin WE, Harris AP, Kaufman JJ, Beal JM: Open, transcolonic ureterointestinal anastomosis; new approach. Surg Gynecol Obstet 97:295–300, 1953.
9. Hendren WH: Nonrefluxing colon conduit for temporary or permanent urinary diversion in children. J Pediatr Surg 10:381–398, 1975.
10. Hill JT, Ransley PG: The colonic conduit: a better method of urinary diversion? Br J Urol 55:629–631, 1983.
11. Jankengt RA: Absorption of urine products in jejunum, ileum and sigmoid loops. Urol Int 22:435–440, 1967.
12. Klein EA, Montie JE, Montague DK, et al: Jejunal conduit urinary diversion. J Urol 135:244–246, 1986.
13. Kronig D: Die Anlegung eines Anus praeternaturalis zur Vermeidung der Colipyelitis bei Einpflanzung der Uretern ins Rektum. Zentrabl Gynak 31:559–561, 1907.
14. Leadbetter WF, Clarke BG: Five years' experience with uretero-enterostomy by the "combined" technique. J Urol 73:67–82, 1955.
15. Lengemann P: Ersatz der extirpierten Harnblase durch das Coecum. Zentralbl Chir 39:1697–1700, 1912.
16. Mathisen W: New method for ureterointestinal anastomosis: preliminary report. Surg Gynecol Obstet 96:255–258, 1953.
17. Mauclaire P: De quelques essais de chirurgie experimentale applicables au traitement de 'exstrophe de la vessie et des anus contre nature complexes. Ann Mal Org Genitourin 13:1080–1081, 1895.
18. Middleton AW Jr, Hendren WH: Ileal conduits in children at the Massachusetts General Hospital from 1955 to 1970. J Urol 115:591–595, 1976.
19. Mogg RA: The treatment of urinary incontinence using the colonic conduit. J Urol 97:684–692, 1967.
20. Morales PA, Whitehead ED: High jejunal conduit for supravesical urinary diversion. Report of 25 cases. Urology 1:426–431, 1973.
21. Myers RP, Rife CC, Barrett DM: Experience with the bowel stapler for ileal conduit urinary diversion. Br J Urol 54:491–493, 1982.
22. Orr JD, Shand JEG, Watters DAK, Kirkland IS: Ileal conduit urinary diversion in children. An assessment of the long-term results. Br J Urol 53:424–427, 1981.
23. Parkhurst EC, Leadbetter WF: A report on 93 ileal loop urinary diversions. J Urol 83:398–403, 1960.
24. Rangel DM, Yakeishi Y, Stevens GH, Fonkalsrud EW: Absorption of urinary contents from isolated segments of jejunum and ileum. Surg Gynecol Obstet 129:1189–1198, 1969.
25. Richie JP, Skinner DG: Ureterointestinal diversion. In PC Walsh, RF Gittes, AD Perlmutter, TA Stamey (eds), Campbell's Urology, Vol 3. Philadelphia, WB Saunders, 1986, pp 2601–2619.
26. Seiffert L: Die "Darm-Siphonblase." Arch F Klin Chir 183:569–574, 1935.
27. Sullivan H, Gilchrist RK, Merricks JW: Ileocecal substitute bladder. Long-term follow-up. J Urol 109:43–45, 1973.
28. Sullivan JW, Grabstald H, Whitmore WF Jr: Complications of ureteroileal conduit with radical cys-

tectomy: review of 336 cases. J Urol 124:797–801, 1980.

29. Turnbull RB Jr, Fazio V: Advances in the surgical technique of ulcerative colitis surgery: endanal proctectomy and two-directional myotomy ileostomy. Surg Annu 7:315–329, 1975.

30. Verhoogen J: Neostomie uretero-caecale. Formation d'une nouvelle pouche vesicale et d'un nouvel uretre. Assoc Franc d'Urol 12:362–365, 1908.

31. Wallace DM: Ureteric diversion using a conduit: a simplified technique. Br J Urol 38:522–527, 1966.

32. Zinman L, Libertino JA: Ileocecal conduit for temporary and permanent urinary diversion. J Urol 113:317–323, 1975.

DAVID A. BLOOM, M.D.
GARY LIESKOVSKY, M.D.

CHAPTER 45   *The Turnbull Loop Stoma*

The first diversionary stomas were accidents of injury or disease, and purposeful stomas did not become a reality until the development of modern surgical techniques. Intentional urinary diversion has progressed from Simon's cutaneous ureterostomy in 1869,[1] Bricker's flush ileal conduit stoma of 1950,[3] the bud stoma of Brooke,[8] and most recently to the loop stoma of Turnbull.[7] Intermittent catheterization has obviated urinary diversion for many patients with neuropathic bladders, and the continent urinary

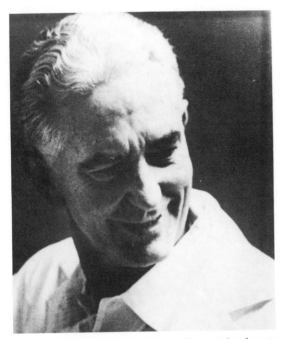

Figure 45–1. *Rupert B. Turnbull, Jr. (October 3, 1913–February 19, 1981). Photograph courtesy of Dr. Ralph Straffon and the Cleveland Clinic Foundation.*

diversions are further diminishing the need for free-draining urinary conduits and collection devices. Nonetheless, there is still a place for external urinary diversion.

The stoma is the weak link of external urinary diversion. The most likely reason for reoperation in patients with external urinary diversion is a stomal problem. Recognizing the susceptibility of the stoma, Turnbull devised a loop stoma that he originally used for fecal diversion in patients with regional enteritis.[9] This type of stoma seemed free from the usual stomal problems, and Turnbull and Hewitt applied the technique to urinary diversion with great success.[7] Turnbull was one of the early leaders in appreciating the problems attendant with fecal and urinary stomas, and he developed, at the Cleveland Clinic, one of the pioneer programs in enterostomal therapy (Fig. 45–1).

Patient selection for the Turnbull stoma has been straightforward; we find this suitable for any patient with a free-draining small bowel urinary conduit. Continent urinary reservoirs are best served by flush stomas, and large bowel diversions are preferably drained by flush or bud stomas, since a loop stoma is excessively bulky in the large intestine.

PREOPERATIVE PREPARATION AND SURGICAL TECHNIQUE

Preoperative selection of stomal location requires examination of the patient in various positions so that the stoma will be away from bony prominences, scars, skin creases, and other factors that prevent proper seating of the future urinary appliance. Factors such as the patient's style of clothing and any physical disabilities, such as hemiparesis, may influence placement to best favor daily maintenance by the patient. The site should be marked by a subdermal injection with methylene blue or another dye, delivered through a 26-gauge needle.

A skin disk is excised at the predetermined stomal site by using the butt end of a 20- or 35-ml syringe plunger as a template. The underlying subcutaneous fat is incised vertically and retracted out of the way with narrow Richardson retractors. This exposes the underlying anterior rectus fascia, which is incised longitudinally for a distance of 2 to 3 cm, and the rectus muscle is bluntly split with curved Mayo scissors. Since the usual stoma site is below the arcuate line, blunt finger dissection is usually all that is required to penetrate the fascia transversalis and peritoneum in order to develop a defect the width of two fingers into the peritoneal cavity. Care must be taken not to injure the inferior epigastric vessels when splitting the rectus muscle or opening the posterior rectus fascia. Multiple absorbable sutures of 2-0 chromic catgut are preplaced along the perimeter of the anterior fascial defect and later secured to the seromuscular layer of the bowel loop. At least six such sutures may be necessary to discourage formation of a parastomal hernia; particular attention should be paid to suture placement along the lateral side of the fascial incision (Fig. 45–2).

The distal end of the conduit is closed with a TA-55 4.8 autosuture stapler. The most mobile part of the distal portion of the loop is identified, and a small Penrose drain is passed through a small mesenterotomy at that location. The drain is pulled through the abdominal aperture, allowing the distal loop of conduit to be gently negotiated out the stomal site. In obese patients with a fat mesentery, additional length of the stomal loop may be obtained by extending the rectus sheath incision in a cephalad or caudal direction. It is important to ensure that the bowel is not twisted as it is brought out through the abdominal wall. We have had

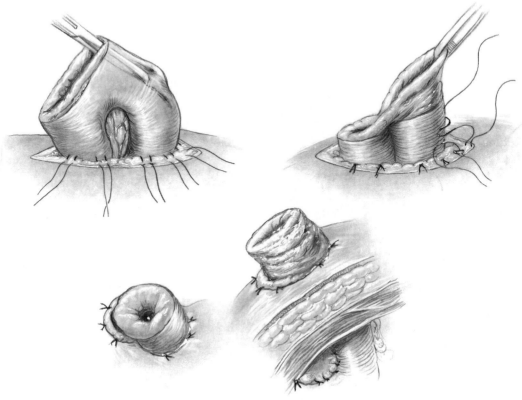

Figure 45–2. *Details of the construction of a Turnbull loop stoma.*

this occur in an obese patient, but fortunately we recognized the abnormal orientation when we tried to bring out the stents. The exposed knuckle of ileum should protrude at least 3 to 4 cm above the skin surface without tension or tendency to withdraw into the abdomen. Once the position of the loop is satisfactory, it is secured in place with the preplaced anterior fascial sutures through seromuscular layers of the conduit. One must avoid placement of suture through the mesentery. Prior to opening the loop, four sutures of 3-0 polyglycolic acid (PGA) are placed in the subdermal tissue: three along the caudal perimeter of the stomal opening and another cephalad in the midline. The cephalad or distal end of the anterior surface of the exposed knuckle is opened transversely about four fifths of the way across the lumen with a clean cut of a sharp Metzenbaum or curved Mayo scissors. The previously placed caudal subdermal sutures are then passed through the adjacent seromuscular layer of the conduit at the skin edge level and, finally, through the caudal or proximal enterostomy edge. The single cephalad subdermal suture is passed through the distal enterostomy edge only and tied. An Allis clamp is then passed proximally through the enterostomy into the lumen of the bowel in order to grasp the anterior luminal surface of the knuckle of conduit just above the level of the previously placed seromuscular 3-0 PGA sutures. A combination of traction on the Allis clamp and eversion of the proximal enterostomy edge forms a protruding nipple stoma. The sutures are then tied, and additional 3-0 PGA sutures are circumferentially placed to secure the remainder of the enterostomy edge to the subdermal skin edge. Ureteral stents, if used, are secured to the stomal lips with fine absorbable sutures. If the ureters are not stented, we recommend the conduit be stented with a No. 16 French fenestrated Robinson catheter and sutured to the stoma to prevent obstruction of the conduit from early postoperative edema or mucus retention. Because the distal end of the conduit has a tendency to prolapse, we have found it necessary to anchor it to the peritoneum and posterior rectus fascia with several extraluminal sutures. These should be made of either synthetic absorbable material or silk. The loop stoma is finally inspected from the peritoneal side to be certain that there are no large defects between the loop and fascia.

A sterile drainage appliance is then placed on the stoma.

DISCUSSION

The Turnbull loop stoma is remarkably free from complications. Stomal stenosis is rare and, in 100 patients with follow-up of over one and up to seven years, there were no instances of stenosis.[2] Encrustations, dermatitis, hemorrhagic stomatitis, and infections are rarely encountered with this diversion. We suspect that stenosis is unlikely due to the nature of the stoma; because it is not a circumferential orifice, it is unlikely to contract centripetally. The loop stoma also favors a very easy and snug fit of the appliance, and it may largely be because of this optimal fit with little contact of exposed skin to the urine in the appliance that the stomal difficulties are minimized. Initial experience with this stoma resulted in a substantial incidence of parastomal herniation (14%). In some patients, prolapse of the redundant end of the stoma is a prelude to parastomal herniation. As we gained experience with this procedure, learned to anchor the distal end of the conduit, and secure the loop circumferentially to the anterior fascia, the incidence of parastomal herniation became much lower.

The usual symptom of a parastomal hernia is a painless bulge at or adjacent to the stomal site. This may progress and make appliance fit difficult. Bowel incarceration is a possibility with a parastomal hernia, but we have not yet seen this in conjunction with the Turnbull loop stoma. A parastomal hernia that complicates appliance care should be corrected. Small hernias can be repaired without stomal relocation by reduction of the hernia, excision of the sac, and repair of the fascial defect.[6] Large or recurrent hernias are best managed by stomal relocation and herniorrhaphy. Kaufman described stomal relocation to the other side of the abdomen without formal laparotomy. He mobilized the conduit through the stomal site and then passed it through the abdominal wall to a new stomal site on the other side of the abdomen. The site of the hernia was then repaired from the outside.[5] Occasionally, parastomal hernias will compromise a loop stoma so severely that conversion to a bud stoma is necessary.

Emmott compared results of Turnbull loop

stomas in 54 patients with those for end stomas in 25 patients (with 27 stomas) over a three-year period.[4] He found stenosis in 44% of the end stomas but in none of the loop stomas. The incidence of parastomal hernia was 2% for the loop stomas and 4% for the end stomas. Virtually no other skin or stomal problems were noted with the loop stoma.[4]

CONCLUSION

We initially began to use the Turnbull stoma for diversion in obese patients but quickly found it a practical and durable stoma for all patients with free-draining small bowel conduits. The favorable experience with this has been shared by other groups, and we continue to advocate the Turnbull loop stoma.

References

1. Abrams JS: Abdominal Stomas. Boston, John Wright PSG, 1984.
2. Bloom DA, Lieskovsky G, Rainwater G, Skinner DG: The Turnbull loop stoma. J Urol 129:715–718, 1983.
3. Bricker EM: Symposium on clinical surgery: bladder substitution after pelvic evisceration. Surg Clin North Am 30:1511–1521, 1950.
4. Emmott D, Noble MJ, Mebust WK: A comparison of end versus loop stomas for ileal conduit urinary diversion. J Urol 133:588–590, 1985.
5. Kaufman JJ: Repair of parastomal hernia by translocation of the stoma without laparotomy. J Urol 129:278–279, 1983.
6. Marshall FF, Leadbetter WF, Dretler SP: Ileal conduit parastomal hernias. J Urol 114:40–42, 1975.
7. Turnbull RB Jr, Hewitt CR: Loop-end myotomy ileostomy in the obese patient. Urol Clin North Am 5:423–429, 1978.
8. Turnbull RB Jr, Weakley FL: Atlas of Intestinal Stomas. St. Louis, CV Mosby, 1967.
9. Turnbull RB Jr, Weakley FL: Ileostomy. In P Cooper (ed), The Craft of Surgery. Boston, Little, Brown, 1971, pp 1141–1148.

DONALD G. SKINNER, M.D.
STUART D. BOYD, M.D.
GARY LIESKOVSKY, M.D.

CHAPTER 46

Creation of the Continent Kock Ileal Reservoir as an Alternative to Cutaneous Urinary Diversion

For the past century urologists and general surgeons have tried to devise an acceptable form of urinary diversion for patients with bladder cancer or malfunction of the lower urinary tract due to congenital anomalies, neurologic disorders, or traumatic injuries.

The incorporation of the intestinal tract for urinary diversion dates back to at least 1888, when Tizzoni and Poggi reported on anastomosing the ureters into isolated ileal segments.[47] There were, however, few clinical applications until pelvic surgeons began an aggressive ablative approach to pelvic malignancy. Ureterosigmoidostomy was the first widely used and accepted method of diversion that followed Coffee's description of transplantation of the ureters into the large intestine.[8] A number of modifications followed in an effort to prevent ascending infection, including the direct elliptical mucosa-to-mucosa anastomosis[33] and finally the technique of Leadbetter,[27] in which a long submucosal tunnel was combined with the Nesbitt elliptical mucosal anastomosis. Despite these modifications, long-term problems surfaced: the syndrome of hyperchloremic metabolic acidosis due to sodium and chloride absorption with potassium and bicarbonate loss from the colon,[10] upper tract deterioration due to reflux or ureteral co-

lonic stenosis,[38] and finally the realization of a more than 300-fold increase in the incidence of colon carcinoma now anticipated in nearly 5% of long-term ureterosigmoid patients.[35] Moreover, ureterosigmoidostomy results in such a restricted lifestyle due to bowel frequency, nocturnal incontinence, and odor that this form of diversion has become the least attractive and rarely seems indicated.[30]

In 1950, Bricker and Eiseman in St. Louis[6] and Gilchrist and associates in Chicago[13] simultaneously reported on their utilization of the ileocecal segment as an alternative method of continent urinary diversion. In this system, the cecum served as a reservoir, the ileocecal valve provided continence, and intermittent catheterization was used to empty the reservoir (Fig. 46–1). Bricker, however, reported that all of their patients had leakage, and when an associate discovered an appliance that could be placed around the ileal stoma to provide true dryness, they quickly abandoned the ileocecal segment and used instead the ileal segment as a more simple conduit.[4, 5] The Bricker operation caught on in the urologic community and has remained the standard form of urinary diversion since 1950. When first introduced, the conduit system, which

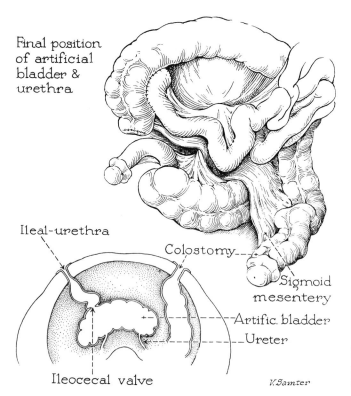

Final position of artificial bladder & urethra

Ileal-urethra

Colostomy

Sigmoid mesentery

Artific. bladder

Ureter

Ileocecal valve

V. Samter

Figure 46–1. *Schematic representation of the continent cecal bladder as developed by Gilchrist and associates. From Gilchrist RK, et al: Surg Gynecol Obstet 90:752, 1950.*

seemed to eliminate the disadvantages of electrolyte imbalance, pyelonephritis, calculus formation, and renal deterioration, rapidly emerged as a more effective procedure for urinary diversion in patients with malignant disease. The long-term results, however, indicate that renal deterioration occurs in a number of patients.[38, 39] The role of reflux, with or without infection, has been blamed for much of this deterioration, and numerous methods have been developed either to prevent reflux in ileal conduits or to use colonic conduits with nonrefluxing anastomoses.[9, 31, 38, 39] Prevention of ureteral reflux has also been achieved by use of an ileocecal conduit utilizing a Nissen wraparound principle on the ileocecal valve.[54] This operation, however, like that for the ileal and sigmoid conduits, has the disadvantage of requiring an external appliance for the collection and storage of urine. Many patients simply are unable to adjust socially, psychologically, or sexually to the wearing of an external appliance to collect waste of any kind.[11, 12, 19, 21]

Ideally, an acceptable urinary diversion should mimic the urinary bladder and be able to effectively collect and store urine without reflux, absorption, or infection problems and permit emptying under voluntary

control at convenient intervals. Throughout the "ileal conduit era," investigators, particularly the Gilchrist group, continued to utilize the ileocecal segment for continent internal diversion, and in 1970 Sullivan and associates reported that continence was achieved in 94% of 40 patients followed for 10 years.[46] However, the operation never caught on and, despite intussusception modifications reported by Zingg and Tscholl, most investigators have had difficulty maintaining competence of the ileocecal valve.[1, 2, 50, 53]

We have used the cecal segment since 1970 for bladder augmentation and lower urinary tract reconstruction.[41] Like Hendren, we have had difficulty preventing reflux unless the mesentery of the terminal ileum is divided and the ileum intussuscepted into the cecum and fixed by staples and a Marlex or polyglycolic acid (PGA) collar.[17, 41] Hendren's technique seems to have largely solved the problem of extussusception, but uninhibited contractions of the intact cecum have resulted in intermittent incontinence, particularly at night.[41, 45]

In 1982, Kock and associates first reported in the United States on their revolutionary technique of urinary diversion via the continent ileal reservoir.[23] Their technique resulted from nearly 20 years of animal experimentation and clinical study.[16, 18, 21, 24, 25, 34, 37, 48] In studies of the functional behavior of different types of bladder substitutes, Kock and associates found that if the ileum is opened and the intestine folded and closed in a special way, the motor activity causes different parts to counteract themselves, giving storage or reservoir properties to the intestinal pouch without the intermittent pressure spikes that occur when cecum is used as a reservoir. This innovative procedure was a modification of the continent ileostomy developed by Kock in the 1960s for patients undergoing proctocolectomy for ulcerative colitis.[22] We believe that an important advantage of the Kock pouch over the cecal reservoir or the isolated intact ileal loop as described by Camey[7] is the observation that filling pressures are consistently lower and the intermittent contractural pressure spikes are not seen, thus increasing reservoir capacity as well as providing better continence and preventing reflux. Pressures within the pouch rarely exceed 15 to 20 cm of water, whereas pressures within either the cecum or ileum often exceed 60 cm of water (Figs. 46–2 through 46–4).[11, 29, 45]

Kock and associates reported their initial experience with 12 patients in the *Journal of Urology*, 1982.[23] This innovative procedure now offers patients requiring cystectomy for bladder cancer, or cutaneous urinary diversion for any reason, an acceptable alternative to the standard ileal conduit, which necessitates wearing an external appliance. Gerber was the first to perform the operation in the United States and in 1983 reported his experience in seven patients operated on between 1979 and 1983.[11] We have used the technique originally described by Kock and have made what we believe to be some important modifications. We began clinical and laboratory trials in 1982 and have previously reported our experience in our original 51 patients.[42, 43] From January 1984 through August 1985, we have performed the procedure in an additional 200 patients. Based on this experience, we believe that the procedure is one of the most innovative advances in the field of urinary diversion. It fulfills the essential criteria of a low-pressure internal reservoir by being truly continent, easy to catheterize and empty, and by preventing reflux. The ileal mucosa used in the pouch appears to adapt well to urine with decreased villus height, and in time a nearly flat mucosa emerges that may decrease absorption.[16, 29] To date, there has been no evidence of late fibrosis or of adverse changes in the morphology or function of the intestinal wall.[16, 20, 29]

PATIENT SELECTION

The majority of candidates for creation of the Kock continent ileal reservoir are those with invasive bladder cancer who need cystectomy. Other candidates are those who have previously undergone urinary diversion but find the wearing of a bag unaccept-

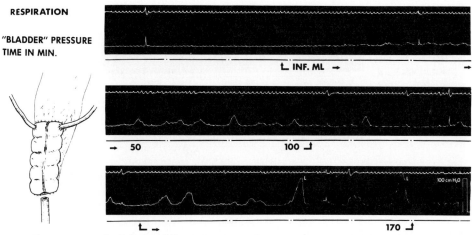

RESPIRATION

"BLADDER" PRESSURE
TIME IN MIN.

L INF. ML →

50   100

170

Figure 46–2. Pressure recording during filling of a cecal bladder reservoir. Note spontaneous pressure spikes in excess of 60 cm water. At the urethra these spikes may result in urinary leakage (L). From Kock NG: Continent ileostomy: historical perspective. In RR Dozois (ed), Alternatives to Conventional Ileostomy. Chicago, Year Book Medical Publishers, 1985, pp 133–145.

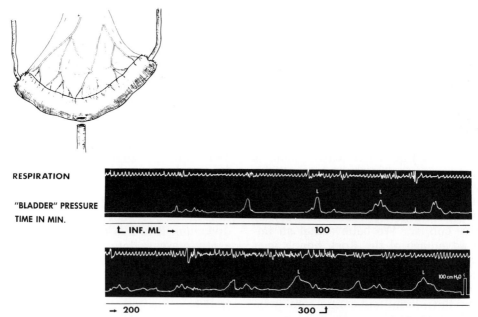

Figure 46–3. Pressure recording during filling of loop ileal reservoir constructed according to the method of Camey.[7] Note spontaneous pressure spikes in excess of 60 cm water. At the urethra these spikes may result in urinary leakage (L), particularly at night. From Kock NG: Continent ileostomy: historical perspective. In RR Dozois (ed), Alternatives to Conventional Ileostomy. Chicago, Year Book Medical Publishers, 1985, pp 133–145.

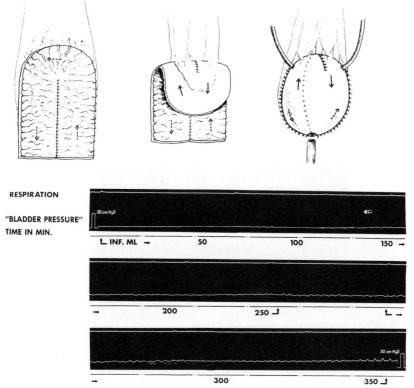

Figure 46–4. Pressure recording during filling of a Kock ileal reservoir. Note lack of motor activity without significant pressure increase to volume in excess of 500 ml water. From Kock NG: Continent ileostomy: historical perspective. In RR Dozois (ed), Alternatives to Conventional Ileostomy. Chicago, Year Book Medical Publishers, 1985, pp 133–145.

able. Patients with neurogenic bladder dysfunction may also become candidates. Prior pelvic radiation does not appear to be a contraindication, although the combination of prior pelvic surgery followed by high levels of radiation may substantially increase the potential for postoperative morbidity.

In order to gain experience with this procedure as well as to understand its limitations, we originally decided that any patient who was a candidate for an ileal conduit could potentially be suitable for a Kock pouch. In our series of 250 patients there were 83 women and 167 men between the ages of 13 and 87. The underlying reason for surgery was varied. A total of 171 of the ileal reservoir patients underwent simultaneous radical cystectomy for cancer. Forty-four of these patients had received radiation therapy to the pelvis at some time in the past. The doses ranged from 1600 rads to greater than 6000 rads. Sixty patients desired conversion from an existing form of urinary diversion: 48 had ileal conduits, 10 had ureterosigmoidostomies, one had a suprapubic cystostomy secondary to traumatic loss of the bladder neck and urethra, and one had bilateral cutaneous ureterostomies. These patients sought conversion to the continent reservoir because of recurrent pyelonephritis, inability to remain dry, or because of the psychosocial stigma associated with their previous type of diversion. Nineteen additional patients had cystectomy and creation of Kock continent reservoirs because of neurogenic bladders or refractory interstitial cystitis.

Our experience has shown us that not all diversion patients, however, make ideal Kock pouch candidates. Patients with prior abdominal operations followed by high levels of radiation therapy obviously have an increased risk of complication. Prior radiation therapy, however, is not a contraindication to the procedure, as some of our most successful results have been achieved in patients undergoing salvage cystectomy following failure of definitive radiation therapy (greater than 6500 rads) for cancer of the prostate or bladder and in patients with fistulas following isotope implants and external beam radiation for cervical or colonic carcinoma.

The obese patient with a thick ileal mesentery is going to present the greatest surgical challenge and postoperatively may experience difficult catheterization problems. Any patient with pre-existing abdominal weakness will also require extra surgical effort to securely fix the efferent limb and nipple because any hypermobility of this valve can make long-term catheterization difficult.

Compromised renal function (creatinine levels greater than 2.0) was once felt to be a contraindication because of electrolyte disturbances secondary to reabsorption. This may not prove to be the case, however, because over time the mucosa of the pouch changes. Kock has observed the finger-like villi of the mucosa flatten, and after two years they may completely disappear in large areas, leaving only smooth mucosa grossly resembling that of the urinary bladder.[29, 37] This reduces the absorptive area, and biopsies show an alteration in the brush-border cell membrane that may also help reduce the potential risk of electrolyte alteration. We have not seen any uncontrollable electrolyte problem in our patients. The important factor in patient selection should be patient motivation and the patient's thorough understanding of the procedure. Any problem or difficulty can be overcome if the patient is willing and eager to work with the diversion team.

PREOPERATIVE PREPARATION

The enterostomal therapist is one of the most valuable members of the diversion team. Good patient instruction by a dedicated therapist prior to and after the surgery makes the postoperative transition and catheterization experience much smoother and easier. The therapist can also provide some needed input into predetermining the general location of the stoma, though the ultimate stomal location may have to be determined by technical factors at the time of surgery. The stoma site can often be lower on the abdominal wall, since avoidance of skin folds for ostomy placement is not a factor. In general, it should be placed where it will be concealed by underwear, several centimeters above the pubis. In young women it can be positioned below the bikini line.

Our preoperative bowel regime is similar to that described for our radical cystectomy technique (Chapter 42). The patient is placed on clear liquids following breakfast the day prior to surgery. A laxative, such as Neoloid, is given by mouth the morning of that pre-operative day, and oral neomycin and erythromycin base are administered that afternoon and evening. Good hydration is maintained by initiating intravenous fluids that night.

OPERATIVE TECHNIQUE

In patients undergoing simultaneous cystectomy, that part of the operation is completed first. In patients undergoing conversion of an existing ileal conduit, it is necessary to take down all intra-abdominal adhesions and to dissect out the existing ileal conduit from the abdominal wall. We have found that the time required for pelvic node dissection with en bloc cystectomy is similar to the time required to dissect out all adhesions and take down an existing ileal conduit in preparation for the creation of the Kock pouch. In patients with existing ileal conduits, the prior small bowel anastomosis is identified and excised along with the area of prior mesenteric division. In patients without prior diversion, the avascular plane between the terminal branch of the superior mesenteric artery and the ileocolic artery is identified and the bowel and mesentery are divided. The mesenteric division extends to the base of the mesentery along the avascular plane to assure good mobility to the efferent limb of the Kock pouch (Fig. 46–5).

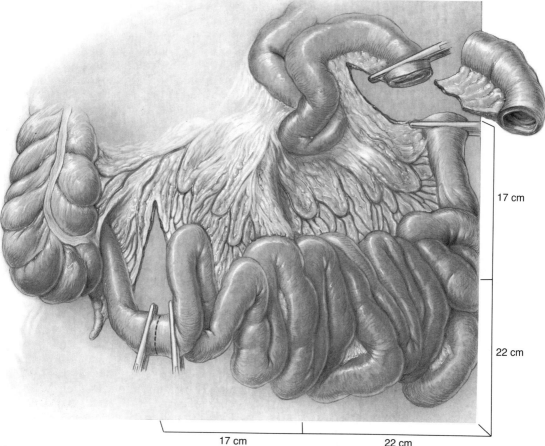

17 cm

22 cm

17 cm   22 cm

Figure 46–5. *Various segments of terminal ileum chosen for creation of the Kock pouch. Note that the distal mesenteric division is usually between the ileocolic artery and terminal ileal branches of the superior mesenteric artery. It extends into the avascular plane of the mesentery. Note that the proximal mesenteric division is quite short to assure a broad vascular supply to the pouch. Usually a small window of mesentery and an additional 3 to 5 cm of small bowel are discarded proximal to the overall segment in order to ensure good mobility to the pouch and to the small bowel anastomosis. The pouch itself is created out of two central 22-cm segments, each with a limb that extends to or away from the pouch and is approximately 17 cm in length. If the patient has an existing ileal conduit, the afferent limb is created from only 13 to 15 cm of small bowel.*

Next, suitable segments of the small bowel are measured and marked with silk sutures: 17 cm for the efferent segment, two 22-cm segments for the pouch itself, and a 17-cm segment for the afferent limb. Approximately 5 cm of ileum proximal to the isolated segment is discarded, along with a small triangular wedge of mesentery (Fig. 46–5). This provides mobility to the pouch and the small bowel anastomosis, and because the mesenteric division is quite short proximally, an excellent blood supply to the pouch is ensured. In patients with existing ileal conduits, an afferent limb of only 13 cm is necessary.

The proximal end of the isolated ileal segment is closed with a running Parker-Kerr suture of 3-0 chromic and a third layer of interrupted 4-0 silk sutures. We are reluctant to use the stapler at this location, proximal to the antireflux valve, because if stones form on the staples they might be difficult to extract and might not pass easily through the antireflux nipple. Obviously, in patients with an existing ileal conduit, this end is left open to be anastomosed to the proximal end of the loop.

A standard small bowel anastomosis is then performed (we use two layers of interrupted 4-0 silk sutures), and the mesenteric trap is closed.

The segment of isolated ileum is then laid out in a U shape, with the lowest point of the U being the marking suture between the two 22-cm segments (Fig. 46–6A). The lowest point should be directed caudally so that subsequently the afferent limb of the pouch can easily be secured to the sacral promontory to facilitate the ureteroileal anastomosis. The two 22-cm segments are then sewn together side-to-side by using running 3-0 PGA sutures, apposing the serosa approximately 1 to 2 cm lateral to the mesentery (Fig. 46–6B).

The bowel is opened just lateral to the serosal suture, using the cautery. This incision along the antimesenteric border of the ileum is extended approximately 3 cm distally beyond the continuous serosal suture, and 1 to 2 cm proximally so that the nipple valves will be staggered and so that subsequent staple fixation of the intussuscepted nipples will not involve the continuous suture line along the pouch's posterior wall (Fig. 46–6B). The incised mucosa is then oversewn with two layers of running 3-0 PGA suture material (Fig. 46–7). This suture

line forms the posterior wall of the pouch, and meticulous, closely placed sutures are essential to make the pouch watertight.

Next, the windows of Deaver are opened along the afferent and efferent limbs of ileum leading to and from the pouch, respectively. The mesentery is divided for approximately 7 to 8 cm proximal to the pouch along the afferent limb of ileum and distal to the pouch along the efferent limb. This is best done with the cautery; an assistant should pick up the individual vessels as they are coagulated (Fig. 46–8). This is a very important part of the operation because when the ileum is intussuscepted into the pouch, mesentery will not be included, thereby preventing late slippage or extussusception of the nipple valve mechanism.

A 2.5-cm strip of doubled PGA mesh is then passed through the window of Deaver just beyond the stripped mesentery, leaving at least one vascular arcade (Fig. 46–9). This mesh will serve as an anchoring collar for the base of the nipple valves. We originally employed Marlex for this purpose but discovered that Marlex was a potential source for erosion into the pouch and subsequent need for reoperation.

The nipples are intussuscepted by passing two Allis forcep clamps approximately two thirds of the way from the open limb toward the anchoring collar, grasping the mucosa, and inverting the ileum into the pouch (Fig. 46–9). Three rows of parallel staples are then applied to the intussuscepted nipples (Fig. 46–10). The TA-55 stapler with 4.8-mm staples is used for this purpose. This size staple is not hemostatic and does not crush the bowel. The full 5.5 cm of the stapler should be utilized to create a nipple longer than 5 cm. The three rows should be placed longitudinally around the anterior 180° of the intussuscepted nipple, leaving the mesenteric or posterior portion free so that a fourth row of staples can subsequently fix the nipple to the back wall of the pouch (Fig. 46–10). It is important to note that the tip of the nipple may appear dusky at the time of creation. There may even be some eventual sloughing of the tip, but the overall length of the valve should always be longer than the needed functional length of 2.5 cm. As depicted, the staples at the base of the nipple valves are the most important for preventing extussusception, and these staples tend to get buried in the mucosa. The staples at the tip of the nipples do not contribute to the

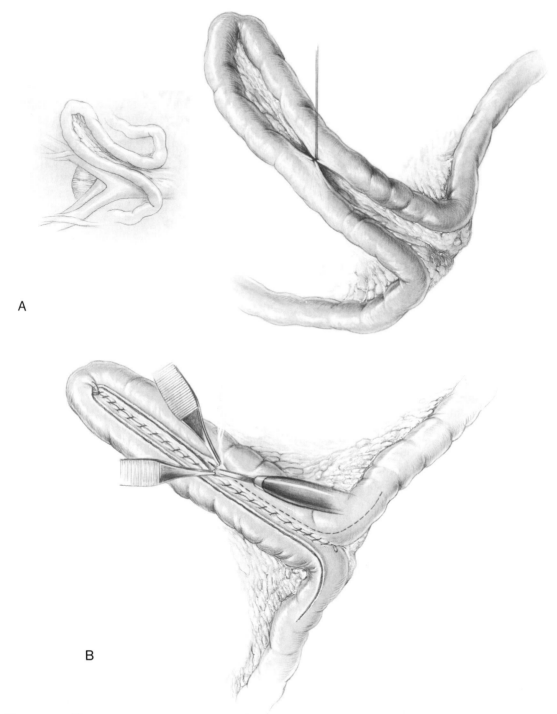

Figure 46–6. *The two 22-cm segments are joined by running 3-0 polyglycolic acid (PGA) continuous suture. The lowest point of the **U** should be directed caudally so that once the pouch is formed the afferent limb will drop readily to the sacral promontory to facilitate the ureteroileal anastomosis (A, inset). The proximal end of the afferent limb is closed with a running Parker-Kerr suture of 3-0 chromic and a third layer of interrupted 4-0 silk imbricating suture. The two 22-cm segments of bowel are then opened immediately adjacent to the continuous serosal suture line so as to form the pouch (B).*

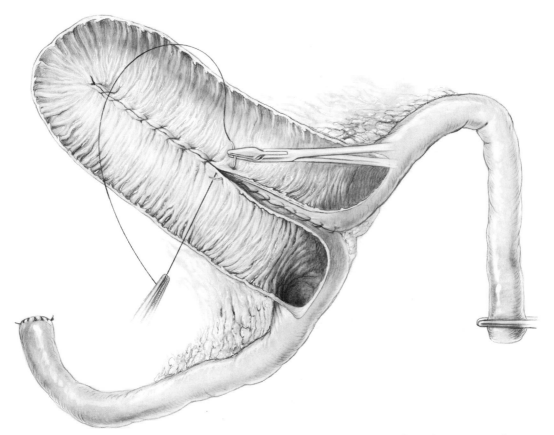

Figure 46–7. Mucosa oversewn with two layers of 3-0 PGA continuous sutures in order to form a watertight suture line. Note that the serosal incision has been extended for several centimeters along the efferent limb and a short distance along the afferent limb so that when the nipples are formed they are separated.

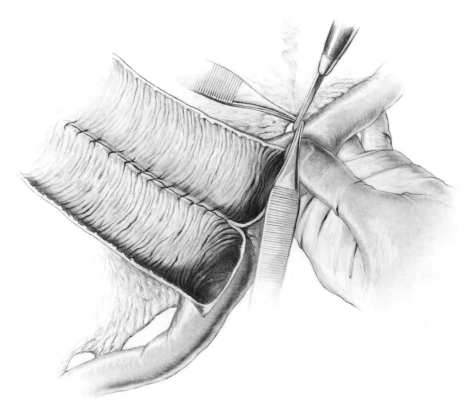

Figure 46–8. The mesentery is next divided immediately adjacent to the serosa of the afferent/efferent limb for a distance of nearly 8 cm. At least one or more vascular arcades should be left, and a 2.5-cm-wide strip of PGA can then be placed through the window of Deaver distal to that arcade. This PGA mesh serves as a collar to fix the afferent/efferent limb to the pouch once the intussusception technique has been accomplished.

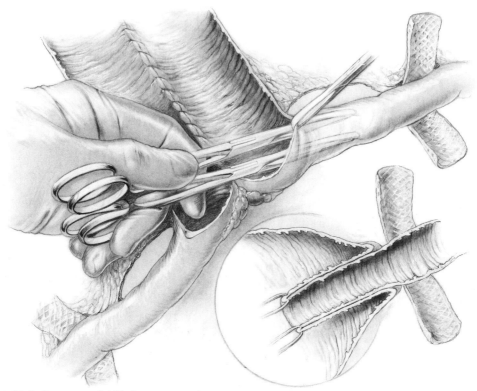

Figure 46–9. By means of Allis forceps passed approximately half way to the PGA mesh, the mucosa is grasped and the ileum is intussuscepted into the pouch so that the PGA mesh now lies adjacent to the pouch and a nipple valve mechanism is created.

662

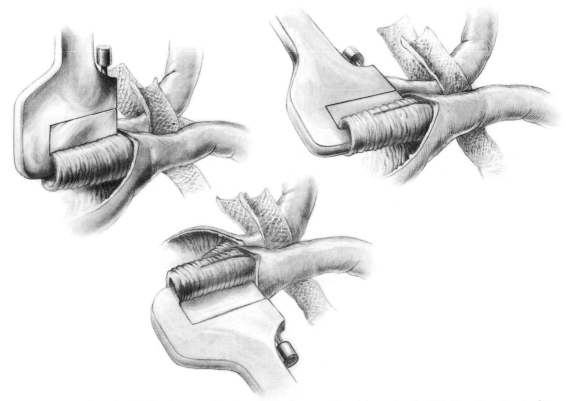

Figure 46–10. Three longitudinal rows of automatic staples are placed by using the TA-55 automatic stapling device and 4.8-mm staples. Note that six staples have been removed from the end of the nipple. These are not required to maintain the intussusception and remain exposed for possible stone formation. The staples at the base of the nipple should not extend beyond the mucosa so as to leave sufficient ileum to close the pouch away from the mesh collar. The three staple lines should be positioned over approximately 180° anteriorly so that the fourth staple row can be placed posteriorly to fix the nipple to the back wall of the pouch and not interfere with the three previously placed staple lines. Holes produced by the pin of the stapler should be closed with 3-0 PGA sutures to prevent possible fistula bypass of the intussuscepted nipple valve.

maintenance of the valve, and these staples tend to remain exposed and become a potential site of stone formation. The distal six staples, therefore, are removed from the corresponding end of the stapler next to the straight arm prior to stapling. These staples can be removed from a standard cartridge by partially firing the device with the jaws separated, extracting six exposed staples, and then gently tapping the remaining staples back into the cartridge with a metal ribbon. Custom cartridges with the six staples removed at the factory are available from V. Mueller Company or may be special-ordered from the US Surgical Company. Equally important, sufficient mucosa and serosa of the pouch must remain beyond the last staple so that the pouch can be closed, leaving the mesh collar away from the mucosa of the pouch.

Next, a fourth row of staples is applied to fix the nipple to the back wall of the pouch.

There are two ways to do this. Whenever possible we slip the anvil of the stapling device along the mesenteric region of the nipple intussusception from the outside (Fig. 46–11B). This keeps staples from being exposed within the pouch and fixes only two walls, one wall of the nipple to the back wall of the pouch. For this technique a standard style cartridge should be used so staples will fix the base of the nipple. The other technique is to make a small opening in the back wall of the pouch approximately 6 cm from the base of the nipple, pass the anvil from the outside to the inside of the pouch, advance the nipple over the anvil, and then fix the nipple, full thickness, to the back wall of the pouch just off the region of the mesentery (Fig. 46–11A). If this procedure is used, a custom stapling cartridge should be utilized. With either technique two additional 3-0 PGA sutures are used to secure the end of each nipple to the back

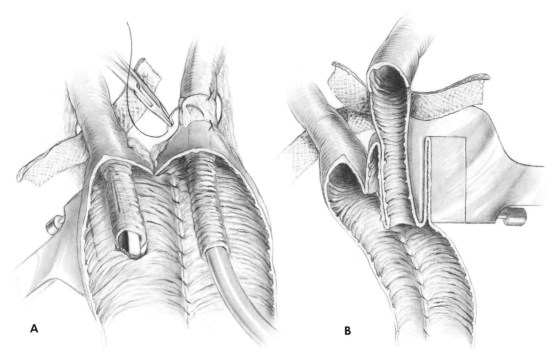

Figure 46–11. *Two methods to fix the nipple valve to the back wall of the pouch. A, A small hole is made in the posterior wall of the pouch several centimeters distant from the nipple. The anvil of the stapling device can be inserted through this hole and the anvil arm of the device can be passed through the nipple. This allows the intussuscepted nipple to be fixed to the back wall of the pouch as further protection against slippage or extussusception. A custom-made cartridge with six staples removed should be used with this method. B, The anvil of the stapler can be inserted into the two walls of the nipple at the region of the mesentery from the outside of the pouch. This will fix the nipple wall to the back wall of the pouch without any staples exposed within the urinary pouch. A standard cartridge with all staples in place should be used with this technique. A also depicts fixation of the PGA mesh at the base of the nipple. A No. 30 Medina tube is inserted through the nipple and on through the PGA mesh so that the mesh can then be positioned around the afferent and efferent limbs. The finger or catheter is used to ensure that the PGA collar is not too tight, in order to avoid the possibility of erosion. The mesh is secured both to the pouch and the respective limb of ileum with interrupted 3-0 PGA sutures.*

wall of the pouch (Fig. 46–12). We believe that secure fixation of the nipple to the pouch wall is an important factor in preventing late extussusception. We have observed that staples allow the nipple to fuse to the pouch wall without causing necrosis since the 4.8-mm staple is nonhemostatic. It is our belief that a suture line or attempts to denude the nipple wall may cause vascular compromise and is not as effective as staple fixation. It is important to suture the pinholes individually at the base of the nipple valve caused by use of the stapling device, since these holes may result in fistulas that bypass the intussusception valve mechanism. The mesh anchoring collar is then fixed to the base of the nipple valves (Fig. 46–12). A small finger or a No. 30 Medina tube can be passed up the intussuscepted nipples and through the mesh site. This will allow the mesh to be affixed circumferentially without being too tight (Fig. 46–11A).

Redundant mesh is excised and the circumferential strip is sutured both to the pouch at the nipple base and to the ileal limb with 2-0 chromic catgut sutures. The collar further helps to maintain the intussusception and serves as the anchoring point for fixing the efferent valve and limb to the abdominal wall. This fixation is obviously important for facilitating long-term catheterization.

The pouch is then closed by folding the ileum in the opposite direction to which it was opened (Fig. 46–13). This method of opening and closing is an important concept that causes the motor activity of the ileum in the different segments of the pouch to counteract themselves, thus creating an extremely low pressure reservoir. The closure is accomplished with a two-layer running 3-0 PGA suture, which is meticulously placed to ensure water tightness. At this point the tip of the closure toward the right side is tucked into the pouch so that the posterior

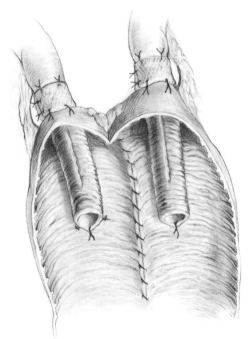

Figure 46–12. Two figure-of-eight 3-0 PGA sutures are used to further fix the ends of each nipple to the back wall of the pouch.

suture line is now visible at a right angle anteriorly off the long continuous anterior suture line. This maneuver places most of the pouch medial to its mesentery and al-

lows the afferent limb to rotate so that it will be ready to fix to the sacral promontory (Figs. 46–14 and 46–15).

Once the pouch closure has been completed, the proximal end of the afferent limb is secured to the sacral promontory. After each ureter has been carefully spatulated, a standard bilateral ureteroileal end-to-side anastomosis is performed using interrupted 4-0 PGA sutures (Fig. 46–15). The distal 12 to 14 cm of No. 8 infant feeding tubes are routinely used as stents. Extra holes are cut (about every 1.0 cm along the length of the tube), and the tube is passed proximally toward the renal pelvis and distally through the afferent nipple, to lie within the pouch. Once the ureteroileal anastomosis has been completed, the trap at the base of the mesentery is closed with interrupted 4-0 silk sutures.

The stoma site is then located and a small plug of skin is removed. The diameter of the stoma should be smaller than that of a standard ileal stoma. Approximate locations of the stoma site can be made preoperatively, but the exact site should be selected after the pouch is created so that the efferent limb can reach the skin in a direction as perpendicular to the pouch as possible. This is especially important in the obese patient. A

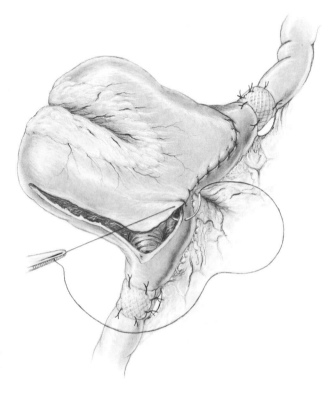

Figure 46–13. The Kock pouch is then closed in the direction opposite to which it was opened. This is done with two layers of continuous 3-0 running PGA sutures to provide a meticulous, watertight closure.

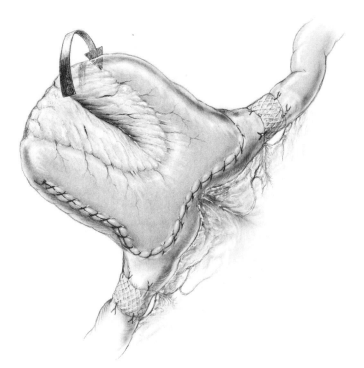

Figure 46–14. *Once the pouch has been closed, the end of the suture line directed toward the right side of the abdomen is tucked into the pouch. This maneuver brings the pouch medial to its mesentery and allows the afferent limb to drop readily toward the sacral promontory to facilitate the ureteroileal anastomosis (see Fig. 46–15).*

vertical incision is made in the subcutaneous fat and the anterior rectal fascia. The rectus muscle is split and a vertical incision just large enough to accommodate two fingers is made in the peritoneum. Two horizontal mattress sutures of No. 1 PGA are then passed through the anterior rectus fascial opening and positioned through both sides of the efferent anchoring collar (Fig. 46–15). Next, a narrow 1.5- to 2.0-cm strip of Marlex is anchored to the abdominal wall just cephalad and lateral to the opening in the peritoneum with 1.0 nylon figure-of-eight sutures. The Marlex strip is then brought through the window of Deaver in the mesentery adjacent to the PGA mesh collar. Redundant ileum from the afferent limb is excised and the ileum brought out through the abdominal wall foramen. Both mattress sutures of No. 1 PGA are then securely fastened, thus fixing the anchoring collar of the pouch and continence valve mechanism to the abdominal wall. Care must be taken at this time to make sure the sutures are not crossed and that there is a straight shot from the end of the ileum to the intussuscepted valve. Next, the Marlex strip is secured to the abdominal wall medial to the mesentery and securely fixed with

another No. 1 nylon figure-of-eight suture (Fig. 46–15, inset). We believe this Marlex strip is an important modification that prevents the development of a peristomal hernia as well as slippage of the continence valve mechanism and helps to eliminate both redundancy of the efferent limb and difficult catheterization problems (Fig. 46–15). All redundant ileum above the skin line should be excised. A flush stoma is finished by sutures made circumferentially to the subcuticular skin with 3-0 PGA.

A No. 30 Medina tube is passed into the pouch and carefully positioned so that the drainage holes are several centimeters beyond the efferent nipple. The tube should allow good irrigation and be positioned away from the suture line closing the pouch. The Medina tube is secured with two No. 1 nylon sutures to keep it in place for three weeks. This tube placement should be done before the abdominal wall is closed.

A one-inch Penrose drain is then passed through a separate stab incision and sewn to the psoas muscle or peritoneum lateral to the rectum with a 3-0 chromic suture several centimeters away from the pouch. This is done to prevent migration of the drain into the pouch.

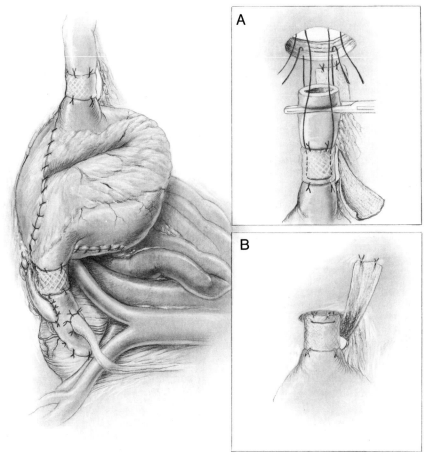

Figure 46–15. *Final location of the pouch with completed ureteroileal anastomosis. Horizontal mattress sutures of No. 1 PGA suture are passed through the anterior rectus fascia, the collar of the efferent limb of the Kock pouch, and back out through the anterior rectus fascia. One suture is placed lateral and one medial to the pouch, and the efferent limb is drawn through the abdominal wall (Inset A). The sutures are then secured so that the PGA mesh is fixed to the anterior rectus fascia, thus affording a very short segment from the PGA mesh collar to the skin. Redundant efferent ileum is excised, providing a flush stoma. Note the use of a narrow Marlex strip fixed to the abdominal wall both lateral and medial to the pouch (Inset B). This strip is passed through the window of Deaver through which the PGA mesh was placed. This strip serving as a strut is important in preventing a parastomal hernia and helps fix the continence valve mechanism to the abdominal wall.*

POSTOPERATIVE FOLLOW–UP

Postoperatively, Medina tubes should be irrigated every four hours with 30 to 60 ml of normal saline, or as often as necessary to prevent obstruction with mucus. By the second or third postoperative day, patients are instructed in self-irrigation techniques. They are usually discharged on the seventh to tenth postoperative day. The Medina tube remains in place for three weeks from the date of operation.

After approximately three weeks, patients return for an overnight admission. On ar-rival, the Medina tube is removed, a "Kock-oscopy" is performed with a standard cys-toscope, and the indwelling ureteral stents are extracted with biopsy forceps. A cysto-gram of the pouch ("Kockogram") is then obtained, followed by intravenous pyelo-gram. If no leaks are observed, the patient is then instructed in self-catheterization tech-nique. Catheterization is begun at two- to three-hour intervals. Parenteral aminogly-cosides are administered during the 24-hour hospitalization. If no difficulties are encoun-tered during the 24-hour stay, the Penrose drain can be removed and the patient dis-charged. The catheterization interval is usually increased by one hour each week.[26] The goal after six to eight weeks is to have patients catheterize themselves only every six hours during the day and be able to sleep eight hours at night. Oral antibiotics are usually maintained until the catheterization schedule is stabilized. All patients wear a small pad over their stoma to prevent spotting of their clothes from small amounts of discharged mucus or urine. The pads are removed for swimming or bathing. Long-term follow-up consists of a check-up every four to six months with a "Kockogram," intravenous urogram, and analysis of serum electrolytes, creatinine, and urine culture.

RESULTS

The average operating time to create a continent Kock reservoir is one to two hours longer than that for creation of a standard ileal conduit. All other operating time is approximately equal, whether it is done in conjunction with cystectomy or as a conversion of an existing ileal conduit. It is tedious surgery in which meticulous attention to every detail is essential. The final stage of the operation, the creation of the stoma and the fixation of the efferent limb, is probably the most crucial to the patient. For them, the ease of catheterization is all important.

EARLY POSTOPERATIVE COMPLICATIONS

Our early complication rates continue to remain similar to those initially reported in our first 51 patients.[42] There were 42 early complications in the 250 patients. This early complication rate is similar to the early complication rate we have observed in other patients undergoing single-stage radical cystectomy and ileal conduit urinary diversion (Chapter 44). Our learning curve in terms of ongoing experience and the various complications are listed in Table 46–1. The series of 250 cases included five operative mortalities, which resulted from sequences of events associated with the cystectomy and were not directly attributed to the Kock pouch. Two of the five had cirrhosis of the liver, which significantly contributed to their mortality.

At the beginning of our series, the importance of drain placement was not appreciated. Two of the original patients developed pelvic abscesses secondary to poor drainage and required reoperation to resolve the abscess. Since that time, Penrose drains have been used, and only one pelvic abscess has been noted subsequently. There were 18 patients who had prolonged drainage of urine, and seven of these required reoperation. Patients who are well drained without evidence of infection should eventually heal without intervention. As noted before, several of the patients were found to have migration of their Penrose drains into the Kock pouch. We now routinely suture the Penrose to the psoas muscle or peritoneum or to the side of the rectum with a 3-0 chromic suture several centimeters away from the base of the afferent limb. In the cases in which the drain was observed in the pouch, all that was needed was to pull the drain out several inches to allow the leak site to close.

Table 46–1. EXPERIENCE IN CONTINENT URINARY DIVERSION (KOCK POUCH), AUGUST 1982 TO AUGUST 1985*

Complication	Patient Group					
	1–51	52–104	105–157	158–200	201–250	Total
Prolonged urine leak—no operation	6	1	2		2	11
Urine leak—reoperated			2†	2	3	7
Pelvic abscess—reoperated	2	1				3
Enterostomy pouch fistula—reoperated			1	1†		2
Enterocutaneous fistula—no operation	1			1		2
Partial small bowel obstruction/ileus pancreatitis—no operation		1	1			2
Pyelonephritis	1				1	2
Gastrostomy leak	1		1†			2
Stent migration		1				1
Other (medical)	1†	1†		4	4	10
Total	12	5	7	8	10	42 (16%)

*Data from 250 patients. Early complications: 42 out of 250 (16%); cystectomy and Kock pouch: 34 out of 189 (18%); conversion to Kock pouch: 8 out of 60 (13%).

†Operative mortality rate: 5 out of 250 (2%).

Reprinted with permission from Skinner DG, Lieskovsky G, and Boyd SD: Continuing experience with the continent ileal reservoir (Kock Pouch): an update after 250 cases. J Urol 137:252, June 1987.

After the first 25 patients, all ureteral anastomoses have been stented. One stent coiled in a hydronephrotic renal pelvis, and this was removed endoscopically. The other early complications included two enterostomy pouch fistulae, of which one closed on its own and one necessitated surgery for Kock pouch conversion to an ileal conduit; two partial small bowel obstructions, which resolved without surgery; two episodes of treatable pyelonephritis; and prolonged drainage from the routinely placed gastrostomy tubes in two patients. The one conversion to an ileal conduit that occurred during the immediate postoperative period was in a woman who received an unknown amount of old-time radiation for an endometrial carcinoma, and she developed an enterocutaneous fistula through the pouch.

LATE COMPLICATIONS

Late complications are often difficult to assess in a population of patients for whom the operation is part of the treatment of malignancy and whose age makes them prey to other serious medical conditions. We have analyzed our data in terms of late complications directly resulting from the operation or as a direct result of this form of urinary diversion. In this context, 77 of the 245 patients surviving the operation have suffered one or more late complications, requiring 85 reoperations. The late complications have mainly involved problems with continence or ease of catheterization. Most of the problems were detected within the first six months of surgery. The late complications and operations required are listed in Table 46–2.

Urinary Leakage

The most common complaint was excessive urine leakage at the stoma, noted in 44 patients (18%). This leakage was often seen in conjunction with difficulty in catheterization. In 18 of these patients, the onset of leakage was sudden and due to acute prolapse of the efferent valve—all in patients who had had perfect continence prior to the event. Chronic stomal leakage was noted in 20 others and was the result of a shortened nipple valve, hypermobility of the nipple, or a split nipple. The other six patients had parastomal hernias that were responsible for, or associated with, their leakage. Overall, 41 of the 44 patients who had this complication have subsequently undergone a total of 55 revisional operations to achieve continence. Three patients have yet to undergo revision; they wear an appliance and intermittently catheterize themselves two to three times during a 24-hour period.

We have found that once significant leakage occurs, or if patients are having difficulty with catheterization, revision should be done promptly, since continence and ease of catheterization can be achieved and should be the goal in all cases. To repair leakage or efferent limb redundancy, we routinely dissect out the efferent limb from the abdominal wall, continuing that part of the

Table 46–2. KOCK POUCH EXPERIENCE 8/82–3/86
SUMMARY OF LATE COMPLICATIONS IN THE FIRST 250 PATIENTS

Complication	I 1–51	II 52–104	III 105–157	IV 158–200	V 201–250	Total 1–250	#Reops
Leak for any reason (18%)	9(1)	9(3)	9(2)	7	10	44(6)	55
Incompetent valve; vascular; split; pinhole	5	4(2)	4	1	6	20(2)	23
Sudden prolapse	2(1)	5(1)	3(1)	6	2	18(3)	18
Parastomal hernia with leak	2	0	2(1)	0	2	6(1)	14
Parastomal hernia without leak	1	0	0	4	1	6	7
Difficult catheter-no leak	3	3	1	1	0	8	9
Marlex erosion	0(3)	1(5)	0(2)	0	0	1(10)	3
Stones in pouch	5(1)	0(1)	0	0	0	5(2)	3
Partial SBO	0	1	0	2	1	4	1
Afferent limb problem	0(1)	0	0(1)	0	1	1(2)	1
Pyelonephritis	1(1)	0	0(1)	0(2)	0	1(4)	1
Hydronephrosis (U-I junction)	1(1)	2	0(1)	0	0	3(2)	3
Electrolyte abnormality	0	1	0(1)	1	0	2(1)	0
Conversion ileal loop	0(1)	2(1)	0	0	0	2(2)	2
	20(9)	19(10)	10(8)	15(2)	13	77(29)	85

( ) = secondary complication asymptomatic or part of another problem.
Reprinted with permission from Lieskovsky G, Boyd SD and Skinner DG: Management of late complications of the Kock pouch form of urinary diversion. J Urol 137:252, June 1987.

dissection through the rectus fascia as far as possible before incising the old midline abdominal incision. Care must be taken not to damage the blood supply to the efferent limb, particularly in the region of its mesentery which is found cephalad. The abdomen is then opened and the pouch dissected off the anterior abdominal wall. Once the efferent limb and pouch have been mobilized, the pouch is opened several centimeters away from the nipple and away from the mesentery of the pouch, allowing the cause of the failure to be determined. If the nipple looks healthy and the cause of leakage was prolapse or hypermobility, the nipple is stapled to the wall of the pouch (Fig. 46–11A) and further fixed with 3-0 PGA sutures securing the muscularis of the nipple to the muscularis of the pouch wall (Fig. 46–12). Since we have started to do this routinely at the time of the initial surgery, this problem is now rarely seen.

Occasionally, a fistula will be found at the base of the nipple, owing to forced catheter false passage, or a split nipple will result in leakage. These valves can be further intussuscepted into the pouch, repaired, restapled, and again fixed to the wall of the pouch over a Medina tube. If the nipple length was found to be inadequate or fibrotic, suggestive of vascular insufficiency or slough of the original nipple, a new efferent limb and nipple needs to be created from an adjacent 15-cm segment of small bowel. This new efferent limb and nipple is then sewn to the pouch as a patch graft at the site where the old limb and nipple were resected. This technique has been successful in six patients.

In patients needing revision who had previously had Marlex used as a collar, we routinely dissect out the foreign material and replace it with PGA mesh. In addition, the afferent antireflux nipple should be checked for evidence of Marlex erosion, as has been seen in two of our patients. When this occurs, the Marlex is dissected out from inside the pouch, but no replacement mesh has been used on the afferent nipple.

The leakage resulting from a parastomal hernia or diastasis in the obese patient is the most difficult to resolve. In this situation, which occurred in six patients, we tried to move the stoma to a new site or, if possible, to strengthen both the anterior and posterior fascia with a sandwich of PGA mesh. Most of these patients required at least one additional surgical procedure to relocate the stoma in order to achieve a satisfactory result. From experience we would recommend against using a sheet of Marlex mesh as a flange around the efferent limb, because of the difficulties encountered at reoperation as well as the ongoing risk of infection. We do recommend the use of a Marlex strip as depicted in Figure 46–15 wherever revision is necessary. We feel this modification will help eliminate further herniation since the region of the mesentery is the usual site for development of a parastomal hernia.

All 41 patients who have undergone revisional surgery are currently dry, although additional surgery was required in several. The remaining three patients with chronic leakage are either awaiting surgery or tolerating the degree of leakage.

Difficult Catheterization

Difficulty catheterizing without associated leakage was noted in eight patients. This problem was corrected by removing the redundancy and angulation of the efferent limb and usually reanchoring the fixation collar to the anterior fascia, especially on the mesenteric side. An infected Marlex collar secondary to erosion was observed twice and corrected by removal of the Marlex and substitution with PGA mesh, which is now routinely used. Again, the Marlex strip should be used in the reoperation to eliminate the tendency for redundancy and creation of a false passage in the region of the mesentery, a common tendency in obese patients with a fat mesentery.

Electrolyte Abnormality

Hyperchloremic metabolic acidosis has been noted to a minor degree in three patients. It has been easily controlled in all with oral bicarbonate. One additional patient who had metabolic hyperchloremic acidosis preoperatively as a consequence of ureterosigmoidostomy was weaned off oral bicarbonate supplement slowly over a period of six months following Kock conversion and now has normal levels of serum electrolytes.

One interesting patient returned on three occasions during the first three months following cystectomy and Kock pouch urinary diversion with symptoms of dehydration, nausea, and vomiting. He also had a serum electrolyte pattern of hyponatremic, hypochloremic, hyperkalemic metabolic acidosis. A careful review of his operative note revealed that at surgery he was found to have a large Meckel's type small bowel diverticulum approximately 10 cm distal to the ligament of Treitz in the proximal jejunum. In order to obviate the need for two small bowel anastomoses, his Kock pouch was created from jejunum. In addition, he had received four cycles of platinum combination chemotherapy before surgery, as his primary urologist felt he had positive nodes on the basis of a pelvic CT scan. This reduced his creatinine clearance to 47 ml/minute, an observation that was not taken into consideration at the time the jejunum was chosen for the pouch. Thus the combination of compromised renal function and a jejunal reservoir resulted in an iatrogenic metabolic condition that could have been avoided or better treated.[14, 32] The patient currently has normal serum electrolyte levels and is maintained on oral sodium chloride supplement.

It should be emphasized that no serious or progressive long-term electrolyte problems have been observed in any patients; the follow-up has now been beyond three years.

Pyelonephritis

Pyelonephritis has been noted in six patients requiring rehospitalization for intravenous antibiotics. Two of these episodes have occurred in patients with reflux, and one has occurred in a diabetic who has now been asymptomatic for over two years. Careful evaluation of the function of the afferent antireflux valve is required if pyelonephritis recurs. In one patient whose Kock pouch was constructed elsewhere, as well as in two of our own patients, we discovered that recurrent bouts of pyelonephritis resulted from prolapse or extussusception of the antireflux nipple when the pouch was full. This prolapse caused reflux and obstructed the afferent limb. When the pouch was drained, the nipple valve reversed itself into the pouch and promptly filled with several hundred milliliters of urine from the afferent limb. The repair of this valve stopped further episodes of pyelonephritis in all four pa-

tients. It is of interest that many of the patients who had undergone previous ureterosigmoidostomy or ileal conduits had suffered recurrent episodes of pyelonephritis. Kock conversion eliminated this problem of febrile episodes despite the fact that most patients have chronic bacteriurea on routine culture of urine from the pouch.

Routine "Kockograms" (cystograms of the Kock pouch) have revealed reflux in only six patients. Reflux by itself is not an indication for revision unless it is associated with recurrent pyelonephritis or upper tract deterioration. To date, only the two patients whose valves extussuscepted have undergone revision.

Hydronephrosis

Hydronephrosis was noted on follow-up intravenous pyelogram (IVP) secondary to ureteroileal anastomotic stenosis in five patients, and three of these have undergone revision. The other two remain stable and are asymptomatic. We have not seen hydronephrosis as a result of afferent nipple stenosis.

Stone Formation

Stone formation in the pouch has been found in seven of the early patients, and five have undergone successful endoscopic removal. The stones tended to form on staples near the end of the nipples, on eroded Marlex collars, or on the heavy 0 PGA sutures we originally utilized that were not absorbed. Since staples are no longer employed on the exposed end of the nipple valve, and the Marlex collar has been replaced by PGA mesh, the anticipated stoma problem has not materialized.

Conversion Back to External Collection

Overall, four patients underwent conversion of the Kock pouch to an ileal conduit, one during the immediate postoperative period as noted previously, and three during the first year following surgery. Of the three conversions, two patients were probably marginal candidates because of ongoing physical and psychologic problems that ultimately made it difficult for them to deal with catheterization and potential further revisional surgery. In both cases the efferent nipple valve was excised and an everted cutaneous nipple was constructed so that the ileal pouch could easily drain into an external appliance.

The third patient had an excellent functional continent pouch for seven months, until he presented with an erythematous recurrent abscess lateral to the stoma and secondary to an infected Marlex collar. After three reoperations to excise the Marlex, all of which resulted in urinary leakage, primary lung cancer with hilar nodal metastasis was diagnosed and the patient requested conversion to an external appliance rather than go through additional surgery to achieve continence.

OTHER LATE COMPLICATIONS

Three delayed small bowel obstructions occurred: two were partial and were managed conservatively with nasogastric suction, and one required reoperation. The latter obstruction occurred in a young exstrophy patient three months following Kock conversion of an ileal conduit at the site of her original small bowel anastomosis. She had originally undergone an ileal conduit diversion at the age of two years. In retrospect we believe that, whenever possible, the old small bowel anastomosis should be excised at the time of Kock pouch conversion and ileum proximal to the old anastomotic site should be used for the ileal pouch. This principle would seem prudent, particularly if the old anastomosis had been done in childhood.

COMMENTS

Our ongoing experience with the Kock continent ileal urinary reservoir has continued to yield encouraging results. The essential criterion of a low-pressure, high-volume internal reservoir that is truly continent, easy to catheterize and empty and prevents reflux has been realized. One only has to look to the patients themselves for encouragement. The most vocal advocates of the procedure remain those Kock pouch patients who previously have had urinary diversion by another method. The mean pouch size

after maturing is between 800 and 1000 ml, with ranges from 500 to 1600 ml. The patients describe a feeling of fullness or slight cramping when the reservoir capacity is reached. Patients with previously irradiated bowel may have a somewhat decreased pouch compliance, but they eventually achieve good pouch capacities. Asymptomatic bacteriuria is routinely noted. Most patients are kept on antibacterial suppression for the first two to three months, but continued prophylaxis is utilized only in the patients with recurrent local symptoms or pyelonephritis. Hyperchloremic acidosis does not appear to be a problem. Currently, only four of our patients are on electrolyte replacement, including one on supplemental sodium and chloride who had his pouch constructed out of jejunum. Only patients with abnormal renal function may eventually require oral bicarbonate supplement.

The long-term question about stone formation is still being examined. Animal laboratory experiments have allowed us to follow dogs with Kock-type diversions utilizing stapled nipple valves for up to 18 months and then to examine the results pathologically. Calculi are a problem only if nonabsorbing material such as the metal staples remain exposed above the mucosa. Care must be taken to bury the staples at the time of surgery. As an alternative, absorbable staples are being studied for this purpose. The presence of any other nonabsorbable material should be minimized, which is why we have stopped using the Marlex anchoring collar and heavy suture material. The presence of calculi or foreign bodies, however, should always be considered whenever there are repeated episodes symptomatic of urinary tract infection in a Kock patient with normal findings on intravenous urogram and "Kockogram." "Kockoscopy" is easily performed, and the pouch can readily be examined for stones, which then can be extracted.

The most important factor in the success of the Kock pouch is creation and maintenance of the nipple valves to prevent reflux and to ensure continence. The principle of an intussuscepted nipple is an old surgical technique described originally by Watsuji in 1899 in the formation of a gastrostomy.[52] Through the years a number of urologists and general surgeons have used this principle. Intussusception techniques were reported in the urologic literature as early as

1949.[3, 15, 27, 29, 35, 44, 51] Other reports have followed, and although Leisinger and associates indicated in 1977 that creation of an intussuscepted nipple valve was simple,[28, 29] experience has shown, in fact, that construction of an effective valve that remains competent is far from easy. Of the original 12 patients reported by Kock and associates, six needed reoperation because of slippage.[23] Turnbull reported that if the surgeon maintained intestinal continuity, up to 8 cm of mesentery could be stripped safely from the ileum without loss of viability.[49] Hendren supported this observation and successfully intussuscepted the terminal 8 cm of ileum into the cecum in an effort to prevent reflux across the ileocecal valve in cases of bladder reconstruction without diversion.[17] Nonetheless, until the availability of nonhemostatic, nonreactive metal staples, the ability to maintain an intussuscepted segment was erratic. The combination of the PGA mesh collar, four rows of staples (one of which fixes the nipple to the pouch wall), and creation of a 5-cm intussuscepted nipple ensures continence and prevents reflux. Careful creation of this valve mechanism is the most important key to a successful, continent internal intestinal reservoir.

As the results indicate, our enthusiasm is still tempered by the need for revisional operations. Our ongoing modifications and fastidious attention to detail reflect our attempt to address the potential complications. Patients must still be aware that complications may occur. High patient motivation and a thorough understanding of the Kock pouch with its potential problems continue to be essential prerequisites to the operation. Further minor refinements will certainly continue to be made, and we anticipate that the long-term revision rate will be minimized. The basic surgical premise as conceived by Kock remains: a low-pressure, high-capacity reservoir with continent and nonrefluxing valves can be constructed from ileum. It is a sound concept that offers an acceptable alternative to the patient who requires cutaneous urinary diversion.

References

1. Ashken MH: An appliance-free ileocaecal urinary diversion; preliminary communication. Br J Urol 46:631–638, 1974.
2. Ashken MH: Continent ileocaecal urinary reservoir. J R Soc Med 71:357–360, 1978.
3. Basso DE: Efficacy and applicability of an intussus-

cepted conical valve in preventing regurgitation and leakage of intestinal contents. Ann Surg 133:477–485, 1951.
4. Bricker EM: Symposium on clinical surgery: bladder substitution after pelvic evisceration. Surg Clin North Am 30:1511–1521, 1950.
5. Bricker EM: Personal communication.
6. Bricker EM, Eiseman B: Bladder reconstruction from cecum and ascending colon following resection of pelvic viscera. Ann Surg 132:77–84, 1950.
7. Camey M, Le Duc A: L'enterocystoplastie avec cystoprostatectomie totale pour cancer de la vessie. Ann Urol 13:114, 1979.
8. Coffey RC: Transplantation of ureters into large intestine. Surg Gynecol Obstet 47:593–621, 1928.
9. Elder DD, Moisey CU, Rees RW: A long-term follow-up of the colonic conduit operation in children. Br J Urol 51:462–465, 1979.
10. Ferris DO, Odel HM: Electrolyte pattern of blood after bilateral ureterosigmoidostomy. JAMA 142:634–640, 1950.
11. Gerber A: The Kock continent ileal reservoir for supravesical urinary diversion. An early experience. Am J Surg 146:15–20, 1983.
12. Gerber A: Improved quality of life following a Kock continent ileostomy. West J Med 133:95–96, 1980.
13. Gilchrist RK, Merricks JW, Hamlin HH, Rieger IT: Construction of substitute bladder and urethra. Surg Gynecol Obstet 90:752–760, 1950.
14. Goldschmidt S, Dayton AB: Studies in mechanism of absorption from intestine, contribution to one-sided permeability of intestinal wall to chlorides. Am J Physiol 48:419, 1919.
15. Grey DN, Flynn P, Goodwin WE: Experimental methods of ureteroneocystostomy: experiences with the ureteral intussusception to produce a nipple or valve. J Urol 77:154–163, 1957.
16. Hannsson HA, Kock NG, Norlen L, et al: Morphological observations in pedicled ileal grafts used for construction of continent reservoirs for urine. Scand J Urol Nephrol 49(Suppl):49–61, 1978.
17. Hendren WH: Reoperative ureteral reimplantation: management of the difficult case. J Pediatr Surg 15:770–786, 1980.
18. Jagenburg R, Kock NG, Norlen L, Trasti H: Clinical significance of changes in composition of urine during collection and storage in continent ileum reservoir urinary diversion. An experimental and clinical study. Scand J Urol Nephrol 49(Suppl):33–42, 1978.
19. Jones MA, Breckman B, Hendry WF: Life with an ileal conduit: results of questionnaire surveys of patients and urological surgeons. Br J Urol 52:21–25, 1980.
20. Kock NG: Evolution of ileostomy surgery. Can J Surg 24:270–276, 1981.
21. Kock NG: Ileostomy without external appliances: a survey of 25 patients provided with intra-abdominal intestinal reservoir. Ann Surg 173:545–550, 1971.
22. Kock NG: Intra-abdominal "reservoir" in patients with permanent ileostomy. Preliminary observations on a procedure resulting in fecal "continence" in five ileostomy patients. Arch Surg 99:223–231, 1969.
23. Kock NG, Nilson AE, Nilsson LO, et al: Urinary diversion via a continent ileal reservoir: clinical results in 12 patients. J Urol 128:469–475, 1982.
24. Kock NG, Nilson AE, Norlen L, et al: Changes in

renal parenchyma and the upper urinary tracts following urinary diversion via a continent ileum reservoir. An experimental study in dogs. Scand J Urol Nephrol 49(Suppl):11–22, 1978.

25. Kock NG, Nilson AE, Norlen L, et al: Urinary diversion via a continent ileum reservoir: clinical experience. Scand J Urol Nephrol 49(Suppl):23–31, 1978.

26. Lapides J, Diokno AC, Silber SJ, Lowe BS: Clean, intermittent self-catheterization in the treatment of urinary tract disease. J Urol 107:458–461, 1972.

27. Leadbetter WF: Consideration of problems incident to performance of uretero-enterostomy: report of a technique. Trans GU Surg 42:39–51, 1950.

28. Leisinger HJ, Sauberli H, Schauwecker H, Mayor G: Continent ileal bladder: first clinical experience. Eur Urol 2:8–12, 1976.

29. Leisinger HJ, Schauwecker H, Sauberli H: Dynamics of the continent ileal bladder. An experimental study in dogs. Invest Urol 15:49–54, 1977.

30. McConnell JB, Stewart WK: The long-term management and social consequences of ureterosigmoid anastomosis. Br J Urol 47:607–612, 1975.

31. Mogg RA: Treatment of neurogenic urinary incontinence using the colonic conduit. Br J Urol 37:681–686, 1965.

32. Morales PA, Whitehead ED: High jejunal conduit for supravesical urinary diversion: report of 25 cases. Urology 1:426–431, 1973.

33. Nesbit RM: Ureterosigmoid anastomosis by direct elliptical connection: preliminary report. J Urol 61:728–734, 1949.

34. Norlen L, Trasti H: Functional behavior of the continent ileum reservoir for urinary diversion. An experimental and clinical study. Scand J Urol Nephrol 49(Suppl):33–42, 1978.

35. Parsons CD, Thomas MH, Garrett RA: Colonic adenocarcinoma: a delayed complication of ureterosigmoidostomy. J Urol 118:31–34, 1977.

36. Perl JI: Intussuscepted conical valve formation in jejunostomies. Surgery 25:297–299, 1949.

37. Philipson BM, Nilsson LO, Norlen L, et al: Mucosal adaptation in ileum after long time exposure to urine. In JWL Robinson, RH Dowling, EO Riecken (eds), Mechanisms of Intestinal Adaptation. Lancashire, England, MTP Press Ltd. 1982, p 613.

38. Richie JP, Skinner DG: Urinary diversion: the physiological rationale for non-refluxing colonic conduits. Br J Urol 47:269–275, 1975.

39. Richie JP, Skinner DG, Waisman J: The effect of reflux on the development of pyelonephritis in urinary diversion: an experimental study. J Surg Res 16:256–261, 1974.

40. Rieger IT, Weisser JR: Substitute bladder operation on paraplegic. US Armed Forces Med J 3:1507–1513, 1952.

41. Skinner DG: Further experience with the ileocecal segment in urinary reconstruction. J Urol 128: 252–256, 1982.

42. Skinner DG, Boyd SD, Lieskovsky G: Clinical experience with the Kock continent ileal reservoir for urinary diversion. J Urol 132:1101–1107, 1984.

43. Skinner DG, Lieskovsky G, Boyd SD: Technique of creation of a continent internal ileal reservoir (Kock pouch) for urinary diversion. Urol Clin North Am 11:741–749, 1984.

44. Smith GI, Hinman F Jr: Intussuscepted ileal cystostomy. J Urol 73:261–269, 1955.

45. Steven K, Klarskov P, Jakobsen H, et al: Transpubic cystectomy and ileocecal bladder replacement after preoperative radiotherapy for bladder cancer. J Urol 135:470–475, 1986.

46. Sullivan H, Gilchrist RK, Merricks JW: Ileocecal substitute bladder. Long-term follow-up. J Urol 109:43–45, 1973.

47. Tizzoni G, Poggi A: Die Wiederherstellung der Harnblase: experimentelle Untersuchungen. Zentralbl Chir 15:921, 1888.

48. Trasti H: Urinary diversion via a continent ileum reservoir. An experimental and clinical study. Scand J Urol Nephrol 49(Suppl):1–71, 1978.

49. Turnbull RB Jr: Personal communication.

50. Turnbull RB Jr, Higgins CC: Ileal valve pouch for urinary tract diversion: preliminary report of eight cases. Cleve Clin Q 24:187–192, 1957.

51. Turner RD, Goodwin WE: Experiments with intussuscepted ileal valve in ureteral substitution. J Urol 81:526–529, 1959.

52. Watsuji H: Eine combinierte Anwendung des hacker- und fontan'schen verfahrens bei der Gastrostomie. Mitt d med Gesellszh zu Tokyo 13:879, 1899.

53. Zingg E, Tscholl R: Continent cecoileal conduit: preliminary report. J Urol 118:724–728, 1977.

54. Zinman L, Libertino JA: Antirefluxing ileocecal conduit. Urol Clin North Am 7:503–512, 1980.

STUART D. BOYD, M.D.

CHAPTER *47*

Management of Male Impotency, Including Technique of Penile Prosthesis Placement

The entire field of sexual rehabilitation of the urologic cancer patient has undergone radical changes in the last 15 years. Not only has a wide variety of penile prostheses been introduced, but the neurovascular anatomy and the neurophysiology of erections have been more fully defined. Even more important to the patient, however, has been the recognition that sexual rehabilitation is a vital aspect in preserving the patient's on-going quality of life and should be integral in the total cancer treatment.

The therapy for prostate and bladder cancer, which often includes radical surgery, radiation therapy, and hormonal manipulation, not only can cause a change in sexual functioning but can obviously be very psychologically intimidating to the patient. Patients have many misconceptions about the potential impact of treatments. The fear of total loss of sexual functioning is the excuse used by many patients to avoid seeking definitive therapy. The concept of sexuality should, therefore, always be included in the earliest treatment plans. A preliminary in-depth discussion, preferably with both the patient and his sexual partner, often can provide everyone with the information needed to help the patient come to terms with his feelings about cancer, its treatment, and its ultimate sexual impact. The patient should specifically be made aware of the different components of sexuality such as desire, arousal, sensation, orgasm, ejacula-tion, and erections. He should be shown how certain aspects can be affected by treatment whereas others are left intact. Just as with the female mastectomy patient, there is no question that the well-informed male urologic patient can better maintain his self-esteem and drive to recover when he continues to feel sexually attractive and functional.

Probably paramount in most men's minds is the question of erectile dysfunction. It is well known that the classical approach to radical prostate and bladder cancer surgery results in near 100% impotency. Even definitive radiation therapy (either external beam or seed implants), though often advertised as potency-sparing, results in anywhere from 20 to 80% eventual loss of functional erections. The identification by Walsh and Donker of the lateral neurovascular bundles that innervate the corpora cavernosa has been one of the major breakthroughs in helping surgeons appreciate the pelvic anatomy and understand the cause of impotency.[7] The surgical sparing of these sacral autonomic nerves in selected cases can result in the maintenance of the preoperative quality of erection in 50 to 80% of patients.[8] Which radical cystectomy or prostatectomy patients will ultimately benefit from this nerve-sparing surgery is still debated. For patients in whom the cancer surgery itself is not compromised, however, this type of surgery will continue to help address this part of the sexual problem.

675

There certainly will continue to be a pool of patients in whom the nerve-sparing surgery is not used, the preoperative erection is of poor quality, or the nerve-sparing surgery is not successful, with postoperative impotence. The need for follow-up radiation therapy will obviously add to this pool. It is to this group of patients that the subject of penile prosthesis implantation is addressed.

PATIENT SELECTION

As noted above, the risk of post-treatment impotency will vary with the type of surgery or radiation used. The risk level for each patient usually can be identified in the pretreatment phase and appropriate counseling given. It is very important that this counseling be afforded to both the patient and his sexual partner, though these discussions can be useful even if the patient is seen alone. It is helpful to understand what the patient's or couple's sexual attitudes are prior to the treatment. This can help to identify the potential role for a prosthesis in the patient's future. Usually a psychologist or psychiatrist who is oriented in sexual rehabilitation is an invaluable member of the counseling team. Psychologic problems should be addressed early in the treatment phase. Problems that could make patients poor candidates for a penile prosthesis include organic brain syndrome, frank psychosis, severe depression, personality disorder, and complicated marital difficulties.[4]

Prior to anticipating any penile prosthetic surgery, several issues concerning patient body image and sexual outlook should be confronted. The patient's mental attitude and physical condition are much more crucial than his age in establishing any implantation criteria. No strict age restrictions need to be applied. Misconceptions about cancer and sexual functioning are common and these should be corrected. For instance, patients often need to be reassured that genital urinary cancers are not spread venereally and that having sex will not diminish their treatment potential. The question of body image is particularly important with bladder cancer patients. Many cystectomy patients feel that if they must wear an ostomy appliance, they are no longer sexually attractive. This problem is addressed with the advent of the new urinary diversion procedures such as the continent Kock ileal reservoir.

Continent diversions help patients better maintain their body image and heighten their interest in continued sexual functioning. Even patients with Stage D prostatic cancer who require early orchiectomy deserve to have the question of sexual rehabilitation raised. Though their sexual desire is likely to diminish, these men certainly still can be sexually aroused and can obtain orgasms.

Some men with impotency can, of course, be treated by means other than penile prosthetic surgery. Included in these options is the new experimental injection of the corpora cavernosa with papaverine hydrochloride and phentolamine mesylate.[9] Patients have been taught to inject themselves with these vasodilators to induce erections on an outpatient basis. This method of drug injection is to be considered, however, both investigational and of limited value at this time.

DEVICE SELECTION

There is a multiplicity of penile prostheses available for implantation today. Essentially these devices fall into three categories. There are malleable (semirigid) rods, inflatable penile prostheses, and newer, cylinder-contained inflatable devices. Unless there are special circumstances dictating that a particular device be used, the choice of prosthesis should be left up to the patient after he has been apprised of the pros and cons of each type. Special circumstances might suggest not using an inflatable prosthesis when manual dexterity is impaired or not using a semirigid rod in a patient with difficulty emptying his bladder or with decreased penile sensation.

A typical malleable prosthesis is depicted in Figure 47–1 (Table 47–1). The original Small-Carrion or Flexi-rod devices are now probably used less frequently than the malle-

Table 47–1. SEMIRIGID RODS

Advantages
1. Technically easy surgery
2. Any surgical approach can be utilized
3. Least expensive

Disadvantages
1. Poor flaccidity
2. Constant pressure on tissues may contribute to pain and erosion
3. Interferes with transurethral endoscopic procedures

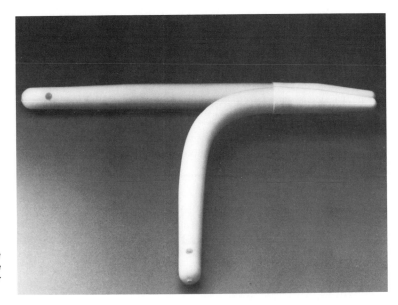

Figure 47–1. The AMS Malleable 600 Penile Prosthesis with the flexibility demonstrated. Courtesy of American Medical Systems.

able wire cylinders. The advantages of these types of prostheses are that technically they are easy to implant, the surgical approach for insertion can be through any of the four incisions (circumcising, penoscrotal, infrapubic, or perineal), and they are the least expensive. Their limitations include poor flaccidity, constant pressure inside the corpora (which increases the incidence of pain and erosion), and interference with transurethral endoscopic procedures.

The inflatable penile prosthesis has been in use for more than 10 years (Fig. 47–2; Table 47–2). It has undergone numerous modifications and improvements, and it is manufactured in slightly varied forms by two different companies. Although it was implanted with mixed results in the 1970s, the inflatable penile prosthesis can now be considered quite reliable. The advantages of this prosthesis are that it allows for a fully controllable erection with full-girth rigidity

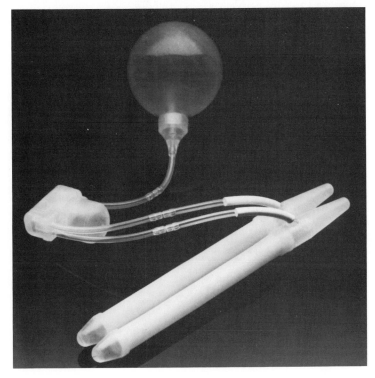

Figure 47–2. The AMS Inflatable 700 Penile Prosthesis. Courtesy of American Medical Systems.

Table 47–2. INFLATABLE PENILE PROSTHESIS

Advantages
1. Controllable erection
2. Full girth erection with good flaccidity
3. Easily concealed
4. Minimal interference with transurethral endoscopic procedures

Disadvantages
1. Most difficult technical surgery
2. More components for mechanical failure
3. More costly than semirigid rods

Table 47–3. HYDROFLEX PROSTHESIS

Advantages
1. Easier surgery than needed for the inflatable penile prosthesis
2. Any surgical approach
3. No separate components other than the cylinders
4. More flaccid than a semirigid rod

Disadvantages
1. Less girth than the inflatable penile prosthesis
2. Less flaccid than the inflatable penile prosthesis
3. As costly as the inflatable penile prosthesis
4. Mechanical failure possible

and excellent flaccidity, it is easily concealed, and it causes minimal to no interference with transurethral endoscopic procedures. Its disadvantages are that it requires the most technically difficult surgery, there are more components for potential mechanical failure, and the device is more costly than the semirigid rods. It also requires some degree of manual dexterity either by the patient or his partner to operate.

The newest type prosthesis consists of self-contained inflatable cylinders of which the Hydroflex (American Medical Systems) is an example (Fig. 47–3; Table 47–3). This device became available for implantation in 1985, although it has been tested at several centers across the United States since 1983. It is designed to allow for rigidity or flaccidity by the transference of fluid back and forth between the portion of the cylinder that occupies the penile shaft and a reservoir in its proximal end. The pump for inflation is built into the head of the cylinder, and

deflation is accomplished by deforming a valve just behind the head (Fig. 47–4). The advantages of this type of device include the fact that it allows for an inflatable erection with more flaccidity than semirigid rods. Any surgical approach to the penis can be used for implantation, and it is much easier technically to implant than the inflatable penile prosthesis because it requires no other components. By its very design, however, there are limitations to this device. Because the cylinders are bulkier than the regular inflatable cylinders, they afford less flaccidity than the inflatable penile prosthesis, especially in the smaller penis. Since the cylinders inflate to a set diameter (11 mm or 13 mm), they also usually afford less girth than the inflatable penile prosthesis. Like the inflatable prosthesis, this is a mechanical device that is potentially prone to mechanical problems, though clinical trials of the most recent design modification have not identified any recurrent defects. The cost

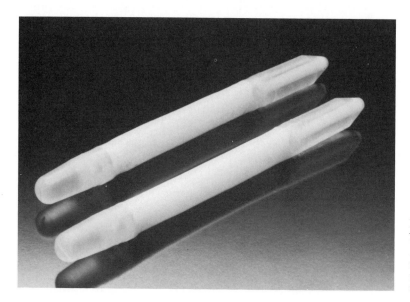

Figure 47–3. The AMS Hydroflex Self-Contained Penile Prosthesis. The pump is contained in the head of the cylinders and the reservoir is in the tail. Courtesy of American Medical Systems.

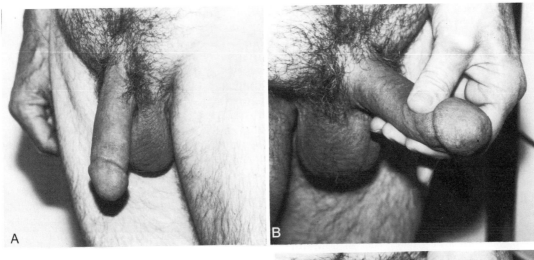

Figure 47–4. A, *Patient with a Hydroflex penile prosthesis in place in the deflated position.* B, *Prosthesis is being inflated to the erected position.* C, *Position of the fingers to deflate the device.*

of the device is about the same as that for the regular inflatable prosthesis.

PREOPERATIVE PREPARATION

The optimal timing of the prosthetic surgery depends on several factors, including the type of cancer surgery, the use of radiation therapy, and the patient's psychologic adjustment. In patients who were already impotent prior to the cancer surgery or in whom it was known that the neurovascular bundle was definitely sacrificed at the time of the pelvic dissection, usually a minimum six-week wait is advised. Penile surgery performed earlier is associated with rather marked pain and edema, especially following a complete pelvic node dissection. A three- to 6-month wait following pelvic radiation therapy is probably also preferable for the same reasons. Following a nerve-sparing procedure for either prostatic or

bladder cancer, at least a one year's observation period should be allowed for assessment of sparing of potency.

Once the surgery time is at hand, prophylaxis against infection must be meticulously provided. It should be established that the patient have sterile urine. Parenteral antibiotics should be started up to 12 hours prior to the surgery. In this age of cost-consciousness, more prostheses are implanted on an outpatient basis, and in these cases, loading doses of broad-spectrum antibiotics such as an aminoglycoside and a cephalosporin should be given approximately one hour before surgery. The patient should be instructed to take an antiseptic shower prior to this. All shaving of the surgical site should be done in the operating room to prevent contamination of any nicks with nosocomial bacteria. A 10-minute scrub with povidone-iodine is used. All potential contamination sites such as the rectum or stomas should be draped with plastic-backed drapes. Extraneous operating room traffic should be eliminated. The environment should be kept as lint-free as possible, and the prosthesis should be handled only on a separate table or stand.

OPERATIVE TECHNIQUE

The operative approach to the penis differs slightly for each device. Suprapubic or penoscrotal incisions can be used for any of the devices. In addition, a subcoronal incision can be used for the semirigid and Hydroflex prostheses. The perineal approach, popularized by Small, is rarely used now by most implanters because of the more difficult dissection and greater risk of contamination.[5] The majority of procedures are performed under general or spinal anesthesia, but the use of local anesthesia is assuming more of a role in outpatient surgery.[2]

Semirigid Prosthesis

Regardless of the approach selected, precise exposure of the corpora cavernosa is necessary for the implantation of any cylinders. The location of both the urethra and the dorsal midline neurovascular bundle should be clearly delineated. Placement of a catheter in the urethra usually is not necessary if one is certain of the dissection. An indwelling catheter often distorts the cosmetic appearance of the glans penis while the dissection and cylinder placement is checked.

The tunica albuginea should be opened longitudinally for a distance of 2 to 3 cm. This incision should be well away from either the urethra or the dorsal bundle. Temporary traction sutures on each side of the incision will aid in exposing the underlying spongy tissue. Dilation of the corpora should be begun by first establishing a plane just under the tunica with the dissecting scissors. The dilation is accomplished by use of the Hegar dilators.

The tips of the dilators should always be directed laterally to avoid accidental perforation of the midline intercorporal septum. If perforation occurs, the tract should be redilated, with the surgeon again being very conscious that the tip of the dilator can always be palpated laterally. Care should be taken to be certain that the dilation is accomplished out to the tip of the corpora under the glans distally and to the crural attachment proximally. Except in unusual circum-

stances of previous trauma, the two corpora should be approximately the same length. The prostheses generally are available in diameters ranging from 9 to 13 mm, and most patients require at least an 11-mm diameter. One should, therefore, usually begin with an 8-mm Hegar dilator and proceed up to a Hegar diameter of 1 mm larger than that of the selected prosthesis. Prostheses of larger diameter afford more rigidity but often at the expense of some decreased malleability.

The proper length of the corpora can be determined by placing the penis on moderate stretch and then measuring both proximally and distally from the traction sutures in the middle of the incisions. It is important not to overestimate the length of the corpora. The cylinders are best placed tail first. Once the cylinders are in position, distal and proximal palpation should be performed to be certain that the tail of the prosthesis extends to the bottom of the crus and that the proximal end supports the glans well. If the cylinders tend to buckle out of the incision, they are too long and should be trimmed appropriately. The incisions should then be closed with a running absorbable suture such as 3-0 PDS (polydioxanone suture). The wound is irrigated well with antibiotic solution and then closed. Most patients are able to be discharged within 24 hours; they are placed on oral antibiotics for one week. Intercourse can commence in four to six weeks after all of the pain and edema have subsided.

Inflatable Penile Prosthesis

The inflatable penile prosthesis is a three-component device consisting of cylinders, a pump, and a reservoir. The device can ordinarily be implanted entirely through either of two incisions, penoscrotal or suprapubic. Both approaches have been well described elsewhere.[1, 6] The urologic cancer patient, however, offers a further challenge. Retropubic fibrosis following radical cystectomy or prostatectomy makes it difficult to reenter this space for placement of the reservoir through either incision. Usually a separate muscle-splitting incision off the iliac crest is required to place the reservoir in a retroperitoneal position. When a thorough pelvic lymphadenectomy has been incorporated with the cancer surgery, the patient will also have markedly prolonged pain and edema in the scrotum after the pump is implanted, requiring much delayed activation of the device.

These unique problems in the cancer patient have led us to develop a new two-stage technique for the implantation of the inflatable penile prosthesis. This is applicable in patients undergoing pelvic surgery in whom it is known that the lateral neurovascular bundles of erection are being sacrificed or in whom the preoperative erection was already of poor quality. The reservoir and pump of the device are implanted during the first stage at the time of the radical cancer surgery, whereas the cylinders are implanted and the device connected electively during the second stage at a later date, usually six to 12 weeks postoperatively. Specifically, toward the end of the cancer surgery and just prior to closing, a retroperitoneal pocket near the left side of the pelvis is created for the reservoir. In cystectomy patients, this is easily accomplished by dissecting the peritoneum off the posterior abdominal fascia low on the left side. The reservoir is placed in this pocket with the reservoir tubing exiting the rectus muscle above the external inguinal ring. In prostatectomy patients in whom the peritoneal envelope has been kept intact, the reservoir is simply placed in the retroperitoneum laterally above the psoas. The reservoir tubing is again brought through the abdominal wall above the external ring, and the tubing is placed in the subcutaneous fat lateral to the midline incision. It is important to keep the reservoir extraperitoneal in order to minimize contamination and to shield it from any intraperitoneal complication or urine leak, especially if reexploration ever becomes necessary. It is easiest to place the reservoir on the left and keep the stomas and other drains on the right. The reservoir is filled with 65 ml of appropriately diluted Hypaque (Winthrop) or Cysto-Conray II (Mallinckrodt) solution, or with sterile saline if the patient is allergic to contrast medium. After the subcutaneous fat above the left external ring is opened, a blunt tunnel is created along the spermatic cord as deep into the scrotum as possible. The pump of the prosthesis is placed low in the scrotum with the deflate side facing laterally. The reservoir tubing from the pump is connected to the reservoir with a straight connector, which is doubly reinforced with 3-0 Prolene ties. The cylinder tubings are shortened appropriately so that they lie in the subcutaneous tissue overlying the pubis; then they are connected

to each other with a right-angle connector in order to cap them off and allow for later easy location. After all the components are well irrigated with antibiotic solution, a Jackson-Pratt drain is placed in the scrotum and subcutaneous tissue and is exited lateral to the midline incision. The Jackson-Pratt drain is left in place for about two days or until drainage is minimal.

The second stage is performed after a minimum six-week waiting period. By this time the scrotal pump will already be well healed and painless, and pumping instructions are easily given. A strong capsule already will have formed around the reservoir. The second stage is easily performed under any type of anesthesia, since neither the abdomen nor the scrotum need be approached. A small vertical incision is made just above the dorsal base of the penis overlying the pubis. The cylinder tubings should be easily located in the subcutaneous fat with the cautery knife. The corpora are exposed just lateral to the dorsal midline neurovascular bundle and opened for a distance of 2 cm proximally. The cylinders are then implanted in the standard fashion.[6] The proper placement of the rear tip extenders and good seating of the cylinder heads into the glans should again be stressed. The incisions are closed with a running 3-0 PDS suture. The cylinders should then be inflated and the quality of erection appraised. Any angulation, bulging, or corporal restrictions should be corrected at this time. After the cylinders are deflated, they are simply attached (with right-angle connectors) to the preplaced cylinder tubings from the pump overlying the pubis. The preplaced cylinder tubings from the pump should first have been disconnected, but the right-angle connector can be kept in one side and used for one of these connections. The whole area is well irrigated with antibiotic solution and the wound is closed in layers with 3-0 Dexon. The patient can usually be discharged within 24 hours. Instructions on use of the pump are given in about two weeks, and sexual activity can begin one month later.

Hydroflex Penile Prosthesis

The surgical technique for the Hydroflex prosthesis is essentially the same as for the semirigid rods. Any comfortable penile incision can be used. The healing of a subcoronal incision, however, may prolong the period before pumping of the device may be initiated, since the incision would overlie the pumping mechanism. The incisions should be at least 3 cm in length in order to simplify the cylinder insertion. Precise dilation and measurement of the corpora is essential, because each cylinder is prefilled and presterilized and cannot be resterilized once it is unpackaged. The Furlow inserter is a convenient measuring device for the corpora, and it can also be used for cylinder placement. The cylinders come in preset lengths of 13, 16, 19, and 22 cm, and 1- or 2-cm rear tip extenders can be used to make up the other lengths. There are two diameter choices: 11 and 13 mm. The corpora must be easily dilated to 13 to 14 mm if the 13-mm cylinder is to be used. For penile lengths of 16 cm or greater, the 13-mm cylinders afford a much superior rigid erection. In the shorter penis, however, the 13-mm device often is too bulky to allow good flaccidity. Insertion of the cylinders is best performed in a standard fashion. The cylinders come loaded with a tip suture that is passed through a Keith needle and placed into the Furlow inserter. After dilation, the insertion tool allows the suture to be placed through the glans at the tip of the corpora. Unlike implanting the inflatable penile prosthesis, however, the head of the device is not pulled up to the glans at this point. The prosthesis is instead rigidly inflated and the rear portion is first pushed down to the crus. The cylinder is then deflated and the traction suture is used to pull the front end into position. The incisions are again closed with a running 3-0 PDS suture. The new AMS Closing Tool is helpful in minimizing the risk of needle damage to the cylinder during closure by keeping the cylinder pushed aside. The wound is well irrigated with antibiotic solution and closed in layers. The patient is usually ready for discharge within 24 hours. Inflation and deflation instructions are begun in two to four weeks after pain and edema have subsided. Intercourse can be instituted in a few weeks as comfort permits.

SPECIAL OPERATIVE TECHNIQUES

For the appropriate patients who desire the inflatable penile prosthesis, the two-stage implantation technique offers numer-ous advantages. The pump and reservoir are very easily implanted during the pelvic surgery and, importantly, do not significantly add to the operative time of the primary procedure. The reservoir is not as easily positioned at a later date. The pump will already be healed when the entire prosthesis is eventually connected, bypassing the initial difficulty of operating the device through the scrotal pain and edema. Psychologically, the patients feel very relieved that their problem with erectile dysfunction is being addressed immediately. The second stage is very easily performed under any type of anesthesia, and the postoperative stay should be lessened. We do not recommend implanting the entire prosthesis at the time of the initial surgery because the increased operative time required to implant and connect the cylinders may add to the morbidity of the primary procedure, the risk of infection to the corpora or cylinders may be greater, and the patient probably will not want to or be able to operate the device for several weeks or months anyway. We have successfully implanted the inflatable penile prosthesis in over 100 cancer patients by using this technique and have not found any increased infection rates, which remain at 2%.

If the patient is also afflicted with Peyronie's disease, the extent of the plaque should be assessed preoperatively and the surgical approach altered appropriately. If the plaque is quite extensive, the malleable, semirigid rods will probably offer the most satisfactory result. In patients with fairly discrete plaques, however, the inflatable devices can still be employed. Usually the plaque can be cracked with the cautery knife at the point of maximum angulation and good straightening will result. If the defect obtained after splitting the affected tunica is quite large, then this defect can be filled with a Gore-Tex graft. The nondistensible type of inflatable cylinders are probably most appropriately used in these cases.

Previous injury, inflammation, or congenital defects may further alter the surgical approach. The most commonly encountered deformity is probably the poorly supported glans penis or so-called SST deformity. This may arise because of improper dilation of the corpora into the glans or too short a prosthetic cylinder. These problems obviously can be corrected by appropriate attention to the details of corporal dilation and cylinder placement. Some patients, however, have this problem because the anatomic septum between the corpora cavernosa and the glans penis is positioned so that the glans will bend despite the correct size of the prosthesis. This problem can be best addressed at the time of the original surgery rather than after the patient is given an opportunity to tolerate it. A technique described by Kaufman offers the easiest and most cosmetic solution.[3] After making a dorsal subcoronal skin incision, horizontal mattress sutures of 3-0 Prolene can be placed into the substance of the glans and then sutured to the tunica albuginea of the corpora on each side of the midline. When these sutures are tied, it has a rein-like effect on the glans, pulling it back onto the cylinders. This technique is also applicable to secondary revisions of the penis, needed when the patient finds the glans too floppy for intercourse.

COMPLICATIONS AND RESULTS

Most of the postoperative complications and difficulties with the prostheses center around infection, prolonged pain, erosion, and mechanical breakdown. The infection rates seem to run about 1 to 3% and do not vary greatly with the various types of prostheses. Prolonged pain is more of a factor with the semirigid rods, although, ultimately, usually less than 1% need to be removed for this reason. Urethral or skin erosion is also more of a problem with the semirigid devices but, again, should occur in less than 1 to 2% of patients. With erosion and removal of one cylinder, several patients have been noted to still continue to have satisfactory intercourse with only one remaining cylinder in place. Mechanical breakdown is a possible risk of the inflatable devices. With the changes in the device in the last few years, however, this rate should be kept below 10%. The mechanical problems include fluid loss, tubing kinks, cylinder buckling, and pump malfunction.

Overall, the results for all of the devices reveal a greater than 90% patient satisfaction rate. Satisfaction is defined as the ability to have intercourse without pain and with adequate rigidity. Patient satisfaction appears to vary greatest with patient expectation. The younger patient, however, is probably going to be most satisfied with the cosmetic result of an inflatable penile prosthesis.

CONCLUSION

The penile prosthesis is now an accepted and integral part of the sexual rehabilitation of the urologic cancer patient. The indications for its use will vary as nerve-sparing surgery establishes its role in the cancer treatment. No one type of prosthesis appears to answer the needs of all patients; there is an acceptable place and function for each device. The cosmetic results will vary with the patient's anatomy and with the skill and experience of the implanter. Maximum patient satisfaction, however, will be achieved by appropriate and intensive counseling both pre- and postoperatively.

References

1. Fishman IJ, Scott FB, Light JK: Experience with inflatable penile prosthesis. Urology 23:86–92, 1984.
2. Kaufman JJ: Penile prosthetic surgery under local anesthesia. J Urol 128:1190–1191, 1982.
3. Kaufman JJ, Lindner A, Raz S: Complications of penile prosthesis surgery for impotence. J Urol 128:1192–1194, 1982.
4. Olsson PA: Penile prosthesis. Med Aspects Human Sexuality, 13:109, 1979.
5. Small MP, Carrion HM, Gordon JA: Small-Carrion penile prosthesis: new implant for management of impotence. Urology 5:479–486, 1975.
6. Stecker JF: Surgical Management of erectile impotence. In DF Paulson (ed), Genitourinary Surgery. New York, Churchill Livingstone, 1984.
7. Walsh PC, Donker PJ: Impotence following radical prostatectomy: insight into etiology and prevention. J Urol 128:492–497, 1982.
8. Walsh PC, Lepor H, Eggleston JC: Radical prostatectomy with preservation of sexual function: anatomical and pathological considerations. Prostate 4:473–485, 1983.
9. Zorgniotti AW, Lefleur RS: Auto-injection of the corpus cavernosum with a vasoactive drug combination for vasculogenic impotence. J Urol 133:39–41, 1985.

DONALD G. SKINNER, M.D.
GARY LIESKOVSKY, M.D.
T. RAND PRITCHETT, M.D.

Technique of Radical Nephrectomy

CHAPTER **48**

INDICATIONS FOR SURGERY ON PATIENTS WITH RENAL CELL CARCINOMA

Radical nephrectomy denotes the removal of Gerota's fascia, with its contents intact, and early ligation of the renal artery and vein. Regional retroperitoneal lymph node dissection is performed routinely, even though there are no solid data supporting its efficacy at improving survival. Obviously, the performance of this procedure as described is dependent upon appropriate patient selection and surgical judgment. Suitable candidates include those with potentially curable lesions (Stages I to III) and those in good medical condition whose life expectancy without cancer of the kidney would be five to 10 years. Radical surgery is probably not advisable for poor-risk patients; rather, simple palliative nephrectomy may be indicated to control pain or bleeding. Age alone is not a contraindication to the procedure, providing that the patient is a reasonable operative candidate. In selected patients with only one or two metastases, aggressive treatment combining radical nephrectomy and simultaneous or subsequent excision of all metastatic lesions seems indicated. This approach is supported by the report of Middleton,[16] who reviewed his experience and that of Skinner and associates[24] and O'Dea and co-workers,[18] demonstrating that 34% of the patients

undergoing nephrectomy and excision of minimal metastases were alive for five or more years after surgery.

SURGICAL TECHNIQUE

We prefer the thoracoabdominal approach for nearly all retroperitoneal tumors and use it in the management of renal cell carcinoma, renal pelvic tumors, and node dissection for testicular tumors. It is particularly useful in the management of massive retroperitoneal disease, including primary tumors, as well as massive metastatic disease from testicular primary lesions.

Sweet[27] and others used the thoracoabdominal approach for gastroesophageal resections as early as 1947. Subsequently, Chute and associates[2] adopted the method for resecting large renal cell carcinomas. Cooper and associates[3] first described use of the approach in retroperitoneal node dissection for testicular tumors. Since then, we have modified it to facilitate a complete retroperitoneal approach in standard procedures or to combine it with an intra-abdominal approach in the treatment of extensive disease or in complicated situations.

We believe there are no absolute contraindications to this approach and use it routinely in the performance of an ileoureteral substitution procedure, radical nephrectomy for renal cell carcinoma, nephroureterectomy for urothelial neoplasms of the upper collecting system, retroperitoneal node dissection for testicular tumors, and resection of all extensive retroperitoneal tumors regardless of origin.

Preoperative Preparation. Preoperative preparation is fairly routine. In older patients, prophylactic preoperative digitalization is usual unless there is a specific contraindication. Our practice is to give 0.5 mg of digoxin early in the day before the operation, followed by 0.25 mg that afternoon and 0.125 mg the evening before surgery. Overnight hydration with Ringer's lactate is routine. In patients with large tumors in whom we anticipate a combined intra-abdominal approach with possible resection of a portion of the colonic mesentery, we initiate a short but effective bowel preparation beginning 24 hours before surgery. Several hours after a routine breakfast the day before surgery, 120 ml of emulsified castor oil is administered, after which the patient is maintained on clear liquids.

Patient Positioning. Patient positioning is extremely important, and attention to detail facilitates all phases of the operation. The patient should be positioned on the ipsilateral side of the operating table with the break of the table located immediately above the iliac crest. The lower of the two legs is flexed 90° at the knee and the hip is flexed approximately 30°. The ipsilateral shoulder is then torqued approximately 30° off the horizontal, and the ipsilateral arm is brought across the chest to be placed in an adjustable arm rest. The pelvis remains nearly supine, perhaps rotated approximately 10° off the horizontal. A sheet roll is then placed longitudinally under the ipsilateral back, and a similar roll is positioned under the contralateral abdomen. The table is then fully hyperextended and the patient secured with wide adhesive tape at the shoulders, hips, and leg. The ipsilateral leg remains extended along the ipsilateral edge of the table, supported by a pillow (Fig. 48–1).

Technique. Generally, an incision is made along the ninth rib, beginning at the midaxillary line, extending across the costochondral junction to the epigastrium, and then directed inferiorly as a midline or paramedian incision. For very large tumors a T-shaped incision is used, extending the horizontal portion of the epigastric incision across to the contralateral costochondral junction and then dropping an ipsilateral

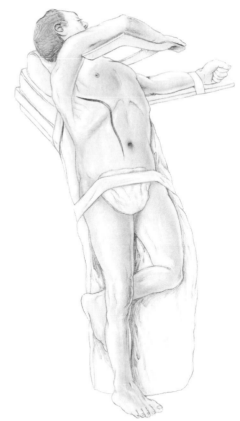

Figure 48–1. Patient positioning for right thoracoabdominal radical nephrectomy. Note that the patient's right side is adjacent to the ipsilateral edge of the operating table.

paramedian or midline extension inferiorly. For tumors associated with a vena caval tumor thrombus, and when control of the vena cava above the diaphragm or at the level of the right atrium is desired, a higher incision resecting the eighth or seventh rib is used.

We prefer rib resection to an intercostal incision. Careful comparison reveals no difference in degree of pain or postoperative requirements for analgesics; rib resection is rapid, easy to close, and allows wider exposure without fracturing adjacent ribs. The muscles overlying the rib and periosteum are incised using cautery, and a subperiosteal resection is performed.

The anterior rectus fascia is incised, the rectus muscle retracted laterally, and the rectus muscle transected in the epigastrium. This prevents denervation of the rectus with resultant diastasis and weakness of the abdominal wall.

The costochondral junction is then divided after bluntly passing a Mayo scissors under the cartilage into the abdominal cavity. This step is important in order to identify the plane between the muscle and fascia of the abdominal wall and the peritoneum, and it is the hallmark to performing a retroperitoneal dissection without entering the peritoneal cavity. However, an exclusively retroperitoneal dissection is applicable primarily for small renal tumors or tumors of the renal pelvis or ureter, since development of the plane between the anterior surface of Gerota's fascia and the colonic mesentery and parietal peritoneum may lead to considerable venous bleeding if the renal artery has not been previously ligated. Therefore, in performing a radical nephrectomy for renal cell carcinoma, we prefer to enter the peritoneum after dividing the costochondral junction. When the peritoneum is opened widely, the pleura is incised and the diaphragm is divided in the direction of its fibers. It is helpful to dissect the peritoneum off the diaphragm posteriorly before dividing, as this facilitates later mobilization of the liver for right-sided tumors or of the spleen for left-sided tumors. A self-retaining Finochietto retractor is then positioned, with the costochondral junction placed through the holes in the blades of the retractor.

Next, attention is directed toward ligation of the renal artery. For right-sided tumors, the cecum is mobilized from the right lower quadrant by incising the avascular line of Toldt and dividing peritoneal attachment to the small bowel mesentery medially up to the ligament of Treitz (Fig. 48–2). Mobilization of the mesentery at the ascending colon overlying the tumor is deferred until the renal artery is ligated. As the small bowel is elevated, the duodenum comes into view and should be elevated along with the pancreas as the dissection continues to the ligament of Treitz. At this point, one can readily palpate the top of the aorta cephalad to the origin of the inferior mesenteric artery. Identification of the aorta is made possible with careful dissection of the fibroareolar lymphatic tissue surrounding it. With right-angled clips, this tissue is then clipped and divided parallel to the aorta, and ipsilateral lumbar arteries are ligated and divided as one dissects in a cephalad direction. A gonadal artery can frequently be identified, clipped, and divided. Immediately cephalad to the gonadal artery, the left renal vein, crossing over the vena cava, should be identified. A Gil-Vernet or vein retractor should elevate this vein, allowing continued dissection of the aorta up to the origin of the

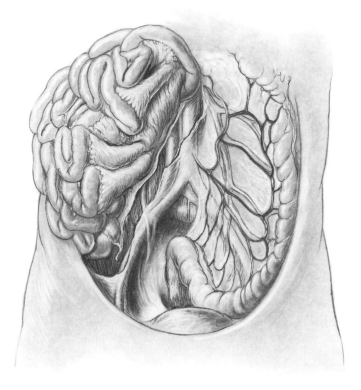

Figure 48–2. Access to the right renal artery. The cecum and ascending colon are mobilized along the avascular line of Toldt. The peritoneal attachments to the small bowel are mobilized from the ileocecal junction proximal to the ligament of Treitz and medial to the descending colonic mesentery. This maneuver elevates the duodenum and pancreas off the retroperitoneal area and allows identification of the inferior mesenteric vein and origin of the superior mesenteric artery from the aorta.

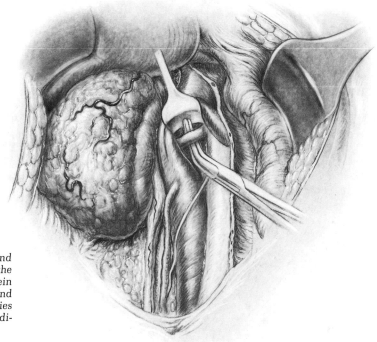

Figure 48–3. Fibroareolar tissue and lymphatic tissue are divided over the top of the aorta. The left renal vein and vena cava have been retracted and the origin of the renal artery or arteries has been identified, ligated, and divided.

superior mesenteric artery. The right renal arteries should then be identified medial to the aorta and behind the left renal vein (Fig. 48–3). These arteries should be ligated and divided at this time.

Next, dissection continues caudally along the top of the aorta distally, sweeping all tissue off the top of the aorta toward the ipsilateral side down to the origin of the inferior mesenteric artery, which should be identified and protected. Ipsilateral lumbar arteries should be ligated and divided, as they may provide additional blood supply to large renal tumors. This dissection sweeps medially to the inferior mesenteric artery and continues along the medial distal aorta, along the common iliac artery, which represents the caudal limits of the dissection. The ureter and gonadal vessels are ligated and divided at this location.

The ascending colon and duodenum are further mobilized off Gerota's fascia and reflected medially. The ascending colon and small bowel contents can then be placed in a Lahey bowel bag and positioned on the chest.

All tissue is then divided over the vena cava, extending in a cephalad direction. The gonadal vein is ligated and divided. If the renal vein is free of tumor extending in the vena cava, it should be ligated and the dis-

section continued along the vena cava up to the insertion of the most inferior hepatic vein, which represents the cephalad extent of dissection. The vena cava should then be completely skeletonized, and the various lumbar veins are ligated individually. Once the vena cava has been skeletonized, it can be elevated with a vein retractor and all tissue from between the aorta and vena cava swept to the ipsilateral side, thus exposing the intervertebral ligaments behind the great vessels. Large hemoclips should be placed on the ascending lumbar venous plexus, which passes posteriorly immediately adjacent to the sympathetic chain.

Attention is finally directed toward the cephalad extent of Gerota's fascia and the adrenal vein. When the peritoneum is mobilized off the diaphragm, the liver can easily be elevated and retracted medially. This maneuver allows one to visualize the adrenal and to dissect Gerota's fascia off the diaphragm, the quadratus lumborum, and psoas muscles from a lateral to medial dissection. The adrenal vein should then be identified and ligated, thus exposing the right crus of the diaphragm. Once this is accomplished, the entire specimen can be removed en bloc with the regional nodes and with Gerota's fascia intact.

The sympathetic grooves should be carefully inspected, as numerous veins interdigitate between these nerves, the lumbar veins, and the ascending lumbar venous trunk. Some of these may require suture ligature. Usually it is possible to preserve the sympathetic chain, but this is of little consequence in most patients afflicted by renal cell carcinoma. The cisterna chyli should be identified and carefully clipped where it passes medial to the right crus of the diaphragm, posterior to the origin of the right renal artery. This will prevent lymph leak during the postoperative period, and inspection of the origin of the superior mesenteric artery may reveal some lymph leak from the dilated lacteals that run parallel to the superior mesenteric artery in this area. These should be individually clipped.

If the primary right renal tumor is small, a radical nephrectomy and regional lymph node dissection can be performed entirely via the retroperitoneal route, the approach of which is described in Chapter 54. The advantage of retroperitoneal dissection is lack of subsequent adhesions and prevention of possible small bowel obstruction. In addition, there is less of an ileus with earlier postoperative return of bowel function.

For small left-sided tumors, it is usually possible to incise the transversalis fascia at the junction of the peritoneum and Gerota's fascia laterally, so that the descending colon and its mesentery can be swept off the anterior surface of Gerota's fascia medially (Fig. 48–4). One looks for the inferior mesenteric vein and can trace it to its junction with the splenic vein in order to identify the superior mesenteric artery. The left renal vein passes immediately caudad to the origin of this artery. The left renal vein is then mobilized by ligation of the adrenal, gonadal, and posterior ascending lumbar veins, allowing early access to the left renal artery.

For large tumors or very vascular tumors, it is best to do this through an intraperitoneal route. The duodenum can be mobilized near the ligament of Treitz, with intraperitoneal identification of the inferior mesenteric vein. Again, one divides all tissue over the aorta extending cephalad to the point where the left renal vein crosses over the aorta. The left renal vein should be mobilized by ligating the gonadal, ascending lumbar, and adrenal veins. It can then be elevated and the renal artery ligated and divided (Fig. 48–5). The left renal vein is then ligated at its insertion into the vena cava. All fibroareolar and lymphatic tissue is then swept off the top of the vena cava medially, thus cleaning the side wall of the vena cava. The ipsilateral

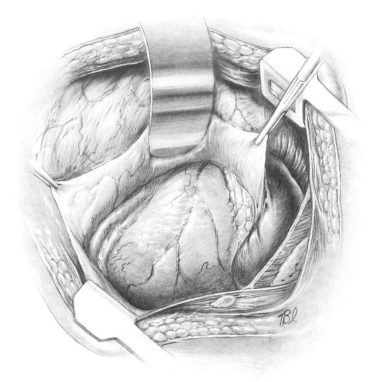

Figure 48–4. For small, left-sided tumors the tranversalis fascia can be divided in the groove between the descending colon and the anterior surface of Gerota's fascia, which allows the descending colon and its envelope of peritoneum to be swept medially off the anterior surface of Gerota's fascia. The inferior mesenteric vein, splenic vein, and origin of the superior mesenteric artery are identified. The left renal vein passes immediately caudal to the origin of this artery.

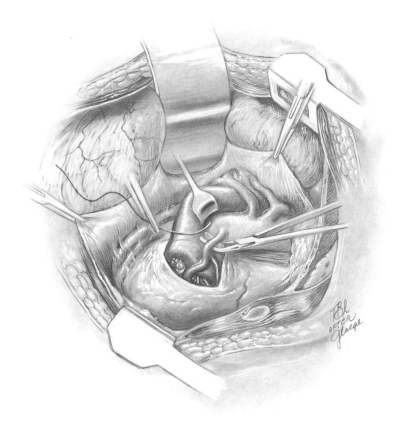

Figure 48–5. *Ligation of the left renal artery. Note relationships with the superior mesenteric artery and the left renal vein.*

lumbar veins are ligated at the point at which they join the vena cava down to the level where the right common iliac artery crosses. The gonadal vessels and ureter are divided where they cross over the left common iliac artery.

Gerota's fascia can be mobilized off the quadratus lumborum and psoas muscles posteriorly. Again, the vascular communications between the adrenal and phrenic vessels are clipped and divided superiorly; the celiac ganglion is also clipped and divided, thus exposing the crus of the diaphragm.

The aorta should then be skeletonized by dividing all fibroareolar and lymphatic tissue immediately over the aorta down to its bifurcation. For most left-sided tumors, the inferior mesenteric artery must be ligated and divided unless there is marked evidence of atherosclerotic disease, in which case such wide regional node dissection is probably not indicated and preservation of the inferior mesenteric artery should be attempted. The uppermost lumbar arteries are ligated off the aorta. Usually, it is not necessary to ligate the lumbar vessels distal to

the inferior mesenteric artery, except in a relatively young patient in whom more aggressive dissection is performed. The aorta can then be elevated and all fibroareolar and lymphatic tissue swept from underneath the great vessels over the intravertebral ligaments to the ipsilateral side, thus allowing complete removal of the kidney within Gerota's fascia en bloc with the regional lymph nodes.

Careful inspection should then be made to ensure that all bleeding is well controlled. We routinely inspect the origins of all lumbar arteries and further secure them with medium-sized hemoclips. We carefully inspect the renal pedicle and the inferior mesenteric artery if it has been ligated, and doubly secure these vessels with a large hemoclip. Retroperitoneal drains are not necessary, but a No. 22 chest tube is routinely inserted. Then, 5 ml of a 0.5% solution of bupivacaine hydrochloride is injected into the intercostal neurovascular bundles of the seventh, eighth, ninth, tenth, and eleventh ribs.[5] This can be done easily by percutaneous injection, with a finger placed within the thorax to ensure proper placement of the needle. Care must be taken not to inject the solution intravascularly. In some cases, an epidural spinal technique is used for anesthesia. If so, the intercostal nerve block is not necessary, and epidural instillation of morphine can be used during the postoperative period for long-term pain relief.

The diaphragm is closed with a running size 0 Dexon or Vicryl suture in two layers. Closure of the remainder of the incision is facilitated by figure-of-eight through-and-through sutures of size 1 nylon, securing all muscular layers of the chest and abdomen in one layer. The knots should be inverted in thin patients. Medially, the diaphragm should be incorporated in several of these sutures.

Several comments concerning this operative technique should be emphasized. Obviously, proper patient selection and surgical judgment are essential prerequisites. The aorta is mobilized unless there is extensive evidence of atherosclerosis, in which case aggressive regional lymph node dissection is probably not indicated. Ligation and division of the lumbar arteries distal to the renal pedicle facilitate aortic mobilization for left-sided tumors, and only ipsilateral lumbar division is performed in right-sided tumors. Bleeding from an avulsed lumbar vessel may occur but can usually be avoided by individual ligation and division of each vessel distal to the renal pedicle. Placement of hemoclips on the distal portion of each vessel facilitates this part of the operation, but it is best to ligate the origins of lumbar arteries and veins from the aorta and vena cava because clips may become dislodged later in the procedure, causing troublesome bleeding from the great vessels. Occasionally, bleeding from a torn lumbar artery or vein may occur despite all precautions, in which case use of an Allis forceps clamp is helpful. In addition, arterial silk sutures should be available at all times.

The cisterna chyli should be identified behind the right renal artery, located in the region medial to the right crus of the diaphragm between the aorta and vena cava. This should be ligated or secured with a large hemoclip to prevent significant loss of protein during the postoperative period and possible chylous ascites. Major hemorrhage from the renal hilum is potentially the most serious complication in the performance of the nephrectomy. Should this occur, it can almost always be controlled by direct compression of the renal pedicle posteriorly against the vertebral bodies. Full dissection of this area will then allow identification of the bleeding vessel.

Postoperative Considerations. The routine use of chest tubes helps to avoid the 30 to 35% incidence of hemopneumothorax, with consequent prolonged hospitalization, that is reported when chest tubes are not used. In general, the tubes are maintained on suction until significant drainage ceases, after which they are removed. Other postoperative complications from radical nephrectomy are similar to those following any major surgical procedure. Several points, however, should be emphasized. With the modified unilateral dissection, the sympathetic ganglia are often removed unilaterally, resulting in a warm ipsilateral leg owing to peripheral vasodilation, compared with the normal but relatively cool contralateral extremity. This event may occasionally cause a frantic call from the intensive care unit; the anxiety can be allayed if the contralateral distal pulses are predictably intact. Occasionally, diarrhea may result from ischemia of the large bowel after ligation of the inferior mesenteric artery. This is rare in younger patients and is usually managed successfully without long-term sequelae.

Concern over possible devascularization of the spinal cord is not warranted, provided that no lumbar arteries are ligated above the renal pedicle. The spinal cord ends at the level of the first lumbar vertebral body. The nutrient arteries to the spinal cord, the longitudinal anterior and posterior spinal arteries, arise from the vertebral arteries and receive additional blood supply from the intercostal and high lumbar arteries through radicular branches.[22]

The main lower anterior radicular artery providing collateral blood supply to the anterior spinal area is called the arteria radicularis magna or artery of Adamkiewicz.[8] This artery originates from the thoracic aorta in 50% of the patients and from the lumbar region in the other 50%.[1, 4] However, it has been demonstrated that in those patients in whom the arteria radicularis magna originates in the lumbar region, there is an important radicular artery from the lower thoracic aorta that is consistently present and provides adequate collateral circulation to the anterior spinal artery.[1, 4]

Although paraplegia after aortic replacement procedures for abdominal aortic aneurysms was not reported before 1960, and

DeBakey's group[6] reported no neurologic deficits in 1432 consecutive patients undergoing abdominal aortic aneurysm resections, 28 cases of paraplegia after abdominal aortic operations were reported in the world literature through March 1975.[8, 10, 15, 26] However, review of these 28 cases revealed that 18 were associated with ruptured aneurysms and prolonged hypotension. Permanent paraplegia occurred in only one of 10 patients who had undergone elective abdominal aortic aneurysm resection. The remaining nine patients recovered function, and all 28 patients showed evidence of extensive atherosclerosis. Therefore, we believe that the evidence supports our contention that extensive aortic mobilization with ligation of the lumbar arteries or aortic replacement is a safe and an appropriate part of the surgical resection of a large renal tumor in patients with life expectancy in excess of five to 10 years without cancer. Obviously, patients with extensive atherosclerotic vessels are not appropriate candidates for the operative procedure described herein and would be best managed with simple nephrectomy.

Ejaculatory failure or retrograde ejaculation commonly results from extensive retroperitoneal lymph node dissection and is seen in approximately 65% of patients undergoing modified unilateral dissection. A young patient of reproductive age may be advised to visit a sperm bank on several occasions preoperatively; ejaculatory fluid can be frozen and stored in the event that subsequent artificial insemination becomes desirable.

Role of Lymphadenectomy

The value of lymphadenectomy in the management of renal cell carcinoma, as in most genitourinary tract cancers, remains controversial. Most would agree that lymphadenectomy not only assists in accurate pathologic staging but also provides valuable prognostic information based on the presence or absence of lymph node involvement. Lymph node dissection has also been recommended to identify those patients who should receive additional therapy. However, such an application is contingent on the efficacy of available therapeutic adjuvants; unfortunately, all have been disappointing so far. Whether there is any significant therapeutic benefit from lymph node dissection with radical nephrectomy remains conjec-

tural. It is our policy to perform lymphadenectomy on all patients for whom radical nephrectomy is potentially curative (i.e., those with disease in Stages I, II, or III). This is based on the premise that, if lymph node dissection were to have any therapeutic benefit, it would be for patients with metastatic foci to only a few lymph nodes. Lacking truly effective adjuvant agents or techniques to predict accurately which patients have nodal involvement, we believe that this approach offers those with regional disease the best possible chance of survival.

Lymphatic drainage of the kidney, although poorly understood, is believed to parallel that organ's vascular architecture. An excellent review by Marshall and Powell[14] indicates that the regional nodes of the right kidney include the lateral caval nodes, the precaval and postcaval nodes, and the interaortocaval nodes, whereas the lymph nodes draining the left kidney consist of the upper left lateral lumbar nodes, the preaortic and postaortic lymph nodes, and the nodes lying on the crus of the left diaphragm posterior and medial to the adrenal vein, as well as those lying along the left renal vein. Unlike the elaborate studies concerning the distribution of nodal metastases reported for testicular cancer,[7] few studies have been done on patients with renal cell carcinoma. Hulten and associates[12] described the distribution of lymph node metastases in 22 patients, seven of whom had evidence of nodal involvement. They concluded that most lymphatic metastases involve the ipsilateral renal hilar nodes, but wide variation in distribution was not uncommon and included involvement of the iliac, mediastinal, or supraclavicular nodes with or without involvement of the renal hilar nodes. Based on their own review, Marshall and Powell[14] recommend that, for right-sided tumors, lymph node dissection should begin at the level of the diaphragm superiorly and include removal of lymph nodes lying on the crus of the diaphragm superiorly, together with removal of all the preaortic and postaortic lymph nodes to the level of the bifurcation of the aorta distally.

Between 18 and 33% of patients undergoing radical nephrectomy with lymph node dissection for renal cell carcinoma have involved nodes identified in the pathologic specimen (Table 48–1).[11, 20, 21, 24, 28] The difference in incidence of nodal involvement is presumably explained by variations in the surgical limits of lymphadenectomy per-

Table 48–1. INCIDENCE OF POSITIVE
NODES IN PATIENTS WITH
RENAL CELL CARCINOMA

First Author	Reference	Percentage of Positive Nodes
Skinner	25	18
Petkovic	20	22
Robson	21	23
Waters	28	24
Guiliani	11	33

formed, as well as in the diligence on the part of the pathologist in identifying all nodal tissue removed. Robson and associates,[21] Middleton and Presto,[17] and Katz and Davis[13] have documented better survival rates for patients treated by radical nephrectomy than for those treated by simple nephrectomy. There is also some evidence that lymph node dissection with radical nephrectomy can improve survival for patients with renal adenocarcinoma. The retrospective study by Robson and associates,[21] as well as our own data,[24] reveals an increasing incidence of lymph node involvement with increasing nuclear grade of the tumor (Grade 1, 12%; Grade 2, 28%; Grade 3, 34%).

Survival rates for the two surgical procedures, taking nuclear grade into account, are compared in Table 48–2. The survival rate after radical nephrectomy with node dissection is higher than that after simple nephrectomy, by a percentage that closely parallels the incidence of lymph node involvement for each grade. However, conclusive statistical data from prospective studies are not available. Thus, the conclusion that radical nephrectomy with regional lymph node dissection improves survival, compared with the results for nephrectomy alone, remains conjectural. In our hands, the addition of en bloc regional lymph node dissection has not affected the postoperative morbidity or mortality, and we recommend it whenever radical nephrectomy is performed for cure.

The collective five-year and 10-year survival rates for patients with involved nodes vary from 14 to 35% and from 3 to 35%, respectively, further emphasizing some therapeutic advantage of lymphadenectomy in conjunction with radical nephrectomy (Table 48–3).[9, 21, 25] The impressive five-year and 10-year survival rates reported by Robson and associates[21] in a highly selected group of patients who underwent extensive preoperative evaluation to exclude metastatic disease are encouraging. These results and those of Guiliani and co-workers[11] may reflect the extent of node dissection performed, because most patients in both series underwent complete retroperitoneal lymph node dissection. However, Simonovitch and associates[23] from the Cleveland Clinic, in their review of 89 patients undergoing either extended (19 patients) or regional (70 patients) lymphadenectomy, found no difference in survival among the eight patients who had evidence of nodal involvement (three in the extended group and five in the regional group). In contrast to Robson and associates,[21] Simonovitch and colleagues[23] believe that a more limited lymphadenectomy should be performed in patients with locally resectable tumor in the absence of distant lymphatic or other parenchymal metastases.

Recently, Peters and Brown[19] reported their comparative five-year survival rates for patients undergoing radical nephrectomy with or without lymph node dissection. Thirty-one of 356 patients reviewed had evidence of Stage III disease, 13 of whom had evidence of node involvement. They reported a five-year survival rate of 44% for all Stage III patients undergoing radical nephrectomy and lymph node dissection, compared with only 25% for Stage II patients undergoing radical nephrectomy alone. Unfortunately, the authors did not distinguish the patients with positive nodes from the rest of the group; thus it is impossible to determine the impact of lymph node dissection on survival in these patients.

Table 48–2. SURVIVAL RATE (%) RELATING TO GRADE AND THERAPY*

Therapy	Grade 1	Grade 2	Grade 3
Incidence of lymph node involvement	12	28	34
Five-year survival following simple nephrectomy	77	31	8
Five-year survival following radical nephrectomy	87	64	40

*Data from Robson CJ, et al: The results of radical nephrectomy for renal cell carcinoma. J Urol 101:297, 1969, and Skinner DG, et al: The surgical management of renal cell carcinoma. J Urol 107:705, 1972, by permission.

Table 48–3. PERCENTAGE SURVIVAL OF PATIENTS WITH METASTATIC RENAL CELL CARCINOMA TO THE REGIONAL LYMPH NODES

| First Author | Reference | Survival Rate (%) | |
		Five-year	Ten-year
Flocks	9	16	16
Robson	21	35	35
Skinner	25	14	3

Because a significant number of patients have only microscopic involvement of lymph nodes at the time of radical nephrectomy, it seems plausible to proceed with lymphadenectomy, as these patients may benefit the most.

SUMMARY

The thoracoabdominal approach to the management of renal tumors has been successfully tolerated in patients of all ages. In a review of more than 300 patients undergoing radical nephrectomy for primary renal parenchymal tumors, we found that the period of postoperative hospitalization, complication rate, morbidity, and mortality accompanying use of the thoracoabdominal approach compared very favorably with the results of transabdominal or lumbar approaches in which the thoracic cavity is not entered. Complications from the procedure can be minimized by careful surgical technique and a thorough knowledge of the anatomy of the retroperitoneum. In qualified hands, the technique is safe and extremely well tolerated by the patient, and it should provide maximum possibility of cure for those afflicted by primary parenchymal tumors of the kidney.

References

1. Adams HD, van Geertruyden HH: Neurologic complications of aortic surgery. Ann Surg, 144:547, 1956.
2. Chute R, Soutter L, Kerr WS: The value of the thoracoabdominal incision in the removal of kidney tumors. N Engl J Med 241:951, 1949.
3. Cooper JF, Leadbetter WF, Chute R: The thoracoabdominal approach for retroperitoneal gland dissection: its application to testis tumors. Surg Gynecol Obstet 90:486, 1950.
4. Coupland GA, Reeve TS: Paraplegia: a complication of excision of abdominal aortic aneurysm. Surgery 64:848–871, 1968.
5. Crawford ED, Skinner DG: Intercostal nerve block with thoracoabdominal and flank incisions. Urology 19:25, 1982.
6. DeBakey ME, Crawford ES, Cooley DA, et al: Aneurysm of abdominal aorta: analysis of results of graft replacement therapy one to eleven years after operation. Ann Surg 160:622, 1964.
7. Donohue JP, Zachary JM, Maynard BR: Distribution of nodal metastases in nonseminomatous testis cancer. J Urol 128:315, 1982.
8. Ferguson LRJ, Bergan JJ, Conn J Jr, Yao JST: Spinal ischemia following abdominal aortic surgery. Ann Surg 181:267, 1975.
9. Flocks RJ, Kadesky MC: Malignant neoplasms of the kidney: an analysis of 353 patients followed five years or more. J Urol 79:196, 1958.
10. Golden GT, Sears HF, Wellons HA Jr, Muller WH Jr: Paraplegia complicating resection of aneurysms of the infrarenal abdominal aorta. Surgery 73:91, 1973.
11. Guiliani L, Martorana G, Giberti C, et al: Results of radical nephrectomy with extensive lymphadenectomy for renal cell carcinoma. J Urol 122:306, 1979.
12. Hulten L, Rosencrantz M, Seeman T, et al: Occurrence and localization of lymph node metastases in renal carcinoma: a lymphographic and histopathological investigation in connection with nephrectomy. Scand J Urol Nephrol 3:129, 1969.
13. Katz SA, Davis JE: Renal adenocarcinoma: prognostics and treatment reflected by survival. Urology 10:10, 1977.
14. Marshall FF, Powell KC: Lymphadenectomy for renal cell carcinoma: anatomical and therapeutic considerations. J Urol 128:677, 1982.
15. Meherz IO, Nabseth DC, Hogan EL, Deterling RA Jr: Paraplegia following resection of abdominal aortic aneurysm. Ann Surg 156:890, 1962.
16. Middleton AW Jr: Indications for and results of nephrectomy for metastatic renal cell carcinoma. Urol Clin North Am 7:711, 1980.
17. Middleton RG, Presto AJ III: Radical thoracoabdominal nephrectomy for renal cell carcinoma. J Urol 110:36, 1973.
18. O'Dea JM, Zincke H, Utz DC, Bernatz PE: The treatment of renal cell carcinoma with solitary metastasis. J Urol 120:540, 1978.
19. Peters PC, Brown GL: The role of lymphadenectomy in the management of renal cell carcinoma. Urol Clin North Am 7:705, 1980.
20. Petkovic SD: An anatomical classification of renal tumors in the adult as a basis for prognosis. J Urol 81:618, 1959.
21. Robson CJ, Churchill BM, Anderson W: The results of radical nephrectomy for renal cell carcinoma. J Urol 101:297–301, 1969.
22. Sher MH, Healy EH: Paraplegia following infrarenal aneurysmorrhaphy. Vasc Surg 5:171, 1971.
23. Simonovitch JP, Montie JE, Straffon RA: Lymphadenectomy in renal adenocarcinoma. J Urol 127:1090, 1982.
24. Skinner DG, Colvin RM, Vermillion CD, et al: Diagnosis and management of renal cell carcinoma: a clinical and pathologic study of 309 cases. Cancer 28:1165, 1971.
25. Skinner DG, Vermillion CD, Colvin RB: The surgical management of renal cell carcinoma. J Urol 107:705, 1972.
26. Skillman JJ, Zervas NT, Weintraub RM, Mayman CI: Paraplegia after resection of aneurysms of the abdominal aorta. New Engl J Med 281:422, 1969.
27. Sweet RH: Carcinoma of the esophagus and the cardiac end of the stomach. JAMA 135:485, 1947.
28. Waters WB, Richie JP: Aggressive surgical approach to renal cell carcinoma: review of 130 cases. J Urol 122:306, 1979.

DONALD G. SKINNER, M.D.
GARY LIESKOVSKY, M.D.
T. RAND PRITCHETT, M.D.

Management of Renal Cell Carcinoma Involving the Vena Cava

CHAPTER 49

Renal cell carcinoma may invade surrounding parenchyma directly and extend through the capsule to invade perinephric fat and contiguous visceral structures, or it may expand into areas of low resistance such as the renal vein and vena cava. Before 1970, patients with vena caval involvement were thought to be incurable, and the few attempts that were made to excise such tumors surgically were associated with high mortality. However, after a careful review of findings in 309 patients treated at Massachusetts General Hospital, it became apparent that tumors with venous extension, even into the vena cava, did not carry an ominous prognosis if they were completely excised and were not associated with perinephric fat, contiguous visceral invasion, or regional nodal or distant metastases.[12, 13] In that study, nearly all patients with vena caval involvement had relatively small tumor thrombi that could be extracted easily without major blood loss.

In 1971, we were confronted with a patient who had tumor extending into the right atrium. This was successfully and fortunately extracted with the aid of a Foley catheter, but without thoughtful control of vena caval inflow.[13] Inasmuch as 5 to 10% of patients who present with renal cell carcinoma are found to have varying degrees of vena caval involvement, the need for devel-

oping a suitable and safe technique for vena caval occlusion and tumor extraction became apparent. Several additional facts now favor the successful surgical removal of these venous tumor extensions. First, the blood supply is derived from the renal artery, not from angiogenesis and the ingrowth of tumor vessels from surrounding structures. This phenomenon can be readily demonstrated in the early phase of the selective renal arteriogram (Fig. 49–1). Therefore, as the tumor thrombus extends it carries with it feeding tumor vessels from the renal hilum and rarely attaches itself to the endothelium of the vena cava (Fig. 49–2).[13] Second, because the type of tumor growth is by expansion along pathways of least resistance rather than by invasion, the wall of the vena cava is rarely involved. Therefore, resection of the vena cava is not necessary and may in fact increase the morbidity of the operation.

Early in our experience, we resected large segments of vena cava with ligation of the left renal vein. However, in half of the patients temporary renal shutdown developed, necessitating renal dialysis and causing a prolonged, difficult postoperative course. McCullough and Gittes[8] reviewed the literature of vena caval resection with ligation of the solitary remaining left renal vein and reported similar findings: three of six pa-

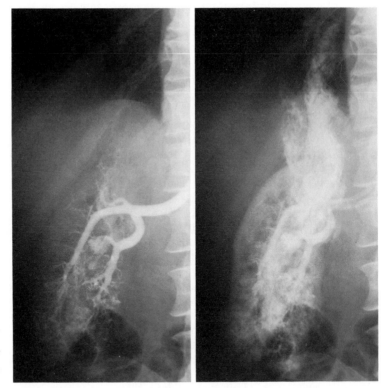

Figure 49–1. *Selective right renal arteriogram showing early and intermediate arterial phase. Note vascular neoplasm occupying the lower pole of the right kidney, with profuse linear striated vessel pattern extending from the level of the renal vein and inferior vena cava to the right atrium. From Skinner DG, et al: Extension of renal cell carcinoma into the vena cava. J Urol 107:712, 1972, by permission of Williams & Wilkins Co.*

tients required temporary dialysis with prolonged hospitalization, averaging 45 days. We believe that every effort should be made to preserve a connection between the left renal vein and the vena cava. In addition, tumors that invade contiguous structures directly (e.g., the wall of the vena cava) have a poor prognosis, and we are unaware of any long-term survivors who had direct invasion of the vena caval wall regardless of the extent of surgical excision. Finally, surgical advances have occurred that make it possible to control the entire vena caval blood flow so that it may be opened without massive blood loss, allowing the tumor thrombus to be safely extracted. Since 1971, sev-

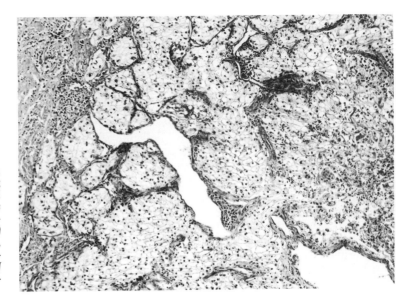

Figure 49–2. *Photomicrograph of tumor thrombus extending into the inferior vena cava and right atrium (× 110). Numerous large endothelium-lined vascular spaces (partially collapsed) are evident. From Skinner DG, et al: Extension of renal cell carcinoma into the vena cava. J Urol 107:714, 1972, by permission of Williams & Wilkins Co.*

eral different techniques and approaches have been reported,[1, 3, 4, 7, 9, 10] and we recently have reviewed our own experience.[6, 11] These patients represent unique and complicated problems that require a great deal of individualization and preoperative planning.

From 1972 to 1983, we operated on 25 patients with renal cell carcinoma extending into the vena cava without evidence of obvious metastatic disease. This series included 15 men and 10 women whose mean age was 60 years (range, 31 to 76). As expected, the right kidney was more commonly involved, but nine (36%) of the 25 patients had tumor originating on the left side. The percentages of patients who had various symptoms or abnormal physical findings at the time of presentation are listed in Tables 49–1 and 49–2. It is notable that only half had evidence of caval obstruction and that a varicocele was found in half of the men.

Because of poor venous flow within the vena cava or complete obstruction caused by the thrombus, many of these patients are in a precarious hemodynamic state at the time of presentation. This fact became vividly clear in one additional patient whose vena cava clotted acutely. Disseminated intravascular coagulopathy developed, and the patient died shortly after admission. An autopsy found that he had a potentially curable tumor completely confined to the vena cava without evidence of metastatic disease, perinephric fat, or regional node involvement. Three other patients had evidence of pulmonary embolism on admission, and two had thrombophlebitis with leg edema that led to the discovery of the renal tumor. Because of this, we routinely start a heparin

Table 49–1. CLINICAL SYMPTOMS OF 25 PATIENTS WITH RENAL CELL CARCINOMA*

Symptoms	Percentage of Patients
Hematuria	52
Pain	44
Manifestations of caval obstruction	36
Weight loss	32
Malaise	24
Dyspnea	16

*Average time from onset of symptoms to diagnosis: 18 weeks; range, one to 104 weeks.

Reprinted with permission from Lieskovsky G, Pritchett TR, Skinner DG: Surgical Management of Renal Cell Carcinoma. 1984 Monographs in Urology, Volume 5, No. 4 July/August.

Table 49–2. CLINICAL SIGNS OF 25 PATIENTS WITH RENAL CELL CARCINOMA

Signs	Percentage of Patients
Abdominal mass	60
Manifestations of caval obstruction	48
Varicocele (males)	47
Peripheral edema	32
Venous collaterals	12
Anemia	12

Reprinted with permission from Lieskovsky G, Pritchett TR, Skinner DG: Surgical Management of Renal Cell Carcinoma. 1984 Monographs in Urology, Volume 5, No. 4 July/August.

infusion immediately after the patient's admission and continue it until 12 hours before surgery.

We have developed a right thoracoabdominal approach that we believe provides optimal exposure to the upper vena cava and allows control of all venous inflow. Experience with the midline transabdominal approach with median sternotomy extension has not been as good, owing to poor exposure of the vena cava and difficulty in getting around the liver. Only a few of these patients have tumor extension into the atrium, which requires cardiopulmonary bypass. Usually, small tumor extensions into the atrium can be handled without the need for bypass. The heparin administration necessary for bypass at the time of an extensive retroperitoneal dissection significantly increases blood loss beyond what is already a bloody operation under the best of circumstances.

For management purposes, we have found it useful to divide these patients into three groups: Group I—those with tumor thrombus extension below the insertion of the hepatic vein (12 patients); Group II—those with intrahepatic tumor thrombus but without extension to the atrium (10); Group III—those with intra-atrial tumor extension (three patients) (Fig. 49–3). Because many of these patients have a completely occluded vena cava, it is often necessary to do a transbrachial venous study of the superior vena cava to determine the precise cephalad extent of tumor extension.

We routinely use a thoracoabdominal approach, excising the eighth rib, extending the incision in the epigastrium to the midline, and then moving inferiorly in a midline or paramedian incision to a level below the umbilicus (Fig. 49–4). For left-sided tumors the transverse portion of the incision in the

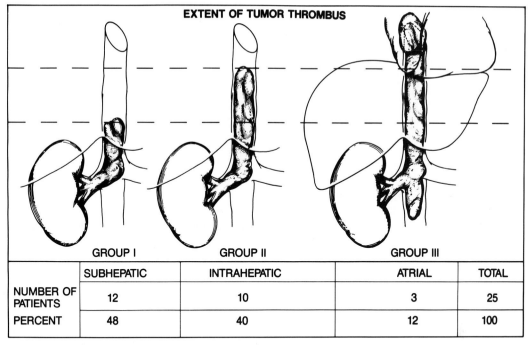

Figure 49–3. Levels at which tumor thrombus may extend into inferior vena cava and number of patients at each level. Reprinted with permission from Lieskovsky G, Pritchett TR, Skinner DG: Surgical Management of Renal Cell Carcinoma. 1984 Monographs in Urology, Volume 5, No. 4 July/August.

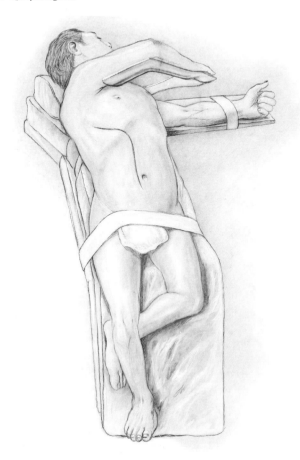

Figure 49–4. Patient positioning for resection of renal cell carcinoma with vena caval extension. Note that the patient's right side is adjacent to the ipsilateral edge of the operating table. A seventh or eighth rib–excising incision is utilized to provide adequate cardiac exposure.

epigastrium is extended to the left costochondral junction, which forms a T-shaped incision. Early ligation of the renal artery is essential to this procedure along with complete isolation of the vena cava by ligating all lumbar veins. This is accomplished by incising the avascular line of Toldt along the ascending colon and peritoneal attachments to the small bowel mesentery so that the bowel, duodenum, and pancreas can be elevated on the superior mesenteric artery pedicle. This allows early ligation of the renal artery. A more detailed description of this surgical approach can be found in Chapter 48. The vena cava can then be mobilized by ligating all lumbar veins and applying a Rumel tourniquet loosely around the distal vena cava and the contralateral left renal vein (for right-sided tumors) or right renal artery (for left-sided tumors). The kidney and Gerota's fascia are then completely mobilized with an en bloc dissection of periaortic and renal hilar lymph nodes. The only remaining attachments are the renal vein and the intracaval thrombus. It is important that the adrenal vein be ligated at this time and the superior vena cava completely skeletonized except for the insertion of the renal vein.

In Groups II and III, a vertical pericardiotomy is performed; the phrenic nerve is avoided and a Rumel tourniquet is applied loosely around the intrathoracic inferior vena cava at this level. Inasmuch as the intrathoracic inferior vena cava is not completely within the pericardium, it is necessary to make a small opening in the pericardium posteriorly so that a clamp and Rumel tourniquet can be passed safely around the vena cava. This dissection should be well above the diaphragm and close to the insertion of the vena cava into the atrium, in order to avoid the large hepatic veins that empty into the vena cava at the level of the diaphragm.

In Group I (subhepatic thrombus) patients, a Rumel tourniquet is placed around the cava below the liver. This maneuver can be facilitated by ligating several of the small inferior hepatic veins, allowing for greater cephalad mobility of the liver. In Groups II and III, the superior mesenteric artery is isolated and occluded with a soft Fogarty vascular clamp. Two Crafoord vascular clamps are placed on the porta hepatis, after which the Rumel tourniquets on the distal vena cava, the contralateral renal vein, and the intrathoracic cava are tightened, isolating the vena cava from all venous inflow (Fig. 49–5). For left-sided tumors, a soft Fogarty vascular clamp is placed on the right renal artery, thus obviating the need to occlude the right renal vein.

In Group III patients with only a small intra-atrial extension, a purse-string suture is placed around the atrial appendage. One of the cardiac surgeons can then usually insert a finger into the atrium and gently milk the thrombus down the cava so that the Rumel tourniquet can be tightened above the thrombus extension where the cava enters into the atrium (Fig. 49–6). If there is large tumor involvement of the atrium, cardiopulmonary bypass will be necessary to prevent intraoperative embolization, which occurred in one of our patients.

If cardiopulmonary bypass seems indicated, it can be readily done through this approach by cannulating the ascending aorta and the superior vena cava through the atrial appendage. One advantage of cardiopulmonary bypass is that the core body temperature can be lowered, protecting the liver from ischemia for a longer time.

A longitudinal incision is then made in the vena cava, extending around the insertion of the involved renal vein and cephalad so that the cava can be widely opened and the tumor thrombus easily dissected out and extracted. Occasionally, the thrombus is adherent to the wall of the vena cava, requiring instrument dissection, but usually it can be bluntly enucleated and slid out easily (Figs. 49–7 and 49–8).

The patient should be placed in a "head-down" position during this part of the operation to prevent subsequent air embolization. Trial occlusion of the vena cava should be done before opening it to make sure that the patient has sufficient intravascular blood volume to sustain the systemic pressure at adequate levels. Obviously, the anesthesiologist must be intimately involved with this sequence of events. We routinely give mannitol prior to occluding the venous inflow into the vena cava. The surgeon has about 20 minutes of safe, warm, hepatic ischemia time, during which the tumor can easily be extracted from the cava and the venacavotomy closed. In patients whose tumor preoperatively completely occludes the vena cava, or who have prior evidence of pulmonary embolism, or in whom clot is encountered in the distal vena cava, we routinely

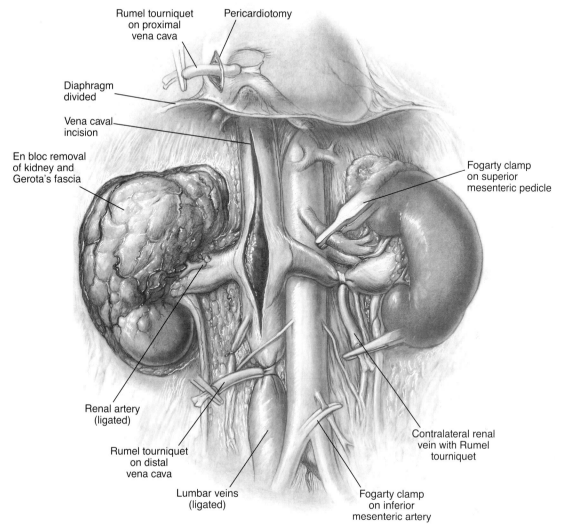

Figure 49–5. *Surgical maneuvers necessary for a safe and effective method of removing all tumor thrombus (See text for details).*

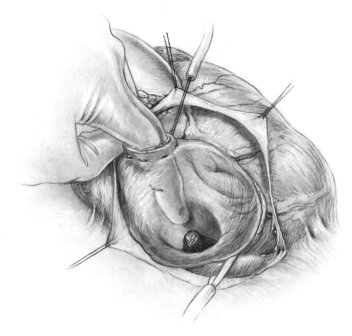

Figure 49–6. The cardiac surgeon can insert a finger through the atrial appendage and into the right atrium in order to ease the tumor thrombus out of the atrium at the time that the primary renal tumor and thrombus are simultaneously extracted from the abdominal vena cava. Once the thrombus has descended out of the atrium into the proximal inferior vena cava, a Rumel tourniquet is tightened around the inferior vena cava at its junction with the atrium. This maneuver provides proximal venous control, prevents intraoperative embolization, and obviates the need for cardiopulmonary bypass.

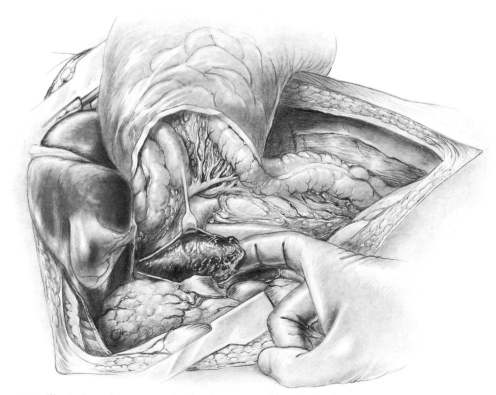

Figure 49–7. Illustration of tumor enucleation by means of longitudinal vena cavotomy extending around the insertion of the right renal vein.

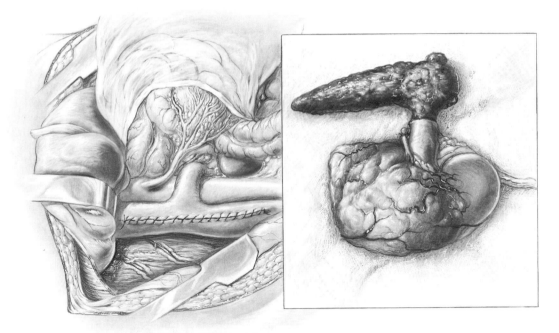

Figure 49–8. Illustration of operative field following tumor removal. We routinely place a partially occluding DeWeese vena caval clip just distal to the renal vein insertion on the vena cava in patients whose tumor preoperatively completely occluded the vena cava, or who had prior evidence of pulmonary embolism, or in whom clot is encountered in the distal vena cava.

place a partially occluding DeWeese vena caval clip just distal to the insertion of the renal vein on the vena cava. It should be emphasized that this may increase venous pressure in the pelvis and increase the risk of postoperative bleeding. Careful attention must be paid to the ligated gonadal veins and ascending lumbar venous plexus to make sure that these vessels are secured. We routinely give these patients the anticoagulant Coumadin for six weeks postoperatively to prevent development of chronic peripheral venostasis and to allow recanalization and the development of collateral circulation.

The morbidity of this operation should not be taken lightly. Our average surgical time was three hours and 45 minutes with a range of one hour and 25 minutes to five hours and 45 minutes. The average estimated blood loss was 3,600 ml, with a range of 600 to 9,500 ml. Our average hepatic ischemia time was 13 minutes, with a range of eight to 20 minutes, and the contralateral renal ischemia time averaged 16 minutes with a range of five to 37 minutes.[11]

One intraoperative death occurred secondary to tumor embolization in a patient who had extension into his atrium and a very friable tumor. This might have been avoided by using cardiopulmonary bypass. We lost no patients secondary to intraoperative blood loss. Overall, three (12%) of the 25 patients died during their hospital stay: one intraoperatively, one of adult respiratory distress syndrome postoperatively (after spontaneous preoperative rupture of his tumor), and one secondary to gastrointestinal tract bleeding that led to development of hepatorenal syndrome. This patient was known to have alcoholic cirrhosis before surgery. One patient had addisonian signs after surgery, with adrenal insufficiency owing to devascularization of the contralateral adrenal gland. The patient subsequently responded well to corticosteroid replacement therapy.

Using the technique described above, we were able to resect the primary renal tumor and vena caval thrombus completely in 24 of 25 patients and to resect all apparent tumor in 20. The remaining four had evidence of additional pulmonary or liver metastases that could not be resected at the time of surgery; none of these patients survived for a year. In comparison, the three-year and five-year survival rates were 50% and 36%, respectively, for patients from whom all apparent tumor was removed.

Table 49–3. SURVIVAL RATES ACCORDING TO LEVEL OF CAVAL TUMOR IN 25 PATIENTS

Level of Caval Involvement	Survival Rate (%)		
	One Year	Three Years	Five Years
Group I—Subhepatic cava (12)	50	42	42
Group II—Intrahepatic cava (10)	60	50	17
Group III—Atrial extension (3)	33	0	0
All patients (25)	52	40	28

Reprinted with permission from Pritchett TR, Lieskovsky G, and Skinner DG: Extension of renal cell carcinoma into the vena cava: Clinical review and surgical approach. J Urol 135:460, 1986.

Survival rates at one, three, and five years, according to level of caval involvement as well as histologic extent, are detailed in Tables 49–3 and 49–4. The extent of tumor thrombus involvement appears to reflect the duration of disease and to affect survival; patients with more extensive tumor thrombi often have concomitant visceral metastases or involvement of the perinephric fat and regional lymph nodes. Nonetheless, when only the vena cava is involved, the three-year and five-year survival rates of 56% and 33%, respectively, indicate the significance of successful removal of these tumors.

Since 1981, three other centers have reported their experience with resection of vena caval tumor thrombi. Kearney and associates,[5] who reported on 24 patients

Table 49–4. SURVIVAL RATES ACCORDING TO STAGE OF TUMOR IN 25 PATIENTS

Histologic Extent	Survival Rate (%)		
	One Year	Three Years	Five Years
Vena cava alone	67	56	33
with perinephric fat	36	29	29
with regional nodes	27	9	9
Cavotomy alone	61	46	31
Caval wall resection	42	33	25
Complete tumor resection	65	50	36
Complete tumor resection impossible because of coexistent visceral (lung, liver) metastases	0	0	0

Reprinted with permission from Pritchett TR, Lieskovsky G, and Skinner DG: Extension of renal cell carcinoma into the vena cava: Clinical review and surgical approach. J Urol 135:460, 1986.

treated over a seven-year period at the Peter Bent Brigham Hospital, were the first to suggest subgrouping of patients according to the level of vena caval involvement. The mean survival for the entire group was just 21 months, but complete resection was possible in only 13. Their only long-term survivors had caval involvement limited to below the hepatic vein insertion and the authors concluded that the level of tumor extension directly related to survival, as did the presence of associated metastatic disease. Of interest, seven (29%) of their 24 patients had oliguria with renal failure in the immediate postoperative period, six of whom required dialysis. All seven had vena caval resection or occlusion of the opposite renal vein as part of the surgical procedure.

Sogani and associates[14] from Memorial Sloan-Kettering Hospital recently reported their experience in 18 patients. Of eight who underwent complete resection and were without evidence of metastases at the time of surgery, half were free of disease for a mean duration of 93 months. On the other hand, the mean survival for those with associated metastases was only 12 months.

Cherrie and associates[2] reviewed the UCLA experience in 27 patients treated over a ten-year period and concluded that vena caval extension alone had only a limited impact on the prognosis (five-year survival of 53% with a median duration of 81 months) but that associated capsular penetration to involve the perinephric fat or extension to regional lymph nodes had a significant influence on survival (two-year survival of 35% with no five-year survivals). Only 5% of their patients with associated distant metastases survived for two years, and none survived for five years.

These results are encouraging for the 5 to 10% of patients undergoing nephrectomy for renal cell carcinoma who have direct vascular extension of tumor into the vena cava. It is apparent that successful removal of these neoplastic thrombi can produce long-term survival for some and certainly can provide prolonged palliation for others. Proper management of these patients is dependent upon complete preoperative assessment of the cephalad extent of the tumor and use of an appropriate operative approach.

A unique approach to the problem of removing extensive intrathoracic venous extension of renal cell carcinoma has recently been reported by Marshall and associates from Johns Hopkins.[7] That group utilized a technique of total body hypothermia with circulatory arrest. Patients are initially placed on cardiopulmonary bypass as the core body temperature is gradually lowered and the head packed in ice. Once core body temperature reaches 19.5°C, the circulation is stopped and a radical nephrectomy, venacavotomy, and atriotomy are performed with the tumor removed in an essentially bloodless field. After closure of the venacavotomy and atriotomy, cardiopulmonary bypass circulation is resumed and the body temperature gradually warmed to 36°C. The heart is then defibrillated and the patient taken off bypass. This technique was initially utilized for patients with severe arterial and venous malformation in the central nervous system. The technique was reported in one patient with renal cell carcinoma under 36 years of age.[7] Whether older patients will tolerate this type of manipulation remains to be seen, but in very advanced Group III tumors in young patients this approach may warrant consideration. In our opinion, cardiopulmonary bypass and systemic heparinization should be avoided whenever possible. Retroperitoneal blood loss is substantially increased by systemic heparinization, and it certainly is not necessary for patients in Groups I and II, or in Group III patients with only a small intra-atrial extension.

We have developed a technique that provides intrathoracic control of the vena cava at its insertion into the atrium to prevent intraoperative tumor embolization, as well as control of the venous inflow into the cava to prevent massive blood loss at the time of the venacavotomy. We believe that this right thoracoabdominal approach is ideally suited to the safe performance of this procedure, but the magnitude of the operation and its technical complexity cannot be underestimated. If resection is successful and complete, the ultimate prognosis depends on known prognostic factors, such as capsular invasion, nodal disease, presence of associated metastases, and the nuclear grade of the tumor. Aggressive surgery in patients with gross nodal disease or known distant metastases is probably unwarranted, owing to the anticipated short tumor-free survival.

References

1. Beck AD: Resection of the suprarenal inferior vena cava for retroperitoneal malignant disease. J Urol 121:112–118, 1979.
2. Cherrie RJ, Goldman DG, Lindner A, deKernion JB: Prognostic implications of vena caval extension of renal cell carcinoma. J Urol 128:910–912, 1982.
3. Clayman RV Jr, Gonzalez R, Fraley EE: Renal cancer invading the inferior vena cava: clinical review and anatomical approach. J Urol 123:157–163, 1980.
4. Cummings KB, Li WI, Ryan JA, et al: Intraoperative management of renal cell carcinoma with supradiaphragmatic caval extension. J Urol 122:829–832, 1979.
5. Kearney GP, Waters WB, Klein LA, et al: Results of inferior vena cava resection for renal cell carcinoma. J Urol 125:769–773, 1981.
6. Lieskovsky G, Pritchett R, Skinner DG: Surgical management of renal cell carcinoma. Monog Urol 5:98–125, 1984.
7. Marshall FF, Reitz BA, Diamond DA: A new technique for management of renal cell carcinoma involving the right atrium: hypothermia and cardiac arrest. J Urol 131:103–107, 1984.
8. McCullough DL, Gittes RF: Vena cava resection for renal cell carcinoma. J Urol 112:162–167, 1974.
9. Novick AC, Cosgrove DM: Surgical approach for removal of renal cell carcinoma extending into the vena cava and the right atrium. J Urol 123:947–950, 1980.
10. Prager RL, Dean R, Turner B: Surgical approach to intracardiac renal cell carcinoma. Ann Thorac Surg 33:74–77, 1982.
11. Pritchett TR, Lieskovsky GL, Skinner DG: Extension of renal cell carcinoma into the vena cava: clinical review and surgical approval. J Urol 135:460–464, 1986.
12. Skinner DG, Colvin RB, Vermillion CD, et al: Diagnosis and management of renal cell carcinoma. Cancer 28:1165–1177, 1971.
13. Skinner DG, Pfister RF, Colvin R: Extension of renal cell carcinoma into the vena cava: the rationale for aggressive surgical management. J Urol 107:711–716, 1972.
14. Sogani PC, Herr HW, Bains MS, Whitmore WF Jr: Renal cell carcinoma extending into inferior vena cava. J Urol 130:660–663, 1983.

MICHAEL M. LIEBER, M.D.
BENAD Z. GOLDWASSER, M.D.

Role of Partial Nephrectomy in Management of Renal Tumors, Including Surgical Technique

CHAPTER 50

The kidneys are located deep in the retroperitoneum, often surrounded by a very thick layer of perinephric fat. As a result, renal cortical tumors, by far the most common tumors of the adult kidney, can reach a large size before becoming symptomatic. In the past, treatment of renal parenchymal tumors has been predicated by the fact that renal tumors commonly have been of large size and often high stage at the time of diagnosis. Simple nephrectomy, often performed through a flank incision, was standard treatment for renal cell carcinoma until the mid-1950s, but more extensive surgical procedures to treat the disease have been popular in the past 30 years, with radical nephrectomy as the treatment of choice.[39]

Radical nephrectomy as used here denotes the en bloc removal of the kidney and renal tumor within the confines of Gerota's fascia, with all the perinephric fat and the ipsilateral adrenal gland, following early ligation of the blood vessels of the renal pedicle. Often a limited or more extensive retroperitoneal lymphadenectomy has been added to the radical nephrectomy.[39] This method of radical nephrectomy for the surgical treatment of renal cortical tumors has been accomplished by an anterior transperitoneal or thoracoabdominal approach to the renal vessels and to nephrectomy, particularly for

large or upper pole tumors and for those tumors with a vena caval tumor thrombus. Such a tactical approach to the treatment of renal cortical cancers was eminently suitable for the vast majority of renal tumors seen during the past 30 years, almost all of which were large and hypervascular, commonly with perinephric fat invasion and occasionally with lymph node metastases.

However, the clinical spectrum of renal cortical tumors coming to the urologist's attention has changed markedly over the past five years and gives every promise of showing continued change in the near future. Many renal parenchymal tumors are being detected by new imaging techniques such as ultrasound, computed tomography (CT) of the abdomen, and magnetic resonance imaging (MRI), which were not available 10 years ago. Many of these renal tumors being discovered have not produced symptoms but have been found during diagnostic tests carried out for nonrenal disorders. Such tumors are smaller, are generally of lower pathologic stage, and should be associated with a more favorable prognosis than were tumors found in prior years as a result of renal symptoms. The extent of the recent dramatic change in presentation of renal cortical tumors is illustrated by the fact that as many renal cell carcinomas now are found incidentally by imaging tests performed for unrelated symptoms as are seen in patients presenting with hematuria, flank pain, or symptoms from metastatic disease.[17] In contrast, a decade ago, 90% of patients presenting with renal cell carcinoma were symptomatic; small asymptomatic renal cell carcinomas were seldom discovered then. This revolutionary change in renal imaging and renal tumor diagnosis has prompted current re-evaluation of appropriate treatment for renal cell carcinoma and other renal cortical tumors, such as oncocytomas.

We have entered a treatment era in which the long-standing urologic surgical practice of automatically performing a radical nephrectomy for every solid renal mass lesion of whatever size may have to be abandoned. A small tumor, particularly if located on one of the poles of the kidneys or superficially on the parenchyma, may be best treated by partial renal resection.

In addition to improved imaging modalities, a significant improvement in our understanding of the pathobiology of renal parenchymal tumors has been seen in the past decade. Ten years ago only six cases of renal oncocytoma had been described in the world's urologic literature. Now it is appreciated that renal oncocytomas are a distinct common clinicopathologic entity and in fact make up 3 to 5% of tumors previously classified as renal cell carcinomas.[19] Renal oncocytomas, even when large, are generally asymptomatic and nearly always have a benign clinical course. It seems likely that almost all renal oncocytomas can be treated adequately by enucleation or partial resection, but the inability to make a preoperative diagnosis has made it difficult to treat them. Now there is evidence that newer diagnostic modalities, such as MRI[38] and perhaps fine-needle aspiration biopsy, may greatly assist in the preoperative diagnosis of renal oncocytomas. The many hundreds of cases of renal oncocytoma now reported in the literature and the increasing evidence that they often are multifocal and commonly bilateral (over time) adds further evidence to the need for renal parenchymal sparing procedures for this special tumor type if renal oncocytomas can be identified pre- or perioperatively.

It is also clear that patients with synchronous bilateral renal cell carcinoma as well as certain patients with asynchronous bilateral tumors have a special tumor biologically and can best be treated by an aggressive surgical approach, often requiring partial resection of one or both kidneys.[14] Along with this special clinical group are the more unusual patients at risk for developing bilateral renal cortical tumors, such as those with von Hippel-Lindau disease, others with the syndrome of familial renal adenocarcinoma associated with a chromosome 3–8 translocation,[5] and patients with angiomyolipomas. Such patients require renal parenchymal sparing procedures as often as these operations can be applied technically.

Finally, patients with solitary kidney (anatomically or functionally) are usually best treated by partial resection of the tumor and adjacent kidney. This has been the group of patients for whom renal parenchymal sparing procedures have been commonly used in the recent past, and is the group of patients providing evidence for the efficacy of this method for treating renal cortical tumors.

RENAL CELL CARCINOMA

Partial Nephrectomy in Patients With a Solitary Kidney or Bilateral Disease

Up to the present time, patients with renal cell carcinoma and a relatively normal contralateral kidney have been treated by total or radical nephrectomy of the tumor-involved kidney. Therefore, most of the clinical knowledge that has accumulated in the use of partial nephrectomy or enucleation for the treatment of renal cell carcinoma has come from experience in treating those patients with tumor in a solitary kidney or those with bilateral renal cell carcinoma. Such patients represent a special challenge to the urologist.

In approximately 2% of patients presenting with renal cell carcinoma, it occurs bilaterally.[49] In the recent past, it was thought that the identification of bilateral renal cell carcinomas, particularly if synchronous, indicated a very poor prognosis. However, the important report by Jacobs and colleagues in 1980,[14] reviewing world experience with the aggressive surgical treatment of patients with bilateral disease, quickly and finally changed our understanding of this specific syndrome. They demonstrated that patients with synchronous bilateral renal cancer treated surgically, often with a radical ne-phrectomy on one side and a partial ne-phrectomy on the other side (but occasion-ally by bilateral partial nephrectomies or bilateral total nephrectomies), showed the same prognosis stage for stage as those pa-tients with unilateral disease treated by rad-ical nephrectomy. Indeed, the five-year sur-vival rate for this entire series (65%) was that seen commonly for the group of patients with Stage I renal cancer in other series.[43] These results confirm for patients with bi-lateral renal cell carcinoma previously pub-lished data from the Mayo Clinic, in which patients with renal cell carcinoma in a func-tionally or anatomically solitary kidney treated by partial nephrectomy were found to have an unexpectedly favorable prog-nosis.[20]

More recently, a number of additional re-ports have documented good prognosis for patients treated by partial nephrectomy for renal cell carcinomas in a solitary kidney or for bilateral renal cell carcinomas. Zincke and associates compared survival in patients who had renal cell carcinoma treated by in situ or extracorporeal partial nephrectomy with that of patients treated by radical ne-phrectomy for unilateral renal cancer in the presence of a contralateral normal kidney.[56] The projected five-year survival rates for the two groups seen at the Mayo Clinic were 78% and 50%, respectively. When deaths due only to cancer were considered, the five-year survival rates for the two groups were 85% and 93%, respectively. Smith and co-workers, reviewing UCLA experience with the same group of patients, reported a five-year survival rate in patients with bilateral renal cell carcinoma or in a solitary kidney of 72%, if patients dying from non-cancer-related causes were excluded.[44] Zincke and Swanson, reporting Mayo Clinic experience with synchronous bilateral renal cell carci-noma, found five-year survival rates to be 78%.[58] Similarly good results have been re-ported by other centers.[48]

All currently published series appear to agree that patients with a low-stage lesion in a solitary kidney, treated by adequate partial nephrectomy, do about as well as patients treated by radical nephrectomy in the presence of a contralateral normal kid-ney. Patients with synchronous bilateral renal tumors treated surgically also appear to have the same favorable prognosis, per-haps because such patients make up a some-

what special syndrome and have lower grade, lower stage tumors at the time of diagnosis.[14] Whether such patients are really biologically different from those with asyn-chronous bilateral renal cancer or represent an artifact of the nature of their clinical presentation remains to be determined. In some series, patients with asynchronous bi-lateral renal cancer have done very poorly, whereas in other series the prognosis of patients with asynchronous bilateral disease has been similar to that seen for synchronous tumors.[22, 44, 48]

Renal cell carcinomas tend to grow as expanding spherical masses in the renal par-enchyma, often with a true pseudocapsule. This is particularly true for low-grade tu-mors and for oncocytomas. Higher grade tumors can be much more invasive with irregular pseudopod-like invasive tumor cell projections that infiltrate throughout the renal parenchyma and make partial renal resection much more difficult or impossible. Finally, some renal cell carcinomas are mul-tifocal throughout the kidney parenchyma, making tumor resection very complicated (Fig. 50–1).

For those patients with localized tumors who have been candidates for treatment by partial nephrectomy, local recurrence has been surprisingly uncommon (Table 50–1). The overall local recurrence rate from a collection of several series of patients with renal cancer in a solitary kidney or bilateral renal cancer treated by partial resection is just 9%.[14, 24, 44, 48, 58] When these results are considered according to the surgical tech-nique used, namely in situ resection versus extracorporeal partial nephrectomy, the lo-cal recurrence rates were 10% and 3%, re-spectively. Smith and colleagues warn against enucleation of renal cell carcinoma because microinvasion of the tumor capsule was common in their experience.[44] Three cases of local recurrence that occurred in Smith's series were those treated by in situ enucleation. In contrast, Novick reports on 15 patients treated by tumor enucleation.[31] Tumors were 1.8 to 7.0 cm in diameter, and all patients were alive three months to six years postoperatively. It was claimed that 87% of all nonmetastatic renal cell carcino-mas with a diameter less than 7 cm have an unperforated pseudocapsule, which pro-vides an ideal plane of cleavage for enuclea-tion. Therefore, Marberger and associates

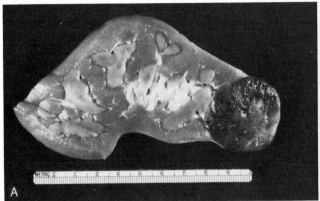

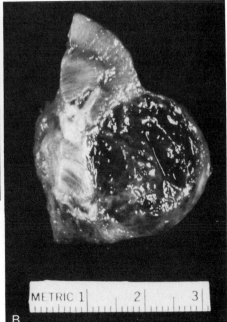

Figure 50–1. *A kidney with a polar solitary tumor (A) that was subsequently diagnosed as an oncocytoma. In the past such tumors were indiscriminately considered an indication for radical nephrectomy. It is now recognized that such tumors may be successfully treated by partial nephrectomy (B).*

recommended that tumors up to 7 cm in diameter be enucleated, whereas larger tumors be excised by partial nephrectomy with frozen sections obtained to verify total tumor removal from the margins.[22] Currently the use of enucleation for renal cell carcinoma is a highly controversial topic and one that will no doubt be further explored in coming decades, when partial renal resection for cortical tumors becomes more common.

At present the prognosis for patients with nonsurgically treated renal cell carcinoma is gloomy. The five-year survival rates for these patients have been 4 to 30%.[8, 21, 33] Wickham found that, of 30 patients with renal cancer in a solitary kidney treated nonsurgically, 75% died within a mean follow-up period of 24 months and all 16 patients with bilat-

eral synchronous tumors died within five months.[54] Unilateral nephrectomy for renal cell carcinoma in a solitary kidney or bilateral nephrectomy for bilateral synchronous renal cancer with postoperative hemodialysis are additional options. However, many of these patients fare poorly, and the majority of them die from dialysis-related complications.[13, 22] Nephrectomy followed by renal transplantation is a more attractive alternative, particularly if performed in patients who were on dialysis for over 15 months following nephrectomy.[34] Of 13 patients with bilateral renal cancer thus treated, six had synchronous tumors and seven had asynchronous tumors.[14, 34, 45, 58] Of the six patients with synchronous tumors, two died of unrelated causes and one died

Table 50–1. LOCAL RECURRENCE FOLLOWING PARTIAL NEPHRECTOMY FOR RENAL CELL CARCINOMA

First Author	Reference	Total (%)	In Situ Surgery (%)	Ex Vivo Surgery (%)
Jacobs	14	6:59 (10)	5:42 (12)	1:17 (6)
Smith	44	3:36 (8.3)	3:32 (19)	0:4 (0)
Topley	48	3:23 (13)	3:19 (16)	0:4 (0)
Marshall	24	1:10 (10)	1:10 (10)	0:7 —
Zincke	56	1:33 (3)	1:26 (4)	0:7 (0)
Total		14:161 (9)	13:129 (10)	1:32 (3)

of metastatic disease. Of the seven patients transplanted following bilateral radical nephrectomy for metachronous renal cell cancer, four died of metastatic disease and one died of sepsis.

Since there are now no exciting systemic nonsurgical treatments for renal cell carcinoma, either chemotherapeutic or immunotherapeutic, it seems likely that surgical therapy will continue to be our primary method for attacking such tumors in the near future. Nevertheless, it is important to note that an occasional patient with very large bilateral renal tumors may have bilateral renal oncocytomas. Such patients have been followed for many years without evidence of tumor progression or metastasis. Bilateral total nephrectomy for a patient with renal oncocytoma or removal of a solitary kidney containing an oncocytoma does not represent a great urologic surgical triumph in 1987. Discriminating use of preoperative diagnostic tests and possibly pre- or intraoperative biopsies are necessary in these difficult cases. There is every reason to think that for the extremely elderly or very poor risk operative candidate, percutaneous needle biopsy diagnosis of renal oncocytoma and nonsurgical treatment (surveillance) might be a reasonable option.

TRANSITIONAL CELL CARCINOMA

Just as radical nephrectomy has been standard treatment for renal cell carcinoma for many decades, radical nephroureterectomy with excision of a cuff of bladder has been standard treatment for transitional cell carcinoma of the upper tract for many years. Indeed, fifty years ago, Kimball and Ferris demonstrated a high rate of tumor recurrence in the bladder and ureteral cuff when nephrectomy alone was performed.[16] Tumors in the ureteral stump developed in 15 to 30% of patients treated with nephrectomy alone,[30, 40, 47] and bladder tumors developed in 30%.[30]

However, it is increasingly recognized that all urothelial tumors of the upper urinary tract are not the same biologically. The natural history of such tumors is now better understood, particularly concerning the difference in behavior of low-grade, low-stage tumors and of more aggressive tumors of

high grade and stage in certain locations. There have been a number of favorable reports recommending conservative treatment for certain ureteral and renal pelvic tumors.[1, 3, 23, 50, 51] Surgical management in these cases may be by pyelotomy with local excision and fulguration, partial nephrectomy, or segmental resection of the ureter. In most cases such procedures are performed in situ. However, in more complex situations, bench surgery and renal autotransplantation may also be required for transitional cell tumors of the renal pelvis.[26, 51]

Most authors recommend conservative surgery in patients with pelvic and ureteral tumors of a solitary kidney, in patients with unilateral tumors and renal insufficiency, in those with bilateral upper tract tumors, and in patients with tumors associated with Balkan nephropathy. Opinions differ markedly, however, as to the proper management of unilateral low-grade, low-stage renal pelvic and ureteral urothelial tumors in the presence of a contralateral healthy kidney. In a Mayo Clinic study the success of conservative treatment was related to the location of the tumor.[57] Whereas the tumor recurred in 23 of 37 patients (62%) with renal pelvic tumors, it recurred in only four of 27 patients (15%) with ureteral tumors. The grade of tumor was also related to the success rate of conservative surgery, particularly in patients with ureteral tumors. Only one of 21 (5%) Grade 1 or 2 ureteral tumors recurred locally after conservative treatment, but three of six (50%) tumors of Grade 3 or 4 recurred locally. Grade of tumor was not so significant a factor for patients with renal pelvic tumors; even for patients with Grade 1 renal pelvic tumors, the local recurrence rate was 50%, and this rate was higher for patients with higher grade tumors. Although survival did not depend significantly on the location of the tumors, nonprogression did. Patients with ureteral tumors fared better than those with renal pelvic tumors. Not surprisingly, urothelial mapping studies of kidneys and ureters removed during nephroureterectomy performed for urothelial tumors of the upper tract have demonstrated a much higher incidence of diffuse urothelial abnormalities, particularly so for patients with high-grade and multiple tumors than for those with low grade tumors.[25] Such field changes in the urothelium make conservative treatment of renal pelvic tumors less likely to be as effective as it is for controlling renal cortical tumors. However, conservative surgery will be more successful for patients with low-grade tumors because the lower incidence of adjacent urothelial abnormalities in these patients makes recurrence less likely. Technical factors related to the ease of surgical exposure, such as the ability to obtain tumor-free surgical margins and accomplish urinary tract reconstruction, very likely account for the greater success of conservative operations for ureteral tumor patients than for patients with renal pelvic tumors. For the same reason, patients with a urothelial tumor in a calyx or infundibulum of the upper or lower pole collecting system may be expected to do better with conservative treatment than are those with tumor in the mid pelvis, because partial resection to remove the upper or lower pole offers a chance for clean surgical margins.

For almost all patients with renal pelvic tumors, total nephroureterectomy and excision of a bladder cuff remains the best treatment. The high rate of recurrence in the ureteral stump when nephroureterectomy is not done, and the low rate (1.5 to 2.0%) of tumor in the contralateral upper urinary tract, convince us that complete nephroureterectomy is usually the treatment of choice even for patients with low-grade tumors in the renal pelvis.[7] In a highly selective group of patients with extensive transitional cell tumors of the renal pelvis in whom every attempt at renal preservation must be done, nephrectomy with excision of all extrarenal pelvis and ureter and autotransplantation of the kidney with pyelocystostomy may be an alternative.[35] This method affords easy follow-up examinations and local treatment by fulguration or intravesical chemotherapy performed transurethrally.

The last few years have witnessed tremendous advances in ureteroscopic instrumentation. Consequently, there is every reason to hope that upper tract tumors, particularly renal pelvic tumors, will be managed by transureteral endoscopic procedures in the future and that the need for partial resection will be markedly reduced. Adaptation of the use of the laser delivered via the ureteroscope may also increase the applicability of conservative endoscopic management of these tumors and reduce the need for open partial resection. However, the common occurrence of extravasation of irrigating fluids during endourologic procedures warrants a word of caution as to the potential hazard of disseminating tumor cells in the retroperitoneum. Finally, the marked recent advances in combination cytotoxic chemotherapy for urothelial cancers suggest that some patients, particularly those presenting with high-grade, high-stage renal pelvic tumors diagnosed by percutaneous fine-needle aspiration biopsy or by transureteroscopic biopsy, will be treated best by intensive systemic chemotherapy in the future rather than by open surgical techniques. Because transitional cell carcinoma is often a diffuse field change disease, partial renal resection in its treatment will never be as useful as it will be for renal cell carcinoma or renal oncocytoma.

PARTIAL NEPHRECTOMY PROCEDURE

Surgical Technique: Preoperative Preparation

Besides the usual measures, preoperative preparation for partial nephrectomy for a renal cortical tumor has a few special features. The best and most sophisticated renal parenchymal imaging modalities need to be applied for patients with renal parenchymal tumors. This usually involves CT scanning of the kidneys. Renal cell carcinomas and renal oncocytomas can be both bilateral and multifocal within one kidney. In addition, ipsilateral or contralateral adrenal metastases can occur and might modify the nature of the planned surgical procedure. In the case of a solitary kidney or bilateral disease, the exact definition of tumor extent and multifocal nature of tumor is important in deciding whether tumor can be operated in situ or whether ex vivo bench surgery and renal autotransplantation are necessary. In our experience, CT scanning of the kidney and renal angiography give a much better index of tumor size, operability, presence or absence of caval tumor thrombus, and multifocal character of the tumor than is often appreciated by direct examination of the kidney at the time of surgery.

Moreover, renal angiography, although not required for a straightforward case, is generally helpful for planning a partial nephrectomy in complex circumstances. The arterial anatomy is a key element in the applicability and success of partial nephrectomy in many cases. Good-quality arteriography, preferably done in multiple planes, allows for a somewhat informed approach to the renal hilum and for easier preservation of known polar vessels. Knowledge of a segmental arterial supply will often permit early and confident division of a segmented vessel supplying only a diseased area. In older patients, occurrence of ipsilateral or contralateral arterial disease can often force modification of a previously planned approach.

Adequate preoperative and intraoperative hydration of the patient should be diligently fostered so that the operated kidney is in the best possible condition to resist acute renal failure if the arterial supply is occluded. For cases that will require prolonged renal ischemia (more than 10 minutes of renal artery occlusion), preparation for cooling the kidney with "slushed" saline or Ringer's lactate should be undertaken. If ex vivo "bench" surgery is a possibility, then the availability of suitable chilled perfusion solutions should be arranged.

In complex cases involving extensive surgery to an anatomically or functionally solitary kidney, a preoperative vascular access procedure is often advisable to ensure convenient hemodialysis in the immediate postoperative period. Alternatively, a Udall catheter introduced through a central line can be used for perioperative dialysis if this is necessary.

Finally, the urine should be cultured preoperatively. Any infection present should be treated vigorously with antibiotics to reduce the incidence of postoperative perirenal and wound infection. Preoperative percutaneous skinny-needle aspiration biopsy may become more common in the future, since preoperative identification of a renal oncocytoma may suggest that tumor enucleation is possible or desirable; alternatively, identification of a definite renal cell carcinoma may argue more in favor of a formal partial resection, taking a margin of normal parenchyma as determined by frozen sections. Such preoperative diagnosis could also make a difference in terms of whether in situ or ex vivo bench surgery is necessary.

Operative Approach

The incision chosen for partial nephrectomy must permit wide exposure so that the kidney can be completely mobilized and adequate access is available to the major vessels in the renal hilum. Partial nephrectomy has the potential for being a very sanguineous procedure, making ready control of the renal artery and vein critical. Whatever incision that the surgeon feels comfortable with and that is capable of permitting these tactical goals will prove satisfactory. Certainly, very small polar or superficial lesions (2 to 4 cm in size) in a previously nonoperated kidney can be treated very successfully through a standard flank incision. However, a kidney that has been operated upon previously or a kidney harboring a large tumor suggests that an anterior transperitoneal approach or even a thoracoabdominal approach will allow a safer and more convenient operation. For patients in whom ex vivo surgery is contemplated with autotransplantation to the pelvis, either an extensive single midline incision or an upper subcostal incision can be used for the nephrectomy and a separate lower transverse or "hockey stick" incision can be used for the autotransplantation.

Operative Techniques

Once the kidney is completely freed from the perirenal fat and the ureter and main renal vessels identified, the surgeon must make his decision as to the operative approach based on location and size of the tumor, ability to perform in situ removal of the tumor or multiple tumors, personal experience, and preoperative imaging studies. When partial nephrectomy is planned, three technical aspects need careful consideration: (1) achieving vascular control, (2) incising through the renal parenchyma, (3) the type of resection.

Vascular Control

The most common complication of partial nephrectomy is hemorrhage. Intraoperative blood loss measured in one series averaged 906 ml.[53] To reduce intraoperative blood loss, a number of techniques have been developed that arrest blood flow to either the entire kidney or that part to be resected. (However, centrally located tumors may not be amenable to in situ partial resection and ex vivo bench surgery may be required.) In nearly every case of partial nephrectomy, the renal artery and vein need to be identified and dissected free, and perhaps have a vessel loop placed around them to permit ready control.

If occlusion of the main renal artery is utilized, regional hypothermia should be considered. Semb showed that with warm ischemia, 11 minutes was the maximum time that could be taken to occlude the renal vessels and result in a minimum functional renal loss.[42] Eighteen minutes of occlusion time produced a moderate reaction, and 50 minutes produced total renal loss. By cooling the kidney with ice-slushed saline, however, safe renal artery occlusion time was increased to 26 minutes. Novick and associates have been able to extend the safe cold ischemia time to three hours by perfusing the in situ kidney through a Swan-Ganz catheter placed preoperatively.[32] Local hypothermia may also be achieved by placing a rubber dam or plastic bag with a drawstring (such as is used for intestinal surgery) around the kidney. Sterile ice-slush saline is then poured into the wound around and over the kidney and allowed to remain for five to 10 minutes prior to renal artery occlusion. In addition, it is helpful for the anesthesiologist to give 25 to 50 gm of mannitol intravenously immediately prior to occluding the renal vascular pedicle.

However, if possible, it is always better to avoid occlusion of the arterial blood supply to the entire kidney if this can be technically performed safely. In the ideal circumstance, the renal lesion to be excised is confined to a polar area supplied by an accessory renal artery or a segmental renal artery branch. If this appears to be the case from preoperative angiography or at the time of renal artery dissection in the hilum, then this branch should be identified, dissected free, and injected with a dilute solution of indigo carmine (0.4%). The dye will stain the segment supplied (Fig. 50–2). If the renal tumor is confined to the stained area, this arterial branch should be ligated and divided (Fig. 50–3), and the natural segmental plane between the stained and normal parenchyma should be utilized for the subsequent resection. As one might suspect, this ideal anatomic circumstance does not often occur.

However, for polar partial nephrectomy a number of other techniques have been described for regional control of blood flow, limiting it to the area resected while at the same time providing adequate arterial circulation to the rest of the kidney. The simplest technique involves having an assistant grasp the waist of the kidney firmly, compressing it between thumb and forefinger (Fig. 50–3). The latter may be associated with inadequate control of hemorrhage and the grasping hand may become fatigued.

The partial nephrectomy clamp described by Storm and associates is a technologically sophisticated instrument (Fig. 50–4) that gives dependable vascular control,[46] but it is bulky and necessitates a somewhat larger incision and mobilization of the entire kidney for its application. Goodwin and Thelen

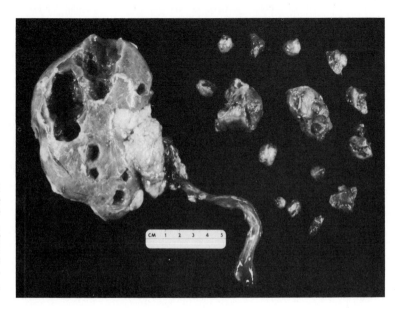

Figure 50–2. *Multifocal renal cell carcinoma throughout the entire kidney parenchyma. In this case of a patient with a solitary kidney, an attempt was made to remove all these tumors by extracorporeal bench surgery. However, even this technique may sometimes be inadequate to remove multiple foci, as happened in this case.*

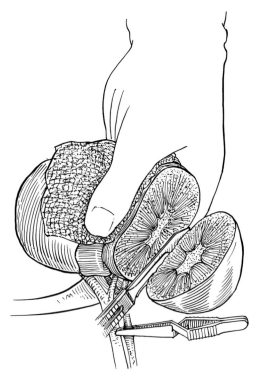

Figure 50–3. Regional control, limiting blood flow to that part of the kidney to be removed, may be achieved by direct compression of the renal parenchyma between thumb and forefinger. However, this is an uncertain way to achieve adequate hemostatic control, subject to human frailty and fatigue.

recommended the use of a rubber band placed proximal to the line of incision, tightened and secured with a clamp.[12] During experimental partial nephrectomies in dogs that were carried out by one of us (B.G.), this technique was found to be inefficient. It was difficult to achieve gradual increase in compression and, conversely, gradual release, which was necessary for identification of bleeders prior to terminating this operation. Recently, a simple instrument was developed, termed the kidney tourniquet (Fig. 50–5).[10] It is made of rubber tubing that is pulled through a clamp to form a noose in a lasso-like fashion. The noose is designed so that by the use of a spring-loaded lever, the lasso may be easily tightened and secured so as not to slip during use. Pulling on the free arm of the tubing will gradually tighten pressure, but the release of pressure must be achieved by the release of the clamp lever. The kidney tourniquet, therefore, attains dependable vascular control, is small, does not necessitate mobilization of the entire kidney,

and is relatively inexpensive. Finally, it may be used for retracting and manipulating the kidney during the resection, it provides secure hemostasis, and there is little chance of dislodgement. These techniques are highly recommended; however, the surgeon should not fail to isolate and control the main renal vessels at the onset of the procedure.

Incising Through the Renal Tissue

Intraoperative and delayed bleeding, urinary fistulae, and secondary nephrectomy were all too common complications of partial nephrectomy that effectively led to its abandonment until the middle of this century. In 1949 and again in 1953, Semb reported a large series of patients who underwent partial nephrectomy with low rates of bleeding and fistula formation.[41] Although this might be attributed to a selection of patients, undoubtedly a major component of this low morbidity must be attributed to the technique he described. Semb advocated dissection within the renal parenchyma by means of the spatulated portion of a scalpel handle and direct ligation of structures encountered, namely blood vessels and calyceal infundibula, during the dissection. Semb's original technique has a number of advantages: little renal tissue is sacrificed, the amount of ischemic tissue left behind to undergo necrosis and atrophy is minimal, and the operating time is short. However, minor vessels are usually severed by the blunt dissection and may cause troublesome bleeding following removal of the pedicle clamp. Recognizing that renal tissue is made of two components, one friable (the renal parenchyma) and one tough and flexible (the blood vessels and collecting system structures), Kim[15] and Williams and associates[55] described a similar technique involving a circumferential No. 1 chromic ligature around the kidney proximal to the line of resection. As the ligature is tightened, the relatively friable parenchyma is cut while the more resistant vessels and collecting system are mass-ligated. The resection is then carried out distal to this ligature. Attention to hemostasis and closure of the collecting system are the same as in all other techniques.

Recognizing the importance of individual

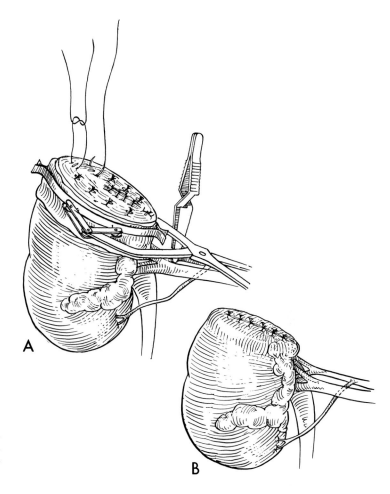

Figure 50–4. The clamp described by Storm, and colleagues[46] gives dependable regional vascular control. However, it necessitates a somewhat larger incision and mobilization of the entire kidney for its application.

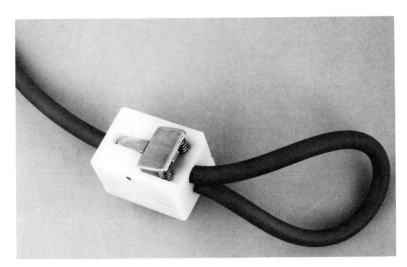

Figure 50–5. This photograph illustrates a new kidney tourniquet made of rubber tubing pulled through a clamp to form a noose in a lasso-like fashion. The use of a spring-loaded lever allows gradual tightening and release of pressure when applied over the kidney.

ligation of the blood vessels and tight closure of the collecting system on the one hand, and the characteristics of the renal substance on the other hand, one of us (B.G.) has devised an instrument that dissects and removes the friable parenchymatous tissue while sparing the blood vessels and collecting system structures (Fig. 50–6).[11] The instrument consists of two parallel arms containing cylindrical blunt teeth. These teeth are evenly spaced and intertwine upon closure of the clamp. The opening and closing is a parallel action, not scissor-like, and ensures uniform pressure on renal tissue. After the capsule is incised and displaced at the line of incision, the clamp is applied by repeated closure and opening over the renal parenchyma (Fig. 50–7A). At this stage the instrument is removed and the incision inspected. The blood vessels and collecting system structures will appear as cord-like bridges coursing across the line of incision with little parenchymatous tissue overlying them (Fig. 50–7B). By means of a small aneurysm needle or a right-angled clamp, ligatures are passed underneath and around the vessels and tied (Fig. 50–7C). The vessels are incised distal to the ligatures; this process is repeated through the entire depth of the renal incision. In both animal studies and human application, this method allowed individual ligation of vessels and collecting system structures, eliminating the need for placing suture ligatures or large figure-of-eight sutures, which contribute to surrounding tissue necrosis. With this instrument, vessels of very small diameter were spared and could be individually ligated. We have found that the combined use of the kidney tourniquet and this new clamp allowed partial nephrectomy to be performed easily with minimal blood loss.[11]

The carbon dioxide laser has been applied to partial nephrectomy.[27] It coagulates vessels smaller than 5 mm in diameter as it amputates, if the blood flow to that area is arrested for the duration of the resection. It causes minimal damage to the underlying parenchyma. The ultrasonic surgical aspirator also has been applied to partial nephrectomy,[4] and recently a technique utilizing a combination of laser surgery and ultrasonic aspiration was presented.[28] However, we believe that the advantage afforded by these two techniques does not justify their expense; therefore they will probably remain in limited use in the near future.

Type of Resection

The two most commonly used methods for polar partial nephrectomy are the wedge and guillotine techniques. The wedge technique is illustrated in Figure 50–8. It is advocated for resections of small amounts of parenchyma and is especially useful for very small polar lesions. Vascular control may be achieved either by occlusion of the renal artery with a bulldog clamp or by placing a kidney tourniquet proximal to the line of incision. Then the wedge of parenchyma may be excised. Occlusion of the blood supply will permit precise, watertight closure of the collecting system and suture ligation

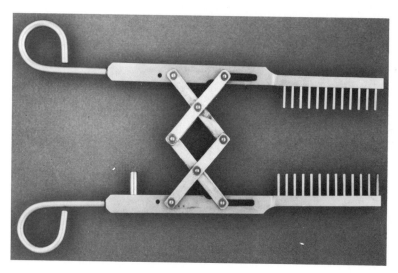

Figure 50–6. The Goldwasser-Carson dissector consists of two parallel arms containing cylindrical, blunt, evenly spaced teeth that intertwine upon closure of the clamp. This instrument dissects and removes the friable renal cortical tissue while sparing most blood vessels and collecting system structures.

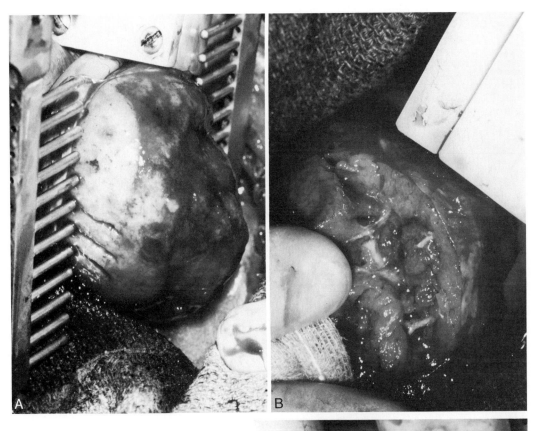

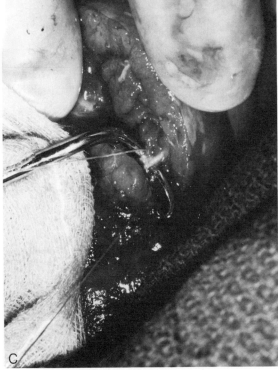

Figure 50–7. For partial nephrectomy, the capsule is incised and retracted off the pole of the kidney. A, With the kidney tourniquet applied and tightened (notice the pale color of the parenchyma), the Goldwasser-Carson dissector is used by repeatedly closing and opening it over the renal parenchyma. At this stage the dissector is removed and the incision inspected. B, Blood vessels may be noted as white cord-like bridges coursing across the line of incision. C, By means of a small aneurysm needle, a ligature is passed underneath and around a blood vessel, which is then tied and severed.

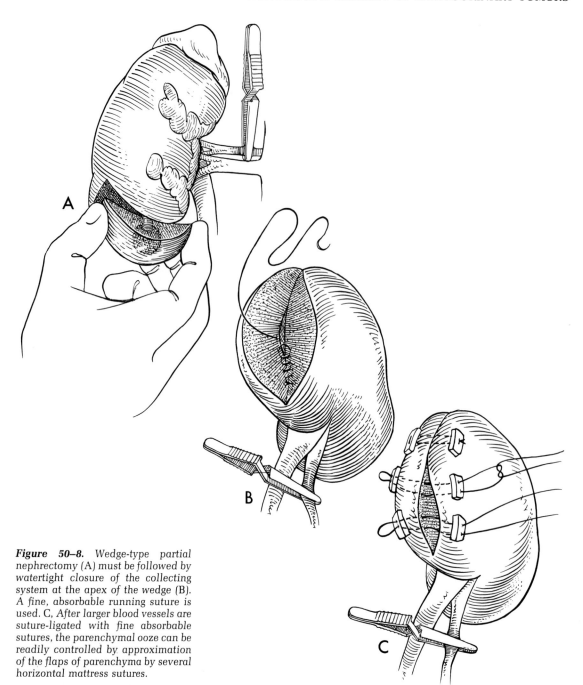

Figure 50–8. Wedge-type partial nephrectomy (A) must be followed by watertight closure of the collecting system at the apex of the wedge (B). A fine, absorbable running suture is used. C, After larger blood vessels are suture-ligated with fine absorbable sutures, the parenchymal ooze can be readily controlled by approximation of the flaps of parenchyma by several horizontal mattress sutures.

or ligation of the larger vessels. The flaps of parenchyma are then commonly approximated with large horizontal mattress sutures, which also control the ooze from the raw surface, although this technique has been criticized because of ischemic necrosis, noted in experimental animals.[29]

For this reason, most authorities now recommend guillotine partial nephrectomy for polar lesions. This approach is illustrated in Figure 50–9. For benign lesions, the renal capsule overlying the diseased portion is generally first dissected free, to be used later to cover the raw area of parenchyma left at the end of the operation. However, when a partial nephrectomy is performed in the treatment of renal cancer, this is not practical or advisable. The renal artery is temporarily occluded and the parenchyma is then divided in a transverse fashion, with care taken to generate a relatively flat surface without divots and crevices. A knife handle

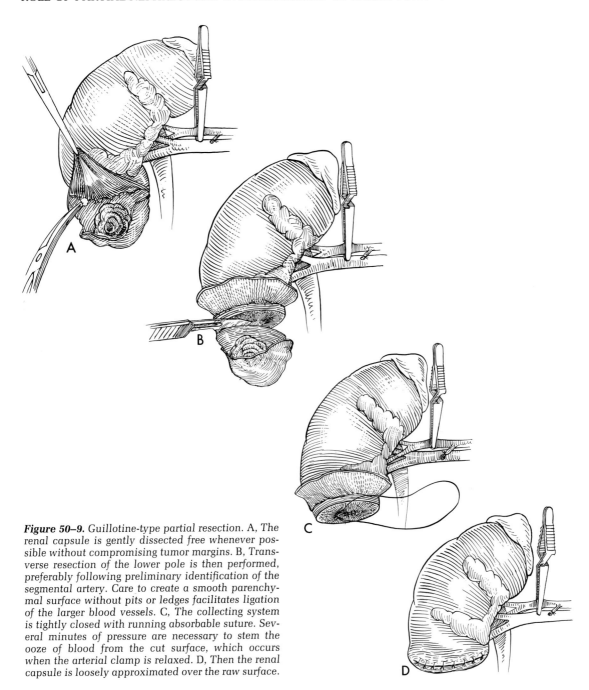

Figure 50–9. Guillotine-type partial resection. A, The renal capsule is gently dissected free whenever possible without compromising tumor margins. B, Transverse resection of the lower pole is then performed, preferably following preliminary identification of the segmental artery. Care to create a smooth parenchymal surface without pits or ledges facilitates ligation of the larger blood vessels. C, The collecting system is tightly closed with running absorbable suture. Several minutes of pressure are necessary to stem the ooze of blood from the cut surface, which occurs when the arterial clamp is relaxed. D, Then the renal capsule is loosely approximated over the raw surface.

or a neurosurgical spatula may be used to divide the parenchyma bluntly, since the larger vessels and collecting system structures will resist it and can be ligated as they are encountered. Alternatively, the Goldwasser-Carson dissector, previously described, may be applied along the line of resection. This will result in preservation of both large and small vessels and collecting system structures, which can then be individually

ligated. Release of the renal artery clamp or tourniquet will then reveal any other large vessels that require control. Watertight closure of the collecting system is performed with a running fine absorbable suture. Dramatic ooze from the raw parenchymal surface is to be expected. This can be controlled easily with gauze-sponge pressure for five minutes before the capsule flaps are reapproximated over the raw area. Recently, microfibrillar collagen has become available as a hemostatic agent, and we have found that this works quite well to stop ooze from the renal parenchyma.

Many substances have been used to cover the raw parenchymal surface of the guillotined parenchyma, including the renal capsule, perirenal fat, free grafts of the peritoneum, and various synthetic plastics.[9, 37] All of these materials appear satisfactory. Many surgeons use nothing at all to cover the raw surface, and these patients appear to do well, with no increased incidence of urinary leakage. If no devitalized tissue is left, the kidney should be expected to heal well. However, multiple drains (Penrose, Hemovac, or Jackson-Pratt) should be left near the kidney to remove any blood or urine that might accumulate in the area.

Techniques for Nonpolar Segmental Lesions

The great majority of localized renal lesions suitable for partial nephrectomy are readily treated by a polar guillotine amputation or equivalent procedure on the lateral superficial parenchyma. However, certain tumors may occur in a nonpolar segment. Unusual local circumstances may demand unusual surgical approaches. Generally, this involves the resection of a large central lesion occurring in a solitary kidney or of such tumors occurring bilaterally. Most problems of this sort can be handled by in situ surgery using renal hypothermia, with careful excision of the tumor and reconstruction of the collecting system. An occasional case of this type will require ex vivo bench surgery for adequate exposure.[2, 6] In such cases, the kidney is excised with the renal vessels as one would do for a donor nephrectomy. The kidney is then perfused with a suitable chilled solution, such as Collins' or Sacks' solution, until the outflow from the renal vein[36] is clear, and a hypothermic state with a parenchymal temperature of about 15°C is achieved.[52] Great care is taken to excise a large tumor involving, for example, the midportion of a solitary kidney, with the required renal pelvic and vascular reconstructions. Usually, the ureter is left intact and the kidney is transplanted back to the ipsilateral iliac fossa. Such techniques require a familiarity with vascular surgery and should be done by surgeons with experience in

renal transplantation. Most renal lesions can be managed by in situ surgery.

Complications

The postoperative complications encountered in 309 partial nephrectomies performed for various indications at the Mayo Clinic from 1957 until 1977 are shown in Table 50–2.[18] The only death occurred in a diabetic patient with a solitary kidney admitted in septic shock, in whom partial nephrectomy was performed for multiple renal abscesses. Major "medical" complications were uncommon. Secondary nephrectomy was necessary in eight patients (2.6%). Three patients had recurrent tumor or infection. The other five had marked perirenal or periureteral fibrosis with a nonfunctioning kidney or urinary fistula. This finding stresses the need for atraumatic dissection and adequate postoperative drainage in an attempt to reduce the incidence of subsequent fibrosis with obstruction to urinary drainage. Most patients with postoperative urinomas or urinary fistulas had had wedge resection with the renal cortex reapproximated with large mattress sutures, strong evidence in favor of a guillotine partial nephrectomy. If no distal urinary obstruction was present, the urinary fistulas healed quite nicely with or without insertion of a ureteral catheter. Almost all wound infections occurred in patients with kidney stones whose urine was not adequately ster-

Table 50–2. POSTOPERATIVE COMPLICATIONS IN 309 PARTIAL NEPHRECTOMIES*

Complication	Number of Patients (%)
Death	1 (0.3)
Delayed nephrectomy	8 (2.6)
Urinoma	3 (1.0)
Urinary fistula	7 (2.3)
Delayed (renal) hemorrhage	2 (0.6)
Abscess	3 (1.0)
Wound infection	15 (5.0)
Ureteral obstruction	3 (1.0)
Postoperative ureteral stone	1 (0.3)
Wound separation	1 (0.3)
Gastrointestinal hemorrhage (gastric ulcer)	1 (0.3)
Pneumonia	1 (0.3)
Pulmonary embolism	2 (0.6)

*Modified from Leach G and Lieber MM: Partial nephrectomy: Mayo Clinic experience 1957–1977. Urology 15:219, 1980.

ilized preoperatively. This complication probably could be eliminated by appropriate preoperative urine cultures and antimicrobial therapy. The best treatment for postoperative complications is prevention.

Murphy and Best describe a similar incidence of major complications (excluding tuberculosis) among 819 patients undergoing partial nephrectomy, reported between 1930 and 1957.[29] Secondary nephrectomies were done in 2.5%; a urinary fistula occurred in 3.9%. However, the secondary hemorrhage rate of 3.4% was higher than the 0.6% found in the Mayo series.

Appropriate case selection, careful preoperative preparation, and major reliance on guillotine-type partial nephrectomy should further reduce the incidence of complications.

FUTURE PERSPECTIVES

There is every reason to believe that current advances in medical electronics and imaging will continue. It is easy to envision a day in the not too distant future when middle-aged patients will go through some abdominal or total body scanning procedure such as magnetic resonance imaging (which does not involve any ionizing radiation exposure) as part of an annual physical examination, just as patients commonly receive an electrocardiogram or chest x-ray in 1987. Widespread use of such screening procedures will reveal many smaller renal parenchymal tumors, tumors of such small size that radical nephrectomy will be immediately apparent as surgical overkill. Partial renal resection for small renal tumors will most likely become the norm, whether such tumors turn out to be oncocytomas or renal cell carcinomas. Further, advanced techniques of tumor classification, such as the application of flow cytometry to quantitation of nuclear DNA content or tumor antigens of renal parenchymal tumor cells removed by percutaneous fine-needle aspiration biopsy, will also no doubt become common in the future. These and even more sophisticated tumor classification techniques will enable us to identify those tumors that are characteristically local growths with limited metastatic potential, perhaps to be generally treated by partial nephrectomy, and to separate out a group of more malignant-behaving tumors that may require more aggressive surgery and perhaps adjuvant chemotherapy, which we hope will be available in the near future.

Whatever form taken by this increasing sophistication in diagnosis and classification of renal tumors, the final result will be that radical nephrectomy will become less commonly used in the future than it has been in the past. Partial nephrectomy will be employed to treat renal cortical tumors much more frequently than in the past 30 years.

References

1. Bloom NA, Vidone RA, Lytton B: Primary carcinoma of the ureter: a report of 102 new cases. J Urol 103:590–598, 1970.
2. Calne RY: Treatment of bilateral hypernephromas by nephrectomy, excision of tumour and autotransplantation. Report of three cases. Lancet 2:1164–1167, 1973.
3. Carroll G: Bilateral transitional cell carcinoma of the renal pelvis. J Urol 93:132–135, 1965.
4. Chopp RT, Shah BB, Addonizio JC: Use of ultrasonic surgical aspirator in renal surgery. Urology 22:157–159, 1983.
5. Cohen AJ, Li FP, Berg S, et al: Hereditary renal-cell carcinoma associated with a chromosomal translocation. N Engl J Med 301:592–595, 1979.
6. Corman JL, Anderson JT, Taubman J, et al: Ex vivo perfusion, arteriography, and autotransplantation procedures for kidney salvage. Surg Gynecol Obstet 137:659–665, 1973.
7. Cummings KB: Nephroureterectomy: rationale in the management of transitional cell carcinoma of the upper urinary tract. Urol Clin North Am 7:569–578, 1980.
8. deKernion JB, Ramming KP, Smith RB: The natural history of metastatic renal cell carcinoma: a computer analysis. J Urol 120:148–152, 1978.
9. Fox M, Henry L, Lomax AH, Rees RWM: The effect of isobutyl-cyanoacrylate monomer adhesive on closure of nephrotomy and partial nephrectomy incisions. Br J Urol 41:539–545, 1969.
10. Goldwasser B, Carson CC, Shalaby NF, Bertram RA: Kidney tourniquet: A new instrument for regional blood control in partial nephrectomy. Urology (in press).
11. Goldwasser B, Carson CC, Shalaby NG, et al: Partial nephrectomy using new dissecting instrument. J Urol 136:54–57, 1986.
12. Goodwin WE, Thelen HM: Preservation of renal function during partial nephrectomy: use of rubber band tourniquet for hemostasis. JAMA 168:179, 1958.
13. Jacobs SC: Role of conservative surgery for patients with bilateral kidney tumors. In WJ Catalona, TL Ratliff (eds), Urologic Oncology. Boston, Martinus Nijhoff, 1984.
14. Jacobs SC, Berg SI, Lawson RK: Synchronous bilateral renal cell carcinoma: total surgical excision. Cancer 46:2341–2345, 1980.
15. Kim SK: New technique of partial nephrectomy. J Urol 92:185–187, 1964.
16. Kimball FN, Ferris HW: Papillomatous tumor of renal pelvis associated with similar tumors of ureter

and bladder: review of literature and report of 2 cases. J Urol 31:257–304, 1934.

17. Konnak JW, Grossman HB: Renal cell carcinoma as an incidental finding. J Urol 134:1094–1096, 1985.

18. Leach GE, Lieber MM: Partial nephrectomy: Mayo Clinic experience 1957–1977. Urology 15:219–228, 1980.

19. Lieber MM, Tomera KM, Farrow GM: Renal oncocytoma. J Urol 125:481–485, 1981.

20. Malek RS, Utz DC, Culp OS, et al: Malignant tumors of solitary kidneys. Mayo Clin Proc 47:180–188, 1972.

21. Marberger M: Organerhaltende Chirurgie beim Nierenkarzinom Aktuelle. Urologie 11:325, 1980.

22. Marberger M, Pugh RC, Auvert J, et al: Conservation surgery of renal carcinoma: the EIRSS experience. Br J Urol 53:528–532, 1981.

23. Marshall FF: The in situ surgical management of renal cell carcinoma and transitional cell carcinoma of the kidney. World J Urol 2:130, 1984.

24. Marshall FF, Walsh PC: In situ management of renal tumors: renal cell carcinoma and transitional cell carcinoma. J Urol 131:1045–1049, 1984.

25. McCarron JP Jr, Chasko SB, Gray GF Jr: Systematic mapping of nephroureterectomy specimens removed for urothelial cancer: pathological findings and clinical correlations. J Urol 128:243–246, 1982.

26. McLoughlin MG: The treatment of bilateral synchronous renal pelvic tumors with bench surgery. J Urol 114:463–465, 1975.

27. Meiraz D, Peled I, Gassner S, et al: The use of the CO_2 laser for partial nephrectomy: an experimental study. Invest Urol 15:262–264, 1977.

28. Melzer R, Landau S, Wood T, Smith JA: Technique of combined ultrasonic aspiration and laser partial nephrectomy. Presented at American Urological Association 80th Annual Meeting, Atlanta, Georgia. May, 1985.

29. Murphy JJ, Best R: The healing of renal wounds: 1. Partial nephrectomy. J Urol 78:504–510, 1957.

30. Murphy DM, Zincke H, Furlow WL: Management of high grade transitional cell cancer of the upper urinary tract. J Urol 125:25–29, 1981.

31. Novick AC: Editorial comment. In WJ Catalona, TL Ratliff (eds), Urologic Oncology. Boston, Martinus Nijhoff, 1984, p. 159.

32. Novick AC, Stewart BH, Straffon RA, et al: Partial nephrectomy in the treatment of renal adenocarcinoma. J Urol 118:932–936, 1977.

33. Patel NP, Lavengood RN: Renal cell carcinoma: natural history and results of treatment. J Urol 119:722–726, 1978.

34. Penn I: Transplantation in patients with primary renal malignancies. Transplantation 24:424–434, 1977.

35. Pettersson S, Brynger H, Henriksson C, et al: Treatment of urothelial tumors of the upper urinary tract by nephroureterectomy, renal autotransplantation and pyelocystostomy. Cancer 54:379–386, 1984.

36. Poutasse EF: Partial nephrectomy: new techniques, approach, operative indications and review of 51 cases. J Urol 88:153–159, 1962.

37. Rathert P, Siemensen H, Theil KH: Experimental and clinical use of cyanoacrylate adhesive and amniotic tissue in partial nephrectomy. J Urol 100:427–432, 1968.

38. Remark RR, Berquist TH, Lieber MM, et al: Magnetic resonance imaging of renal oncocytoma. Urology (in press).

39. Robson CJ, Churchill BM, Anderson W: The results of radical nephrectomy for renal cell carcinoma. J Urol 101:297–301, 1969.

40. Rubenstein MA, Walz BJ, Bucy JG: Transitional cell carcinoma of the kidney: 25-year experience. J Urol 119:594–597, 1978.

41. Semb C: Partial resection of kidney: operative technique. Acta Chir Scand 109:360–366, 1955.

42. Semb C: Conservative renal surgery. J R Coll Surg Edinb 10:9–30, 1964.

43. Skinner DG, Colvin RB, Vermillion CD, et al: Diagnosis and management of renal cell carcinoma. A clinical and pathologic study of 309 cases. Cancer 28:1165–1177, 1971.

44. Smith RB, deKernion JB, Ehrlich RM, et al: Bilateral renal cell carcinoma and renal cell carcinoma in the solitary kidney. J Urol 132:450–454, 1984.

45. Spees EK, Light JA, Smith EJ, et al: Transplantation in patients with a history of renal cell carcinoma: long-term results and clinical considerations. Surgery 91:282–287, 1982.

46. Storm FK, Kaufman JJ, Longmire WP: Kidney resection clamp: new instrument. Urology 6:494–495, 1975.

47. Strong DW, Pearse HD, Tank ES Jr, et al: The ureteral stump after nephroureterectomy. J Urol 115:654–655, 1976.

48. Topley M, Novick AC, Montie JE: Long-term results following partial nephrectomy for localized renal adenocarcinoma. J Urol 131:1050–1052, 1984.

49. Vermillion CD, Skinner DG, Pfister RC: Bilateral renal cell carcinoma. J Urol 108:219–222, 1972.

50. Vest SA: Conservative surgery in certain benign tumors of ureter. J Urol 53:97–121, 1945.

51. Wallace DMA, Wallace DM, Whitfield HN, et al: The late results of conservative surgery for upper tract urothelial carcinomas. Br J Urol 53:537–541, 1981.

52. Ward JP: Determination of the optimum temperature for regional renal hypothermia during temporary renal ischaemia. Br J Urol 47:17–24, 1975.

53. Wein AJ, Carpiniello VL, Mulholland SG, Murphy JJ: Partial nephrectomy: review of 80 cases, emphasizing its role in management of localized renal stone disease. Urology 10:193, 1977.

54. Wickham JE: Conservative renal surgery for adenocarcinoma. The place of bench surgery. Br J Urol 47:25–36, 1975.

55. Williams DF, Schapiro AE, Arconti JS, Goodwin WE: A new technique of partial nephrectomy. J Urol 97:955–960, 1967.

56. Zincke H, Engen DE, Henning KM, McDonald MW: Treatment of renal cell carcinoma by in situ partial nephrectomy and extracorporeal operation with autotransplantation. Mayo Clin Proc 60:651–662, 1985.

57. Zincke H, Neves RJ: Feasibility of conservative surgery for transitional cell cancer of the upper urinary tract. Urol Clin North Am 11:717–724, 1984.

58. Zincke H, Swanson SK: Bilateral renal cell carcinoma: influence of synchronous and asynchronous occurrence on patient survival. J Urol 128:913–915, 1982.

DAVID F. PAULSON, M.D.

Technique of Radical Perineal Prostatectomy

CHAPTER 51

Multiple modalities currently are used in the treatment of prostatic adenocarcinoma. Treatment selection is based on the stage of the disease and both patient and physician bias. The treatment philosophy that promotes radical surgery is based on the observation that the human malignancies confined to a single anatomic site fare better if that site can be segregated from the host. The anatomic location of the prostate presents technical problems in removal of the organ without damage to adjacent organ structures. Two popular approaches to the prostate have been developed for radical prostatectomy, the radical retropubic prostatoseminal vesiculectomy and the perineal prostatoseminal vesiculectomy. The radical perineal prostatoseminal vesiculectomy has certain advantages as it provides a relatively avascular field, good exposure for reconstruction of the vesicourethral anastomosis, and dependent postoperative drainage.[1-5] It is well tolerated in the elderly patient in whom an intra-abdominal approach might compromise postoperative pulmonary function. The principal disadvantage is that it does not afford simultaneous exposure of the pelvic lymphatic drainage of the prostate. Two incisions are required if pelvic lymphadenectomy is to be accomplished. In addition, preservation of the anatomic innervation of erection may be more difficult. Contraindications are ankylosis of the hips or previous open prostatic surgery that fixes the prostate and bladder in the pelvis and makes reconstruction of the vesicourethral

junction difficult. The excessively obese patient may have so much limitation of diaphragmatic movement in the exaggerated lithotomy position that this position cannot be achieved.

POSITIONING OF PATIENT

The sacrum is brought to the edge of the table with the buttocks extending several inches over the edge of the table (Fig. 51–1). Padded shoulder braces are placed against the acromial processes to prevent stretch or pressure injury to the brachial plexus. The sacrum may be raised on sand bags or folded towels to assist in positioning. The legs are padded to prevent damage to the nerves and vessels. Correct positioning will place the perineum parallel to the floor and provide optimum exposure.

ENTRY TO THE PROSTATE

With the patient in the exaggerated lithotomy position, a Lowsley prostatic tractor is passed retrograde through the urethra into the bladder and the blade opened (Fig. 51–2). If the Lowsley tractor cannot be passed into the bladder, a sound or a Foley catheter may be used. A ureteral catheter can be used to bypass false passages or strictures and can be secured to the end of the Lowsley. The ureteral catheter will guide the Lowsley into the bladder. The skin in-

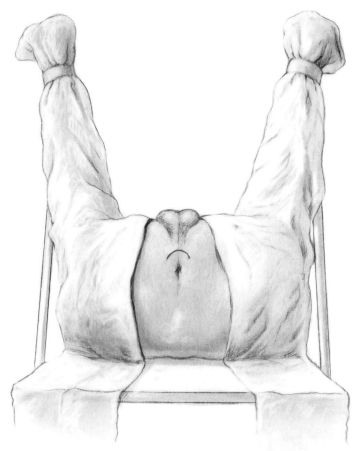

Figure 51–1. *Exaggerated lithotomy position for radical perineal prostatectomy. Line of incision is indicated.*

cision is made 1.0 cm anterior to the anal verge and curved posterolaterally on either side within the medial borders of the ischial tuberosities. The skin incision should be extended laterally to the posterior anal margin. The superficial perineal fascia is incised using the cautery and the ischiorectal fossa developed. The superficial central muscles of the perineum then are divided with the cautery (Fig. 51–3). The rectal sphincter will be visualized as an arch overlying the rectum (Figs. 51–4 and 51–5). A retractor then can be placed beneath this musculature and elevated. Blunt dissection may be necessary to reveal the glistening anterior rectal fascia. The fascia of the rectum can be used as a guide, and with blunt resection the rectum can be mobilized on either side of the rectourethralis muscle. The surgeon should recognize that the rectum is pulled forward by the retourethralis (Fig. 51–6). Division of this muscle permits posterior displacement of the rectum (Figs. 51–7 and 51–8).

THE CLASSIC PROSTATECTOMY

The rectum may be separated from the posterior surface of the prostate by blunt dissection between Denonvilliers' fascia anteriorly and the rectal fascia posteriorly. After the rectum is displaced posteriorly, it may be protected by a folded moist gauze and retraction maintained with a weighted posterior retractor. During dissection of the rectum to the level of the prostate and during division of the rectourethralis, the rectum may be identified by placing a finger in it. Blunt dissection then will permit exposure of the lateral and anterior margins of the prostate (Fig. 51–9). The fascia overlying the prostate should be white and glistening. This fascia is incised (the two leaves of Denonvilliers' fascia) to reveal a plane between it and the prostatic capsule. However, this fascia may be carried with the specimen, using

Text continued on page 728

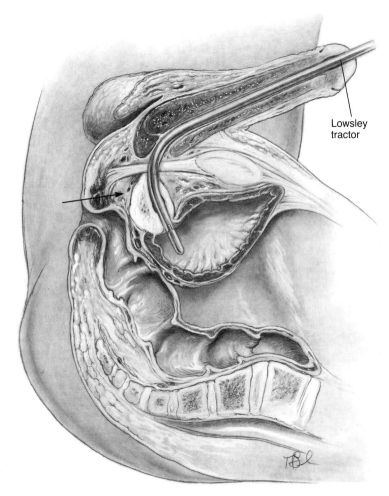

Lowsley
tractor

Figure 51–2. *Positioning of the Lowsley tractor. The approach to the prostate is indicated by the arrow.*

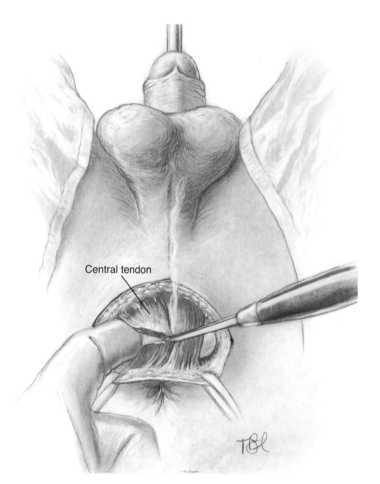

Central tendon

Figure 51–3. The central tendon is the muscular sheet that extends anterior to the rectum and is superficial to the external anal sphincter. Incision of the central tendon alone, with division of the projection of the external sphincter to the perineal body, will permit the dissection to be carried out beneath the triangle formed by the superficial external anal sphincter.

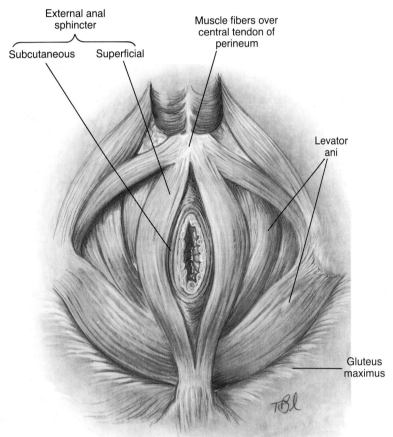

External anal
sphincter

Subcutaneous   Superficial

Muscle fibers over
central tendon of
perineum

Levator
ani

Gluteus
maximus

Figure 51–4. *The fibers of the external anal sphincter can be seen following division of the central tendon. A retractor can be placed in the triangle formed by the superficial external anal sphincter and those muscle fibers elevated to provide visualization of the rectal wall.*

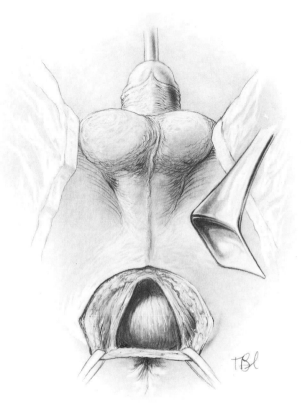

Figure 51–5. *The anterior retractor has been removed for this diagrammatic representation of the subsphincteric approach. The anterior rectal fascia can be followed to the level of the rectourethralis muscle.*

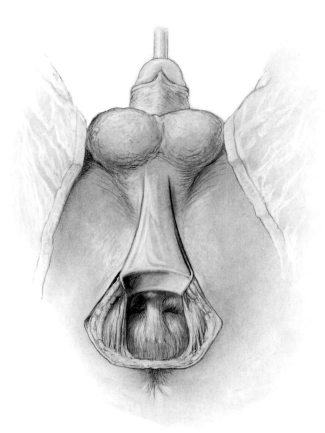

Figure 51–6. With the sphincter retracted superiorly (lateral retractor can be placed beneath the muscle to produce additional exposure) the rectourethralis can be visualized. The extent of development of this muscle is variable.

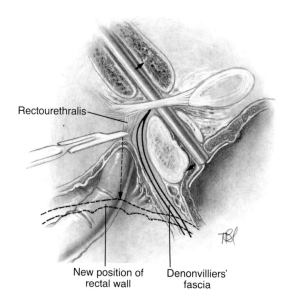

Rectourethralis

New position of rectal wall

Denonvilliers' fascia

Figure 51–7. Lateral view of the rectourethralis. The surgeon's finger has been placed in the rectum to assist in identification of the rectal wall.

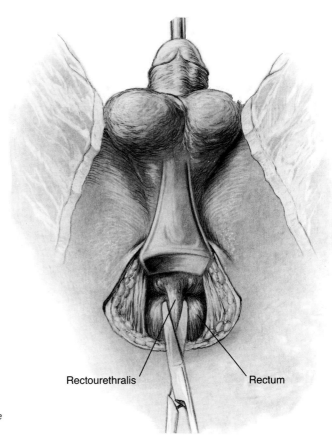

Rectourethralis   Rectum

Figure 51–8. The line of incision of the rectourethralis is identified.

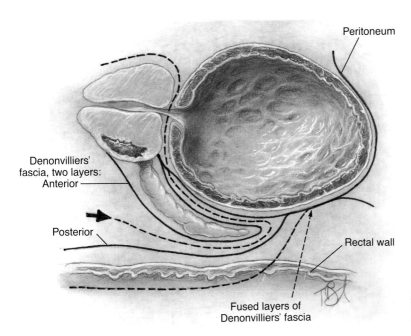

Peritoneum

Denonvilliers' fascia, two layers:
Anterior

Posterior

Rectal wall

Fused layers of
Denonvilliers' fascia

Figure 51–9. Limits of dissection for the radical prostatectomy. Solid arrow with dashed line indicates surgical route.

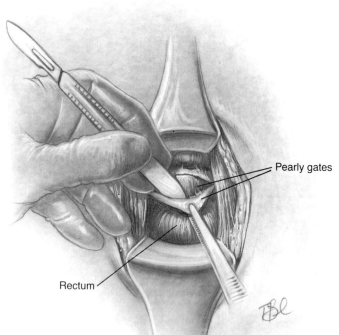

Pearly gates

Rectum

Figure 51–10. *Incision of the overlying fascia ("the pearly gates") to expose the true capsule of the prostate.*

the anterior rectal fascia to protect the rectum (Figs. 51–10 and 51–11).

A line of cleavage is developed on either side of the membranous urethra just distal to the prostatic apex. A curved clamp or finger then is placed around the membranous urethra distal to the prostatic apex, the Lowsley tractor removed, and the urethra sharply divided (Fig. 51–12). Care is taken to divide the urethra distal to the apex of the prostate. A Young prostatic tractor or Foley catheter is passed through the prostatic urethra into the bladder and the blades extended (or the balloon inflated). With pressure on the retractor to displace the prostate posteriorly and with sharp dissection, a plane can be developed beneath the venous plexus and between the bladder and the prostate anteriorly (Fig. 51–13). As the prostate is displaced from the bladder neck anteriorly, a "horse collar" of bladder neck fibers is identified at the bladder neck between 10 and two o'clock (Fig. 51–14). The bladder is entered beneath this horse collar of fibers at 12 o'clock and the incision carried from 12 to two o'clock and from 12 to 10 o'clock, preserving continuity of these bladder neck fibers. At this point, the Young tractor can be withdrawn and a Foley cath-

eter of any appropriate size passed through the prostatic urethra and brought out superiorly through the line of incision between the prostate and bladder neck. Traction on this catheter will permit the prostate to be displaced posteriorly (Fig. 51–15). Downward traction on this catheter will define the line of cleavage between the bladder neck and prostate. This margin should be sharply divided until the prostate is attached only between five and seven o'clock at the posterior bladder neck. When visualization is difficult, digital examination will allow the posterior bladder neck to be identified as a ridge by palpation. The trigonal fibers should be divided just distal to the bladder neck as they course down into the prostatic urethra. A transverse incision is made at the level of the bladder neck and is carried across the posterior aspect of the specimen to separate the bladder neck fibers from the prostate. The posterior bladder neck can be grasped with an Allis clamp and elevated. Dissection now proceeds between the bladder anteriorly and the seminal vesicles posteriorly. The prostate now is attached only by a few bladder fibers at five and seven o'clock. These fibers can be sharply divided and the prostate cut away from the bladder

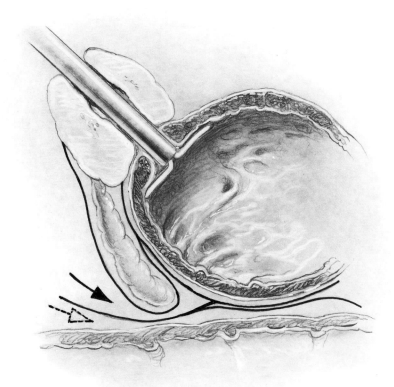

Figure 51–11. The solid arrow identifies the preferred plan of dissection above the anterior rectal fascia (the posterior fascia of Denonvilliers) and the fascia of the rectovesical septum (the anterior layer of Denonvilliers' fascia). The broken arrow indicates a line of dissection beneath the rectal fascia, which carries hazard of rectal perforation.

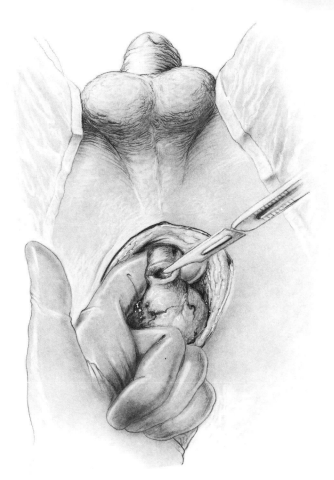

Figure 51–12. The apex of the prostate is identified and the membranous urethra is sharply divided.

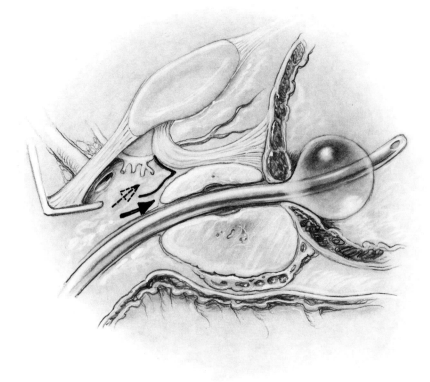

Figure 51–13. The solid arrow indicates the proper plane of dissection beneath the anterolateral fascia and beneath the venous plexus. Dissection above this fascia (dotted arrow) carries the hazard of disruption of the venous sinus and troublesome bleeding.

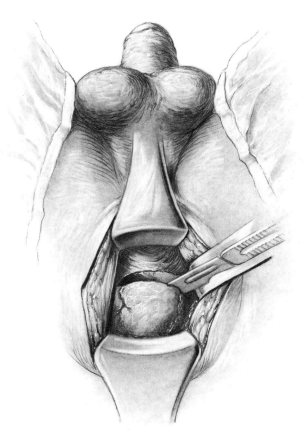

Figure 51–14. The prostate has been dissected off the bladder neck anteriorly, the bladder neck identified, and the prostate cut away from the bladder at this level.

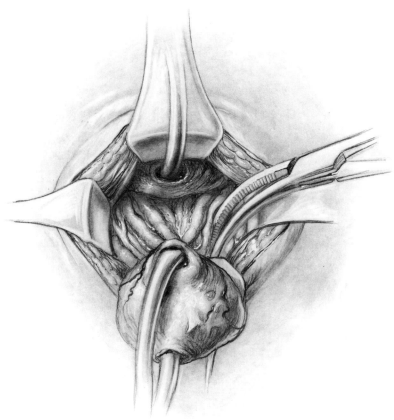

Figure 51–15. The posterior bladder neck has been cut away and the bladder allowed to retract separately. A plane is then developed between the bladder anteriorly and the prostate and seminal vesicles posteriorly.

neck without fear of encountering excessive bleeding. The prostate and the seminal vesicles will remain secured posterolaterally by the vascular pedicles, but free from the bladder (Fig. 51–15). These pedicles can be isolated at their point of egress from the specimen at five and seven o'clock behind a right-angle clamp and controlled either with metallic surgical clips or with absorbable sutures. Following division of the vascular pedicles bilaterally, the specimen is retained only by the seminal vesicles and the vas deferens. The vasa deferentia are exposed for a distance of approximately 3 cm, cross-clamped, divided, and ligated with absorbable sutures. The vas deferens can be occluded with metallic surgical clips, but care must be taken not to cut through the duct during application of these clips. The seminal vesicles are removed with the specimen by using sharp and blunt dissection. The fibrofilamentous tissue overlying the seminal vesicles, which may contain small feeding vessels, can be divided with the cutting cautery. The glistening surface of the sem-

inal vesicles will assist in identification of the proper plane of dissection and, as these investing fibers are severed, the seminal vesicles will be exposed (Fig. 51–16).

After hemostasis is secure, the vesicle neck should be reconstructed and continuity established between the reconstructed bladder neck and the membranous urethra. This is done by a direct anastomosis between bladder neck and urethra, supported by a modification of the Vest traction sutures. This provides alignment between the reconstructed bladder neck and the membranous urethra and places minimum tension on the direct anastomosis. The bladder neck is closed from six to 12 o'clock with a running 0 chromic suture (Fig. 51–17). This permits the vesicourethral anastomosis to be done superiorly at maximum distance from the ureteral orifices. The closure can be conducted by moving from 12 to six o'clock and making the vesicourethral anastomosis inferiorly. This, however, rolls the posterior bladder neck and trigone into a tube and may occlude the ureteral orifices by incor-

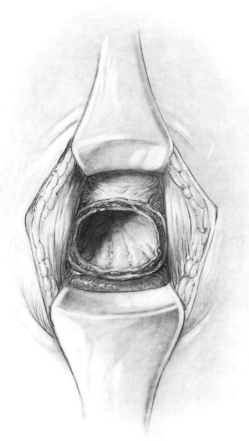

Figure 51–16. View of the bladder after removal of the specimen. The bladder neck fibers are preserved anteriorly but may be sacrificed posteriorly and laterally as necessary for removal of the tumor.

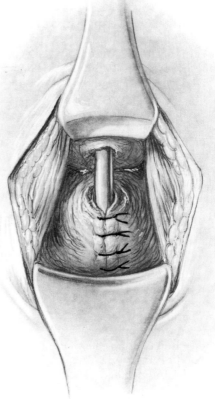

Figure 51–17. Closure of the bladder neck from six o'clock.

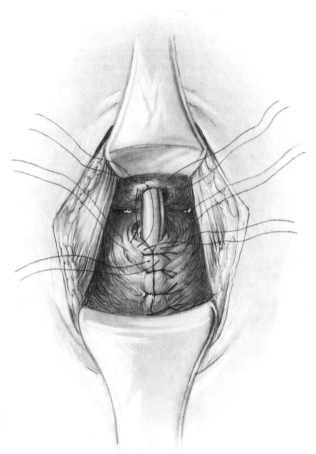

Figure 51–18. Vest sutures of size 0 chromic catgut, placed at two, five, eight, and 10 o'clock for the direct anastomosis.

porating the ureteral orifices in the bladder closure.

The closure of the bladder neck should be carried out, moving from 6 to 12 o'clock until the reconstructed bladder neck admits snugly a No. 18 French Foley catheter (Fig. 51–18). The Foley catheter then is removed from the bladder and mattress sutures of 0 chromic catgut are placed about the reconstructed bladder neck at two, five, seven, and 10 o'clock, outside-in, inside-out approximately 5 mm from the margin of the newly constructed bladder neck, tied loosely, and left long for subsequent placement beneath the perineal skin. Four sutures of 2-0 chromic catgut now are placed in the membranous urethra at two, four, eight, and 10 o'clock. A No. 18 French Foley catheter is passed through the urethra and into the bladder, and the balloon is inflated. The previously placed 2-0 chromic catgut sutures at one, four, eight, and 10 o'clock then are placed in the reconstructed bladder neck in these positions. As these sutures are secured, the reconstructed bladder neck is approximated to the membranous urethra. The 0 chromic catgut traction sutures, previously placed about the bladder neck, are drawn

through on each side of the perineal body and tied subcutaneously to support the direct anastomosis between the bladder neck and urethra. This anastomosis should be made without tension. The wound is drained with a Penrose drain, which may be brought out either through a stab wound or through the lateral aspect of the incision. During closure, the levator ani musculature should be approximated in the midline with absorbable suture material. Reconstruction of this area supports the new bladder neck and reduces the likelihood of vesical and rectal incontinence.

References

1. Belt E: Radical perineal prostatectomy in early carcinoma of the prostate. J Urol 48:287–297, 1942.
2. Dees JE: Radical perineal prostatectomy for carcinoma. J Urol 104:160–162, 1970.
3. Jewett JH: The case for radical perineal prostatectomy. J Urol 103:195–199, 1970.
4. Ray GR, Cassady JR, Bagshaw MA: External-beam megavoltage radiation therapy in treatment of post-radical prostatectomy residual or recurrent tumor: Preliminary results. J Urol 114:98–101, 1975.
5. Weyrauch HM (ed): Surgery of the Prostate. Philadelphia, WB Saunders, 1959.

GARY LIESKOVSKY, M.D.

Technique of Radical Retropubic Prostatectomy (Campbell's Procedure) with Limited Pelvic Lymph Node Dissection

Radical retropubic prostatectomy in association with a limited bilateral pelvic iliac lymph node dissection has once again achieved popularity among urologists as the preferred treatment for patients with cancers clinically confined to the prostate (Stages A_2, B_1, and B_2), and occasionally for selected patients with clinical evidence of extracapsular extension (Stage C) but without clinically evident pelvic nodal metastases. We continue to feel as our Nobel laureate Charles Huggins stated so well 16 years ago, "Radical prostatectomy is for the surgeon who cares, for cancer is safest when completely removed and preserved in pickle."[10]

Since 1974 we have utilized the antegrade approach for radical retropubic prostatectomy as first described by Campbell in 1959[4] and subsequently modified by Mittemeyer and Cox.[16] This technique offers two major advantages over procedures in which the dissection is initiated at the apex. First, early development and division of the vasculolymphatic pedicles minimizes blood loss and prevents vigorous prostatic manipulation, which may result in iatrogenic dissemination of tumor cells. Second, it permits accurate placement of sutures in the membranous urethra at the time it is transected, providing for a precise, tension-free vesicourethral anastomosis and significantly di-

minishing the risk of urinary incontinence or anastomotic strictures.

We recognize, however, that patients undergoing radical prostatectomy using this approach will have postoperative erectile dysfunction. We offer implantation of a penile prosthesis to those individuals expressing interest in resuming normal sexual activity following recovery from their operation. Since most of our patients opt to have an inflatable penile prosthesis, we have developed our own two-stage implantation technique for facilitating the insertion of this device (see Chapter 47). The technique involves the first-stage implantation of the reservoir and pump of the device at the time of the radical prostatectomy, with later elective second-stage insertion and connection of the cylinders. The first stage can be accomplished without significant increase in operative time or additional morbidity. This approach allows one to immediately address the psychologic sequelae of impotency and provides certain technical advantages over implantation of an inflatable device as a single-stage procedure at a later date. Staging the prosthesis in this manner not only obviates the need to reenter an adherent pelvis for positioning of the reservoir but allows the scrotal pump adequate time to heal, enabling easy and knowledgeable operation once the second stage is completed. This technique has been highly successful and well accepted.

Recently Walsh and associates, and others,[6, 11, 19–21] have developed and utilized a surgical technique of radical retropubic prostatectomy that attempts to preserve the pelvic plexus of nerves innervating the corpora cavernosa, thereby allowing for maintenance of postoperative sexual function. We feel this is the preferred approach for selected patients with early stage disease and utilize the technique described by Walsh in Chapter 53 for patients with clinical Stage B_1 disease desiring maintenance of potency. However, we believe that Campbell's technique, as described herein, is a better operation for those with Stage B_2 disease because of the issue of the implication of extracapsular tumor extension. Catalona and Dresner[5] and Eggleston and Walsh[6] have enhanced our knowledge of the incidence of extracapsular extension of cancer of the prostate according to clinical stage, ranging from 18% in patients with Stage A and B_1 disease to 57% among patients with clinical Stage B_2 disease. Both groups feel that one can perform the nerve-sparing operation without significantly increasing that incidence, compared with the results of standard radical prostatectomy performed by the perineal or Campbell's retropubic approach. Nonetheless, concern has been expressed as to whether this retrograde approach may compromise the surgical margin, converting a surgically confined lesion into one that demonstrates extension to the surgical margin. Walsh and associates[20] refute these concerns and believe that in those patients with close or positive resection margins, the compromise was felt to be related to local tumor extension outside the prostate rather than to reduction in the amount of periprostatic tissue removed or the adequacy of resection. Certainly there is vast appeal to the potency-sparing operation and the implication is that perhaps more patients with clinical Stage B_2 and possibly even early Stage C disease may be considered for the operation or some modification of it if results of the pelvic lymph node dissection are negative.

In a recent analysis of 64 men undergoing the nerve-sparing radical retropubic prostatectomy, Walsh and Mostwin[21] report that only 50% of patients with clinical Stage B_2 disease were potent one year after surgery, compared with greater than 90% for those with earlier clinical stage lesions. Microscopic penetration of the prostatic capsule or involvement of the seminal vesicles, however, reduced the potency rate at one year to 69% and 25%, respectively. Historically, with long-term follow-up and large numbers of patients, Belt and Schroeder[2] reported that pelvic recurrence occurred in only 6% of patients undergoing radical perineal prostatectomy if the cancer was confined to the prostate (12 out of 185). However, when capsular penetration occurred or the seminal vesicles were involved (pathologic Stage C), pelvic recurrence was noted in 22% (59 out of 267). Byar and Mostofi and the Veteran's Administration Cooperative Urological Research Group in their report noted a profound effect on prognosis in patients with capsular penetration or with seminal vesicle involvement, all of whom had had radical prostatectomy.[3] Of 33 patients with penetration of the capsule, only 33% survived seven years, compared with a 70% survival rate in those when tumor only extended to or invaded the prostatic capsule. A similar significant reduction in the seven-year survival rate was also observed in patients with invasion of the seminal vesicle, compared with the rate for those in whom this feature was absent (33% and 66%, respectively). Unfortunately, this report was prior to the era of staging pelvic lymphadenectomy, and therefore some of the adverse prognostic effect of local extension could be attributed to unsuspected nodal disease.

Since 1972, it has been our policy to deliver 4500 to 5000 rads of external beam radiation through a limited portal to encompass the prostatic bed for patients with capsular penetration, positive surgical margin, or seminal vesicle involvement as a means of preventing pelvic recurrence. Using this approach we have observed only one of 45 such patients to show recurrence of disease in the pelvis and feel this approach provides excellent local control.

Recently, Gibbons and associates reported similar results for their patients followed beyond five years.[9] Among 45 patients with capsular penetration or positive surgical margins, 22 received 5000 rads and 23 were followed conservatively. The local control rate was 95% among patients receiving adjuvant radiation and 70% among those not treated. So far, there has been insufficient follow-up from authors performing the nerve-sparing operation to know the incidence of pelvic recurrence and its relationship to the development of metastatic disease. The Stanford group also has achieved long-term (10-year) disease-free survival in 57% of patients with positive margins following radical prostatectomy who were treated with full-dose external-beam radiation therapy within four months of resection.[1] We and others, however, have observed increased complications from that dose of radiation without any proven benefit and believe that 4500 to 5000 rads is sufficient to sterilize microscopic residual disease without increasing morbidity.

Our limited experience with the nerve-sparing operation has revealed that those patients who were potent following the operation, and subsequently received 4500 to 5000 rads because of pathologic Stage C disease, became impotent following the radiation. Walsh does not recommend postoperative radiation for patients with extraprostatic extension and to date has not observed a significant incidence of pelvic recurrence, but follow-up is short.

However, we must emphasize caution regarding the significance of extracapsular extension, seminal vesicle involvement, or a positive surgical margin until we have at least 10 to 15 years of follow-up. We believe adjuvant radiation therapy will reduce the anticipated local recurrence rate in patients with these unfavorable pathologic findings, unfortunately at the expense of rendering most of them impotent following a successful nerve-sparing operation. Until more accurate noninvasive techniques become available to assess local extension, we have limited our indications for the nerve-sparing, potency-preserving radical retropubic prostatectomy to those patients with clinical stage B_1N (Jewett nodule) or B_1 (tumor involving only one lobe) disease and away from the apex, for whom there is a high probability of cure with surgery only and retention of erectile function. All other patients undergo the Campbell radical retropubic approach with limited pelvic node dissection, a description of which follows.

PREOPERATIVE PREPARATION

All patients undergoing radical retropubic prostatectomy and limited pelvic lymphadenectomy receive preoperative hydration with intravenous Ringer's lactate or 5% dextrose with 0.5 normal saline at a rate of 125 ml/hr beginning the afternoon prior to surgery. Patients with significant bacteriuria, and all those undergoing implantation of the pump and reservoir portion of an inflatable penile prosthesis, receive parenteral antibiotics including an aminoglycoside starting 12 hours before surgery and continued for a minimum of five days, after which oral antibiotics are administered. In patients undergoing salvage retropubic prostatectomy for radiation failure, a neomycin retention enema (200 ml of a 1% solution) is administered the night before surgery and the morning of the operation in case of an inadvertent rectotomy. A combination of general and continuous epidural anesthesia is routinely employed; the latter appreciably diminishes blood loss during the prostatectomy and also assists in alleviating postoperative discomfort. This further promotes better coughing and deep breathing and lessens early postoperative pulmonary complications.

OPERATIVE TECHNIQUE
Pelvic Lymphadenectomy

The patient is placed in the extended supine position with 10 to 20° Trendelenburg. Following preparation of the external genitalia and abdomen, the operative site is draped and the bladder is drained by an indwelling Foley catheter that is connected to gravity drainage.

Through a lower midline extraperitoneal incision extending from the pubis to just above the umbilicus, the anterior rectus fascia is incised, the rectus muscles are retracted laterally, and their pubic insertions are partially divided. The retropubic space is entered and the peritoneum bluntly dissected off the posterior rectus fascia medially and the transversus abdominis muscle and transverse fascia laterally. Additional exposure is provided by dividing the posterior rectus fascia above the arcuate line.

The peritoneum is then mobilized from the area of the femoral canal and freed from the spermatic cord, which is retracted laterally after the vas deferens has been clipped and divided. Before the pelvic lymphadenectomy is begun, the peritoneum should be mobilized above the point at which the ureter crosses the common iliac artery.

A self-retaining Finochietto or Balfour retractor is then positioned and an Israel retractor is placed under the distal rectus muscle to provide exposure to the femoral canal. Care should be taken not to injure the inferior epigastric vessels in this region by too vigorous retraction of the muscle. For cancer of the prostate, dissection is initiated just distal to the place where the ureter crosses the common iliac artery (Fig. 52–1). At this point the lymphatics on the medial aspect of the common and external iliac artery are clipped and divided without compromising the lymphatic channels draining the most lateral lymph nodes (Fig. 52–2). The nodal tissue overlying the hypogastric artery is cleanly dissected and swept distally. At this point the proximal lymphatics surrounding the external iliac vein are circumferentially clipped and divided, allowing the vein to be stripped of its loose fibroareolar lymphatic tissue. A finger positioned between the external iliac artery and vein exposes a thin fascia overlying the psoas muscle. This is incised just medial to the genitofemoral nerve. Occasionally a small vein can be identified draining from the psoas muscle into the external iliac vein and should be clipped and divided. After completion of the proximal dissection, attention is then directed distally to the area of the femoral canal. The lymph node of Cloquet or Rosenmüller represents the distal limits of the dissection in this area (Fig. 52–3). Lymphatics draining into this node and surrounding the external iliac vein are carefully clipped

and divided to prevent the accumulation of lymph and the loss of protein. Once again, care should be exercised during the dissection of this area not to interfere with the drainage of the lymphatic vessels coursing along the lateral aspect of the external iliac artery. These are preserved to lessen the potential morbidity that may follow complete skeletonization of these vessels, especially in patients who may receive postoperative adjuvant radiotherapy.[12] After sweeping the tissue proximally, the surgeon commonly encounters an accessory obturator vein inserting into the posterior wall of the external iliac vein, just proximal and medial to the circumflex iliac vein itself. The accessory obturator vein should be ligated to prevent bothersome bleeding should the vein be avulsed.

Following completion of the proximal and distal lymphatic dissection, the loosely adherent fibroareolar lymphatic tissue anterior to the external iliac vein is incised, thereby joining the distal and proximal dissection, which divides the specimen in such a way that half is swept medial to the vein and the other half lateral into the obturator hypogastric fossa. This is accomplished by retracting the external iliac artery laterally and then passing a gauze sponge between the artery and vein in order to sweep the lateral specimen into the obturator fossa (Fig. 52–4A and B). At this point retraction of the external iliac vein laterally allows for retrieval of the gauze sponge with one's left hand and permits dividing any remaining attachments

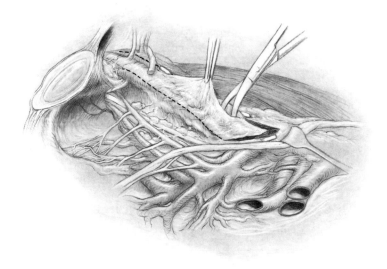

Figure 52–1. Proximal incision of the fibroareolar tissue loosely adherent to the adventitia of the pelvic vessels begins just distal to where the ureter crosses the common iliac artery. Medial and lateral dotted lines indicate line of division anterior to the iliac vein and artery, respectively.

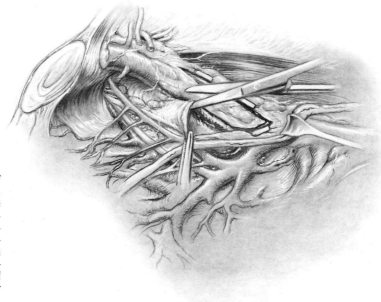

Figure 52–2. Completion of proximal limits of dissection. Note the parallel row of clips applied to the divided lymphatic tissue anterior to the external iliac artery to prevent protein loss. Also note preservation of the continuity of the lymphatic channels along the lateral aspect of the external iliac artery to diminish lymphedema.

of the specimen from the posterior wall of the external iliac vein. This maneuver assists in exposing the obturator nerve, which can then be dissected free from the specimen (Fig. 52–4C). Any residual attachments to the proximal hypogastric artery and vein are then clipped and divided, with the posterior extent of the dissection represented by the ventral aspect of the hypogastric vein and artery deep within the pelvis. In most situations the obturator vessels coursing through the obturator canal are removed with the specimen and their proximal origins secured by hemoclips.

Finally, a well-defined, thin fascial plane separating the bladder and prostate from the loose, fatty areolar pelvic nodal tissue facilitates removal of the entire specimen from the obturator hypogastric fossa, which can then be removed en bloc and submitted to the pathology laboratory. A similar dissection is then performed on the contralateral side prior to proceeding with radical retropubic prostatectomy.

Radical Retropubic Prostatectomy

A key to the safe performance of the antegrade approach for radical retropubic pros-

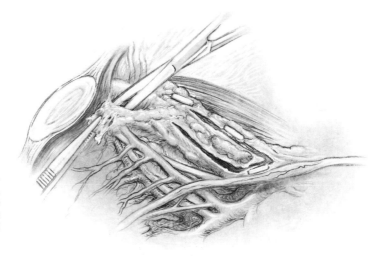

Figure 52–3. Distal limit of dissection is the lymph node of Cloquet, lying just medial to the external iliac vein and directly anterior to Cooper's ligament in the area of the femoral canal.

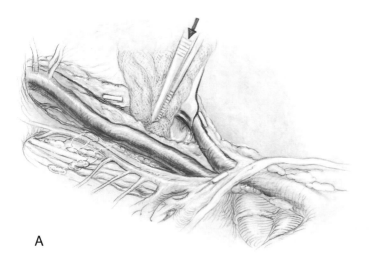

A

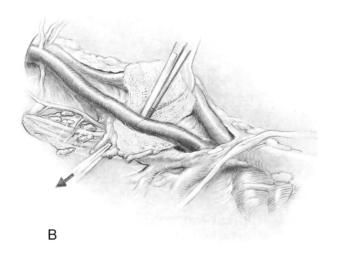

B

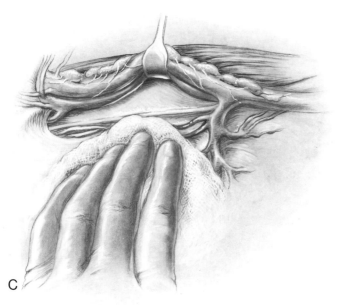

C

Figure 52–4. A, The proximal and distal limits of dissection have been joined, allowing a portion of the fibroareolar tissue to pass medial toward the bladder and the remainder to pass between the external iliac vein and artery. A gauze sponge is used to push the lateral tissue between the artery and vein, sweeping the fibroareolar tissue off the psoas muscle into the obturator fossa.

B, This maneuver is facilitated by lateral retraction of the external iliac artery. Once the gauze has been tucked into the obturator hypogastric fossa with the aid of tissue forceps, it is retrieved beneath the iliac vessels, thus dissecting all fibroareolar tissue from the lateral pelvic wall.

C, Lateral retraction of the pelvic vessels, together with medial traction on the gauze sponge, allows exposure of the obturator nerve.

tatectomy is a thorough understanding of the vascular supply to the prostate and seminal vesicles. The main arterial blood supply to the prostate and seminal vesicles and base of the bladder is derived from the inferior vesicle artery, a branch of the hypogastric artery. The artery is reported to divide into two major components:[7] One group, the internal or urethral branches, is located just beneath the posterior bladder wall lateral to the vesicoprostatic junction at approximately the five- and seven-o'clock positions and supplies the vesical neck and the periurethral portion of the prostate. We have defined this vascular supply to the prostate as the lateral pedicle, since its origin and location is lateral to the tips of the seminal vesicle, which it also supplies. The external or capsular branches course along the posterior lateral surface of the prostate, giving off branches both ventrally and dorsally to supply the outer surface of the gland, including the apex and the urethroprostatic junction. An additional supply of blood is provided by the middle rectal and branches of the internal pudendal vessels, located in these posterior pedicles that run perpendicular from the anterior rectal wall to the posterior inferior aspect of the prostate. Lymphatic channels draining the prostate closely parallel this vascular network within these pedicles.

A small gauze sponge may be used to sweep the loosely adherent fibrofatty tissue from the anterior and lateral aspects of the prostate and bladder neck into the obturator fossa, which provides excellent exposure to the vesicoprostatic junction and endopelvic fascia on either side. Two hemostatic sutures, preferably 2-0 chromic, are placed in the midline at the bladder neck and just distal in the prostatic capsule to control bleeding from the superficial branch of the deep dorsal vein complex. A transverse incision using diathermy is made just cephalad to the vesicoprostatic junction between the previously placed bladder neck sutures and is extended laterally for a distance of 2 to 3 cm (Fig. 52–5). Laterally, veins derived from the deep dorsal vein and pudendal and vesical plexus form a periprostatic network that courses through a superficial fibroareolar layer as it drains into the internal hypogastric vein (Fig. 52–6). By developing a plane between this layer of tissue and the prostatic capsule, the surgeon is able to clip and divide these veins and thereby prevent troublesome bleeding should the vessels be inadvertently torn (Fig. 52–7). The circumferential bladder neck incision is then continued with the cautery after the capsular veins have been controlled. A curved tonsil clamp placed on the tip of the exposed Foley catheter facilitates caudal retraction of the

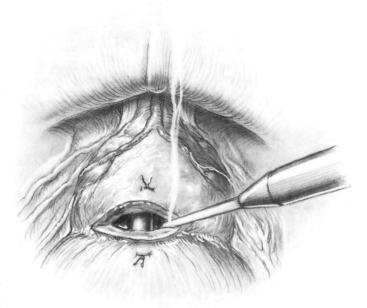

Figure 52–5. The transverse bladder incision is made between midline hemostatic sutures just proximal to the vesicoprostatic junction.

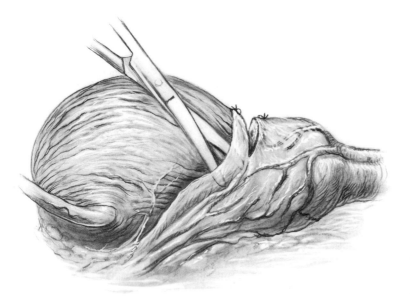

Figure 52–6. Development of the plane between the prostatic capsule and the periprostatic network of veins.

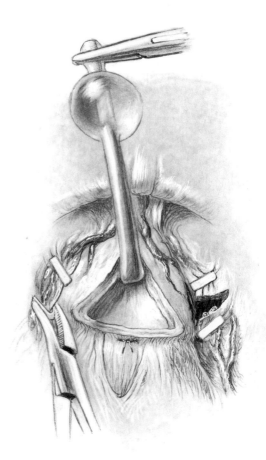

Figure 52–7. Application of clips to the venous plexus provides excellent hemostasis after these are divided.

bladder neck and prostate and provides excellent exposure of the ureteral orifices and trigone. An Allis clamp placed on each corner of the divided bladder neck incision, together with retraction of the proximal anterior bladder neck ,by using one's middle finger or a narrow Deaver retractor, facilitates stretching of the posterior bladder neck and trigone into a horizontal plane.

A transverse incision of 2 to 3 cm in the posterior bladder wall, distal to the carefully protected ureteral orifices, is made perpendicular to this horizontal plane and is carried through the full thickness of the posterior detrusor, thereby exposing the ampullae of the vasa and anterior surface of the seminal vesicles (Fig. 52–8). The remaining detrusor muscle attachments are divided laterally, thereby completely dismembering the bladder neck from the prostate. The bladder is then swept cephalad to further expose the ampullae of the vas deferens and seminal vesicles. Immediately adjacent to the lateral border of each seminal vesicle is a layer of tissue that includes a leash of vessels extending from the tip of the seminal vesicle to their origin from the hypogastric artery; this we have previously defined as the lateral pedicle. Autonomic parasympathetic nerves innervating the corpora cavernosa are also presumed to course within this pedicle, and their preservation is essential when the Walsh radical prostatectomy is performed.

Development of the lateral pedicle is assisted by first placing a curved right-angled clamp under each ampulla of the vas and dividing them between large hemostatic clips. Attention is then directed at exposing the tips of each seminal vesicle, facilitated by superior traction of the divided proximal ends of the vas and posterior lip of bladder neck achieved with an Allis clamp, together with counter-traction applied inferiorly to the distal ends of the divided vasa. By using the left hand with the palm directed cephalad, the right pedicle can be developed by positioning the index finger lateral and the second finger medial to the tip of the seminal vesicle, while the palm of the hand keeps the bladder in place superiorly. Dual large straight hemoclips are then placed on this pedicle approximately 1 cm apart and then divided. An identical procedure is then performed on the contralateral side, thereby completing division of the lateral pedicles bilaterally.

The next important step is the development of the posterior vasculolymphatic pedicles. Because the development of these pedicles is based on a thorough understanding

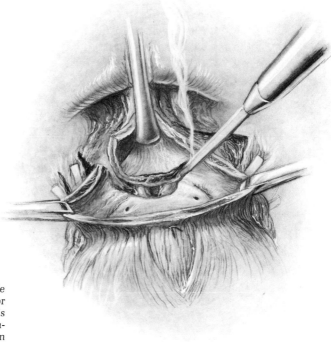

Figure 52–8. A transverse incision is made through the full thickness of the posterior detrusor just distal to the trigone. This is facilitated by caudal retraction on the catheter tip and simultaneous lateral retraction of the bladder neck by Allis clamps.

of the formation and relationship of Denonvilliers' fascia to the pelvic organs, a brief review is necessary.

According to Shackelford's description,[18] Denonvilliers' fascia is formed by the fusion of the anterior and posterior peritoneal reflections in the region of the cul-de-sac, which then extends distally to the urogenital diaphragm (Fig. 52–9). Others feel that there are two distinct layers: a loose areolar posterior layer closely associated with the anterior rectal wall, and the thicker, more membranous layer associated with the posterior surface of the bladder, prostate, and seminal vesicles. In either case, identifying Denonvilliers' space lying behind the membranous or fused layer is important anatomically because it facilitates sweeping the posterior surface of the prostate and seminal vesicles off the anterior rectal wall caudally to the level of the membranous urethra.

Development of Denonvilliers' space at the time of surgery is accomplished by placing an Allis clamp on the previously divided distal ends of the ampulla and retracting them inferiorly. Incising the membranous layer of Denonvilliers' fascia lying immediately behind the divided ampulla allows for entrance into Denonvilliers' space, which is generally heralded by a fibroareolar fatty tissue (Fig. 52–10). Then the space is developed further by bluntly and gently sweeping the rectum off Denonvilliers' fascia by using the tips of the fingers directed in a posterior motion. The posterior pedicles so formed, one on either side, are defined easily as they course from the posterior lateral aspect of the surface of the prostate and seminal vesicles to the anterior lateral rectal wall. Placing an Allis clamp on the tip of the seminal vesicle allows one to then divide the right posterior pedicle by positioning the index finger of the left hand medial and the second finger lateral to this pedicle while at the same time protecting the rectum posteriorly from inadvertent injury. Then the pedicle is clipped and divided down to the urogenital diaphragm by large right-angle hemoclips (Fig. 52–11). A similar maneuver is then performed on the contralateral side, thereby completing the division of the lateral and posterior pedicles to the prostate.

Terminal attachments of the endopelvic fascia to the apex of the prostate are then divided, thereby completely freeing the specimen except for the membranous urethra and posterior rectourethralis muscle, the periurethral pillars, and the anterior puboprostatic ligaments. These ligaments are in turn separated by placing a finger between them and depressing the deep dorsal vein complex posteriorly. This stretches the ligaments, allowing them to be divided close to their attachment to the undersurface of the pubis. Occasionally, veins closely associated with these ligaments can cause troublesome bleeding, which may be prevented by clipping the ligaments prior to division. Finally, with the surgeon's finger on either side of the prostatic apex, the deep dorsal vein complex can be circumscribed by a right-angle clamp and ligated. It can then be

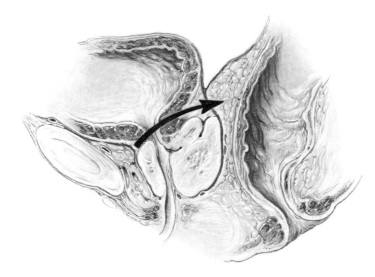

Figure 52–9. Illustration of the formation of Denonvilliers' fascia. It is believed to be derived from fusion of the anterior and posterior peritoneal reflections, and that Denonvilliers' space lies behind the fascia. Arrow indicates how access to Denonvilliers' space is achieved using the antegrade (Campbell's) approach. (Adapted with permission from Shackelford, R. T.: Surgery of the Alimentary Tract. Philadelphia, W. B. Saunders, 1982.)

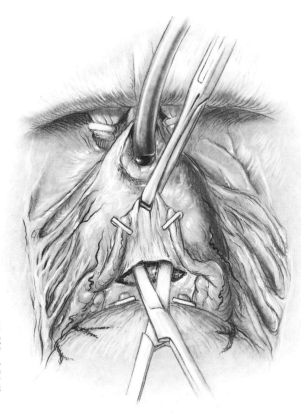

Figure 52–10. After the seminal vesicles and ampullae of the vasa are exposed by retracting the bladder cephalad, entry into Denonvilliers' space is accomplished by incising the membranous Denonvilliers' fascia behind the divided ampullae which are shown retracted with an Allis clamp.

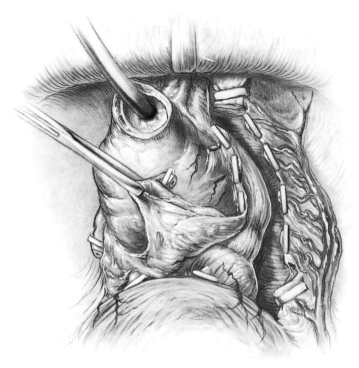

Figure 52–11. Contralateral traction by an Allis clamp placed on the tip of the right seminal vesicle and edge of Denonvilliers' fascia assists in defining the right posterolateral pedicle, which has been clipped and divided exposing the anterior rectal wall.

sharply transected and the distal end further secured with a No. 883 2-0 catgut suture for additional hemostasis. This then exposes the membranous urethra together with the peri-urethral pillars, lateral to the urethra itself. These in turn are sharply divided, exposing the entire membranous urethra, which is stretched 2 cm above the urogenital diaphragm.

With the urethra stretched, a sharp transverse incision is made along the anterior aspect of the membranous urethra immediately distal to the apex of the prostate, exposing the previously placed Foley catheter (Fig. 52–12). The continuity of the posterior membranous urethra is preserved until anterior sutures of 2-0 chromic are positioned accurately in the urethra and their direction of placement tagged appropriately with either curved or straight hemostats (Fig. 52–13). Additional sutures of 2-0 chromic catgut are placed as the remaining posterior urethral attachment is severed. After deflat-

ing the catheter balloon and removing the Foley, the entire en bloc specimen is removed. A total of approximately six to eight sutures are placed circumferentially to help create a water-tight vesicourethral anastomosis.

After thorough inspection of the area for hemostasis, attention is redirected to the trigone and bladder neck. Prior to closure of the bladder neck, a portion is excised and sent to the pathology laboratory for frozen section. Temporary No. 5 infant feeding tubes are then passed up each ureter to facilitate identification of the orifices during closure of the bladder neck (Fig. 52–14). With interrupted 2-0 figure-of-eight chromic catgut sutures, the posterior bladder wall is approximated in a vertical fashion until the vesical neck accommodates one finger easily (Fig. 52–15).

After closure of the bladder neck, the ureteral stents are removed and a new No. 22 French 5 ml Foley catheter is repositioned

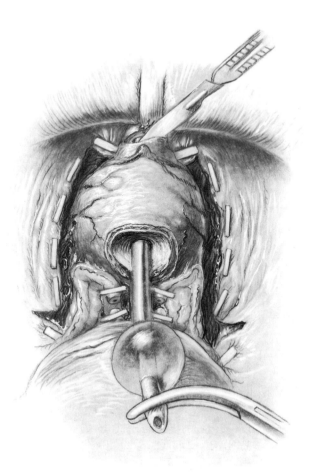

Figure 52–12. *After the major vasculolymphatic pedicles and the periurethral lateral pillars have been divided, and the deep dorsal vein complex secured and divided, the exposed anterior urethra is sharply transected exposing the Foley catheter.*

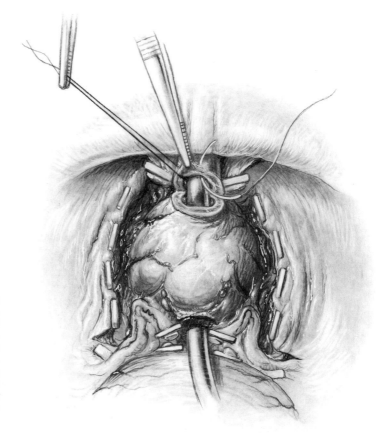

Figure 52–13. Sutures of 2-0 chromic are circumferentially positioned in the anterior urethra and subsequently in the posterior urethra prior to dismembering the prostate from the urethra. Preplacement of these sutures prevents retraction of the urethra into the urogenital diaphragm frequently encountered when this step is eliminated.

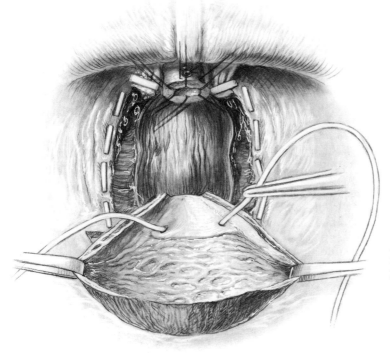

Figure 52–14. The en bloc specimen has been removed and circumferential sutures preplaced in the urethra. No. 5 infant feeding tubes are routinely placed into each ureter: (1) to make sure a ureteral injury has not occurred, and (2) to prevent damage to either orifice during reconstruction of the vesical neck.

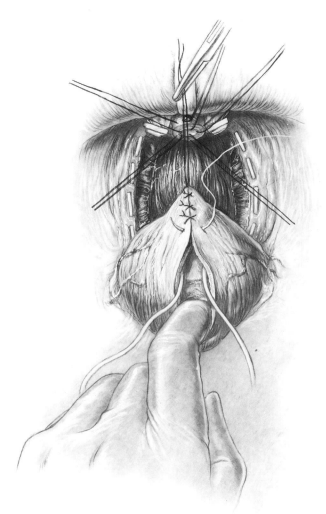

Figure 52–15. The vesical neck is reconstructed using figure-of-eight, 2-0 chromic catgut suture in a posterior to anterior direction. This should easily accommodate one finger. Note the temporary indwelling infant feeding tubes used to protect the ureteral orifices during closure of the bladder neck.

through the urethra into the bladder. At this point the balloon of the catheter is not inflated, in order to decrease the potential for inadvertent puncture of the balloon during placement of the urethral sutures into the bladder neck. In order that the knots of the sutures are extraluminal, the ends of the sutures that have been placed inside out in the urethra are rethreaded on an empty curved No. 5 Mayo needle. Then each of the previously placed circumferential urethral sutures are placed accurately in the bladder neck, beginning with the posterior sutures and followed by the lateral and anterior ones.

When all the urethral sutures have been positioned in the new bladder neck, the Foley catheter balloon is inflated 5 to 7 ml and the vesical neck approximated to the severed membranous urethra by a combination of gentle traction on the Foley catheter

and pressure directed inferiorly on the anterior bladder wall by using a long Allis clamp (Fig. 52–16). Beginning with the posterior sutures, each is tied without tension and the integrity of the vesicourethral anastomosis tested by irrigating the Foley catheter. If there is significant extravasation, and only if it is technically feasible, additional sutures are carefully placed.

After the radical prostatectomy is completed and the vesicourethral continuity is established, drainage of the retropubic space is accomplished through a separate stab incision using a one-inch Penrose drain placed near the anastomosis. If there is excessive venous bleeding from the operative site, it is our preference to use a large Hemovac tube connected to suction for 24 to 48 hours.

The catheter is connected to a gravity drainage apparatus and the drainage tubing secured to the thigh in such a manner that

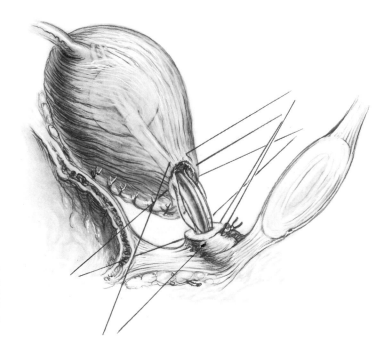

Figure 52–16. A new Foley catheter has been inserted into the bladder and the previously placed urethral sutures have been positioned in the newly reconstructed bladder neck and are ready to be tied.

abduction of the leg will not cause tension on the catheter. In order to prevent the catheter from being dislodged inadvertently after the operation, we secure the catheter routinely at the level of the urethral meatus to the distal penile shaft. After the foreskin has been retracted and the distal 2 to 3 cm of the penile skin prepped with tincture of benzoin, one-inch adhesive is circumferentially applied over the skin proximal to the base of the glans. Two sutures of 2-0 silk are tied around the catheter at the level of the urethral meatus and two of the strands positioned over the adhesive, after which they are covered by an additional layer of tape. The opposing ends of the silks are then tied, providing additional insurance that the catheter will not become dislodged should the balloon fail postoperatively. In addition, the neck of the valve line is reinforced with a heavy silk tie as additional insurance against deflation of the balloon secondary to a leaky valve.

POSTOPERATIVE MANAGEMENT AND COMPLICATIONS

Postoperatively, we continue to believe that prophylactic anticoagulation, unless specifically contraindicated, is important in all patients undergoing pelvic node dissection whether it is in conjunction with radical cystectomy or radical prostatectomy. It had been our practice to utilize parenteral crystalline warfarin sodium (Coumadin). A dose of 10 mg of Coumadin was first administered in the recovery room. Thereafter, subsequent parenteral doses were ordered on a daily basis according to each day's prothrombin time (PT), with optimal prophylactic anticoagulation aimed at maintaining a PT between 18 and 22 seconds, or one and one half to two times the control. If the patient's PT exceeded 25 seconds, anticoagulation was reversed with parenteral vitamin K (AquaMEPHYTON), as the complications of excessive anticoagulation exceeded its possible benefit. By using this protocol we have completely eliminated postoperative thromboembolic complications.[13] Due to current unavailability of parenteral Coumadin, we now administer 15 mg of crushed oral Coumadin through a nasogastric tube in the recovery room and subsequently titrate doses on a daily basis to achieve a therapeutic level of anticoagulation. We have yet to see development of thrombophlebitis or pulmonary embolism in patients who have achieved therapeutic levels using oral Coumadin; however, this later protocol has only recently been initiated and only time will indicate if its efficacy equals our previous experience with parenteral Coumadin.

Nasogastric suction is usually required only for the first 24 to 48 hours and is thereafter discontinued. By the third or fourth postoperative day, most patients have resumed oral feeding, and analgesics and antibiotics can be administered by mouth. In patients undergoing the first stage of insertion of an inflatable penile prosthesis, parenteral antibiotics are given for a minimum of five days to decrease the risk of infection. In all other cases, patients are placed on a broad-spectrum oral antibiotic such as a combination trimethoprim-sulfamethoxazole or a cephalosporin. In both circumstances, maintenance antibiotics are prescribed at discharge, usually six to eight days following surgery, and are given until the Foley catheter is removed. The catheter is generally removed three weeks following surgery. Gravity cystograms are unnecessary since late anastomotic leaks are rare. Prior to catheter removal we instill the bladder with 100 ml of a sterile solution, remove the catheter, and instruct the patient to initiate and terminate his urinary stream on command. In the majority of cases, even at this early stage, most patients can stop and start their stream, providing positive reinforcement that their external sphincter mechanism is intact. Many patients will have transient incontinence, mostly stress-related, for a period of four to six weeks or longer; this condition steadily disappears with time.

In 1979 we reported our complications among 65 patients undergoing conventional pelvic lymph node dissection followed by a variety of methods of radical prostatectomy, including three that were performed through a perineal approach. In this group there were 18 early (28%) and nine late (14%) complications, similar to the results in other reports. The most significant late complication was penile, scrotal, or leg edema, which occurred twice as often in patients receiving postoperative adjuvant radiation for a positive margin or pathologic Stage C disease (20%) as it did in those patients undergoing only combined radical prostatectomy and pelvic node dissection (7%). Interestingly, of 17 patients undergoing pelvic lymphadenectomy only as a staging procedure followed by definitive external beam radiation therapy, seven (41%) had chronic lymphedema. Since employing a limited pelvic node dissection prior to radical retropubic prostatectomy, we have to date eliminated this late complication of lymphedema.

Of the 65 patients previously reported, two were totally incontinent. One had an incidental proctotomy at the time of radical perineal prostatectomy, which resulted in a rectourethral fistula and subsequent incontinence. The other patient had an uneventful radical retropubic prostatectomy, but on the third postoperative day failure of the balloon caused the indwelling catheter to become dislodged. This necessitated replacement of the catheter, which resulted in a false passage and development of contracture of the bladder neck. Subsequently, this was repaired perineally, but the patient became incontinent. A third patient with a positive urethral margin and microscopic involvement of the seminal vesicles received postoperative radiation. Though continent initially, after radiation therapy he developed stress incontinence, which was alleviated by insertion of a Kaufman prosthesis.

From June 1978 to August 1982, 30 additional patients underwent radical retropubic prostatectomy with a limited pelvic node dissection for adenocarcinoma of the prostate using the technique described in this article. Significant early complications occurred in four patients (13%). One patient required a ureteral reimplantation at the time of surgery because of recognized ureteral injury during lymphadenectomy.

A second patient developed significant postoperative bleeding, which required reoperation later on the day of surgery. At reoperation the source of bleeding was never identified and was attributed to a bleeding diathesis secondary to chronic ingestion of aspirin for osteoarthritis. In this patient routine anticoagulation with Coumadin was not initiated, and he developed a documented pulmonary embolus five days later. Despite systemic heparinization he continued to have repeated pulmonary emboli, necessitating the insertion of a transvenous umbrella. The patient eventually made a slow recovery and was discharged from the hospital totally continent.

A third patient developed a probable retroperitoneal hematoma resulting in a prolonged ileus, perhaps secondary to anticoagulation. This resolved after reversal of anticoagulation and the initiation of conservative measures. The final patient sustained a laceration to the common iliac artery that was treated at the time of surgery by angioplasty and showed an initial uneventful recovery. Two weeks later, however, he returned to the hospital with swelling of the lower abdomen and hypotension. Immediate reexploration revealed bleeding from the original site of injury. It was repaired again, this time without further sequelae.

Since August 1982 thru August 1985, an additional 99 patients have undergone radical retropubic prostatectomy and limited pelvic lymphadenectomy using the Campbell's approach. In this group, eight early complications occurred in seven patients (7%). Four required reoperation for postoperative bleeding. An arterial source of the bleeding was identified in three patients (inferior epigastric, accessory obturator, and anterior rectal artery) and easily controlled without major sequelae in two of the three patients. The third patient also had an incidental rectotomy, closed primarily, and required extended intensive care and ventilatory assistance, from which he recovered with discharge 30 days following surgery and without sequelae from the rectotomy. One other patient also had an inadvertent rectotomy for a small clinical Stage C lesion, which was repaired in three layers with interrupted 4-0 silk; the patient was discharged on the seventh postoperative day. No sequelae developed from his inadvertent rectotomy. One patient with chronic renal failure (creatinine of 6.0 mg/dl) underwent radical prostatectomy for a pathologic B_2 tumor without intraoperative complication. On the fifth postoperative day feculent drainage was observed from the indwelling Foley catheter. Cystourethrography confirmed a rectourethral fistula, and an immediate diverting colostomy was performed. Subsequent anoscopy revealed a small fistula between the vesicourethral anastomosis and anterior rectal wall, presumably due to a poorly placed posterior urethral suture. Follow-up cystourethrography failed to reveal the fistulous communication, and the catheter was withdrawn. Fortunately, continence was maintained, following which bowel continuity was reestablished. One other patient underwent surgery for a pathologic Stage D_1 prostatic cancer. On the fourth postoperative day the patient mistakenly received a 10-fold excess of 50 mg of parenteral Coumadin, which was quickly reversed by administration of vitamin K. Subsequently, therapeutic levels of anticoagulation were never achieved. Five days following discharge the patient developed bilateral pulmonary emboli requiring rehospitalization and systemic heparinization.

A comparison of the early complication rate over the past 14 years for three separate study periods reflects our ongoing effort to virtually eliminate postoperative morbidity through strict attention to perioperative details and operative technique (Table 52–1).

As previously reported, the rate of incontinence of the first 95 patients was 3.2%, similar to the long-term rate of 2.4% reported by Middleton, who utilized a similar approach.[15] Analysis of our last 99 patients reveals two with total and two with stress incontinence. Both patients with total incontinence are scheduled for corrective surgery employing an artificial external urinary sphincter, whereas those with only stress incontinence manage well with an occasional daytime anti-incontinence pad.

The role of pelvic lymph node dissection remains controversial. Currently, it is recommended as an aid in accurate pathologic staging and, in some centers, in selecting those who are candidates for radical prostatectomy based on the presence or absence of unsuspected nodal metastasis. In patients with grossly positive pelvic nodes confirmed by biopsy, lymphadenectomy primarily serves as a predictor of prognosis without itself providing any therapeutic benefit. In these situations it is our policy not to perform a radical prostatectomy but to proceed with immediate bilateral orchiectomy or an alternative means of withdrawing androgen support. Dispute, however, continues as to whether or not pelvic lymph node dissection in patients with minimal lymph node metastasis, when combined with resection of the primary tumor alone or when combined with other adjuncts, has any therapeutic benefit over a more conservative approach.

Table 52–1. COMPARISON OF EARLY COMPLICATION RATES IN PATIENTS UNDERGOING CAMPBELL'S RADICAL PROSTATECTOMY AND PELVIC LYMPHADENECTOMY

Year	Number of Patients	Early Complication Rate (%)
1971–1977	65*	(18/65) 28
1978–1982	30	(4/30) 13
1982–1985	99	(7/99) 7

*Three underwent radical perineal prostatectomy.

Since approximately one third of patients with nodal disease harbor only microscopic metastasis, usually to one or two lymph nodes,[8, 14] it is our contention that the patients who benefit the most from a pelvic lymphadenectomy when combined with a radical prostatectomy are those with unsuspected metastasis limited to a few lymph nodes. Paulson has reported that even in patients with only one positive lymph node, the median time to failure was unchanged whether or not patients underwent radical prostatectomy, definitive radiation therapy, or delayed hormone therapy.[17] On the other hand, Zincke and the Mayo Clinic group have reported that adjunctive bilateral orchiectomy in patients with regional nodal involvement, who have also undergone radical prostatectomy and pelvic lymphadenectomy, offers a distinct therapeutic advantage, compared with the rates for those patients not undergoing bilateral orchiectomy.[22] It has been our policy over the past 10 years, in patients with unsuspected microscopic nodal metastases, to implement adjuvant cytotoxic chemotherapy utilizing either cyclophosphamide, 1 gm/m^2, monthly for six months, or alternating cyclophosphamide 1 gm/m^2, with 5-fluorouracil, 1.0 gm monthly for 6 months. The preliminary trend suggests a definite advantage for those receiving cytotoxic chemotherapy, compared with results for historic controls, but sufficient long-term analysis is required before this aggressive form of therapy demonstrates statistical advantage over alternative forms of treatment.

In conclusion, an analysis of our experience with the modified Campbell's technique indicates that it can be performed with an acceptably low rate of morbidity and remains the optimal procedure for the management of cancer clinically confined to the prostate and in selected patients with clinical evidence of extracapsular extension.

References

1. Bagshaw MA, Ray GR, Cox RS: Radiotherapy of prostatic carcinoma: long- or short-term efficacy (Stanford University experience). Urology 25 (Suppl 2):17–23, 1985.
2. Belt E, Shroeder FH: Total perineal prostatectomy for carcinoma of the prostate. J Urol 107:91–96, 1972.
3. Byar DP, Mostofi FK: Carcinoma of the prostate:

4. Campbell EW: Total prostatectomy with preliminary ligation of the vascular pedicles. J Urol 81:464–467, 1959.
5. Catolona WJ, Dresner SM: Nerve-sparing radical prostatectomy: extraprostatic tumor extension and preservation of erectile function. J Urol 134:1149–1151, 1985.
6. Eggleston JC, Walsh PC: Radical prostatectomy with preservation of sexual function: pathological findings in the first 100 cases. J Urol 134:1146–1148, 1985.
7. Flock RH: The arterial distribution within the prostate gland: its role in transurethral resection. J Urol 37:524–548, 1937.
8. Fowler JE Jr, Whitmore WF Jr: The incidence and extent of pelvic lymph node metastases in apparently localized prostatic cancer. Cancer 47:2941–2945, 1981.
9. Gibbons RP, Cole BS, Richardson RG, et al: Adjuvant radiotherapy following radical prostatectomy: results and complications. J Urol 135:65–68, 1985.
10. Huggins CB: Commentary on the treatment of prostate cancer. J Urol 102:119–120, 1969.
11. Lepor H, Gregerman M, Crosby R, et al: Precise localization of the autonomic nerves from the pelvic plexus to the corpora cavernosa: a detailed anatomical study of the adult male pelvis. J Urol 133:207–212, 1985.
12. Lieskovsky G, Skinner DG, Weisenburger T: Pelvic lymphadenectomy in the management of carcinoma of the prostate. J Urol 124:635–638, 1980.
13. Lieskovsky G, Skinner DG: Technique of radical retropubic prostatectomy with limited pelvic node dissection. Urol Clin North Am 10:187–198, 1983.
14. McLaughlin AP, Saltzstein SL, McCullough DL, Gittes RF: Prostatic carcinoma: incidence and location of unsuspected lymphatic metastases. J Urol 115:89–94, 1976.
15. Middleton AW Jr: Pelvic lymphadenectomy with modified radical retropubic prostatectomy as a single operation: technique used and results in 50 consecutive cases. J Urol 125:353–356, 1981.
16. Mittemeyer BT, Cox HD: Modified radical retropubic prostatectomy. Urology 12:313–320, 1978.
17. Paulson DF: Pelvic lymphadenectomy is not essential to staging accuracy in all patients with localized prostate cancer. Semin Urol 3:204–211, 1983.
18. Shackelford RT, Zuidema GD (eds): Surgery of the Alimentary Tract, Vol 3, Chap 8. Philadelphia, WB Saunders, 1982, pp 327–380.
19. Walsh PC, Donker PJ: Impotence following radical prostatectomy: insight into etiology and prevention. J Urol 128:492–497, 1982.
20. Walsh PC, Lepor H, Eggleston JC: Radical prostatectomy with preservation of sexual function: anatomical and pathological considerations. Prostate 4:473–485, 1983.
21. Walsh PC, Mostwin JL: Radical prostatectomy and cystoprostatectomy with preservation of potency. Results using a new nerve-sparing technique. Br J Urol 56:694–697, 1984.
22. Zincke H, Utz DC: Radical surgery for stage D_1 prostate cancer. Semin Urol 1:253–260, 1983.

prognostic evaluation of certain pathologic features in 208 radical prostatectomies. Examined by the step-section technique. Cancer 30:5–13, 1972.

PATRICK C. WALSH, M.D.

Technique of Radical Retropubic Prostatectomy with Preservation of Sexual Function—An Anatomic Approach

CHAPTER 53

Because impotence has been a common complication of radical prostatectomy, affecting over 90% of treated patients, the surgical management of localized prostatic cancer has never gained widespread popularity. In 1982 Walsh and Donker[18] suggested that impotence was produced by injury to the pelvic nerve plexus that provides autonomic innervation to the corpora cavernosa. Based on this observation, the technique of radical retropubic prostatectomy was modified in a minor way.[19] Although the branches of the pelvic plexus that innervate the corpora cavernosa are microscopic in size, they can be recognized intraoperatively because of their rather constant association with the capsular vessels of the prostate.[9, 11, 19] These neurovascular bundles are located in the leaves of the lateral pelvic fascia and previously were injured unknowingly during standard radical prostatectomies. However, once the precise location of these neurovascular bundles was determined, the technique of radical prostatectomy could be modified in a way that enabled the surgeon to visualize these bundles intraoperatively and decide whether it was safe to preserve the neurovascular bundles or necessary to sacrifice them with the specimen. This approach has resulted in preservation of sexual function in a large majority of the patients.[3, 20]

This chapter describes an anatomic approach to radical retropubic prostatectomy, emphasizing reduced blood loss, improved visualization, and accurate resection of involved structures. This technique reduces the morbidity of the procedure to a minimum without altering its therapeutic efficacy. It is hoped that these advances may lead to widespread acceptance of radical prostatectomy as the most effective form of treatment for the management of localized prostatic cancer. When performed correctly, the side effects of this procedure should be equal or less than those associated with radiation therapy. A film depicting the surgical technique is available.[17]

SURGICAL ANATOMY

If one hopes to minimize the morbidity of radical prostatectomy, it is necessary to understand fully the anatomic relationships of the prostate to its adjacent structures. The prostate is confined to a small recess in the pelvis where it is surrounded by the levator ani musculature and pubis and other more vulnerable structures such as the rectum, the urogenital diaphragm with the external sphincter, Santorini's plexus, and the autonomic branches of the pelvic plexus to the corpora cavernosa.

753

Pelvic Fascia

The prostate is covered with two distinct and separate fascial layers: Denonvilliers' fascia and the lateral pelvic fascia. Denonvilliers' fascia is a filmy delicate layer of connective tissue that is located between the anterior wall of the rectum and the prostate; this fascial layer extends cranially to cover the posterior surface of the seminal vesicles and lies snugly against the posterior prostatic capsule (Fig. 53–1A). The fascia is most prominent and dense near the base of the prostate and seminal vesicles and thins dramatically as it extends caudally to its termination at the rectourethralis musculature. Microscopically, it is impossible to discern a "posterior" and "anterior" layer to this fascia.[7] For this reason, to obtain an adequate surgical margin one must excise this fascia completely. In addition to Denonvilliers' fascia, a second important prostatic layer of fascia, the lateral pelvic fascia, covers the pelvic musculature (Fig. 53–1A). This fascia has also been called the prostatic fascia or the parietal layer of the endopelvic fascia. Anteriorly and anterolaterally this fascia is in direct continuity with the true capsule of the prostate. The major tributaries of the dorsal vein of the penis and Santorini's plexus travel within this fascia (Fig. 53–1A). Posterolaterally, the lateral pelvic fascia separates from the prostate to travel immediately adjacent to the pelvic musculature surrounding the rectum. The prostate receives its blood supply and autonomic innervation through the leaves of this fascia. In an effort to avoid injury to the dorsal vein of the penis and Santorini's plexus during radical perineal prostatectomy, the lateral pelvic fascia should be reflected off the prostate (Fig. 53–1B). This accounts for the reduced blood loss associated with radical perineal prostatectomy. As described by Young and Davis,[23] once the posterior surface of the prostate has been exposed, "the next proce-

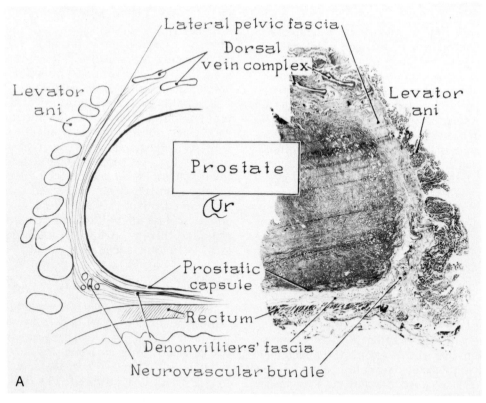

Figure 53–1. A, Cross section through an adult prostate, demonstrating the anatomic relationships between the lateral pelvic fascia, Denonvilliers' fascia, and the neurovascular bundle. B and C, The surgical plane (dashed line) employed in radical perineal and retropubic prostatectomy. Note the site for incision in the lateral fascia that avoids injury to the neurovascular bundle. Reprinted with permission from Walsh PC, Perlmutter AD, Gittes RF, et al.: Campbell's Urology. 5th ed. Philadelphia, WB Saunders, 1986.

Illustration continued on opposite page

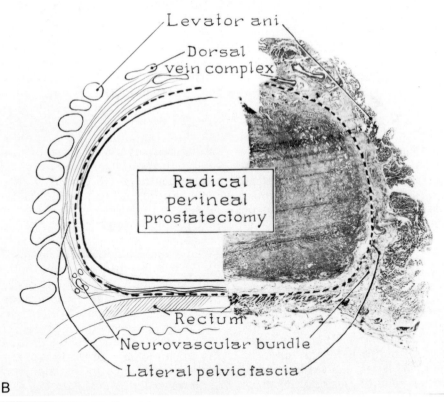

Levator ani

Dorsal
vein complex

Radical
perineal
prostatectomy

Rectum

Neurovascular bundle

Lateral pelvic fascia

B

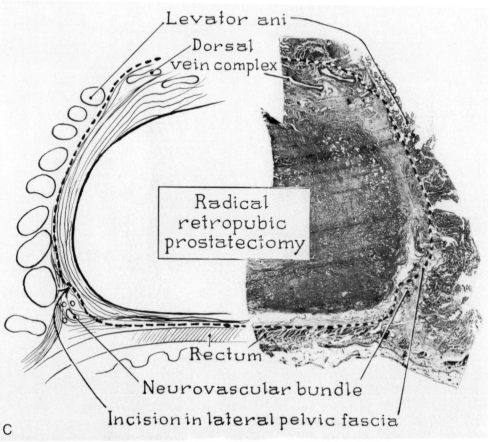

Levator ani

Dorsal
vein complex

Radical
retropubic
prostatectomy

Rectum

Neurovascular bundle

Incision in lateral pelvic fascia

C

Figure 53–1 Continued

755

dure is to search for the point along the lateral surface of the prostate where the fascia coming from the lateral wall of the pelvis divides to encircle the prostate. By making an incision through the posterior layer close to the prostate one can then by blunt dissection easily separate the anterior layer from the prostate on each side until the membranous urethra is reached." In a radical retropubic prostatectomy, the prostate is approached from outside the lateral fascia (Fig. 53–1C); for this reason the dorsal vein complex must be ligated and the lateral pelvic fascia must be divided.

Arterial Supply and Venous Drainage

The prostate receives its arterial blood supply from the inferior vesical artery, which has also been termed the prostatovesicular artery. According to Flocks,[4] after the inferior vesical artery provides small branches to the inferior, posterior extent of the seminal vesicle and the base of the blad-

der and prostate, the artery terminates in two large groups of prostatic vessels: the urethral and capsular groups. The urethral vessels enter the prostate at the posterolateral vesicoprostatic junction, providing arterial supply to the vesical neck and periurethral portion of the gland. The capsular branches run along the pelvic side wall in the lateral pelvic fascia traveling posterolateral to the prostate, providing branches that course ventrally and dorsally to supply the outer portion of the prostate. The capsular vessels terminate as a small cluster of vessels that supply the pelvic floor. Histologically, the capsular group of vessels is surrounded by an extensive network of nerves (Fig. 53–2).[9, 11, 19] The capsular vessels, both arteries and veins, provide the macroscopic landmark that aids in the identification of the microscopic branches of the pelvic plexus that innervate the corpora cavernosa.

The venous drainage of the prostate is into the plexus of Santorini. It is necessary to have a complete understanding of these veins in order to avoid excessive bleeding and to ensure a bloodless field when expos-

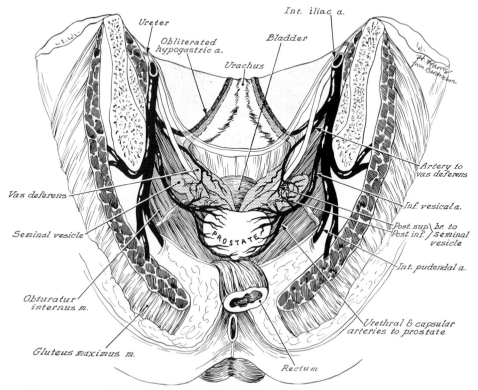

Figure 53–2. Posterior view of the arterial supply to the prostate. The rectum has been removed to expose the posterior surface of the prostate and pelvis. Reprinted with permission from Weyrauch HM: Surgery of the Prostate. Philadelphia, WB Saunders, 1959.

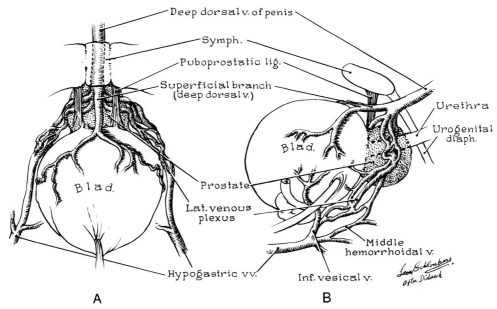

Figure 53–3. Santorini's venous plexus. A, View of trifurcation of dorsal vein of penis with patient in supine position; relationship of venous branches to puboprostatic ligaments is depicted. B, Lateral view shows anatomic relationships at trifurcation. In this schematic illustration, the pelvic fascia has been removed. In reality, these structures are never visualized in this skeletonized manner because they are encased by the lateral pelvic fascia. Reprinted with permission from Reiner WG, Walsh PC: An anatomical approach to the surgical management of the dorsal vein and Santorini's plexus during radical retropubic surgery. J Urol 121:198–200, 1979.

ing the membranous urethra and apex of the prostate. The deep dorsal vein leaves the penis under Buck's fascia between the corpora cavernosa and penetrates the urogenital diaphragm, dividing into three major branches: the superficial branch and the right and left lateral venous plexuses (Fig. 53–3A).[16] The superficial branch, which travels between the puboprostatic ligaments, is the centrally located vein overlying the bladder neck and prostate (Fig. 53–3B). This vein is easily visualized early in retropubic operations and has communicating branches over the bladder itself and into the endopelvic fascia. The superficial branch lies outside the pelvic fascia; the common trunk and lateral venous plexuses are covered and concealed by this fascia. The lateral venous plexuses traverse posterolaterally (Fig. 53–3B) and communicate freely with the pudendal, obturator, and vesical plexuses. These plexuses interconnect with other venous systems to form the inferior vesical vein, which empties into the internal iliac vein. With the complex of veins and plexuses anastomosing freely, any laceration of these rather friable structures can lead to considerable blood loss.

Pelvic Plexus

The autonomic innervation of the pelvic organs and external genitalia arises from the pelvic plexus, which is formed by parasympathetic visceral efferent preganglionic fibers, nervi erigentes, that arise from the sacral center and sympathetic fibers from the thoracolumbar center (T-11 to L-2) (Fig. 53–4A).[18] The pelvic plexus in men is located retroperitoneally beside the rectum and forms a fenestrated rectangular plate that is situated in the sagittal plane. The branches of the inferior vesical artery and vein that supply the bladder and prostate perforate the pelvic plexus. For this reason, ligation of the so-called lateral pedicle in its midportion not only interrupts the vessels but also transects the nerve supply to the prostate, urethra, and corpora cavernosa. The pelvic plexus provides visceral branches that innervate the bladder, ureter, seminal vesicles, prostate, rectum, membranous urethra, and corpora cavernosa. In addition, branches that contain somatic motor axons travel through the pelvic plexus to supply the levator ani, coccygeus, and striated urethral musculature. The nerves

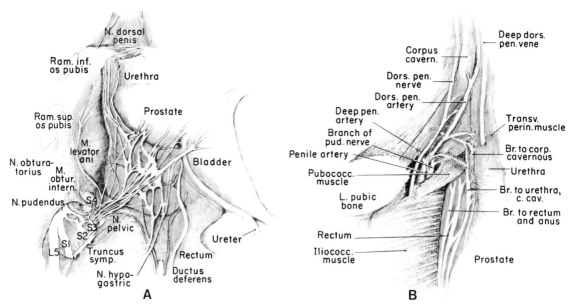

Figure 53–4. A, Dissection of left pelvic plexus in male newborn with peritoneum, pelvic vessels, pelvic fascia, and pubic symphysis removed. B, Close-up view of the dissection, demonstrating the anatomic location of the branches of the pelvic plexus that innervate the corpora cavernosa. Reprinted with permission from Walsh PC, Donker PJ: Impotence following radical prostatectomy. J Urol 128:492–496, 1982.

innervating the prostate travel outside the capsule of the prostate and Denonvilliers' fascia until they perforate the capsule where they enter the prostate. The branches to the membranous urethra and corpora cavernosa also travel outside the prostatic capsule in the lateral pelvic fascia. It has been demonstrated that the branches that innervate the corpora cavernosa are located dorsolaterally in the lateral pelvic fascia between the prostate and rectum.[9, 11, 18] At the level of the membranous urethra they travel at three and nine o'clock. After piercing the urogenital diaphragm they pass behind the dorsal penile artery and dorsal penile nerve before entering the corpora cavernosa (Fig. 53–4B). Although these nerves are microscopic in size, their anatomic location can be estimated intraoperatively by using the capsular vessels as a landmark. For this reason, throughout the remainder of the chapter, I will refer to this structure as the neurovascular bundle (Fig. 53–1).

SURGICAL TECHNIQUE

Preoperative Preparation

Surgery is deferred for six to eight weeks following the needle biopsy of the prostate.

This delay enables inflammatory adhesions or hematoma that result from the needle biopsy to resolve so that the anatomic relationships between the prostate and surrounding structures are returned to a more normal state prior to surgery. This is especially important if one hopes to preserve the neurovascular bundles intraoperatively and to avoid rectal injury. If a needle aspiration of the prostate has been done as a diagnostic procedure or if the patient can be operated on within a week after the needle biopsy, there is no reason for delay.

Since transfusions are frequently required in the perioperative period, during the six to eight week delay patients are offered the opportunity to donate three units of blood for autotransfusion. This can avoid the need for heterologous transfusion.[15] Patients are advised to avoid taking aspirin or other nonsteroidal anti-inflammatory agents that interfere with platelet function. They are admitted to the hospital the day before surgery and undergo standard preoperative evaluation. The night before surgery they are given a Fleet enema.

Special Instruments

Unlike radical perineal prostatectomy, radical retropubic prostatectomy requires very few special instruments. A fiberoptic headlight is most useful because much of the procedure is performed beneath the pubis in an area in which visualization can be difficult. A standard Balfour retractor with a malleable center blade is useful during the lymph node dissection and subsequently during the radical prostatectomy to provide cranial and posterior retraction on the peritoneum and bladder, respectively. Coagulating forceps, vessel loops, and bulldog clamps are the only other specialized instruments that should be available.

Anesthesia, Incision, and Lymphadenectomy

A spinal or epidural anesthetic is preferable for this procedure. Conduction anesthesia is safer and seems to be associated with less blood loss.[15] The patient is placed in the supine position with the table broken in the midline to extend the distance between the pubis and umbilicus. The table is then tilted in the Trendelenburg position until the legs are parallel to the floor. The skin is prepared and draped in the usual way. A No. 22 catheter with a 30-ml balloon is passed into the bladder and the catheter is connected to sterile closed continuous drainage. A right-handed surgeon always stands on the left side of the patient. A midline extraperitoneal lower abdominal incision is made extending from the pubis to the umbilicus. The rectus muscles are separated in the midline and the transverse fascia is opened sharply to expose the space of Retzius. Care is taken to incise the anterior fascia down to the pubis and to incise the posterior fascia above the semicircular line to the umbilicus. Laterally, the peritoneum is mobilized off the external iliac vessels to the bifurcation of the common iliac artery. This maneuver is facilitated by isolating, dividing, and ligating the vas deferens bilaterally. At this point a self-retaining Balfour retractor is placed and the staging pelvic lymphadenectomy on the right side is commenced. Exposure is facilitated by using the malleable blade attached to the Balfour retractor to retract the peritoneum superiorly.

The lymphadenectomy is considered a staging and not a therapeutic procedure. Its value is to identify those patients with occult metastases to pelvic lymph nodes in whom a radical prostatectomy would be of little benefit. For this reason the modified technique of Whitmore and associates is utilized.[22] The dissection is initiated along the external iliac vein. The lymphatics overlying the external iliac artery are preserved. The dissection proceeds inferiorly to the femoral canal, where care is taken to ligate the lymphatic channels at the node of Cloquet. Next, the obturator lymph nodes are removed with care to avoid injury to the obturator nerve. The obturator artery and vein are usually left undisturbed and are not ligated unless excessive bleeding occurs. Because the internal pudendal artery occasionally arises from the obturator artery, sacrifice of the obturator artery could reduce arterial blood flow to the corpora cavernosa. The dissection then proceeds superiorly to the bifurcation of the common iliac artery, where the lymph nodes in the angle between the external iliac and hypogastric arteries are removed. At the completion of the dissection, the vasculature in the hypogastric and obturator fossa should be neatly skeletonized (Fig. 53–5). These lymph nodes are sent for frozen section and a similar procedure is carried out on the left side. The pathologist is requested to section all lymph nodes and perform frozen sections only on those lymph nodes that look suspicious. Using this procedure, I have experienced a 3% false-negative rate for frozen section evaluations. In all cases, the lymph nodes that were falsely classified were 4 mm or less in diameter. For this reason, I feel that frozen section analysis of lymph nodes is of great value. To reduce blood loss during the remainder of the procedure, the hypogastric arteries are encircled with vessel loops, and bulldog clamps are placed proximal to the origin of the obliterated umbilical artery.[15]

Incision in Endopelvic Fascia

At this point, the malleable blade is repositioned to retract the bladder. If the balloon on the Foley catheter is positioned in the dome of the bladder beneath the well-padded malleable blade, maximal cranial and posterior displacement of the bladder will be achieved, providing excellent exposure of the anterior surface of the prostate. The fibroadipose tissue covering the prostate is carefully dissected away to expose the pelvic fascia, puboprostatic ligaments, and superficial branch of the dorsal vein. The

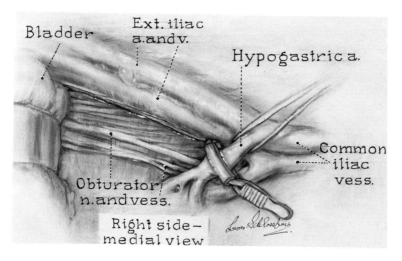

Figure 53–5. View of the right pelvis following completion of the staging lymph node dissection. Note that the fibrofatty tissue overlying the external iliac artery has not been disturbed and that a bulldog clamp has been placed on the hypogastric artery. From Walsh PC: Radical retropubic prostatectomy. In PC Walsh, et al (eds), Campbell's Urology, 5th ed. Philadelphia, WB Saunders, 1986, pp 2754–2775.

endopelvic fascia is entered where it reflects over the pelvic side wall, well away from its attachments to the bladder and prostate (Fig. 53–6). At this site the visceral pelvic fascia, which covers the anterior surface of the prostate and encases the main trunk of the dorsal vein complex, attaches to the parietal pelvic fascia covering the pelvic musculature. At the point where the fascia is incised, it is often transparent, revealing the underlying levator ani musculature. After the fascia has been opened, one can usually visu-

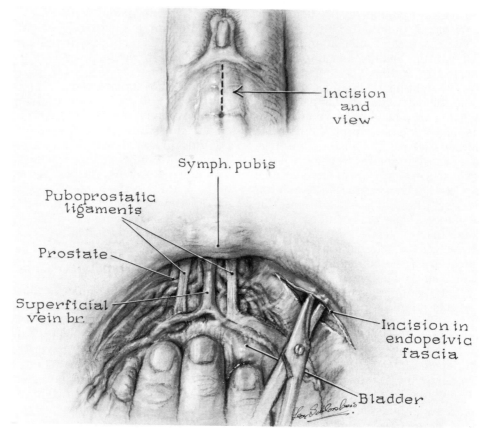

Figure 53–6. The incision in the endopelvic fascia is made at the junction with the pelvic side wall, well away from the prostate and bladder. From Walsh PC: Radical retropubic prostatectomy. In PC Walsh, et al (eds), Campbell's Urology, 5th ed. Philadelphia, WB Saunders, 1986, pp 2754–2775.

alize the bulging lateral venous plexus of Santorini, which is located medially. The lateral venous plexuses traverse adjacent to the prostate and the lower portion of the bladder. Therefore, an incision in the endopelvic fascia adjacent to the bladder or the prostate risks laceration of these important structures with potential severe blood loss. Beneath this venous complex lies the prostatovesicular artery and the branches of the pelvic plexus that course toward the prostate, urethra, and corpora cavernosa. The incision in the endopelvic fascia is then carefully extended in an anteromedial direction toward the puboprostatic ligaments, enabling the surgeon to palpate the lateral surface of the prostate.

Division of the Puboprostatic Ligaments

The fibrofatty tissue covering the superficial branch of the dorsal vein and pubopros-

tatic ligaments is gently teased away to prepare for division of the ligaments without inadvertent injury to the superficial branch of the dorsal vein. This maneuver enables the surgeon to incise the puboprostatic ligaments sharply at their attachment to the pubis. Care must be taken to dissect the superficial branch of the dorsal vein away from the medial edge of the ligaments before they are divided. According to Albers and associates,[1] the puboprostatic ligaments consist mostly of collagen and contain no vessels. They should be incised close to the pubis, and care should be exercised not to injure the superficial branch of the dorsal vein. Thus, there is no need to ligate them. Once the puboprostatic ligaments are transected, the superficial branch of the dorsal vein is readily apparent over the bladder neck in the midline. This vein should be dissected carefully from the undersurface of the pubis, thereby exposing the trifurcation of the dorsal vein over the region of the prostatourethral junction (Fig. 53–7).

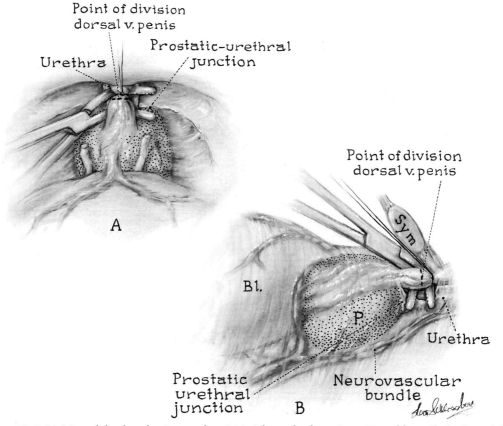

Figure 53–7. Division of the dorsal vein complex. A, A right-angle clamp is positioned beneath the ligated dorsal vein at the time of division. B, Separation of the lateral pelvic fascia between the dorsal vein complex and urethra. After Walsh PC: Radical retropubic prostatectomy. In PC Walsh, et al (eds), Campbell's Urology, 5th ed. Philadelphia, WB Saunders, 1986, pp 2754–2775.

Ligation of Dorsal Vein Complex

The lateral wall of the urethra is identified by palpating the indwelling catheter. Anterior to the catheter is a thick complex composed of the main trunk of the dorsal vein with its surrounding pelvic fascia (Fig. 53–7B). The complex is easily identified by palpating its distinct, sharp, shelf-like edge just anterior to the urethra. Utilizing a right-angle clamp, the surgeon perforates the lateral pelvic fascia and passes the clamp through the avascular plane between the anterior surface of the urethra and the posterior surface of the dorsal vein complex (Fig. 53–7B). At this level the complex with its associated fascia is 1 to 2 cm thick. A 0 silk ligature is then passed around the dorsal vein. A large right-angle clamp is next used to widen the opening between the dorsal vein complex and urethra, facilitating subsequent isolation of the urethra. Because the neurovascular bundle is posterior to the urethra, it cannot be damaged during this maneuver. When frozen sections confirm the absence of metastatic disease in the pelvic lymph nodes, the ligature is tied (Fig. 53–7A). The dorsal vein complex with its investment of fascia is then transected on the bladder side of the ligature with a No. 15 blade on a long handle (Fig. 53–7A). Generally, there is little or no backflow from the untied lateral plexus at this point, because of the valves in the venous system. This is especially true in patients under epidural or spinal anesthesia; in patients under general anesthesia there may be more back bleeding as a result of the increased venous pressure associated with increased intrathoracic pressure. If backbleeding is a problem, the venous channels over the anterior surface of the prostate can be oversewn with a 2-0 chromic catgut suture, or small gauze packs can be placed in the obturator and hypogastric fossa to compress the vesical venous plexus and hypogastric veins.

Division of Urethra

At this point it is essential to use a sponge stick for downward displacement of the prostate so that the prostatourethral junction can be seen (Fig. 53–8). Absolute control of venous bleeding from the dorsal vein complex is mandatory during this stage of the procedure so that visualization can be achieved in a bloodless field. If the ligature has fallen off the dorsal vein or if there is significant oozing, a 2-0 chromic catgut suture on a large needle can be used to oversew the fascial edges of the ligated distal vein so that hemostasis can be perfected. With posterior displacement of the prostate by a sponge stick, the prostatourethral junction should be well visualized. Intact bands of lateral fascia are present on either side of the urethra (Fig. 53–9). These fascial bands must not be disturbed, since they contain the branches of the pelvic plexus that innervate the corpora cavernosa. In the past these fascial bands were routinely divided in an effort to skeletonize the urethra and mobilize the apex of the prostate, and this was a major reason why most patients were impotent following this procedure. The plane between the urethra and the lateral fascia is next developed by using sharp dissection, and an umbilical tape is passed around the urethra with care not to injure the adjacent fascia (Fig. 53–9). The anterior wall of the urethra is then incised at its junction with the apex of the prostate. This permits the Foley catheter to be brought through this incision, clamped, and divided. Next, the posterior wall of the urethra is divided (Fig. 53–10). Some authors advocate placing sutures in the distal urethra at this point in the procedure for later use during the anastomosis. However, in my experience these sutures are often pulled out during the subsequent maneuvers, and I have never had great difficulty replacing them later in the procedure.

Division of the Rectourethralis Muscle and Lateral Fascia

Utilizing upward traction on the divided catheter, the surgeon incises the rectourethralis muscle in the midline, freeing the apex of the prostate from the underlying rectum (Fig. 53–10). At times this can be done with ease utilizing blunt finger dissection, but frequently the rectourethralis musculature is thickened and sharp dissection is necessary. With traction on the catheter, one can often (but not always) visualize bands of skeletal muscle and fibrous tissue that tether the apex of the prostate to the pelvic floor musculature (Fig. 53–11A). These bands are most often prevalent in older patients who have large prostates. When viewed laterally, these bands travel

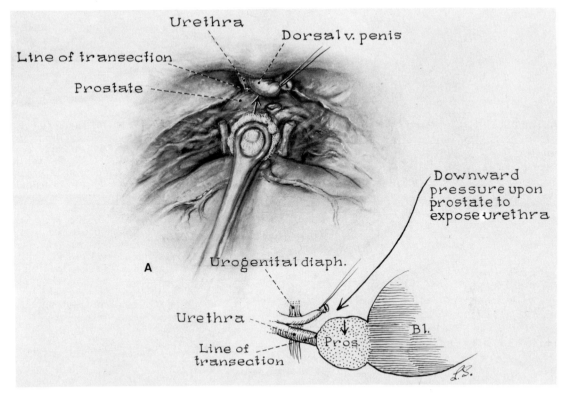

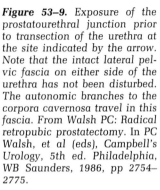

Figure 53–8. The dorsal vein has been transected, and a sponge stick is used to displace the prostate posteriorly to expose the prostatourethral junction. From Walsh PC: Radical retropubic prostatectomy. In PC Walsh, et al (eds), Campbell's Urology, 5th ed. Philadelphia, WB Saunders, 1986, pp 2754–2775.

Figure 53–9. Exposure of the prostatourethral junction prior to transection of the urethra at the site indicated by the arrow. Note that the intact lateral pelvic fascia on either side of the urethra has not been disturbed. The autonomic branches to the corpora cavernosa travel in this fascia. From Walsh PC: Radical retropubic prostatectomy. In PC Walsh, et al (eds), Campbell's Urology, 5th ed. Philadelphia, WB Saunders, 1986, pp 2754–2775.

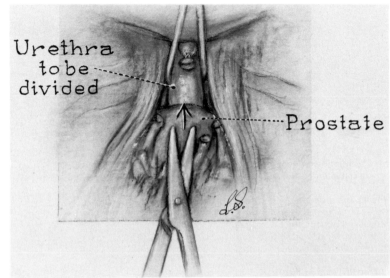

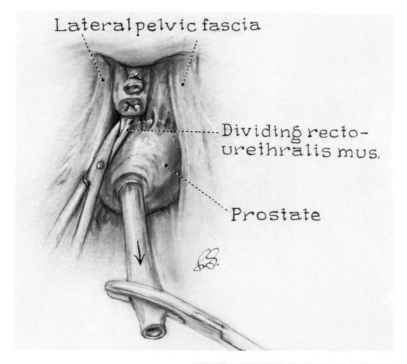

Figure 53–10. The urethra has been transected and the divided catheter, which has been clamped, is used to retract the apex of the prostate superiorly, exposing the rectourethralis muscle. The muscle is divided to open the plane posteriorly between the anterior rectal wall and Denonvilliers' fascia, which covers the posterior prostatic surface. From Walsh PC: Radical retropubic prostatectomy. In PC Walsh, et al (eds), Campbell's Urology, 5th ed. Philadelphia, WB Saunders, 1986, pp 2754–2775.

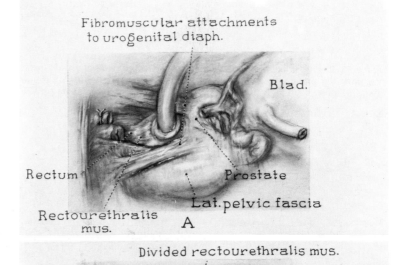

Figure 53–11. Preparation of the apex of the prostate prior to division of the lateral pelvic fascia. A. Apex of the prostate is often tethered to the urogenital diaphragm by fibromuscular bands that travel anteriorly, outside the lateral pelvic fascia. B, After the fibromuscular bands have been severed, the rectourethralis muscle fibers can be divided under direct vision. From Walsh PC: Radical retropubic prostatectomy. In PC Walsh, et al (eds), Campbell's Urology, 5th ed. Philadelphia, WB Saunders, 1986, pp 2754–2775.

outside the lateral pelvic fascia, anteriorly. Consequently, they can be divided without fear of injury to the neurovascular bundles that are inside the lateral pelvic fascia (Fig. 53–11B). Once this has been accomplished, division of the rectourethralis muscle can be completed under direct vision, with care not to injure the neurovascular bundles located at the edges of this muscle bilaterally (Fig. 53–11B). With finger dissection, the plane between the anterior wall of the rectum and the prostate with its investment of Denonvilliers' fascia is developed (Fig. 53–1C). After this plane has been established, a right-angle clamp is used to separate the lateral pelvic fascia from the lateral surface of the prostate at the apex (Fig. 53–12). At this point, the lateral fascia is usually quite thin and transparent. The lateral fascia is then incised at a point sufficiently anterior to preserve the neurovascular bundle, and the incision is carried cranially up to the area of the prostatic pedicle (Fig. 53–12). Recall that the neurovascular bundles are located dorsolateral to the prostate. In the past, this incision in the lateral fascia was made at random with blunt dissection. Although the neurovascular bundles were usually not removed with the specimen, they were injured during the dissection. With the technique described herein, the incision in the lateral fascia is made with precision and with

knowledge of the location of the neurovascular bundle. If the induration on the side of the nodule appears to extend into the lateral pelvic fascia or neurovascular bundles, the fascia is divided wherever necessary to excise all evident tumor (see later). The primary objective of the surgical procedure is the removal of all tumor, and in this setting preservation of potency is of secondary concern. Indeed, it may only be necessary to preserve the neurovascular bundles on one side to preserve potency (see below).

Once the lateral pelvic fascia has been divided, the neurovascular bundles can be seen at the posterolateral edge of the prostate. The lateral pelvic fascia is made up of multiple leaves, with the neurovascular bundle imbedded in them. Up to this point only the superficial leaves of the lateral pelvic fascia, those adjacent to the pelvic musculature, have been divided. The neurovascular bundles are imbedded in deeper leaves of the fascia and are attached to the prostate by the vessels that supply it. Because the neurovascular bundles supply few vascular branches to the distal third of the prostate, the bundles can usually be teased away from the prostate at this point. However, at the midpoint of the prostate, small arterial and venous branches are usually first to be visualized (Fig. 53–13). These first branches should be ligated individually with fine su-

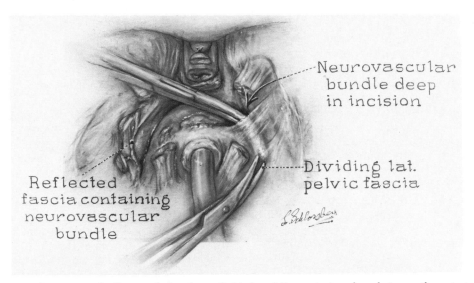

Figure 53–12. The rectourethralis muscle has been divided and the posterior plane between the anterior rectal wall and prostate has been developed. A right-angle clamp is passed between the prostatic capsule and the transparent lateral pelvic fascia, identifying the site for the initial incision in the fascia, anterior to the neurovascular bundle. From Walsh PC: Radical retropubic prostatectomy. In PC Walsh, et al (eds), Campbell's Urology, 5th ed. Philadelphia, WB Saunders, 1986, pp 2754–2775.

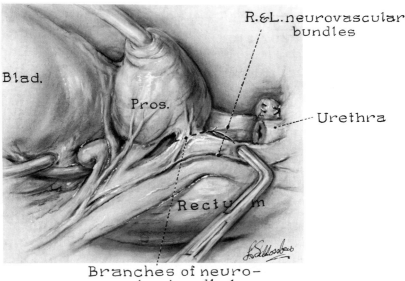

Figure 53-13. *The lateral pelvic fascia has been divided bilaterally, releasing the apex of the prostate. The neurovascular bundles are intact. At the midpoint of the prostate, small arterial and venous branches are usually first visualized. These branches are ligated individually, using fine sutures or clips and avoiding mass ligatures, which could produce inadvertent tenting of the bundle into the ligature and subsequent injury. After Walsh PC: Radical retropubic prostatectomy. In PC Walsh, et al (eds), Campbell's Urology, 5th ed. Philadelphia, WB Saunders, 1986, pp 2754–2775.*

tures or clips; mass ligatures that could produce inadvertent tenting of the bundle into the ligature with subsequent injury should be avoided (Fig. 53–13). As one approaches the base of the prostate, the bundles travel further posteriorly, and this is less of a problem.

At this point the attachment between the rectum and Denonvilliers' fascia should be divided in the midline posteriorly, exposing the posterior surface of the seminal vesicles, and the plane between the lateral edges of the seminal vesicles and the overlying lateral pelvic fascia should be developed (Fig. 53–14). This enables the lateral pedicles to be divided, on the lateral surface of the seminal vesicles near their junction with the prostate, with interrupted 2-0 silk sutures (Fig. 53–15). The neurovascular bundles should be in full view, and care should be exercised to avoid injuring these structures by ligating the pedicles too far posteriorly.

Excision of the Lateral Pelvic Fascia and Neurovascular Bundle

In certain circumstances it may be necessary to excise the lateral pelvic fascia and

neurovascular bundles completely on one or both sides. This decision can be made either preoperatively or intraoperatively based on a variety of clinical findings: (1) surgery on an impotent patient, (2) induration involving the lateral sulcus found on preoperative physical examination, (3) induration in the lateral pelvic fascia found intraoperatively after the endopelvic fascia has been opened, or (4) fixation of the neurovascular bundle to the capsule of the prostate detected once the lateral pelvic fascia has been divided. In these situations the lateral pelvic fascia and neurovascular bundle can be isolated, ligated, and divided under direct vision, out at the apex of the prostate lateral to the urethra (Fig. 53–16A). Next, the lateral pelvic fascia can be divided posterior to the neurovascular bundle on the posterolateral surface of the rectum. Once again this can be performed under direct vision, with the dissection terminating at the tip of the seminal vesicle, at which point the neurovascular bundle is again ligated and divided (Fig. 53–16B). In this way the neurovascular bundle and lateral pelvic fascia can be excised under direct vision in a more complete way than previously possible. Once this has been accomplished, the rectum is dissected

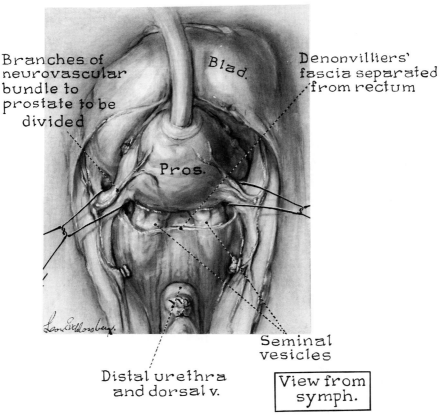

Branches of neurovascular bundle to prostate to be divided

Blad.

Denonvilliers' fascia separated from rectum

Pros.

Distal urethra and dorsal v.

Seminal vesicles

View from symph.

Figure 53–14. The attachment between the rectum and Denonvilliers' fascia has been divided in the midline posteriorly, exposing the posterior surface of the seminal vesicles. The plane between the lateral edges of the seminal vesicles and the overlying pelvic fascia has been developed, thus enabling the lateral pedicles to be divided on the lateral surface of the seminal vesicles near their junction with the prostate by using interrupted 2-0 silk sutures. Illustrated as viewed from the symphysis pubis.

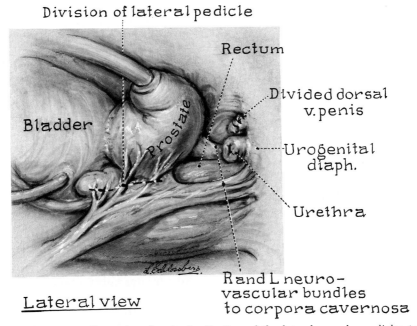

Division of lateral pedicle

Rectum

Divided dorsal v. penis

Bladder

Prostate

Urogenital diaph.

Urethra

R and L neurovascular bundles to corpora cavernosa

Lateral view

Figure 53–15. A lateral view illustrating the site for ligation of the lateral vascular pedicles to the prostate, alongside the seminal vesicles and anterior to the neurovascular bundles. After Walsh PC: Radical retropubic prostatectomy. In PC Walsh, et al (eds), Campbell's Urology, 5th ed. Philadelphia, WB Saunders, 1986, pp 2754–2775.

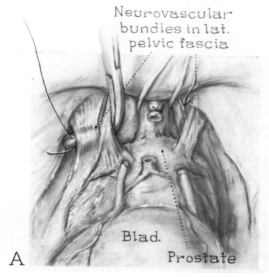

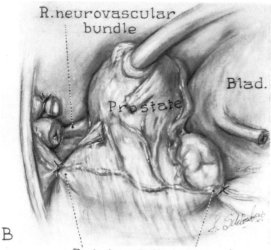

Figure 53–16. Steps in wide excision of the lateral pelvic fascia and neurovascular bundle. A, Ligature placed around lateral pelvic fascia and neurovascular bundle at apex of prostate lateral to urethra. B, Points of division of neurovascular bundle at apex and tip of seminal vesicle. Lateral pelvic fascia will be divided posterior to neurovascular bundle on lateral surface of rectum. From Walsh PC: Radical retropubic prostatectomy. In PC Walsh, et al (eds), Campbell's Urology, 5th ed. Philadelphia, WB Saunders, 1986, pp 2754–2775.

free from the posterior surface of the prostate over to the lateral pelvic fascia on the contralateral side. In doing this, the contralateral neurovascular bundle can be clearly delineated and skeletonized, enabling it to be preserved in its entirety. Indeed, it may be necessary only to preserve one neurovascular bundle to preserve potency (see further on). Following a dissection such as this, the excised specimen demonstrates abundant soft tissue covering the lesion (Fig. 53–17A), wide excision of all soft tissue on the ipsilateral side of the rectum, and preservation of the contralateral neurovascular bundle (Fig. 53–17B).

Division of the Bladder Neck and Excision of the Seminal Vesicles

At this point in the procedure the prostate has been mobilized almost completely. The anesthesiologist is requested to give the patient an ampule of indigo carmine dye to aid later in identification of the ureteral orifices. The bladder neck is incised anteriorly at the prostatovesicular junction (Fig. 53–18). The anterior fibromuscular stroma of the prostate contains little or no glandular tissue, and for this reason there should be little fear that tumor is present at this site. The incision is

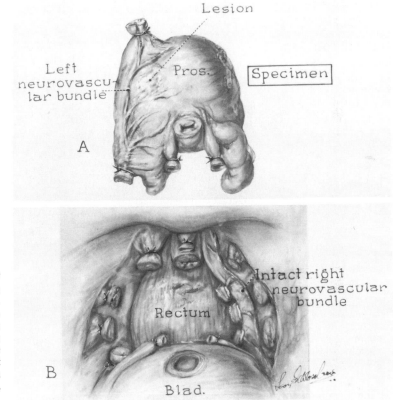

Figure 53–17. Appearance of radical prostatectomy specimen (A) and operative field (B) following unilateral complete excision of lateral pelvic fascia and neurovascular bundle. From Walsh PC: Radical retropubic prostatectomy. In PC Walsh, et al (eds), Campbell's Urology, 5th ed. Philadelphia, WB Saunders, 1986, pp 2754–2775.

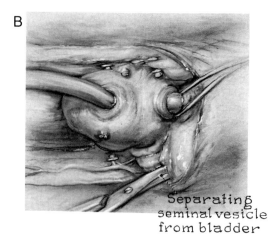

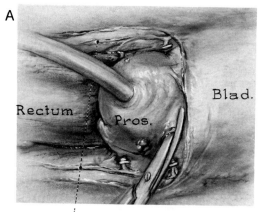

Figure 53–18. Technique for division of the bladder neck. A, The bladder neck is incised anteriorly. B, The lateral fascia and pedicles overlying the seminal vesicles have been fully divided. This facilitates identification of the plane between the bladder and seminal vesicles at the level of the prostatovesicular junction and avoids inadvertent dissection within the layers of the trigone. C, An Allis clamp is used to elevate the posterior bladder neck during dissection of the plane between the posterior bladder wall and the seminal vesicles, exposing the vasa deferentia and seminal vesicles.

carried down to the mucosa, the mucosa is incised, the Foley balloon is deflated, and the two ends of the catheter are clamped together to provide traction. The mucosa overlying the posterior bladder neck is next incised, and the plane between the posterior bladder wall and seminal vesicles is developed. Care must be taken to avoid inadvertent dissection within the layers of the trigone, resulting in ureteral injury. The correct plane of dissection can often be identified laterally, especially if the prostatic pedicles have been fully divided (Fig. 53–18). In this case, it is fairly easy to develop a lateral plane between the bladder and seminal vesicles at the level of the prostatovesicular junction. Once this has been accomplished, the vasa deferentia are divided in the midline and the seminal vesicles are dissected free from surrounding structures (Fig. 53–18). Residual vascular pedicles along the lateral surface of the seminal vesicles are divided and ligated, facilitating exposure of the tips of the seminal vesicles. Previously, the lateral pedicles to the prostate were divided on the lateral surface of the seminal vesicles near their junction with the prostate. Thus, during the process of dissecting out the seminal vesicles, they will be located in a pocket formed by the posterior wall of the bladder and the lateral pelvic fascia with the neurovascular bundle. Care should be exercised not to damage the neurovascular bundles during this step in the operation. As the tips of the seminal vesicles are dissected free, the small arterial branch at the tip of each seminal vesicle should be identified, divided, and ligated. Any residual attachments of Denonvilliers' fascia are divided, and the specimen is removed. The specimen is inspected carefully to identify any area in which the margin of resection is uncertain. If such a region is found, biopsies of the adjacent area or wider resection is indicated. The bulldog clamps are removed, and the operative site is inspected carefully for bleeding. Small bleeding vessels on the neurovascular bundle should not be cauterized for fear of coagulating the fine nerve bundles. Bleeding from these small vessels usually ceases spontaneously.

Bladder Neck Closure and Anastomosis

The bladder neck is reconstructed using interrupted sutures of 2-0 chromic catgut to approximate full thickness mucosa and muscularis. The efflux of indigo carmine from the ureteral orifices is noted while the sutures are placed; ureteral catheters are seldom necessary. This is usually accomplished by reapproximating the posterolateral margins of the bladder neck on both sides (Fig. 53–19). Care is taken to include the posterior vesical musculature that may have been dissected off the posterior wall of the bladder during excision of the seminal vesicles. The bladder neck is narrowed until it is approximately the diameter of the fifth finger. With interrupted 4-0 chromic catgut sutures, the mucosa of the bladder is advanced over the raw mus-

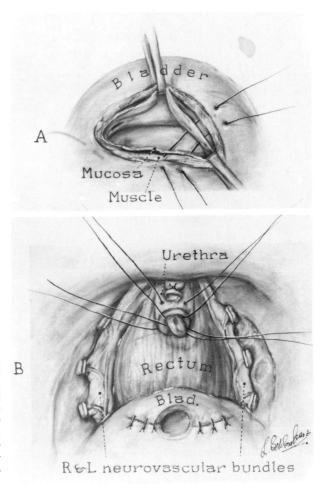

Figure 53–19. *A, The bladder neck is closed with 2-0 chromic catgut. The closure is performed at the posterolateral margins of the bladder neck bilaterally. B, The vesicourethral anastomosis is performed by using 2-0 chromic catgut sutures on ⅝-circle tapered needles. Note that the sutures in the distal urethra do not penetrate the skeletal musculature of the external sphincter. From Walsh PC: Radical retropubic prostatectomy. In PC Walsh, et al (eds), Campbell's Urology, 5th ed. Philadelphia, WB Saunders, 1986, pp 2754–2775.*

cular edges of the bladder neck and sutured to the perivesical fascia (Fig. 53–20). In this way, a nice rosette of mucosa is present at the bladder neck. When the urethral anastomosis is completed, this rosette should permit accurate coaptation of the bladder neck mucosa to the urethral mucosa, thus avoiding a bladder neck contracture.

For cases in which the bladder neck has been resected more widely, the "tennis racket" closure may be used (Fig. 53–20). The closure is initiated in the midline by using a running or interrupted 2-0 chromic catgut suture approximating full thickness layers of the bladder (Fig. 53–20). The closure proceeds anteriorly until the bladder neck is once again narrowed to approxi-

mately the diameter of the fifth finger. The mucosal edges are again advanced over the raw bladder neck edges with interrupted 4-0 chromic catgut suture material (Fig. 53–20). The second layer of the closure is accomplished by approximating the lateral bladder fascia in the midline with interrupted 2-0 chromic catgut sutures (Fig. 53–21). Utilizing the bladder fascia for this closure avoids the risk of inadvertent injury to the ureters, which are located more medially in the bladder musculature. A new Foley catheter (No. 20 French, 5 ml balloon) is placed through the urethra, with the tip positioned just inside the pelvis (Figs. 53–19 and 53–21). The edges of the urethra can be visualized more easily if a silk ligature is

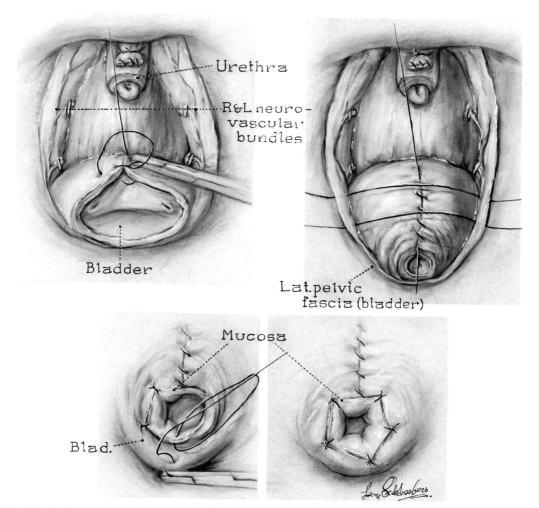

Figure 53–20. "Tennis racket" technique for bladder neck closure. In the upper drawings the closure is initiated in the midline by using a running interrupted 2-0 chromic catgut suture approximating full thickness layers of the bladder. In the lower drawings the bladder mucosa is advanced over the raw bladder neck edges by using interrupted 4-0 chromic catgut suture material.

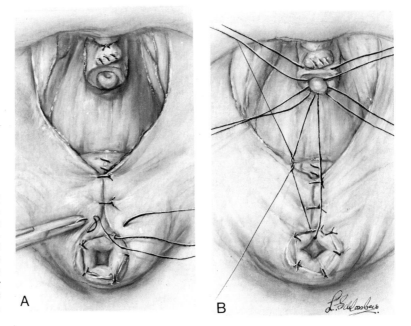

Figure 53–21. A, The second layer of the closure is accomplished by approximating the lateral bladder fascia in the midline, using interrupted 2-0 chromic catgut sutures. B, Five sutures have been placed in the distal urethra. The posterior midline suture at 6 o'clock has been placed in the bladder neck.

placed through the holes in the catheter and the catheter is pulled back and forth through the distal end of the urethra, facilitating identification of the urethral mucosa for more accurate placement of sutures. In addition, a sponge stick is used to displace the rectum posteriorly. Using a 2-0 chromic catgut suture on a ⅝ circle tapered needle, the surgeon reapproximates the bladder neck to the urethra with five sutures (one o'clock, five o'clock, six o'clock, seven o'clock, and 11 o'clock) (Fig. 53–21). Initially, the two anterior sutures (one o'clock and 11 o'clock) are placed by passing the needle from inside the urethral lumen alongside the catheter to the outside of the urethral stump without incorporating the striated pelvic floor musculature. If the sutures are placed deep in the pelvic floor musculature, they may damage the branches of the pelvic plexus to the corpora cavernosa as they travel laterally through the striated musculature to innervate the corpora cavernosa. With traction on the two anterior sutures and with downward displacement on the sponge stick, it is usually quite easy to place the two posterior sutures. At this point, care should be taken to avoid incorporation of the neurovascular bundles into these two sutures. Next, a final suture is placed at six o'clock from outside the urethra to the inside. The needle on this suture is then passed through the bladder neck posteriorly from inside to outside. The other four sutures must be placed in their

corresponding positions in the bladder neck, using a separate needle.

After the five sutures are placed, the balloon and the valve on the catheter are tested, the catheter is positioned in the bladder, and the sutures are tied. The right posterior and anterior sutures are tied initially. Next, the midline posterior suture is tied. One should not attempt to tie this suture initially, because there is little fascia in the urethra posteriorly and the suture will become dislodged. Finally, the two sutures on the left are tied. The balloon is then inflated with 15 ml of saline, and the catheter is irrigated. Small suction catheters are placed, the operative site is irrigated vigorously with saline, and the incision is closed with absorbable sutures and skin clips. The catheter is carefully taped to the thigh.

POSTOPERATIVE MANAGEMENT

The postoperative recovery of men who undergo radical retropubic prostatectomy is usually quite smooth, and the patients ambulate immediately. Intravenous fluids are administered until the patients can tolerate fluid intake by mouth. This usually occurs on the first or second postoperative day. The closed suction tubes are left in place until they cease to function, usually on the third or fourth postoperative day. Occasionally, patients will have moderate amounts of urinary leakage for seven to 10 days. This usually is of no consequence. Patients are discharged from the hospital with a Foley catheter in place, ordinarily within 7 to 10 days, and return three weeks after the procedure for removal of the catheter. Initially, most patients have significant amounts of stress incontinence. This usually resolves within the first or second postoperative month.

COMPLICATIONS

Radical retropubic prostatectomy is a procedure that is well tolerated with minimal morbidity and a low mortality rate (0 to 1.7%). The complications can be divided into those occuring intraoperatively, early in the postoperative period, and late.

Intraoperative Complications

The most common intraoperative problem during radical retropubic prostatectomy is hemorrhage, usually arising from venous structures. This may occur during the pelvic lymphadenectomy if one of the branches of the hypogastric vein is inadvertently torn. Venous injury such as this should be repaired with cardiovascular silk sutures. Hemorrhage also can occur during the incision in the endopelvic fascia if the incision is made too close to the prostate, during division of the puboprostatic ligaments if the ligaments are not dissected free from the superficial branch of the dorsal vein, and during exposure of the apex of the prostate with transection of the dorsal vein complex. However, if one understands fully the anatomy of the dorsal vein complex, this bleeding is usually satisfactorily controlled once the dorsal vein has been ligated and divided. It is imperative to obtain excellent hemostasis before the apex of the prostate is approached so that the anatomy can be viewed in a bloodless field. Most often, blood loss during the procedure occurs gradually from venous back bleeding, resulting in an average accumulated loss of one to three units. This loss can be reduced by temporary occlusion of the hypogastric arteries by means of bulldog clamps and through the use of spinal or epidural anesthesia.[15] Less common complications include injury to the

obturator nerve during the pelvic lymph node dissection, rectal injury, and ureteral injury. If the obturator nerve is inadvertently severed, an attempt should be made at reanastomosis using very fine nonabsorbable sutures. Rectal injury is an infrequent but serious complication that may occur during dissection at the apex of the prostate and when the plane between the rectum and Denonvilliers' fascia is developed. The rectum should be closed in two layers after the edges of the incision have been freshened. It seems wise to interpose omentum between the rectal injury and the vesicourethral anastomosis to reduce the possibility of a vesicourethral fistula. At the conclusion of the procedure the anal sphincter should be dilated widely. In addition, it is probably judicious to perform a proximal diverting colostomy. Ureteral injuries occur secondary to inadvertent dissection within the layers of the trigone while attempts are being made to identify the proper cleavage plane between the bladder and seminal vesicles. If this occurs, ureteral reimplantation should be undertaken.

Early Postoperative Complications

Thrombophlebitis and pulmonary embolism are two of the most common and potentially serious complications of the procedure. Thrombophlebitis has been reported to occur in 3 to 12% of patients and pulmonary emboli in 2 to 5%. Some authors have advocated postoperative anticoagulation, achieved by the use of either warfarin sodium[10] or minidose heparin. However, the efficacy of minidose heparin has yet to be established, and it appears to be associated with an increase in the incidence of prolonged lymphatic drainage or lymphocele formation.[2] My own approach to the prevention of thrombophlebitis has been careful attention both intraoperatively and postoperatively to avoid venous stasis. Intraoperatively, patients are placed in the Trendelenburg position to provide adequate venous drainage of the lower extremities. Postoperatively, patients are made to walk about on the first postoperative day, they are encouraged to perform dorsiflexion exercise 100 times every hour while awake, and for three to four weeks postoperatively they are not permitted to sit with their legs in the dependent position. Utilizing these measures, we have achieved an incidence of pulmonary emboli of less than 1% in over 300 consecutive cases.

Disruption of the urethrovesical anastomosis can be a disastrous complication that may lead to permanent incontinence. This occurs most frequently when the Foley catheter is inadvertently removed in the early postoperative period. To avoid this complication, the balloon and valve on the catheter should be tested immediately before the catheter is placed in the bladder. Some authors have advocated making a small cystotomy incision, passing a nylon suture through the eye of the catheter, and tying the suture over a button on the anterior abdominal wall. The catheter should be taped carefully to the thigh, and the anchorage of the catheter should be examined each postoperative day. If the catheter does inadvertently fall out prematurely, we usually make one attempt to pass a catheter of smaller caliber into the bladder. If this is not successful on the first attempt, the patient undergoes cystoscopy, and the catheter is placed under direct vision.

Late Postoperative Complications

Contracture of the bladder neck has been reported to occur in 3 to 12% of cases. It is usually caused by poor mucosa-to-mucosa apposition of the bladder to the urethra at the time of the anastomosis, but it can also be caused by overzealous reconstruction of the bladder neck. Patients with bladder neck contracture usually complain of a dribbling stream, but at times it may be difficult to make the diagnosis if the patient's only complaint is overflow incontinence. In any patient who complains of incontinence, a catheter should always be passed to make certain that there is no obstruction or significant residual urine. Bladder neck contractures usually respond to one or two dilations. If this fails, I have found that dilation under anesthesia with injection of triamcinolone acetonide (200 mg) directly into the area of the stricture has been beneficial in permanently resolving this complication.

Fortunately, urinary incontinence is an infrequent complication of radical retropubic prostatectomy, occurring in 0 to 4% of reported series. However, incontinence is more frequent when a pubectomy is performed[13] or when vest sutures are utilized.[8] There are several mechanisms of urinary continence in men: the vesical neck, the passive urethral mechanism, and the external sphincter–pelvic floor mechanism. All passive mechanisms, such as the bladder neck and the intrinsic urethral mechanism, are most effective when elevated by the tonic activity of the pelvic floor.[6] In patients who are incontinent after radical prostatectomy, the cause in many cases can be related to rigidity of the remaining posterior urethra and nonelevation of the bladder base after voluntary cessation of urination.[6] Consequently, to achieve continence after radical retropubic prostatectomy, it is mandatory to avoid injury to the pelvic floor mechanism, to reconstruct the vesical neck so that it will provide a passive mechanism of continence, and to coapt the bladder neck to the urethra accurately to avoid stricture formation.

PRESERVATION OF POTENCY

For years it was assumed that most if not all patients who underwent radical prostatectomy would be impotent postoperatively. For this reason, many patients and their physicians selected less effective forms of treatment. However, the etiology of impotence following radical prostatectomy was unclear. For this reason we undertook a study of the etiology of impotence following radical prostatectomy and concluded that impotence results from injury to the pelvic nerve plexus that provides autonomic innervation to the corpora cavernosa.[18] Based on these anatomic studies, it appeared that injury to the pelvic plexus occurred in at least two ways: (1) at the time of apical dissection with transection of the urethra and the adjacent lateral pelvic fascia through which the branches to the corpora cavernosa travel and (2) during division of the lateral pelvic fascia and lateral pedicle. These conclusions led to the minor modifications of the procedure that have been outlined in great detail in this chapter. This modified technique of radical retropubic prostatectomy has now been utilized in operations on over 300 men between the ages of 34 and 72 years with Stages A and B adenocarcinoma of the prostate. Follow-up evaluation of three months or longer has been published on the first 64 consecutive men who were potent preoperatively and who had sexual partners.[20] At three and six months after surgery, 30 to 40% of patients were potent. At nine months postoperatively, 60% were potent, and after one year 86% of patients experienced the return of sexual function. The gradual return of sexual function in this group of patients is similar to the pattern for the return of potency in patients following pelvic fracture with urethral injury and suggests that surgical manipulation may induce temporary nerve injury that necessitates regeneration. The major determinant in return of sexual function is the clinical and pathologic stage of the disease. In patients with low-stage disease (A_2, B_1N, and B_1) the return of sexual function at one year was 92 to 100%. This was distinctly greater than in patients with Stage B_2 lesions, in whom only 50% of patients were potent by one year. These data suggest that in more advanced lesions attempts at excision of all tumor resulted in injury to the neurovascular bundles. In all surgical procedures, every attempt was made to excise all tumor, and there is no evidence that this procedure, when performed correctly, compromises the adequacy of the removal of the cancer.

The development of the nerve-sparing technique for radical retropubic prostatectomy was originally based upon sound anatomic and pathologic principles. First, it was recognized that the branches of the pelvic plexus to the corpora cavernosa travel outside the capsule of the prostate and outside Denonvilliers' fascia.[18] Second, it was determined that the neurovascular bundles travel within the leaves of the lateral pelvic fascia and that during standard radical perineal prostatectomy the lateral pelvic fascia was reflected off the prostate in an effort to avoid injury to the dorsal vein of the penis and Santorini's plexus.[19, 23] Thus, it must be recognized that the excellent long-term control of disease that has been reported following radical perineal prostatectomy (control of both local and distant metastases) has been achieved without routine resection of the lateral pelvic fascia and neurovascular bundles. Indeed, originally we examined prostatic specimens removed by the standard radical perineal technique, the standard radical retropubic technique, and the

nerve-sparing modification to determine the amount of periprostatic tissue and skeletal muscle that was removed.[19] These findings confirmed the anatomic observations and suggested that there was less periprostatic tissue and skeletal muscle removed with the radical perineal technique than with either retropubic approach. Also, based upon the descriptions of radical retropubic prostatectomy that are available in standard textbooks, there is no evidence that the neurovascular bundles were completely resected during the retropubic approach either.[12, 14,] Instead, the neurovascular bundles were inadvertently and unknowingly injured during apical dissection of the prostate, transection of the urethra, and mobilization of the prostate from the rectum with division of the lateral pelvic fascia and ligation of the lateral pedicles. These portions of the procedure were often performed rather blindly and bluntly without precise identification and resection of the neurovascular bundles located posterolaterally. During the nerve-sparing technique, all of these structures are clearly visualized and depending on the findings at surgery, a deliberate decision can be made as to whether the structures can be preserved or must be resected widely with the specimen. Based upon this knowledge, the entire neurovascular bundle can be resected, if necessary, by dividing the fascia and enclosed neurovascular bundle lateral to the urethra and resecting the fascia lateral to the rectum. In this way, a wider margin of resection can be achieved. Furthermore, the amount of periprostatic tissue removed by any of the techniques of radical prostatectomy is markedly limited. It must be remembered that the prostate is located deep in the pelvis and is surrounded by many vulnerable structures such as the urogenital diaphragm, pelvic side wall, rectum, bladder neck, and trigone, which limit true "radical" removal of the prostate. Recently, we published an extensive anatomic evaluation of the male pelvis that focused on the relationships between the prostate, neurovascular bundles, and surrounding structures.[9] Careful scrutiny of the whole-mount cross sections examined in this study demonstrates that at many sites the true surgical margins surrounding the prostate are only 1 to 2 mm from the gland. The term radical in cancer surgery usually refers to any operation that removes several centimeters of clinically uninvolved tissue around the evident tumor. Because radical prostatectomy often provides only 1 or 2 mm of such tissue, it might be more appropriate to call all of these operations total prostatectomies rather than radical prostatectomies because of the scant amount of adjacent tissue that can be removed. We have recently evaluated the pathologic findings in the first 100 consecutive patients who underwent a radical retropubic prostatectomy in which the neurovascular bundles were accurately identified and were preserved or sacrificed, depending upon the findings intraoperatively. In the first 100 patients the surgical margins of resection were positive in only seven patients, and in all of them there was extensive periprostatic involvement by tumor; in five of the seven there was involvement of the seminal vesicles, and in none of the seven were the surgical margins positive only at the site of the nerve-sparing modification. Based upon these findings there is no indication that the modified surgical procedure compromises the adequacy of the removal of the cancer, which is determined primarily by the extent of the tumor rather than the operative technique.

Utilizing the anatomic approach to radical prostatectomy outlined in this chapter, one should be able to avoid unnecessary injury to the lateral pelvic fascia at the level of the distal urethra and to make an informed decision about the extent of resection of the lateral pelvic fascia and lateral pedicles of the prostate. In performing all procedures, the primary goal of surgery is to remove all tumor. Potency is of secondary concern. It is not clear how often patients will be potent if the neurovascular bundle is sacrificed on one side. In my limited experience at this time, several patients in whom the neurovascular bundle was sacrificed on one side are potent. In patients undergoing radical extirpation of tumors of the sacrum it has been shown that sacrificing the sacral nerve routes on one side does not affect sexual performance adversely.[5] With further experience it may be possible with confidence to sacrifice the neurovascular bundles more often on one side and thus widen the margins of excision. The primary goal should be reduction in the morbidity of radical prostatectomy without reducing its efficacy as the most effective form of treatment for localized prostatic cancer. It is hoped that these efforts will encourage more urologists to take a greater interest in offering this option to the young, healthy, sexually active patient, who is often the ideal candidate for the procedure.

References

1. Albers DD, Faulkner KK, Cheatham WN, et al: Surgical anatomy of the pubovesical (puboprostatic) ligaments. J Urol 109:388–392, 1973.
2. Catalona WJ, Kadmon D, Crane DB: Effect of minidose heparin on lymphocele formation following extraperitoneal pelvic lymphadenectomy. J Urol 123:890–892, 1980.
3. Eggleston JC, Walsh PC: Radical prostatectomy with preservation of sexual function: pathological findings in the first 100 cases. J Urol 134:1146–1148, 1985.
4. Flocks RH: Arterial distribution within prostate gland: its role in transurethral prostatic resection. J Urol 37:524–548, 1937.
5. Gunterberg B, Petersen I: Sexual function after major resections of the sacrum with bilateral or unilateral sacrifice of sacral nerves. Fertil Steril 27:1146–1153, 1976.
6. Hinman F: Male incontinence: relationship of physiology to surgery. J Urol 115:274–276, 1976.
7. Jewett HJ, Eggleston JC, Yawn DH: Radical prostatectomy in the management of carcinoma of the prostate: probable causes of some therapeutic failures. J Urol 107:1034–1040, 1972.
8. Kopecky AA, Laskowski TZ, Scott R Jr.: Radical retropubic prostatectomy in the treatment of prostatic carcinoma. J Urol 103:641–644, 1970.
9. Lepor H, Gregerman M, Crosby R, et al: Precise localization of the autonomic nerves from the pelvic plexus to the corpora cavernosa: a detailed anatomical study of the adult male pelvis. J Urol 133:207–212, 1985.
10. Lieskovsky G, Skinner DG: Technique of radical retropubic prostatectomy with limited pelvic node dissection. Urol Clin North Am 10:187–198, 1983.
11. Lue TF, Zeineh SJ, Schmidt RA, Tanagho EA: Neuroanatomy of penile erection: its relevance to iatrogenic impotence. J Urol 131:273–280, 1984.
12. McLaughlin AP III: Radical retropubic prostatectomy. In JH Harrison, RF Gittes, AD Perlmutter, et al (eds), Campbell's Urology, 4th ed. Philadelphia, WB Saunders, 1979, pp 2315–2326.
13. Middleton AW Jr: A comparison of the morbidity associated with radical retropubic prostatectomy with and without pubectomy. J Urol 117:202–205, 1977.
14. Peters PC: Radical retropubic prostatectomy. In JF Glenn (ed), Urologic Surgery, 3rd ed. Philadelphia, JB Lippincott, 1983, pp 949–955.
15. Peters CA, Walsh PC: Blood transfusion and anesthetic practices in radical retropubic prostatectomy. J Urol 134:81–83, 1985.
16. Reiner WG, Walsh PC: An anatomical approach to the surgical management of the dorsal vein and Santorini's plexus during radical retropubic surgery. J Urol 121:198–200, 1979.
17. Walsh PC: Radical retropubic prostatectomy and cystoprostatectomy: surgical technique for preser-

vation of sexual function. A film produced by Aegis Productions Inc, New York, NY, and distributed by Norwich Eaton Pharmaceuticals, Norwich, NY, 1984.

18. Walsh PC, Donker PJ: Impotence following radical prostatectomy: insight into etiology and prevention. J Urol 128:492–497, 1982.

19. Walsh PC, Lepor H, Eggleston JC: Radical prostatectomy with preservation of sexual function: anatomical and pathological considerations. Prostate 4:473–485, 1983.

20. Walsh PC, Mostwin JL: Radical prostatectomy and cystoprostatectomy with preservation of potency: results using a new nerve-sparing technique. Br J Urol 56:694–697, 1984.

21. Weyrauch HM: Surgery of the Prostate. Philadelphia, WB Saunders, 1959, p 27.

22. Whitmore WF Jr: Interstitial I-125 implantation in the management of localized prostatic cancer. In KH Kurth, FMJ deBruyne, FH Schroeder, et al (eds), Progress and Controversies in Oncological Urology. New York, Alan R Liss, 1984, pp 513–527.

23. Young HH, Davis DM: Young's Practice of Urology, Vol 2. Philadelphia, WB Saunders, 1926, pp 463–466.

PHILLIP G. WISE, M.D.
PETER T. SCARDINO, M.D.

Thoracoabdominal Retroperitoneal Lymphadenectomy for Testicular Cancer

CHAPTER 54

The role of retroperitoneal lymph node dissection (RLND) in the management of testicular cancer remains controversial. With the availability of dramatically effective chemotherapy, many physicians abandoned the operation in all but a few selected patients, recommending expectant management after orchiectomy for those without evidence of metastases and combination chemotherapy for all others. Lymph node dissection was reserved for the removal of any residual retroperitoneal mass after intensive chemotherapy. Recently, however, the wisdom of surveillance has been questioned because of reports of high relapse rates (especially among patients in certain high-risk groups), late relapsers (three years or more after orchiectomy), high-stage disease at relapse (resulting in possible preventable deaths due to cancer), and resistance of teratoma to chemotherapy (necessitating eventual surgical resection despite chemotherapy). Furthermore, refinements in the technique of RLND for patients with low-stage disease allow preservation of the sympathetic nerves responsible for ejaculation and emission in most patients, whereas essentially all of the nodes at risk of harboring metastases can be removed.

In this chapter we will describe the history of the development of RLND, the rationale for its use in staging and therapy, the current indications for the operation, the margins of the dissection we now use for patients with negative and positive nodes intraoperatively, and the complications and results of the operation, illustrating in detail our modified technique for left thoracoabdominal RLND for low-stage (A and B_1) tumors.

HISTORICAL DEVELOPMENTS

Following the early work of Most in 1898[25] and Cuneo and Marcille in 1901,[4] Jamieson and Dobson[13] mapped the lumbar nodes in what has become the classic description of testicular lymphatic drainage. By injecting dye into the testicles of stillborn fetuses, they determined that the primary sites of drainage from the right testicle are interaortocaval, preaortic, and precaval nodes, and from the left testicle drainage sites are the left para-aortic and preaortic nodes. Despite this information, retroperitoneal lymphadenectomy was not employed routinely for treatment of testicular tumors until 1948, when Lewis reported 192 operations without a single mortality[19] and later noted a five-year survival rate of 46% among 28 patients with nonseminomatous tumors

779

treated by orchiectomy, retroperitoneal lymphadenectomy, and radiation therapy.[20]

Cooper, Leadbetter, and Chute[2] developed the thoracoabdominal approach to retroperitoneal lymphadenectomy because of the wide exposure of the primary lymph nodes near the renal hilum. Thoracoabdominal RLND was further refined by Skinner and Leadbetter,[40] who in 1971 reported a series of 58 consecutive cases without an operative mortality and a survival rate of 90% if the nodes were negative and 56% if the nodes were positive.

The transabdominal approach was popularized by Mallis and Patton,[24] Staubitz,[44] and Whitmore[48] but was insufficient for gross or suprahilar nodal disease until refined by Donohue, who developed an extended bilateral suprahilar node dissection using a transperitoneal midline incision with full mobilization of the pancreas.[6] Basing his conclusions on this extended dissection in 100 patients, Donohue definitively mapped the distribution of retroperitoneal nodal metastases in patients with grossly negative (Stage B_1), grossly positive (Stage B_2), and massive (Stage B_3) left- and right-sided tumors (Fig. 54–1).[9] This landmark work provided the data for rational modifications of the dissection appropriate to the extent of each patient's disease.

The stimulus for such modifications arises from concern about the loss of ejaculation which often results from standard retroperitoneal lymphadenectomy.[12] But the operation can be modified to preserve the nerves responsible for emission and ejaculation[10, 18, 32, 36] (Fig. 54–2) while still removing the nodes at high risk of harboring metastases (Fig. 54–3).

The low morbidity and mortality of the operation, its efficacy in staging and in controlling retroperitoneal metastases, and the likelihood of preserving fertility in patients with low-stage disease suggest that retroperitoneal lymph node dissection will continue to play an important role in the management of early stage nonseminomatous testicular cancer.

RATIONALE FOR RETROPERITONEAL DISSECTION

Retroperitoneal lymph node dissection is not simply a staging procedure but is thera-

peutic as well. There are many reasons why the operation remains an integral part of the modern management of nonseminomatous tumors.

Staging
(Table 54–1)

In nonseminomatous testicular cancer, the retroperitoneal lymph nodes are the first site of metastases in nearly 90% of patients. If the nodes are negative, only 7% to 15% of patients will subsequently relapse, invariably outside the field of dissection, indicating that the first site of metastatic disease lay elsewhere.[7, 10, 21, 32, 39, 44, 48] Retroperitoneal nodal metastases are most accurately detected by systematic, complete dissection. The most sensitive modern staging studies fail to detect nodal metastases in 15 to 25% of patients yet are falsely positive in 15 to 20%.[3, 15, 30–33, 35, 43, 45]

The pattern of nodal metastases is variable, so a complete dissection is necessary for accurate identification of nodal metastases.[9, 13, 34] Selective node biopsy exposes the patient to the same operative risk of morbidity and mortality as a thorough dissection but offers limited staging information and no therapeutic efficacy. This approach, recommended by Javadpour,[14] is condemned by virtually all authorities in the field.

Retroperitoneal lymph node dissection is an extensive technical procedure, but in the hands of experienced surgeons it is safe, with rare mortality and minimal morbidity.[8, 38, 41, 48]

And, finally, the status of the retroperitoneal nodes (surgical stage) most accurately indicates the prognosis of patients with early stage disease.[3, 21, 37–39, 42, 48] The relapse rate (without adjuvant chemotherapy) is approximately 10% for pathologic Stage A and 45% for pathologic Stage B tumors,[7, 21, 38, 42, 49] varying from about 25% for pathologic Stage B_1 to 60% for Stage B_2.

Therapy
(Table 54–2)

The therapeutic benefits of retroperitoneal dissection for nonseminomatous testicular cancer have been clearly documented. The operation is not simply a staging procedure. Long-term disease-free survival, before the era of combination chemotherapy, has been

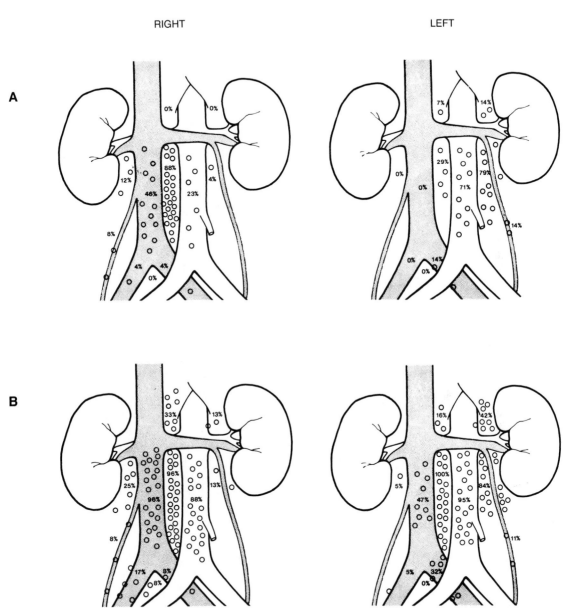

Figure 54–1. Distribution of retroperitoneal nodal metastases in early-stage, nonseminomatous testicular cancer, when the nodes appear grossly negative (A, Stage B₁) and grossly positive (B, Stage B₂) during the operation. Reproduced with permission from Donohue JP, Zachary JM, Maynard BR: Distribution of nodal metastases in nonseminomatous testis cancer. J Urol 128:315–320, 1982, © by Williams & Wilkins, 1982.

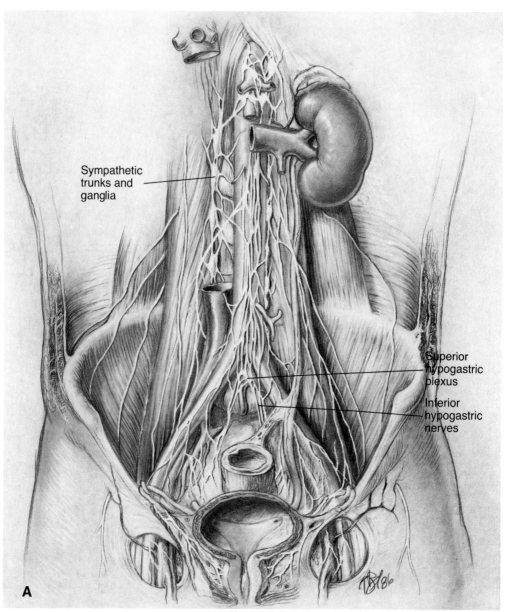

Figure 54–2. *Distribution of sympathetic nerves in the retroperitoneum and pelvis. A, Anterior view of bilateral sympathetic chains and the aortic and hypogastric plexus.*

Illustration continued on opposite page

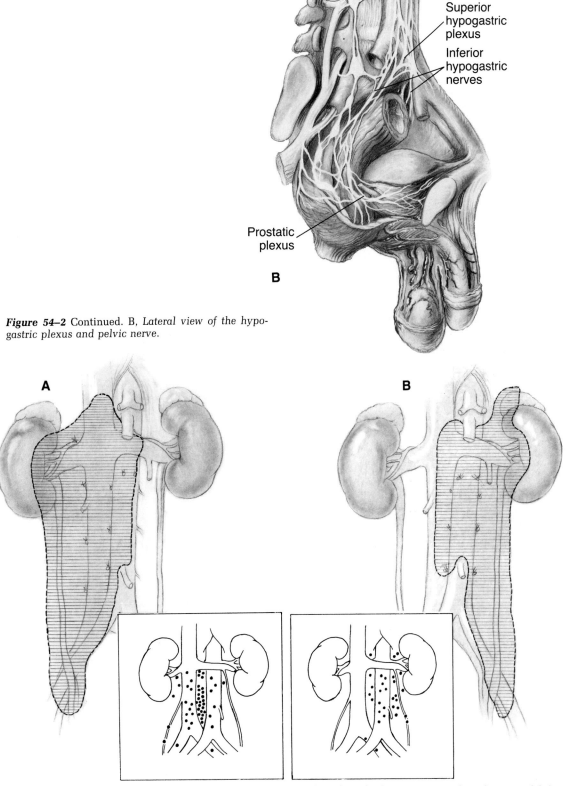

Aortic
plexus

Superior
hypogastric
plexus

Inferior
hypogastric
nerves

Prostatic
plexus

B

Figure 54–2 Continued. B, *Lateral view of the hypo-gastric plexus and pelvic nerve.*

A

B

Figure 54–3. Limits of modified nerve-sparing retroperitoneal lymph node dissection on right side (A) and left side (B) for patients with grossly negative nodes. The dissection is designed to remove all nodes likely to contain metastases (see Fig. 54–1) yet preserve the contralateral sympathetic chain and hypogastric plexus. Insets show margins of dissection overlaid on distribution of nodes in Stage B_1.

Table 54–1. RATIONALE FOR THE USE OF
RLND FOR STAGING

1. RLN are usually the first site of metastases; the retroperitoneum is a difficult site to assess accurately.
2. Nodal metastases are most accurately detected by RLND:
   15 to 25% false-negative clinical results
   15 to 20% false-positive clinical results
3. Pattern of nodal metastases is variable; node biopsy inaccurate.
4. RLND causes low morbidity and rare mortality.
5. Status of RLN most accurately predicts prognosis.

reported in 63% of patients with positive nodes.[48] In testicular cancer, the retroperitoneal nodes are often, therefore, the *only* site of metastases.

Under surveillance, nodal metastases will progress, requiring aggressive treatment.[15, 29, 33, 35, 43] Complete removal of positive nodes facilitates chemotherapy, so relapse rates are extremely low with limited chemotherapy. The Intergroup Testicular Tumor Study compared the results of two three-week cycles of cisplatin, vinblastine, and bleomycin with results of no adjuvant therapy in over 200 patients. With limited adjuvant therapy, the relapse rate was 6% and there was one death; without adjuvant chemotherapy, the relapse rate was 45% and the mortality rate was 5%.

With a properly performed lymph node dissection, retroperitoneal recurrence is rare, occurring in less than 2% of patients with positive nodes.[21, 32, 39, 42, 44, 48] Even then, recurrence is almost always outside the field of dissection.

INDICATIONS

Despite the advantages of RLND, it is a formidable operation. If the operation could be avoided without placing the patient at

Table 54–2. RATIONALE FOR THE USE OF
RLND FOR THERAPY

1. RLN are often the only site of metastases.
2. Most patients with nodal metastases can be cured with RLND alone.
3. The retroperitoneum is a difficult site to monitor for recurrence; retroperitoneal recurrence is rare after RLND.
4. Complete RLND combined with limited adjuvant chemotherapy results in almost uniform cure.

greater risk of death from cancer or subjecting him to even more morbid treatment (such as intensive combination chemotherapy), RLND would soon be abandoned. Although we continue to recommend RLND for most patients with early stage tumors, others favor *surveillance* rather than *RLND* for patients in clinical Stage A and *chemotherapy* rather than *RLND* for those in clinical Stage B (B_1 and B_2).

Surveillance vs. RLND for Clinical Stage A

If a patient is to be considered a candidate for surveillance, he must undergo a rigorous, thorough staging evaluation (Table 54–3). These studies should be performed and interpreted by the most experienced personnel available. Even in centers that specialize in the treatment of testicular cancer, understaging occurs in 20 to 30% and overstaging in 15 to 20% of patients.[3, 15, 31, 33, 35, 39, 43, 45] About 30% of clinical Stage A patients followed in a surveillance program progress to a higher stage; their tumors are understaged initially. Two thirds of these tumors (20%) will progress in the retroperitoneum.[3, 8, 14, 15, 29, 33–35, 41, 43] At the same time, among those patients considered in Stage B, approximately 15 to 20% will have negative nodes if RLND is performed, for a false-positive rate of 15 to 20%.[30, 31, 33] If patients are included who have a CT scan of the abdomen or lymphogram that is equivocal or whose markers fall too slowly or are not monitored sufficiently after orchiectomy (on at least days 2 and 7 postoperatively), the progression rate in a surveillance program will be even higher.[11, 15]

Table 54–3. MINIMUM ESSENTIAL STAGING
STUDIES AND RESULTS NEEDED FOR
CONSIDERING A PATIENT A CANDIDATE
FOR SURVEILLANCE

Procedure	Results
Radical inguinal orchiectomy	Negative margins
Markers (hCG, AFP, LDH)	If elevated, fall to normal at expected half-life
Abdominal CT scan	No suspicious nodes
Chest CT or lung tomograms	No suspicious metastases
Lymphogram	No suspicious nodes

The results of surveillance programs throughout the world consistently show a progression rate of approximately 30% (22 to 44%).[15, 16, 29, 33, 35, 43] Several deaths have occurred in surveillance programs, but the overall results are good, with disease-free survival rates of 98 to 99%, since almost all relapsing patients can be salvaged with intensive combination chemotherapy.

A surveillance program has several advantages. It is certainly attractive to patients and to physicians. It is easy to carry out, and the survival rate is excellent (99%). There is no risk of loss of ejaculation, and the overall morbidity is low *for the patients whose disease does not progress*. Nevertheless, there are also disadvantages. The level of commitment to follow-up for patients and physicians is lower. Meticulous staging is mandatory initially and must include a technically successful lymphogram. The retroperitoneum is the site of relapse in 20% of these patients but is very difficult and somewhat expensive to monitor accurately. Among the patients who relapse and require chemotherapy, many will become infertile; others who require RLND (most will)[33, 43] will lose ejaculation because the margins of dissection must be wider. But perhaps the greatest disadvantage of surveillance is that the tumor may progress to an advanced stage despite careful monitoring, and the patients will then require intensive chemotherapy and, often, surgery as well. Several recent studies report that recurrent tumor is first discovered in an intermediate or advanced stage in more than 80% of the patients.[15, 33, 43] Surveillance, therefore, becomes a *gamble* for the patient, a case of "double or nothing."

On the other hand, retroperitoneal lymph node dissection provides accurate staging and prognostic information and materially affects the need for additional therapy. If the nodes are negative, fewer than 10% of patients will have recurrence, and adjuvant chemotherapy is unnecessary. A retroperitoneal recurrence is unlikely, so monitoring the patient requires only a chest x-ray, measurement of tumor markers, and a careful physical examination. If the nodes are positive, appropriate adjuvant chemotherapy can be given with almost uniformly effective results, or the patient can be monitored with little concern for occult retroperitoneal recurrence. The patient and his physician are fully aware of his prognosis; treatment can be assigned more rationally, and both are committed to regular follow-up. Finally, recent modifications in the technique for retroperitoneal dissection allow virtually complete removal of the nodes at significant risk of harboring metastases but will leave the nerves responsible for ejaculation undisturbed in most patients.[1, 10, 17, 18, 32, 36, 47]

Nevertheless, RLND has a number of disadvantages. The operation provides little therapeutic benefit if the nodes are negative, as they are in 50 to 70% of patients. Some patients (7 to 10%) relapse in spite of a properly performed dissection. Loss of ejaculation and the resulting infertility still occur in some patients even with the modified operation. And most patients, if treated in a surveillance protocol, will not relapse—for them, an operation was truly unnecessary.

Both surveillance and RLND for clinical Stage A patients have disadvantages if applied as a uniform rigid policy. Recently, certain risk factors have been identified (Table 54–4), which allow many patients to be assigned to a group at "high risk" or "low risk" for relapse.[5, 11, 27, 29, 33] Those with teratoma or teratocarcinoma, whose primary tumor is confined to the testis (T1) without vascular or lymphatic invasion, have less than a 10 to 15% risk of relapse and may need no further therapy. Those with embryonal carcinoma (or choriocarcinoma), extension of tumor into the spermatic cord (T4), or with vascular or lymphatic invasion, appear to have a risk of relapse greater than 50% and would seem poor candidates for a surveillance program.

Chemotherapy vs. RLND for Clinical Stage B
(Table 54–5)

Combination chemotherapy is so effective for advanced disease that in some centers patients with limited, readily resectable

Table 54–4. PROGNOSTIC FEATURES FOR CLINICAL STAGE A PATIENTS AT "LOW RISK" AND "HIGH RISK" FOR RELAPSE IN A SURVEILLANCE PROGRAM

Prognostic Feature	Low Risk	High Risk
Cell type	Teratoma	Embryonal carcinoma
Local extent	Confined to testis	Invading cord
Vascular invasion	Absent	Present
Lymphatic invasion	Absent	Present

Table 54–5. COMPARISON OF TREATMENT MODALITIES FOR PATIENTS WITH CLINICAL STAGE B_1 AND B_2 NONSEMINOMATOUS TUMORS*

Treatment	Number of Patients	Patients Undergoing RLND (%)	Patients Undergoing Chemotherapy (%)	Survival Rate (%)
Primary chemotherapy	54	22	100	96
RLND, with or without chemotherapy†	91	100†	52	98

*From Pizzocaro G: Surgery for stage II nonseminomatous testicular cancer. Workshop on Testicular Cancer, University of Copenhagen, Denmark, 1986.

†In this group, 22% were overstaged clinically and had negative lymph nodes at RLND.

Stage B tumors (B_1 and B_2) are treated with chemotherapy initially, reserving RLND for those patients with a retroperitoneal mass after chemotherapy.[23, 27] In this approach testicular cancer is viewed as no different than lymphoma: a systemic disease requiring systemic therapy. Because chemotherapy is so effective, the survival rate is just as good as with the traditional approach of RLND (with or without adjuvant chemotherapy). But to achieve these results, intensive chemotherapy has been used (e.g., four cycles of cisplatin, vinblastine, and bleomycin), with a substantial increase in toxicity compared with that in treatment programs relying on initial RLND. With chemotherapy, all patients are subjected to the substantial morbidity and occasional mortality (1 to 2%) of cisplatin-based combination chemotherapy. Some of these patients (Peckham reports 22%)[28] will need RLND after chemotherapy, when the operation is more difficult and when preservation of ejaculation is rarely possible. And, perhaps most worrisome, is that about 20% of clinical Stage B patients (40% of B_1 and 10% of B_2) are *overstaged*.[31] If RLND is done, these patients will have *negative* nodes and would have been grossly overtreated with a full course of chemotherapy.

With RLND, staging is far more accurate. Adjuvant chemotherapy can be offered on the basis of the status of the nodes, which is the most important prognostic feature for these patients.[37, 42] Two thirds of patients with positive nodes will never relapse after RLND, even if adjuvant chemotherapy is not used.[7, 48] Relapse almost never occurs in the retroperitoneum, which is difficult to monitor accurately, but usually is seen in the lungs, where recurrence can be identified early.[42] Such relapse responds completely to chemotherapy in more than 90% of patients. On the other hand, limited adjuvant chemotherapy after RLND for patients with positive nodes (Stages B_1 and B_2) in the Intergroup Study lowered the relapse rate to 6% and the mortality rate to less than 1%.

We have used limited adjuvant chemotherapy for all patients with positive nodes.[37, 42] Beginning three to four weeks after the operation, as soon as the patient has substantially recovered, we now give two three-week cycles of cisplatin, etoposide (VP-16), and bleomycin.

In summary, intensive chemotherapy results in overtreatment of patients with clinical Stage B_1 and B_2 disease. Although survival rates are excellent, morbidity remains substantially greater than with RLND, with or without adjuvant chemotherapy, in the hands of experienced practitioners. Until less toxic chemotherapy becomes available, or studies demonstrate that less intensive chemotherapy (e.g., two cycles of therapy) is equally effective, we will continue to recommend RLND for patients with clinical Stage B_1 and B_2 tumors.

MARGINS OF DISSECTION

The margins of RLND can be based logically on the known pattern of lymphatic drainage from the testis and the consequent distribution of nodal metastases from left- and right-sided primary tumors. A meticulous, thorough removal of all node-bearing tissue within the appropriate boundaries results in a very low incidence of relapse in the retroperitoneum and provides highly accurate prognostic information on which to base a decision regarding adjuvant chemotherapy.[38, 39, 49]

Distribution of Nodal Metastases

Donohue has performed the definitive investigation of the distribution of nodal metastases, relating the nodal distribution to the extent of tumor apparent to the surgeon at the time of the operation (Fig. 54–1).[9] After 275 extended bilateral retroperitoneal dissections, Donohue analyzed the distribution of nodal metastases by side and by extent in 100 patients with positive nodes. There were 40 Stage B_1 and 43 Stage B_2 tumors. If the nodes appeared negative intraoperatively (Stage B_1), the most common sites of nodal metastases from right-sided primary tumors were the interaortocaval (88%), precaval (46%), preaortic (23%), and right paracaval (12%) zones. In no case were suprahilar nodes positive, nor were the left para-aortic (4%) or left iliac (4%) nodes positive in the face of negative interaortocaval or paracaval nodes. Hence, a complete dissection within the margins outlined in Figure 54–3A would always correctly stage the patient and would remove 96% (48 out of

50) of the nodes harboring metastases from right-sided tumors.

When the nodes are grossly positive intraoperatively (Stage B_2), a more extensive operation is necessary to completely remove all node-bearing tissue at risk (Fig. 54–1B). The dissection should include both suprahilar regions and the left para-aortic area (Fig. 54–4A).

For left-sided tumors, Donohue found that if the nodes appeared negative on gross inspection (Stage B_1) the predominant areas for metastases were the left para-aortic (79%), preaortic (71%), and interaortocaval (29%) zones. In contradistinction to the dissection for right-sided tumors, the margins for left-sided Stage B_1 tumors must include both suprahilar zones (at least immediately above the right renal artery). Such a dissection for left-sided primary tumors, outlined in Figure 54–3B, would remove 94% (29 out of 31) of the positive nodes in Stage B_1. If the nodes are grossly positive (Stage B_2), then an extended dissection is necessary if all positive nodes are to be removed (Fig. 54–4B). The lower aorta cannot be spared

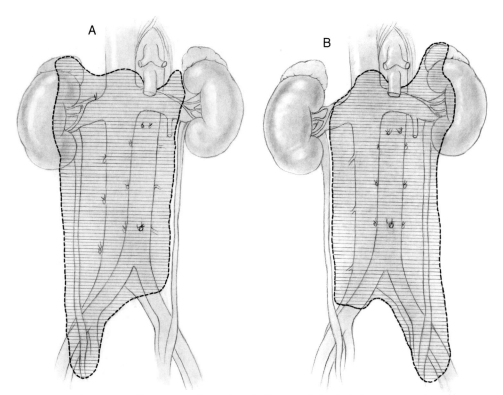

Figure 54–4. Extended limits of dissection for right-sided (A) or left-sided (B) tumor if the nodes are grossly positive (Stage B_2). No attempt at nerve sparing is made. Modified from Scardino PT: Thoracoabdominal retroperitoneal lymphadenectomy for testicular cancer. In ED Crawford, TA Borden (eds), Genitourinary Cancer Surgery. Philadelphia, Lea & Febiger, 1982, pp 271–289, with permission.

without leaving positive nodes in many patients (Fig. 54–1B).

Donohue's findings are consistent with other reports showing that the surgeon's judgment about the presence or absence of positive nodes at the time of the operation is 90% accurate.[10, 17, 32, 34]

Preservation of Ejaculation

Infertility and loss of ejaculation are a major source of concern for patients with testicular cancer and for their physicians. In a disease with greater than 85% cure rates (greater than 95% for early stages), focus on the quality of life, especially reproductive capacity, is natural. With the standard or extended retroperitoneal dissection, permanent dry ejaculation occurs in two thirds or more of patients.[8, 18, 26, 38, 41, 46] Although the neuroanatomy and physiology of ejaculation are not completely understood,[1, 22] several investigators have reported preservation or recovery of ejaculation after modified retroperitoneal dissection.[10, 17, 18, 23, 36] The margins of dissection differ substantially in these reports, however.

Lange[17] recommends preservation of the lumbar sympathetic chains bilaterally, carefully dissecting the tissue overlying them. His dissection extends to the lateral aspect of the contralateral great vessel above the inferior mesenteric artery but remains ipsilateral below it, avoiding the tissue beneath or between the iliac arteries. He reports that 51% of stage A and B₁ patients experienced spontaneous return of ejaculation.[17] Fossa recommends avoiding the suprahilar areas and limiting the dissection to the midaorta for both right- and left-sided tumors. In a series of 36 patients she reported preservation of ejaculation in 78%.[10] But reference to Donohue's study indicates that 29% of positive nodes may lie outside the limits of this dissection for left-sided Stage B₁ tumors. Pizzocaro[32] performs a similar dissection for Stage B₁ with preservation or recovery of ejaculation in 53 (87%) of 61 patients. Here again, the dissection for left-sided tumors does not include the interaortocaval area. This limited dissection appears to result in a relapse rate of approximately 15% for pathologic Stage A, higher than those in series using an extended node dissection.

Which nerves must be preserved if emission and ejaculation are not to be lost? Uni-

lateral lumbar sympathectomy itself seldom disturbs ejaculation. Even bilateral sympathectomy from T12 to L3 leaves nearly half of the patients able to ejaculate.[47] However, resection of the hypogastric plexus in the presacral area between the iliac arteries, the "final common pathway" of sympathetic innervation for contraction of the bladder neck and vasa differentia, invariably results in dry ejaculation.[1]

These considerations have led us to outline the margins of a modified retroperitoneal lymph node dissection that allows removal of 90 to 95% of the nodes at risk of harboring metastases in Stage B₁ tumors while preserving ejaculation in most patients (Fig. 54–3). The interaortocaval nodes are removed for left- and right-sided tumors. Contralateral dissection below the inferior mesenteric artery is limited to several centimeters for left-sided tumors. The contralateral sympathetic chain in the paravertebral groove is preserved in each case, but the ipsilateral chain is taken, since in our experience it has not been feasible to leave the ipsilateral sympathetic chain and remove the node-bearing tissue completely. The tissue anterior and posterior to the aorta below the inferior mesenteric artery and that in the interiliac area is preserved. Note, however, that this dissection is used only if the nodes appear grossly normal during the operation, regardless of the clinical stage preoperatively.

SURGICAL TECHNIQUE

We have previously described in detail our technique of thoracoabdominal RLND.[38, 49] Currently we use this "extended" operation only in patients with positive nodes intraoperatively. In the following section we describe the modified operation we use for those whose nodes appear negative intraoperatively.

Preoperative Preparation

The patient is admitted to the hospital the day before the operation for a complete history and physical examination, hemogram, and evaluation of electrolytes, creatinine, LDH, hCG, and α-fetoprotein levels, as well as a chest x-ray. Two units of packed red blood cells are reserved. The patient is hydrated overnight with 5% dextrose and 0.45% saline plus 20 mEq KCl per 1000 ml at 150 ml/hr. A urethral catheter is inserted after the patient is anesthetized on the morning of the operation.

Position
(Fig. 54–5)

The position of the patient is crucial. After induction of endotracheal anesthesia with the patient in the supine position, he is

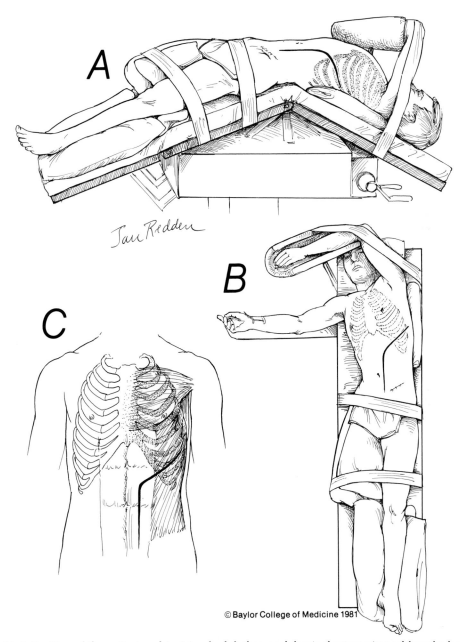

© Baylor College of Medicine 1981

Figure 54–5. Position of the patient and incision for left thoracoabdominal retroperitoneal lymphadenectomy. A, The break in the table is placed directly under the soft tissue of the flank. B, The left arm is elevated on a well-padded Kraus support. C, The midpoint of the incision is on the paramedian line, halfway between the xiphoid and the umbilicus, with arms of equal length extending caudad to the pubic region and laterally over the eighth or ninth rib to the posterior axillary line. From Scardino PT: Thoracoabdominal retroperitoneal lymphadenectomy for testicular cancer. In ED Crawford, TA Borden (eds), Genitourinary Cancer Surgery. Philadelphia, Lea & Febiger, 1982, pp 271–289, with permission.

moved so that his costovertebral angle is over the break in the table. His ipsilateral side is brought flush with the edge of the operating table, and the contralateral leg is flexed 90°. The ipsilateral leg lies straight, over the contralateral ankle, and all pressure points are padded. The hips are nearly flat on the table, but the thorax is rotated approximately 20 to 30° and supported by a small roll. A Kraus arm support, attached to the contralateral side of the table, is used to support the ipsilateral arm, permitting easy adjustments in the position of the table. The contralateral arm is extended on an arm board. Wide adhesive tape is used to secure the patient to the table after it is maximally flexed (hyperextended). The table is tilted in Trendelenburg position until the abdomen is horizontal.

Incision
(Figs. 54–5 and 54–6)

The incision is started over the eighth, ninth, or tenth rib at the posterior axillary line, crosses the costochondral cartilage, and continues toward a point midway between the xiphoid and the umbilicus. Just short of the midline, it is brought inferiorly as a paramedian incision (Fig. 54–5). The subcutaneous tissue and muscles over the rib are incised with electrocautery. The rib is then resected in the standard fashion (Fig. 54–6A). Heavy scissors are used to excise a 1- to 2-cm segment of costochondral carti-

lage (Fig. 54–6B), and the soft tissues are gently spread to identify the peritoneum, which bulges up into the wound, facilitating further development of the retroperitoneal plane (Fig. 54–6C). The rectus abdominis muscle is then divided and retracted laterally after division of the anterior rectus sheath. With electrocautery the external and internal oblique muscles are divided in turn. The transversus abdominis is divided bluntly in the direction of its fibers. The posterior rectus sheath is all that remains over the peritoneum, which is mobilized from it bluntly (Fig. 54–6D).

Mobilization of the Peritoneum
(Fig. 54–7)

A combination of blunt and sharp dissection is used to free the peritoneum from the muscles and fascia of the abdominal wall. The surgeon, with palm facing upwards, uses a sweeping motion of the fingers against the abdominal wall. The peritoneum can be mobilized anteriorly to the linea alba, to which it is firmly adhered.

Next, the peritoneum is mobilized from the diaphragm (Fig. 54–7A). The bed of the resected rib is incised, opening the pleural cavity. The diaphragm is incised in the direction of its fibers as the peritoneum is mobilized from it. The dissection is easier if the assistant places traction anteriorly on the edge of the wound and the surgeon retracts the peritoneum posteriorly and in-

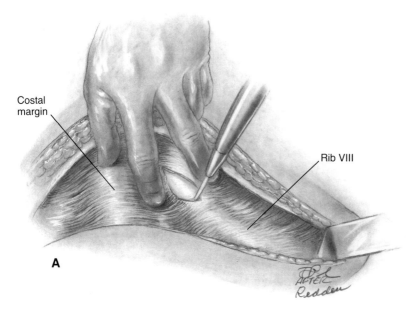

Costal
margin

Rib VIII

A

Figure 54–6. Thoracoabdominal incision: A, Subperiosteal excision of the eighth rib, using the electrocautery.

Illustration continued on opposite page

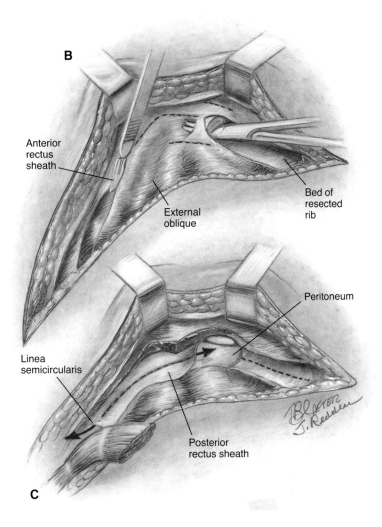

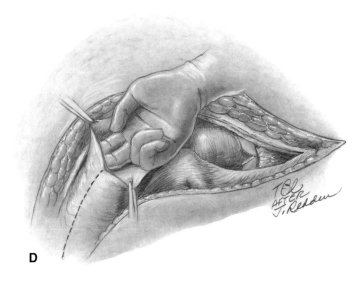

Figure 54–6 Continued. B, *Division of anterior rectus sheath and external oblique muscle to the costal margin. Scissors are inserted under the costal cartilage and a segment is resected. C, The peritoneum bulges through this defect and can be completely mobilized from the posterior sheath. An incision in the bed of the rib opens the pleural cavity and exposes the lung. D, The peritoneum is mobilized from the posterior sheath bluntly. Modified from Scardino PT: Thoracoabdominal retroperitoneal lymphadenectomy for testicular cancer. In ED Crawford, TA Borden (eds), Genitourinary Cancer Surgery. Philadelphia, Lea & Febiger, 1982, pp 271–289, with permission.*

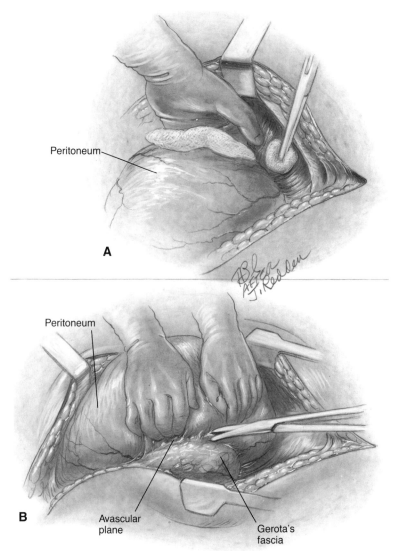

Figure 54–7. Mobilization of the peritoneum to accomplish an extraperitoneal dissection: A, With retraction inferiorly on the peritoneum and superiorly on the costal margin, the diaphragm can be swept off the peritoneum with a moistened sponge stick. B, Once the central tendon of the diaphragm is exposed and Gerota's fascia is completely mobilized from the lumbar muscles posteriorly to the level of the aorta, the peritoneum is dissected away from Gerota's fascia anteriorly in the avascular plane. Modified from Scardino PT: Thoracoabdominal retroperitoneal lymphadenopathy for testicular cancer. In ED Crawford, TA Borden (eds), Genitourinary Cancer Surgery. Philadelphia, Lea & Febiger, 1982, pp 271–289, with permission.

feriorly while the peritoneum is swept from the diaphragm with a moistened sponge stick. Sharp dissection along the smooth surface of the peritoneum is necessary whenever dense adhesions are encountered. Annoying bleeding results if the diaphragmatic muscle bundles are cut, and the peritoneum tends to shred if the dissection is carried into it. The peritoneum must be mobilized superiorly to the central tendon of the diaphragm (Fig. 54–7B) and inferiorly to the iliac vessels. A self-retaining retractor (Finochietto or Fodor) is placed at the cut margin of the costal cartilage and secured with towel clips. At this time the left lung can be palpated for nodules and any suspicious areas can be excised for biopsy.

Gerota's fascia and the perirenal fat, together with the thin fascia covering the lumbar muscles, are elevated to expose the quadratus lumborum and psoas muscles. The dissection continues bluntly and rapidly until the aorta is identified. The peritoneum is then lifted up and, with sharp and blunt dissection, is separated from Gerota's fascia along the avascular plane (Fig. 54–7B). The dissection is carried medially along the course of the left renal vein to the inferior vena cava, mobilizing the duodenum and pancreas anteriorly. There are often large retroperitoneal lymphatics here that join with the lacteals draining the intestinal tract. These must be meticulously clipped along the base of the superior mesenteric artery to avoid excessive lymphatic leakage.

The retroperitoneum is now completely

exposed and it is possible to proceed to the lymph node dissection itself.

Superior Margin of Dissection
(Fig. 54–8)

The operation begins at the base of the superior mesenteric artery (SMA). The lymphatics overlying the root of the SMA are elevated with a fine right-angle clamp, clipped, and divided until the anterolateral wall of the aorta is exposed (Fig. 54–8A).

Once the lateral wall of the aorta and the left crus of the diaphragm are in view, the suprahilar dissection can be performed as the surgeon retracts the mobilized kidney inferiorly. This maneuver places tension on the band of tissue between the adrenal gland and the aorta. This tissue is clipped and divided, mobilizing the upper pole of the kidney and allowing ready identification of the left renal artery as it comes off the aorta (Fig. 54–8B).

The superior margin of dissection contin-

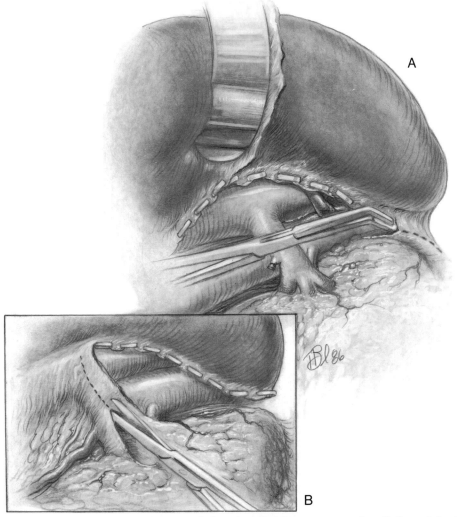

Figure 54–8. *The peritoneum and its contents, including the left colon, are retracted medially and the duodenum is mobilized, exposing the left renal vein and the vena cava. A, The dissection begins at the base of the superior mesenteric artery. Numerous small lymphatics in this area must be clipped and divided until the anterolateral wall of the aorta is exposed. B, The suprahilar dissection is best performed by retracting the kidney and adrenal inferiorly, then clipping and dividing the tissue overlying the left crus of the diaphragm and the aorta laterally. The superior margin of dissection is continued medially to the right side of the vena cava at the level of the right renal vein. Modified from Scardino PT: Thoracoabdominal retroperitoneal lymphadenectomy for testicular cancer. In ED Crawford, TA Borden (eds), Genitourinary Cancer Surgery. Philadelphia, Lea & Febiger, 1982, pp 271–289, with permission.*

ues to the right side over the aorta, across the vena cava to the origin of the right renal vein.

Lateral Margins of Dissection and Exposure of the Great Vessels
(Figs. 54–9 and 54–10)

Now the left adrenal and spermatic veins are ligated and divided so that the renal vein can be retracted anteriorly, exposing the left renal artery. The tissue overlying the aorta is divided inferiorly to the level of the inferior mesenteric artery (IMA) (Fig. 54–9A). This dissection is facilitated by insertion of a finger between the adventitia of the aorta and the thick envelope of fibroareolar tissue.

If the nodes appear grossly normal, the right lateral margin of the dissection is the lateral wall of the inferior vena cava (IVC) above the level of the IMA. The fibroareolar tissue overlying the IVC is clipped and divided (Fig. 54–10A). The aorta is then mobilized by identifying and dividing all of the lumbar arteries from the renal vessels to the

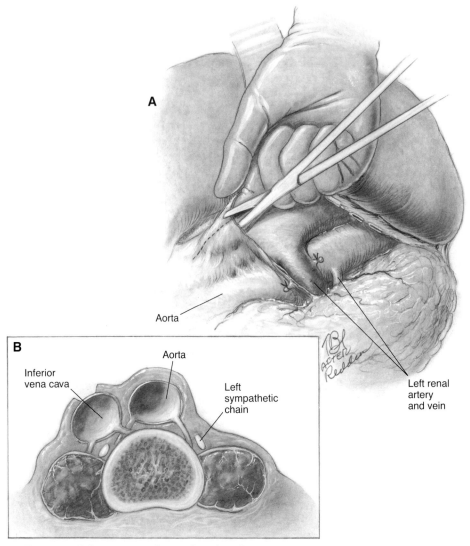

Figure 54–9. *Exposure of the great vessels. A, The adrenal and spermatic venous branches of the left renal vein are divided so that the vein can be retracted inferiorly and the origin of the left renal artery identified. The node-bearing tissue over the aorta is divided inferiorly to the inferior mesenteric artery. B, This cross-sectional view below the renal hilum illustrates the dissection. From Scardino PT: Thoracoabdominal retroperitoneal lymphadenectomy for testicular cancer. In ED Crawford, TA Borden (eds), Genitourinary Cancer Surgery. Philadelphia, Lea & Febiger, 1982, pp 271–289, with permission.*

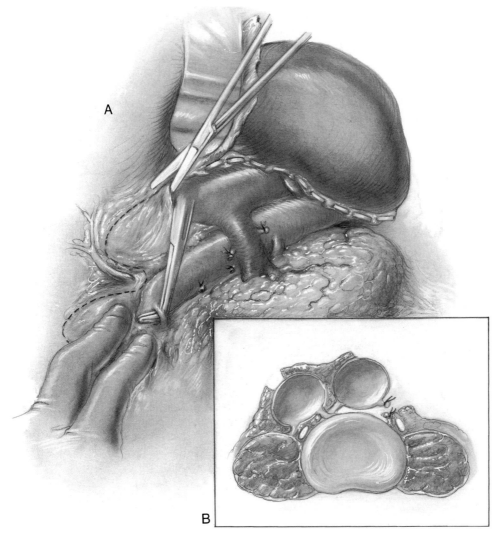

Figure 54–10. Defining the margins of the dissection: A, The superior margin of dissection has been established. The tissue along the right lateral border of the vena cava is clipped and divided inferiorly to the level of the inferior mesenteric artery (IMA). Mobilization of the aorta requires ligation and division of all lumbar arteries between the renal artery and the IMA. Below the IMA only the left lumbar arteries are divided. B, Cross-sectional view.

Illustration continued on following page

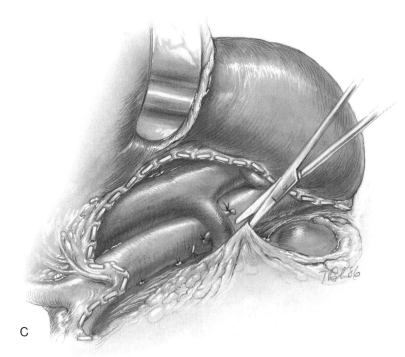

C

Figure 54–10 Continued. C, The hilum is fully exposed by dividing the tissue over the renal vein and artery. Completely skeletonizing the vessels and the renal pelvis is facilitated by full mobilization of the kidney so that the dissection can be performed anterior and posterior to the vessels. Modified from Scardino PT: Thoracoabdominal retroperitoneal lymphadenectomy for testicular cancer. In ED Crawford, TA Borden (eds), Genitourinary Cancer Surgery. Philadelphia, Lea & Febiger, 1982, pp 271–289, with permission.

IMA. Below the level of the IMA, the tissue anterior to the aorta and between the aorta and vena cava is spared, to avoid damage to the sympathetic nerves responsible for ejaculation and emission.

Next, attention is turned to the renal hilum. With the kidney mobilized, the tissue surrounding the artery, vein, ureter, and renal pelvis can be dissected both anteriorly and posteriorly. The lymph nodes of the left renal hilum are the most frequent sites of metastases and must be completely removed.

Interaortocaval Dissection
(Fig. 54–11)

Next, the left renal vein is retracted inferiorly, exposing the right renal artery (Fig. 54–11). The interaortocaval tissue at the level of the right renal artery is clipped, divided, and swept inferiorly. The posterior margin of the dissection is the white fascial fibers of the prevertebral ligaments, which can be seen as the tissue is removed.

To retract the vena cava to the right, the *left* lumbar veins are divided. The lateral margin of dissection beneath the vena cava is along the *right* lumbar veins and the sympathetic chain in the paravertebral

groove. These structures are left intact. The dissection continues inferiorly to the level of the IMA and the tissue is passed beneath the mobilized aorta (Fig. 54–11B and C).

Completion of the Dissection
(Fig. 54–12)

Dissection continues along the left paravertebral groove. The left sympathetic chain cannot be spared if all of the node-bearing tissue is to be removed.

The ureter is identified, bluntly freed from the specimen, and retracted laterally. The left spermatic vessels are dissected to the internal inguinal ring and removed below the ligature left at the time of the inguinal orchiectomy. Finally, the nodes anterior and lateral to the common iliac artery are removed. The inferior margin of dissection should be 3 to 4 cm below the bifurcation of the left iliac artery. The lateral margin of the pelvic dissection is the genitofemoral nerve (Fig. 54–12).

Now the margins of the dissection are inspected for lymphatic leakage. The lymphatics should be secured with clips or ligatures rather than electrocautery. The renal arteries are inspected for adequate flow, and all lumbar arteries and veins are checked.

Figure 54–11. Dissection of the interaortocaval tissue: A, After the left lumbar veins are divided, the vena cava and left renal vein are retracted to expose the right renal artery. Once this artery is freed, the tissue just superior to it can be mobilized as a packet, clipped, divided, and swept inferiorly along the prevertebral fascia. B, The lateral margin of the dissection is established beneath the vena cava by clipping and dividing just to the left of the right lumbar veins. The interaortocaval and periaortic tissue can then be passed beneath the mobilized aorta. C, The tissue anterior, medial, and posterior to the vena cava is taken, but the right sympathetic chain and right lumbar veins are left intact. All of the interaortocaval tissue is removed down to the level of the inferior mesenteric artery. The aorta is lifted anteriorly, allowing the specimen to be passed beneath it as the dissection continues along the prevertebral fascia. Modified from Scardino PT: Thoracoabdominal retroperitoneal lymphadenectomy for testicular cancer. In ED Crawford, TA Borden (eds), Genitourinary Cancer Surgery. Philadelphia, Lea & Febiger, 1982, pp 271–289, with permission.

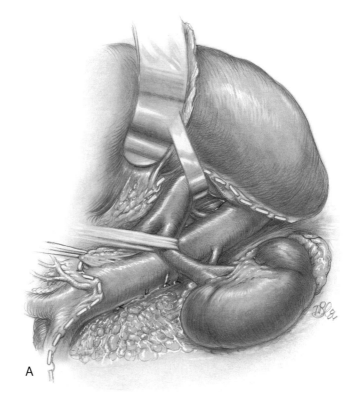

A

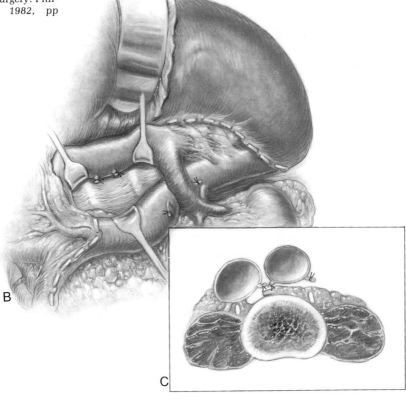

B

C

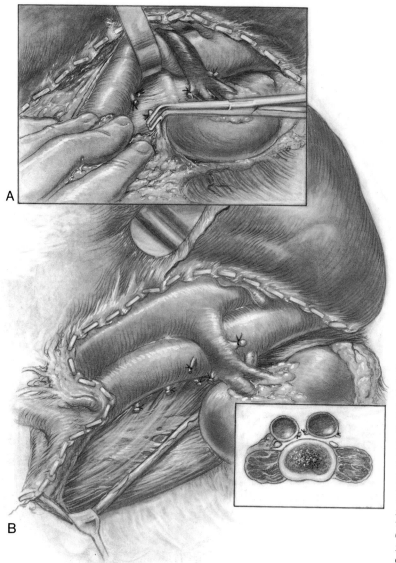

Figure 54–12. Completion of the dissection: A, The small perforating vessels along the left paravertebral groove must be clipped as the specimen is removed. The left sympathetic chain cannot be spared if all of the periaortic nodes are to be removed. B, Overview and cross section of the field after the specimen is removed. Modified from Scardino PT: Thoracoabdominal retroperitoneal lymphadenectomy for testicular cancer. In ED Crawford, TA Borden (eds), Genitourinary Cancer Surgery. Philadelphia, Lea & Febiger, 1982, pp 271–289, with permission.

Closure of the Incision

A No. 32 Argyle chest tube is placed one interspace above or below the incision and left for 48 to 72 hours, or until drainage is less than 100 ml/day. The intercostal nerves are blocked by infiltration with 0.5% Marcaine (bupivacaine hydrochloride without epinephrine), 5 ml at each of five intercostal nerves. The table is straightened to relieve the tension, and the diaphragm is closed securely in two layers with running 2-0 polyglycolic (Dexon) or coated polyglactin (Vicryl) sutures. A watertight closure is necessary in order to prevent prolonged serous drainage of retroperitoneal contents through the thoracotomy tube. We prefer 1 Dexon or coated Vicryl figure-of-eight, all-layer interrupted sutures to close the thoracic portion of the incision. Near the costal margin medially the sutures are passed through the diaphragm as well as through the chest wall, to completely seal the pleura from the retroperitoneal space. All sutures are individually placed before any are tied. The abdominal part of the incision is closed in layers in a routine manner using 1 Dexon or Vicryl. There is frequently accumulation of retroperitoneal fluid, which is reabsorbed in a matter of days. Drains to this area are discouraged.

Postoperative Care

The patient should be kept well hydrated. With the extensive retroperitoneal dissection, third-space fluid loss can be significant. Although blood loss averages less than 1000 ml, there is profound water loss from the large surface area exposed during this lengthy procedure and protein loss from cut lymphatics. These patients require colloid replacement equivalent to 1000 to 1500 ml during the operation and 500 to 1000 ml per day for one to two days afterward. Continuous assessment of the volume status of the patient is necessary. Infusions of 5% dextrose and saline at 150 ml/hr and 5% albumin at 50 ml/hr are routinely administered for 18 to 24 hours. When urine output, vital signs, and serial hematocrits reflect reaccumulation of retroperitoneal fluid (usually on the third postoperative day), the parenteral fluids can be reduced. The nasogastric tube may be removed in one or two days, as tolerated. A chest x-ray is routinely obtained in the recovery room to assure full expansion of the lung and correct placement of the tube.

COMPLICATIONS

Intraoperative complications are rare. However, the most serious have been injuries to the renal vessels, requiring either bypass graft or nephrectomy. During the dissection around the aorta, avulsion of small arteries is not uncommon. Therefore, fine, synthetic monofilament sutures such as 6-0 Prolene should be available to repair the defect.

Dissection of the renal artery often causes intense spasm. To avoid ischemic injury to the kidney, we routinely give 25 gm mannitol intravenously before dissecting the artery. If arterial spasm persists after the dissection, topical papaverine or lidocaine will promote dilatation.

Minor postoperative complications have been reported in 3% of patients and major complications in 3%.[21, 41] The latter include wound infection, prolonged atelectasis or pneumonia, prolonged thoracotomy tube drainage, and prolonged ileus. Delayed bleeding, lymphoceles, thrombophlebitis, and pulmonary emboli have been rare. Pancreatitis is rarely seen after the thoracoabdominal procedure, although it appears more commonly after extended transabdominal RLND.

The average hospital stay is 11 days.[41] The mortality rate is very low, with only one operative death in over 900 cases reported.[38]

FOLLOW-UP CARE

The patient must be followed closely after a lymphadenectomy whether or not adjuvant chemotherapy is administered. The patient should return to the office every two months for the first year and every three months for the second year, every four months for the third year, every six months for the fourth and fifth years, and annually thereafter. The office visit should include a chest x-ray, serum levels of human chorionic gonadotropin and α-fetoprotein, and a physical examination with special emphasis on examination of the supraclavicular nodes, breast, abdomen, and remaining testicle.

CONCLUSION

RLND is a safe and effective procedure for patients with early stage (A, B_1, and B_2) nonseminomatous testicular cancer. The major disadvantage of the operation, permanent loss of ejaculation, can now be avoided in 90% of patients with grossly negative nodes at the time of operation. RLND eliminates the retroperitoneum—a difficult area to monitor—as the site of relapse, and provides highly accurate prognostic information for the rational selection of patients for adjuvant chemotherapy. The long-term results of treatment with RLND are unexcelled (99 to 100% for patients in Stage A, 96 to 98% for those in Stages B_1 and B_2) and have set the "gold standard" for the treatment of testicular cancer.

References

1. Chiou RK, Fraley EE, Lange PH: Newer ideas about fertility in patients with testicular cancer. World J Urol 2:26–31, 1984.
2. Cooper JF, Leadbetter WF, Chute R: Thoracoabdominal approach for retroperitoneal gland dissection: its application to testis tumors. Surg Gynecol Obstet 90:486–496, 1950.
3. Crawford ED, Scardino PT: Testicular carcinoma: an overview. *In* ED Crawford, TA Borden (eds),

Genitourinary Cancer Surgery. Philadelphia, Lea & Febiger, 1982, pp 249–261.

4. Cuneo B, Marcille M: Topographie des ganglions ilia-pelviens. Bull Soc Anat, Paris, 6s III-653, 1901.

5. DeWys WD, Paulson D, Spaulding J, Jacobs EW: Intergroup Testicular Study: Selection of testicular cancer patients for a protocol omitting retroperitoneal node dissection. Proc Am Soc Clin Oncol 3:157 (abstr), 1984.

6. Donohue JP: Retroperitoneal lymphadenectomy: the anterior approach including bilateral suprarenal-hilar dissection. Urol Clin North Am 4:509–521, 1977.

7. Donohue JP, Einhorn LH, Williams SD: Is adjuvant chemotherapy following retroperitoneal lymph node dissection for nonseminomatous testis cancer necessary? Urol Clin North Am 7:747–756, 1980.

8. Donohue JP, Rowland RG: Complications of retroperitoneal lymph node dissection. J Urol 125:338–340, 1981.

9. Donohue JP, Zachary JM, Maynard BR: Distribution of nodal metastases in nonseminomatous testis cancer. J Urol 128:315–320, 1982.

10. Fosså SD, Klepp O, Ous S, et al: Unilateral retroperitoneal lymph node dissection in patients with nonseminomatous testicular tumor in clinical stage I. Eur Urol 10:17–23, 1984.

11. Herr HW, Whitmore WF Jr, Sogani PC, et al: Selection of testicular tumor patients for omission of retroperitoneal lymph node dissection. J Urol 135:500–503, 1986.

12. Hinman F: The operative treatment of tumors of the testicle. JAMA 63:2009, 1914.

13. Jamieson JK, Dobson JF: The lymphatics of the testicle. Lancet 1:493, 1910.

14. Javadpour N, Moley J: Alternative to retroperitoneal lymphadenectomy with preservation of ejaculation and fertility in stage I nonseminomatous testicular cancer: a prospective study. Cancer 55:1604–1611, 1985.

15. Jewett MA: Nonoperative approach for the management of clinical stage A nonseminomatous germ cell tumors. Semin Urol 2:204–207, 1984.

16. Johnson DE, Lo RK, von Eschenbach AC, Swanson DA: Surveillance alone for patients with clinical stage I nonseminomatous germ cell tumors of the testis: preliminary results. J Urol 131:491–493, 1984.

17. Lange PH, Narayan P, Fraley EE: Fertility issues following therapy for testicular cancer. Semin Urol 2:264–274, 1984.

18. Lange PH, Narayan P, Vogelzang NJ, et al: Return of fertility after treatment for nonseminomatous testicular cancer: changing concepts. J Urol 129:1131–1135, 1983.

19. Lewis LG: Radical orchiectomy for tumors of the testis. JAMA 137:828–832, 1948.

20. Lewis LG: Radioresistant testis tumors: results in 133 cases; 5-year follow-up. J Urol 69:841–844, 1953.

21. Lieskovsky G, Weinberg AC, Skinner DG: Surgical management of early-stage nonseminomatous germ cell tumors of the testis. Semin Urol 2:208–216, 1984.

22. Lipshultz LI, McConnell J, Benson GS: Current concepts of the mechanisms of ejaculation. Normal and abnormal states. J Reprod Med 26:499–507, 1981.

23. Logothetis CJ, Samuels ML, Selig DE, et al: Primary chemotherapy followed by a selective retroperitoneal lymphadenectomy in the management of clinical stage II testicular carcinoma: a preliminary report. J Urol 134:1127–1130, 1985.

24. Mallis N, Patton JF: Transperitoneal bilateral lymphadenectomy in testis tumors. J Urol 80:501–503, 1958.

25. Most I: Ueber maligne Hoden Geschwulste und ihre Metastaten. Arch Pathol Anat Physiol Klin Med 154:138, 1898.

26. Narayan P, Lange PH, Fraley EE: Ejaculation and fertility after extended retroperitoneal lymph node dissection for testicular cancer. J Urol 127:685–688, 1982.

27. Peckham MJ (ed): The Management of Testicular Tumours. London, E. Arnold, 1981.

28. Peckham MJ, Hendry WF: Clinical stage II nonseminomatous germ cell testicular tumors. Results of management by primary chemotherapy. Br J Urol 57:763–768, 1985.

29. Peckham MJ, Barrett A, Husband JE, Hendry WF: Orchidectomy alone in testicular stage I nonseminomatous germ-cell tumours. Lancet 678–680, 1982.

30. Pizzocaro G: Retroperitoneal lymph node dissection in clinical stage IIA and IIB nonseminomatous germ cell tumours of the testis. Int J Andrology (in press).

31. Pizzocaro G, Musumeci R: The relative value of lymphangiography (LAG) and computed tomography (CT) in diagnosing small retroperitoneal metastases. In S Khoury (ed): Testicular Cancer. New York, A. R. Liss, 1985, p 261.

32. Pizzocaro G, Salvioni R, Zanoni F: Unilateral lymphadenectomy in intraoperative stage 1 nonseminomatous germinal testis cancer. J Urol 134:485–489, 1985.

33. Pizzocaro G, Zanoni F, Salvioni R, et al: Surveillance or lymph-node dissection in clinical stage-I non-seminomatous germinal testis cancer. Br J Urol 57:759–762, 1985.

34. Ray B, Hadju SI, Whitmore WF Jr: Distribution of retroperitoneal lymph node metastases in testicular germinal tumors. Cancer 33:340–348, 1974.

35. Read G, Johnson RJ, Wilkinson PM, Eddleston B: Prospective study of follow-up alone in stage I teratoma of the testis. Br Med J [Clin Res] 287:1503–1505, 1983.

36. Richie JP, Garnick, M: Modified lymph node dissection in clinical stage I disease. Societe Internationale 'd Urologie, Abstract 79, June 23, 1985.

37. Scardino PT: Adjuvant chemotherapy is of value following retroperitoneal lymph node dissection for nonseminomatous testicular cancer. Urol Clin North Am 7:735–745, 1980.

38. Scardino PT: Thoracoabdominal retroperitoneal lymphadenectomy for testicular cancer. In ED Crawford, TA Borden (eds), Genitourinary Cancer Surgery. Philadelphia, Lea & Febiger, 1982, pp 271–289.

39. Scardino PT, Skinner DG: Germ-cell tumors of the testis: improved results in a prospective study using combined modality therapy and biochemical tumor markers. Surgery 86:86–93, 1979.

40. Skinner DG, Leadbetter WF: The surgical management of testis tumors. J Urol 106:84–93, 1971.

41. Skinner DG, Melamud A, Lieskovsky G: Compli-

cations of thoracoabdominal retroperitoneal lymph node dissection. J Urol 127:1107–1110, 1982.

42. Skinner DG, Scardino PT: Relevance of biochemical tumor markers and lymphadenectomy in management of non-seminomatous testis tumors: current perspective. J Urol 123:378–382, 1980.

43. Sogani PC, Whitmore WF Jr, Herr HW, et al: Orchiectomy alone in the treatment of clinical stage I nonseminomatous germ cell tumor of the testis. J Clin Oncol 2:267–270, 1984.

44. Staubitz WJ, Early KS, Magoss IV, Murphy GP: Surgical management of testis tumor. J Urol 111:205–209, 1974.

45. Tesoro-Tess JD, Pizzocaro G, Zanoni F, Musumeci R: Lymphangiography and computerized tomogra-phy in testicular carcinoma. How accurate in early stage disease? J Urol 133:967–970, 1985.

46. Thachil JV, Jewett MAS, Rider WD: The effects of cancer and cancer therapy on male fertility. J Urol 126:141–145, 1981.

47. Whitelaw GP, Smithwick RH: Some secondary effects of sympathectomy with particular reference to disturbance of sexual function. N Engl J Med 245:121–130, 1951.

48. Whitmore WF Jr: Surgical treatment of adult germinal testis tumors. Semin Oncol 6:55–68, 1979.

49. Wise PG, Scardino PT: Thoracoabdominal retroperitoneal lymphadenectomy for nonseminomatous testicular cancer. Urol Clin North Am 10:371–379, 1983.

JOHN P. DONOHUE, M.D.
RANDALL G. ROWLAND, M.D.
RICHARD BIHRLE, M.D.

Transabdominal Retroperitoneal Lymph Node Dissection

CHAPTER 55

HISTORIC NOTES

The initial approach to the "lumbar ganglia" that drained the testis was via a flank incision. As a student, Chevassu described this in a thesis at the turn of the century.[1, 2] Frank Hinman, Sr., described the procedure well and employed it with clinical success in the 1930s and later.[11] During the Second World War, Lloyd Lewis and colleagues described and perfected an anterior transabdominal approach. This became further improved and was still better described in the writings of Patton, Van Buskirk, Whitmore, and Young.[15, 20, 22, 23] In the early 1950s, Cooper, Leadbetter, and Chute described an alternative extended thoracoabdominal approach.[3] Two decades later, an extended anterior approach was described that permitted access in the high retroperitoneum on either side.[4]

Each approach has its advocates. Each is quite effective because adequate exposure can be provided in the retroperitoneal space by approaching either through midline anterior or thoracoabdominal incisions. Although it is difficult to estimate the usage of each, we believe that the anterior midline approach is employed more commonly, whereas the thoracoabdominal approach has several strong supporters who use it well.[9, 17] Briefly, the anterior midline approach provides rapid opening and closing of the wound and establishes satisfactory exposure for low-stage as well as higher stage disease. Several experienced groups use the midline incision to good effect, even in postchemotherapy, bulky dissections. On the other hand, excellent exposure also is afforded by the thoracoabdominal approach, and it is actually preferred in cases with mass or bulky lesions that are high in the retroperitoneal space, particularly when there is retrocrural involvement.

CURRENT STATUS

Significant changes are underway in the evolution of the technique of retroperitoneal lymphadenectomy. For low-stage disease, a number of workers both here and abroad have described techniques that permit ejaculation postoperatively in up to 90% of cases.[12, 16, 21] The postganglionic fibers of the lumbar sympathetic chain can be identified and preserved, particularly when there is no clinical evidence of disease in cases that appear to be of Stage I classification. Also, in clinically advanced disease the distribution of nodes has been well described,[6] and a template for dissection that will include these is readily achieved by experienced groups. Finally, the role of surgery in still

802

further advanced disease is now well established as "postchemotherapy," and the nature and extent of such surgery has been thoroughly described.[5, 8] Briefly, it involves an extended bilateral (as opposed to a modified unilateral) dissection, which has become feasible in low-stage disease, as noted above.

SURGERY FOR LOW-STAGE DISEASE

Quite understandably, surgery itself for low-stage disease has been questioned. This is appropriate in view of the fact that in our series and in the experience of many others, about 70% of clinically negative patients will indeed have negative lymph nodes. Assuming only a slight pathologic sampling error, this implies that there was no therapeutic effect to the retroperitoneal lymph node dissection (RPLND) surgery. The arguments and pro and con for surgery in low-stage disease have been well developed and discussed elsewhere. Patients who relapse in surveillance studies do so most often in the retroperitoneum, as one would expect (Table 55–1). Unfortunately this area is difficult to monitor and will require even more aggressive and frequent study in the future (e.g., having abdominal CT scans every six weeks as opposed to every three months, as has been suggested). If the patients are carefully selected on the basis of primary testicular (pT) pathologic characteristics, and if all patients who show suspicious results on any clinical parameter (e.g., lymphangiogram) are excluded, there is no question that satisfactory data can be obtained. In fact,

most (but not all) patients can be salvaged at clinical relapse, with the salvage rate now estimated to be in the 95th percentile.[10] Unfortunately, this is not an improvement in survival statistics but in fact is lower in terms of absolute survival, which was in excess of 99% if one accepts the data from the largest American series.[22] The only positive thing that can be said for surveillance is that patients who were truly negative were spared an operation that offers no therapeutic benefit.

Improvements in technique of staging RPLND now render moot the primary argument against the procedure. This argument is that young men become sterile from ejaculatory impotence after operation, at a time of life prior to marriage when this is most threatening. It is of great interest that worldwide data are being generated regarding preservation of ejaculation, and thus of fertility, following RPLND surgery. Therefore, the main emotional and social argument against RPLND in low-stage disease has been defused by the nerve-sparing modifications emerging on both sides of the Atlantic.[12, 16, 21]

Recent modifications include preservation of the lower preaortic postganglionic fibers, particularly those below the level of the inferior mesenteric artery. The modified template for dissection is described graphically in Figures 55–1 A and B. It should be mentioned that the primary focus of right-sided drainage is in the interaortacaval nodes, and this area must be cleared when staging for low-stage, right-sided disease. Although right pericaval nodes may also be involved in clinical Stage I disease, usually they are not. It is the interaortacaval group, high and below the level of the renal vein

Table 55–1. SURVEILLANCE DATA FOR PATIENTS RECEIVING ORCHIECTOMY ONLY FOR MANAGEMENT OF NONSEMINOMATOUS GERM CELL TUMOR OF THE TESTIS*

| | Site of Relapse | | | |
Institution	Retroperitoneum Only	Outside Retroperitoneum	Markers Only	Total
Christie Hospital	1	2	0	3
Royal Marsden	5	3	1	9
Princess Margaret	12	0	0	12
Memorial Sloan–Kettering	5	2	1	8
MD Anderson	3	5	2	10
Total	26	12	4	42

*Data courtesy of D. Swanson, M.D. (personal communication). As expected, most relapses in the surveillance protocol occur in the retroperitoneum, because testicular cancer spreads primarily through the lymphatics. This area is more difficult to monitor and is not as ideal a model for chemotherapy as, for example, chest disease. Already two out of 46 patients followed for over 36 months have succumbed in the longest surveillance series reported in the United States.

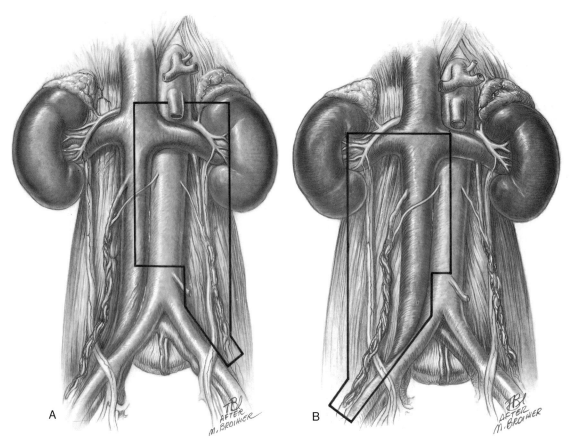

Figure 55–1. A, Template or boundaries for retroperitoneal lymph node dissection patients who have left-sided primary tumors but no clinical evidence of disease (clinically negative). This designation also implies no gross disease at the time of exploration. B, Boundaries or template for clinically negative patients with right-sided primary tumors. The primary zone of spread is the interaortocaval group of nodes. For both right- and left-sided primary tumors, care is taken to spare the preaortic tissues below the level of the inferior mesenteric artery, where the postganglionic sympathetic fibers course.

and extending down the length of the cava, that must be accounted for. Therefore, a "unilateral" node dissection for right-sided disease implies clearance of the interaortacaval (i.e., centrally placed) nodes. On the other hand, a left-sided primary tumor may permit clearance of the left periaortic nodes exclusively, if the early experience of German and Norwegian workers[8, 21] can be confirmed in larger series over time. Our own bias is to include right periaortic (interaortacaval) nodes in left-sided cases, at least down to the origin of the inferior mesenteric artery (Fig. 55–1B. This opinion is based on our earlier distribution studies. With these modifications, ejaculatory potency is preserved in a great majority of patients.

Surgical Technique

The technique of the surgery has been thoroughly described in early publications cited.[4] This exposure is obtained by making a midline incision from xiphoid to pubis. Drapes and a circular plastic wound protector are placed, and currently we are using a self-retaining ring retractor that is affixed to the table. After careful exploration of the abdomen, the root of the small bowel is divided. For low-stage disease it is not necessary to divide the right posterior colonic mesentery and to mobilize the bowel completely, placing it in a bowel bag on the patient's chest. Rather, the viscera can be retracted in wet laparotomy pads, exposing the interaortacaval and the periaortic groups of nodes. We also divide the inferior mesenteric vein between suture ligatures in order to better mobilize the left colonic mesentery and permit improved elevation and mobilization of the pancreas. This is not necessary in staging RPLND for clinically negative patients, particularly those with right-sided primary tumors. On the other hand, in those with left-sided primary tumors, this vein should be divided and the colonic mesentery mobilized to facilitate retraction and exposure in this area. The basic principle of dividing the nodal and adventitial packages as they surround the great vessels in a longitudinal manner is indicated in Figures 55–2A through E. This is most easily accomplished at the 12 o'clock position over both the vena cava and aorta. It is also done over the renal vein in order to begin the dissection with a transverse unfurling of the nodal package, establishing the superior margin of dissection.

For low-stage disease, care must be taken when dividing the nodal package at the 12 o'clock position to avoid the preaortic tissues below the inferior mesenteric artery, providing all tissue appears completely negative for tumor. This will permit the patient to ejaculate postoperatively. Therefore, the preaortic "split" is confined to the level of the inferior mesenteric artery takeoff, and then the tissue is rotated laterally off the great vessels. The lumbar vessels are ligated between 2-0 silk sutures in continuity, then divided. We also place a small vascular clip proximal to the ligatures for added security before dividing them, allowing mobilization of the great vessels off the posterior body wall. It also permits better exposure, ensures better vascular control, and lowers inadvertent blood loss that may occur in the absence of this prospective exposure approach. Of course, it is not necessary to divide the lumbar vessels when doing a node dissection for low-stage disease; however, in our experience, this facilitates exposure and completeness of lymphatic clearance.

SURGERY FOR HIGH-STAGE DISEASE

An algorithm of the progress of a patient who presents with advanced Stage III or advanced abdominal disease is shown in Figure 55–3. Normally platinum-based con-

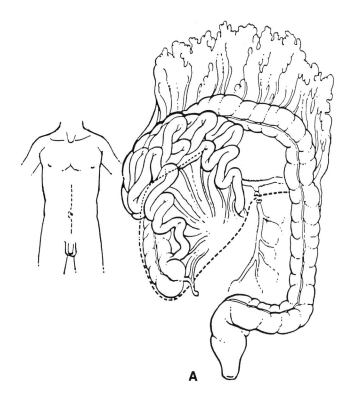

Figure 55–2. A, Posterior mesenteric attachments are divided (right mesocolon from the foramen of Winslow, around the cecum, and then up the root of the small bowel to the ligament of Treitz). Then the inferior mesenteric vein is divided between ligatures near its drainage into the splenic vein. The pancreas is mobilized cephalad and the mesentery of the left colon is mobilized as needed.

Illustration continued on following page

A

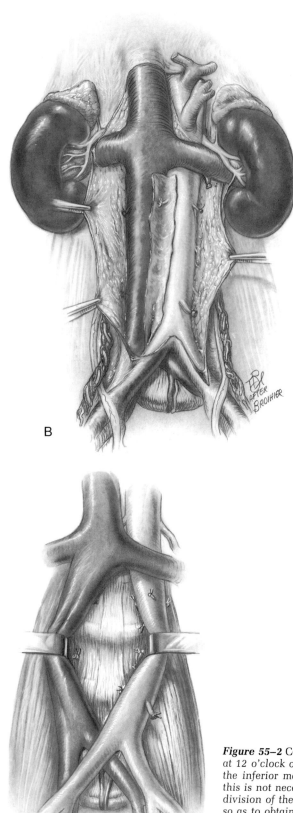

B

C

Figure 55–2 Continued. B, The anterior "split" of the nodal package at 12 o'clock over the great vessels is demonstrated. In this drawing the inferior mesenteric artery is also divided. In low-stage disease, this is not necessary. C, View of the anterior spinous ligaments after division of the lumbar vessels permits retraction of the great vessels so as to obtain complete clearance of the more lateral and posterior lymphatics.

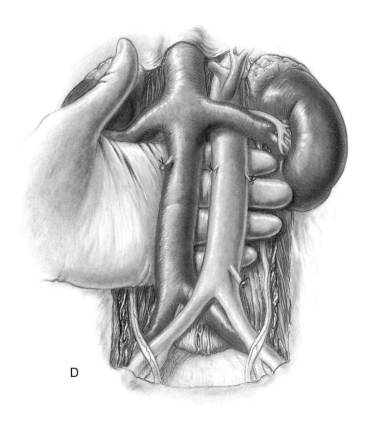

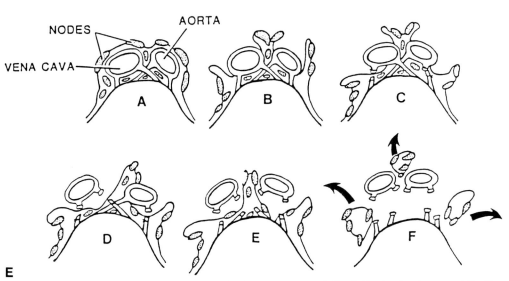

Figure 55–2 Continued. D, *Vessels elevated in hand, demonstrating mobility following lumbar vessel ligation and division. E, Axial view, showing anterior split in B, and then lumbar vessel division in D through E. This permits removal of the nodal tissue from the posterior body wall. Lumbar vessels at the foramina can be secured at this time.*

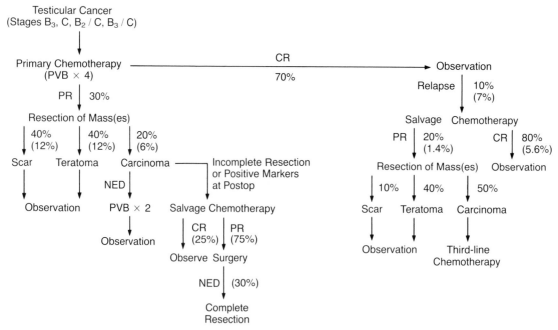

Figure 55–3. *Treatment scheme for disseminated testicular cancer, as used at Indiana University. Percentages in parentheses indicate percentages of original population. Key: CR = complete clinical remission; PR = partial clinical remission; NED = no evidence of disease.*

solidation chemotherapy is given to reduce or eliminate the tumor burden, and then the patient is reevaluated. If the tumor has been eliminated to the extent that a complete remission (CR) is obtained, we simply follow the patient, secure in the knowledge that 10% or fewer of such patients will relapse. Furthermore, they tend to relapse by metastasizing into the chest, and therefore retroperitoneal lymphadenectomy is unnecessary in someone who has truly negative results on CT scan of the abdomen *after* completion of chemotherapy. When analyzing recurrence in this group, we have found that only one in four patients who does relapse actually will have recurrence in the belly. Therefore, retroperitoneal lymphadenectomy in this group is unwarranted *if* they have a solid, complete remission after chemotherapy. Unfortunately, about 30% of patients do not obtain complete remission but eventually require postchemotherapy surgery. Any residual mass lesion following chemotherapy should be excised for both histologic assessment and assignment of further therapy in the event of persistent malignant elements. The approach to patients with advanced disease after chemotherapy has been extensively described.[7]

Patients with bulky, teratomatous tumors present a difficult problem, particularly if the tumor is massive, and even more so if it contains abundant immature elements. The significance of a resected teratoma and its relapse potential is the subject of much interest and current study.[13] Regression analysis studies reveal that primary factors in postchemotherapy relapse in teratoma patients are (1) site, (2) tumor burden, and (3) histologic features of the surgical specimen. There is a significant difference between primary mediastinal tumor relapse and that of lung *or* abdomen, or lung *and* abdomen. There is also a significant difference between small versus moderate versus massive disease resected after chemotherapy. Those with the most bulky disease relapse most commonly. Usually relapse is outside the field of resection, but it also is not uncommon to have relapse occur within the field of dissection, particularly related to posterior body wall foramina, gastrointestinal viscera, or deep pelvic or mediastinal nodes. This has been described in earlier communications.[13, 14] Finally, those patients with cancer in the histologic surgical specimen represent a more difficult group who have responded less well to the chemotherapy. If the resection is complete, they still have a fair chance of cure with the addition of salvage chemotherapy. One of the most difficult subsets in this histologic analysis are those with sarcomatous elements in the resected surgical specimen. Analysis reveals these people to be at particularly high risk for relapse. Of considerable interest also, when reviewing histologic findings, is the occasional patient with non–germ cell elements in resected tumor. Ulbright and associates[19] have described such elements as adenocarcinoma, embryonal rhabdomyosarcoma, and so forth in these tumors. Of interest is the fact that in most cases these non–germ cell elements were found in the primary tumors. In three of 11 patients, primary mediastinal tumor was found to have these elements initially. Another primary retroperitoneal tumor was found to have non–germ cell elements and, of the remaining 11 cases, seven were found to have primary non–germ cell elements coexistent with the primary testicular tumor. The heterogeneity among germ cell tumors in the testis is becoming well recognized. New insights are provided by study of tumors resected following chemotherapy. In reviewing 269 cases of teratoma seen at Indiana University Medical Center from 1974 to 1982, 11 patients with nonseminomatous germ cell tumors (NSGCT) were found to have elements of non–germ cell malignancies as noted above. Apparently platinum-based combination chemotherapy eliminated the more sensitive germ cell elements, unmasking the remaining non–germ cell elements that persisted following chemotherapy.

The technique of resecting the retroperitoneum following chemotherapy is well described in earlier publications.[18] The basic strategy of postchemotherapy RPLND for residual bulk disease is shown in Figures 55–4A through C. Not only should the tumor itself be excised, but tissues within the original retroperitoneal template of nodal drainage from the testis should be removed as well. Therefore, with few exceptions, a full bilateral RPLND is indicated in postchemotherapy dissection. Normally, the exposure is the same as described for low-stage disease. In most cases not only is the root of the small bowel mesentery incised, but also the posterior attachments to the cecum and the mesocolon of the right side are divided, and bowel is mobilized up and away from

the anterior aspect of Gerota's fascia and placed on the chest in a bowel bag. Such cases commonly require additional exposure; therefore, we usually divide the inferior mesenteric vein between silk ligatures and then mobilize the left colonic mesentery. The inferior mesenteric artery is usually divided in order to complete mobilization of the left colonic mesentery and retract this away from the tumor and the retroperitoneal nodes. Of course, the lumbar postganglionic fibers will be dissected during the preaortic dissection, and most of these patients will not be able to ejaculate if a complete dissection has been accomplished in the lower periaortic zone.

A basic strategy is to begin anterior to the great vessels either in the iliac or left renal venous area. The longitudinal split is made over the great vessels, sometimes with the need to retract tumor laterally as one does so. Dividing the lumbar vessels allows retraction of the great vessels off and away from the tumor and, when this is accomplished, the tumor can then be resected from the posterior body wall. At this point the lumbar vessels are controlled at the foramina with clips, suture ligatures, or both. Bovie cautery, using an extender if necessary, is usually quite helpful in postchemotherapy dissection. This strategy is depicted graphically in Figures 55–2C through E.

One should note particularly the need for specialized vascular techniques in some patients. We have resected the vena cava in 18 patients in our series, usually because of involvement with tumor. In a number of cases the tumor extended inside the cava and was found to be inseparable from it in the course of the dissection. Of interest is the fact that in some postchemotherapy patients, the intracaval tumor may be cystic and teratomatous, reflecting changes wrought by chemotherapy. The patients with caval resection are at high risk for postoperative ascites and leg lymphedema, both of which are reversible in time. Care should be taken to avoid a subadventitial plane of cleavage on the aorta, particularly any extended dissection on this plane. The vascularity of the wall of the aorta is much impaired in patients who are left with an extensive subadventitial dissection. We have noted difficulty in repairing arteriotomies, and there is a tendency for a vessel to leak or rupture postoperatively if hypertension develops. In five patients (from over 200

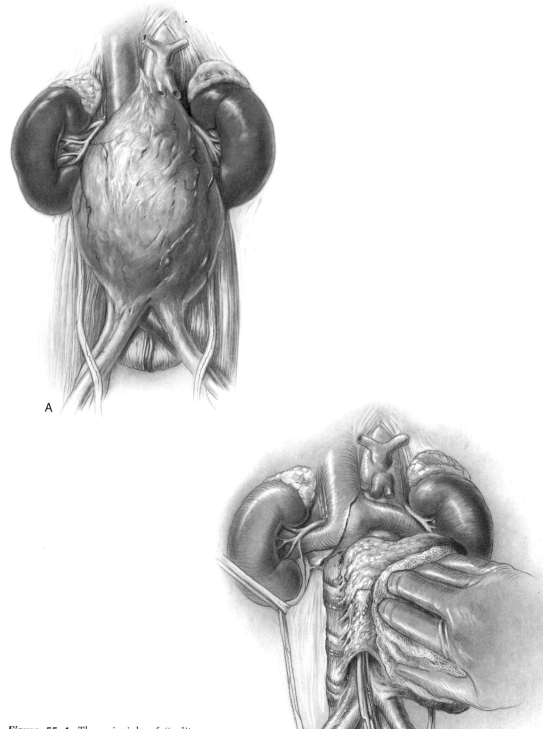

A

B

Figure 55–4. The principle of "split and roll" still applies in bulky disease. The cava in A can be split anteriorly through the subadventitial plane. We usually use Bovie cautery over a dissecting clamp.

Illustration continued on opposite page

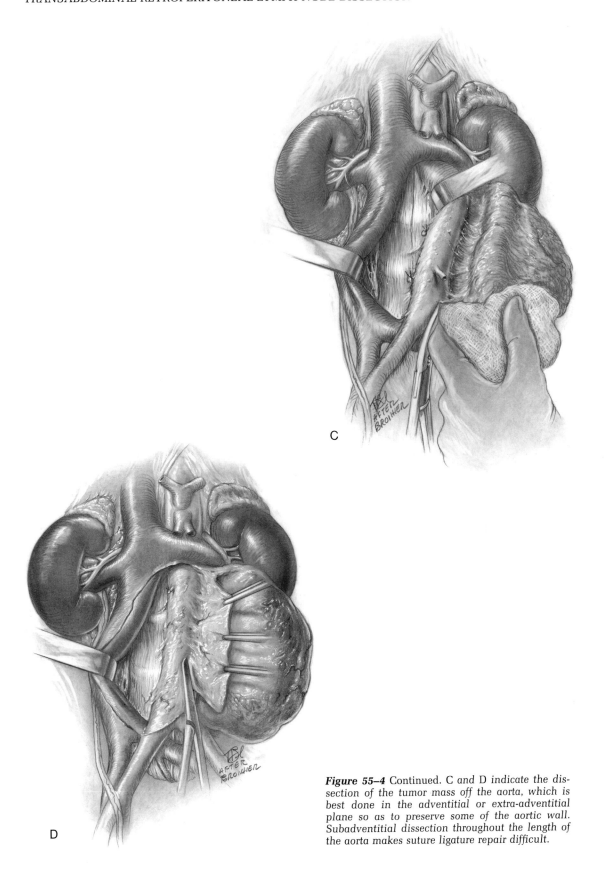

Figure 55–4 Continued. C and D indicate the dissection of the tumor mass off the aorta, which is best done in the adventitial or extra-adventitial plane so as to preserve some of the aortic wall. Subadventitial dissection throughout the length of the aorta makes suture ligature repair difficult.

postchemotherapy patients) it has been necessary for us to replace such damaged areas with knitted Dacron graft material. In each case the graft was well tolerated and the immediate outcome was favorable.

Another word of caution relates to suprahilar disease, which can take two forms. Direct extension from a massive infrahilar tumor may project into the suprahilar zone. In this case, it is usually precrural and can be rolled down and away from the great vessels. Occasionally it needs to be removed en bloc, with one kidney or the other being inseparable from the renal hilum. The usual path of lymph flow into the chest from the retroperitoneum is periaortic and posterior. CT scans have taught us that most suprahilar positive nodal disease is in the retrocrural zone (Figs. 55–5, 55–6). If this enlarges, it becomes expedient to use a thoracoabdominal approach, reflecting the essential nature of a posterior mediastinal fixed tumor. With early and low bulk involvement, this part of the dissection can be done through the anterior approach, even if it requires splitting the crus for a few centimeters. This can always be repaired by direct suture reapproximation of the crura and the posterior ligamentous attachments of the spine. The cisterna chyli is based anywhere from L-1 to T-10 in the posterior periaortic retrocrural space, together with the azygos and hemiazygos venous systems, and it can usually be recognized. This must be handled with great care and suture-ligated or clipped at its base so as to avoid leakage and subsequent ascites. About 1% of our advanced cases will develop postoperative ascites; they usually can be managed conservatively with hyperalimentation and then oral feedings with medium and short chain lipoprotein diets. Surgical intervention with peritoneal venous shunting, for example, is a rarely needed alternative to conservative management.

SUMMARY

Concerning low-stage disease, it would seem that the honeymoon is over for surveillance in the United States. Many patients have presented to our institution with advanced disease, having escaped any notice in the academic community or in the avenues of reporting. Sadly, several have died

and probably will not appear in any report. Surveillance simply will not work if applied on an ad hoc basis at the community level. The busy physician has not the retrieval and fail-safe methods to detect someone in his practice who is not compliant with follow-up testing. Once such patients ultimately present with advanced disease, it is sometimes too late to retrieve them even with state of the art chemotherapy or surgery. In the best of hands, with meticulous selection at entry and very careful follow-up, two of 46 patients who relapsed have succumbed in a very well done study here in the United States.[10] It must be emphasized that staging RPLND as performed today does little harm. It establishes accuracy of pathologic stage and is therapeutic for those with positive nodes by virtue of the lymphadenectomy itself. The challenge remaining is to determine accurately by clinical methods the patients who are to be classified in Stage I. Refinements in imaging techniques, tumor markers, and even fine-needle aspiration, for example, may provide an alternative to RPLND staging surgery. But, since surgery itself is much less an insult today with the modifications noted earlier, we recommend RPLND in clinical Stage I disease.

Concerning high-stage disease, RPLND remains a great challenge. The selection of cases for surgery depends on clinical studies. One could argue that CT scan is much too insensitive in these postchemotherapy patients, but it is reasonably accurate. Our retrospective analysis suggests that of those who achieve a complete remission with chemotherapy alone, less than 5% will ever relapse in the retroperitoneum following chemotherapy. With close follow-up and repeat CT scans, these patients will be detected. This is quite different from the clinical Stage I model who has not had chemotherapy, for in the best of hands, 20% or more of this clinical Stage I group will have positive nodes and relapse clinically. Furthermore, without prior chemotherapy, the relapse in this same group tends to be rapid and fulminating. If relapse occurs in the retroperitoneum in the postchemotherapy group, it usually is delayed in its presentation. Therefore, our own practice is to permit clinical staging in the postchemotherapy patients in order to direct selection of patients for surgery. Those with a radiographic lesion in the retroperitoneum

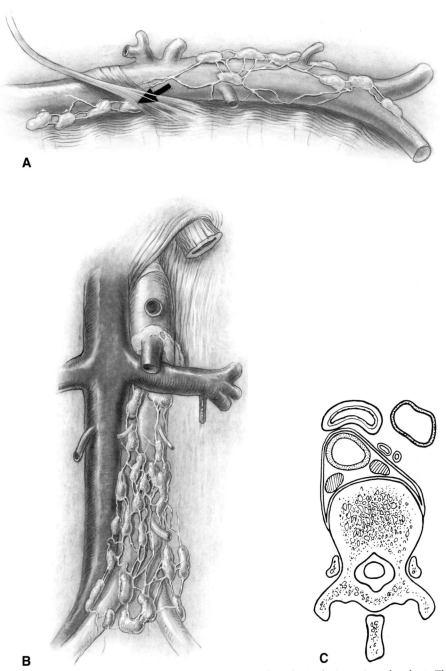

Figure 55–5. A, *Lateral view of the lymphatic flow of para-aortic lymphatic drainage into the chest. The drainage passes through the diaphragm in the aortic hiatus bounded on either side by the crus of the diaphragm. It drains posterior and lateral to the aorta, into the cisterna chyli, and then into the posterior mediastinal nodes. B, Anterior view of the para-aortic nodes and their relationship to the two renal veins. The stippled nodes above the renal vein are posterior to the aorta, since drainage below the renal vein goes cephalad into the chest below the crura of the diaphragm. C, Axial view showing the relationship of the crus of the diaphragm, the aorta, and the para-aortic nodes, which parallel the azygos and hemiazygos venous systems.*

Suprahilar tumor anterior
to diaphragmatic crura

Aorta

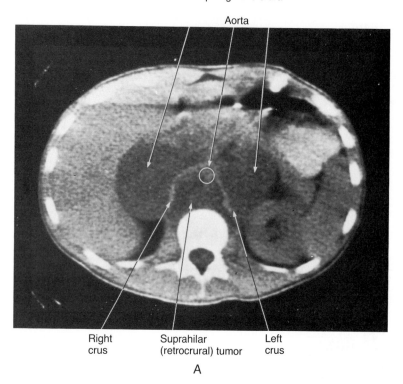

Right   Suprahilar   Left
crus   (retrocrural) tumor crus

A

Aorta

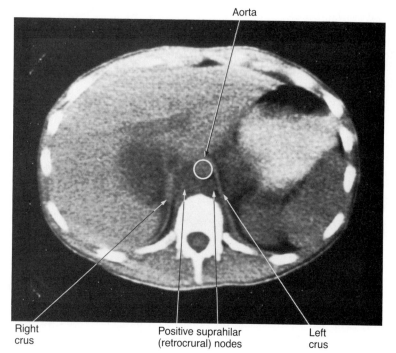

Right   Positive suprahilar   Left
crus   (retrocrural) nodes   crus

B

Figure 55–6. A, CT scan of the suprarenal hilar zone, showing both precrural and retrocrural tumor. The tumor anterior to the crura arises by direct extension from a larger abdominal tumor, centered below the renal hilus. B, Retrocrural nodes drain para-aortic lymphatics from the abdomen. This CT scan reveals adenopathy in the suprahilar zone, above the renal vessels. This zone then continues to become the posterior mediastinal nodal chain in the chest.

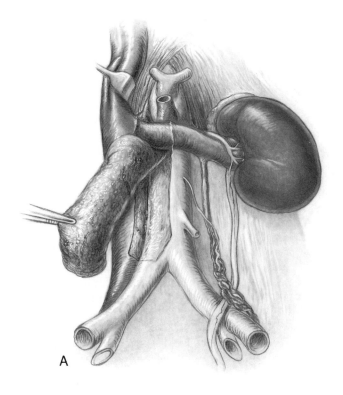

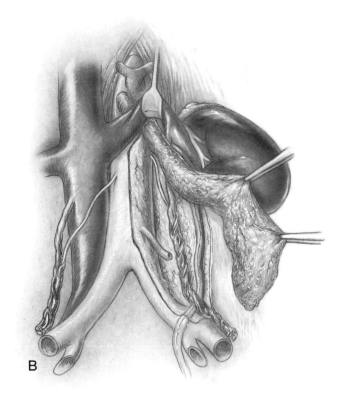

Figure 55–7. Schematic representation of the extension of suprahilar nodes from the infrahilar nodal package. On both the right and left sides these run beside the aorta and posterior to the renal vessels. They also run retrocrurally as they continue to drain up into the posterior mediastinum. Elevating the renal vessels allows examination and clearance of these nodes. In A, the primary zone of spread on the right side is shaded; in B, shading denotes the primary zone of spread on the left side.

undergo a complete bilateral retroperitoneal lymphadenectomy. Patients in Stage II or Stage III who achieve completely negative results are followed with interval CT scans (about every three months in the first year postchemotherapy, every four to six months in the second year, and yearly thereafter for those enjoying continuing CR). The same is true for chest disease. We resect persistent radiographic lesions and give salvage chemotherapy for those with any residual malignancy in the resected specimen. If there is scar necrosis or simple teratoma in the resected specimen, we withhold salvage chemotherapy. At the present time, we are undecided as to whether those with abundant immature elements in a resected teratoma should have further or salvage chemotherapy. So far, we have chosen to withhold additional chemotherapy and later, if patients relapse, we treat them with chemotherapy or surgery.

RPLND for low-stage disease has been scaled down (Fig. 55–7) with coincident increase in preservation of ejaculation. At this time it seems the safest and least risky approach for Stage I clinical disease. RPLND for high-stage disease is usually extended bilaterally and at times requires extensive combined chest and pelvic procedures. Therefore, there is a wide spectrum in the technical demands of RPLND surgery, depending on the clinical presentation.

References

1. Chevassu M: Tumeurs du testicule (Thesis). Paris, 1906.
2. Chevassu M, Prique: Teratoma du testicule. Bull Soc d Chir (Paris) 14–60, 1898.
3. Cooper JF, Leadbetter WF, Chute R: Thoracoabdominal approach for retroperitoneal gland dissection: its application to testis tumors. Surg Gynecol Obstet 90:486–496, 1950.
4. Donohue JP: Retroperitoneal lymphadenectomy: the anterior approach including bilateral suprarenal-hilar dissection. Urol Clin North Am 4:509–521, 1977.
5. Donohue JP, Einhorn LH, Williams SD: Cytoreductive surgery for metastatic testis cancer: considerations of timing and extent. J Urol 123:876–880, 1980.
6. Donohue JP, Zachary JM, Maynard BR: Distribution of nodal metastases in nonseminomatous testis cancer. J Urol 128:315–320, 1982.
7. Donohue JP, Rowland RG: The role of surgery in advanced testicular cancer. Cancer 54:2716–2721, 1984.
8. Fossa SD, Klepp O, Ous J, et al: Unilateral retroperitoneal lymph node dissection in patients with nonseminomatous testicular cancer in clinical state I. Eur Urol (in press).
9. Fraley EE: Transthoracic retroperitoneal lymphadenectomy for testicular cancer. In: JP Donohue (ed). Testis Tumors, Vol 7. International Perspectives in Urology. Baltimore, Williams & Wilkins, 1983, p 169.
10. Herr H, Segani P, Whitmore W, et al: Non-operative management of selected clinical stage I patients with non-seminomatous testicular cancer. J Urol 135:500, 1986.
11. Hinman F: Operative treatment of tumors of the testicle. JAMA 63:2009, 1914.
12. Lange PH, Narayan P, Fraley EE: Fertility issues following therapy for testicular cancer. Semin Urol 11:264, 1984.
13. Loehrer PJ, et al: Teratoma following cis-platinum based combination chemotherapy for non-seminomatous germ cell tumors: a clinicopathologic correlation. J Urol (submitted).
14. Loehrer PJ, Sledge GW, Einhorn LH: Heterogeneity among germ cell tumors of the testis. Semin Oncol 12:304–316, 1985.
15. Patton JF, Mallis N: Tumors of the testis. J Urol 81:457, 1959.
16. Richie J, Garnick M: Modified lymph node dissection in clinical stage I testis cancer (Abstr 179). Societe Int. d'Urologie, Vienna, June 23–28, 1985.
17. Skinner DG: Mangement of non-seminomatous tumors of the testis. In DG Skinner, JB deKernion (eds). Genitourinary Cancer. Philadelphia, WB Saunders, 1978, pp 470–493.
18. Skinner DG, Fraley EE, Donohue JP, Staubitz W: VIII. Surgical standing of testicular tumors. IX. Historical perspectives on node dissection. XI. Transabdominal lymphadenectomy. In JP Donohue (ed). Testis Tumors. Vol 7. International Perspectives in Urology. Baltimore, Williams & Wilkins, 1983, pp 145–206.
19. Ulbright TM, Loehrer PJ, Roth LM, et al: The development of non–germ cell malignancies within germ cell tumors: a clinicopathologic study of 11 cases. Cancer 54:1824–1833, 1984.
20. Van Buskirk KE, Young JG: Evolution of the bilateral antegrade retroperitoneal lymph node dissection in the treatment of testicular tumors. Milit Med 133:575, 1968.
21. Weisbach L, Boedefeld E: Modified lymph node dissection to preserve fertility. (Abstr 180) Societe Int. d'Urologie, Vienna, June 23–28, 1985.
22. Whitmore WF Jr: Treating germinal tumors of the testis. Cont Surg 6:17, 1975.
23. Young JD Jr: Retroperitoneal surgery. In JF Glenn, WH Boyce (eds). Urologic Surgery, 2nd ed. New York, Harper & Row, 1975, p 848.

E. DAVID CRAWFORD, M.D.

Technique of Ilioinguinal Lymph Node Dissection

CHAPTER 56

Radical ilioinguinal lymphadenectomy remains the optimal treatment in the management of tumor-bearing ilioinguinal nodes. Genitourinary neoplasms with the propensity for lymphatic drainage to iliac or inguinal chains include carcinomas of the penis, distal urethra, scrotum, and testis with scrotal invasion. Since these neoplasms are relatively rare in the United States, this radical surgical procedure is not routine in the spectrum of operative management of the general urologist. The most frequent indication for ilioinguinal lymphadenectomy is penile cancer with biopsy-proven or clinically suspected lymphatic involvement.

HISTORIC PERSPECTIVE

Although reports of surgical intervention in the treatment of penile cancer date back to the time of Celsus, it was not until 1886 that MacCormac[15] advocated bilateral inguinal lymphadenectomy in addition to penectomy. Young [19] supported the combined surgical approach, reporting a series of 23 cases in 1907. However, the alarming operative and postoperative morbidity and mortality led to judicious application of the operation. In 1948, with Daseler's precise anatomic outline of the inguinal lymphatic chain[4] and Baronofsky's advancements in transplanting the sartorius muscle over the femoral vessels as a protective cover and surface for skin flaps,[1] surgical techniques were greatly refined. Kuehn and Roberts[12] extended Young's en bloc inguinal node dissection to include iliac nodes. Cabanas' series[3] demonstrated a specific lymph node center designated the "sentinel lymph node," which appears to be the initial echelon of lymphatic drainage in penile cancer. Hardner and associates,[9] Skinner and co-workers,[17] Fraley and Hutchens,[7] and de-Kernion[5] have reviewed surgical results of radical ilioinguinal lymphadenectomy. Terms used to describe, but not always synonymous with, ilioinguinal lymph node dissection include groin dissection, pelvic-inguinal lymphatic excision, inguinofemoral dissection, superficial inguinal dissection, and inguinal lymphadenectomy.[11] A number of surgical incisions and techniques to execute this procedure have been described by Block, Fraley, Gray, Young, and others.[2, 7, 8, 11, 19] Refinements in surgical techniques accompanied by advancements in perioperative management have resulted in a significant decrease in the postoperative complications associated with ilioinguinal lymphadenectomy.

INDICATION

Regional lymph node metastases in the absence of documentable distant metastases from penile carcinoma are a clear indication for ilioinguinal lymphadenectomy. Appropriate management of the ilioinguinal nodes without biopsy-proven metastases is controversial and is discussed in Chapter 37.

817

Jackson's Staging System (Table 56–1) indicates that Stage I clinical tumors confined to glans, prepuce, or both, although frequently accompanied by adenopathy, are pathologically metastatic to nodes in only 5 to 10% of cases.[6, 11] The incidence of lymphatic involvement in tumors of clinical Stage II approaches 40%.[6] For both Stage I and II tumors, subjecting all patients to radical ilioinguinal lymphadenectomy is unnecessary. However, the argument for routine employment of ilioinguinal lymphadenectomy is quite impressive for the clinical Stage II presentations (Chapter 37). Patients with Stage III tumors, defined as having operative inguinal node metastases, are managed with the aggressive operative procedure subsequently described, and a subset of 30 to 40% of these patients will be cured by lymphadenectomy.[6] The management of Stage IV penile carcinoma, including inoperable lymphatic metastases or distant metastases, demands a multimodality intervention. However, in a select group of Stage IV patients, an improved quality of life may justify prophylactic lymphadenectomy for local control or prevention of femoral artery hemorrhage.

As carcinoma of the penis with nodal metastases is uniformly fatal if management consists of penectomy alone,[10] removal of involved nodes is indicated. Palpable lymph nodes in the presence of a primary penile carcinoma may be a sign of infection, which should resolve within one month with a trial of adequate antibiotics. In patients with questionable adenopathy, sentinel node biopsy may prove of value in developing a therapeutic plan.[3] Proper patient selection for lymphadenectomy remains confusing and controversial.[10, 11] Until these issues are resolved, I recommend bilateral ilioinguinal lymphadenectomy for penile carcinoma in the presence of one or more of the following conditions:

1. Lymphadenopathy persisting more than four weeks after penectomy and adequate antimicrobial treatment.

2. Pathologic confirmation of nodal metastasis(es).
3. Subsequent development of adenopathy in a patient with a history of penile carcinoma in the absence of any other inflammatory or infective process.
4. Extensive lesion at the base of the penis at presentation.
5. Any lesion involving the corpora cavernosa.

A less common indication for a bilateral ilioinguinal lymphadenectomy is the male or female patient with carcinoma of the urethra demonstrating regional adenopathy. Regional node dissection similarly is indicated in the patient with carcinoma of the scrotum accompanied by clinically or pathologically involved nodes. The necessity of bilateral dissection remains controversial.[14] However, I recommend it in all patients who are not prohibitive surgical risks.

ANATOMIC CONSIDERATION

Complete surgical removal of the inguinal and iliac node chains is of paramount importance in the cure of patients with locally advanced carcinomas of the penis, distal urethra, scrotum, or testis with scrotal involvement. Essential to the success of this radical surgical procedure is the comprehensive identification and removal of the ileal and inguinal lymph node echelons. Precise identification of the fascial planes of the lower abdomen and thigh, the femoral canal, and the corresponding lymph node distribution within the fascial planes and femoral canal is necessary in the performance of a meticulous ilioinguinal lymphadenectomy. The superficial fascia of the thigh consists of two layers. Superficial branches of the inferior epigastric artery, external pudendal artery, and the circumflex iliac artery supply the skin and subcutaneous tissues of the region. These blood vessels coursing in the fatty or superior layer of the superficial fascia run parallel to the inguinal ligament.

The deeper or membranous layer of the superficial fascia of the thigh is known as Camper's fascia. In consideration of the horizontal course of the blood vessels in the superficial fascia, vertical incisions are avoided to ensure adequate blood supply to the margins of the incision. Deep to Camper's fascia is the fascia lata, which envelops the thigh and gluteal region. This fascia is

Table 56–1. JACKSON'S STAGING SYSTEM

Stage I	Tumor confined to the glans prepuce
Stage II	Invasion into the penile shaft or corpora
Stage III	Proven, operable regional (groin) node metastasis(es)
Stage IV	Tumor extending off the shaft of the penis with inoperable groin nodes or distant metastasis(es)

attached superiorly to the posterior surface of the iliac crest, sacrum, coccyx, sacrotuberous ligament, ischium, inferior pubic ramus and arch, pubic symphysis and crest, and inguinal ligament. Distally, it is attached at the knee to the condyles of both the femur and tibia and to the head of the fibula. The fascia lata is thinnest on the medial side of the thigh and thickest on the lateral aspects of the thigh. Both Camper's and Scarpa's fasciae compose the superficial fascia of the lower abdomen. The most superficial, Camper's fascia, continues uninterruptedly onto the thigh. Scarpa's fascia fuses with the fascia lata approximately 1 cm below the inguinal ligament, forming the groin crease or Holden's line. Originating from the medial aspect of the dorsal venous arch of the foot, the greater saphenous vein ascends to the anterior medial thigh after passing posteriorly to the knee. Removal of both layers of the superficial fascia results in visualization of the saphenous opening where the

greater saphenous vein pierces the deep fascia. This saphenous opening is formed by the fascia lata, with the superior portion also being formed by a bundle of connective tissue arising from the medial portion of the inguinal ligament (Fig. 56–1A). The saphenous opening is covered by the cribriform fascia.

Prior to entering the femoral vein, the greater saphenous vein pierces not only the deep fascia (fascia lata and cribriform fascia) but also the femoral sheath (Fig. 56–1B). This femoral sheath is approximately 4 cm in length and consists of three distinct compartments: the medial channel containing lymphatics and lymph nodes, the intermediate channel containing the femoral vein, and the lateral channel containing the femoral artery. The femoral sheath is formed by the inferior migration of layers of the fascia from the posterior abdominal wall as the blood vessels exit the abdomen to enter the thigh. The anterior wall of the femoral

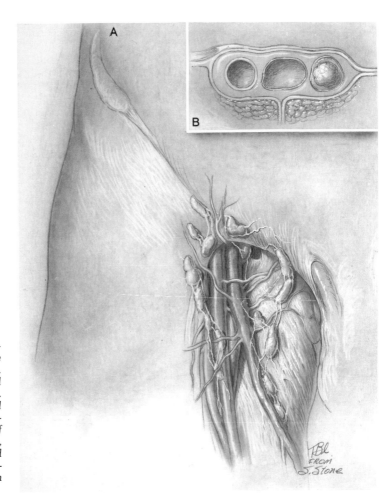

Figure 56–1. A, The superficial fascia has been removed, exposing the saphenous vein and its tributaries. The saphenous opening is formed by condensation of the fascia lata. B, Transverse section of the femoral sheath depicts the fascial encasement and the anatomic position of the femoral artery, femoral vein, and lymph node channels. Modified from Crawford ED: Radical ilioinguinal lymphadenectomy. Urol Clin North Am 11:543, 1984.

sheath is formed by condensation of the transverse fascia, whereas the posterior wall is an extension of the iliac fascia. The femoral nerve, which is lateral to the femoral canal, is not located within this sheath, as it exits the abdomen in the subserous fascia.

The anatomic area designated the femoral triangle is bound superiorly by the inguinal ligament, laterally by the sartorius muscle, and medially by the long adductor muscle. The femoral nerve is the most lateral structure in the femoral triangle approximated by the femoral artery, femoral vein, genitofemoral nerve and, finally, the most proximal structure, the ilioinguinal nerve.

The lymph nodes in the groin are divided into two groups by a horizontal line crossing the thigh at the point where the greater saphenous vein enters the femoral vein. Lymph nodes above the horizontal line are designated superficial inguinal; those below are the subinguinal nodes. However, the deep layer of the subinguinal nodes, gener-

ally containing three nodes, is located under the fascia lata within the femoral sheath. The first of the three nodes in this set is located inferior to the saphenofemoral junction, the second in the femoral canal, and the third at the femoral ring (node of Cloquet or Rosenmüller). Anatomically, the majority of the lymph nodes removed during the inguinal lymphadenectomy are not inguinal but are, more accurately, subinguinal nodes. Table 56–2 outlines the afferent and efferent branches associated with these lymph node chains.

The inguinal lymph nodes are classically bordered superiorly by the inguinal ligament, inferiorly by a line crossing the point of intersection of the sartorius and adductor muscles, laterally by a line dropped vertically from the anterior iliac spine, and medially by a similar line commencing at the pubic tubercle. However, as Daseler has pointed out,[4] all potential cancer-bearing nodes are not located within these bounda-

Table 56–2. SOURCE OF AFFERENT LYMPHATICS AND DESTINATION OF INTERCONNECTING EFFERENT LYMPHATICS OF THE ILIOINGUINAL REGION*

Lymph Node Group	Afferent Channels From	Efferent Channels To
Superficial inguinal and subinguinal:	1. Superficial lymphatics of lower extremity 2. Scrotum 3. Vulva 4. Penis (or clitoris) 5. Anus and perianal skin 6. Skin of perineum and buttocks 7. Skin of anterior abdominal wall below umbilicus	1. External iliac nodes 2. Deep inguinal nodes
Prepubic:	1. Penis (or clitoris)	1. Superficial inguinal nodes
Deep subinguinal:	1. Deep lymphatics of lower extremity 2. Superficial inguinal nodes	1. External iliac nodes

External iliac:	1. Superficial inguinal nodes
	2. Deep inguinal nodes
	3. Deep lymphatics of abdominal wall
	4. Lymphatics of medial thigh accompanying obturator artery
	5. Part of drainage from:
	  a. Dome of bladder
	  b. Prostate
	  c. Ductus deferens
	  d. Seminal vesicles
	  e. Membranous and prostatic urethra
	  f. Cervix and uterus
	  g. Vagina
	  h. Glans penis
	  i. Hypogastric (internal iliac) nodes
		1. Common iliac nodes

*In Spratt JS Jr, Shieber W, Dillard BM: Anatomy and Surgical Technique of Groin Dissection. St. Louis, C. V. Mosby Co., 1965, with permission.

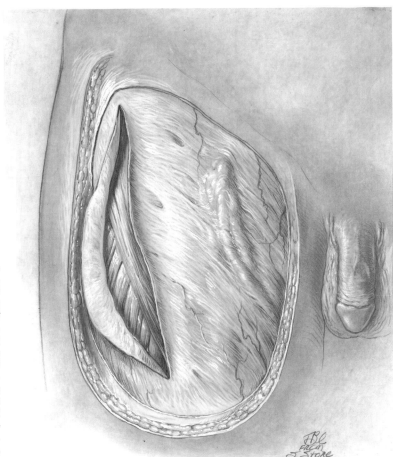

Figure 56–2. Anatomic depiction of the quadrilateral area as defined by Daseler (right thigh).[4] The fascial layers encountered include the superficial layer of the superficial fascia, the membranous layer of the superficial fascia (Camper's fascia), and the fascia lata. The superficial and subinguinal lymph nodes are located between the membranous layer of the superficial fascia and the fascia lata. Modified from Crawford ED: Radical ilioinguinal lymphadenectomy. Urol Clin North Am 11:543, 1984.

ries. He outlines an area of dissection as a quadrilateral area bounded superiorly by a line 12 cm in length parallel to and 1 cm above the inguinal ligament; medially by a line 15 cm in length dropped perpendicularly downward from the pubic tubercle; laterally by a 20-cm line dropped from the lateral limits of the superior boundary; and inferiorly by a transverse line 11 cm in length connecting the lower limit of the lateral and medial borders (Fig. 56–2). The superficial inguinal and subinguinal lymph nodes are located deep to the membranous fascia (Camper's fascia of the thigh). These superficial lymphatics send their efferent vessels into glands of deeper position situated along the femoral vessels (deep subinguinal) and then into the retroperitoneal iliac chain. Because of their expansive field, the superficial glands offer a more difficult surgical dissection, whereas the deeper glands are clustered along the iliac and femoral vessels in simple chains. An average

of 8.25 lymph nodes per extremity were reported by Daseler, who characterized their location into zones (Fig. 56–3). By creating a horizontal line at the saphenofemoral junction, four quadrants corresponding with Daseler's four zones are outlined. Daseler's fifth zone was the saphenous femoral junction. Lymph nodes in Quadrant 1 are intimately associated with the superficial circumflex iliac vein. Nodes from Quadrant 2 are located in the superior medial quadrant and cluster along the terminal portions of the superior epigastric and superficial external pudendal veins. An important discovery in Daseler's dissections was that lymph nodes were occasionally observed in several specimens 1 cm superior to the inguinal ligament. Quadrant 3 is inferomedial in position and contains nodes clustered around the greater saphenous vein. The inferior lateral lymph nodes from the fourth quadrant are grouped around the lateral accessory saphenous vein and termination of the superficial circumflex

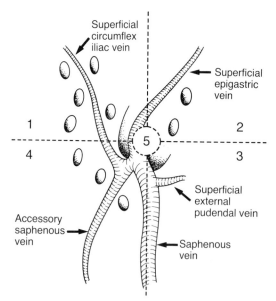

Figure 56–3. Relationship of the saphenous vein and its tributaries to the inguinal lymph nodes. These lymph nodes are separable into five groups. Modified from Daseler EH, et al: Radical excision of the inguinal and iliac lymph glands. Surg Gynecol Obstet 87:679–694, 1948.

iliac vein. Daseler's fifth zone is the central presaphenous region immediately overlying the saphenofemoral junction. Each quadrant may contain several lymph nodes or be completely void of nodes. The node most frequently encountered in Daseler's study was one located at the angle formed by the bifurcation of the lateral accessory saphenous from the greater saphenous vein.

As previously mentioned, the deep inguinal lymph nodes follow the course of the femoral artery and vein. Several lymph nodes cluster around the femoral sheath in fat-filled connective tissue, with the most constant and largest of this group being the lymph node of Cloquet or Rosenmüller.

In summary, any anatomic dissection of the groin should encompass all these node-bearing areas and include dissection within the femoral sheath.

The next echelon of drainage is the iliac region. Nodes of the iliac region are intimately associated with the external iliac, internal iliac, and common iliac blood vessels. The external iliac nodes range from eight to 10 in number; the hypogastric and iliac glands range from four to six. The external iliac nodes generally reside along the medial aspect of either the artery or the vein or in the sulcus between these vessels.

The hypogastric nodes are similarly related to the hypogastric vessels. The common iliac node chain may reside medially or even partially concealed posterior to the vessels.

The following discussion will describe anatomic cleavage planes and boundaries that will facilitate the removal of all potentially cancer-laden lymph nodes.

SURGICAL PROCEDURE

Broad-spectrum antibiotic coverage and intravenous volume expanders are initiated the evening prior to the surgical procedure. With the patient placed supine on the operative table, adequate endotracheal anesthesia is obtained and the kidney rest is elevated under the lumbar spine to provide slight hyperextension. Antiembolic material is then wrapped around both legs. The leg on the ipsilateral side is abducted at the thigh, flexed at the knee, and rotated externally. Urethral catheterization is performed. The entire lower abdomen and upper thighs are prepped for the procedure, and the patient is draped in the usual fashion.

Pelvic Lymph Node Dissection

A midline incision is extended from the symphysis pubis lateral to the umbilicus, terminating superior to the umbilicus (Fig. 56–4A). The subcutaneous tissue and anterior rectus sheath are divided with the rectus muscles retracted laterally (Fig. 56–4B). The layer immediately deep to the rectus muscles is the fascia of the rectus abdominis muscle (Fig. 56–4C). This fascia is contiguous with the transversalis fascia. The fascia is entered sharply, lateral to the midline, in order to expose the underlying retroperitoneal structures. The dissection is then carried inferiorly and laterally until the external iliac vessels are identified. Inadvertent injury to the inferior epigastric vessels often is associated with a failure to remain deep to this fascia.

The peritoneal reflection is identified, with the vas and spermatic vessels coursing in its medial aspect. The spermatic vessels are dissected free from this reflection, and the vas divided (Fig. 56–5). The obliterated processus vaginalis will be adherent to the internal ring and is sharply divided (Fig. 56–6). At this point in the procedure, the

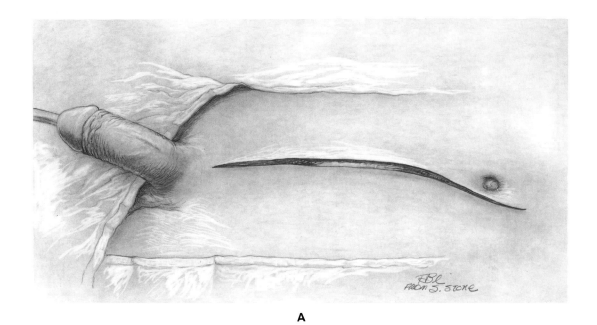

A

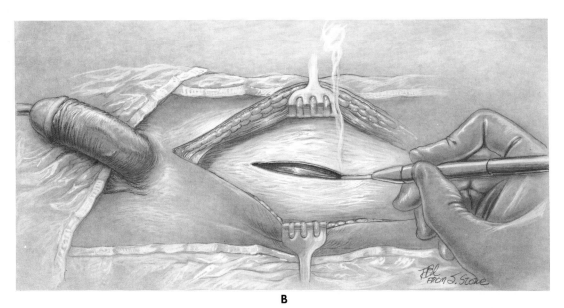

B

Figure 56–4. A, *The patient is positioned for a pelvic lymphadenectomy. Modified after Crawford ED: Radical retropubic prostatectomy: modified Campbell technique. In ED Crawford, TA Borden (eds), Genitourinary Cancer Surgery. Philadelphia, Lea & Febiger, 1982, with permission.* B, *Rectus fascia is divided, exposing rectus muscles.*

Illustration continued on following page

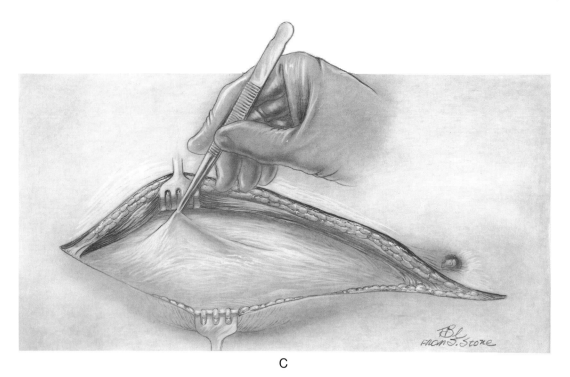

C

Figure 56–4 Continued. C, *The incision has been carried through the rectus fascia, and the rectus muscles have been retracted laterally. An incision is made in the investing fascia of the rectus abdominis muscle, exposing the retroperitoneal connective tissue. Modified after Crawford ED: Radical retropubic prostatectomy: modified Campbell technique. In ED Crawford, TA Borden (eds), Genitourinary Cancer Surgery. Philadelphia, Lea & Febiger, 1982, with permission.*

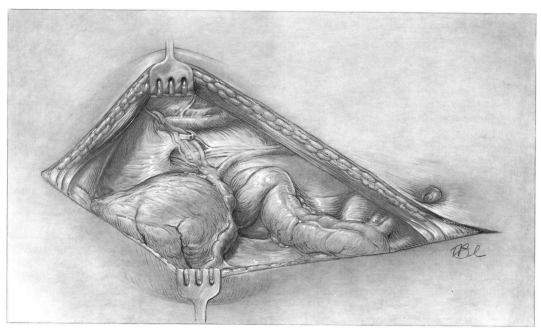

Figure 56–5. The vas is separated from spermatic vessels and divided.

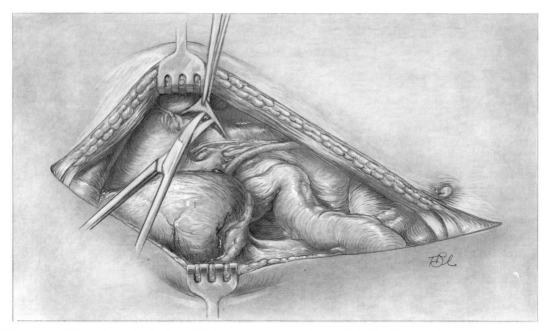

Figure 56–6. The peritoneal reflection with the vas and spermatic vessels is identified, and an incision is made at the internal ring lateral to the spermatic vessels. Modified after Crawford ED: Radical retropubic prostatectomy: modified Campbell technique. In ED Crawford, TA Borden (eds), Genitourinary Cancer Surgery. Philadelphia, Lea & Febiger, 1982, with permission.

peritoneum is easily mobilized, providing excellent exposure for pelvic lymphadenectomy. With a retractor placed in the wound, the dissection is first carried out on the ipsilateral side, employing the technique of bilateral pelvic lymphadenectomy as described in Chapter 51, with the following modifications:

All fat and node-bearing connective tissue should be removed from around the distal common iliac artery, the internal iliac artery and its major branches, the external iliac vessels, and the obturator fossa; if metastases are noted at the level of the common iliac vessels or extensively in the lower pelvis, then the procedure is terminated; if metastatic involvement is absent, then a contralateral pelvic dissection is performed. This dissection is more encompassing than the staging pelvic lymph node dissection for prostate cancer, as the lymph nodes down to and behind the inguinal ligament are removed and the femoral canal region is dissected (Fig. 56–7).

I do not advocate en bloc removal of the pelvic and inguinal lymph nodes but rather remove the pelvic lymph glands as a separate specimen. The inguinal ligament is then sutured to Cooper's ligament to prevent a postoperative hernia. Upon completion of this procedure, the wound is closed in a routine fashion without any drains.

Ilioinguinal Node Dissection

A curvilinear incision is made in the groin parallel to the inguinal ligament (Fig. 56–8). This should be approximately 5 to 10 cm below the ligament, with the medial aspect near the scrotum (mid thigh) and lateral aspect extending toward the anterior superior iliac spine. At its highest point, the incision should be approximately 2 to 4 cm from the inguinal canal. The dissection will then encompass all areas in the quadrilateral area as defined by Daseler. Development of viable skin flaps is essential at this point. The flaps must be developed superficial to Camper's fascia, preserving a generous amount of subcutaneous adipose tissue. The skin edges are handled meticulously and are easily maneuvered with skin hooks. The skin flaps are developed to 2 cm above the inguinal ligament and 1 cm below the apex of the femoral triangle. The dissection is carried laterally over the sartorius muscle and medially to the edge of the adductor longus. As the flaps are developed, meticulous hemostasis is employed.

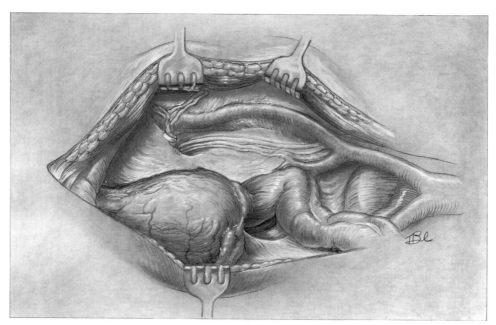

Figure 56–7. Lateral view of right pelvis at the termination of pelvic lymphadenectomy. All fat and node-bearing connective tissue has been removed from around the distal common iliac artery, the internal iliac artery and all its major branches, the external iliac vessel, and obturator fossa. Modified after Lieber JJ: Pelvic lymphadenectomy. In ED Crawford, TA Borden (eds), Genitourinary Cancer Surgery. Philadelphia, Lea & Febiger, 1982, with permission.

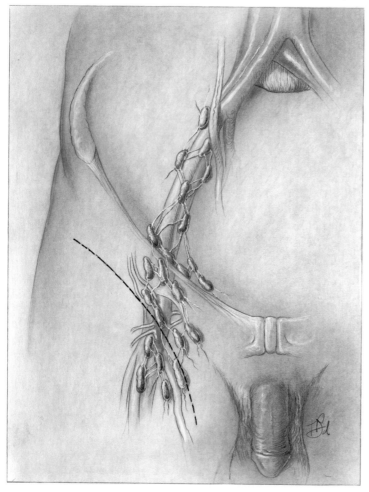

Figure 56–8. Relationship of the inguinal lymph nodes to the proposed incision site on the right thigh.

The lymph node dissection is begun superiorly, sweeping all tissue from the aponeurosis of the external oblique downward to the inguinal ligament (Fig. 56–9). All the divided tissue in this area may be hemoclipped or electrocoagulated. Dissection is then carried inferiorly and medially over the femoral canal (Fig. 56–10). Node-bearing tissue in Quadrant 2 is stripped from the long adductor muscle. The medially located preputial node is identified and swept inferiorly and laterally. As the procedure develops laterally, the femoral vessels are identified; when the femoral vein is encountered, the overlying fascia is removed from the vein. Dissection proceeds laterally to the femoral artery, and the tissue overlying the artery is sharply entered and stripped. Several small cutaneous branches of the femoral artery are preserved if possible. The profunda femoris vessel arises posteriorly and laterally approximately 2 cm distal to the inguinal ligament. It is essential not to injure or ligate this vessel. As the dissection proceeds laterally, the femoral nerve is identified (Fig. 56–11). No nodal tissue resides in this area, so it is not necessary to strip the nerve meticulously. Several small cutaneous branches of the nerve need not be preserved.

The upper portion of the dissection continues laterally to the iliac spine, exposing the origin of the sartorius muscle. The thickened lateral portion of the fascia lata is incised from this point down to the inferior margin of the dissection.

The superior and lateral margins of the dissection have now been defined. The adventitia surrounding the femoral artery and vein is dissected inferiorly. There is no node-bearing tissue posterior to the artery and vein; therefore, dissection in this area should be avoided in order to prevent injury to the deep femoral and profunda femoris artery. In proceeding distally over the femoral vessels, the insertion of the saphenous vein will be observed. Recently I have preserved this vessel, although most surgeons ligate it. Preservation may decrease postoperative venous and lymphatic stasis. The fascia lata of the thigh now can be adequately reflected medially from the sartorius, iliac, and pectineal muscles. The medial portion of the dissection is defined over the long adductor muscle and the thin layer of the fascia lata is incised inferiorly. The fibrofatty and nodal tissue overlying and between the femoral vessels is dissected inferiorly to the apex of the femoral triangle by incising

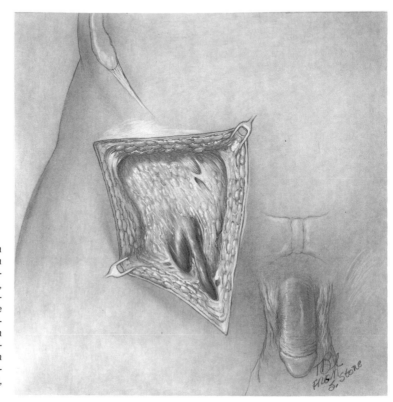

Figure 56–9. Skin flaps have been developed and are handled with skin hooks. The lymph node dissection is commenced superiorly, sweeping all tissue from the aponeurosis of the external oblique downward to the inguinal ligament. Modified after deKernion JB: Ilioinguinal lymphadenectomy. In ED Crawford, TA Borden (eds), Genitourinary Cancer Surgery. Philadelphia, Lea & Febiger, 1982, with permission.

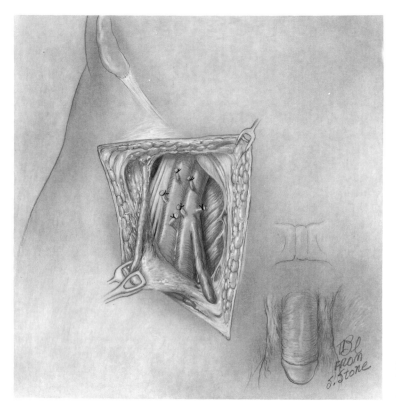

Figure 56–10. The greater saphenous vein is identified as it enters the femoral vein. Several cutaneous branches are ligated and divided at their junction with the femoral vein. Modified from Crawford ED: Radical ilioinguinal lymphadenectomy. Urol Clin North Am 11:543, 1984.

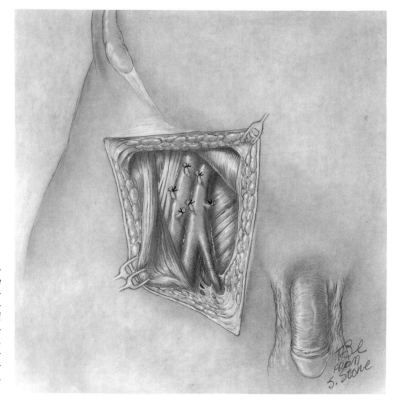

Figure 56–11. The superior, lateral, and medial portions of the dissection are completed, exposing the underlying muscles, femoral nerve, femoral artery, and femoral vein. The greater saphenous vein has been preserved. Modified from Crawford ED: Radical ilioinguinal lymphadenectomy. Urol Clin North Am 11:543, 1984.

the fascia lata. At this point in the procedure, all the margins have been defined. The inferior margin is dissected free, and the specimen is removed en bloc (Fig. 56–12).

WOUND CLOSURE

In order to minimize postoperative wound complications, meticulous closure of the surgical incision is performed. The wound is inspected carefully for lymphatic or vascular oozing. After adequate hemostasis is achieved, the sartorius muscle is sharply dissected at its origin from the iliac spine and sutured to the inguinal ligament as described by Baronofsky.[1] The blood supply enters the muscle approximately 10 cm distal to its origin and is preserved (Fig. 56–13).

A suction catheter is inserted under the distal flap and attention given to subcutaneous closure (Fig. 56–14). The subcutaneous tissues are closed and anchored to the corresponding underlying muscles with 4-0 polyglycolic acid (PGA) sutures in order to eliminate any dead space, which discourages fluid collection.

Excess skin is frequently present after removal of the underlying nodal tissue. Several millimeters of this may have to be removed prior to closure. I suggest employment of the technique as described by Smith and Middleton,[18] using fluorescein to ascertain the viability of the skin edges. With an intravenous injection of 10 ml of fluorescein, the skin flaps are observed 15 minutes later under a Wood's light. Poorly vascularized areas will have a bluish hue, whereas well-vascularized areas will exhibit a yellow-green fluorescence. The devascularized area is trimmed and the superficial subcutaneous tissue is approximated with 4-0 PGA sutures. The skin edges are approximated with 4-0 nylon skin sutures. Dry, sterile dressings are applied without pressure, as pressure may compromise vascularity of the flaps.

POSTOPERATIVE CARE AND COMPLICATIONS

The patient is maintained on bed rest with lower extremity antiembolic wrapping and elevation for seven days. Suction catheters are routinely observed for patency and are removed when the patient begins to walk about.

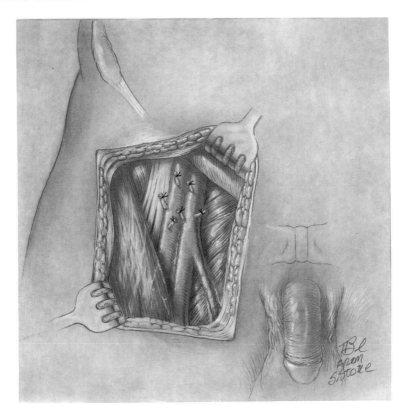

Figure 56–12. Completed lymph node dissection. Modified from Crawford ED: Radical ilioinguinal lymphadenectomy. Urol Clin North Am 11:543, 1984.

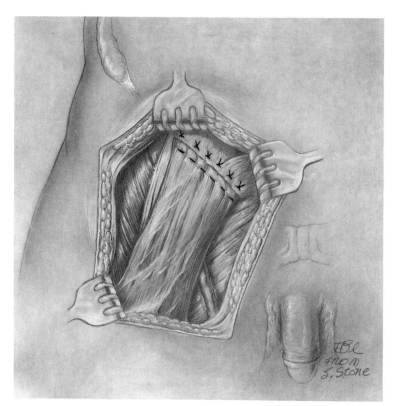

Figure 56–13. The transposed sartorius muscle is sutured to the inguinal ligament. Potential dead spaces are obliterated by approximating the subcutaneous tissues to the underlying muscles with 4-0 polyglycolic acid sutures. Modified from Crawford ED: Radical ilioinguinal lymphadenectomy. Urol Clin North Am 11:543, 1984.

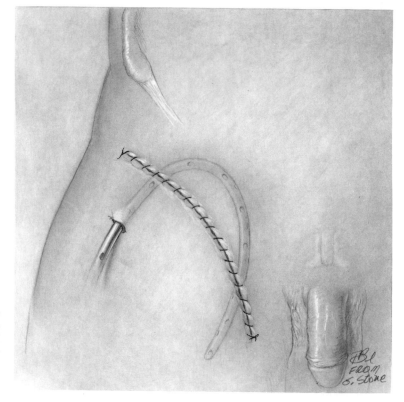

Figure 56–14. A suction catheter is inserted under the lower flap and coiled under the upper and lower flaps. Modified from Crawford ED: Radical ilioinguinal lymphadenectomy. Urol Clin North Am 11:543, 1984.

Postoperative anticoagulation in these and other high-risk surgical patients has been widely discussed. In the past, we routinely employed 5000 units of heparin subcutaneously every 12 hours, but recently we have been impressed with adjusting minidose heparin levels to the activated partial thromboplastin times as suggested by Leyvraz and associates.[13] This approach seems appropriate for postlymphadenectomy management, as tissue thromboplastin levels frequently override the effect of minidose heparin. Dihydroergotamine heparin has recently been approved to prevent deep venous thrombosis, and its therapeutic benefit is currently undergoing evaluation at our institution in comprehensive urologic procedures associated with thromboembolic phenomena.[16]

Although flap necrosis can occur anywhere along the incisional line, the most common site is over Scarpa's triangle; this may occur between the fifth and twelfth postoperative days. Precise development and manipulation of the flaps accompanied by a proper closure may decrease this complication.

Wound infections are uncommon, unless the surgical procedure was carried out in an ulcerated or an infected groin. Necrosis of the flaps will frequently be associated with wound infections. Lower extremity edema is reported in 2 to 40% of patients.[11] This edema may be transient or permanent and frequently involves the thighs and less often the lower leg. This complication appears to be circumvented by postoperative immobilization, lower extremity elevation, and use of support stockings. Careful ligation of the lymphatics and postoperative suction decreases the incidence of lymphorrhea and seroma.

Life-threatening hemorrhage from the femoral vessels is a rare occurrence with the transposition of the sartorius over the denuded vessels. Hematomas of varying sizes may develop and are managed in the usual manner. Employing the technique of suturing the inguinal ligament to Cooper's ligament decreases the incidence of incisional hernia.

Morbidity following the ilioinguinal lymphadenectomy can be high and is generally attributable to local wound complications. Appropriate patient selection, accompanied by precise operative technique and vigorous perioperative support, will result in decreased postoperative complica-tions and, importantly, will result in better patient survival.

Acknowledgments

The author gratefully acknowledges the medical illustrations prepared by Ms. Sheryl Stone (Veterans Administration Medical Center) and the editorial assistance provided by Ms. Marilyn Davis, M.S.

References

1. Baronofsky ID: Technique for inguinal node dissection. Surgery 24:555–567, 1948.
2. Block NL, Rosen P, Whitmore WF Jr: Hemipelvectomy for advanced penile cancer. J Urol 110:703, 1973.
3. Cabanas RM: An approach for the treatment of penile carcinoma. Cancer 39:456–466, 1977.
4. Daseler EH, Anson BJ, Reimann AF: Radical excision of the inguinal and iliac lymph glands: a study based upon 450 anatomical dissections and upon supportive clinical observations. Surg Gynecol Obstet 87:679–694, 1948.
5. deKernion JB: Ilioinguinal lymphadenectomy. In ED Crawford, TA Borden (eds): Genitourinary Cancer Surgery. Philadelphia, Lea & Febiger, 1982, pp 317–323.
6. deKernion JB, Tynberg P, Persky L, Fegen JP: Carcinoma of penis. Cancer 32:1256–1262, 1973.
7. Fraley EE, Hutchens HC: Radical ilio-inguinal node dissection: skin bridge technique. A new procedure. J Urol 108:279–283, 1972.
8. Gray DB, Bailey HA: A new technique for radical ilio-inguinal dissection. Ann Surg 145:873–885, 1957.
9. Hardner GJ, Bhanalaph T, Murphy GP, et al: Carcinoma of the penis: analysis of therapy in 100 consecutive cases. J Urol 108:428–430, 1972.
10. Hoppmann HS, Fraley EE: Squamous cell carcinoma of the penis. J Urol 120:393–398, 1978.
11. Hovnanian AP: The evolution and present status of pelvi-inguinal lymphatic excision. Surg Gynecol Obstet 124:851–865, 1967.
12. Kuehn CA, Roberts RR: Amputation and radical lymph gland dissection in carcinoma of the penis: an operative technique. J Urol 69:173–180, 1953.
13. Leyvraz PF, Richard J, Bachmann F, et al: Adjusted versus fixed-dose subcutaneous heparin in the prevention of deep-vein thrombosis after total hip replacement. N Engl J Med 309:954–958, 1983.
14. Lowe FC: Squamous cell carcinoma of the scrotum. J Urol 130:423–427, 1983.
15. MacCormac W: Five cases of amputation of the penis for epithelioma. Br Med J 1:343–345, 1886.
16. Multicenter Trial Committee: Dihydroergotamine-heparin prophylaxis of postoperative deep vein thrombosis. A multicenter trial. JAMA 251:2960–2966, 1984.
17. Skinner DG, Leadbetter WF, Kelley SB: The surgical management of squamous cell carcinoma of the penis. J Urol 107:273–277, 1972.
18. Smith JA Jr, Middleton RG: The use of fluorescein in radical inguinal lymphadenectomy. J Urol 122:754–756, 1979.
19. Young HH: A radical operation for the cure of cancer of the penis. J Urol 26:285–294, 1931.

THOMAS E. PALMER, M.D.
DAVID L. McCULLOUGH, M.D.

Endourologic Management of Obstructive Problems in the Cancer Patient

CHAPTER 57

Although metastases to the ureter are uncommon,[1, 15] ureteral obstruction due to direct extension or external compression by pelvic malignancy or lymph nodes is not. Urologists frequently care for patients with advanced malignancy in whom death due to uremia is inevitable if palliative urinary diversion is not performed. These patients are often seriously ill and are poor surgical risks owing to malnutrition, sepsis, fluid and electrolyte imbalance, and the hematologic and immunologic consequences of previous antineoplastic therapy. One must carefully balance the merits of prolonging life and the associated potential for considerable pain, suffering, and expense against death due to uremia. Previous studies dealing with this problem have shown that open surgical diversion, primarily by nephrostomy, has been associated with significant morbidity and mortality. Life-threatening complications have been reported to be as high as 45%,[6, 13] with only 31% having a routine postoperative recovery.[21] Forty-nine per cent of these patients required additional surgery after the initial diversion.[21] Complications were the cause of death in 3 to 8% of patients and contributed to the death of another 29 to 34 per cent.[13, 21]

Survival rates following urinary diversion have been historically poor. In a series of three reports totalling 327 cases, the majority of patients undergoing diversion by various surgical techniques had a postoperative survival of less than six months.[4, 13, 21] Between 35 and 41% did not leave the hospital prior to their death,[4, 21] and almost one third of the survival time for the entire group was spent in hospital.[21] In contrast, however, approximately 50% of these patients returned home for two months or longer with minimal or well-controlled pain and acceptable mental function.[13]

If postoperative complications that cause or contribute to the patient's demise could be minimized, more patients could return home for longer periods and spend less survival time confined to the hospital. Percutaneous or endoscopic urinary diversions have far less potential for complication than open surgical diversions. These procedures can often be performed on critically ill patients under local anesthesia, thereby avoiding the risk associated with general anesthesia. Displaced or dislodged drainage tubes can usually be repositioned or replaced without an open surgical procedure. The reported rates of morbidity and mortality following percutaneous nephrostomy have been 4% and 0.2%, respectively,[23] with previously reported deaths occurring due to hemorrhage in patients with underlying bleeding disorders.

Recent reports with endoscopically placed stents for ureteral obstruction secondary to cancer have been encouraging. Gibbons and associates reported 17 patients treated with placement of a Gibbons stent. Nine of them were uremic. Eighty-eight per cent of these patients were discharged from the hospital and lived longer than two months.[8] Hepperlin and associates reported that 85% of their patients diverted with a pigtail ureteral stent returned home and lived longer than two months (average survival of 277 days in 20 patients).[12] These two series also illustrated that with advances in techniques, guide wires, and catheters, more urinary diversions can be created with self-retaining ureteral stents cystoscopically placed or via a previously placed percutaneous nephrostomy. As a result, fewer patients require external collection devices, an important factor since only 13% of patients with surgically placed open nephrostomy tubes had their tubes removed following additional anticancer therapy.[13]

PROGNOSTIC FACTORS

Data available from previous reports concerning prognostic indications are conflicting. Possibly, different series may have involved patients of varying surgical risk at different points in the natural history of their disease. One would expect that patients who have been found to have ureteral obstruction before they become symptomatic or uremic will live longer after diversion than will those in the more terminal stages of various malignancies. Previous therapy, different cell types and stages, age, and other concurrent medical disorders influence survival. However, certain trends have emerged in reviewing the literature.

Holden, McPhee, and Grabstald[13] found that patients with localized tumors have a better prognosis than do patients with metastatic lesions. They divided patients into three stages, regardless of cell type. Stage A patients had tumors confined to the organ of origin and represented 8% of the total. This group had a two-year survival of 88%. Stage B patients had direct extension of the tumor or positive regional nodes and represented 31% of the total. Stage C patients (61% of total) had disseminated disease. Stage B and C patients had two-year survival rates of 18% and 2%, respectively. Further evidence that these patients had a poorer prognosis than those in Stage A is substantiated by the fact that 32% of Stage B patients and 49% of

Stage C patients did not live two months after diversion.

The degree of renal failure at the time of diversion does not have prognostic significance.[6, 19] Three series reveal that the duration of disease from time of original diagnosis to development of ureteral obstruction is not indicative of survival after diversion,[4, 13, 21] with the possible exception of cervical cancer. Meyer and associates[19] found that patients who survived for longer than six months after diversion had an average interval of 2.6 years after completion of treatment and subsequent nephrostomy, whereas those who survived less than six months had an interval of only 1.25 years (p <0.05).

Patients with cancer of the prostate have the most favorable prognosis when compared with patients having tumors of other cell types. Prostate cancer patients have an average survival after diversion of one year.[4, 6] This is especially true in patients who have not had prior hormonal manipulation. Khan and Utz reported on a group of patients with bilateral obstruction secondary to prostate cancer who had serum creatinine levels that ranged from 2.0 to 28.4 mg/dl.[14] They found a one-year survival of 38% of those with previous hormonal therapy, in contrast to 78% survival at one year for those who had not received hormonal therapy. Michigan and Catalona had a similar group of patients and showed that 88% of patients treated with orchiectomy showed improvement, with 94% of those patients alive at one year and 70% surviving two years.[20] Patients receiving radiation therapy did not respond as well, and no patient who failed endocrine treatment or who had a relapse after a previous response to endocrine treatment improved with radiation therapy.[20] Although not specifically dealing with patients who underwent palliative urinary diversion, these two reports support the efficacy of hormonal therapy in patients with ureteral obstruction due to prostatic cancer. One of the authors of this chapter (DLM) has had several patients with prostatic cancer who were hormonal failures but have lived over three years following ureteral reimplantation. The dome of the bladder was used as the reimplantation site.

Cervical cancer patients have had a favorable prognosis as well. Fallon and associates[6] found an average survival rate of 18 months following nephrostomy. Twenty per cent of their patients returned home with little or no pain, were alert, had no limitation in activity, and survived for at least two months. Another 67% were discharged from the hospital with moderate limitation in activity and pain controlled by analgesics.[6] In another report, 41% lived six months or longer, with an average survival after diversion of 11.0 months.[19] These patients were described as having a "reasonable quality of life."[19]

Survival after palliative urinary diversion in patients with bladder cancer has historically been poor, with an average survival of approximately 4.5 months.[4, 6, 16] One half of the patients reported by Fallon, Olney, and Culp[6] were confined to the hospital or had a persistent decline in status. Early results with combination chemotherapy for advanced transitional cell carcinoma are encouraging, however, and may contribute to longer survival in this group of patients.[27]

Patients with primary malignancy of the breast, colon, or rectum have had poor survival after diversion.[6, 10, 24] Ulm and Klein reported an average survival of three months for 10 patients with obstruction due to cancer of the rectosigmoid. Only one patient of a group of seven who underwent nephrostomy for metastatic carcinoma of the breast survived longer than four months in a series by Grabstald and Kaufman.[10]

FACTORS THAT INFLUENCE THE DECISION TO DIVERT

Although the physician must rely upon personal judgment according to the individual clinical situation, there are factors that influence the decision for or against palliative urinary diversion in the cancer patient. Foremost among these are the wishes of the patient and the family. The physician should assist in this decision through care and understanding with open, honest discussion of the patient's prognosis and chance for reasonable quality of life after diversion. There are times when the patient may wish to prolong life for legal or financial reasons. Many times the patient will want to live as long as possible despite an unfavorable outlook. We believe that these wishes should be honored in most instances, except when death is so imminent that diversion would be an exercise in futility.

Another factor to consider is the possibility of additional anticancer therapy. Patients who develop obstruction prior to exhausting all therapeutic options are generally good candidates for palliative diversion. This is especially true in patients who present with uremia and a previously undiagnosed malignancy, or in patients with prostatic cancer who have not had the benefits of hormonal manipulation. On the other hand, it is difficult to recommend diversion in patients who have had all possible modes of treatment and continue to have progression of their disease.

The cell type of the primary malignancy may also influence the decision. As has been shown, patients with prostatic or cervical cancer tend to have a longer life expectancy after diversion than do patients with colorectal, bladder, or breast cancer.

One must also consider the presence or absence of other serious, potentially life-threatening medical diseases. Although age has not generally been found to be of prognostic significance, one study found that all patients over 80 years of age died soon after diversion. The amount of pain that the patient has and the physician's ability to control this pain with analgesics is an important factor. Uremia and the oblivion it affords may be a more humane course in patients with severe, poorly controlled pain. Obstruction associated with flank pain, sepsis, or fistula is usually an indication for palliative urinary diversion.

Although percutaneous nephrostomy usually is a safe, uncomplicated procedure, there are times when its performance is unwise. This occurs in patients with bleeding disorders, renal vascular malformations or aneurysms, or large vascular perirenal or renal tumors. One should remember that the previously reported deaths secondary to percutaneous nephrostomy have all occurred in patients with underlying clotting disorders. Open diversion with visual control of any bleeding would be more advisable in this circumstance.

PERCUTANEOUS NEPHROSTOMY

Early efforts at supravesical diversion of the urine were fraught with complications and mortality. In 1950, Bricker described the ureteroileocutaneous urinary diversion, which continues to be used extensively.[3] As early as 1955, Goodwin and associates reported the first percutaneous nephrostomy performed by the trocar method.[9] Approximately 10 years later, percutaneous nephrostomy became somewhat more simplified after Bartley and associates reported insertion of a percutaneous nephrostomy using the Seldinger technique.[2] Percutaneous drainage of the upper urinary tract gained in popularity in the mid 1970's[11] and has been the subject of extensive publication in recent urologic literature.

Anatomy

The ability to safely bypass obstruction with percutaneous techniques is founded upon the knowledge not only of the gross and surface anatomy of the kidneys but also upon the anatomy of the intrarenal vascular and collecting structures. The kidneys are usually paired retroperitoneal organs that lie lateral to the vertebral column at approximately the area from the twelfth thoracic rib to the third lumbar vertebral body; the right kidney is slightly lower than the left. The twelfth rib crosses the kidney at a 45° angle posteriorly, with one half to two thirds of the kidney inferior to the rib. Also, the kidney does not lie in the true coronal plane of the body. The medial aspect is anterior to the lateral aspect, thus placing the kidney at an angle of about 30° to the coronal plane. It is important to position the patient correctly when directing the initial puncture for percutaneous nephrostomy.

The intrarenal collecting systems and renal pelves vary in size, shape, and number. Generally, there are four to 12 calyces, with eight being the most frequently seen. The calyces are usually compound in the upper and lower poles. The remainder of the calyces are arranged in anterior and posterior rows. The posterior group of calyces lies at an angle of 20° from the frontal plane of the kidney, which lies, as previously described, at an angle of 30° to the coronal plane of the body. Because of this, on the anterior-posterior views of a standard intravenous urogram the anterior calyces are projected to be more lateral whereas the posterior group appears "end-on."

Vascular Anatomy

The renal artery arises from the aorta and is most often single, lying between the renal vein, which is anterior, and the renal pelvis,

which is posterior. The main renal artery divides into an anterior branch, which gives off segmental branches to the apical, upper anterior, middle anterior, and lower renal segments, and a posterior branch, which supplies the posterior renal segment. These are end arteries. The usual junction between the anterior and posterior arterial divisions is 1 to 2 cm behind the lateral border of the kidney—the so-called Brödel's bloodless line of incision. Because this line of incision leads into the posterior calyceal group and the lowermost calyx in this group is below the twelfth rib and thus the pleura, it is obvious that this is the safest route by which one may gain percutaneous access to the upper urinary tract.

Localization and Placement of the Percutaneous Needle

Fluoroscopy is the best imaging mode for localization of the collecting system. It readily permits one to visualize the needles, catheters, guide wires, and dilators used for the safe insertion and proper positioning of a nephrostomy tube. It is also a technique with which the urologist is familiar. When the patient has acceptable renal function, the collecting system may be opacified with intravenous injection of contrast medium. However, many patients with urinary obstruction do not have acceptable renal function. In this case, a portable ultrasound machine may be used for antegrade pyelography so that the initial puncture may be guided rather than performed "blind." The definitive placement of the nephrostomy tube can then be performed under fluoroscopic control. Later, the nephrostomy tube usually can be inserted under local anesthesia with lidocaine or bupivacaine coupled with intravenous sedation and analgesia with diazepam and meperidine. Many uremic patients require no sedation. Preoperative antibiotics are given prophylactically.

The patient is placed in the prone position and is then rotated to an oblique position of 30 to 45°. This places the posterior calyceal group at approximately a 90° angle with the fluoroscopic table. The skin is prepped and draped. The skin is anesthetized and a 22-gauge spinal or Chiba needle is inserted medial and inferior to the twelfth rib. This needle should be inserted at a 90° angle to the table or parallel to the beam of the fluoroscopic unit. Repeated attempts are sometimes necessary; however, owing to the small size of these needles, trauma is minimal. Aspiration of urine proves entry into the collecting system and may require extension tubing and a syringe. Dilute contrast medium is then injected in an antegrade fashion. The use of dilute rather than concentrated contrast medium facilitates easier visualization of the guide wire, dilators, and catheters. Overdistention should be avoided, as this can force infected urine into the general circulation and can also result in extravasation of contrast, which could obscure the field of view. The 22-gauge needle should be left in place during the definitive puncture to allow for injection of additional contrast medium if necessary.

Definitive Nephrostomy Tube Placement

With the patient in the prone position and rotated obliquely to an angle of 45°, the desired site of entry into the calyceal system is chosen. The most inferior calyx of the posterior group is usually the proper choice in cancer patients with ureteral obstruction, as this affords good drainage and provides relatively easy access to the ureter for later antegrade insertion of a ureteral stent. The posterolateral course allows the percutaneous nephrostomy to pass through the renal parenchyma in Brödel's bloodless line of incision, avoiding major renal segmental arteries and permitting the parenchyma to stabilize the catheter. Except in experienced hands and unusual circumstances, the definitive puncture should be made below the twelfth rib to prevent a pneumothorax.

A small skin incision is made after injection of local anesthesia. Under fluoroscopic control a No. 18 French trocar needle is inserted into the collecting sytem, taking care to keep the path of the needle parallel to the x-ray beam. The proper depth of insertion can usually be determined by the depth required to perform the earlier localization puncture. After the calyx is entered, urine is aspirated and cultured and a small amount of dilute contrast medium is injected to confirm proper placement. At this point, a 0.038-inch J- or "floppy"-tip guide wire is inserted through the needle. Ideally, for maximum stabilization, the guide wire is passed down the ureter. Unfortunately, many times this is not possible, and the guide wire curls in the renal pelvis. This step prevents accidental dislodgement of the guide wire during dilation of the tract. The needle is then removed and the dilators are passed sequentially over the guide wire to enlarge the tract. One must be certain that the guide wire is held straight and taut during the dilation of the tract and insertion of the nephrostomy tube, otherwise there may be kinking of the guide wire and loss of access to the collecting system. The nephrostomy tube is passed over the guide wire after the tract has been dilated. The optimal position for the tip of the catheter is usually the renal pelvis, especially if one is using a pigtail or self-retaining catheter. This is verified with irrigation of a small amount of dilute contrast medium to ensure that drainage is not impaired. The nephrostomy tube is then secured to the skin with nylon sutures or to the plastic disk (supplied in the commercially available kits), which is then taped to the skin. Antibiotic ointment and a bulky dressing are applied.

When one intends to use the percutaneous nephrostomy as a long-term or permanent method of drainage, the tube probably should be irrigated with normal saline periodically to prevent sludging and obstruction. Also, the nephrostomy should be replaced approximately every two to three months. This can easily be accomplished as an outpatient procedure by inserting the guide wire down the nephrostomy, removing the tube, and inserting a new catheter over the guide wire. Proper position is again ascertained with fluoroscopy. If the tract is well formed, successively larger catheters may be inserted without a guide wire until the catheter of the desired size has been placed. Fascial dilators, like the Amplatz or Olbert balloon dilator, have been used with percutaneous stone extraction to obtain a tract that will accept a catheter of No. 26–28 French. However, this size is not necessary for long-term drainage in the cancer patient and is uncomfortable and cumbersome. A nephrostomy of No. 12–14 French is usually more than adequate.

Results and Complications

A recent series of 1207 patients by Staples presented a success rate of 98%, a complication rate of 4%, and a mortality rate of 0.2%.[23] This series involved nephrostomies placed for various indications in patients with varying degrees of illness or surgical risk. Four deaths were reported following percutaneous nephrostomy, and all were due to hemorrhage in patients with a coagulopathy or uremia from malignant disease. Apparently, complications and mortality are more frequent in the patient with ureteral obstruction secondary to cancer. A distinct advantage of the percutaneous nephrostomy is that the insertion is much safer in poor-risk patients than is open surgical placement of a nephrostomy tube. The patients can be stabilized for further treatment of their tumors with various chemotherapeutic agents, including those with potential nephrotoxicity or with radiation therapy.

URETERAL STENTS

Urologists are familiar with ureteral stents and methods of cystoscopic insertion. They were originally described by Brown and Harrison[5] in 1951. Zimskind, Fetter, and Wilkerson used silicone tubing placed over a No. 4 French catheter to bypass ureteral obstruction in 1967.[28] These stents frequently migrated or required an external collection device after being secured to a ureteral catheter. In 1974, the "shepherd's crook" self-retaining ureteral catheter was developed by McCullough. This catheter was used to bypass malignant ureteral obstruction in a woman with breast cancer.[18]

Within the past 10 years, major advances

have occurred in this area, both in configuration and composition, that allow the patient more comfort and freedom of movement without the necessity of an external drainage appliance. The biologically inert materials currently in use make long-term maintenance within the urinary tract possible. There are three basic indwelling ureteral stents currently available: the Gibbons ureteral stent,[7] the double-J silicone stent,[17] and the polyethylene double pigtail stent[22] (Fig. 57–1). There are, of course, modifications of these according to the designer and manufacturer.

The advantages of the indwelling ureteral stent over those of a nephrostomy tube are obvious. The stents are more physiologically compatible and better tolerated by the patient, and urologists are familiar with the basic techniques necessary for proper insertion.

The Gibbons ureteral stent is composed of silicone and is available in lengths of 15, 23, and 29 cm and diameters of No. 7 and No. 9 French.[7] The stent consists of tubing with several drainage holes along the length of the stent, radiopaque dentate protrusions that prevent distal migration, and a distal radiopaque collar with a tail that prevents proximal migration and facilitates removal. This stent is used primarily in patients with distal ureteral obstruction. Estimation of the length of the stent to be inserted is not as important as with other stents, and less foreign body is left in the bladder, thus decreas-

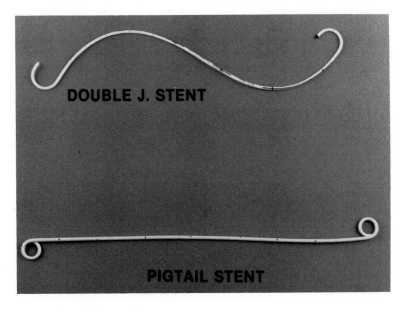

Figure 57–1. Double-J and pigtail stents.

ing irritative bladder symptoms. This stent is not a good choice in proximal ureteral obstruction.

The "double-J" stent is composed of silicone and has self-retaining J-hooks on each end to prevent either distal or proximal migration when properly placed (Fig. 57–1). The stent is available commercially in diameters of Nos. 6, 7, and 8.5 French. Lengths vary from 16 to 30 cm. There are drainage holes every centimeter.

The double pigtail ureteral stent is composed of polyethylene and has a pigtail configuration at each end to prevent migration in either direction. This stent is commercially available in diameters of Nos. 5, 6, 7, and 8 French, in varying lengths from 8 to 30 cm. The double pigtail stent is supplied with both ends of the catheter open. These stents have side hole patterns to facilitate drainage.

Methods of Placement

There are various methods for cystoscopic insertion of catheters. The length of the stent is determined by estimation of ureteral length from a retrograde or intravenous pyelogram. Insertion of the double pigtail stent and the Gibbons stent requires prior insertion of either an angiographic guide wire or a No. 4 French ureteral catheter endoscopically. Frequently, it is necessary to dilate the ureter prior to passage of the desired indwelling ureteral stent. This can be accomplished by inserting a smaller conventional ureteral catheter for three to four days for "soft dilatation." Many times, however, one may pass a guide wire to the renal pelvis and coaxially dilate the ureter over the guide wire with successively larger ureteral catheters. In the case of the Gibbons ureteral stent, after a ureteral catheter of the same size as the desired Gibbons stent has been advanced through the point of obstruction, this catheter is removed and a No. 4 French ureteral catheter is inserted. The Gibbons ureteral stent is then placed over the No. 4 French ureteral catheter and is inserted in a retrograde fashion up the ureter. This maneuver can be facilitated with the use of sterile mineral oil injected through the lumen of the given stent prior to passage over the catheter. Care is taken to leave the distal flange portion of the stent at the level of the ureteral orifice inside the bladder. The stent is then stabilized with the push catheter and

the No. 4 French ureteral catheter is gently withdrawn, leaving the stent in place.

A similar method of insertion can be used with both the pigtail ureteral stent and the double-J stent. An angiographic guide wire is initially passed in a retrograde fashion to the level of the renal pelvis. Successive dilatation is performed if necessary, and then the stent is passed over the guide wire with the push catheter and inserted into the ureter. Approximately 4 cm should be visible cystoscopically with either stent to allow formation of the distal configuration. By stabilizing the stent with the push catheter, the angiographic guide wire can then be gently removed, leaving the stent in proper position. Placement is then verified radiographically. The alligator forceps may be used to "fine-tune" the position of the stent.

One advantage that the double-J stent has over the other two stents is that it can be placed without prior catheterization or placement of a guide wire in the ureter. To do this, the proper size and length is estimated as described previously. The distal end of the stent is sharply removed; however, the proximal end remains closed. The stylet wire provided by the manufacturer is then inserted through the stent and the stent is inserted by using the stylet wire and push catheter in the same fashion as one would insert a conventional ureteral catheter in a retrograde fashion. Again, care must be taken to leave approximately 4 cm in length visible in the bladder to allow formation of the distal configuration. After proper placement is verified, the push catheter again is used to stabilize the stent and the stylet wire is removed.

These maneuvers can be performed on a conventional cystoscopic operating table, and proper placement can be verified with static x-rays. However, fluoroscopy can be utilized both during and after the insertion to verify proper placement. For hospitals in which overhead fluoroscopy is not available in the cystoscopic suite, a C-arm can be used. Patency of internal ureteral stents can be checked with a retrograde cystogram.

Antegrade Insertion

Occasionally, the ureteral orifice cannot be located cystoscopically because of involvement of the trigone by tumor or previous radiation therapy. Even if the ureteral orifice is visible, one may encounter difficulty due to ureteral kinking, tortuosity, or stricture. It is often possible to advance a guide wire into the bladder in an antegrade fashion from a previously placed percutaneous nephrostomy. Placement of the percutaneous nephrostomy in the posterior lower-pole calyx usually provides a gentle curve to the ureteropelvic junction and proximal ureter, thus making antegrade insertion of the guide wire less difficult.

After placement of a percutaneous nephrostomy, the angiographic guide wire is inserted through the nephrostomy tube. Often the guide wire advances into the ureter without difficulty. There are times, however, when the guide wire coils in the renal pelvis. This can usually be avoided by passing an angle-tipped angiographic catheter over the guide wire and then using the angle of the catheter to direct the guide wire through the ureteropelvic junction. The guide wire is then advanced gently down the ureter in an antegrade fashion. It may be helpful to pass the angiographic catheter down the ureter also. The guide wire should always be passed before the catheter to prevent possible perforation of the ureter by the catheter. Passage of the guide wire and catheter down the ureter is usually quite simple; however, resistance is occasionally encountered. When this happens, contrast medium should be injected into the collecting system to allow visualization of the area of obstruction. This dilute contrast medium allows visualization of the catheter and guide wire. An obstruction is infrequently complete, and it may be traversed by using the guide wire in a gentle probing fashion. Occasionally, the resistance will cause kinking of the guide wire and catheter. When this happens, a No. 12 French Teflon dilator may be passed over the catheter into the renal pelvis or upper ureter in order to stabilize the catheter and guide wire and permit applied force to the area of obstruction. After the obstruction is bypassed, the guide wire and catheter can be advanced antegrade into the bladder.

The guide wire may be retrieved cystoscopically, using an alligator forceps or stone basket, and then advanced antegrade through the urethra and out the urethral meatus. At this point, the guide wire may be used to facilitate retrograde passage of the three available stents. Smith and associates have described the technique for insertion of a Gibbons stent in this situation.[22] The double-J silicone stent is difficult to use

when placed over the guide wire, as the surface "drag" prevents removal of the guide wire without displacement of the stent. Therefore, the polyethylene stent should be used. After retrograde advancement of the stent and proper placement is confirmed fluoroscopically, the push catheter is inserted over the guide wire through the flank and is used to stabilize the stent in the renal pelvis. The guide wire is then gently removed, leaving the stent in the renal pelvis with formation of the pigtail configuration to prevent migration. The push catheter is then removed, and the stent is thus internalized.

At times, owing to local growth of a pelvic malignancy or to prior radiation therapy, advancement of the cystoscope transurethrally may not be possible. In this instance, the polyethylene double pigtail stent may be inserted in an antegrade fashion without cystoscopic control. The stent is placed over the guide wire and is inserted in an antegrade fashion using the push catheter for insertion through the skin, perirenal tissue, and renal parenchyma. It is helpful to loop a small nylon suture through a proximal drainage hole and out the end of the stent to allow one to pull the stent back into the renal pelvis in case it is inserted too far distally to allow formation of the proximal pigtail configuration. After proper placement is verified fluoroscopically, the push catheter is used to stabilize the stent, at which time the nylon suture is cut and removed. The guide wire is then gently removed also, and the stent is internalized.

The antegrade insertion of the stent can be used in patients who have ileal conduit urinary diversions with obstructive ureters. However, a recent article by Walther and associates[26] reported that these stents can rapidly become obstructed by the mucus secreted by the intestinal segment, possibly resulting in death.

Complications

Since these stents are made of relatively inert materials, they are well tolerated by the patient. Some patients may experience irritative bladder symptoms, which can be managed with antispasmodic drugs. Infections occur but can usually be resolved with antibiotics if the stent has not become encrusted. Encrustation can be avoided or minimized with formation of dilute acid urine. Proximal migration may occur as a result of improper placement. The stent can usually be retrieved by using No. 5 French grasping forceps or a small stone basket to entrap the stent. Percutaneous nephrostomy is rarely necessary to remove the stent.

URETEROSTOMY IN SITU

Ureterostomy in situ is a procedure for supravesical diversion described in 1953 by Vose and Dixey.[25] This procedure requires less time and dissection than does formal open nephrostomy and can be utilized in remote locations where percutaneous nephrostomy may not be available. Local anesthesia will suffice in a patient who is at prohibitive risk for general anesthesia.

The patient is positioned on the operating room table according to the surgeon's choice of incision. A muscle-splitting incision is made subcostally with the patient in the flank position, or approximately one inch medial to the anterior superior iliac spine if the patient is supine. The peritoneum is reflected medially and the ureter is identified in the retroperitoneum. Minimal mobilization of the ureter is required. A small longitudinal ureterotomy is made between two stay sutures. A No. 12 French Robinson catheter is inserted into the ureter and is brought out through a separate stab wound below the surgical incision to ensure that the path of the catheter is a gentle curve without kinking. Additional holes in the catheter may facilitate drainage. The ureterotomy is closed with 4-0 chromic suture. One may wish to secure the catheter loosely to the ureter with an absorbable stitch. A Penrose drain is placed near the incision in the ureter and the stent is anchored to the skin with a nonabsorbable suture. (We prefer nylon, since there is less skin reaction.)

After four to six weeks a tract will have formed that permits tube change if necessary. It is helpful to inject contrast material in a retrograde fashion to confirm proper placement.

SUMMARY

As more advancements are made in oncology, urologists may see more patients with ureteral obstruction related to cancer.

The decision to recommend palliative urinary diversion in these patients involves many philosophical and ethical questions. There are times when uremia and the relatively painless death it affords will be the more humane course. On the other hand, many patients can survive with good quality of life after diversion. We have presented certain guidelines that we believe can aid in this decision-making process. Previous reports have involved open surgical diversion that have resulted in a high rate of complications and death. Percutaneous and endoscopic methods of diversion hold promise for patients who previously would have had their lives shortened by open surgery. In addition, recently developed, self-retaining ureteral stents allow internal diversion without the added nuisance of an external collection device; these new stents can obviously improve the patient's quality of life after diversion.

References

1. Abrams HL, Spiro R, Goldstein N: Metastases in carcinoma: analysis of 1000 autopsied cases. Cancer 3:74–85, 1950.
2. Bartley O, Chidekel N, Radberg C: Percutaneous drainage of the renal pelvis for uraemia due to obstructed urinary flow. Acta Chir Scand 129:443–446, 1965.
3. Bricker EM: Symposium on clinical surgery: bladder substitution after pelvic evisceration. Surg Clin North Am 30:1511–1521, 1950.
4. Brin EN, Schiff M Jr, Weiss RM: Palliative urinary diversion for pelvic malignancy. J Urol 113:619–622, 1975.
5. Brown HP, Harrison JH: The efficacy of plastic ureteral catheters for constant drainage. J Urol 66:85, 1951.
6. Fallon B, Olney L, Culp DA: Nephrostomy in cancer patients: to do or not to do? Br J Urol 52:237–242, 1980.
7. Finney RP: Double-J and diversion stents. Urol Clin North Am 9:89–94, 1982.
8. Gibbons RP, Correa RJ Jr, Cummings KB, Mason JT: Experience with indwelling ureteral stent catheters. J Urol 115:22–26, 1976.
9. Goodwin WE, Casey WC, Woolf W: Percutaneous trocar (needle) nephrostomy in hydronephrosis. JAMA 157:891–894, 1976.
10. Grabstald H, Kaufman R: Hydronephrosis secondary to ureteral obstruction by metastatic breast cancer. J Urol 102:569–576, 1969.
11. Harris RD, McCullough DL, Talner LB: Percutaneous nephrostomy. J Urol 115:628–631, 1976.
12. Hepperlin TW, Mardis HK, Kammandel H: The pigtail ureteral stent in the cancer patient. J Urol 121:17–18, 1979.
13. Holden S, McPhee M, Grabstald H: The rationale of urinary diversion in cancer patients. J Urol 121:19–21, 1979.

14. Khan AU, Utz DC: Clinical management of carcinoma of prostate associated with bilateral ureteral obstruction. J Urol 113:816–819, 1975.
15. Klinger ME: Secondary tumors of the genito-urinary tract. J Urol 65:144–153, 1951.
16. Kohler JP, Lyon ES, Schoenberg HW: Reassessment of circle tube nephrostomy in advanced pelvic malignancy. J Urol 123:17–18, 1980.
17. Mardis HK, Kroeger RM, Hepperlen TW, et al: Polyethylene double-pigtail ureteral stents. Urol Clin North Am 9:95–101, 1982.
18. McCullough DL: "Shepherd's crook" self retaining ureteral catheter. Urologist's Lett 32:54, 1974.
19. Meyer JE, Green TH Jr, Yatsuhashi M: Palliative urinary diversion in carcinoma of the cervix. Obstet Gynecol 55:95–98, 1980.
20. Michigan S, Catalona WJ: Ureteral obstruction from prostatic carcinoma: response to endocrine and radiation therapy. J Urol 118:733–738, 1977.
21. Sharer W, Grayhack JT, Graham J: Palliative urinary diversion for malignant ureteral obstruction. J Urol 120:162–164, 1978.
22. Smith AD, Lange PH, Miller RP, Reinke DB: Introduction of the Gibbons ureteral stent facilitated by antecedent percutaneous nephrostomy. J Urol 120:543–544, 1978.
23. Staples DP: Percutaneous nephrostomy: techniques, indications and results. Urol Clin North Am 9:15–29, 1982.
24. Ulm AH, Klein E: Management of ureteral obstruction produced by recurrent cancer of the rectosigmoid colon. Surg Gynecol Obstet 110:413–418, 1960.
25. Vose SN, Dixey GM: Ureterostomy-in-situ. J Urol 69:503–506, 1953.
26. Walther PJ, Robertson CN, Paulson DF: Lethal complications of standard self-retaining ureteral stents in patients with ileal conduit urinary diversion. J Urol 133:851–853, 1985.
27. Yagoda A: The chemotherapy for advanced urothelial cancer. Semin Urol 1:60–74, 1983.
28. Zimskind PD, Fetter TR, Wilkerson JL: Clinical use of long-term indwelling silicone rubber ureteral splints inserted cystoscopically. J Urol 97:849, 1967.

BALFOUR M. MOUNT, M.D., F.R.C.S.(C)
JOHN F. SCOTT, M.D.

Palliative Care of the Patient With Terminal Cancer

CHAPTER **58**

There are three goals in the treatment of malignant disease: to cure, to prolong life, and to improve the quality of survival. In recent decades, interest and financial resources have been focused on improving our skills in investigating, diagnosing, curing, and prolonging survival. Although a high percentage of our urologic oncology patients will die of their carcinomas, little effort has gone into sharpening our skills in treating patients with incurable disease. There is increasing evidence that these patients and their families experience a wide variety of critical problems that usually go unrecognized by those responsible for their care. The terminally ill patient, instead of receiving sympathetic understanding and expertise in meeting medical and emotional needs, may encounter isolation and depersonalization.[4, 8, 9, 16]

Hinton[6] has commented, "We emerge deserving of little credit; we who are capable of ignoring the conditions which we make muted people suffer. The dissatisfied dead cannot noise abroad the negligence they have experienced."

DEFINING APPROPRIATE THERAPY

The current tendency to equate excellence of medical care with aggressive investigation and therapy is a natural outcome of the recent rapid expansion of medical knowledge. The result is a generation of physicians conditioned to see their role exclusively as "employed by the patient to fight for his life."[5] Failure to recognize that further investigation and active treatment may be inappropriate in the presence of advanced disease has frequently resulted in unnecessary suffering. We have too often failed to recognize that the capacity to act does not, in itself, justify the action.

When therapy to prolong life is still appropriate, unproven therapeutic modalities are justifiable only as part of carefully designed and supervised clinical trials. Accepted forms of treatment may be justified only after a consideration of attendant morbidity, probability of response, and mean duration of response, in consultation with the patient and family.

When palliative care becomes the only appropriate goal, further investigations should be carried out only if they lead to improved symptom control. Investigations for research purposes are justifiable in this setting only when informed consent has been obtained from the patient.

The decision that therapy should be restricted to palliative care is made more easily if the physician's perception of his or her mandate embraces the broader concept of alleviating suffering rather than simply "fighting for life." The physician's need to treat and the family's need to treat are unacceptable rationales for further therapy. Such a decision should be associated not with a pessimistic attitude that "nothing more can be done" but with a positive statement that although therapy can no longer be expected to make an impact on the disease process, much can be done to control symptoms and assist the patient in living as fully as possible. It may be helpful to remind the patient that many medical problems, such as diabetes, arteriosclerotic vascular disease, and multiple sclerosis, cannot be cured and yet we can learn to live within such situations in spite of decreasing resources. The patient and family are left with the concept of an appropriate shifting in therapeutic goals by a physician who remains interested and actively involved. The statement "nothing more can be done" reflects a tragic ignorance of the multidimensional needs of these patients and their families and the creative therapeutic responses to these needs that are now possible.

THE NATURE OF THE NEED

Our traditional preoccupation with pathophysiology alone is woefully inadequate in the arena of advanced disease. Although the medical needs may be undeniably complex and will be of great concern, added to them are the complicating factors of the psychologic stress for the patient and family, strained interpersonal relationships, frequent financial problems, and the ever-present metaphysical questions that these patient/family units are forced to face. "Why me? Why this suffering? Why is this allowed? Is this all there is?" Experience suggests that if suffering is to be successfully alleviated, intervention must be directed at all levels: physical, psychological, metaphysical or spiritual, and social.

CHRONIC PAIN: ITS NATURE AND MANAGEMENT

When intractable pain is present, its treatment is the central problem in the palliative care of patients with advanced malignant disease.

The Nature of Chronic Pain

Pain is a somatopsychic phenomenon. Although it arises in a physical stimulus, its perception is always modified by the mind. That it is not proportional to the degree of injury is the experience of daily life, as seen with the athlete who does not realize that he has been injured until after the game, the anxious patient whose pain is alleviated by the reassuring news from a physician that the underlying problem is not serious, and the pain of childhood injury that is so greatly helped by a mother's hug.

It has long been known that pain is modified by the patient's perception of its cause.[13] Four hundred years ago Michel Eyquem de Montaigne (1533–1592) observed that "the pain of fatal illness is doubly painful because it threatens us with death." Indeed, a wide variety of factors has been shown to influence pain threshold. Fatigue, anxiety, depression, the poor control of other symptoms, mental or social isolation, and similar adverse factors have been shown to lower the pain threshold, resulting in an increase in perceived pain. Conversely, a good sleep, an empathic environment, companionship, the control of other symptoms, and similar supportive influences are known to raise the pain threshold, thus decreasing perceived pain.

Moreover, cultural factors (pertaining to beliefs, values, and customs as transmitted from one generation to another) and social factors (interrelationships between individuals or groups, including occupational and family roles and social class) strongly influence pain perception.[7, 18]

Finally, one must note the important differences between acute and chronic pain. Acute pain has a beginning and an end. It has a useful purpose in that it draws attention to the injured area and the need for a therapeutic response. It can be classified as mild, moderate, or severe. Chronic pain, however, can be characterized as part of a vicious circle with no end in sight. The fearful anticipation of chronic pain leads to anxiety, depression, and insomnia, which in turn accentuate the pain.[13] Leshan[10] suggests that meaninglessness, helplessness, and hopelessness are characteristic of the nightmare world inhabited by the patient with chronic pain.

Saunders[22] has coined the term *total pain* to describe the all-consuming nature of chronic pain and our need to attack all of its components: physical, psychological, social, and spiritual. Pain forcefully reminds the patient with advanced malignant disease of his prognosis and thus further accentuates his agony.

The Management of Chronic Pain

General Principles[24, 28]

Identify the Cause of Each Pain. Table 58–1 lists the causes of pain in cancer patients. Clarification of the cause is an essential step in pain control, since it may lead to specific therapy such as focal irradiation for a bony metastasis, extraction of a carious tooth, or bowel care for pain due to constipation.

Twycross studied 100 consecutive patients with pain in the presence of advanced malignant disease and found that 11% had constipation as the cause of one of their pains, whereas approximately half the patients (48%) had musculoskeletal or arthritic pain. None of the pains were due to the malignancy in 6% of cases.[29]

Adequate assessment involves obtaining an accurate history, carrying out a thorough physical examination, and being able to differentiate specific pains, since 80% of advanced cancer patients have more than one pain and one third have four or more pains.[29]

Enhance the Patient's Sense of Personal Control. The presence of advanced malignant disease is usually associated with a spiralling sense of loss of control for the patient. This is aggravated when medical therapy is planned without the patient's permission or participation. Carefully informing the patient in familiar, nonmedical terms about the extent of the disease, the mechanism of each pain, and the treatment options, will give the patient a greater sense of control.

Focus on Whole Family. The patient and family must be considered as a unit if optimal pain control is to be achieved. A sense of helplessness, anxiety, and anger is engendered in the family when they are poorly informed or treated as passive bystanders. The patient's pain is invariably aggravated as a result. If, however, the collaborative input of the family is sought and they are included both as care recipients and caregivers, misunderstandings, uncertainty, and dysfunctional reactions are minimized.

Family-related considerations relevant to pain assessment and therapy include the meaning of pain and accepted manner of expressing pain in the family, ethnic group, and religion involved; family coping styles evident in past crises; and the impact of the patient's pain and disease on family communication, roles, and financial resources. Family meetings may be an extremely useful vehicle for promoting trust, diminishing uncertainty, and nurturing family resources so that they can more effectively support the patient.

Utilize Team Approach. The complexity of pain frequently demands a team for effective therapy. The genitourinary cancer patient and family as the core of this team may require the assistance of physicians (urologist, family physician, internist, oncologist, radiation therapist, general surgeon, neurosurgeon or neurologist, anesthetist, psychiatrist), nurses (hospital, home care), social worker, pharmacist, chaplain, physiotherapist, occupational therapist, dietitian, psychologist or allied professional such as a music therapist, diversional therapist, and volunteers.

Although only part of this extended team is likely to be required for any one case, the availability of such an array of disciplines should be established. Such a team requires

Table 58–1. CAUSES OF PAIN IN CANCER PATIENTS*

Caused by Cancer	Related to Cancer	Related to Therapy	Unrelated to Cancer or Therapy
Bone infiltration, with or without muscle spasm	Muscle spasm	Postoperative acute pain	Musculoskeletal
Nerve compression or infiltration	Constipation	Postoperative neuralgia	Headache (migraine, tension)
Visceral involvement	Bedsore	Phantom limb pain	Arthritis
Soft tissue infiltration	Lymphedema	Postirradiation inflammation or fibrosis	Cardiovascular
Ulceration, with or without infection	Candidiasis	Postirradiation myelopathy	
Raised intracranial pressure	Herpetic neuralgia	Postchemotherapy neuropathy	
	Deep vein thrombosis	Necrosis of bone	
	Pulmonary embolus		

*From Scott JF (ed): Cancer Pain, a Monograph on the Management of Cancer Pain. Ottawa, Canada, Health and Welfare, 1984. Reprinted with permission.

coordination, communication, documentation, and frequent team conferences to achieve best results.

Use Multiple Methods. Effective therapy utilizes a combination of methods; they (1) modify disease (surgery, radiation therapy, hormonal therapy, or chemotherapy), (2) modify pain perception (education, psychologic support, relaxation, drugs), (3) interrupt pain transmission (TENS, nerve blocks, neurosurgery), and (4) modify lifestyle (physical and occupational therapy aids, homemaking services).

Control Other Symptoms. Improved control of other symptoms raises the pain threshold and eases the patient's pain.

Use Environment to Modify Pain. Environment has a dramatic impact on pain perception. This important clinical observation may be used as an effective adjunct to other modalities in cancer pain management. Even as positive influences in the patient's psychological and social "environment" may ameliorate pain, so too may changes in the physical environment. For many the preferred environment is the home. An institution can never hope to duplicate the therapeutic milieu that is created by the supportive presence of persons, sights, smells, sounds, and things that are familiar and personally selected.

Conversely, when "home" is a focus of interpersonal stress, uncontrolled noise, and heightened anxiety, the hospital may represent an oasis of tranquillity and safety. To know which is better for a given patient and family presupposes having taken the effort to assess the resources of that family system. However resourceful, the family attempting to give home care to a terminally ill loved one in pain will need the input of easily available around-the-clock professional consultation, as from a visiting nursing service.

A therapeutic milieu may be created in a hospital ward, but it demands attention to detail concerning all aspects of the physical, emotional, and interpersonal setting. This may include use of high staffing levels using selected, trained support personnel; flexibility that allows personalization regarding routines such as visiting (children and pets), timing of baths and meals, decor (photographs and favorite keepsakes from home), diversional therapy, and a balance between privacy and community; controlled ward traffic, noise, temperature, and odors; and carefully selected physical environment fea-

tures. These may include orientation devices (clocks and calendars); natural light, plants, access to outside; architectural innovations in handling space, lighting, color, textures, and shapes; optional music and TV (as controlled by patient); paintings, colorful quilts and curtains, and other decorative features; and homelike features such as facilities for a family member to stay overnight, a family kitchen on the ward, a quiet area, or a tank for tropical fish.

The effect of a comforting, reassuring, positive environment frequently leads the newly admitted patient in a hospice or palliative care unit to comment, "I don't know what it is, but I feel better just being here." The environment is an important factor in pain control.

ANALGESICS[17, 24, 28]

Table 58–2 suggests an analgesic of choice and alternatives at varying levels of pain severity. Table 58–3 gives analgesic equivalences for a variety of narcotic analgesics. The wide variety of analgesics on the market can lead to confusion. It is wise to be familiar with the three basic analgesics—aspirin, codeine, and morphine—as well as one or two alternatives for each pain level. It is better to know a few drugs well than to have uncertain familiarity with a long list.

With mild or moderate pain, a non-narcotic is used initially. Aspirin and the nonsteroidal anti-inflammatory drugs decrease the inflammatory reaction caused by tumor and tissue-injury release of pain-producing algogenic substances, including the prostaglandins, histamine, bradykinin, and other chemicals.

Analgesic use for cancer pain has undergone radical change and improvement in the past decade. Current concepts often run counter to traditional beliefs about narcotic utilization. The following issues deserve attention:

Acute or Chronic Pain? Acute pain (postoperative, recent fracture, painful procedures) will call for a standard dose of a relatively short-acting narcotic followed by doses as needed to cover the rapidly changing requirements. Chronic pain, however, requires the regular administration of individually optimized doses of a narcotic at intervals dependent on the kinetics of the chosen narcotic in that individual (although

Table 58–2. ANALGESIC THERAPY*

Pain Severity	Drug of Choice	Alternatives
I: Mild	Acetylsalicylic acid	Acetaminophen
		Nonsteroidal anti-inflammatory drugs
II: Mild to moderate	Acetylsalicylic acid and codeine	Codeine with or without acetaminophen
III: Moderate to severe	Codeine	Oxycodone
	Morphine	Levorphanol
		Anileridine
		Oxymorphone
IV: Severe	Morphine	Hydromorphone
		Methadone

*From Scott JF (ed): Cancer Pain, a Monograph on the Management of Cancer Pain. Ottawa, Canada, Health and Welfare, 1984. Reprinted with permission.

as-needed scheduling may supplement this baseline). There is no place for "prn" analgesic orders as the basis for treating intractable pain!

Pain Severity? When pain is continuous, the tachycardia, perspiration, pallor, and diagnostic clinical features of altered expression and daily activity associated with acute pain may no longer be in evidence. Pain severity can only be determined by carefully listening to the patient.

Prognosis and Analgesic Choice. The fear of "running out of effective drugs" in the patient expected to live for an extended period has frequently curtailed the early introduction of narcotics. Apparent life expectancy should have no influence on the choice of analgesic. Severe pain demands narcotic administration regardless of prognosis. It is reassuring to know that psychologic dependence does not occur, physical dependence is not clinically significant, and

tolerance is an infrequent occurrence when oral narcotics are utilized according to techniques described in this chapter.

Changing Analgesics: When and How. If an analgesic fails to provide total pain relief, (1) check that it is being administered regularly around the clock; (2) ensure that the interval between doses approximates the duration of action of that analgesic; (3) increase the dose to the upper limits of the range of effectiveness (acetylsalicylic acid, 650 mg every four hours; codeine, 60 mg every four hours; morphine, no clear upper limit); (4) reconsider the possible use of adjunct approaches—either pharmacologic (e.g., combinations such as acetaminophen plus codeine; use of nonsteroidal anti-inflammatory drugs, steroids, or benzodiazepines) or nonpharmacologic (as discussed under general principles above); and (5) only then consider switching to another analgesic.

Tables of analgesic equivalence, such as

Table 58–3. ANALGESIC DRUGS AND DOSE EQUIVALENTS TO STANDARD INTRAMUSCULAR MORPHINE DOSE OF 10 MG*

Drug	Equivalent Dose (mg)	
	Intramuscular	Oral
Agonists		
Morphine sulfate	10	20–30
Codeine phosphate	120	200
Hydromorphone (Dilaudid)	2	4
Levorphanol (Levo-Dromoran)	2	4
Oxycodone (Percodan, Percocet)		10–15
Anileridine (Leritine)	25	75
Meperidine (Demerol)	75	300
Oxymorphone (Numorphan)	1.5	5 (suppository)
Methadone	10	20
Heroin	5–8	10–15
Agonist-Antagonists		
Pentazocine (Talwin)	60	180
Nalbuphine (Nubain)	10	
Butorphanol (Stadol)	2	
Buprenorphine (Temgesic)	0.4	0.8 (can be sublingual)

*From Scott JF (ed): Cancer Pain, a Monograph on the Management of Cancer Pain. Ottawa, Canada, Health and Welfare, 1984. Reprinted with permission.

Table 58–3, are largely derived from single-dose, acute pain studies and thus should be considered as only a rough guide to dose when changing from one analgesic to another.

Ten Cardinal Rules of Narcotic Use in Chronic Cancer Pain

1. *Use pure agonists as first line therapy.* There is a higher incidence of psychotomimetic effects (dysphoria, hallucinations), nausea, and vomiting with the narcotic agonists-antagonists. Their theoretical advantage over agonists in terms of respiratory depression is not significant if agonists are used optimally as described.

2. *Never mix agonists with agonist-antagonists.* Because of competitive binding and blockage of opioid receptors, mixing drugs from these two classes will not help pain and may lead to a loss of analgesia and withdrawal reactions.

3. *Do not mix two antagonists.* It makes no pharmacologic sense to mix two weak narcotics or two strong narcotics. Occasionally, a patient receiving a strong narcotic regularly will also take a weaker narcotic "as required" for intermittent "breakthrough" pain. However, it would be better to take an extra dose of the regular strong narcotic in such situations.

4. *Do not stay with weak narcotics if pain is not relieved.* When a weak narcotic (with or without a non-narcotic analgesic) is given regularly at maximal doses and fails to relieve the pain, do not try an alternative weak narcotic but move immediately to a strong narcotic.

5. *Use oral route whenever possible.* The oral administration of narcotics gives a more useful plasma concentration curve and prolonged analgesia and avoids the toxicity that may occur with parenteral administration (Fig. 58–1A). The oral route eliminates parenteral injections, enables the patient to maintain control of the drugs, and allows mobility for home care and travel.

6. *Around-the-clock regular dosing.* Most narcotics have a duration of analgesic action of four to six hours. Therefore, control of chronic pain requires four to six doses spaced equally throughout the 24-hour period. It is especially important to ensure that pain is not allowed to cause insomnia. Painful, sleepless nights will lower pain thresh-

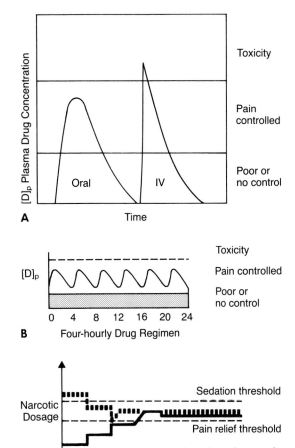

Figure 58–1. Plasma narcotic concentrations. A, By route of administration; B, with continuous pain relief; C, alternative methods of drug dosage adjustment. Solid line in C indicates sequential increments in narcotic dose at intervals of two days; dashed line indicates an initially high dose, sequential decrements until pain disappears, followed by a slight increase in dose in order to provide analgesia without sedation.

old and lead to more pain. Once analgesia has been consistently achieved, the scheduled dose at night may be discontinued, usually with augmentation of the bedtime dose to one and one half to two times the usual daytime dose. Patients requiring high doses of morphine (60 mg or more) usually need to be awakened for medication during the night to prevent morning pain.

7. *Never "prn."* When the physician orders narcotics for chronic pain on an "as required" or "prn" basis, a vicious circle is instituted. Pain initiates despair, which gives rise to more pain. A destructive roller-coaster effect is set in motion. (A) The patient feels pain and calls the nurse or other

caregiver to ask for an analgesic, a process that characteristically involves delays and the perpetuation and escalation of pain. (B) The decision must then be made by patient, family, and caregiver whether the next dose is "really necessary." Uncertainty and the potential for mistrust enter the equation. (C) The relative overdose needed to control the resultant augmented pain state is likely to leave the patient "snowed," sedated, and stuporous, until the point several hours later when pain recurs and the cycle is repeated.

Continuous pain requires continuous analgesia. The aim is to adjust the dose in order to reliably just prevent the resurgence of pain rather than to treat it repeatedly.

Waiting for pain to reappear, as with "on demand" narcotic orders, is illogical and cruel and perpetuates the fear and memory of pain. Such an order should only be written to cover the possibility of "breakthrough" pain not covered by the baseline, regularly scheduled narcotic dose.

8. *Individually optimize dose.* There is no standard or set dose of narcotics in cancer pain because there is a great variation between individuals in analgesic efficacy. The correct dose of a narcotic is that which gives pain relief for at least three and preferably four or more hours. As pain changes through various stages of disease and treatment, narcotic dosage must be adjusted to match pain intensity.

"Recommended" doses are derived from acute, intramuscular, single-dose pain studies and are not applicable to chronic cancer pain. The dose of the strong narcotics (except meperidine and the agonists-antagonists) can be increased almost indefinitely without reaching a ceiling or plateau of maximum effect.

9. *Consider adjuvant medications.* The addition of a second drug that relieves pain by a different mechanism is preferable to raising the dose of narcotic indefinitely. For example, in bone pain and other pains in which inflammation or prostaglandins are postulated to be involved, the use of acetylsalicylic acid or a nonsteroidal anti-inflammatory drug along with a narcotic is a logical combination. When pain is due to brain, cord, or peripheral nerve compression by an adjacent tumor mass or related tissue edema, steroids may be beneficial. When anxiety or depression augment pain, psychotropic drugs may be useful.

Other drugs can indirectly relieve pain by preventing narcotic side effects (constipation, nausea) and by relieving other cancer symptoms (cough, insomnia).

10. *Use narcotics as one part of the total treatment plan.* Despite their central importance, narcotics can never be more than one part of a comprehensive approach to pain control, which will include anticancer treatment, nondrug measures, and psychosocial support as suggested by the aforementioned general principles.

In difficult cases of cancer pain, admission to a hospital, hospice, or a palliative care unit may be required both for investigation and treatment.

ORAL MORPHINE ADMINISTRATION

Morphine is the strong narcotic of choice for cancer pain. Moderate to severe chronic pain can be relieved in the vast majority of patients when morphine is regularly administered by mouth.

Traditional fears related to narcotic use that have contributed to a documented endemic deficiency in pain control are now recognized as outdated and unjustified when current techniques of utilization are employed. These include the fear that morphine use inevitably leads to (1) respiratory depression, (2) addiction (psychologic dependence), (3) rapid tolerance with attendant dose escalation, (4) euphoria, and (5) a clouded sensorium.

It is now recognized that analgesia occurs at a lower narcotic dose (serum concentration) than that necessary for respiratory or other central nervous system depression (Fig. 58–1). Furthermore, with consistent pain prevention (Fig. 58–1B), the analgesic dose has been found to plateau, with significant tolerance rarely being encountered even when administration is continued for periods extending to many years. In general, increased morphine requirement means an increase in pain, not tolerance. Finally, the analgesia associated with careful dose titration occurs without affective change secondary to the narcotic. In short, the patient is left alert, pain-free, clear of mind, and able to relate to loved ones.[14, 28]

For most patients, pain relief can be obtained with 5 to 10 mg of morphine every four hours, although in small or elderly patients as little as 2.5 mg may be effective. The usual four-hourly morphine dosage range is 2.5 to 30 mg, but doses of 200 mg have been used. In establishing the optimal dose, the usual increment is 5 to 10 mg per dose. For excruciating pain, an alternative method is to start with a relatively high narcotic dose, subsequently adjusting the dose in sequential decrements until analgesia without sedation is achieved.

Careful observation of the patient's condition over a complete 24-hour period may suggest augmentation of one or two specific doses at periods of peak activity.

If parenteral medication becomes necessary, the equivalent dose of morphine is roughly half the previous oral dose. Thus, a patient whose pain has been controlled with 30 mg of morphine taken orally would require about 15 mg intramuscularly.[14, 18, 28]

If oral morphine is not providing complete pain relief, the following possibilities should be considered: (1) the morphine dose should be increased; (2) the pain is relatively unresponsive to morphine, such as that seen with nerve injury ("plexopathy," "deafferentation pain"); (3) the psychologic, social, and spiritual components of the patient's "total pain" require attention; (4) there are acute spasms of pain; (5) there is poor compliance (living alone, fear, misunderstanding); (6) there is inadequate dose delivery (drooling, coughing up or vomiting the solution); (7) a co-analgesic is required; and (8) a nondrug measure is required.

Spasmodic acute pain in the patient whose chronic pain is well controlled may occur from many causes, as with spasms involving bowel, bladder, or biliary tract, sudden movement aggravating general bone pain or a pathologic fracture, a painful dressing change, or fecal disimpaction. In such situations a nitrous oxide–oxygen mixture in a bedside tank equipped with a mask or mouthpiece having a patient-triggered demand valve may offer safe, effective control of the transient severe pain.

Nerve injury pain is incompletely relieved with narcotic analgesics. Although dose escalation will initially result in amelioration of the pain, beyond a certain point further increases in dose are ineffectual, leaving untouched the dysesthetic, burning, or hyperesthetic component. When this occurs, the dose of morphine should be lowered until the smallest dose providing the maximum narcotic effect is determined. The four-

hourly dose is then continued at this level. Steroids (to decrease perineural edema), phenytoin sodium (Dilantin) or similar agents (to decrease nerve irritability), and low doses of amitriptyline (25 to 50 mg given at bedtime to enhance analgesia, perhaps by potentiating the pain-inhibiting effects of the serotonergic descending pain pathway) have been added as a tripartite approach to the residual pain, with some benefit in a proportion of these patients. Transcutaneous electrical nerve stimulation and cordotomy have also provided relief in some. However, deafferentation pain remains problematic and demands attention to detail, diligent and patient persistence, and employment of all the nonpharmacologic approaches outlined if optimal relief is to be attained. Further research is clearly needed in this area.

Side Effects of Narcotic Administration

Drowsiness. When morphine is initiated, transient sedation frequently occurs. This is partly a direct effect of the drug on the central nervous system, but the exhaustion and sleep deprivation of chronic pain is another major factor. When pain is finally relieved, the patient may sleep for long periods. Drowsiness usually clears two to five days after a steady dose is achieved. Much anxiety for both patient and family can be avoided if they are forewarned about the possibility of sedation and reassured regarding its transience.

Continuing drowsiness may indicate a need to decrease morphine dose or, if it is felt that the co-analgesic being used may be a contributing factor, to change that medication. Sedation may also be a sign of disease progression and not always a side effect of therapy.

The elderly and frail should be warned of possible dizziness and unsteadiness because of postural hypotension. They require very cautious dose titration.

Nausea and Vomiting. When narcotics are initiated, nausea and vomiting may occur. This is short-lived, frequently lasting only two to three days, then subsiding. Several separate factors may contribute to this, including (1) stimulation of the chemoreceptor trigger zone in the medulla, (2) delayed gastric emptying related to the direct effect of narcotics on the gastrointestinal tract, (3) increased vestibular sensitivity, (4) anxiety (starting morphine may have been seen as an ominous death-heralding event), and (5) the taste of the oral morphine solution.

When oral morphine is initiated, a regular antiemetic should be prescribed (for several days to two weeks) unless the patient has previously been taking codeine or another narcotic for some time (Table 58–4). Since narcotics and the phenothiazines are synergistic, the dose of only one variable (the narcotic or the phenothiazine) should be changed at a time, should a phenothiazine be chosen as the antiemetic. Even small dose alterations may lead to profound changes in analgesia and sedation.

Constipation. If not carefully monitored and prevented, constipation may be just as difficult to control as the pain itself. Morphine binds to receptors in the gastrointestinal tract, causing decreased peristalsis and diminished secretions. In cancer patients, decreased liquid intake, less exercise, and poor diet all aggravate the problem. As in pain control, the aim of bowel care should be to prevent rather than treat the problem (Table 58–5).

Confusion. Morphine may cause or increase confusion, dysphoria, and hallucinations in a small number of patients (especially the elderly). However, confusion in the cancer patient with pain may also be due to brain metastases; hepatic, renal, or respiratory insufficiency; or other metabolic changes associated with advancing disease.

Urinary Retention. Morphine increases vesical outflow resistance, increases the tone of the detrusor muscle, and depresses the central response to sensory messages from the bladder. In a few patients this may lead to urinary retention.

Table 58–4. NARCOTIC-INDUCED NAUSEA AND VOMITING*

Mechanism	Drug of Choice
Chemoreceptor trigger zone stimulator	Prochlorperazine, 5 to 10 mg three times daily Haloperidol, 0.5 to 1 mg twice daily
Gastric stasis or delayed emptying	Metoclopramide, 10 mg four times daily
Vestibular stimulation	Dimenhydrinate, 100 mg four times daily, or another antihistamine

*From Scott JF (ed): Cancer Pain, a Monograph on the Management of Cancer Pain. Ottawa, Canada, Health and Welfare, 1984. Reprinted with permission.

Table 58–5. BOWEL MANAGEMENT*

1. Check previous bowel and laxative habits.
2. Record bowel movements daily.
3. Examine rectum to rule out impaction (in presence of diarrhea or fecal incontinence, this also rules out impaction overflow).
4. Encourage intake of fluids, juice, fruit, and bran.
5. Use stool softener (e.g., docusate sodium), one to nine capsules per day for all patients on strong narcotics.
6. If not effective, add a peristaltic stimulant (e.g., senna concentrate) or substitute a combination drug (e.g., Peri-Colace, Regulex-D, Dorbanex). Titrate dose.
7. If not effective, try rectal suppository of glycerine or bisacodyl (Dulcolax). Titrate dose.
8. If suppository is ineffective, use a phosphate enema (Fleet), with or without a soapsuds enema.
9. Use raised toilet seats, footstools, slipper pans and commodes for comfort and improved ability to defecate.
10. Generally avoid bulk laxatives, especially as fluid intake is decreased.

*After Twycross RG, Lack SA: Symptom Control in Far Advanced Cancer, Vol 1, Pain Relief. New York, Pitman, 1983. From Scott JF (ed): Cancer Pain, a Monograph on the Management of Cancer Pain. Ottawa, Canada, Health and Welfare, 1984. Reprinted with permission.

OTHER NARCOTICS

Morphine is the standard narcotic against which all other analgesics are compared. Other narcotics, however, are available as alternatives.

Meperidine (Demerol) has a chemical structure that is quite different from that of morphine, but it binds to the opioid receptors to produce essentially the same type of analgesic effect. Meperidine is widely used in acute and postoperative pain, partially because of its decreased spasmogenic effect on smooth muscle. However, in chronic cancer pain it is a poor analgesic because (1) duration of action is short (two to three hours), (2) it is of low analgesic potency when given by mouth, and (3) it may produce central nervous system excitation or convulsions with repeated large doses (due to accumulation of toxic metabolite, normeperidine).

Hydromorphone (Dilaudid) is a derivative of morphine. Its properties and effects closely resemble those of morphine, except it is much more soluble. A concentrated form of hydromorphone is an attractive alternative for patients requiring regular intramuscular injections of narcotic over an extended period, since a large quantity of the drug can be delivered in a small volume. It can be given orally, sublingually, parenterally, and by rectal suppository. Given intramuscularly, a 2-mg dose has the same analgesic effect of 10 mg of morphine.

Methadone is a synthetic molecule with a pharmacologic action similar to that of morphine. It is well absorbed orally with little gastrointestinal intolerance. It has a longer serum half-life, permitting less frequent administration than morphine (every six to eight hours). It is highly soluble, so large doses can be given in small volumes, both by mouth and by intramuscular injection. When other narcotic solutions are poorly tolerated, even large doses of methadone may be injected into an empty gelatin capsule in a small volume, rendering a convenient, taste-free oral formulation. This preparation should be made immediately before administration at the bedside so that the gelatin capsule remains intact until swallowed.

One major concern associated with the use of methadone is accumulation. The pharmacokinetics of methadone are complex. Although the analgesic action lasts four to eight hours, its serum half-life is very long (average, 25 hours). It may take from four days to three weeks for a steady state to be reached. Particular caution is required for the elderly and those patients with hepatic or renal dysfunction.

Diamorphine (heroin) is widely used in the United Kingdom for cancer pain. After administration, heroin is very rapidly hydrolyzed to 6-monoacetyl morphine and then to morphine. After intramuscular injection, heroin has a slightly quicker peak effect and slightly shorter duration of action when compared with morphine. Other than its very high solubility, there have been no proven advantages of heroin over other strong narcotics.

Levorphanol (Levo-Dromoran) is an effective morphine alternative for moderate to severe pain. Its long duration of action (four to eight hours), its tablet formulation, and its relative freedom from side effects (causing less nausea than is seen with morphine in one study) make it a good choice in ambulatory, nonhospitalized patients.

Oxycodone (Percodan, Percocet, Supeudol) is a morphine derivative closely resembling codeine in structure. It is available for oral and rectal administration. Tablets may contain the narcotic combined with a small dose of caffeine and either acetylsalicylic acid or acetaminophen, but tablets of pure oxycodone are also available. It is a good oral analgesic for moderate levels of cancer pain.

Anileridine (Leritine) is similar in structure to meperidine. Although its intramuscular serum half-life is two to four hours, it is an effective oral analgesic when given every four hours for moderate cancer pain.

Pentazocine (Talwin) is a narcotic agonist-antagonist. When given by mouth in the marketed 50-mg dosage, pentazocine produces an analgesic effect equal to, but not greater than, that of aspirin or acetaminophen. It should not be used because of erratic oral absorption and its high incidence of adverse reactions at therapeutic doses in cancer patients (including sedation, drowsiness, nausea, and vomiting). Remember *never* to combine pentazocine (or any agonist-antagonist) with morphine or any other agonist narcotic analgesic.

OTHER ROUTES OF NARCOTIC ADMINISTRATION

In cancer pain, the oral route of administration is generally the most effective and efficient means of delivering analgesia. In certain situations, however, other routes can be used.

Rectal. Ambulatory, nonhospitalized patients or patients receiving nursing care in their homes may experience periods when oral analgesia is difficult or impossible to administer. Examples of such times are when there is vomiting after chemotherapy treatments, severe nausea from advancing disease, difficulty in swallowing, soreness in the mouth, and aversion to the taste of the oral analgesic. In such cases the use of rectal suppositories should be considered.

Intramuscular. This route is usually associated with treatment of acute pain (especially postoperative), since peak effect is more rapid and serum level more predictable. Most analgesic studies and most comparative tables are based on the intramuscular route.

There may be situations in which a cancer patient with chronic pain will require intramuscular narcotic administration. These include the inability to swallow or the occurrence of severe vomiting, a severe and sudden exacerbation of chronic pain, development of a secondary acute pain (e.g., fracture), and occurrence of a terminal event, with profound weakness and clouded consciousness.

In general, the intramuscular route should be avoided or used only for short periods until oral, rectal, or another form of analgesia can be established.

Subcutaneous. When oral or rectal administration is difficult or impossible, a constant subcutaneous infusion of morphine can be used with a butterfly needle connected to either a standard intravenous infusion set or to a portable syringe pump, which can be filled and cared for by the patient or a family member in the home.

Intravenous. For patients who already have an intravenous infusion running and who are unable to take oral analgesics, intravenous administration of narcotics can avoid repeated intramuscular or subcutaneous injections. Whenever possible a constant infusion of narcotic should be used instead of intermittent bolus injections. In this way, peaks and troughs in serum level can be avoided, thus decreasing risk of toxicity and probably decreasing the total daily dose.

Epidural or Intrathecal. Following the discovery of opiate receptors in the dorsal horn of the spinal cord, several researchers have demonstrated analgesia when narcotics were administered directly to specific spinal cord segments. Morphine, delivered to low thoracic and lumbosacral regions both epidurally and intrathecally, has caused periods of analgesia ranging from four to 24 hours. Local anesthetic agents and steroids may be injected by the same catheter.

These techniques are still experimental. A few cases of late respiratory depression have been reported after the administration of epidural morphine in patients not previously on narcotics. To date, this has not been reported in cancer patients already on narcotics. Further study is needed to define the risks and indications of this type of therapy.

Co-analgesics

A variety of drugs may be effective in pain relief when taken alone or with analgesics.

Although not true analgesics in the pharmacologic sense, they should be considered for the treatment of all types of cancer pain. Table 58–6 lists co-analgesics of use in specific pain syndromes.

Corticosteroids constitute the first-line approach to pain due to increased intracranial pressure. Concurrent use of diuretics may be beneficial in this setting and in the presence of pain due to head and neck tumors and lymphedema. Corticosteroids may also be useful with nerve compression, hepatomegaly, intrapelvic or retroperitoneal tumor, or metastatic arthralgia.

Nondrug Therapies

Usually, cancer pain requires systemic analgesic therapy (with or without coanalgesic drugs). However, in many situations nondrug measures may be extremely important adjuncts (Table 58–7).

Modify the Pathologic Process. Whenever possible, specific therapy aimed at the underlying disease will achieve the most satisfying pain relief.

Radiotherapy. Radiation treatments have an important role to play in relieving pain due to malignant disease. Many tumors, although not curable with radiotherapy, will shrink enough to improve a patient's symptoms.

Radiation directed to bone at the site of an impending or established pathologic fracture can provide partial or complete relief of pain in about 90% of patients.

The tumors most commonly associated with bone metastases are breast, lung, prostate, kidney, thyroid, and malignant melanoma. The bones most commonly affected are vertebrae, proximal end of the femur, pelvis, ribs, proximal humerus, and the skull.

Radiation therapy is often of benefit to patients suffering from cervical or lumbar plexopathies secondary to tumor invasion. Local expanding masses and ulcerating tumors may frequently be controlled, and superior vena caval, bronchial, ureteric, or biliary obstructions may be relieved. The therapist may utilize an external beam, local implantation, or systemically administered isotopes, depending on the circumstances. A single-dose schedule is preferable, except where danger of cord compression or nausea and vomiting necessitate fractionation of dose over days or weeks.

Table 58–6. CO-ANALGESICS FOR SPECIFIC PAIN SYNDROMES*

Type of Pain	Co-analgesic
Bone pain	Acetylsalicylic acid or nonsteroidal anti-inflammatory drugs
Raised intracranial pressure	Corticosteroids
Nerve pressure pain	Corticosteroids, phenytoin and
Postherpetic neuralgia	Tricyclic antidepressants (e.g., amitriptyline, 20 to 100 mg at bedtime)
Superficial dysesthetic pain	Amitriptyline; carbamazepine, 200 mg three times daily
Intermittent stabbing pain	Valproate sodium, 200 mg three times daily; carbamazepine, 200 mg three times daily; nitrous oxide-oxygen inhalation
Gastric distention pain	Simethicone after meals; metoclopramide, 10 mg every four hours
Rectal or bladder tenesmic pain	Chlorpromazine, 10 to 25 mg every four to eight hours
Muscle spasm pain	Diazepam, 5 mg twice daily, or other benzodiazepine; baclofen, 10 mg three times daily
Lymphedema	Dexamethasone; diuretic
Skin ulceration (malignant, decubitus, or infected)	Acetaminophen, acetylsalicylic acid, or nonsteroidal anti-inflammatory drugs; if infected, metronidazole, 250 to 400 mg three times daily, or alternative antibiotic after a culture is taken; for painful dressing change, nitrous oxide-oxygen inhalation or lidocaine aerosol spray
Stomatitis	For candidiasis, nystatin, 100,000 units four times daily; lidocaine cream or jelly; artificial saliva
Pain and depression	Tricyclic antidepressant (avoid benzodiazepine)
Pain and anxiety	Benzodiazepine or phenothiazine

*From Scott JF (ed): Cancer Pain, a Monograph on the Management of Cancer Pain. Ottawa, Canada, Health and Welfare, 1984. Reprinted with permission.

Chemotherapy and Hormonal Therapy. Chemotherapy and hormonal drugs may often control pain if the tumor is sensitive to the drugs chosen. When cure or prolongation of survival is the aim of therapy, the toxic effects of some of these agents are usually acceptable. When the only aim of therapy is palliative pain control, the toxic effects of chemotherapy are often not justifiable.

Surgery. Palliative forms of surgery can relieve pain in a number of situations. These include relieving bowel or urinary obstruction, decompression laminectomy, prophylactic nailing of impending pathological fractures, internal fixation (or replacement arthroplasty) of established fractures, drainage of abscesses, and debulking friable tumors.

Interrupt Pain Transmission

Nerve Stimulation. Certain neurons in the dorsal horn, when activated through direct electrical stimulation or through stimulation of large fibers not conventionally associated with pain (e.g., with vibration, touch, and pressure), inhibit the propagation of pain.

The gate-controlling physiology of the dorsal horn explains the ancient observation that gentle rubbing of a painful part (counterirritation) or the application of ice, heat, or pressure eases the discomfort. More specific techniques of nerve stimulation have been developed, including transcutaneous electrical nerve stimulation (TENS) and acupuncture. The TENS apparatus consists of a battery-powered pulse generator and electrodes that are applied to the skin at empirically determined trigger points, or acupunc-

Table 58–7. NONDRUG THERAPIES
FOR PAIN*

Type of Pain	Nondrug Therapy
Nerve pressure pain	Surgical decompression
	Radiotherapy
	Nerve block
	TENS
Bone pain	Radiotherapy
	Fixation for pathologic fracture (established or impending)
Raised intracranial pressure	Elevate head of bed (avoid lying flat)
Muscle spasm	Massage
	Exercises
	Hot or cold packs
Lymphedema	Elastic stockings
	Elevate foot of bed
	Compression cuff
Activity-precipitated pain	Splints
	Slings
	Collars
	Corsets
	Walkers
	Crutches
Visceral pain of pancreatic cancer	Celiac plexus block

*From Scott JF (ed): Cancer Pain, a Monograph on the Management of Cancer Pain. Ottawa, Canada, Health and Welfare, 1984. Reprinted with permission.

ture points. They may lie adjacent to the painful region or may be located some distance proximal to the pain. TENS is well tolerated by most patients, although skin irritation is sometimes experienced.

Several hours of pain relief may be achieved after as short a time of stimulation as five to 20 minutes. About two thirds of patients obtain short-term relief and one eighth realize some long-term benefit, although information on its use in cancer pain is only anecdotal.

Nerve Block. Peripheral nerve transmission of pain can be interrupted temporarily (using local anesthetics) or permanently (using a neurolytic, sclerosing agent such as alcohol or phenol). Theoretically, local anesthestic blocks are temporary, but in practice they may provide partial or complete pain relief for a prolonged period.

Some possible applications of nerve blocks in cancer pain include local anesthetic blocks (often with corticosteroid) for solitary rib metastases, painful trigger points, and other skeletal secondary tumors involving bony prominences, and neurolytic blocks for pain in the celiac plexus (for cancer of the pancreas), intrathecal pain, and blockage of sympathetic fibers (in treatment of causalgic types of pain or intrapelvic pain).

Destructive procedures must be avoided if anticancer therapy is likely to succeed or if the patient is expected to survive for several years. In all cases, an anesthetist or physician skilled in nerve blocks is required.

Neurosurgery. With proper use of medication and other measures, recourse to neurosurgical techniques to relieve cancer pain should be uncommon. However, if drugs and other methods are ineffective, neurosurgical intervention should not be needlessly delayed.

Percutaneous cordotomy is indicated for unilateral pain in segments from the mid-thoracic region downwards and in which all other forms of pain control are unsuccessful. Rarely, bilateral cordotomy is performed, but interruption of motor fibers to the diaphragm may occur in high cervical procedures, leading to sleep apnea.

Other forms of neurosurgical ablation or stimulation are experimental and are restricted to pain research centers.

Physiotherapy. A wide variety of physical therapies are important adjuncts in the management of cancer pain. *Therapy of muscle spasm* includes the use of massage, the application of cold or heat (or both), the use of special collars or traction, passive exercise, and positioning of the chair or bed. *Counterirritation* aids are mentholated ointments, heat or cold, and pressure, vibration, and rubbing. *Mobilization* therapy involves exercises to strengthen and prevent contractures and spasms, compression cuffs used to suppress lymphedema, and aids for transferring the patient (such as a board or bar) and helping the patient to walk (such as walkers, crutches, and canes). *Immobilization* therapy teaches techniques to avoid strain or fatigue and utilizes aids such as collars, corsets, splints, slings, and traction. Finally, *general relaxation* techniques include breathing exercises, distraction or imagery exercises, music therapy, prayer, and hypnosis.

CONTROL OF PHYSICAL SYMPTOMS OTHER THAN PAIN

The shifting symptom complexes and diminishing resources of the terminally ill require regular and frequent reassessment for symptom control. Such a practice will pay rich dividends in the avoidance of potentially serious problems and unnecessary hospitalization. The implied message that the physician has a continuing interest in the patient's welfare is a reassuring factor of major importance to both patient and family.

It is interesting to note that a physician's visit will be remembered as being longer in duration and of greater meaning if the physician sits down at the bedside so that there is eye contact on the same level. How often we look down on our patients! Touching the patient, in general, brings with it reassurance. However, it may represent an intrusion of privacy to a few. It requires sensitivity to meet patients where they are rather than where we feel they should be.

Table 58–8 outlines methods commonly employed in the control of physical symptoms other than pain.

Of particular note is the significant experience at St. Christopher's Hospice, London[2] in the symptomatic medical management of malignant bowel obstruction. Occurring in one in 23 patients dying from carcinoma at their institution, obstruction rises to an incidence of 25% in series of patients with ovarian carcinoma.[26]

Obstrution in a patient with extensive abdominal or pelvic malignancy is rarely caused by a single occluding lesion. Instead, multifocal partial obstruction due to tumor or adhesions is combined with degrees of functional deficit (pseudo-obstruction) due to tumor infiltration of gut muscle or autonomic nerve supply, thereby interfering with peristalsis.

Although surgery should be considered in each case of malignant bowel obstruction, the results are disappointing in terms of mean survival and symptom control. Surgery is recommended when there is "good evidence of a single block in a relatively fit patient."[2]

In the absence of surgery, intravenous fluids and nasogastric suction (the traditional management of a patient admitted with bowel obstruction) yield poor long-term results in terms of sustained response. Furthermore, the patient develops symptoms related to the nasogastric tube itself and has activities restricted by the intravenous line.

Medical management of malignant bowel obstruction rests on three observations:

1. Such obstruction is usually temporary. Most obstructions will open up, in time, to allow the passage of flatus and stool.

2. Vomiting is well tolerated in the absence of nausea.

3. Unlike mechanical bowel obstruction, malignant bowel obstruction generally is not associated with ischemia, resultant bacteremia, and sepsis. One can thus afford to be conservative.

Malignant bowel obstruction may be managed with rigorous mouth care to control thirst, oral intake as desired, careful titration of medications to control nausea as per Table 58–4, the use of softening laxatives such as dioctyl sodium sulfosuccinate (Dioctyl Forte one or two tablets, three times daily), and reassurance to minimize the psychologic trauma of vomiting. A combination of diphenoxylate hydrochloride and atropine (Lomotil, two tablets four times daily) may be used to control painful colic. The frequency of vomiting will depend on the level of the bowel obstruction. In the majority of cases, malignant bowel obstruction resolves to some extent even if it has persisted for prolonged periods (up to 26 days in the author's personal experience). This approach provides patient comfort without resorting to colostomy, nasogastric suction, or intravenous fluids.[2]

When death is imminent, a standing order for scopolamine, 0.4 mg to be given subcutaneously as required, is of great assistance in controlling the noisy respirations or "death rattle" that is so distressing to the relatives, if not to the patient, during the final hours of life. Morphine and chlorpromazine given intramuscularly are useful in relieving distress stemming from a major crisis such as hemorrhage or massive pulmonary embolus. Their use in this setting, for the control of symptoms only, differs significantly from the prescribing of drugs with the intent of shortening life. If their use leads to an insignificant shortening of life, this is an accepted risk, taken in the interest of relieving suffering. A clear understanding of these goals will alleviate anxiety on the part of the nursing staff in this situation.

MENTAL DISTRESS IN THE SETTING OF TERMINAL ILLNESS AND ITS MANAGEMENT

The terminally ill patient is nearly always either consciously or unconsciously aware

Table 58–8. METHODS OF MANAGEMENT OF SYMPTOMS OTHER THAN PAIN*

Symptom	Comment	Therapy
Anorexia	Very common Important effect on general status and morale Reassure patient and compulsive family that large intake is unnecessary	Glucocorticoids (prednisone, 5 mg three times daily) Small food helpings on small plates Patient's preferred foods

Nausea and Vomiting	Variety of causes, including bowel obstruction, tumor bleeding, metabolic upset, psychologic, drugs, radiation
	Vomiting is well tolerated in the absence of nausea
		Control subliminal nausea
		If related to oral narcotics, switch narcotics; try suppository (e.g., oxycodone) or use with phenothiazine (prior to parenteral); once nausea is controlled, try oral route again
		Phenothiazine (in order of ascending sedative effect)
		  (a) Prochlorperazine, 5 to 10 mg
		  (b) Promazine, 25 mg
		  (c) Chlorpromazine, 10 to 25 mg (orally, intramuscularly, or rectally)
		For further control, one or both of the following may be added to the phenothiazine (Table 58–4)
		  (a) an antihistamine
		  (b) metoclopramide
		Small meals of favorite foods
		See text concerning bowel obstruction

Dysphagia	Varies from mild and occasional to pronounced and present with all oral intake	Eliminate nonessential drugs
		Use oral liquid drugs or suppositories
		Crush tablets and mix with ice cream
		Small liquid or soft meals of favorite foods
		Honey solutions and iced carbonated drinks
		Use local anesthetics, with care (topical application or rinse and spit out)
		  (a) Viscous lidocaine
		  (b) Diphenhydramine hydrochloride mixed in equal parts with aluminum and magnesium hydroxide (antacid)

Dry mouth: thirst, dehydration	N.B.: Thirst—symptom (unpleasant)
	      Dehydration—metabolic state (can be asymptomatic)
	      Often drug related
	      Intravenous fluids and nasogastric tubes are generally not justifiable!
		Scrupulous and frequent mouth care
		Treat candidiasis with nystatin suspension or vaginal suppositories taken orally
		Mouth wash every two hours; use lip salve or bland cream for lips
		Remove encrustations with water-soluble (catheter) lubricant followed by gauze swab wipe-out
		Eliminate causative drugs if possible
		Give lemon candies, pineapple chunks, artificial saliva

Symptom	Comment	Treatment
	Dry mouth is common; watch for and treat	Remove foreign objects from mouth Treat candidiasis as for dysphagia Treat stomatitis due to chemotherapy with astringent mouth wash and topical anesthetic Give ice chips, favorite drink, water sips (by syringe or eyedropper if too weak to use straw)
Hiccoughs	Irritating and exhausting	Rebreathing into paper bag Chlorpromazine, 25 mg orally or intramuscularly Breath-holding

Dyspnea	Often associated with anxiety
	Common causes are pleural effusion, lymphangitic tumor spread
	Less common are bronchial obstruction, massive ascites, or abdominal tumor
		Calm, quiet reassurance with frequent observation, open window, fan
		Positioning in bed or reclining chair
		Mouth care
		Oxygen? (often of little help)
		Thoracentesis and instillation of chemotherapeutic agents or sclerosing irritant for malignant pleural effusion
		Bronchodilators (as required, bronchospasm)
		  (a) Oxtriphylline (Choledyl), 200 mg four times orally
		  (b) Salbutamol (Ventolin), by inhaler
		  (c) Aminophyllin suppositories, 500 mg one or two as needed, also intravenously, orally at lower doses
		Glucocorticosteroids
		  (a) Prednisone, 10 to 15 mg three times daily, tapering to 5 mg three times daily
		Antibiotics, for symptomatic control in presence of purulent sputum
		  (a) Trimethoprim and sulfamethoxazole
		  (b) Ampicillin
		  (c) Chloramphenicol
		Narcotics
		  Low doses to suppress respiratory center and relieve restlessness
		  Oral morphine (see text concerning pain) or parenteral narcotic with phenothiazine or diazepam or alone

Terminal airway secretions ("death rattle")	Often disturbing for families, rarely for patients themselves	Scopolamine, 0.4 mg as needed
Cough	Tiring, particularly at night N.B.: If patient is already receiving significant dose of narcotic for pain, do not add narcotic (e.g., codeine) for cough	Linctus codeine or other narcotic, at night particularly Bronchodilators, antibiotics, physiotherapy, hydration, where appropriate Expectorants are of questionable benefit

Table continued on following page

Table 58–8. METHODS OF MANAGEMENT OF SYMPTOMS OTHER THAN PAIN Continued

Symptom	Comment	Therapy
Anxiety	Common factor in escalating pain and analgesic requirements	Discussion and support are the primary therapies Diazepam, 2 to 5 mg three times daily orally; 10 mg intramuscularly (unreliably absorbed) or intravenously (slowly) in acute panic states Promazine, 25 mg orally three times daily Chlorpromazine, 10 to 25 mg three times daily orally
Depression	Not all depression requires medication: anticipatory grief is an integral component of the normal response to life-threatening illness	Attention to physical and mental distress Tricyclic antidepressants (a) Imipramine, 25 to 100 mg (b) Amitriptyline, 25 to 100 mg Both are given upon retiring, starting at low dose and increasing as needed
Confusion and restlessness	Variety of etiologic factors requiring careful evaluation Often correctable by nonpharmacologic means Hypercalcemia may be masked by low serum albumin	Reality reinforcement, including calendars, clocks, orientation tours, repeated identification of familiar objects and events, photographs, social interaction Haloperidol, 1 to 4 mg every four to six hours, may be useful Elevated intracranial pressure: dexamethasone trial, 4 mg four times daily If agitated, chlorpromazine, 10 to 25 mg (mild) or 25 to 50 mg (severe), intramuscularly Hypercalcemia: consider mithramycin, 25 μg/kg (approx. 1.5 mg) slowly over two hours
Insomnia	Adequate sleep important with diminished reserves	Attention to physical and mental distress Rituals: warm water bottle, hot drink, "well-timed bedpan," change of position, quiet, shaded lights, alcohol Nonbarbiturate hypnotics Chlorpromazine, 25 to 50 mg Tricyclic antidepressants or narcotic analgesics, if already in use, but not simply as hypnotics Waken for regular four-hourly narcotic dose if analgesia is inadequate throughout the night
Urinary symptoms		Take to bathroom frequently Leave urine bottle close by

Condition	Comments	Management
Incontinence		Condom for nocturnal incontinence Catheter for constant incontinence or for retention, with maintenance urinary antiseptic if symptomatic Treat symptomatic infections only
Constipation	Debilitation, dehydration, drugs, immobility all contribute Common Prevent rather than treat	Increased fluid and bulk (bran) if tolerated Glycerine suppositories, disposable phosphate enema Stool softener (e.g., dioctyl sodium sulfosuccinate) and peristaltic agent (e.g., senna) Digital disimpaction
Diarrhea	Rule out constipation with overflow	Codeine, 15 to 60 mg three times daily, or Lomotil, two tablets four times daily Bismuth subgallate, 500 mg three times daily, may be useful for unpleasant colostomy or fistula odors
Fungating growths	Need not be offensive	Scrupulous cleanliness Frequent dressing change Wash with dilute Dakin's or peroxide solution Malodorous infections may respond to yogurt applications Rarely, systemic antibiotics for infection with associated foul discharge
Pruritus	Common with obstructive jaundice; may be intolerable	Rule out sensitivity to linen Calamine lotion with phenol up to 1% Discontinue steroids if healing is poor Hydrocortisone cream Oral antihistamines
Decubitus ulcers	Common in older patients Rare in young patients even if very cachectic and immobile	Prevent with mobilization, physiotherapy, frequent position change, massage, reclining chairs Camp air mattress on bed, half-filled with water, is an excellent, economic water bed; alternately, foam or alternating pressure mattress If ulcers are small and shallow, frequent cleansings with Dakin's solution If deep, 20% benzoyl peroxide-soaked pad to stimulate granulation, packed into wound under airtight cellophane dressing; surrounding intact skin protected with Vaseline or silicone cream (Barriere), ultraviolet light, physiotherapy

*From Scott JF (ed): Cancer Pain, a Monograph on the Management of Cancer Pain. Ottawa, Canada, Health and Welfare, 1984. Reprinted with permission.

that death is close.[1, 8] Kubler-Ross has suggested that there is a series of mental adjustments that we may go through in coming to terms with the fact that we have a serious or life-threatening disease. These may include denial, anger, bargaining, depression, and, finally, acceptance. Whatever the sequence in a given patient, one can usually find a subtle balance between a realistic acceptance on the one hand and simultaneous rejection on the other. In dying, we are challenged to adapt not to a single loss but rather to a series of losses: job, mobility, strength, physical and mental capacity, plans for the future, and, ultimately, existence itself.

It is helpful to recognize that the patient's family will also go through a similar series of mental adjustments. An understanding of this process will assist the physician in accepting the anger of the patient or a relative when it is redirected at him, and in mediating more skillfully when anger is directed at a family member. Depression may call for a lengthy discussion and a listening ear rather than a consultation from a neurologist or psychiatrist, or the ordering of antidepressant medications.

Through understanding the dynamics of adjusting to death, the physician may realize more clearly the degree to which he or she shares in the same series of mental adjustments as the patient's death is faced. The physician may then recognize with greater perception that avoidance of contact with the patient reflects one's own despair. The physician's attitude toward his or her own death has been found to be an important variable in determining how the patient's needs are perceived: 84% of the physicians at the Royal Victoria Hospital who felt they would want to know their own prognosis if they were fatally ill thought that their patients also desired direct communication of prognosis, whereas only 45% of the physicians not wanting to know their own prognosis thought their patients desired honesty of communication.[20] Our skill at "hearing" our patients will also depend on our recognition that they use plain language, figurative speech, and nonverbal communication in expressing their fears and needs to us.[8]

Fears of the Dying

A realistic appraisal of potential problems and reassurance that they will be dealt with will go a long way toward allaying relevant anxieties and will dispel a host of irrelevant concerns that are linked in the patient's mind to the fearful term *cancer*. There are at least seven common fears. The fear of pain and mutilation is frequently encountered. As already noted, the intractable pain of advanced malignant disease can generally be controlled by using oral narcotics, thereby leaving the patient alert and pain-free.

A second fear is that of a loss of control and of increasing dependency. This is particularly a problem for the previously self-reliant individual. It is important to recognize the process of depersonalization that we impose on our patients, a "stripping" process by which the person is incorporated into the institution, eliminating all sense of autonomy, identity, and individuality. The process starts in the admitting department with the inevitable delay and is quickly reinforced by hospital regulations requiring a limitation in personal effects, a restriction of visiting hours, the necessity of obtaining permission for leaving the ward, the regulation of contacts with the outside world, and the confiscation of medications taken at home.

A third area of fear is for the future of the patient's loved ones. "What will happen to them after I die?"

A fourth anxiety has been termed reflected fear, which the patient sees in the eyes of those around him. This was commented on by a young cancer patient who stated, "I never knew what fear was until I saw it in the eyes of those caring for me."

A fifth important fear is that of isolation. Patients with advanced disease are likely to encounter decreasing interest and few visits from their physicians and members of the nursing staff if they are hospitalized, and from friends if they are at home. Reassurance that the physician will continue to supervise the patient's care with interest and concern, and the facilitation of family discussions and expression of feeling, are effective weapons in combating isolation.

Two further fears commonly seen in the terminally ill are the fear of the unknown and a concern that life will have been meaningless. The former tends to center on practical questions, "How will I die? Will I suffer? What will happen after death?" The latter, more philosophical in orientation, is concerned particularly with major metaphysical issues. If it is recognized that such questions are of central importance for the terminally ill patient, the perceptive physician will find the opportunity to help the patient express these questions and formulate his or her own answers. If we argue as physicians that our sole concern is with the medical needs of our patient, we ignore the significance of our position in the patient's support system. The physician may well be the only individual with an opportunity to help the patient explore these vital areas. While the physician may not be comfortable as a religious counselor, he or she may assist through active listening and a gentle probing of the patient's own views, fears, and hopes.

Urologic cancers are frequently associated with serious threats to the patient's body image and concept of self. Problems requiring particular understanding and supportive discussion include impotence induced by radical pelvic surgery, exogenous estrogen therapy, or anxiety alone; sterility in the young testicular tumor patient following retroperitoneal lymph node dissection; the loss of one or both testicles; gynecomastia due to hormonal therapy; the necessity of urinary diversion; penile amputation; and the loss of hair and other side effects of irradiation and chemotherapy. Time must be taken to talk through the implications of each of these problems and the anxieties that they produce.

The Conspiracy of Silence

Uncertainty leads to anxiety. The frequently encountered reluctance of patient, family, and physician to frankly discuss the reality facing them has been referred to as "the conspiracy of silence." A candid, honest, yet supportive approach to the reality facing the patient will produce less anxiety in the long run than well-intentioned dishonesty or a lack of communication. The "conspiracy of silence" hinders the patient's relationships with those around them. Furthermore, it is a spreading process, with dishonesty regarding diagnosis and prognosis leading to the need for distortions in other matters.

The physiologic explanation of "out of body" experiences described by some individuals near death remains uncertain. Such experiences are often disturbing to the patient, who may fear he is losing touch with reality and thus may tell no one of the event. On the other hand, the patient may be deeply impressed by the experience and describe it in detail to relatives and friends, thus heightening *their* anxiety. The knowledge that such dramatic occurrences may be a part of an encounter with death for emotionally stable, objective, and reliable individuals is reassuring to all concerned.[15]

The Need for Hope

Although there is a need for supportive honesty in dealing with the terminally ill, the physician must not break down a patient's need for denial. The physician must also honor the need for hope. It is important, however, that we not misunderstand what the patient is hoping for. A plea for cure or a longer life may in fact be an expression of fear long after the patient realizes that these are no longer reasonable goals. For most terminally ill patients, a desire for longer life gives way to other hopes: hope for an end to suffering and for a family and physician who will stay at hand until the end. A family's well-meaning plea, "Don't tell him," must be met with a careful examination of the reasons for this request. Such a statement provides a useful opportunity for further exploration of fears and relationships. To simply accept it at face value may be to reinforce problems in communication and to miss the opportunity to promote understanding and thus, invariably, lessen anxiety.

At the Time of Death

Most patients do not fear death itself, but pain in dying. In reality, however, when death comes, it is usually painless and peaceful for a patient dying of malignant disease. Mental and physical pain commonly recede during the last few days, and almost always in the last hours. The reassurance that this will be the case may encourage a family to keep their loved one at home when their anxiety would otherwise necessitate hospitalization. The family will need particular support and guidance if the patient is to die at home. The assistance of a home-care nurse to supervise the administration of medications during the final days is invaluable. It is also important that the family be aware of the community resources available to them. A social worker may be of great assistance in this regard. The patient should, as much as possible, be included in such discussions and in the planning for the family's future. Anxieties are lessened if the family has discussed funeral arrangements before the death.

Saunders[22] reminds us that the family's distress and corresponding need for a listener may be even greater than that of the patient. Grief, feelings of guilt, and old unresolved tensions may make them withdraw from real contact and communication with the patient, thus increasing the suffering on both sides.

It is often expected that the physician will come to the bedside when the patient dies at home. Although this is not always possible, it should be a definite goal for the physician primarily involved in the case. An important contribution toward the resolution of the family's immediate problems and future "grief work" can be made if the physician is present at that critical point.

When the patient dies in hospital, close communication between family and staff is required. It is important that the family be present when the patient dies. The presence of a mature staff member who reacts to the situation with calm and poise may have a great stabilizing influence on the family. Following the death, family members should be encouraged to see the body. A natural, unobtrusive act such as straightening the hands or touching the hair of the deceased carries with it the implied message that it is all right and not frightening to touch the body. A brief commemorative act on the part of the physician or nurse present at the time of death declares that something of significance has happened. A prepared statement or memorial prayer can be useful in this regard. After quietly stating to the family that such is the practice of the ward and asking whether they approve, the staff member may proceed. This tends to ease the tension of the moment and has, in the writer's (and others') experience, invariably been meaningful regardless of the family's religious background.

Bereavement

Although the needs of the patient end with death, the family's needs continue. In normal grief there is an initial period of numbness. This immediate panic reaction, which may be hours to days in duration, gives way to a recurrent syndrome of somatic symptoms. This is characterized by episodes of pining and yearning with sensations of tightness in the throat, choking, sighing respirations and shortness of breath, an empty feeling in the abdomen, anorexia, and weakness. These symptoms occur in waves. As time passes, these episodes, which may be precipitated by any reminder of the deceased, become less frequent.

A sense of unreality and a withdrawal of interest from daily affairs characterizes the thoughts and feelings of the bereaved, preoccupied as they are with the deceased. It is important to recognize that visual and auditory hallucinations in which the grieving person sees and even hears the deceased loved one speaking may be part of the *normal* grief reaction.

Our experience supports the observation, made by others, that bereavement follow-up by a nurse or physician involved in the death makes an important difference to the successful resolution of the family's grief.[21] Lindemann[11] has observed that normal grief is essentially therapeutic. The grieving person is learning to live with the memory of the loved one. The funeral plays an important part in the early grief experience as a dramatization of the loss. Parkes observed that people who express their feelings early in the bereavement tend to have an earlier resolution of their grief. The physician can assist this process by including the family in the nursing care of the patient and by promoting honesty of communication between family members. A long preparation time prior to the death of the loved one was a further factor in easing the resolution of grief.[21]

Freud's term *grief work* refers to the task facing all bereaved people as their emotional investments shift while they attempt to reestablish a balance in their psychologic economy. Lindemann noted six needs of the bereaved: (1) to confront and accept the loss sustained; (2) to live with the memories of the deceased; (3) to develop a new focus and new goal in life; (4) to express and gain insight into authentic feelings about the deceased, including feelings of anger and guilt; (5) to have support; and (6) to have a meaning to life. Once again the physician may assist in the expression and working out of these needs.

The importance of psychologic, spiritual, and interpersonal considerations, in addition to the complex medical needs of terminally ill patients, places special demands on the urologist acting as a thanatologist. Such a physician is required to be an internist skilled in the fine titration of medications against symptoms, a psychiatrist, a philosopher, and a social worker. The end of life is a time of unparalleled potential for personal and interpersonal growth for both patient and family. Having assisted in the realization of this potential, the physician may find that he or she has shared in the growing process.

The last decade has made it clear that higher standards in the care of the terminally ill must be attained if we are to write an end to the unnecessary and largely unrecognized suffering of the 70% of North Americans who die in institutions. In striving for this goal, we will be erecting a monument, not to incurable disease, but to human dignity.

References

1. Bahnson CB: Psychologic and emotional issues in cancer: the psychotherapeutic care of the cancer patient. Semin Oncol 2:293–309, 1975.
2. Baines MJ: Control of other symptoms. In C Saunders (ed), The Management of Terminal Malignant Disease. London, Edward Arnold, 1984.
3. Catalano RB: The medical approach to management of pain caused by cancer. Semin Oncol 2:379–392, 1975.
4. Duff RS, Hollingshead AB: Dying and Death in Sickness and Society, Chap 15. New York, Harper & Row, 1968.
5. Epstein FH: The dying patient: the role of the physician in the prolongation of life. In FJ Ingelfinger, RV Ebert, M Finland, AS Relman (eds), Controversy in Internal Medicine. Philadelphia, WB Saunders, 1974, pp 103–109.
6. Hinton J: Dying. 2nd ed. Harmondsworth, England, Penguin, 1972, p 159.
7. Jacox AK: Sociocultural and psychological aspects of pain. In AK Jacox (ed), Pain: A Source Book for Nurses and Other Health Professionals. Boston, Little, Brown, 1977, pp 57–87.
8. Kubler-Ross E: On Death and Dying. New York, MacMillan, 1969.
9. Lasagna L: Physicians' behavior toward the dying patient. In OG Brim, HE Freeman, S Levine (eds), The Dying Patient. New York, Russell Stage, 1970.
10. LeShan L: The world of the patient in severe pain of long duration. J Chronic Dis 17:119–126, 1964.
11. Lindemann E: Symptomatology and management of acute grief. Am J Psychiat 101:141–148, 1944.
12. Marks RM, Sachar EJ: Undertreatment of medical inpatients with narcotic analgesics. Ann Intern Med 78:173–181, 1973.
13. Melzack R: The Puzzle of Pain. New York, Basic Books, 1973.
14. Melzack R, Ofiesh JG, Mount BM: The Brompton mixture: effects on pain in cancer patients. Can Med Assoc J 115:125–129, 1976.
15. Moody RAJ: Life After Life. New York, Bantam, 1976.
16. Mount BM: The problem of caring for the dying in a general hospital: the palliative care unit as a possible solution. Can Med Assoc J 115:119–121, 1976.
17. Mount BM: Narcotic analgesics. In RG Twycross, V Ventafidda (eds), The Continuing Care of Terminal Cancer Patients. Oxford, Penguin Press, 1980, pp 97–116.
18. Mount BM: Psychological and social aspects of cancer pain. In PD Wall, R Melzack (eds), Textbook of Pain. New York, Churchill Livingstone, 1984, pp 460–471.
19. Mount BM, Ajemian I, Scott JF: The use of the Brompton mixture in treating the chronic pain of malignant disease. Can Med Assoc J 115:122–124, 1976.
20. Mount BM, Jones A, Patterson A: Death and dying: attitudes in a teaching hospital. Urology 4:741–747, 1974.
21. Parkes CM: Bereavement Studies of Grief in Adult Life. London, Tavistock Publications, 1972.
22. Saunders C: The Management of Terminal Illness. London, Hospital Medical Publishers, 1967.
23. Saunders C: Care of the dying—6: The nursing of patients dying of cancer. Nurs Times 72:1203–1205, 1976.
24. Scott JF (ed): Cancer Pain, a Monograph on the Management of Cancer Pain. Ottawa, Canada, Health and Welfare, 1984.
25. Shephard DAE: Principles and practice of palliative care. Can Med Assoc J 116:522–526, 1977.
26. Tunca JC, Buchler DA, Mack EA, et al: The management of ovarian-cancer-caused bowel obstruction. Gynecol Oncol 12:186–192, 1981.
27. Twycross R: Clinical experience with diamorphine in advanced malignant disease. Int J Cin Pharmacol 7:184–198, 1974.
28. Twycross RG: Relief of pain. In C Saunders (ed), The Management of Terminal Malignant Disease, 2nd ed. Baltimore, Edward Arnold, 1984, pp 64–90.
29. Twycross RG, Fairfield S: Pain in far-advanced cancer. Pain 14:303–310, 1982.
30. Twycross RG, Lack SA: Symptom Control in Far Advanced Cancer, Vol 1, Pain relief. New York, Pitman, 1983.

Index

Note: Page numbers in *italics* indicate illustrations; those followed by t indicate tables.